PRINCIPLES OF NUCLEAR MEDICINE

Edited by HENRY N. WAGNER, Jr., M.D.

Professor of Radiology and Radiological Science,
Associate Professor of Medicine,
The Johns Hopkins Medical Institutions

W. B. SAUNDERS COMPANY, Philadelphia, London, Toronto

W. B. Saunders Company: West Washington Square,
Philadelphia, Pa. 19105

12 Dyott Street
London, W.C.1

1835 Yonge Street
Toronto 7, Ontario

Reprinted May, 1968, October, 1968 and May, 1969

Principles of Nuclear Medicine

TO ANNE

CONTRIBUTORS

WILLIAM H. BEIERWALTES, M.D.
> Professor of Medicine, Director of Nuclear Medicine and of the Thyroid Research Laboratory, University of Michigan Medical School, Ann Arbor, Michigan

NATHANIEL I. BERLIN, M.D., Ph.D.
> Clinical Director, National Cancer Institute; Chief, Metabolism Branch, National Cancer Institute, National Institutes of Health, Bethesda, Maryland

GORDON L. BROWNELL, Ph.D.
> Associate Professor, Massachusetts Institute of Technology, Cambridge, Massachusetts; Applied Physicist, Massachusetts General Hospital, Boston, Massachusetts

LUIGI A. DONATO, M.D.
> Professore Incaricato, Facoltà di Medicina e Chirurgia; Aiuto, Clinica Medica Generale; Vice Direttore, Centro di Medicina Nucleare, Università de Pisa, Pisa, Italy

WILLIAM H. ELLETT, M.Sc.
> Honorary Research Assistant, Royal Postgraduate Medical School, University of London; Medical Physics Department, Hammersmith Hospital, London, England

DAVID A. GOODWIN, M.D.
> Research Fellow in Nuclear Medicine, The Johns Hopkins Medical Institutions, Baltimore, Maryland

C. CRAIG HARRIS, B.S. in E.E., M.S.
> Research Staff Member, Oak Ridge National Laboratory, Oak Ridge, Tennessee

RICHARD A. HOLMES, M.D.
> Fellow in Nuclear Medicine, The Johns Hopkins Medical Institutions, Baltimore Maryland

JOHN A. JACQUEZ, M.D.
> Associate Professor of Physiology, Medical School; Associate Professor of Bio-

statistics, School of Public Health, The University of Michigan, Ann Arbor, Michigan

SHIGEKOTO KAIHARA, M.D.
Fellow in Nuclear Medicine, The Johns Hopkins Medical Institutions, Baltimore, Maryland

ARTHUR KARMEN, M.D.
Associate Professor of Radiological Science, The Johns Hopkins Medical Institutions, Baltimore, Maryland

RALPH M. KNISELEY, M.D.
Associate Chairman, Medical Division, Oak Ridge Institute of Nuclear Studies, Oak Ridge, Tennessee

DONALD R. KORST, M.D.
Associate Professor of Internal Medicine, University of Wisconsin Medical School; Director of Education in Medicine, Madison General Hospital; Research Associate, Nuclear Medicine Section, University Hospitals, Madison, Wisconsin

HENRY H. KRAMER, Ph.D.
Group Leader, Nucleonics Program, Union Carbide Corporation, Sterling Forest Research Laboratory, Tuxedo, New York

DAVID E. KUHL, M.D.
Associate Professor of Radiology, School of Medicine, University of Pennsylvania; Chief, Nuclear Medicine Section, Department of Radiology, Hospital of the University of Pennsylvania, Philadelphia, Pennsylvania

VINCENT LOPEZ-MAJANO, M.D.
Instructor in Radiology, The Johns Hopkins Medical Institutions, Baltimore, Maryland

ALFONSE T. MASI, M.D., Dr.P.H.
Professor of Medicine, University of Tennessee College of Medicine; John Gaston Hospital, Memphis, Tennessee

TIMOTHY MERZ, M.D.
Associate Professor, School of Hygiene and Public Health, Assistant Professor, School of Medicine, The Johns Hopkins Medical Institutions, Baltimore, Maryland

FRED MISHKIN, M.D.
Fellow in Nuclear Medicine, The Johns Hopkins Medical Institutions, Baltimore, Maryland

NORMAN F. MOON, M.D.
Department of Orthopaedic Surgery, Lovelace Clinic; Attending Orthopedic Surgeon, Bataan Memorial Methodist Hospital, Bernadillo County-Indian Hospital, and Veterans Administration Hospital, Albuquerque, New Mexico; Formerly Instructor, Section of Orthopaedic Surgery, The University of Michigan Medical Center, Ann Arbor, Michigan

WIL B. NELP, M.D.
Associate Professor of Medicine and Radiology, University of Washington School of Medicine; Head, Division of Nuclear Medicine, University Hospital; Consultant in Internal and Nuclear Medicine, Veterans Administration Hospital, United States Public Health Service Hospital, King County Hospital, Providence Hospital, Seattle, Washington

RALPH S. PENNER, M.D.
Assistant Professor, The Johns Hopkins Medical Institutions; Associate Radiologist, Mercy Hospital, Baltimore, Maryland

E. JAMES POTCHEN, M.D.
Associate Professor of Radiology, Washington University School of Medicine; Director, Nuclear Medicine Division, Mallinckrodt Institute of Radiology, St. Louis, Missouri; Advanced Fellow in Academic Radiology, James Picker Foundation; National Institutes of Health—National Research Council

RICHARD C. REBA, M.D.
Assistant Professor of Radiology, Internal Medicine, and Radiological Science, The Johns Hopkins Medical Institutions; The Johns Hopkins Hospital, Baltimore, Maryland

BUCK AUSTIN RHODES, B.S.
Instructor in Nuclear Medicine and Radiological Science, School of Hygiene and Public Health, The Johns Hopkins University, Baltimore, Maryland

ROBERT H. ROHRER, Ph.D.
Professor and Chairman, Department of Physics, Emory College; Professor (Radiological Physics), Department of Radiology, Emory University School of Medicine, Atlanta, Georgia; Consultant, Oak Ridge National Laboratory, Oak Ridge, Tennessee

D. A. ROSS, M.D., Ph.D.
Research Staff Member, Oak Ridge National Laboratory, Oak Ridge, Tennessee

WALTON W. SHREEVE, M.D., Ph.D.
Senior Scientist, Medical Research Center; Attending Physician, Hospital of the Medical Research Center, Brookhaven National Laboratory, Upton, New York

EDWARD M. SMITH, D.Sc.
Assistant Professor of Radiology, Division of Nuclear Medicine, University of Miami School of Medicine, Coral Gables, Florida

DONALD E. TOW, M.D.
Assistant Professor of Radiology, The Johns Hopkins Medical Institutions, Baltimore, Maryland

ROBERT L. VOUGHT, M.D., M.P.H.
Senior Epidemiologist, Epidemiology and Field Studies Branch, National Institute of Arthritis and Metabolic Diseases; Attending Physician, Clinical Center, National Institutes of Health, Bethesda, Maryland

HENRY N. WAGNER, Jr., M.D.
Professor of Radiology and Radiological Science, Associate Professor of Medicine, The Johns Hopkins Medical Institutions; Physician and Radiologist, The Johns Hopkins Hospital, Baltimore, Maryland

WERNER WAHL, Ph.D.
Union Carbide Corporation, Neisler Laboratories, Inc., Upton, New York

THOMAS A. WALDMANN, M.D.
Senior Investigator, Metabolism Branch, National Cancer Institute, National Institutes of Health, Bethesda, Maryland

WILLIAM W. WALTON, Jr., Ph.D.
Member of the Technical Staff, Research Analysis Corporation

FOREWORD

Seldom in medical history has a medical discipline shown such spectacular growth as nuclear medicine. From its early beginnings shortly before World War II when artificially produced radionuclides first became available, nuclear medicine has developed into one of the most exciting and important components of modern biomedical science.

Nuclear methods have found application in both the diagnosis and treatment of disease. With the passage of time, however, it is increasingly evident that diagnostic techniques are receiving an increasingly large share of the attention of clinical investigators.

The potential of nuclear methods to detect clinical changes in anatomical structure, physiology, and biochemistry is almost limitless. Although nuclear techniques are similar to roentgenological methods in terms of the format of the information they yield, the use of radiopharmaceuticals in which the radioactive tracer becomes an integral part of the living system under study often allows the acquisition of quantitative information not obtainable by other means.

The progress of nuclear medicine has been so swift that the question may be raised concerning future growth of this discipline. Are the advances in the years ahead likely to be as great as those achieved in the recent past? The answer is almost certainly yes. The surface has been hardly scratched in the application of short-lived radionuclides to biomedical problems. Furthermore, new developments in the field of radiopharmacology indicate a continuing availability of new, biologically significant compounds of substantial research and clinical interest. Hence, it appears that within a very few years, a large portion of the population will have the benefit of nuclear methods in the evaluation of their disease.

The preparation of a text in a field that is growing as rapidly as nuclear medicine poses many difficulties. If discussion is centered principally on methods that are well established, the book is outdated well before publication. On the other hand, if excessive attention is directed to the frontiers of the science, the reader may find trouble in applying his new-found knowledge to practice. In this book, the authors have continually born in mind the need to provide a balance between these extremes. Hence, the book should serve both as a text for the student and as a reference for the specialist; it can be used for fundamental as well as for advanced training in the clinical and research applications of radioactive tracers.

Throughout the book an attempt has been made to present the techniques of nuclear medicine in light of the diagnostic problem at hand. Since the breadth of the field makes it difficult for a single person to cover all subjects in sufficient depth for the book to be useful as a text, contributions have been gathered from several authors. It is hoped that the house officer and medical student will use the book to obtain answers to questions concerning the application of tracer techniques in the management of their patients, that it will help them to appreciate how radionuclides can be applied to medical diagnosis, and that it will provide them with a working knowledge of the advantages and limitations of these methods.

RUSSELL H. MORGAN, M. D.

ACKNOWLEDGMENTS

In preparing this book, in addition to the valuable contributions of the other authors, I have had the valuable aid of Lt. Cdr. Thomas Mitchell and Mr. Edward Buddemeyer, who reviewed several of the chapters and helped in the preparation of the Appendix. I am also indebted to Dr. Owsei Temkin, who reviewed the first chapter, to Sister Austin Marie, O.S.F., and Mrs. Julia Buchanan, who aided in checking the bibliography, to Miss Mary Louise Mehring and Mrs. Sally Donovan, who aided in preparation of the manuscript, and to the publisher's staff for continual encouragement during the entire preparation of the book.

HENRY N. WAGNER, JR., M.D.

CONTENTS

CHAPTER I

INTRODUCTION

HENRY N. WAGNER, Jr.

Not only is medicine an art, calling for the exercise of talent and creativity, but it is also a science—a body of knowledge, techniques, and skills that can be systematically studied and improved. Radioactive tracers have had, and undoubtedly will continue to have, a profound effect on medical science. Several tracer techniques are widely used in clinical medicine; others are carried out only in research laboratories. But, as in other special areas of medicine, procedures that are now considered ancillary will probably become an important part of the routine medical examination. Such a commonplace test as the hematocrit, for example, was introduced into the medical examination as late as 1891, but since then it has become so routine that it is now virtually part of the physical examination. It is probable that the same thing will happen with procedures now being developed and applied in nuclear medicine.

WHAT IS NUCLEAR MEDICINE?

Nuclear medicine is the application of radioactive materials to the diagnosis and treatment of patients and the study of human disease. The field can be symbolized by a triangle with *radiopharmaceuticals, instruments,* and *biomedical problems* at the three corners, and with the patient at the center.

The field had its beginning in 1661 when in the *Sceptical Chymist* Robert Boyle conceived of an "element" as a substance that cannot be decomposed into simpler constituents—modernizing the ancient atomic concept of Democritus. More than a century later, Lavoisier, using an improved balance, extended Boyle's criterion and introduced a distinction between *element* and *compound*.

In 1803, Dalton advanced his chemical theory of atoms to explain the laws of chemical combination. His postulates, published in 1808 in his *New System of Chemical Philosophy*, were these:

1. All matter is composed of atoms.
2. Chemical combinations take place between these atoms.
3. The atoms are indivisible.
4. All atoms of the same element are identical in properties, including weight.
5. Atoms of different elements have different properties and different weights.
6. Chemical compounds are made of small numbers of atoms.

The laws of conservation of mass, constant composition, and multiple proportions were consequences of Dalton's theory.

Despite the value of Dalton's theory during the century following its introduction, we now know that only the first two of his postulates are correct. The existence of isotopes nullifies Dalton's postulation that all atoms of the same element have the same atomic weight. Boltwood discovered the element ionium and found that its chemical properties are so similar to those of thorium that if the two elements are mixed no chemical process will separate them. Similar efforts of other talented chemists confirmed the chemical identity of substances such as mesothorium and radium. Subsequently, more and more radioactive elements were found to be chemically inseparable from each other or from their stable elements. Not only were these atoms alike in their chemical behavior, but they yielded visible light and x-ray spectra that were identical.

To classify these chemically identical elements in the periodic table, Soddy, in 1913, proposed the name *isotopes* for these inseparable substances "because they occupy the same place in the periodic table. They are chemically identical, and, save only as regards relatively few physical properties, which depend upon atomic mass directly, physically identical also."

The question then arose, were these isolated cases, or are there isotopic forms of all elements? The answer was soon forthcoming. We now know that most elements consist of at least two isotopes, the atomic weight of any element being the mean of the weights of the different isotopes and the relative amounts of each.

Our present image of atoms as consisting of a nucleus surrounded by a cloud of electrons is so widely accepted that it has almost become the symbol of our time. It is easy to forget that a little over half a century ago it was believed that an atom consisted of a definite number of electrons "enclosed in a sphere of uniform positive electrification." Rutherford, in 1911, showed that this atomic model could not account for the observed scattering of alpha particles when they were shot through thin films of matter, and he proposed that the atom consists of a very small positively charged nucleus in which is concentrated practically all the atomic mass and which, like the sun, is surrounded by "planetary" electrons.

Bohr, working with Rutherford at the University of Manchester, conceived the first clear-cut idea of the orbital structure of the atom. Working with the simplest element, hydrogen, he utilized quantum theory to establish the fundamental laws governing the motion of electrons around the nucleus, and proved the correctness of these views by predicting the spectral lines emitted by elements made luminous by heating or electrical excitation. According to the Bohr model, electrons circling the atomic nucleus may move only along certain "quantized" orbits; i.e., their behavior is restricted to a series of discrete values. For example, when hydrogen is in the so-called ground state, a single electron revolves around the heavy positive nucleus in a distinct orbit about 10^{-8} (a hundred-millionth) of a centimeter in diameter. If energy is supplied to the atom by heating or electrical excitation, the electron may leave this orbit and jump momentarily to an orbit farther from the nucleus. The uniqueness of Bohr's theory was the postulate that only certain orbits are possible for the electron. It may travel in any one of these but is never permitted anywhere else within the atom. Soon after its leap to the higher orbit, the electron is attracted by the positive charge of the nucleus and jumps back to the ground state through one or more successive orbital states. Each inward jump releases energy, which we see as light, the pattern of spectral lines corresponding to the particular atom under study. Every type of atom emits light of characteristic frequencies or colors. When electrons are revolving in the ground state, or in stable orbits, no energy is radiated.

In describing the spectrum of hydrogen, Bohr extended the quantum theory, originated by Max Planck at the turn of the century. Planck had advanced the radically new hypothesis that energy can be radiated only in discrete packets or quanta, the energy of which is directly proportional to the frequency of the radiation. Bohr made the assumption that the angular momentum of the electrons is also "quantized," and that the electron is restricted to orbits that correspond to integer multiples of $h/2\pi$, where h is Planck's constant.

The quantum theory is applicable to another phenomenon of electromagnetic radiation, the photoelectric effect. If a beam of light of a suitable frequency falls upon a metal surface, it causes the emission of electrons, known as photo-electrons. In 1905, Einstein proposed that the photoelectric process could be explained on the assumption that a quantum of light is absorbed by each electron and converted into the kinetic energy with which the electron is expelled from the surface. Einstein suggested that a beam of light consists of packets of energy (photons), some of which are reflected from the surface of the metal, and others of which enter the metal and are completely absorbed. The entire energy of a packet or quantum of light is given up to a single orbital electron in an atom of the metal. As the more energetic electron springs out of the metal, one can measure its kinetic energy. This energy is somewhat less than the original energy added, since a certain amount of energy is spent in order for the electron to leave the metal.

If one experiments with various beams of light of different frequencies, measuring the kinetic energy of electrons emitted under the impact of each frequency, and if the electron energy is plotted against the frequency of the light, one finds that the points will lie along a straight line that has the slope of h, Planck's constant; this confirmation of basic theory is one of the milestones in the history of physics.

Subsequent work was required to extend Bohr's simple model to explain the electron orbits of more complex atoms. It was necessary to introduce additional quantized relationships, until finally there were four, representing (1) the size of the orbit, (2) its shape, (3) its orientation in space with respect to an applied electromagnetic field, and (4) the electron spin.

Another milestone in quantum physics is the exclusion principle of Pauli.

It had been found that, regardless of the charge of an atomic nucleus, the overall size of atoms remains approximately the same. It was to explain this apparent contradiction of the laws of classic physics that Pauli postulated that each quantum orbit may hold no more than two electrons, or, stated in other terms, no two electrons with the same spin occupy identical orbits. Thus, in atoms with the stable configuration associated with the lowest possible energy level, an increase in the number of orbits is counterbalanced by smaller orbital diameters, the size of the atom remaining nearly the same as before. The main orbital shells are designated by the principal quantum numbers, 1, 2, 3, 4, 5, 6, and 7, and also by the letters K, L, M, N, O, P, and Q.

The importance of Pauli's exclusion principle is that it provides the basis for the chemical identity of an atom by explaining the principles governing the electron orbits, and by explaining the sequence of atomic species in the periodic table of elements, first described by Mendeléeff.

Were it not for the fact that electron orbits are quantized, there would be an infinite number of atoms rather than the 100-odd elements of which the world is made. If the electron of the hydrogen atom could revolve around the nucleus in any orbit whatsoever, and not just in a limited number of orbits (one corresponding to the normal state and the others to transient excited states), hydrogen would not be the distinctive element that it is—nor would carbon, oxygen, iron, or gold.

ELEMENTARY PARTICLES

In 1932, only four particles were considered to be elementary: the electron, proton, neutron, and photon. Photon has now replaced the term *quantum* in referring to electromagnetic radiations, such as light, x-rays, and gamma rays. The electron, proton, and neutron are the building blocks of atoms; the photon is the building block of the electromagnetic field. The photon is never at rest and always travels with the velocity of light. Because of its motion, it possesses energy. Therefore according to the famous relation of Einstein, $E = mc^2$, the photon also possesses mass, which (in this case) exists only by virtue of the motion. Since the electron, proton, and neutron can be at rest, each has a mass when at rest and a corresponding energy at rest. When in motion, these particles have additional energy and mass.

The electron is the lightest particle with any rest mass, and is taken as the basic unit in atomic physics. In these units, the proton has a mass of about 1836.1 and a charge of plus one; the neutron has a mass of about 1838.6 and no charge. The photon has no rest mass and no charge, although it is the carrier of electromagnetic energy.

The electron and the photon suffice to explain all the chemical or external properties of atoms; the proton and neutron account for the charge of each nucleus and approximately for its mass. A neutron alone cannot serve as the nucleus of an atom, but it combines with protons and other neutrons to form various composite nuclei.

In addition to these, a large number of other "elementary" particles have been discovered, many of them after their existence had been predicted on theoretical grounds. For example, extending Pauli's principle, Dirac predicted the existence of the positive electron, or *positron*, which was subsequently discovered, and which, as we shall see subsequently, has had a considerable number of medical applications. The positron is an example of an "antiparticle," so called because it cancels out an ordinary electron, resulting in annihilation radiation. Dirac postulated the possible existence of a positron when his wave equation for the electron was solved and yielded a negative as well as a positive frequency. The existence of the positron was subsequently proved by Anderson.

At present, elementary particles fall into four groups: (1) heavy particles, consisting of the nucleons (proton and neutron) and their antiparticles; (2) mesons, or particles of intermediate weight; (3) light particles, consisting of the electron and neutrino and their antiparticles; and (4) in a class by themselves, photons. These particles behave according to the general laws of physics, i.e., the laws of conservation of energy, of angular momentum, of charge, and of nuclear matter. The latter refers to the fact that the number of nucleons remains constant.

Although it is heretical to the modern physicist, the nonphysicist can form a mental picture (however inaccurate) of the electrons spinning in their quantized orbits. As yet, no one has a mental picture of the inside of the atomic nucleus. We know that it is quite small, having a diameter of a few ten-trillionths of a centimeter. As Hofstadter has stated, if an atom could be expanded so that its outer electrons enclosed an area the size of New York City, the nucleus at its center would be as big as a baseball. Its existence was discovered by Rutherford when he observed scattering of alpha particles. Since nearly all the weight of the atom is in the nucleus, its density is so great that it is beyond comprehension, approximately 10^{14} g./cc. By all known laws of physics, the charged protons in the nucleus should repel one another, instead of clinging together so strongly that one must use enormously energetic machines to pull them apart. The force that holds the nucleons together must be radically different from any yet known. To get an approximation of the strength of these forces, one can measure the energy set free or consumed in various nuclear reactions. By using Einstein's relation $E = mc^2$, we know that the binding energy is equal to the mass defect in the nucleus multiplied by the square of the velocity of light. The mass defect refers to the fact that the mass of the nucleus is slightly less than the sum of the masses of the component nucleons. By these two methods, it has been determined that the binding energy holding each particle in a heavy nucleus is between 6 and 8 million electron volts, or roughly a million times the energy that holds atoms together in a molecule.

We know that these tremendous nuclear forces are of exceedingly short range. At a distance of about 10^{-13} centimeters, the nuclear force of attraction between two protons is about 40 times as strong as the electric force of repulsion between them. At four times that distance the nuclear force has dropped off to the same strength as the electrical force; at 25 times that distance, the electrical force is a million times stronger.

The number of orbital electrons in the atom is equal to the number of protons in the nucleus. The arrangement of the electrons in the orbits and the laws governing their motion are responsible for the chemical properties, such as solubility, reactivity, electrical conductivity, crystal structure, hardness, strength,

and so on. All atoms of a given element (there are 103 different types) are chemically identical, even though the weight of their nuclei may differ. The differences
in nuclear weight among the isotopes of a given element result from differences
in the number of neutrons in the nucleus. The neutron has an electrical charge
of zero, does not participate in chemical reactions, and can move readily through
the barrier of electrical charge surrounding the nucleus; i.e., it can move readily
through matter. On the other hand, it enters readily into the nucleus, where it
participates in nuclear (rather than chemical) reactions.

The discovery of the neutron in 1932 by Chadwick confirmed Rutherford's
prediction of the existence of a particle with a mass very similar to that of a
proton but with no electrical charge. The protons provide the positive charge of
the nucleus, and the neutrons provide the additional mass. Neutrons exist in the
nucleus of every atom except hydrogen.

Neutrons may be freed from atomic nuclei in several ways. Frederic Joliot and
his wife, Irene Curie, directed alpha particles from a radium salt against beryllium
metal. When this is done, a small number of alpha particles encounter the
beryllium nuclei and expel a neutron. For about every 5000 bombarding alpha
particles emitted by the radium, one neutron is emitted. Neutrons may also be
released by bombardment of a light element with fast particles, such as deuterons,
or with gamma rays. But the easiest and most common source of neutrons is the
chain-reacting atomic pile. Nuclear fission results in the release of great numbers
of neutrons.

NUCLEAR FISSION

Shortly after Chadwick discovered the neutron, Fermi and his associates
exposed many elements to these particles. Fermi wondered what would happen
if one exposed uranium, the last substance in the periodic table, to neutrons. In
view of what was known from other reactions of neutrons with nuclei, one should
obtain an element with an atomic number of 93; but no such element was known
to exist. The experiment was conducted and the investigators set out to define
the nuclear reaction that had occurred. After studying the chemical properties
of the substances produced, Fermi concluded that the resultant chemical substances were not any of the elements between atomic numbers 86 and 92. After
many efforts to identify the resultant substances, Hahn and Strassmann in 1939
finally proved beyond doubt that the union of a neutron with a uranium atom
results in the splitting off of a barium atom, which subsequently decays to
lanthanum. Under neutron bombardment uranium had split into two lighter
fragments. This momentous discovery was another milestone in the history of
science.

Nuclear fission provides a ready source of neutrons because in the process
of fission of the large unstable transuranic elements an average of 2.5 neutrons
are released per bombarding neutron. This results in a chain reaction which, if
controlled in a nuclear reactor, can be a major source of useful radioactive
elements. These are obtained either by chemical separation of fission fragments
that have mass numbers from about 70 through 160, or by the process of neutron
bombardment of other elements exposed to the neutrons produced during the
fission process.

The same year that Hahn and Strassmann described nuclear fission (1939), the information was relayed by way of the physicists Meitner, Bohr, Szilard, and Einstein to Franklin D. Roosevelt, President of the United States, who organized the Manhattan Project to develop atomic energy for military use. Fermi and his associates developed the first atomic "pile" within an abandoned football stadium at the University of Chicago. On December 2, 1942, the first nuclear reactor was operated successfully.

RADIONUCLIDE PRODUCTION

On June 14, 1946, in the journal *Science,* an announcement was made by the Manhattan Project Headquarters, Washington, D.C., that "Production of tracer and therapeutic radioisotopes has been heralded as one of the great peacetime contributions of the uranium chain-reacting pile. This use of the pile will unquestionably be rich in scientific, medical and technological applications."

On August 2, 1946, the first shipment of radioisotopes was sent out from Oak Ridge. A compound labeled with carbon-14 was sent to the Barnard Free Skin and Cancer Hospital in St. Louis. This signaled the present era of widely available radioisotopes produced at reasonable cost for use by persons with the ability to use these new tools safely. By 1962, the Oak Ridge National Laboratory alone had made over half a million shipments of radioisotopes, totaling 1,600,000 curies of radioactivity. On July 31, 1964, there were 1085 physicians in the United States licensed to use radioisotopes in private practice and some 1201 medical institutions licensed to handle radioisotopes.

The capacity of the nuclear reactor to produce large quantities of radioactive tracers led to rapid growth of the field of nuclear medicine, despite the fact that reactors were limited to relatively few nuclear reactions. Isotopes that in the past had been made with difficulty in the cyclotron were available at low cost and in great quantity, and the time was at hand to build upon the pioneering work of the medical teams of Lawrence and others, who in 1936 had administered the artificially produced radioactive isotope, phosphorus-32, to a patient with the express purpose of treating his disease, a major event in the practice of medicine.

THE TRACER PRINCIPLE

Although we have come quite a long way from the time when a small amount of cyclotron-produced radioactive iodine was administered and a Geiger counter tube was held directly over the thyroid gland to measure its iodine uptake, the basic principles remain essentially the same.

As long ago as 1923 (or as recently, depending on the viewpoint), Hevesy used a naturally occurring radioactive isotope of lead to obtain information regarding certain aspects of calcium metabolism in plants. Following Urey's isolation of deuterium, the tracer principle was extended to man by Schoenheimer and his associates (1942). In 1937 radioactive sodium was used by Stone and Hamilton, and the next year Hertz and Evans carried out their early studies of thyroid physiology using iodine-131.

What types of information do radioactive tracers provide that can be used to solve problems in medical diagnosis? Since the next chapter (and much of the entire book) deals specifically with this question, only the briefest outline will be given here. Implicit in the process of medical diagnosis is the assumption that it is possible and useful to classify patients' diseases into categories. Predicting the outcome of the illness, altering the natural progression of the disease, and elucidating its cause are among the reasons for attempting to derive an abstraction (the diagnosis) from the reality of the patient's illness.

Diagnosis is the process of identifying the patient's disease, and it is an ancient practice. Temkin (1963) has pointed out that when Job was smitten with illness, he complained: ". . . wearisome nights are appointed to me. When I lie down, I say, When shall I arise, and the night be gone? and I am full of tossings to and fro unto the dawning of the day. My flesh is clothed with worms and clods of dust; my skin is broken, and become loathsome. . . . When I say, My bed shall comfort me, my couch shall ease my complaint; then thou scarest me with dreams, and terrifiest me through visions: So that my soul chooseth strangling, and death rather than my life." Job, the sick man, tried to express how he felt. The narrator puts it more briefly: "Satan . . . smote Job with sore boils from the sole of his foot unto his crown." He made the diagnosis of a disease: "generalized boils" caused by Satan.

Modern physicians are aware that each patient is an individual person who is, in many respects, unique. He has specific parents, was born in a particular place and culture, is from a certain racial stock, eats special types of food, and is exposed to his individual environment. Yet as a patient he is suffering from a disease process that has certain features in common with those of other patients. In making "the diagnosis," the physician, in the philosophical sense, abstracts the disease from the myriad characteristics of the patient as a person. He has learned to deal with multiple factors that vary so greatly from one patient to another than their differences greatly outnumber their similarities. So he must for the present dismiss from consideration most aspects that are singular about the patient, and much that makes the patient a fascinating and unique individual, until he is left with a handful of manifestations that specific diseases have in common. He is then able to make judgments about the nature of the process, and the probable outcome of the disease; and usually he is better able to plan treatment.

As Kerr (1962) has stated, "All of our thinking is done in a roundabout way. Instead of leaping to conclusions in the presence of single objects, we circle such objects warily, keeping a discreet distance from them, squinting our eyes so that we shall blur what is 'real' about them and see only what is general or 'universal' about them—until their repeated essentials can be added up in the countinghouse of the abstract."

Although Kerr was referring to the evaluation of a work of art, his description is also applicable to the manner of the physician in making a diagnosis—he sees the patient both as an individual and as a member of a group; neither aspect tells the whole story or the same story; neither can be substituted for the other. The physician searches for the universal in the particular, for the disease in his patient.

Throughout history, diseases have been looked at in one of two ways: as an entity that befalls a healthy person, or as a deviation from normality. The "ontological" doctrine, which regards diseases as specific entities, has alternated with the "physiological" view, which considers a disease as simply an abnormal state experienced by a given individual organism at a given time. In one form or another, the ontological attitude has usually been dominant among both laymen and physicians. It assumes that disease is a thing in itself, essentially unrelated to the patient's personality, his bodily constitution, or his mode of life. This concept reasserts itself repeatedly in everyday language when it is said that the patient *has* a disease.

Dubos (1965) has pointed out that, regardless of their level of education and sophistication, patients are prone to blame their illness on something they "caught" or ate, or that happened to them. Physicians are inclined to such ways of thinking also, particularly since they can see the "cause" of disease as something they can attack and destroy.

According to Dubos, there is no more spectacular phenomenon in the history of medicine than the rapidity with which the germ theory of disease became accepted by the medical profession. This acceptance was only partly due to the personalities of its two leading proponents, Louis Pasteur and Robert Koch. The triumph of the germ theory would not have been as immediate and decisive if the medical profession had not been prepared for it by the observations and reflections of several great clinicians throughout the early part of the nineteenth century. From the previously haphazard accumulation of clinical facts, these physicians derived generalizations that made it possible to classify diseases as if they were well defined biological entities.

By relating clinically and conceptually the characteristics of each disease to a particular cause, physicians were prepared to accept the teachings of microbiology, and were ready to accept the doctrine of specific causes. This acceptance was consonant with two great themes of early nineteenth century biology: the Linnean classification of plants and animals, and the acceptance of determinism instead of vitalism. On this dual basis, it became possible to construct the theory that each particular disease has its particular cause, and that each noxious agent exerts a characteristic pathological effect. Later, nutritional deficiencies were added to infectious diseases as another type of pathological category, which was again consistent with the doctrine of specific etiology. The more recent categories —biochemical lesions, molecular pathology, congenital anomalies, and genetic disorders—are direct linear descendants of the doctrine of causal specificity.

But, as Dubos has emphasized, few pathological states can be classed as true biological entities. A single noxious agent can express itself in a variety of ways, and different agents can elicit similar reactions.

The doctrine of specificity has not been discredited; rather it is now being enlarged to include not only the operations of external agents but also the factors that govern the responses of the individual. Simple cause-effect relationships involving only one variable are rarely sufficient to account for the phenomenon referred to as a disease. We now accept the concept of multifactorial causation as an extension of the doctrine of specificity.

Thus, instead of focusing on only a few noxious factors of the external world, we now try to study as many as possible of the internal mechanisms through which the body and mind respond to environmental stimuli and stresses. Disease categories are based upon alterations in the normal functions and structures of the body. We try to measure as many as possible of the individual's activities, mental and physical—from thoughts and dreams to eructation and flatulence, from hopes and fears to respiration and urination. A large amount of data is obtained from each individual patient, and the total body of data will fit one individual only. Today, as in ancient times, we compare the behavior and characteristics of our patients with our picture of healthy persons. By observing large numbers of persons, we try to establish standards of what is normal, and to develop tests that will detect and express the deviation from the norm. Thus, the history of medicine has involved an ever lengthening chart of data accumulating in the course of examination of the patient: pulse rate and temperature, x-ray images, chemical, bacteriological, and immunological tests, and now measurements with radioactive tracers.

The modern physician has at his disposal a vastly greater number of sources of objective data concerning a particular patient than the ancient doctor could ever dream of. He is harvesting technological advances in all fields of science, adapting to his problems the methods of physics and chemistry and biochemistry. One of the most productive areas has been the application of radioactive tracers to the care of patients and the study of disease.

Tracer techniques are being developed in great numbers and there is now a need for the physician to be able to interpret and synthesize these advances into his medical practice. Although the history of a new field is almost always marked by an early and enthusiastic acclaim, which is often followed by a period of disappointment, these in turn are usually followed by a more realistic appraisal of the range of usefulness of the new field.

The field of nuclear medicine provides additional information concerning the structure and function of the human body, information that in the past could be obtained only in experimental animals, but now can be obtained in man himself. The delicate and complex responses of the body to noxious stimuli can be observed in ways not possible before. Previously unobtainable details of the gross structure of organs or the detailed chemical behavior of individual types of cells can now be obtained. We have new methods of studying hour-to-hour variations as well as variations between individuals. The specific ways these are employed in nuclear medicine is the subject of this book.

REFERENCES

Dubos, R.: Man Adapting. Yale University Press, New Haven, 1965.
Fermi, E.: Elementary Particles. Yale University Press, New Haven, 1951.
Hevesy, G.: Radioactive Indicators. Interscience Publishers, Inc., New York, 1948.
Hofstadter, Robert: The Atomic Nucleus. *Sci. Amer.* 195:55 1956.
Kerr, W. The Decline of Pleasure. Simon & Schuster, New York, 1962.
Temkin, O.: The Scientific Approach to Disease. *In* Crombie, A. (ed.): Scientific Change—Historical Studies in the Intellectual, Social and Technical Conditions for Scientific Discovery and Technical Invention from Antiquity to the Present. Basic Books, Inc., New York, 1963.

BIBLIOGRAPHY

Prepared by Asa Seeds, M.D.

The following is an historical bibliography for the period 1815 to 1942. With a few exceptions, references throughout the book cover the period after 1942.

YEAR	AUTHOR	REFERENCE		SUBJECT
1815	Prout, W.	*Ann. Phil.*	6:269	Suggested relationship of elements
1869	Mendeléeff, D.	*J. Prakt. Chem.* (2nd Ed.)	106:251	An early example of periodic table
1886	Goldstein, E.	*Berlin Ak. Sber*	39:691	Protons first observed as positive "canal" rays in a discharge tube
1891	Stoney, G. J.	*Dublin Soc. Sci. Trans.*	4:563	First used term "electron"
1896	Becquerel, H.	*Compt. Rend.*	122:420, 559, 1086	Discovered radioactivity of uranium
1897	Thomson, J. J.	*Phil. Mag. 5th series*	44:293	Generally given credit for the identification of the orbital electron
1898	Curie, P., Mme. Sklodowska-Curie	*Compt. rend. acad. d. sc.*	127:175	Identified radium
1899	Giesel, F. O.	*Ann. Phys. Chem.*	69:834	Radiation could be deflected by magnetic field
1901	Planck, M.	*Ann. Physik.*	4:553	Energy absorption and emission; Planck's (universal quantum theory) constant
1903	Rutherford, E.	*Phil. Mag. 6th series*	5:177	Alpha particles in magnetic field
	Strutt, R. J.	*Proc. Roy. Soc.*	72:208	Determined that some radiations could not be deflected and were highly penetrating; called them gamma rays
	Crookes, W.	*Proc. Roy. Soc.*	71:405	Spinthariscope for study of activity by fluorescent screen
	Rutherford, E. Cooke, H. L.	*Phys. Rev.*	16:183	First studies of "background" irradiation leading to concept of cosmic rays
1905	Einstein, A.	*Ann. Physik.*	17:132	Proposed famous equation
1907	Thomson, J. J.	*Phil. Mag. 6th series*	13:561	First measurements of protons
1908	Rutherford, E.	*Proc. Roy. Soc. A*	81:141	First work on ionization phenomena in high voltage vacuum tube
1911	Wilson, C. T. R. Rutherford, E.	*Proc. Roy. Soc. A* *Phil. Mag.*	85:285 21:669	Cloud chamber Identification of protons
1913	Hevesy, G.	*Chem. News*	108:166	Radioelements as tracers in chemistry and physics
	Soddy, F.			Proposed the name *isotopes*
1916	Field, C. E.	*Med. Rec.*	89:135	Physiological and chemical properties of radium
1923	Compton, A. H.	*Phys. Rev.*	21:483	Principle of Compton effect; Compton scatter
	Hevesy, G.	*Biochem. J.*	17:439	Introduction of tracer techniques using early form of Geiger counter
1924	Hevesy, G.	*Compt. rend. acad. d. sc.*	179:291	Tracers of lead

YEAR	AUTHOR	REFERENCE		SUBJECT
1925	Martland, H. S. Conlon, P. Knef, J. P.	*J.A.M.A.*	85:1769	Danger in the use and handling of radioactive substances
	Martland, H. S.	*Amer. J. Cancer*	15:2435	The occurrence of malignancy with radiation
1926	Stevens, R. H.	*Amer. J. Roentgen.*	16:155	The use of intravenous injections of radium chloride in malignant lymphomas
1928	Geiger, H.	*Phys. Z.*	29:839	Detector tube
1929	Geiger, H. Müller, W.	*Phys. Z.*	30:489	Geiger-Müller tube
1930	Bothe, W. Becker, H.	*Z. Physick*	66:289	Basic work for Chadwick's discoveries
	Cockcroft, J. D. Walton, E.	*Proc. Roy. Soc. A*	129:477	Acceleration of protons
	Lawrence, E. O. Edlefsen, N.	*Science*	72:376	Magnetic accelerator
	Bothe, W. Becker, H.	*Z. Physick*	66:307	Discovered the radiation from light elements when bombarded by alpha rays
	Rutherford, E. Chadwick, J. Ellis, C. D.	Macmillan Co.		Radiations from radioactive substances
	Hevesy, G. Wagner, O. H.	*Arch. Exp. Path.* *Pharmakol.*	149:336	Tracer studies
1931	Lawrence, E. O. Livingston, M. S.	*Phys. Rev.*	38:834	Cyclotron
	Curie, I.	*Compt. rend.* *acad. d. sc.*	193:1412	Basic work for Chadwick's discoveries
	Joliot, F.	*Compt. rend.* *acad. d. sc*	193:1415	Basic work for Chadwick's discoveries
	Van de Graff, R. J.	*Phys. Rev.*	38:1919	Accelerator
	Sloan, D. Lawrence, E. O.	*Phys. Rev.*	38:2021	Linear accelerator
	Curie, M. Debierne, A. Eve, A. S. Geiger, H. Hahn, O. Lind, S. C. Meyer, St. Rutherford, E. Schweidler, E.	*Rev. Mod. Phys.*	3:427	Radioactivity and the laws of radioactive decay
1932	Chadwick, J.	*Nature*	129:312	Discovered a particle without a charge; proposed existence of neutron
	Urey, H. C., et al.	*Phys. Rev.*	39:164	Discovered deuterium
	Cockcroft, J. D. Walto, E. T. S.	*Proc. Roy. Soc.*	136:619	High-velocity positive ions
	Lawrence, E. O. Livingston, M. S.	*Phys. Rev.*	40:19	Cyclotron

YEAR	AUTHOR	REFERENCE		SUBJECT
1933	Swann, W. F. G.	*Phys. Rev.*	43:217	Cosmic rays
	Oppenheimer, J. R. Plesset, M. S.	*Phys. Rev.*	44:53	Electron orbital potentials
1934	Curie, I. Joliot, F.	*Nature*	133:201	Artificial production of a new kind of radioactive element
	Fermi, E.	*Nature*	133:757, 898	Radioactivity by neutron bombardment; extensive work on uranium family by neutron capture
	Livingston, M. S. Henderson, M. C.	*Proc. Natl. Acad. Sci. U.S.A.*	20:470	Radioactivity induced by neutron bombardment
1936	Yukawa, H. Sakata, S.	*Proc. Phys. Math. Soc. Japan*	18:128	Electron capture by positron-emitting nuclei
	Lawrence, E. O. Cooksey, D.	*Phys. Rev.*	50:1131	Multiple acceleration of ions to high speed
	Gingrich, N. S.	*Rev. Sci. Instrum.*	7:207	
	Gamow, G. Teller, E.	*Phys. Rev.*	49:895	Atomic structure
	Gingrich, N. S. Evans, R. D. Edgerton, H. E.	*Rev. Sci. Instrum.*	7:450	Count rate meters
1937	Crane, H. R. Moutzon, J. C.	*Rev. Sci. Instrum.*	8:351	Simple design for a cloud chamber
	Martin, L. C. Wilkins, T. R.	*J. Opt. Soc. Amer.*	27:340	Photographic emulsion for recording particle tracks
	Bethe, H.	*Rev. Mod. Phys.*	9:69	Explanation of nuclear reactions
	Bethe, H. Placzek, G.	*Phys. Rev.*	51:450	Neutron reactions
	Hamilton, J. G. Stone, R.	*Radiology*	28:178	Clinical use of radioactive sodium
	Lauritsen, C. C. Lauritsen, T.	*Rev. Sci. Instrum.*	8:438	Quartz fiber electrometer
1938	Hertz, S. Roberts, A. Evans, R. D.	*Proc. Soc. Exp. Biol. Med.*	38:510	Radioactive iodine in the study of thyroid physiology
	Wilkins, T. R. St. Helens, H.	*Phys. Rev.*	54:783	Photographic emulsion for recording particle tracks
	Hahn, O. Strassmann, F.	*Naturwissenschaften*	26:755	Discovered fission of uranium
	Feather, N.	*Proc. Cambridge Phil. Soc.*	34:115	Measured beta particle energy by maximum range in aluminum
	Hamilton, J. G.	*Amer. J. Physiol.*	124:667	Absorption of the radioactive isotopes of sodium, potassium, chlorine, bromine, and iodine in normal human subjects
1939	Lawrence, J. H. Scott, K. G.	*Proc. Soc. Exp. Biol. Med.*	40:694	Metabolism of phosphorus in normal and lymphomatous animals
	Hahn, O. Strassmann, F.	*Naturwissenschaften*	27:11, 89	Fission of uranium

YEAR	AUTHOR	REFERENCE		SUBJECT
	Lawrence, J. H. Scott, K. G. Tuttle, L. W.	*Internat. Clin.*	3:33	Studies of leukemia with radio-active phosphorus
1940	Hamilton, J. G. Soley, M. H.	*Amer. J. Physiol.*	131:135	Studies in iodine metabolism by thyroid gland in situ by use of radioiodine in normal subjects and in patients with various types of goiter
	Turner, L. A.	*Rev. Mod. Phys.*	12:1	Nuclear fission
	Fermi, E.	*Phys. Rev.*	57:485	Radioactivity bombardment with neutrons
	Taylor, L. S. Singer, G.	*Amer. J. Roentgen.*	44:428	Internal dosimetry
	Lawrence, J. H.	*Radiology*	35:51	Preliminary report on a new method of treatment of leukemia and polycythemia
1941	Hamilton, J. G.	*J. Appl. Phys*	12:440	Applications of radioactive tracers to biology and medicine
	Urey, H. C.	*J. Appl. Phys.*	12:270	Preparation and use of stable isotopes
1942	Hertz, S. Roberts, A.	*J. Clin. Invest.*	21:31	Application of radioactive iodine, to the therapy of Graves' disease
	Hamilton, J. G. Lawrence, J. H.	*J. Clin. Invest.*	21:624	Therapeutic applications of radiophosphorus and radioiodine
	Hamilton, J. G.	*Radiology*	39:541	The use of radioactive tracers in biology and medicine
	Treadwell, A. de G. Low-Beer, B.V.A. Friedell, H. L. Lawrence, J. H.	*Amer. J. Med. Sci.*	204:521	Metabolic studies of neoplasms of bone with the aid of radioactive strontium
	Schoenheimer, R.	Harvard University Press		The dynamic state of body constituents

CHAPTER II

THE DIAGNOSTIC PROCESS

HENRY N. WAGNER, JR.

WILLIAM W. WALTON, JR.

Improvements in medical diagnosis can be closely correlated with the development of new instruments. The invention of the compound microscope in 1830 was a milestone of special significance in medical history. Since that time, many instruments and methods have emerged that are now indispensable to the modern practice of medicine. The ophthalmoscope, invented by Helmholtz in 1851, and x-rays, discovered by Röntgen in 1895, are two of numerous examples. These highly developed instruments and techniques at times provide the sole means for making an accurate diagnosis.

To give reliable results, diagnostic aids must, of course, be properly employed; but they are frequently misused. One type of error is to ignore new diagnostic methods completely; another is to ascribe to them a diagnostic importance, reliability, or specificity they do not merit. To minimize these errors, one must view these techniques in the light of the entire diagnostic procedure. Only in this way can their full value be realized.

Medical diagnosis is the process of identifying a disease by studying its manifestations. Implicit in this definition is the assumption that it is both possible and desirable to classify diseases. Were this not possible—if each person manifested a disease in a unique way—there would be an infinite variety of nonspecific diseases, and medical diagnosis as we know it could not exist.

The Hippocratic school was among the first to group patients according to similarities in the manifestations of their diseases. Sydenham advanced this concept of *syndromes* much further by classifying patients into major disease categories.

A widely accepted classification of diseases (*Standard Nomenclature of Diseases,* 1952) is based on the portion or system of the body involved (topographical) and the cause of the disorder (etiological). Its main *topographical* divisions are:

0—Body as a whole
1—Integumentary system
2—Musculoskeletal system
3—Respiratory system
4—Cardiovascular system
5—Hematological system
6—Digestive system
7—Urogenital system
8—Endocrine system
9—Nervous system
X—Organs of special sense

These major topographical divisions are further subdivided to specify a particular organ or part of an organ, e.g., the pylorus of the stomach.

The major classifications of *etiology* are:

— 0 Prenatal influences
— 1 Lower plant or animal parasites
— 2 Higher plant or animal parasites
— 3 Intoxication (noxious substances)
— 4 Trauma or physical agents
— 5 Circulatory disturbances
— 6 Disturbances of innervations or of psychic control
— 7 Mechanical abnormalities
— 8 Disorders of metabolism, growth, and nutrition
— 9 New growths (neoplasms)
—10 Diseases of undetermined cause

As in the topographical classification, the major etiological groups are further subdivided to specify particular etiological agents, e.g., poisoning by a specific substance.

Although this system was designed primarily for keeping medical records, many physicians think along these same lines of topographical-etiological relationships when making a diagnosis.

The diagnostic process is frequently quite complex. The number of facts that can be collected concerning a person's medical history and present state of health are practically limitless. Therefore every question that the physician asks in obtaining the medical history, every maneuver that he performs in the physical examination, and every subsequent laboratory procedure that he orders should be selected because of the likelihood that the new fact will alter the estimate of probability that the patient has a particular disease or diseases.

An essential feature of the diagnostic process is its statistical or probabilistic nature. Rarely can a medical diagnosis be made with absolute certainty. In many cases it must be stated in terms of the most likely diagnosis together with alternative diagnoses.

The relationship between a disease and its manifestations must be considered probabilistic, since it is usually not possible to state with certainty that a particular manifestation or set of manifestations will be exhibited by a patient with a specific disease. The physician can only state the likelihood or conditional probability of observing particular manifestations in a patient with a particular disease.

Another important characteristic of the diagnostic procedure is that it cannot be conducted in a completely standardized fashion for every patient. In his approach to establishing the diagnosis, the physician should try to be sequentially logical from start to finish. He should be concerned with why he asks one question rather than another, why he examines one area of the body in more detail than another, and why he tests a particular chemical constituent of the blood or requests a particular type of x-ray examination rather than another. He should try to avoid the error of continually ordering a battery of expensive laboratory tests on the grounds that there is a *possibility*, however remote, that the patient has a certain disease.

In his management of a patient's illness, the physician must continually make complex decisions: first, in establishing the diagnosis and then in selecting appropriate therapy. Recently, statisticians and mathematicians have been trying to obtain at least a partial answer to the basic question of how decisions are, and should be, made. The necessary conditions for the existence of a decision problem are a decision maker, one or more objectives, and at least two possible courses of action. Game theory, utility theory, and value theory are recent developments that attempt to explain how a decision maker chooses between alternative courses of action.

Physicians must continually choose from among alternative courses of action, most of which are initially directed toward establishing which disease or diseases a patient may have. If these were known with certainty, it would be much easier to select the most desirable course of action. Conflicting objectives arise since, in the process of identifying the patient's disease, the physician wishes to avoid exorbitantly high costs in making the diagnosis whether the cost is considered in terms of expense or discomfort or risk to the patient, as in exploratory surgery.

One important consideration is whether the decision-making process is carried out under conditions of certainty or uncertainty (Luce and Raiffa, 1957). If each alternative course of action leads to a specific and invariant outcome, the decision can be made with certainty. The physician frequently prefers and chooses a given diagnostic procedure because he knows which procedures are most specific for the diagnosis of particular diseases. Rather than order a large number of tests in an unselective manner, his aim should be to approach systematically the procedure of greatest diagnostic value under the circumstances.

Often, however, the specificity of disease manifestations is not sufficiently great to permit absolute certainty of diagnosis, and the physician is faced with making a decision under conditions of uncertainty. Under these circumstances, he may defer his decision and continue in a logical fashion to collect additional data until a more definite diagnosis can be made. His success can be measured by how efficiently and effectively he proceeds.

Figure 2-1 is a schematic representation of a logical system of medical diagnosis. The patient's syndrome (S_j) results from the existence of a particular disease (D_i) or diseases. The physician's aim is to establish with a high degree of certainty that the syndrome is the result of a particular disease or diseases.

The physician's first step is to construct the patient's *syndrome*. An essential part of the procedure is the evaluation and "weighing" of manifestations according to their diagnostic reliability and specificity in relation to particular diseases. Symbolically, the syndrome can be represented as the sum of the disease manifestations multiplied by the diagnostic significance or "weight" of the individual manifestations:

$$S_j = \Sigma_j(m_j w_j)$$

where $S_j =$ the patient's syndrome; $m_j =$ the manifestation; and $w_j =$ the weight of the manifestation, m_j.

The reason for integrating the manifestations to form a syndrome rather than considering each manifestation separately is that in combination a group of manifestations often provide a specificity that none would have alone. For example, exophthalmos and hyperthyroidism in combination form the specific syndrome, Graves' disease.

Given a complicated diagnostic problem, it is helpful to divide the diagnostic process according to two major aims: (1) to increase progressively the probability of finding that the patient's illness is a particular disease or diseases; and (2) to decrease progressively the probability that his illness is some other disease. Initially the physician obtains a full medical history, including a review of each major organ system, to reduce the possibility of overlooking manifestations. A thorough physical examination is then performed. These procedures lead to the exclusion of many diagnostic possibilities. On the other hand, particularly in obtaining the history of the present illness, the physician elicits more and more manifestations (m_j) and begins to form a picture of the patient's syndrome. This is supplemented by findings of the physical examination. The aim is eventually to classify the patient's evolving syndrome in the light of *medical knowledge*, represented in Figure 2-1 as $P(S_j/D_i)$. The symbol $P(S_j/D_i)$ represents the probability of the occurrence of syndrome S_j, given a particular set of diseases D_i.[1] The expression $P(D_i/S_j)$ is the probability of the patient's having the set of diseases D_i, given the syndrome S_j. Thus, one may consider medical knowledge as being represented by $P(S_j/D_i)$, i.e., knowledge of the conditional probability of the occurrence of certain syndromes given particular diseases (or in the initial stages of the diagnostic process, classes of diseases). To be an effective diagnostician, the physician must know not only the average or "classic" manifestations of diseases, but also the variations in syndromes that may exist in particular diseases. The term $P(D_i)$ is the *a priori* probability that the patient has a particular set of diseases, D_i, as estimated by the prevalence of D_i in the population from which the patient is a sample. A medical aphorism used to express this type of consideration is that "common diseases occur commonly."

One way to determine the probability that the patient has a particular disease, given his syndrome, is to use Bayes' theorem of inverse probability:

$$P(D_i/S_j) = \frac{P(S_j/D_i) \times P(D_i)}{\Sigma_i[P(S_j/D_i) \times P(D_i)]}$$

---

[1] The set of diseases may, and frequently will, be only one disease.

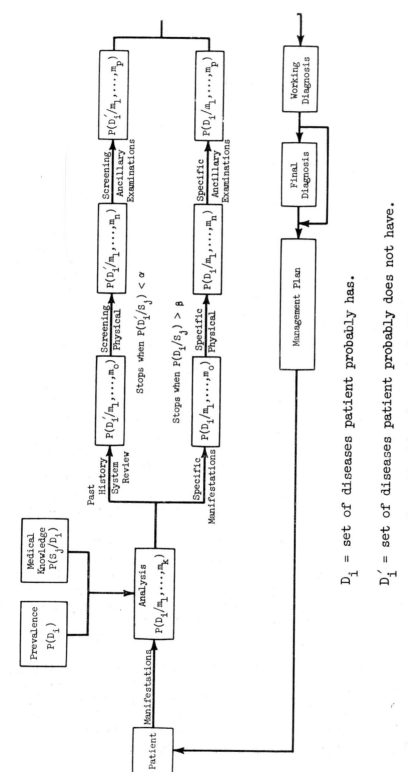

FIGURE 2-1. A logical system of medical diagnosis.

D_i = set of diseases patient probably has.

D_i' = set of diseases patient probably does not have.

This equation states that the probability that a patient with a given syndrome, S_j, has a particular disease, D_i, is directly proportional to the probability of occurrence of his syndrome in that disease multiplied by the *a priori* prevalence of that disease, and inversely proportional to the probability of occurrence of his syndrome in all other diseases. This use of Bayes' theorem in medicine was first suggested by Ledley and Lusted (1959) and has subsequently been used by others.

The physician can apply Bayes' theorem as he forms a dichotomy consisting of a set of diseases that the patient may have (symbolized as D_i) and a set that he probably does *not* have (symbolized as $D_í$). He continues to elicit additional manifestations that will increase the probability that the patient's disease is a certain specific one. He increases progressively the probability of the presence of the primary set of diseases D_i, while decreasing progressively the probability of the secondary set of diseases, $D_í$.

In performing the physical examination of the patient, the physician examines in great detail the parts of the body thought from previous data to be possibly diseased; he also performs a systematic physical examination to reduce the likelihood of missing relevant physical signs not indicated by the patient's symptoms. Similarly, ancillary laboratory tests are of two types, those suggested by previous data and those obtained as screening tests to lower further the probability of diseases $D_í$.

Working diagnoses may be reached at several stages: after the description of the present illness is obtained, after the past history has been reviewed, after the physical examination, or after the initial ancillary tests have been completed. Working diagnoses are those diseases (or classes of diseases, initially) that have a progressively higher probability as the analysis proceeds, and as the manifestations are collected to form the complete syndrome, S_j. This sequential approach to decision problems was initially proposed by Wald (1947), who introduced the concept of waiting to make a decision until a sufficient amount of information is available to warrant a decision. Thus, the physician may at any stage of the process make a decision, or he may defer until more information is obtained.

How sure does the physician have to be of the diagnosis? This varies with the disease, and can be expressed in terms of *thresholds*. The physician must make the diagnosis with a degree of certainty that exceeds a definite threshold value, which is a function of the losses that will result from diagnostic errors and the gains associated with a correct diagnosis. For example, the threshold would be low for diseases such as pernicious anemia or subacute bacterial endocarditis —in which the losses associated with missing the diagnosis are exceedingly high, whereas the costs of treatment are relatively low. Consequently, a decision to treat would be reached if the probability of either disease was greater than, say, 10 per cent. This means, of course, that one must be willing to treat a fairly large number of patients unnecessarily.

Another threshold value is the probability below which one is willing to state that a disease is not present; this is a measure of how certain one must be before one is willing to accept the risk of making the decision that the patient is free of a given disease. By making a definite effort to establish the low probability of presence of diseases other than the final diagnosis, one avoids the error of completely ignoring certain diseases as possibilities.

An important part of a systematic approach to medical diagnosis is knowing when to proceed from the patient's history to the physical examination, and from the physical examination to ancillary examinations, and when to conclude the diagnostic process. One criterion is to continue each category of examination for as long as the probability of the patient's having certain diseases is increasing at a significant rate. On the other hand, if further history taking, or further physical examination, is not significantly altering the probabilities, one should proceed logically to a new set of tests as a new source of manifestations.

DIAGNOSTIC ERRORS

These may be classified as follows:

(1) Data concerning the patient's illness may be *incomplete;* i.e., insufficient manifestations have been elicited to permit definition of the patient's syndrome.

(2) Data may be *incorrect,* leading to construction of an erroneous syndrome.

(3) The physician may persistently consider manifestations only as isolated phenomena, rather than as parts of syndromes.

(4) The physician's medical knowledge may be incomplete; i.e., he may not be sufficiently familiar with the frequency of particular syndromes in particular diseases, or with the variability of syndromes in particular diseases.

(5) He may not consider certain diseases or may be unaware of the particular incidence of certain diseases in the population of which the patient is a sample.

(6) He may not systematically follow the diagnostic leads obtained in the course of the diagnostic process, e.g., during the eliciting of the present illness, the physical examination, or as a result of laboratory procedures.

(7) He may ignore the necessity of making a positive effort to reduce the probability of all other diseases as sources of the illness; i.e., he is not sufficiently thorough and comprehensive in using his screening questions, general physical examination, and screening ancillary examinations effectively in the process of eliminating possibilities.

(8) Instead of using a systematic and logical approach, the physician uses an unthinking approach that is at best inefficient and costly, and at worst ineffective.

USE OF ANCILLARY EXAMINATIONS

How do ancillary examinations, such as radioisotope techniques, fit into the diagnostic system? How do they permit more effective diagnosis?

First, ancillary examinations provide *new* data, permitting more precise definition of the patient's syndrome. For example, the use of radioactive iodine may provide the new manifestation that the patient is incorporating iodide into his thyroid gland at an abnormally rapid rate.

Second, they provide more *reliable* data. For example, the use of ^{51}Cr-labeled red blood cells in patients with acute blood loss provides a better index of the patient's red blood cell volume than does the estimation of the volume of packed red blood cells (hematocrit).

Third, they provide diagnostically *more specific* manifestations, those that rapidly increase the probability of the patient's having a specific disease. For example, the use of radioactive vitamin B_{12} alone and in combination with gastric intrinsic factor can establish the diagnosis of pernicious anemia.

Fourth, they provide *objective, quantitative* data that will increase greatly the probability of the patient's having a specific disease, thereby confirming the diagnosis. For example, the demonstration of an abnormally rapid removal of labeled erythrocytes from the circulation can establish the diagnosis of hemolytic anemia.

Fifth, they provide useful *screening* procedures that decrease the probability that the patient has some other possible disease. For example, the use of brain scanning can decrease the probability of brain tumor in a patient suspected of having a cerebrovascular occlusion.

Sixth, they decrease the cost of obtaining data necessary to confirm or eliminate the likelihood of a disease. For example, radioisotope studies of the kidneys may obviate the necessity of renal arteriography.

Seventh, they raise the likelihood of a disease to a high enough level to warrant a procedure that is more costly in terms of expense or, especially, risk for the patient. For example, the use of pulmonary scanning may obviate the need for pulmonary arteriography, or may increase the probability that pulmonary arteriography will provide useful information.

Eighth, they provide quantitative data useful for practical care and clinical management of the patient, e.g., in the assessment of the magnitude of intracardiac shunt.

REFERENCES

Ledley, R. S., and Lusted, L. B.: Reasoning Foundations of Medical Diagnosis. *Science* 130:9, 1959.
Luce, R. D., and Raiffa, H.: Games and Decision. John Wiley & Sons, Inc., New York, 1957.
Standard Nomenclature of Diseases and Operations. McGraw-Hill Book Co., New York, 1952.
Wald, A.: Sequential Analysis. John Wiley & Sons, Inc., New York, 1947.

CHAPTER III

MATHEMATICS

HENRY N. WAGNER, Jr.
WILLIAM W. WALTON, Jr.
JOHN JACQUEZ

INTRODUCTION

Medical knowledge consists largely of an impressive collection of empirical data, much of which has resulted from careful observation and investigation of patients. Medicine still does not have the coherent structure of a fully developed science. In the physical sciences, mathematics has been the foundation upon which a scientific structure has been built. Unfortunately, biologists in general and physicians in particular have been hesitant to fully utilize mathematics in the solution of their problems. To some extent, this has resulted from the occasional misuse of mathematics, particularly when theoretical analysis has rested on erroneous assumptions or on questionable experimental data. An equally grave error is to ignore mathematics completely.

Mathematics in medicine relies largely on statistics and probability theory, two fields which have been developed to study nondeterministic processes, i.e., processes in which an exact cause and effect relationship does not exist. In most biomedical investigations, multiple factors influence the particular parameter of interest. For example, although it is impossible to predict the course of the illness of a specific patient, generalizations can be made to describe a large population of such patients. Similarly, although it is impossible to predict when an individual radioactive atom will decay, if one considers an extremely large number of radioactive atoms and measures the number decaying over constant periods of time, one can use a statistical approach to determine the average rate of decay. Thus, we can formulate laws that describe the behavior of a *popula tion* of atoms, rather than the behavior of a single atom.

STATISTICS

Henry N. Wagner, Jr.

William W. Walton, Jr.

PROBABILITY DISTRIBUTIONS

The laws of probability are useful whenever the occurrence of an anticipated event is dependent to some degree upon chance. Two fundamental concepts necessary to study nondeterministic processes are the probability *distribution function,* $F(x)$, and the probability *distribution density function,* $f(x)$. A distribution function $F(x)$ is defined as the probability that the random variable (X) assumes a value equal to or less than x; i.e., $F(x) = P(X \leq x)$. The first derivative of the distribution function is the more familiar *distribution density function,* $f(x)$, which is a graph of the frequency with which one observes progressively increasing values of x.

The distribution density can be described by various parameters, such as the mean and standard deviation. For example, if one measures the number of radioactive atoms disintegrating per minute over one minute intervals, one will not obtain exactly the same number in each interval, but will observe that the results tend to be grouped around a value, referred to as the average value, or mean. Symbolically, this is indicated by $\bar{x}$, which is equal to $\sum_{i=1}^{n} \frac{x_i}{n}$, that is, the sum of the number of disintegrations in all intervals divided by the number of intervals n. The standard deviation is a measure of the variability or spread of the observations around this central value. $\bar{x}$ is an estimate of the true population mean μ, obtained from a sample of size n. The reliability of the estimate $\bar{x}$ increases as the sample size increases.

Normal distribution

The most frequently encountered probability distribution in the biomedical field is the normal or Gaussian distribution. Examples encountered in everyday life which follow this distribution are height, weight, and temperature. For example, if we were to measure the body temperature of a large cross section of the population and plot the number of times each particular value was observed on the vertical axis and the temperature on the horizontal axis, we would obtain the well known symmetrical curve, frequently described as "bell-shaped." We would observe a few low temperatures and a few high temperatures, but most would be clustered around the average value 98.6° F. The Gaussian distribution is usually observed under circumstances in which large numbers of factors are influencing the variable and in which these factors are independent of one another. What can be learned from such a graph? First, it tells us the mean or the most probable value that we would obtain if we collected more observations. This corresponds to the maximum point on the curve. We cannot predict exactly what the next individual result will be; however, it is possible to determine the probabilities that one will obtain certain individual results if one continues to make observations. This knowledge gives us information about the degree of variability of the observations, at times referred to as the degree of "spread" of the data. We can describe the degree of deviation from the most probable or mean value. If one determines the deviation of each individual value from the mean value $(\bar{x})$, symbolized $(x_i - \bar{x})$, squares these values to cancel out the plus and the minus signs and then takes the square root of the sums of these squares, and divides by the number of observations, n, one obtains a value referred to as the *standard deviation*.

Symbolically,

$$s = \sqrt{\frac{\sum_{i=1}^{n}(x_i - \bar{x})^2}{n}}$$

For smaller samples, where n is less than 30, one usually divides by the number of observations minus one, i.e., n — 1. It is common practice to use s to designate the standard deviation obtained from a sample and to use $\jmath$ to denote the true standard deviation of the population.

The standard deviation, σ, determines what portion of our observations can be expected to fall between a specified interval on either side of the mean. The probability density for the normal distribution is given by the expression:

$$f(x) = \frac{1}{\sigma\sqrt{2\pi}} \cdot e^{-\frac{1}{2}\left(\frac{x-\bar{x}}{\sigma}\right)^2}$$

Since the integral of $f(x)$ does not have a simple functional form, we must exhibit the distribution function as an integral, i.e.,

$$f(x) = \frac{1}{\sigma\sqrt{2\pi}} \int_{-\infty}^{x} e^{-\frac{1}{2}\left(\frac{x-\bar{x}}{\sigma}\right)^2} dx$$

This function gives the probability that x will lie between minus infinity and x. To evaluate this integral numerically is a long and tedious task. Fortunately, this has already been done and complete sets of tables are available.

For example, in a normally distributed set of values of x, a range of

$\bar{x} \pm 1\,\sigma$ will include 68.3 per cent of the population
$\bar{x} \pm 2\,\sigma$ will include 95.4 per cent of the population
$\bar{x} \pm 3\,\sigma$ will include 99.7 per cent of the population

The standard deviation of a measurement is an estimation of the *precision* of the measurement. It tells us how reproducible the results have been. Precision must be differentiated from *accuracy*. The latter tells us how close we have come to making an estimate of the true value we are seeking. If our measuring device has a systematic error (so called because it is not random) we may obtain precise data that are quite inaccurate.

The standard deviation is sometimes expressed as a percentage of the mean value, that is

$$\frac{\sigma}{\overline{x}} \cdot 100$$

This value is referred to as the *relative standard deviation,* with units of per cent. It may also be referred to as the *standard error* of the measurement. $\frac{\sigma}{\sqrt{n}}$ is referred to as the standard deviation of the mean.

POISSON DISTRIBUTION

Another distribution frequently encountered in medicine, particularly in nuclear medicine, is the Poisson distribution. In contrast to the normal distribution which deals with *continuous* variables, the Poisson distribution is applicable only to the study of *discrete* variables. Our previous example of a continuous variable was the temperature of individuals. This measurement can assume an infinite number of values. An example of a discrete variable is the number of patients with thyrotoxicosis who have exophthalmos. In this case, as with other discrete variables, only a finite number of values can be assumed by the variable under consideration.

The Poisson distribution, along with the binomial distribution, forms the cornerstone for the study of discrete processes just as the normal distribution does for continuous processes. The Poisson distribution can be derived as a convenient approximation of the binomial distribution or it can be derived independently on the basis of mathematical assumptions that match certain physical processes. The physical process of radioactive disintegrations matches very closely the assumptions necessary to derive this distribution. The required physical assumptions are that the conditions of the experiment remain constant over the time interval of interest and that each time interval be independent of the preceding and succeeding intervals so that the number of events observed in any one interval does not reveal any information about the number of events that may be observed in another. Hence a radioactive substance emits α particles and the distribution of the number of particles reaching a given portion of space in time t obeys the Poisson distribution. This is true only for substances such as radium which decay very slowly, so that for relatively short periods of time conditions may be considered relatively constant. The derivation, which is not given here, would lead to the following expression for the probability of observing n particles in time t where λ is the average number of particles observed over many intervals t.

$$P(n) = (\lambda t)^n e^{-\lambda t}/n!$$

When n becomes very large the probability computations using this expression become very lengthy and tedious and hence this distribution is frequently approximated by the normal distribution. For an excellent discussion of this the reader is referred to Feller, *An Introduction to Probability Theory and Its Applications* (1957).

An important characteristic of the Poisson distribution is that the standard deviation is equal to the square root of the mean. That is,

$$\sigma = \sqrt{\lambda}$$

Increasing the number of observations will increase the absolute value of the variability but will decrease the variability expressed as a percentage of the mean. Other examples of events that follow the Poisson distribution are blood cell counts.

Although the normal distribution is most frequently used in biomedical statistics, the Poisson distribution is widely used in radioisotope methodology. Since, when derived as an approximation of the binomial, it is based on the assumption that the *frequency* of an individual event is small whereas the *total number* of events is large, it describes exactly the decay of millions of atoms from among a population of billions.

LAWS OF PROBABILITY

In the practice of medicine, the physician constantly applies the laws of probability, either consciously or subconsciously. The term probability is usually defined as the limit of the relative frequency of occurrence of an event. For example, the probability with which one might observe persons with pernicious anemia in a given population is given by the equation:

$$P = n_A/n$$

where n_A is the number of persons with pernicious anemia and n is the number of persons in the whole population. The quantity n_A is the *absolute* frequency. The probability P is the *relative* frequency with which this disease occurs. If, in a population of 1,000,000 persons, there were 1000 cases of pernicious anemia, in a random sample of 1000 persons we would *not* expect to observe precisely one case. We would observe a frequency of exactly 0.001 only under the limiting condition, that is, if the whole population were sampled.

In the present text, we need not be concerned with a rigorous and abstract discussion of probability theory, but will consider certain fundamental mathematical rules of probability that are of particular value in medical diagnosis.

Simultaneous Occurrence of Two Events. A common problem is the calculation of the probability of the simultaneous occurrence of two events when one knows the probability of occurrence of each event separately. For example, one might consider the problem of the incidence of pernicious anemia in Negroes. Let *event A* be pernicious anemia, and let *event B* represent a Negro. P(A) is the probability of observing A; P(B) is the probability of observing B. P(AB) is the probability of simultaneous occurrence of both events and is computed as:

$$P(AB) = n_{AB}/n \tag{1}$$

where n = the total number of persons in the population and n_{AB} equals the total number of Negroes in the population with pernicious anemia.

If, and only if, A and B are independent of each other, then

$$P(AB) = P(A) \times P(B) \tag{2}$$

The importance of the necessary condition of independence of the two variables in the application of this rule of probability is well illustrated by the example. If the relationship described by equation 2 is not demonstrated by the observed data, one can conclude that events A and B are not independent, but related. Since the incidence of pernicious anemia is much lower in Negroes than in Caucasians, the probability of observing a Negro with pernicious anemia would be much less than the combined probabilities of observing a Negro in the population, and the probability of observing a person with pernicious anemia.

A second fundamental rule of probability describes the probability of occurrence of *either* event A or event B or *both* occurring in a given sample. This rule is referred to as the general rule of addition of probabilities:

$$P(A + B) = P(A) + P(B) - P(AB)$$

Conditional Probability. We have just seen that the probability of observing pernicious anemia depends upon whether or not the patient is a Caucasian or Negro (as well as upon many other factors). This introduces the concept of *conditional probability*. The probability of observing pernicious anemia in a patient can be expressed as

$$P(A) = n_A/n \tag{3}$$

where n_A equals the total number of patients with pernicious anemia and n equals the total number of patients in the population. If it is now specified that the patient is a Negro, we must now consider the conditional probability of observing pernicious anemia, conditioned by the fact that the patient is a Negro. The probability is now written as:

$$P(A/B) = \text{probability of A, given B} = n_{AB}/n_B \tag{4}$$

where n_{AB} equals the total number of Negroes with pernicious anemia and n_B equals the total number of Negroes in the population. This probability is clearly different from that given in equation (3).

An important relationship in the use of conditional probabilities is as follows:

$$P(AB) = P(B) \, P(A/B) = P(A) \, P(B/A) \tag{5}$$

This equation states that the probability of the simultaneous occurrence of events A and B is equal to the probability of B times the probability of A given the occurrence of event B. Similarly, the simultaneous occurrence of both events equals the probability of A times the probability of B given the occurrence of event A.

STATISTICS OF MEDICAL DIAGNOSIS

The systematic approach to medical diagnosis that we have proposed can be characterized as follows: (1) the diagnostic process is expressed in mathematical terms based on its statistical or probabilistic nature; (2) manifestations of disease are weighted in accordance with their specificity, sensitivity, and reliability and collected into syndromes; (3) the system is based on sequential analysis, and the physician may at any point defer his diagnosis until additional information is collected; and (4) sequential actions are based on a theory ot thresholds related to the costs of alternative courses of action, in terms of various diseases that the patient may have.

RELATIONSHIP AMONG MANIFESTATIONS, SYNDROMES, AND DISEASE

A manifestation is defined as a symptom, physical sign, radiographic finding, or result of a laboratory test. These fall into one of two groups. The first consists of manifestations which can be measured along a continuous scale, such as age, temperature, and blood pressure. The second consists of manifestations which can only assume a finite number of values. They are discrete, such as sex or the presence or absence of pain. Discrete manifestations cannot be expressed quantitatively; only their presence or absence can be noted. Occasionally, an attempt at quantitation is made, e.g., by grading the manifestations between zero and four plus. Nevertheless, they are basically discrete variables.

Since many manifestations are not specific when considered as isolated phenomena, it is useful to consider groups of manifestations. Such groups are referred to as syndromes, and may be quite specific. We have previously defined a syndrome (S) as the sum of the weighted manifestations (m_j) of a disease, i.e.,

$$S = \sum_{j=0}^{n} m_j w_j$$

where w_j = the weight of each manifestation, m_j, and n = the number of manifestations.

Just as we can speak of the probability of observing (or not observing) certain manifestations in a patient with a given disease, so also can we speak of the probability of observing specific *syndromes* in a patient with a given disease. This is represented by the histogram shown in Figure 3-1.

Each S_j represents a different patient syndrome, and consists of the sum of n weighted manifestations, each of which forms a part of the syndrome. The weight of each manifestation is depicted graphically by the size of the cells that form S_j. In the figure, S_j is the syndrome most frequently observed for the disease, D_i. Syndrome S_{j-1} or S_{j+1} may contain one more or one less of the manifestations that formed S_j, or they might even consist of a completely different set of manifestations. This figure, when completed for all possible syndromes, sum-

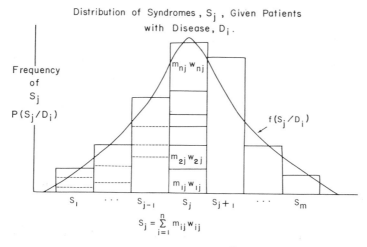

FIGURE 3-1.   Histogram of syndromes of disease.

marizes the medical knowledge about the probabilistic relationship between disease D_i and the set of m syndromes observed with this particular disease. The quantities S_j assume discrete values and consequently are discrete random variables. However, since they are formed by summing several random variables, which are binomially distributed, they can be approximated by a normal distribution. Therefore the conditional probability density of S_j, given a disease, D_i, i.e., $f(S_j/D_i)$, can be represented by the smooth curve that has been superimposed on the histogram.

The diagnostic process requires that this type of information be available for all diseases under consideration.

DEFINITION OF THE NORMAL RANGE

Relationship between Populations with and without a Disease. We have previously defined medical knowledge as knowledge of the conditional probability of observing certain manifestations and syndromes in particular diseases. This includes knowledge of the probability of occurrence of individual manifestations or syndromes in the population of individuals who are apparently not sick. The physician must compare his particular patient with the healthy population as well as with persons known to have particular diseases. He must first answer the question, is the patient sick? and then the question, what is the identity of the sickness?

Just as it is necessary for the physician to be aware of what is and what is not a normal finding, so also is it a primary task of a laboratory performing diagnostic tests to define clearly the normal ranges of its results. Laboratory results frequently follow a Gaussian distribution, and thus one can characterize the normal values by establishing the mean value and the standard deviation. After this has been done, an important decision must be made regarding the establishment of the operational *range of normality*.

In many instances, if one examines a large number of patients with a particular disease, a Gaussian distribution of the results will also be observed, but with a different mean value and standard deviation from that observed in healthy persons. For example, the diseased population may have generally higher values of the variable than the healthy population. Nearly always the two populations, the healthy and the diseased, overlap to some extent. Some values will be found that could belong to either population. If there were no overlap, the physician could determine with certainty to which population the patient belonged. The overlap between the healthy and diseased populations introduces the possibility of errors.

Type I and Type II Errors. One type of error is to conclude that a healthy person has the disease. This is usually referred to as a *false positive* or Type I error. The second type of error is to conclude that a sick person is well, referred to as a *false negative* or a Type II error. These errors are inversely related and their respective magnitudes will depend on where one sets the upper limit of the healthy population, i.e., the range of normality. For example, if one sets this upper limit at a low value, many healthy persons will be considered sick; i.e., false positive errors will be frequent. Conversely, if the normal limit is set high, false negative errors will be encountered frequently.

Wald (1947) has proposed a solution to this dilemma. He has suggested that the relative costs resulting from each type of error are the most important considerations. The total expected costs can be expressed as follows:

Total expected cost = probability of Type I error $\times$ cost of Type I error + probability of Type II error $\times$ cost of Type II error

Wald's decision rule states that one should set the limit of normality to minimize the total expected cost. For example, the cost of calling a patient with pernicious anemia normal would be quite high in view of the serious consequences of leaving this disease untreated. Therefore, we would make every effort to avoid false negative (Type II) errors. On the other hand, we cannot restrict the limits of normality too much or the cost of the error of calling many normal people abnormal (Type I error) will become exorbitant. Scheff (1963) has analyzed the possible consequences of this type of error. He points out that physicians usually assume that judging a sick person well is more to be avoided than judging a well person sick, that it is far more culpable to dismiss a sick patient than to retain a well one. This decision rule may often place patients in the "sick role" who could otherwise have continued in their normal pursuits. Undoubtedly the decision rule, "When in doubt, diagnose illness," is frequently extremely helpful. One need only cite the occasional tragic occurrence of an undetected subdural hematoma to emphasize the point. Occasionally, however, this rule can lead to errors. Garland reported that in the examination of 14,867 chest x-rays for signs of tuberculosis, there were 1216 positive readings that turned out to be clinically negative (Type II error) and only 24 negative readings that turned out to be clinically positive (Type I error). This report provides objective evidence of the frequent application of the decision rule, "better safe than sorry."

What is one to do when faced with the dilemma of where to set normal values for a laboratory procedure? One can be guided by Wald's decision rule and should consider carefully the *costs* of *both* types of error rather than only the *number* of possible errors. Then the levels of normality can be established that will minimize *total* expected *costs*.

Specificity and Sensitivity. The possibility of diagnostic errors results not only from overlap of manifestations between patients with a particular disease and the healthy population, but also from overlap between various diseases. The degree of overlap is expressed by the term *specificity*, which is related to the probability that a particular manifestation will be observed in the healthy population or in patients with diseases other than the primary disease in which one finds the manifestation of interest. For example, if a manifestation occurs in 5 per cent of healthy persons, or persons with other diseases than the one of interest, its specificity for the disease of interest would be 0.95. A specificity of 1.00 indicates that the manifestations occur only in the disease of interest and never in the rest of the population.

Specificity should be differentiated from *sensitivity*. The latter is defined as the probability that the manifestation will be observed in the particular disease of interest. Thus, a manifestation that is present in half the patients with a given disease will have a sensitivity of 0.50. A manifestation that occurs in every patient with a given disease has a sensitivity of 1.00. At times a manifestation may have a high specificity and a low sensitivity, e.g., the presence of LE cells in the blood of patients with lupus erythematosus. Observation of this sign permits diagnosis with a high degree of certainty. Its absence does not eliminate the probability of the patient's having the disease. On the other hand, a decreased rate of accumulation of radioactive iodine is a sensitive test for hypothyroidism, but it is not specific since it may occur under other circumstances, e.g., following ingestion of iodine-containing medications. Observation of this manifestation cannot be used as conclusive evidence that the patient has hypothyroidism.

Ancillary diagnostic tests can be divided into two major categories, *screening* tests and *definitive* tests. The former are characterized by having a high sensitivity, the latter by a high specificity. A perfect test would be one that was completely sensitive and completely specific, a phenomenon rarely, if ever, encountered in medicine.

Gains and Losses. An important characteristic of the system of medical diagnosis presented in Chapter II was its sequential nature; serial actions were governed by a theory of thresholds related to the costs and gains of subsequent courses of action. At the completion of the history and physical examination, it was suggested that the physician form a set of conditional probabilities as to which diseases or at least which classes of diseases the patient may have. For example, he may decide that the patient has disease of either the endocrine or hematologic system. The information available at this stage of the diagnostic process may not be sufficient to establish the diagnosis with a sufficiently high probability. Under these circumstances, ancillary tests can be used to provide additional manifestations. How can one decide the proper sequence in which these tests should be performed?

A fundamental assumption is that there are gains and losses associated with the performance of each test. The losses include danger to the patient, discomfort associated with the test, and financial cost. Gains include the value of making a correct diagnosis, a minimum delay in the onset of therapy, and return of the patient to his usual activities. Also to be considered are efficient use of physician time, laboratory facilities, and hospital beds, as well as gains resulting from minimizing the period of illness with its important consequences to the patient and his family. It is frequently helpful for the physician to construct a table of the gains and losses associated with each course of action, that is, with each diagnostic procedure that is contemplated, and then analyze all possible courses of action before reaching a decision. This may help to avoid the error of failing to utilize fully the information available from the history and physical examination prior to the selection of laboratory tests.

Decision Criteria. After the physician has constructed a table of the gains and losses associated with alternate courses of action, how is he to proceed? One useful decision rule is an extension of Bayes' theorem of inverse probability discussed in Chapter II. This rule states that one should minimize the *total expected Bayes' loss*. Bayes' loss is computed for *each* possible course of action by multiplying the probability of the patient's having a particular disease times the losses that would result from taking that course of action. This is done for all possible diseases that the patient may have. The decision rule is to select the course of action that would minimize this *total* expected loss, i.e., the course of action for which the sum is minimum. Another way of stating this decision rule is that the *total* expected *gains* should be maximized.

ANALYTICAL TECHNIQUES

Numerous statistical techniques have wide applicability in the field of medicine. Examples of their usefulness are to describe the parameters of a population, to define whether a particular value in a diagnostic test is within the normal range, and to determine relationships which may exist among variables of a population. Among the most useful are: (1) maximum likelihood; (2) regression analysis; (3) least squares; and (4) correlation analysis. A complete discussion of these methods is beyond the scope of this chapter, but simple examples will be cited.

METHOD OF MAXIMUM LIKELIHOOD

A frequently encountered problem is the estimation of the parameters of a distribution of values. R. A. Fisher developed the method of maximum likelihood as a means of dealing with this problem. This method can be used to find the maximum likelihood estimate of the parameter λ of a Poisson distribution for which a random sample $x_1, x_2, \ldots, x_n$ has been collected. It can be shown that the maximum likelihood estimate of λ is the mean. Thus if a population follows the Poisson distribution, the parameter that describes the probability density function is the mean. We have stated previously that an important characteristic of the Poisson distribution is that the variance is equal to the mean and that the square root of the mean is equal to the standard deviation.

In addition to its general usefulness as a statistical tool in defining the parameters of a distribution, the method of maximum likelihood has been successfully used in the general process of medical diagnosis, but is less useful than Bayes' rule of minimizing total expected loss.

REGRESSION ANALYSIS

Regression is another highly useful statistical tool. It is concerned with determining the relationship that exists among two or more variables. In its simplest form, the relationship between two variables may be linear, in which case regression analysis is particularly convenient. Regression analysis was devised by Galton to clarify the relationship between the heights of parents and of their children. He reasoned that if tall parents had tall children and short parents had short children, the world would eventually be full of giants and midgets. By plotting the heights of parents against the heights of their children, he was able to determine that children *regressed;* that is, tall parents usually had shorter children and shorter parents had taller children. In this process he developed this important analytical technique.

An example encountered in medicine is the determination of the effect of age on a particular physiological parameter. Another example is the relationship between plasma protein-bound iodine and the rate of accumulation of radioactive iodine. If there is a linear relationship between two variables, the relationship can be illustrated by graphing one variable against the other. The sample points form a pattern grouped around a straight line. The relationship can be expressed by the equation $Y = AX + B$. Instead of fitting a line to the data by eye, one may use regression analysis to determine the constants A and B. The pairs $(x_1, y_1), (x_2, y_2), \ldots, (x_n, y_n)$ are assumed to be random independent variables and the conditional densities of each y_i for a specific x_i are:

$$f(y_i/x_i) = \frac{1}{\sqrt{2\pi}\sigma} e^{-\frac{1}{2}\left[\frac{y_i - (Ax_i + B)}{\sigma}\right]^2}$$

The values x_i are considered to be constants and the analysis is viewed as the regression of y on x. The method of maximum likelihood can be used to estimate the regression coefficients A and B and the standard deviation, σ. σ^2 is called the "standard error of estimate" and measures the error incurred by using the regression equation to estimate values of y for given values of x. Partially differentiating the likelihood function with respect to A, B, and σ, and equating these derivatives to zero, we get three simultaneous equations which can be solved for A, B, and σ. The final equations are:

$$A = \frac{n\sum_i x_i y_i - \sum_i x_i \sum_i y_i}{n\sum_i x_i^2 - (\sum x_i)^2}$$

$$B = \frac{\sum_i x_i^2 \sum_i y_i - \sum_i x_i \sum_i x_i y_i}{n\sum_i x_i^2 - (\sum_i x_i)^2}$$

$$\sigma = \sqrt{\frac{1}{n} \sum_i [y_i - (Ax_i + B)]^2}$$

where n equals the number of observations, i.e., pairs of (x_i, y_i). Regression analysis can be extended to three or more variables. For example, we might want to obtain a regression,

$$y = AX + BZ + C$$

A similar procedure can be employed to estimate the regression coefficients A, B, and C. The technique is identical to the two variable analysis, but the complexity increases rapidly as more variables are added. With modern computing facilities, standard regression routines can perform all the computations with ease.

LEAST-SQUARES ANALYSIS

In regression analysis, the distribution of points around the line of regression was assumed to be normal. The method of least squares is independent of the form of the distribution. Least-squares analysis determines a line described by the expression $y = AX + B$, by minimizing the sum of the squares of the vertical distances between the sample points and the line. The coefficients A and B are determined so that the quantity

$$\sum_{=1}^{n} [y_i - (AX_i + B)]^2$$

is a minimum. Differentiating this expression with respect to A and B and equating the derivatives to zero gives the following two equations:

$$\sum_{i=i} (-2)[y_i - (AX_i + B)] = 0$$

$$\sum_{i=1}^{n} (-2)[y_i - (AX_i + B)] = 0$$

When these equations are solved for A and B, the resultant equations are exactly the same as those obtained in regression analysis (see the preceding section). Least squares is a maximum likelihood estimate of the regression line when the form of the distribution of errors is normal. The least-squares method can also be used to estimate the parameters of a nonlinear relationship such as

$$y = AX^2 + BX + C$$

In addition to its usefulness as an analytical technique, the method of least squares is a useful concept in medical diagnosis. For example, the diagnosis of hypothyroidism is frequently confirmed by measuring the radioiodine (^{131}I) accumulation by the thyroid. Suppose one also measures the red cell uptake of triiodothyronine. In patients with hypothyroidism the red cell uptake is usually lower than in persons with normal thyroid activity. Let us assume both tests have been made on a sufficient number of individuals known to have hypothyroidism and a second group known to have normal thyroid activity. The problem is to determine whether a patient whose test results are represented by x, y (where x is the thyroidal accumulation of radioiodine, and y is the triiodothyronine red cell uptake result) is normal or hypothyroid.

The least-squares criterion can be applied as follows: One determines the distance between the values observed for the new patient and all the paired values in patients known to have hypothyroidism. One then squares these distances and adds the results. One also determines the distance between the values observed for the new patient and the paired values observed in normal persons, and similarly sums the squared distances. The smallest sum of the squared values determines to which population the patient is assigned.

The calculation for computing the sums of the squares of these distances is:

$$\sum_{i} [(x - x_i')^2 + (y - y_i')^2]$$

where x_i' = the radioiodine uptake of each patient known to have hypothyroidism and y_i' = the triiodothyronine red cell uptake result in such patients; and

$$\sum [(x - x_i)^2 + (y - y_i)^2]$$

where x_i = the radioiodine uptake of each person known to be normal and y_i = the triiodothyronine red cell uptake result in normal persons. Most computing facilities have packaged programs for making the necessary computations, even when more than two variables are considered.

CORRELATION ANALYSIS

Correlation analysis is also used to study relationships between two or more random variables. The correlation coefficient for a set of paired data (x_1, y_1),

$(x_2, y_2), \ldots, (x_n, y_n)$ is estimated by maximum likelihood methods and can be expressed as follows:

$$\text{The correlation coefficient} \quad R = \frac{\sum_i (x_i - \mu_x)(y_i - \mu_y)}{\sqrt{\sum (x_i - \mu_x)^2} \ \sqrt{\sum (y_i - \mu_y)^2}}$$

where $\mu_x = \sum_i \dfrac{x_i}{n}$, i.e., mean value of x.

$\mu_y = \sum_i \dfrac{y_i}{n}$, i.e., mean value of y.

When the two random variables are uncorrelated, i.e., x and y are independent, R will be zero. When x and y are totally dependent, R will be one. Of course, R can assume intermediate values.

This concept can also be applied to medical diagnosis. Correlation analysis is particularly useful in establishing the relationship between a particular manifestation and a disease. When $R = 1$, the manifestation is an extremely sensitive index of the presence of the disease.

STATISTICS OF NUCLEAR MEASUREMENTS

INTRODUCTION

Fundamental to the application of radioisotope methodology is the determination of the quantity of radioactivity under a variety of circumstances. As in any physical or chemical measurement, errors arise from human factors, instrument drift, instrument "noise," fluctuations resulting from the random nature of radioactive decay, and many other factors not under the control of the observer. Such errors are referred to as *random* errors, and should be distinguished from *systematic* or constant errors that can usually be avoided by proper experimental procedures.

Certain errors, such as those introduced by volumetric or gravimetric determinations, can be minimized by proper selection of equipment and by careful attention to manipulative techniques. These types of errors are not peculiar to nuclear measurements, but are present in all physical or chemical determinations. In this section, we are concerned with errors that are the result of the random nature of radioactive decay. In nearly every case, these errors may be minimized by sufficiently long counting times and are of fundamental importance if one wishes to enhance precision while minimizing the time allotted to carrying out the procedures.

Measurements of radioactivity can be described by the Poisson probability distribution, which we have previously described as being characterized by the fact that the standard deviation σ is equal to the square root of the mean $\bar{x}$. Mathematically this is indicated by $\sigma = \sqrt{\bar{x}}$

A frequent problem in nuclear measurements is to determine how many counts are needed for a desired precision. Suppose one wishes a relative standard deviation of 1 per cent. Then $\sigma/N = 0.01$, where $N =$ the number of counts. Therefore $\dfrac{\sqrt{N}}{N} = 0.01$ and $N = 10,000$. Since the Poisson distribution and hence radioactive decay can be approximated by the Gaussian distribution, there is a 68 per cent chance of being within one standard deviation, or in this case, within 1 per cent of the true value, since 10,000 counts were observed. If we wished to be even more certain of being within 1 per cent of the true value, we would have to set $2\sigma/N = 0.01$ and N would then equal 40,000. We would then have a 95 per cent chance of being within 1 per cent of the true value. This is usually described as being within the 95 per cent *confidence* level.

If we wish to express the results in terms of counting rate rather than total number of counts, the standard deviation

$$\sigma_R = \frac{\sqrt{N}}{t} = \frac{\sqrt{Rt}}{t} = \sqrt{\frac{R}{t}}$$

since the counting rate R = N/t, where t = the counting time, and the relative

standard deviation $= \frac{\sigma_R}{R} \times 100$.

Propagation of Errors and Selection of Sample and Background Counting Times

When two quantities are added or subtracted, the error of the result is not the simple sum of the errors of the individual values but is

$$e = \sqrt{e_1^2 + e_2^2}$$

where e = the error of the sum of the corresponding individual errors. This rule is referred to as propagation of errors, and is particularly important in measurement of radioactivity.

When determining the amount of radioactivity in an unknown sample, one observes not only the disintegrations that result from the unknown sample, but also the counts that result from the presence of ionizing radiation in the environment of the counter. Such environmental radiation, or background radiation, is composed of alpha, beta, gamma, and cosmic radiations. The source of such background may be the radiation detector itself, the shielding material surrounding the detector, radioactive material in the earth or building material, and the atmosphere. Background radioactivity also follows the Poisson distribution; that is, the standard deviation of the counts equals the square root of the observed counts.

By the rule of propagation of errors, when one determines the counting rate in the sample, referred to as the *combined* counts since one is measuring the net counts in the sample plus the simultaneously measured background, the standard deviation for the sum of two or more count rates is given by the following equation:

$$\sigma_s = \sqrt{\sigma_1^2 + \sigma_2^2 + \sigma_3^2 + \ldots}$$

The standard deviation of the difference between two count rates is given by:

$$\sigma_d = \sqrt{\sigma_1^2 + \sigma_2^2}$$

where: $\sigma_1, \sigma_2, \ldots$ = the standard deviations of the count rates being combined
σ_s = the standard deviation of the sum of several count rates
σ_d = the standard deviation of the difference of two count rates

and the standard deviation is calculated as follows:

$$\sigma_R = \frac{\sqrt{N}}{t} \text{ and } R = \frac{N}{t}$$

then

$$\sigma_R = \sqrt{\frac{R}{t}}$$

where: N = the number of counts collected in time t
       R = the count rate
      σ_R = the standard deviation of the count rate.

An example of the use of these equations is as follows: 400 background counts C_b were collected in 20 minutes and 900 sample counts C_{s+b} were collected in one minute. The combined standard deviation is calculated as follows:

$$\sigma_b = \frac{\sqrt{C_b}}{t} = \frac{\sqrt{400}}{20} = 1.0$$

and $R_b = 20 \pm 1.0 = 20 \pm 5$ per cent

$$\sigma_{s+b} = \frac{\sqrt{C_{b+s}}}{t} = \frac{\sqrt{900}}{1} = 30$$

and $R_{s+b} = 900 \pm 30 = 900 \pm 3.3$ per cent.
The net counting rate

$$R_s = R_{s+b} - R_b = 900 - 20 \pm \sqrt{30^2 + 1^2}$$
$$R_s = 880 \pm 30 = 880 \pm 3.4 \text{ per cent.}$$

Consider also the following example: 900 background counts were collected in 30 minutes and 1600 sample counts were collected in 40 minutes. The combined standard deviation is calculated as follows:

$$\sigma_b = \frac{\sqrt{C_b}}{t} = \frac{\sqrt{900}}{30} = 1.0$$

and $R_b = 30.0 \pm 1.0 = 30.0 \pm 3.3$ per cent

$$\sigma_{s+b} = \frac{\sqrt{C_{b+s}}}{t} = \frac{\sqrt{1600}}{40} = 1.0$$

and $R_{s+b} = 40.0 \pm 1.0 = 40 \pm 2.5$ per cent.
The net count rate $R_s = R_{s+b} - R_b = 40.0 - 30.0 \pm \sqrt{1^2 + 1^2}$
$$R_s = 10.0 \pm 1.4 = 10.0 \pm 14 \text{ per cent.}$$

The large relative standard deviation is an excellent illustration of why one must keep the background as low as possible and wisely distribute the available counting time between counting the sample and counting background.

To determine the standard deviations for quotients and products the following equations are used:
    for products

$$\frac{\sigma_P}{R_P} = \sqrt{\left(\frac{\sigma_1}{R_1}\right)^2 + \left(\frac{\sigma_2}{R_2}\right)^2 + \cdots}$$

for quotients

$$\frac{\sigma_Q}{R_Q} = \sqrt{\left(\frac{\sigma_1}{R_1}\right)^2 + \left(\frac{\sigma_2}{R_2}\right)^2}$$

where: σ_P = the standard deviation of the product R_P
 σ_Q = the standard deviation of the quotient R_Q

One may obtain graphically the precision of the net count rate by use of the nomographs of the *Radiological Health Handbook*. The precision data contained in these nomographs are expressed in terms of the "90 per cent confidence level" and "95 per cent confidence level." The 95 per cent confidence level corresponds approximately to plus or minus two standard deviations. If the net count rate were reported to be 10.0 ± 2.7 counts/min. at the 95 per cent confidence level, it would mean that the range 7.3 to 12.7 counts/min. would include the true count rate in 95 per cent of the sample determinations.

To obtain the maximum precision in the net count rate for a given counting time, one must divide the counting period wisely between counting the sample and background. The expression which gives one the optimum distribution of counting time may be derived as follows:

$$R_s \pm \sigma_s = R_{s+b} - R_b \pm \sqrt{\sigma_{s+b}^2 + \sigma_b^2}$$

and

$$R_s = R_{s+b} - R_b$$

$$\sigma_{s+b} = \sqrt{\frac{R_{s+b}}{t_{s+b}}}$$

$$\sigma_b = \sqrt{\frac{R_b}{t_b}}$$

where R_s = net count rate with standard deviation σ_s
 R_{s+b} = gross count rate obtained in time t_{s+b} with a standard deviation of σ_{s+b}
 R_b = background count rate obtained in time t_b with a standard deviation of σ_b
 t = $t_b + t_{s+b}$ = total counting time

then

$$\sigma_s = \left(\frac{R_b}{t_b} + \frac{R_{s+b}}{t_{s+b}}\right)^{\frac{1}{2}}$$

$$\sigma_s^2 = \frac{R_b}{t_b} + \frac{R_{s+b}}{t_{s+b}}$$

The differential of this function is:

$$2\sigma_s d\sigma_s = -\frac{R_b}{t_b^2} dt_b - \frac{R_{s+b}}{t_{b+s}^2} dt_{b+s}$$

For σ_s to be a minimum $d\sigma_s = 0$
and $t = t_b + t_{b+s}$ = constant
 $dt = 0 = dt_b + dt_{b+s}$
 $dt_b = - dt_{b+s}$

then   therefore

$$\frac{R_b}{t_b^2} = \frac{R_{s+b}}{t_{s+b}^2} \qquad\qquad \frac{t_{s+b}}{t_b} = \sqrt{\frac{R_{s+b}}{R_b}}$$

To use the last equation one must have an estimate of R_{s+b} and R_b. For example, if one has 1 hour to count a sample which has an approximate count rate of 35 counts/min. and a background of 25 counts/min.

$$\frac{t_{s+b}}{t_b} = \sqrt{\frac{35}{25}} = 1.18$$

$t_{s+b} + t_b = 60; \ t_b = 60 - t_{s+b}$
$t_b = 60 - 1.18 \ t_b$
$t_b = 27.5$ min.
$t_{b+s} = 32.5$ min.

Having determined the optimum allocation of time to background and sample measurements, one might wish to determine the expected error when optimum times are used. An expression for this minimum error can be found by inserting the derived expressions for t_b and t_{b+s} into the original equation for σ_s. The resulting expression can be referred to as $\sigma_s(\text{opt.})$

$$\sigma_s(\text{opt.}) = \left(\frac{R_b}{t_b} + \frac{R_{s+b}}{t_{s+b}}\right)^{\frac{1}{2}}$$

when

$$\frac{t_{s+b}}{t_b} = \sqrt{\frac{R_{s+b}}{R_b}}$$

and since

$$t_{s+b} + t_b = t$$

$$\frac{t_{s+b}}{t - t_{s+b}} = \sqrt{\frac{R_{s+b}}{R_b}}$$

$$t_{s+b} = \frac{t\sqrt{\dfrac{R_{s+b}}{R_b}}}{1 + \sqrt{\dfrac{R_{s+b}}{R_b}}}$$

Similarly

$$t_b = \frac{t}{1 + \sqrt{\dfrac{R_{s+b}}{R_b}}}$$

Substituting both these expressions and simplifying leads to:

$$\sigma_s(\text{opt.}) = \frac{\sqrt{R_{s+b}} + \sqrt{R_b}}{\sqrt{t}}$$

From this expression, one can see that the optimum error is inversely related to the square root of the total sampling time and it is clear that if one wished to reduce this error to one half, the total sampling time would have to be four times as large. One must of course still observe the proper ratio between time observed on the sample and background as already given.

It is also interesting to investigate the optimum relative standard deviation. This is given by:

$$\text{opt. relative } \sigma \quad = \frac{\sigma_s(\text{opt.})}{R_{b+s} - R_b} = \frac{\sqrt{R_{b+s}} + \sqrt{R_b}}{\sqrt{t}\,(R_{b+s} - R_b)}$$

This demonstrates mathematically the well known practical fact that when the background is large in comparison to the sample, such that the quantity $R_{b+s} - R_b$ becomes small, even very large sampling times may not increase the precision to an acceptable level.

From this expression it is readily seen that the relative standard deviation even when the background radiation is reduced to zero is:

$$\text{opt. relative } \sigma = \frac{1}{\sqrt{R_{s+b}t}}$$

One may also calculate the time necessary to count a sample and the background to obtain a stated precision in the net count rate. For example, what is the total counting time if a sample has a count rate of approximately 100 counts/min. and the background 20 counts/min., to obtain a 5 per cent relative standard deviation for the net count rate?

$R_s = 100 - 20 = 80$

$0.05 = \dfrac{\sigma_s}{80}$

$\sigma_s = 4$

$\dfrac{t_{b+s}}{t_b} = \sqrt{\dfrac{R_{b+s}}{R_b}} = \sqrt{\dfrac{100}{20}} = 2.236$

$t_{b+s} = 2.236\, t_b$

$\sigma_s = \sqrt{\dfrac{R_b}{t_b} + \dfrac{R_{b+s}}{t_{b+s}}} = \sqrt{\dfrac{20}{t_b} + \dfrac{100}{2.236\, t_b}}$

$16 = \dfrac{65.2}{t_b}$

$t_b = 4$

$t_{b+s} = 2.236 \times 4 = 9$

$t_{b+s} + t_b = 13$

The required total counting time would be 13 minutes.

Loevinger and Berman (1951) have provided a convenient method that is useful for the determination of minimum combined counting times (Fig. 3-2). One decides the percentage error that is permissible and makes an approximate measurement of the sample-to-background ratio. The use of the figure may be illustrated by a numerical example. Suppose one wishes to determine the sample counting rate to an error of 3 per cent. Suppose that the approximate sample-to-background ratio r = 1.5. Then, from the graph, the horizontal 3 per cent line crosses the r = 1.5 curve at the vertical line for 18,000 total counts. This point of intersection lies halfway between the background-counts curves for 8000 and 12,000. Hence, by interpolation, the total background count is about 10,000. For a counter with an ordinary background of 50 to 100 counts/min. these counts will run to many hours, so that the use of the optimum-time graph is well worth while. A practical procedure would be to count background and sample for about 300 counts, or 5 minutes each, and then estimate R_b and r as a basis for assigning the number of counts to be taken. It would be appropriate in such a case to take half the background counts before, and half after, the sample count.

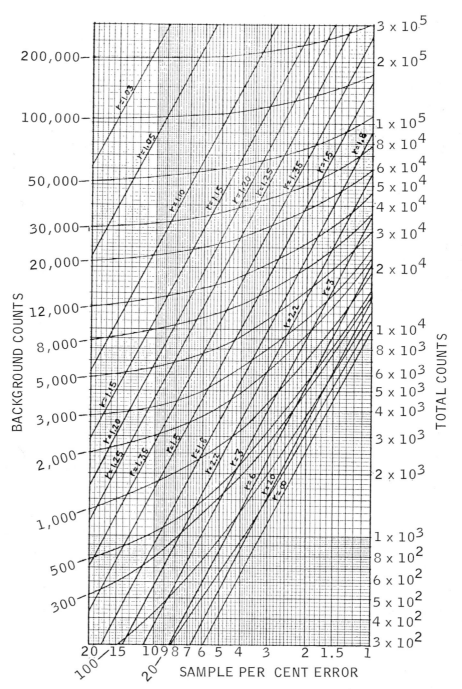

FIGURE 3-2. Loevinger and Berman method of determining minimum combined counting times. (From Loevinger and Berman, 1951.)

The statistical error of a count rate meter reading

We have previously shown that the optimum relative standard deviation is given by $\sigma = \dfrac{1}{\sqrt{R_{s+b}t}}$. For a rate meter, the counting time is twice the time constant of the meter or 2rc. Therefore:

$$\frac{\sigma_{R_s}}{R_s} = \frac{1}{\sqrt{R_s(2rc)}}$$

where R equals the count rate in counts per second, and rc equals the time constant; r equals resistance in ohms, c equals capacitance in farads; rc units are seconds. Therefore

$$\sigma_{R_s} = \sqrt{\frac{R_s}{2rc}}$$

Thus the error of the rate meter is similar to that obtained by making scaler counts during an interval of time twice the time constant.

It may be seen that as the time constant increases, the standard deviation decreases. From a statistical viewpoint, it would be desirable to use a long time constant. Frequently this is not possible since one may wish to observe rapid changes in count rate. In this case, precision must be sacrificed.

Comparison of detection systems or detection parameters

One is frequently faced with the problem of choosing the conditions under which a nuclear measurement is to be made. In most cases, statistical considerations are of paramount importance. For example, one has the decision of whether to count the entire gamma ray spectrum (integral counting) or to count only photons of a narrow energy range (differential counting). Several criteria have been proposed for use in making these types of decisions. Some have been discussed in Chapter V.

Loevinger and Berman have proposed use of a *figure of merit*, defined as R_s^2/R_b, where R_s = the net counting rate (sample counting rate minus background counting rate) and R_b = the background counting rate. They have shown that in measuring weak samples the shortest overall counting time, i.e., combined background and sample counting time, is obtained when the figure of merit is maximum. This can be illustrated by an example. Assume that one wishes to count low levels of radioactivity from cesium-137. One wishes to know the optimum photon energy range over which to make the measurements. An efficient way to determine this is to use a pulse-height analyzer in which the lower-level discriminator can be progressively lowered while counts are made both of background and of a ^{137}Cs standard. One notes that both the sample counts and the background counts increase steadily as the lower-level discriminator is lowered and photons of progressively lower energy are recorded. One then graphs the integral spectrum of both the standard ^{137}Cs and the background, and can obtain graphically the count rates for all possible combinations of lower- and upper-level discriminator. This is done by subtracting the count rate at the upper energy level of a prospective window from the count rate at the setting of the lower level. Typical results can be seen in the following table:

TABLE 3-1. WIDTH OF WINDOW

%	MEV. RANGE	Δ ^{137}Cs COUNT	Δ BKG.	R	R^2/BKG. FIGURE OF MERIT
1	0.65–0.67	10.0	1.5	8.5	48.17
2	0.64–0.68	18.0	3.0	15.0	75.00
3	0.63–0.69	28.0	5.0	23.0	105.80
4	0.62–0.70	37.0	8.5	28.5	95.56
6	0.60–0.72	54.0	10.0	44.0	193.60
8	0.58–0.74	61.0	12.0	49.0	200.08
10	0.56–0.76	45.0	7.0	38.0	206.29
12	0.54–0.78	75.0	17.0	58.0	197.88
14	0.52–0.80	83.0	19.0	64.0	215.58
16	0.50–0.82	89.0	21.0	68.0	220.19
18	0.48–0.84	92.0	23.0	69.0	207.00
20	0.46–0.86	97.5	25.5	72.0	203.29
22	0.44–0.88	101.0	28.0	73.0	190.32

It may be seen that the figure of merit was highest (220) when a window was selected that was 16 per cent of the total photon energy spectrum. Consequently for low-level counting of cesium, this would be the optimum use of the pulse-height analyzer.

For measurement of samples containing relatively large amounts of radioactivity, efficiency rather than the figure of merit should be maximized. Efficiency is defined by the calibration factor, f, which is equal to counts per second per disintegrations per second.

Other criteria have been used in evaluating detection systems. One is to determine the *minimal detectable activity*, defined as the amount of activity (disintegrations per unit time) that produces a response which differs from the background reading by three times the standard deviation of the background reading.

$$\text{minimum detectable activity} = \frac{3\sigma_{\text{s}}}{f}$$

where f = calibration factor (counts/sec. divided by disintegrations/sec.).

The National Bureau of Standards has defined a term *background equivalent activity*, the amount which produces a response of the instrument which is equal to its background reading.

$$\text{background equivalent activity} = R_b/f$$

This is an adequate criterion for strong samples, but is not useful for comparing the response of detection systems designed for weak samples.

TRACER KINETICS

JOHN A. JACQUEZ

INTRODUCTION

Radioactive tracers make possible study of the kinetics of bodily constituents without interfering with the normal functions of the body. To derive maximum benefit from this new capability requires full utilization of modern analytical techniques. In this section mathematical techniques useful in the measurement of rate processes are presented.

TERMINOLOGY AND DEFINITIONS

The term *specific activity* refers to a measure of radioactivity per unit mass or per mole of a substance. Any convenient set of units, such as counts per micromole or microcurie per gram, can be used so long as these are clearly stated. When using the terms *radioactivity* or *specific activity*, it will be assumed that corrections have been made for radioactive decay.

An amount of a material which behaves as if it were a homogeneous, kinetically distinct component is called a *compartment* or *pool*. A compartment may or may not correspond to an actual physiological space. It may refer to a particular chemical or a labeled substance in one physiological space or in a number of physiological spaces. We will represent a *space* or a *compartment* diagrammatically by a rectangular box and when necessary use S and C to distinguish between a space and a compartment, respectively; arrows between compartments represent the *processes* which exchange material between them; one-sided arrows will be used to designate chemical reactions, and full arrows to designate spatial transfers such as might result from diffusion or a transport process.

To clarify the distinction between space and compartment, consider the following examples. Suppose compound A exchanges between two *physiological spaces* by diffusion—this is a *two compartment* system and is represented diagrammatically by Figure 3-3. Suppose that A undergoes a reaction with another compound B to form AB. This system is shown in Figure 3-4. If A is labeled with a tracer, this system is representable as a *four compartment* system as in Figure 3-5. However, as is not unusual, if A exchanges between spaces S_1 and S_2 extremely slowly but AB exchanges very rapidly and the reaction $A+B \rightleftharpoons AB$ is a slow reaction, this system may act kinetically like the three compartment system shown in Figure 3-6 in which the third compartment consists of AB in S_1 and S_2. The exchange of a slowly dissociating weak acid, HA, between intracellular and extracellular phases would be a good example of this; in such cases, the anion A^- often exchanges so much more slowly than does the

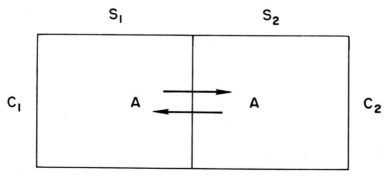

FIGURE 3-3. Two compartment system (C_1, C_2); exchange of A between two spaces (S_1, S_2).

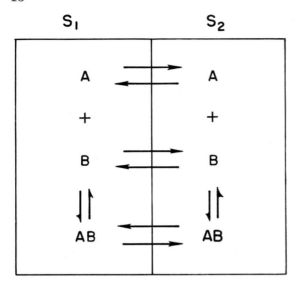

FIGURE 3-4. Transfer of A, B, and complex AB between two spaces.

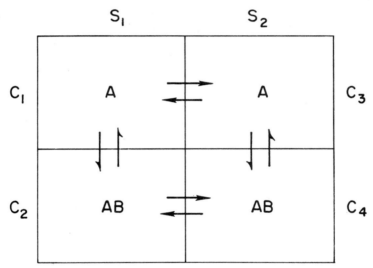

FIGURE 3-5. Four compartment system; two kinetically distinct forms of A (A and AB) in each of two spaces.

undissociated acid HA that the intracellular phase can be treated as being impermeable to it.

If the amounts of material in the various compartments of a system are constant, their rates of change (derivatives with respect to time) must be zero and the system is in a *steady state*. If a substance in a compartment is in a steady state and is neither produced nor destroyed, then the rate at which it enters the compartment equals the rate at which it leaves; this rate is the *turnover rate* and has the dimensions of mass/time. The *turnover time* is the total mass of the substance in the compartment divided by its turnover rate. If the compartment is not in a steady state, the term *turnover rate* is sometimes

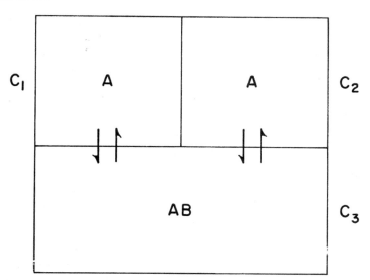

FIGURE 3-6. Three compartment system; C_1 is A in S_1, C_2 is A in S_2, and C_3 is AB in S_1 and S_2.

used to mean the lesser of the two one-way rates. However, it is preferable to reserve the term turnover for steady states and to identify the two one-way rates as such in nonsteady-state situations.

LINEAR SYSTEMS

FIRST ORDER PROCESSES

Physical systems are described mathematically in terms of quantities such as temperature, pressure, and the concentration of various molecular species. Such quantities are commonly called the *state variables* of the system. Suppose that $x_1, x_2, \ldots, x_n$ are state variables of a system. The basic laws governing changes in such systems are often given by equations which tell how the rate of change of one variable depends on the values of the other variables, as in equation 6 for example.

$$\frac{dx_i}{dt} = f_i(x_1, x_2, \ldots, x_n) \tag{6}$$

This is a differential equation. The function on the right side of equation 6 is usually a sum of terms which represents the various basic processes going on in the system. To illustrate, consider the reaction shown by equation 7.

$$A + B \underset{k_2}{\overset{k_1}{\rightleftharpoons}} AB \tag{7}$$

Let x_1, x_2, and x_3 be the concentrations of A, B, and AB, respectively. Two basic processes occur in this system, the forward reaction whose rate is v_f and the backward reaction whose rate is v_b.

$$\begin{aligned} v_f &= k_1 x_1 x_2 \\ v_b &= k_2 x_3 \end{aligned} \tag{8}$$

The order of a process is defined as follows. For each term in the equation for a process (v_f and v_b each have only one term) add the exponents of each of the state variables; this sum for the term having the highest such sum is the *order* of the process. Thus v_b is a first order process and v_f is a second order process.

The rates of change of the state variables x_1, x_2, and x_3 are all expressed in terms of these two processes, as in equation 9.

$$\frac{dx_1}{dt} = v_b - v_f = k_2 x_3 - k_1 x_1 x_2 \tag{9}$$

Many common processes, such as the following, are first order.

Radioactive Decay.   Consider a large number of atoms of a single radioactive isotope which decays to a nonradioactive isotope. At the atomic level the process can be described only in terms of a probability that an atom will decay in any period of time. As a result, if the number of atoms present is not large, the number decaying per unit of time will show the random fluctuations we expect from chance occurrences. However, if the number is very large, these fluctuations will be small in comparison to the number of atoms decaying, and we can say that the number decaying per unit of time is directly proportional to the number present at that time; thus this is a first order process. Let N be the number present at time t and N_0 the number present at $t = 0$. Equation 10 describes this first order process.

$$\frac{dN}{dt} = - \lambda N \tag{10}$$

This is a *first order linear differential equation*. It is first order because the highest derivative appearing in it is a first derivative. The degree of a term is the sum of the exponents of all *dependent variables* and of the exponents of their *derivatives* in that term. A differential equation is said to be linear if no term is of degree greater than one.

Starting with equation 10,

$$\frac{dN}{dt} = -\lambda N$$
$$\frac{dN}{N} = -\lambda dt \tag{11}$$

$$\int_{N_0}^{N} \frac{dN}{N} = \int_{0}^{t} - \lambda dt \tag{12}$$

$$\ln N - \ln N_0 = - \lambda t$$
$$N = N_0 e^{-\lambda t} \tag{13}$$

which is the usual expression for radioactive decay.

Growth. Some portion of the growth curve of many biological systems, such as cultures of microorganisms, tissue cultures, and transplantable animal tumors, is describable as a first order process. For that portion of the growth curve for which this is true, the rate of increase of the mass, m, of the system is proportional to the mass. Thus equation 14 is, except for the sign, the same as equation 10.

$$\frac{dm}{dt} = km \tag{14}$$

The solution to this equation is similar to that used in equations 12 and 13 and leads to:

$$m = m_0 e^{kt} \tag{15}$$

In this case, k is called the specific growth rate and m_0 is the mass at the arbitrarily chosen zero of the time scale.

Uniform, Instantaneous Mixing. Let Figure 3-7 represent a chamber of constant volume V with constant volume inflow and outflow rates of v. Mixing in such a chamber is often sufficiently rapid in comparison to other processes under study so that one can assume that there is instantaneous and complete mixing of inflowing material in the chamber. Let x(t) be the concentration of some material in the chamber, x(0) being the concentration at t = 0, and let f(t) be the concentration in the liquid flowing into the chamber. The rate at which material leaves the chamber is vx, a first order process; the rate at which it enters is vf(t), a zero order process but time dependent. Then v[f(t)−x] must be the rate at which the total amount of material in chamber changes.

$$V\frac{dx}{dt} = v[f(t) - x] \tag{16}$$

If f(t) = 0, the equation is the same as that of radioactive decay; if f(t) is a constant, c, and x_0 = 0, the concentration builds up to the level x = c. The results are given in Table 3-2.

Diffusion. The random motion due to thermal agitation of atoms and molecules in solutions and gases tends to obliterate differences in concentration between different parts of the solution or gas. At the macroscopic level, the effects of this thermal agitation are seen as the process of diffusion. Consider a cylinder of solution in which there is a concentration gradient along the axis

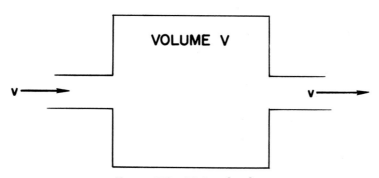

FIGURE 3-7.   Mixing chamber.

TABLE 3-2.   SOLUTIONS OF EQUATION FOR A MIXING CHAMBER

x(0)	f(t)	SOLUTION
x_0	0	$x = x_0 e^{-\frac{v}{V}t}$
0	c	$x = c[1 - e^{-\frac{v}{V}t}]$
x_0	c	$x = x_0 e^{-\frac{v}{V}t} + c[1 - e^{-\frac{v}{V}t}]$
x_0	f(t)	$x = x_0 e^{-\frac{v}{V}t} + \int_0^t f(s)e^{-\frac{v}{V}(t-s)}ds\,*$

* where s is a dummy variable.

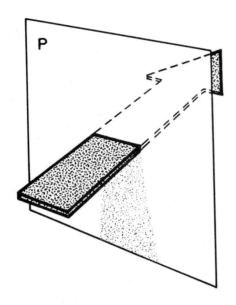

FIGURE 3-8.

of the cylinder. In Figure 3-8, P is a plane of area A perpendicular to the direction in which the concentration changes. We will use the symbol Δ (preceding a variable) to indicate a small change in a quantity; let Δc be the change in concentration in distance Δx, perpendicular to the plane in Figure 3-8. Fick's law states that the amount of material, Δq, crossing the plane by diffusion in time Δt is proportional to the product of the area, A, and the concentration gradient, Δc/Δx, across the plane (equation 17).

$$\frac{\Delta q}{\Delta t} = -\, DA \, \frac{\Delta c}{\Delta x} \tag{17}$$

This may also be given as a differential equation (equation 18).

$$\frac{dq}{dt} = -\, DA \, \frac{\partial c}{\partial x} \tag{18}$$

The constant D is the diffusion coefficient. The negative sign in equations 17 and 18 is needed because there is a positive transfer of material when the gradient is negative.

Let us apply equation 17 to the diffusion of a compound between two spaces (also compartments in this case) with use of the assumption that the material crosses a boundary (a membrane for example) between the two compartments slowly compared to the rates of diffusion and of mixing within the compartments. This is equivalent to assuming that the concentrations inside each of the two compartments is uniform at all times. Let c_1 and c_2 be the two concentrations. Then the rate at which material crosses from compartment 1 to compartment 2 is given by equation 19.

$$\frac{dq}{dt} = - DA \frac{(c_2 - c_1)}{\delta} \tag{19}$$

where δ is the thickness of the membrane. The ratio $k = D/\delta$ is the *permeability constant* and is usually given in the units cm./sec. or cm./min. Thus, the rate of transfer of material between the two compartments is given by the difference between two first order processes, kAc_1, and kAc_2. If the transfer equation is written per unit of membrane area, as in equation 20, the resulting quantity is a *net flux*, F, and the two first order processes are the one way fluxes F_{12} and F_{21}.

$$F = \frac{1}{A} \frac{dq}{dt} = kc_1 - kc_2 = F_{12} - F_{21} \tag{20}$$

If the volume V of compartment 1 is constant, $\frac{dq}{dt} = V \frac{dc_1}{dt}$, and equation 20 may be written

$$\frac{dc_1}{dt} = \frac{kA}{V} (c_1 - c_2) \tag{21}$$

With minor changes, this is the same equation as 16. If the concentration c_2 is held constant and $c_1 = 0$ at $t = 0$, the solution is given by equation 22 which is the same as the second case in Table 3-2.

$$c_1 = c_2 \left[1 - e^{-\frac{kAt}{V}}\right] \tag{22}$$

Again, the solution is given in terms of an exponential function.

First Order Chemical Reaction. As a final example, consider the reversible monomolecular reaction shown in equation 23.

$$A \underset{k_2}{\overset{k_1}{\rightleftharpoons}} B \tag{23}$$

If x_1 and x_2 denote the concentrations of A and B, respectively, from the law of mass action one obtains equation 24.

$$\frac{dx_1}{dt} = -k_1 x_1 + k_2 x_2 \tag{24}$$

Again, the rate of change of x_1 is given by the difference between two first order processes, the rate at which B is converted into A, $k_2 x_2$, and the rate at which A is converted into B, $k_1 x_1$. If the total amount of A and B in the system is fixed, $x_1 + x_2 = S = x_1(0) + x_2(0)$, where $x_1(0)$ and $x_2(0)$ are initial concentrations. Then, equation 24 may be rearranged to give 25.

$$\frac{dx_1}{dt} = k_2 S - (k_1 + k_2) x_1 \tag{25}$$

This, with some rearrangement, is the same equation as equation 16, and corresponds to case 3 of Table 3-2. The solution is equation 26.

$$x_1 = x_1(0)e^{-(k_1+k_2)t} + \left(\frac{k_2S}{k_1 + k_2}\right)(1 - e^{-(k_1+k_2)t}) \qquad (26)$$

These examples illustrate the importance of first order processes. The rates of first order processes are no more than first order in all state variables. The solutions can generally be written as sums of a finite number of exponential terms.

MORE COMPLEX SYSTEMS

If the rates of change of *all* of the *state variables* of a system can be written as sums of processes none of which is of higher than first order, the system is a *linear system* and is described by a set of *linear differential* equations. Let us consider a few examples of linear compartmental systems and then present the general case.

Two Compartment System with Excretion. Figure 3-9 represents a two compartment system; these have fixed volumes V_1 and V_2, respectively. These compartments are assumed to be well mixed, and to have uniform concentrations x_1 and x_2 with a diffusional exchange across an area A and an excretion, proportional to x_2, from compartment 2. The total amounts of material in the two compartments are $q_1 = V_1x_1$ and $q_2 = V_2x_2$. First let us write the equations in terms of the total material in each of the compartments. For the sake of generality we will assume that k_{12} and k_{21} are not equal. Then equations 27 give the rates of change of q_1 and q_2 in terms of the constituent processes.

$$\frac{dq_1}{dt} = -k_{12}Ax_1 + k_{21}Ax_2$$

$$\frac{dq_2}{dt} = k_{12}Ax_1 - k_{21}Ax_2 - kx_2 \qquad (27)$$

Substitute

$$\frac{k_{12}A}{V_1} = \lambda_{12}, \frac{k_{21}A}{V_2} = \lambda_{21}, \text{ and } k/V_2 = \lambda_{20}.$$

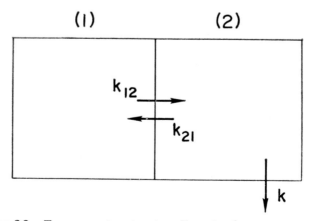

FIGURE 3-9.   Two compartment system. Excretion from compartment 2.

Note that the k's and λ's are defined to be non-negative. Equations 27 then become 28.

$$\frac{dq_1}{dt} = -\lambda_{12}q_1 + \lambda_{21}q_2$$

$$\frac{dq_2}{dt} = \lambda_{12}q_1 - \lambda_{21}q_2 - \lambda_{20}q_2 \tag{28}$$

On the other hand if these first order differential equations are written in terms of concentrations as in equations 29, the symmetry in the coefficients in equations 28 is lost.

$$\frac{dx_1}{dt} = -\frac{k_{12}A}{V_1} x_1 + \frac{k_{21}A}{V_1} x_2$$

$$\frac{dx_2}{dt} = \frac{k_{12}A}{V_2} x_1 - \frac{k_{21}A}{V_2} x_2 - \frac{k}{V_2} x_2 \tag{29}$$

Let us solve equations 28 and then give the λ actual values so that we may exhibit the nature of the solutions graphically. This will serve to illustrate a method of solution which works well for two and three variable problems although the algebra becomes cumbersome for larger problems.

In general, for any system of first order linear differential equations, the solution for each variable may contain as many exponential terms as there are first order differential equations in the system. (The exceptions will be mentioned later.) For the set given by equations 28, assume that the solutions are equations 30.

$$q_1 = Ae^{m_1 t} + Be^{m_2 t}$$

$$q_2 = Ce^{m_1 t} + De^{m_2 t} \tag{30}$$

The constants A, B, C, D, and m_1 and m_2 are to be determined. Substituting equations 30 into set 28, equations 31 are obtained.

$$(m_1 A + \lambda_{12}A - \lambda_{21}C)e^{m_1 t} + (m_2 B + \lambda_{12}B - \lambda_{21}D)e^{m_2 t} = 0$$

$$[(m_1 + \lambda_{21} + \lambda_{20})C - \lambda_{12}A]e^{m_1 t} + [(m_2 + \lambda_{21} + \lambda_{20})D - \lambda_{12}B]e^{m_2 t} = 0 \tag{31}$$

Equations 31 can hold for all t only if the coefficients of the exponential terms are identically zero. From the first two, C and D are determined in terms of A and B (equations 32).

$$C = \frac{(m_1 + \lambda_{12})}{\lambda_{21}} A; \quad D = \frac{(m_2 + \lambda_{12})B}{\lambda_{21}} \tag{32}$$

A and B will be determined by the initial values of q_1 and q_2. Substituting the equation for C in the first coefficient of the second of equations 31 gives equation 33.

$$[(m_1 + \lambda_{21} + \lambda_{20})(m_1 + \lambda_{12}) - \lambda_{12}\lambda_{21}]A = 0 \tag{33}$$

which gives the quadratic, 34

$$m^2 + (\lambda_{12} + \lambda_{21} + \lambda_{20})m + \lambda_{12}\lambda_{20} = 0 \tag{34}$$

in which we drop the subscript on m. Substituting the value for D in the

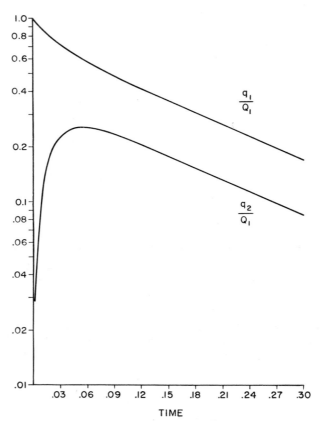

FIGURE 3-10. Two compartment model. Fraction of injected material remaining in compartments 1 and 2 as function of time. Injection into compartment 1.

second coefficient of the second one of the equations 31 gives the same equation as 34 for m_2. Equation 34 is called the *characteristic equation* for the system. It has two roots which are m_1 and m_2. If we define α and β as in equations 35,

$$\alpha = \frac{\lambda_{12} + \lambda_{21} + \lambda_{20}}{2}$$

$$\beta = \frac{\sqrt{(\lambda_{12} + \lambda_{21} + \lambda_{20})^2 - 4\lambda_{12}\lambda_{20}}}{2}$$

(35)

then the roots are given by equation 36.

$$m_1 = -(\alpha + \beta); \quad m_2 = -(\alpha - \beta)$$ (36)

Substituting into equations 30, the solutions become 37.

$$q_1 = Ae^{-(\alpha+\beta)t} + Be^{-(\alpha-\beta)t}$$

$$q_2 = \left(\frac{m_1 + \lambda_{12}}{\lambda_{21}}\right) Ae^{-(\alpha+\beta)t} + \left(\frac{m_2 + \lambda_{12}}{\lambda_{21}}\right) Be^{-(\alpha-\beta)t}$$

(37)

The two arbitrary constants, A and B, are determined by the initial conditions, that is, the values of q_1 and q_2 for $t = 0$.

A NUMERICAL EXAMPLE. Let $\lambda_{12} = 15$, $\lambda_{21} = 20$, $\lambda_{20} = 15$. Then $\alpha + \beta = 45$, $\alpha - \beta = 5$.

Case I. At $t = 0$, a tracer is injected into compartment 1; the initial conditions are then $q_1(0) = Q_1$, $q_2(0) = 0$. Substituting into equation 37 one obtains 38.

$$\frac{q_1}{Q_1} = 0.25e^{-45t} + 0.75^{-5t}$$

(38)

$$\frac{q_2}{Q_1} = 0.375[e^{-5t} - e^{-45t}]$$

These two functions are plotted on a semilogarithmic scale in Figure 3-10.

Case II. If, on the other hand, the tracer is injected into compartment 2 at $t = 0$, $q_1(0) = 0$, $q_2(0) = Q_2$ and the equations become equations 39.

$$\frac{q_1}{Q_2} = 0.5[e^{-5t} - e^{-45t}]$$

(39)

$$\frac{q_2}{Q_2} = 0.75e^{-45t} + 0.25e^{-5t}$$

For comparison with the previous, these are plotted in Figure 3-11.

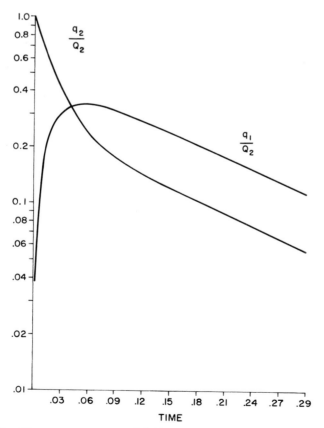

FIGURE 3-11. Two compartment model. Fraction of injected material remaining in compartments 1 and 2 as function of time. Injection into compartment 2.

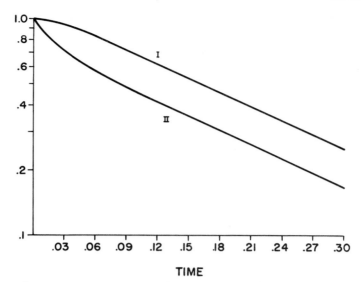

FIGURE 3-12. Two compartment model. Fraction of amount injected remaining in system after injection into compartment 1 or 2.

Suppose, however, that only the total radioactivity in the system can be measured. The use of a total-body counter to measure total radioactivity in an animal might be an example of this. The results obtained for injection into compartments 1 or 2 are shown in curves I and II, respectively, of Figure 3-12.

Two Compartments Exchanging with a Third Compartment with Excretion from the Third. This situation is shown diagrammatically in Figure 3-13. The system is described by equations 40.

$$\frac{dq_1}{dt} = -\lambda_{13}q_1 + \lambda_{31}q_3$$

$$\frac{dq_2}{dt} = -\lambda_{23}q_2 + \lambda_{32}q_3 \tag{40}$$

$$\frac{dq_3}{dt} = \lambda_{13}q_1 + \lambda_{23}q_2 - (\lambda_{30} + \lambda_{31} + \lambda_{32})q_3$$

The characteristic equation for this system is a cubic equation. Suppose that the roots are $-\alpha_1$, $-\alpha_2$, and $-\alpha_3$. The solutions are given by equations 41.

$$q_1 = \lambda_{31}\left[\frac{A}{\lambda_{13} - \alpha_1}e^{-\alpha_1 t} + \frac{B}{\lambda_{13} - \alpha_2}e^{-\alpha_2 t} + \frac{C}{\lambda_{13} - \alpha_3}e^{-\alpha_3 t}\right]$$

$$q_2 = \lambda_{32}\left[\frac{A}{\lambda_{23} - \alpha_1}e^{-\alpha_1 t} + \frac{B}{\lambda_{23} - \alpha_2}e^{-\alpha_2 t} + \frac{C}{\lambda_{23} - \alpha_3}e^{-\alpha_3 t}\right] \tag{41}$$

$$q_3 = Ae^{-\alpha_1 t} + Be^{-\alpha_2 t} + Ce^{-\alpha_3 t}$$

The constants A, B, and C are determined by the initial values $q_1(0)$, $q_2(0)$, and $q_3(0)$.

The General Linear System. In the general case of an n compartment system, we assume that each compartment may interchange with any other and that there may be an intake into and an excretion from each compartment. Referring to Figure 3-14, which represents the ith compartment of such a system, I_i is the rate of input from the environment, $\lambda_{io}q_i$ the excretion rate, $\lambda_{ij}q_i$ the rate of transfer of material from compartment i to compartment j, and $\lambda_{ji}q_j$ the rate of transfer from compartment j into i. Equation 42 gives the rate of change of q_i with respect to time.

$$\frac{dq_i}{dt} = I_i + \sum_{\substack{j=1 \\ j \neq i}}^{n} \lambda_{ji}q_j - \left[\sum_{\substack{j=0 \\ \neq i}}^{n} \lambda_{ij}\right] q_i \qquad (42)$$

If we define $\lambda_{ii} = -\sum_{j \neq i} \lambda_{ij}$, equation 42 may be rewritten in the more symmetrical form of equation 43.

$$\frac{dq_i}{dt} = \sum_{j=1}^{n} \lambda_{ji}q_j + I_i \qquad (43)$$

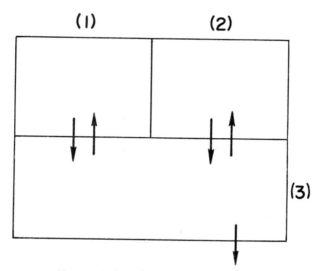

(1) **(2)** **(3)**

FIGURE 3-13.   Three compartment system.

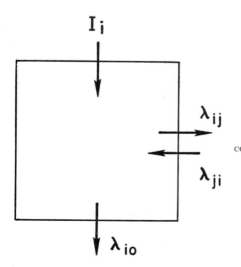

I_i

λ_{ij}

λ_{ji}

λ_{io}

FIGURE 3-14. Schematic diagram of one compartment of a general linear system.

Thus the system is described by a set of *first order linear differential equations.* The λ_{ji} and I_i may be functions of time and the set is still said to be linear. However, such a set is easily solvable as a finite sum of exponential terms only if the λ_{ji} and I_i are constant. The problem is not much more difficult if the I_i are functions of time so long as the λ_{ji} are constant. If the I_i are all zero, the set of equations 43 is said to be *homogeneous.* Corresponding to a set of n simultaneous homogeneous equations of the type of 43, if the λ_{ji} are constants, there is generally one characteristic equation which is of degree n. If the roots of the characteristic equation are all distinct, the solution is a sum of exponential terms as shown in the previous example (equations 37). The solutions are more complicated if the characteristic equation has multiple roots. This occurs rarely enough in practice so that we need not consider the details. If there are no isotope fractionation effects, the time course of the concentrations of the isotope in different compartments will still be given by linear differential equations, but all of the rate constants will no longer be the same as for the normal isotope. Agnew (1960) gives a good exposition of the methods for solving linear differential equations. The general case is best discussed in the language of matrix algebra. References recommended for advanced reading are Berman and Schoenfeld (1956), Berman, Shahn, and Weiss (1962), Berman, Weiss, and Shahn (1962), Shemin and Rittenberg (1946), and Sheppard and Householder (1951).

Two general types of systems commonly referred to are the catenary and mamillary. In a catenary system, the compartments are arranged in a series, each one, other than the end compartments, exchanging with only the two adjacent compartments (Fig. 3-15). In a mamillary system each of a set of peripheral compartments exchanges only with a central compartment (Fig. 3-16). Many physiological systems are interpretable as a mamillary system in which the central compartment represents the plasma. Figure 3-17 shows a mixed system which can be used in the interpretation of many experiments

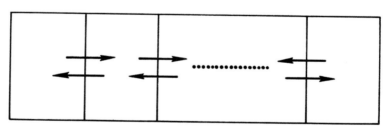

FIGURE 3-15.   Schematic drawing of a catenary system.

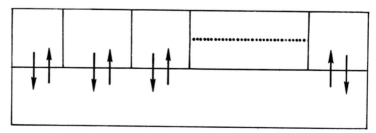

FIGURE 3-16.   Mamillary system

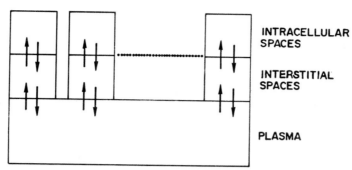

FIGURE 3-17. A compartmental model of the relation between plasma and intracellular and interstitial spaces in different capillary beds.

on exchange of a material between intracellular and interstitial space of different capillary beds and the plasma.

NONLINEAR SYSTEMS: THE STEADY STATE

GENERAL

Although linear systems have mathematical properties which make them desirable, many, if not most, processes in living things are not first order. Such systems cannot be described by linear differential equations; nonlinear differential equations are required. Why, then, the emphasis on linear compartmental systems? First, no uniform techniques are available for solving sets of nonlinear differential equations. More important, however, from the standpoint of radio-isotope methodology is the fact that *for all systems, if the system is in a steady state, the equations which describe the distribution of a tracer amount of a radioactive isotope will be linear differential equations.*

The use of linear differential equations to describe the kinetics of radio-isotope distribution for nonlinear systems depends on two important assumptions. These are: (1) the system is in a steady state, and (2) the system can be treated as a set of compartments in each of which there is complete mixing of labeled and unlabeled material and this mixing is rapid in comparison with the rates of any transfers between the compartments. The assumption of negligible isotope fractionation effects is usually also made. The latter is required in order to make valid estimates of transfer rates and turnover times; it is not needed to obtain linear differential equations for the distributions of the isotope under steady-state conditions. We will demonstrate these points first with a general argument and then with two examples.

Let q_i be the total amount of material in the ith compartment. In general, the rate of change of q_i is given by a sum of terms which represent transfers of material from compartment i to other compartments and from other compartments to compartment i. Let f_{ji} $(q_1, q_2, \ldots, q_n; k_1, k_2, \ldots, k_m)$ represent the rate of transfer of material from the jth to the ith compartment; this is a function of the amounts $q_1, q_2, \ldots, q_n$ and also of the parameters $k_1, k_2, \ldots, k_m$ which stand for the pertinent reaction rate constants, diffusion and permeability constants. Let the values of the parameters for the isotope be $k_1', k_2', \ldots, k_m'$.

Let $\phi_{ij}(q_1, q_2, \ldots, q_n; k_1, k_2, \ldots, k_m)$ be the rate of transfer of material from the ith to the jth compartment. Then the rate of change of q_i is given by equation 44.

$$\frac{dq_i}{dt} = \sum_{\substack{j=i \\ j \neq i}}^{n} [f_{ji}(q_1, q_2, \ldots, q_n; k_1, k_2, \ldots, k_m) - \phi_{ij}(q_1, q_2, \ldots, q_n; k_1, \ldots, k_m)] \quad (44)$$

Suppose we add a *trace* amount of one radioisotope to some compartment or compartments of the system. Let ϵ_i be the total amount of labeled material in the ith compartment (this is measured in the same units as is q_i). If r_i is the conversion factor from mass units to radioactivity, the specific activity of compartment i is $a_i = r_i \epsilon_i / q_i$. Then if any labeled material which is added to a compartment is mixed rapidly with the contents of the compartment in comparison to the rate at which material enters or leaves, the rate at which radioactivity goes from compartment j to i is the specific activity, a_j, multiplied by the rate at which material goes from j to i, i.e., $a_j f_{ji}$; but since this represents isotope which is transferred, the parameters have the values for the isotope. Taking into account the conversion factor to mass units, the rate of transfer of labeled material from j to i must be $\frac{a_j}{r_j} f_{ji} (q_1, \ldots, q_n; k_1', k_2', \ldots, k_m')$. We write f_{ji}' and ϕ_{ij}' to indicate that the parameters refer to the isotope. Thus the net rate of change of labeled material in i must be given by equation 45.

$$\frac{d\epsilon_i}{dt} = d\frac{\left(\dfrac{a_i q_i}{r_i}\right)}{dt} = \sum_{\substack{j=1 \\ j \neq i}}^{n} \left[\frac{a_j}{r_j} f_{ji}' - \frac{a_i}{r_i} \phi_{ij}'\right] \quad (45)$$

If chemical reactions are present which involve more than one molecule of a reactant, the transfer rates f_{ji}' and ϕ_{ij}' may have to be multiplied by stoichiometric coefficients. If the system is in a *steady state*, all the q_j are constant and so are the f_{ji}, ϕ_{ij}, and f_{ji}' and ϕ_{ij}'. Then equation 45 can be written either in terms of total radioactive material or in terms of specific activity: equations 46 and 47.

$$\frac{d\epsilon_i}{dt} = \sum_{i \neq i} \left[\epsilon_j \left(\frac{f_{ji}'}{q_j}\right) - \epsilon_i \left(\frac{\phi_{ij}'}{q_i}\right)\right] \quad (46)$$

$$\frac{da_i}{dt} = \sum_{j \neq i} \left[a_j \left(\frac{r_i}{r_j}\right)\left(\frac{q_j}{q_i}\right)\left(\frac{f_{ji}'}{q_j}\right) - a_i \left(\frac{\phi_{ij}'}{q_i}\right)\right] \quad (47)$$

These are, of course, linear differential equations. Note that $\frac{f_{ji}'}{q_j}$ and $\frac{\phi_{ij}'}{q_i}$ are fractional transfer rates; that is, $\frac{f_{ji}'}{q_j}$ represents the fraction of compartment j transferred to i per unit of time. However, the transfer rates for the normal isotope will be estimated correctly only if the isotopes have the same rate constants so that $f_{ji} = f_{ji}'$ and $\phi = \phi_{ij}'$. Usually the r_j are all the same.

EXAMPLES

Bimolecular Reaction. Assume that compounds A and B undergo reaction according to equation 48.

$$A + B \underset{k_2}{\overset{k_1}{\rightleftharpoons}} AB \tag{48}$$

Let A' represent the isotope which partakes in a similar reaction with constants k_1 and k_2. Let z_1 and z_2 be the concentrations of A and AB, respectively, ζ_1 and ζ_2 the concentrations of A' and $A'B$, and y the concentration B. The rate equations for z_1 and ζ_1 are given by equations 49 and 50.

$$\frac{dz_1}{dt} = k_2 z_2 - k_1 z_1 y \tag{49}$$

$$\frac{d\zeta_1}{dt} = k_2' \zeta_2 - k_1' \zeta_1 y \tag{50}$$

Suppose that the reaction takes place in a closed vessel of constant volume V. We rewrite equations 49 and 50 in terms of total amounts. Let q_1 and q_2 be the total amount of A and AB; then by conservation of mass, $Q = q_1 + q_2$ is constant. Let ϵ_1 and ϵ_2 be total amount of A' and $A'B$; also by conservation, $\epsilon = \epsilon_1 + \epsilon_2$. Furthermore the total amount (molecular) of B, AB, and $A'B$ is constant, $P = y + q_2 + \epsilon_2$. Because we assume that only tracer amounts of the radioisotope are present, ϵ may be neglected in comparison to y and q_2. Taking these into account, we can rewrite equations 49 and 50.

$$\frac{dq_1}{dt} = k_2 q_2 - \frac{k_1 q_1}{V} [P - Q + q_1] = k_2 [Q - q_1] - \frac{k_1 q_1}{V} [P - Q + q_1] \tag{51}$$

$$\frac{d\epsilon_1}{dt} = k_2' \epsilon_2 - \frac{k_1' \epsilon_1}{V} (P - Q + q_1) \tag{52}$$

In this case the conversion unit from molecular (molar) amounts to units of radioactivity will be the same for the two compartments, $r = r_1 = r_2$, and the specific activities are $a_1 = r\epsilon_1/q_1$, $a_2 = r\epsilon_2/q_2$. Equations 51 and 52 hold whether or not the system is in a steady state. But if the system is in a steady state, $\frac{dq_1}{dt} = 0$, q_1 and q_2 are constant, and equation 52 may be rewritten in terms of specific activity as in 53.

$$\frac{da_1}{dt} = k_2' \left(\frac{q_2}{q_1} \right) a_2 - \frac{k_1'}{V} a_1 [P - Q + q_1] \tag{53}$$

Note that equations 52 and 53 could have been written directly from 46 and 47, for $\frac{f_{21}'}{q_2}$ is $\frac{k_2' q_2}{q_2}$ and $\frac{\phi_{12}'}{q_1}$ is $\frac{k_1' q_1}{V q_1} [P - Q + q_1]$. Equations 52 and 53 can be further simplified by taking into account the relation $\epsilon = \epsilon_1 + \epsilon_2$; if we write $a = \frac{r\epsilon}{Q}$, $a_2 q_2 = aQ - a_1 q_1$ where aQ is the amount of radioactive isotope added to the system.

$$\frac{d\epsilon_1}{dt} = k_2' \epsilon - \epsilon_1 \left\{ k_2' + \frac{k_1'}{V} (P - Q + q_1) \right\} \tag{54}$$

$$\frac{da_1}{dt} = k_2' \frac{aQ}{q_1} - a_1 \left\{ k_2' + \frac{k_1'}{V} (P - Q + q_1) \right\} \tag{55}$$

If $k_1' = k_1$, $k_2' = k_2$, then the measured fractional transfer rates give the true fractional transfer rates for the normal isotope in this steady state.

Dimerization. If the reaction is a dimerization, the problem becomes considerably more complex. Let A be the normal isotope and A' the radioactive isotope. Now we must consider the three reactions given in equation 56.

$$A + A \underset{k_2}{\overset{k_1}{\rightleftharpoons}} A_2$$

$$A' + A \underset{k_2'}{\overset{k_1'}{\rightleftharpoons}} A'A \tag{56}$$

$$A' + A' \underset{k_2''}{\overset{k_1''}{\rightleftharpoons}} A_2'$$

Let z_1 and z_2 be concentrations of A and A_2, ζ_1 and ζ_2 be concentrations of A' and A_2' and ξ be the concentration of the mixed dimer A'A. The rate equations for z_1, ζ_1, and ξ are equations 57 to 59.

$$\frac{dz_1}{dt} = 2k_2 z_2 - 2k_1 z_1^2 \tag{57}$$

$$\frac{d\zeta_1}{dt} = k_2' \xi - k_1' z_1 \zeta_1 + 2k_2'' \zeta_2 - 2k_1'' \zeta_1^2 \tag{58}$$

$$\frac{d\xi}{dt} = k_1' z_1 \zeta_1 - k_2' \xi \tag{59}$$

Again, we will assume that the system is closed and of constant volume, V. Let q_1 and q_2 be the total (molar) amounts of A and A_2. Let ϵ_1, η_1 and η_2 be total amounts of A', AA' and A_2', respectively. The conservation relationships for this closed system are given by equations 60.

$$Q = q_1 + 2q_2 + \eta_1$$

$$\epsilon = \epsilon_1 + \eta_1 + 2\eta_2 \tag{60}$$

Q and ϵ are constants. The total amount of radioisotope in dimer forms is $\epsilon_2 = \eta_1 + 2\eta_2$. Equations 57 to 59 may be rewritten in terms of total amounts as in 61 to 63.

$$\frac{dq_1}{dt} = 2k_2 q_2 - \frac{2k_1}{V} q_1^2 \tag{61}$$

$$\frac{d\epsilon_1}{dt} = k_2' \eta_1 - \frac{k_1'}{V} q_1 \epsilon_1 + 2k_2'' \eta_2 - \frac{2k_1''}{V} \epsilon_1^2 \tag{62}$$

$$\frac{d\eta_1}{dt} = \frac{k_1'}{V} q_1 \epsilon_1 - k_2' \eta_1 \tag{63}$$

In the steady state $\dfrac{dq_1}{dt} = 0$ and q_1 and q_2 are constant. If tracer amounts are used, η_2 and ϵ_1^2 will be the same order of magnitude and will be negligible in comparison to ϵ_1 and η_1. If terms in η_2 and ϵ_1^2 are neglected, the last two terms of equation 62 can be dropped: rewriting equation 62 in terms of specific activities gives equation 64.

$$\frac{da_1}{dt} = k_2' \left(\frac{q_2}{q_1} \right) a_2 - \frac{k_1'}{V} q_1 a_1 \tag{64}$$

This may be arrived at in another way. Let $k_2'' = k_2' + \Delta\, k_2'$ and $k_1'' = k_1' +$

$\Delta k_1'$ where Δk_2 and $\Delta k_1'$ will generally be small in comparison to k_1' and k_2'. Then equation 62 may be rearranged to give 65.

$$\frac{d\epsilon_1}{dt} = k_2'(\eta_1 + 2\eta_2) - \frac{k_1'}{V}\epsilon_1(q_1 + 2\epsilon_1) + 2\Delta k_2'\eta_2 - \frac{2\Delta k_1'}{V}\epsilon_1^2 \qquad (65)$$

But $\eta_1 + 2\eta_2$ is the total radioisotope in dimer form. Thus, if we neglect the last two terms in equation 65 and the factor $2\epsilon_1$ in the second term, equation 66 is obtained.

$$\frac{d\epsilon_1}{dt} = k_2'\epsilon_2 - \frac{k_1'}{V}q_1\epsilon_1 \qquad (66)$$

which gives equation 64 when expressed in terms of specific activity. If there is an appreciable isotope fractionation effect and the concentration of A_2' is of interest and can be measured independently, the full equations 61 to 63 must be retained. Then even if the major components A and A_2 can be considered to be in equilibrium, the kinetics of formation of A_2' will be nonlinear.

Returning to a comparison of equations 61 and 66, note that $\frac{f_{21}'}{q_2} = 2k_2'$ and $\frac{\phi_{12}'}{q_1} = \frac{2k_1q_1}{V}$. The stoichiometric coefficient (2) is missing from equation 61 because the primary reaction involving the radioisotope is $A' + A \rightleftharpoons AA'$ and only one molecule of tracer disappears for each molecule of dimer formed. If there is any doubt as to which stoichiometric coefficient to use in tracer kinetics, it is best to write out all possible reactions as in 56, the rate equations corresponding to 61 to 63, and then to make the appropriate approximations.

EXPERIMENTAL DESIGN AND ANALYSIS OF DATA

THEORY TO DATA AND BACK

Given a specific model of a compartmental system, values for the various rate and transfer constants, and a set of initial conditions, a unique solution (in terms of sums of exponentials) can be found for linear systems. This is not the usual problem which confronts the biologist; given the data he must somehow generate a plausible model. We must recognize that some prior knowledge about the system is almost always an important factor in the decision as to what data to collect. The major types of problems can be classified as follows:

Parameter Estimation When the System is Known. Occasionally the system is so well explored that the experimenter can say with considerable assurance that he has a completely determined model and wants only to quantify the parameters of the system. As a general rule, the experiments used for the estimation should cover as wide a range of *initial conditions* as possible. Not only will this provide better estimates than will many replications of a more limited range of experiments, but it will provide a more critical test of the validity of the model. However, one must not allow the range of experimentation to become so large that an inadequate sample size is obtained to permit accurate estimation of the parameters. The minimum number of determinations required can be obtained by considering equation 43. Assume there are n compartments and that reliable measurements of each of the rates $\dfrac{dq_i}{dt}$ and of all the concentrations q_j and the inputs I_i can be obtained; then there are n^2 of the λ_{ij} to be determined. If the excretion rates can also be determined there will be $n(n - 1)$ parameters to be determined. Only $n - 1$ of the n equations of the form of 43 are independent so that in effect enough experiments must be performed to provide $n - 1$ more sets of such $n - 1$ equations.

Parameter Estimation When the System is Partly Unknown. This is a far more common problem. The investigator is usually interested primarily in a particular part of the total system for which a well defined model may exist. His major concern is to fill in details of the model with respect to the part under investigation and to treat the remainder of the system as simply as possible.

Curve Fitting: The Search for a Model. In many situations little information may be available concerning a complex system, at least initially. The problem then is to examine one or more curves of data from an experiment and see whether the curves are exponential in nature, and if so, to determine how many exponential components are required to obtain an "adequate" fit.

GRAPHICAL METHODS

Before attempting more complicated methods of analysis, graphical methods should always be tried first. Graphical methods have two important advantages. First, the investigator often may have considerable data of a qualitative nature to guide him; simple visual examination of a graph may permit the investigator to decide whether the data fit the body of knowledge available to him or whether there is something grossly "wrong" with the data. Secondly, exponential decay constants estimated from a graph can often serve as good first approximations, particularly for trial and error calculations made on a digital computer.

Graphical methods for estimating exponential decay constants are most useful if no two constants are close in value and if there are not too many components. The use of more than three components creates nearly hopeless problems, and often results merely in "an exercise in curve fitting" rather than a source of physical knowledge.

A useful technique for two and occasionally for three components follows. Suppose that equation 67 represents the curve.

$$y = C + A_1 e^{-\lambda_1 t} + A_2 e^{-\lambda_2 t} \tag{67}$$

We assume $\lambda_1 > \lambda_2$. The first requirement is that data be obtained for a sufficiently long time for the exponential components to become negligible in comparison to the constant C. The estimate of y, when t is very large, will be $y_\infty = C$. One proceeds then to plot $y - C$ on semilogarithmic paper or to plot $\log [y - C]$ against t on arithmetic paper.

$$\log [y - C] = \log [A_1 e^{-\lambda_1 t} + A_2 e^{-\lambda_2 t}] \tag{68}$$

If λ_1 is sufficiently greater than λ_2, after some period of time say for $t > \tau$, $A_1 e^{-\lambda_1 t}$ will be quite small in comparison with $A_2 e^{-\lambda_2 t}$, then equation 68 becomes 69 and will give a straight line of slope $-\lambda_2$ and intercept of $\log A_2$ at

$$\log (y - C) \simeq \log A_2 - \lambda_2 t \tag{69}$$

$t = 0$. This is shown for a particular case in Figure 3-18 in which Z_1 is equation 67 and log Z_2 is equation 68. Knowing A_2 and λ_2, $A_2 e^{-\lambda_2 t}$ can be subtracted from $y - C$. Then equation 70 is obtained.

$$\log [y - C - A_2 e^{-\lambda_2 t}] = \log A_1 - \lambda_1 t \tag{70}$$

This is shown in Figure 3-18 as Z_3 and allows estimation of A_1 and λ_1.

Although theoretically quite simple, there are many pitfalls in this technique of "stripping" or "peeling" components of a multiexponential curve. Errors of measurement introduce scatter in the points so that a number of approximately equally good fits can be obtained. This is particularly true if the decay constants differ by less than a factor of two. A discussion of this problem may be found in Riggs, 1963.

ANALOG COMPUTATIONS

In the simulation of compartmental systems by means of an analog computer, an electronic circuit is connected so that a particular voltage corresponds to each of the variables of the compartmental system. Differential equations,

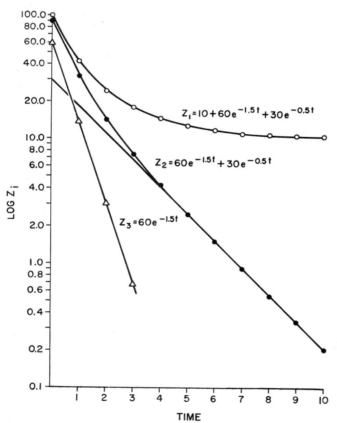

$$Z_1 = 10 + 60e^{-1.5t} + 30e^{-0.5t}$$

$$Z_2 = 60e^{-1.5t} + 30e^{-0.5t}$$

$$Z_3 = 60e^{-1.5t}$$

LOG Z_i

TIME

FIGURE 3-18. Illustration of the graphical "peeling technique" for estimating exponential decay constants.

identical to those of the system under study, describe the time variations of these analog voltages. Variable potentiometers usually represent the transfer constants λ_{ji} of equation 43. By varying the λ_{ji} one attempts to fit a particular experimental curve. In effect, then, this is a way of fitting the differential equation of the compartmental system.

DIGITAL COMPUTATIONS

The solution of systems of differential equations as given by equations 43 or the fitting of a curve by a sum of exponentials can be done most expeditiously with a digital computer. Two approaches can be used.

Fitting the Solutions. The common approach used is to assume that the solution for the variables under study is given by a sum of a certain number of exponentials as in equation 71.

$$y = A_0 + \sum_{1}^{n} A_j e^{-\gamma_j t} \tag{71}$$

The A_j and γ_j in the equation are determined by a least-squares fit (which will be discussed) of equation 65 to the data. Unfortunately, the methods do not always converge on the solution unless relatively good *initial estimates* of the A_j and γ_j are available. Furthermore, the assumption that equation 71 represents the solution implies that all of the roots of the characteristic equation for the system of equations 43 are distinct.

Fitting the Differential Equations. The second approach is to fit the differential equations by the following technique. Initial estimates of the λ_{ji} are used to obtain solutions of the differential equations by numerical integration. The sum of squares of the deviations of the solutions from the data is calculated and the λ_{ji} are changed to minimize the sum of squares. This technique is longer than that of fitting the solutions but does not depend on the assumption of distinct roots of the characteristic equation of equations 43.

Many programs have been written for fitting sums of exponentials and for solving linear differential equations. One of the most extensive is the program written by Berman, Weiss, and Shahn, 1962. This program, originally written in FORTRAN for the IBM 7090 can handle nonlinear differential equations as well and can also fit sums of Gaussian curves as well as sums of exponentials.

STATISTICAL CONSIDERATIONS

LEAST SQUARES

Let us suppose that equation 72 represents the time course of some variable of a system.

$$y = f(t, \lambda) \tag{72}$$

The parameter λ is to be determined. The data obtained at times $t_1, t_2, \ldots, t_n$ are $y_1, y_2, \ldots, y_n$, respectively. Suppose the value of λ which gives the best least-squares fit is λ^*. This is the best estimate available for the value of λ. We assume that a measured value y_i consists of the "true" value $f(t_i, \lambda)$ plus an error ϵ_i which is assumed to be a normally distributed random variable with zero mean and variance σ_i^2. Thus equation 73 describes the measurements.

$$y_i = f(t_i, \lambda) + \epsilon_i \tag{73}$$

Let $\eta_i = \dfrac{\epsilon_i}{\sigma_i}$; then the η_i are normally distributed random variables with mean zero and variance 1. Thus we can write equation 74

$$\frac{1}{\sigma_i} [y_i - f(t_i, \lambda)] = \eta_i \tag{74}$$

Squaring equation 74 and summing over all i, gives equation 75.

$$\sum_{i=1}^{n} \frac{1}{\sigma_i^2} [y_i - f(t_i, \lambda)]^2 = \sum \eta_i^2 \tag{75}$$

If we choose $\lambda = \lambda^*$, which minimizes this sum of squares, we obtain the best estimate of λ, in the least-squares sense. Thus we seek to minimize the sum given by the left side of equation 75.

In practice σ_i is replaced by the experimentally obtained estimate of the

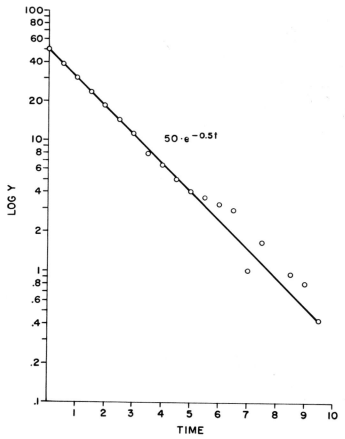

FIGURE 3-19. Plot on a semilogarithmic scale of a one component exponential decay with constant error variance.

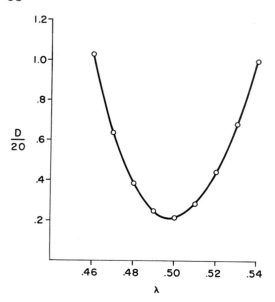

FIGURE 3-20. Sum of squares of deviations of fitted curve from experimental points for different values of parameter λ.

experimental error (standard error). The standard error at each point should be determined by obtaining complete replicates: this means a replicate in which every procedure involved in a measurement is repeated independently, not just another reading on the same sample. Too often, calculated counting errors or an estimated instrumental error is used instead of a good estimate of error of the entire experimental technique—often the former not only markedly underestimates the experimental error but also shows a different dependence on the value y_i than does the experimental error.

Having obtained a least-squares solution, it is often useful to examine the sum of squares surface near the minimum values, to see if the minimum is a sharp minimum in the various parameters. This gives a measure of the sensitivity of the solution to variation in the fitted parameters. Some insight into this can be gained by holding all the parameters but one at their "least-squares" values and seeing how the sum of squares varies with this one parameter.

Some of these points are best illustrated with an example. The function $y = 50\ e^{-0.5t}$ was calculated for each of 20 values of t. To each value an error was added. The error was determined by drawing from a symmetrical distribution which was a discrete approximation to a normal distribution. Figure 3-19 gives the usual plot on semilog paper; this illustrates a typical finding. The variation due to errors is markedly accentuated at low values of the ordinate on a semilogarithmic plot; nonetheless the error distribution function is the same for all points in this example. Figure 3-20 gives the sum of squares (divided by 20) as a function of λ for A held constant at A = 50.

How MANY POINTS

Many experimenters underestimate their observational error and use too few points in fitting curves. At least three points are needed to fit a straight line and obtain an estimate of error and this only when it is known that the data must fall on a straight line. If a decision has to be made as to whether the data can be fitted by a straight line, a minimum of four points is required and the larger the experimental error, the more points should be added. Even if a fit by eye seems adequate, and it often is if there are enough data points, for estimating parameters, it is often useful to calculate the sum of squared deviations for a few values of the parameters.

POPULATION DISTRIBUTIONS OF PARAMETERS

Consider a hypothetical process in a living system in which the variable y depends on the values of a number of parameters, $\lambda_1, \lambda_2, \ldots, \lambda_n$. Suppose the time course is given by equation 76.

$$y = f(t_1, \lambda_1, \lambda_2, \ldots, \lambda_n) \tag{76}$$

The values of these parameters will vary from one individual to another according to some distribution. For simplicity, let us consider only one parameter, λ, and use the subscript i to indicate an individual from the population. Thus in individual i, the parameter has the value λ_i and the variable y_i follows a time course given by equation 77.

$$y_i = f(t, \lambda_i) \tag{77}$$

Of course, the independent variable need not be time. We suppose that λ has some distribution in the population under study with mean μ, variance σ^2. Suppose a sample of n individuals is drawn from the population. How does the time course of the sample mean, $\frac{1}{n} \Sigma y_i$, differ from that of individuals? Indeed, does the mean have the same sort of functional dependence on time as does the process in individuals? This is important! It is fairly common to find attempts to fit a mean curve for a sample and to estimate population parameters therefrom (Furchner and Richmond, 1959). Let $Y_n(t)$ represent the mean $\frac{1}{n} \sum_1^n y_i$. First we suppose that we may expand $f(t, \lambda_i)$ in a Taylor's series about μ as in equation 78.

$$f(t, \lambda_i) = f(t, \mu) + (\lambda_i - \mu)\frac{\partial f}{\partial \mu} + \frac{(\lambda_i - \mu)^2}{2}\frac{\partial^2 f}{\partial \mu^2} + \frac{(\lambda_i - \mu)^3}{3!}\frac{\partial^3 f}{\partial \mu^3} + \cdots \tag{78}$$

Here $\frac{\partial^n f}{\partial \mu^n}$ means the nth derivative of $f(t, \lambda)$ with respect to λ, evaluated at $\lambda = \mu$. Taking the average,

$$Y_n = \frac{1}{n}\Sigma y_i = f(t, \mu) + \frac{\partial f}{\partial \mu}\Sigma\frac{(\lambda_i - \mu)}{n} + \frac{1}{2}\frac{\partial^2 f}{\partial \mu^2}\Sigma\frac{(\lambda_i - \mu)^2}{n} + \cdots \tag{79}$$

although we cannot predict the exact value for this for any particular sample, the expected value (the mean for a large number of samples of size n) for this expression can be calculated. This is given by equation 80 where μ_3 is the third central moment of the population.

$$Y_n = f(t, \mu) + \frac{\sigma^2}{2}\frac{\partial^2 f}{\partial \mu^2} + \frac{\mu_3}{3!}\frac{\partial^3 f}{\partial \mu^3} + \cdots \tag{80}$$

This shows that in general the sample mean *does not* follow the same curve as does the process in an individual. If the distribution curve for λ is very narrow so that the moments of the distribution of λ are quite small, the terms after the first may only be small corrections to $f(t, \mu)$.

There is only one case in which the sample mean of a sample of size n follows the same curve as the individuals and this is when y is linear in the parameters. Suppose

$$y_i = m_i f(t) + b_i \tag{81}$$

where m_i and b_i have some independent distributions in the population and $f(t)$ is some function of time. Then the mean value Y_n will be given by equation 82.

$$Y_n = \frac{1}{n} \sum y_i = \left[\frac{1}{n} \sum m_i \right] f(t) + \frac{1}{n} \sum b_i \tag{82}$$

As an example, let us consider a process given by the double exponential decay given by equation 83.

$$y_i = A_i e^{-\alpha_i t} + B_i e^{-\beta_i t} \tag{83}$$

We assume the parameters A, B, α, and β have independent distributions in the population. If instead of gathering sufficient data to fit each of a number of individuals (i) and determining A_i, B_i, α_i, and β_i, suppose we determine only the mean value for a sample mean of size n. Then the sample mean is given by equation 84.

$$Y_n = \bar{A} e^{-\bar{\alpha} t} \left\{ \frac{1}{n} \sum a_i e^{-\Delta \alpha_i t} \right\} + \bar{B} e^{-\bar{\beta} t} \left\{ \frac{1}{n} \sum b_i e^{-\Delta \beta_i t} \right\} \tag{84}$$

Here $a_i = A_i / \bar{A}$; $b_i = B_i / \bar{B}$, $\Delta \alpha_i = \alpha_i - \bar{\alpha}$, and $\Delta \beta_i = \beta_i - \bar{\beta}$. The $\bar{A}$, $\bar{B}$, $\bar{\alpha}$, and $\bar{\beta}$ are the population means for the respective parameters. Note that the bracketed terms are functions of time. It is quite possible to find that a sum of three or four exponential terms gives a very good fit to such a sample mean.

The moral is obvious: whenever possible obtain enough data on each individual. Fit the curves for *each individual* and obtain the population distribution for the fitted parameters.

NONLINEAR SYSTEMS: NONSTEADY STATE

FLUXES

It is possible to measure one-way fluxes between two compartments in a nonsteady state by injecting labeled tracer amounts of material into compartment i and measuring the rate of appearance of tracer in compartment j. Compartment j need not be well mixed; Wrenshall (1955) and Schachter (1955) have shown that as long as compartment i is well mixed, extrapolating the measured flux from i to j back to the time of injection gives a good measure of the flux from i to j. However, the assumption that there is no isotope fractionation must still be used. Furthermore, it is presumed that the transfer from i to j is direct and does not involve intermediate compartments. The presence of intermediate compartments small in comparison to i and j is not easy to rule out although sometimes this can be done by obtaining measurements on many compartments and determining the precursor relationships (Solomon and Gold, 1955).

KINETICS

Not infrequently a tracer is used to follow the distribution and metabolism of a compound such as a drug which is not normally found in the body. In this case one cannot assume that a steady state exists, and if the drug undergoes metabolic changes or enters transport processes in the body, it is likely that its kinetics will be nonlinear. Even if the drug enters only first order processes in the peripheral tissues, the early time course of its distribution in the circulation is a difficult problem. Because of the closed-loop nature of the circulation, the concentration at any one point in the circulation will undergo oscillations in the first few circulation times after injection. Furthermore there is evidence for uneven perfusion of some peripheral capillary beds (Renkin, 1959). More detailed considerations about blood flow will be found in McDonald (1960) and Sheppard and Martin (1950).

In practice, nonlinear systems are usually treated by attempting to construct as simple a model as possible to fit the system. This involves making reasonable hypotheses about the structure of the system and the processes going on. The system is then described by a set of differential equations supplemented with some equations of material balance. Such equations are usually not solvable by analytical techniques and numerical solutions must be obtained with use of a digital or analog computer (Aronoff, 1956, and Bellman et al., 1960). If a fairly good fit of theory to experiment is obtained, it is a good idea to test the sensitivity of the predictions of the theory to variation in each of the parameters in the theory. Such a sensitivity study is necessary to guide the design of more experiments to test the theory critically.

CONCLUSION

ADVICE TO COMPARTMENT SEEKERS

It is very popular these days to seek a compartmentalized system to represent experimental data. This may not always be appropriate. Insight into life processes is our goal, not a uniform method of representation. If a compartmental system does not provide physical insight, discard it. However, if it is used, the following precautions should be remembered:

It is often not difficult to fit curves of the type found in biological research with a sum of a few exponential terms. The fact that this is possible tells very little about the basic processes going on. The results of such a curve fitting are significant only when interpreted in the light of other knowledge about the system.

All too often the basic assumptions underlying the application of linear differential equations to a description of tracer kinetics in nonlinear systems is forgotten. Whenever possible, the steady-state assumptions must be tested by sampling the various compartments and showing that the amounts of material in them are constant or nearly so over the period of the experiment. In intact normal animals, homeostatic mechanisms will usually maintain steady states but even here one must demonstrate that the steady-state assumption holds. In *in vitro* studies of isolated organs, tissue slices, or cell suspensions, the experimenter *must prove* that his steady-state assumption is valid; such preparations are often not in a steady state, but deteriorate slowly during the experiment. Furthermore, violations of the assumptions of uniform mixing and of the absence of isotope fractionation must be considered.

TESTING HYPOTHESES

At times a number of possible hypotheses are tenable and it is necessary to devise tests to choose among these alternatives. The following general principles should be followed.

In compartmentalized systems, whenever possible, the experiments should be rerun with the isotope injected initially into each of the different compartments of the system.

If the steady state can be altered, the various experiments should be rerun in each of a number of different steady states.

REFERENCES

Agnew, R. P.: Differential Equations. Ed. 2. McGraw-Hill Book Co., New York, 1960.

Aronoff, S.: Techniques of Radiobiochemistry. Iowa State College Press, Iowa City, 1956.

Bellman, R., Jacquez, J. A., and Kalaba, R.: Some Mathematical Aspects of Chemotherapy: 1. Organ Models. *Bull. Math. Biophys.* 22:181, 1960.

Berman, M., and Schoenfield, R.: Invariants in Experimental Data on Linear Kinetics and the Formulation of Models. *J. Appl. Phys.* 27:1361, 1956.

Berman, M., Shahn, E., and Weiss, M. F.: The Routine Filling of Kinetic Data to Models: A Mathematical Formulation for Digital Computers. *Biophys. J.* 2:275, 1962.

Berman, M., Weiss, M. F., and Shahn, E.: Some Formal Approaches to the Analysis of Kinetic Data in Terms of Linear Compartmental Systems. *Biophys. J.* 2:289, 1962.

Feller, W.: An Introduction to Probability Theory and Its Applications. Vol. I. John Wiley and Sons, Inc., 1957.

Fisher, R. A.: Statistical Methods for Research Workers. Oliver L. Boyd, Ltd., Edinburgh, 1954.

Garland, L. H.: Studies of the Accuracy of Diagnostic Procedures. *Amer. J. Roentgen.* 82:25, 1959.

Loevinger, R., and Berman, M.: Efficiency Criteria in Radioactivity Counting. *Nucleonics* 9:26, 1951.

McDonald, D. A.: Blood Flow in the Arteries. Monograph 7 of the Physiological Society. Edward Arnold, Ltd., London, 1960.

Radiological Health Handbook. Revised Ed. U.S. Department of Health, Education and Welfare, Division of Radiological Health, Washington 25, D.C., 1960.

Renken, E. M.: Exchangeability of Tissue Potassium in Skeletal Muscle. *Amer. J. Physiol.* 197:1211, 1959.

Riggs, D. S.: The Mathematical Approach to Physiological Problems. Williams and Wilkins Co., Baltimore, 1963.

Schachter, H.: Direct Versus Tracer Measurement of Transfer Rates in a Hydrodynamic System Containing a Compartment Whose Contents Do Not Intermix Rapidly. *Canad. J. Biochem.* 33:940, 1955.

Scheff, T. J.: Decision Rules, Types of Errors, and Their Consequences in Medical Diagnosis. *Behav. Sci.* April, 1963.

Shemin, D., and Rittenberg, D.: The Life Span of the Human Red Blood Cell. *J. Biol. Chem.* 166:627, 1946.

Sheppard, C. W., and Householder, A. S.: Tracer Experiments in Closed Steady-State Systems. *J. Appl. Physiol.* 22:510, 1951.

Sheppard, C. W., and Martin, W. R.: Cation Exchange Between Cells and Plasma of Mammalian Blood. I. Methods and Application to Potassium Exchange in Human Blood. *J. Gen. Physiol.* 33:703, 1950.

Solomon, A. K., and Gold, G. L.: Potassium Transport in Human Erythrocytes: Evidence for a Three Compartment System. *J. Gen. Physiol.* 38:371, 1955.

Wald, A.: Statistical Decision Functions. John Wiley and Sons, Inc., New York, 1947.

Wrenshall, G. A.: Working Basis for the Tracer Measurement of Transfer Rates of a Metabolic Factor in Biological Systems Containing Compartments Whose Contents Do Not Intermix Rapidly. *Canad. J. Biochem.* 33:909, 1955.

GENERAL REFERENCES

Bellman, R., Jacquez, J. A., and Kalaba, R.: Mathematical Models of Chemotherapy. Proceedings of the Fourth Berkeley Symposium on Mathematical Statistics and Probability. Vol. IV. University of California Press, Berkeley, 1960.

Berger, E. Y., and Steele, J. M.: The Calculation of Transfer Rates in Two Compartment Systems Not in Dynamic Equilibrium. *J. Gen. Physiol.* 41:1135, 1958.

Bowen, H. J. M.: Biological Fractionation of Isotopes. *Int. J. Appl. Radiat.* 7:261, 1960.

Brownell, G. L., Cavicchi, R. V., and Perry, K. E.: An Electrical Analog for Analysis of Compartmental Biological Systems. *Rev. Sci. Instrum.* 24:704, 1953.

Chance, B.: Analogue and Digital Representations of Enzyme Kinetics. *J. Biol. Chem.* 235:2440, 1960.

Chance, B., Garfinkel, D., Higgins, J., and Hess, B.: Metabolic Control Mechanisms. V. A Solution for the Equations Representing Interaction Between Glycolysis and Respiration in Ascites Tumor Cells. *J. Biol. Chem.* 235:2426, 1960.

Chance, B., Higgins, J. J., and Garfinkel, D.: Analogue and Digital Computer Representations of Biochemical Processes. *Fed. Proc.* 21:75, 1962.

Cornfield, J., Steinfeld, J., and Greenhouse, S. W.: Models for the Interpretation of Experiments Using Tracer Compounds. *Biometrics* 16:212, 1960.

Dobson, E. L., and Warner, G. F.: Measurement of Regional Sodium Turnover Rates and Their Application to the Estimation of Regional Blood Flow. *Amer. J. Physiol.* 189:269, 1957.

Furchner, J. E., and Richmond, C. R.: Comparative Metabolism of Radioisotopes in Mammals. II. Retention of Iodine[131] by Four Mammalian Species. *Health Phys.* 9:277, 1959.

Gardner, D. G., Gardner, J. L., Lausk, G., and Meinke, W. W.: Method for the Analysis of Multicomponent Exponential Decay Curves. *J. Chem. Phys.* 31:978, 1959.

Garrett, E. R., Thomas, R. C., Wallach, D. P., and Alway, C. D.: Psicofuranine: Kinetics and Mechanisms in Vivo with the Application of the Analog Computer. *J. Pharmacol. Exp. Ther.* 130:106, 1960.

Ginsberg, J. M., and Wilde, W. S.: Distribution Kinetics of Intravenous Radiopotassium. *Amer. J. Physiol.* 179:63, 1954.

Gold, G. L., and Solomon, A. K.: The Transport of Sodium into Human Erythrocytes In Vivo. *J. Gen. Physiol.* 38:389, 1955.

Hart, H. E.: Analysis of Tracer Experiments in Non-Conservative Steady-State Systems. *Bull. Math. Biophys.* 17:87, 1955.

Hearon, J. Z.: The Kinetics of Linear Systems with Special Reference to Periodic Reactions. *Bull. Math. Biophys.* 15:121, 1953.

Johnson, C. L.: Analog Computer Techniques. McGraw-Hill Book Co., New York, 1956.

Landahl, H. D.: Note on the Interpretation of Tracer Experiments in Biological Systems. *Bull. Math. Phys.* 16:151, 1954.

Moir, I. W., Pritchard, W. H., and Ford, A. B.: The Early Disappearance of I[131] Albumin from the Circulation of Edematous Subjects and its Implications in the Clinical Determination of the Blood Volume. *J. Lab. Clin. Med.* 47:503, 1956.

Perl, W.: A Method for Curve-Fitting by Exponential Functions. *Int. J. Appl. Radiat.* 8:211, 1960.

Reiner, J. M.: The Study of Metabolism Turnover Rates by Means of Isotopic Tracers. I. Fundamental Relations. *Arch. Biochem.* 46:53, 1953.

Reiner, J. M.: The Study of Metabolic Turnover Rates by Means of Isotopic Tracers. II. Turnover in a Simple Reaction System. *Arch. Biochem.* 46:80, 1953.

Robertson, J. S.: Theory and Use of Tracers in Determining Transfer Rates in Biological Systems. *Physiol. Rev.* 37:133, 1957.

Sangren, W. C., and Sheppard, C. W.: A Mathematical Derivation of the Exchange of a Labeled Substance Between a Liquid Flowing in a Vessel and an External Compartment. *Bull. Math. Biophys.* 15:387, 1953.

Sheppard, C. W.: Basic Principles of the Tracer Method. John Wiley and Sons, Inc., New York, 1962.

Solomon, A. K.: Equations for Tracer Experiments. *J. Clin. Invest.* 28:1297, 1949.

Solomon, A. K.: The Kinetics of Biological Processes; Special Problems Connected with the Use of Tracers. *Advances Biol. Med. Phys.* 3:65, 1953.

Worsley, B. H., and Lax, L. C.: Selection of a Numerical Technique for Analyzing Experimental Data of the Decay Type with Special Reference to the Use of Tracers in Biological Systems. *Biochim. Biophys. Acta* 59:1, 1962.

Worsley, B. H., Reid, D. B., and Lax, L. C.: On the Calculation of "Turnover Time" and "Turnover Rate" from Experiments Involving the Use of Labeling Agents. *J. Gen. Physiol.* 26:325, 1943.

CHAPTER IV

BASIC PHYSICS OF
NUCLEAR MEDICINE

ROBERT H. ROHRER

INTRODUCTION

The major advantage of radioisotope techniques in nuclear medicine is that if proper techniques are used, we can determine not only *where* a radioactive material is in the body but *how much* of *what kind* is there at the time. This provides means of measuring the function of different organs or even parts of organs of the body and also lets us build up pictorial representations of the distribution of the radioactivity. Such images help in the localization of areas of malfunction and in locating abnormal concentrations of radioactive tracers.

But there are problems and limitations in the use of these radioactive materials and in the detection of the radiations they emit. For example, the most ideal conditions for external detection would be those in which all the radiations being emitted reached the detector without being absorbed or deflected from their original path; and, for highest efficiency, all radiation reaching the detector should be detected. Hopefully, the radiation would be detected in such a way that the identity of the nuclide could be established.

If these criteria could be met, we could use extremely small quantities of radioactive atoms. Each event detected would be an indication of one radioactive process from one atom. The number of events counted would give the exact number of atoms within view of the detector. The radiation from the atoms, not being absorbed, would do no damage to body tissue. If there were no scattering within the body and if the detector could tell from what direction the radiations came, there would be no doubt of the location of the source. If the detector has spectroscopic capabilities, we can observe several different physiological processes at one time. Such feats would be possible if each radioactive decay process were uniquely associated with a distinctly different kind of radiation. But such is not the case. Atoms emit radiation in all directions. When one radiation quantum is emitted, its chances of being intercepted by the detector are very small—unless, of course, the detector surrounds the source. Fortunately, it is not difficult to calculate the probability that a quantum will be intercepted.

Once a radiation quantum leaves a source, even if it should start out in the direction of the detector, it may be either absorbed or scattered and thus be prevented from reaching the detector.

We would like to dispense with absorption and scattering when we are trying to propagate radiation from the source to the detector, but we need absorption for the detection of radiation.

In addition to being concerned with the effect of scattering radiation *out of* a beam directed toward a detector, we must be equally aware that radiation not originally headed toward the detector can be deflected *into* it by scattering. This can lead to a false indication of the quantity or location of the source material.

In order to obtain quantitative data, one must take these factors into account, as well as the possibilities that the radiation may not be efficiently detected upon reaching the detector. Armed with the knowledge of interaction probabilities for various kinds of radiation and some idea of the structures that the radiation must penetrate, we can make good approximations of the corrections that must be applied.

To understand the problems of propagation and detection of nuclear radiations, we need a background in the basic physics of nuclear radiation.

Models

An understanding of radioactivity and of the interaction of radiation with matter is possible only if we have some concept of the nature of the atom. Individual atoms are too small to be seen with any known technique, but we are able to observe things that atoms do. From these observations we can devise models that are our guesses of what atoms might be like. We can explain the behavior of atoms in simple terms if we use simple models and go so far as to use *different* models to describe different characteristics of the *same* atom. Even the most sophisticated of physicists stoop to this practice when it makes understanding easier.

The fundamental particles of the atom

For our purposes we can consider atoms as made up of three fundamental particles: *electrons, protons,* and *neutrons.* Their properties are given in Table 4–1. Electrons appear to be nebulous bodies somewhat larger than protons and neutrons but much lighter in weight. Electrons all have the same mass and they all carry the same negative charge, e (1.6×10^{-19} coulombs), which appears to be the smallest charge of electricity that exists in nature. The only force that electrons seem to experience in encountering other particles is the force due to their electrical charge. Because of their cloudlike consistency, if they run into particles like neutrons and protons, they simply keep going as if no material

TABLE 4-1. THE ATOMIC PARTICLES

NAME	SYMBOL	MASS (grams)	(a.m.u.)*	(Mev.)†	CHARGE ‡	RADIUS (cm.)
Electron	e^-	0.9108×10^{-27}	0.000549	0.511	$-e$	2.82×10^{-13}
Proton	p	1.6724×10^{-24}	1.00728	938.22	$+e$	1.45×10^{-13}
Neutron	n	1.6747×10^{-24}	1.00867	939.23	0	1.45×10^{-13}

* The atomic mass unit (a.m.u.) is $\frac{1}{12}$ the mass of an atom of the nuclide carbon-12.

† The fifth column gives the mass of the particle expressed in energy units, million electron volts. This is the mass-energy equivalent of the "rest mass" of the particle from the Einstein relation, E (Mev.) = mc^2.

‡ The unit of charge, e, is 4.8×10^{-10} electrostatic units (e.s.u.) or 1.6×10^{-19} coulombs.

objects had been in their paths. Protons are quite different. They are small, dense bodies carrying a positive charge that is equal to the charge carried by the electron. They can be pictured as spheres similar to glass marbles with the added features of being electrically charged and having cohesive coatings on their surfaces. In collisions with other protons or with neutrons, a proton will experience collision and sticking forces. Neutrons are very much like protons except that they carry no charge and are slightly heavier than protons. They collide and stick on contact with other neutrons or with protons. Because neutrons have no electrical charge, they experience no forces when they encounter electrons. Protons, with their positive charges, exert pulling forces on negatively charged electrons. The neutron has in the past been pictured as being a proton in combination with an electron, but there is evidence that this is not a reasonable model. As can be seen in Table 4-1, the mass of the neutron is greater than the sum of the masses of the proton and the electron. There are other more sophisticated arguments against the electron-proton model of the neutron.

THE STRUCTURE OF THE ATOM

The atom consists of a small central nucleus approximately 10^{-12} cm. in radius, positively charged, and very dense. Surrounding the nucleus is a spherical region that is mostly empty space occupied by electrons moving about rapidly and held in the atom by the pull of the positive charge of the nucleus. The "atmosphere" of electrons extends about 10^{-8} cm. outward from the nucleus.

The nucleus is a mass of protons and neutrons held tightly packed together by cohesive forces. The number of neutrons in the nucleus is symbolized by the letter N, the *neutron number*. The number of protons in the nucleus is symbolized by Z, called by two names, the *proton number* and the *atomic number*. The sum of N and Z we call A, the *mass number*. Because neutrons and protons make up the atomic nucleus, they are called *nucleons*. The charge of the nucleus is the sum of the charges of the protons. Using e to represent the charge of one proton, the total nuclear charge can be given as + Ze. This charge limits the number of electrons that an atom can have under normal circumstances. Each nuclear proton attracts one electron into the atom. Atoms usually have the same number of electrons as they have protons. It follows that the proton number, Z, is also the electron number of the atom in its normal state. Since chemists number their atoms according to the number of electrons they have, Z is known as the atomic number.

The mass of the nucleus can be approximated by multiplying the number of nucleons (the mass number A) by 1.67×10^{-24} g. This is a good estimate of the mass of the atom as well, because the mass of electrons does not make a noticeable contribution to the atomic mass. The radius of the nucleus is given by the approximation

$$R_n \cong 1.45 \times 10^{-13} A^{\frac{1}{3}} \text{ cm.} \tag{1}$$

This expression is based on the model that the nucleus is a sphere whose volume must be proportional to the number of nucleons in it. Experiments have proved it to be very nearly correct. Nuclear radii vary from 1.45×10^{-13} cm. to 9.2×10^{-13} cm. (The largest nucleus has a mass number of 257.)

The approximate radius of the atom is given by the expression

$$R_a \cong 0.6 \times 10^{-8} (A/\rho)^{\frac{1}{3}} \text{ cm.} \tag{2}$$

where ρ represents the mass density of the elemental material in its solid form expressed in grams per cubic centimeter. This expression is based on the concept that in solids, atoms are in contact with each other and the distance between their centers is twice their radii. Atomic sizes estimated in this way vary from 0.9×10^{-8} cm. (carbon) to 1.6×10^{-8} cm. (lead). There is not much variation in size from one atom to another. Using these data we must conclude that even in solids, the atomic nuclei occupy only one part in 3×10^{13} of the total volume of the solid. The remaining space is occupied by the atomic electrons which must be widely spaced because electrons are about the same size as atomic nuclei and each atom contains Z electrons. This picture helps us understand how particles of atomic radiation can penetrate many layers of atoms without undergoing interactions.

The electrons are assigned to the atom in a definite pattern. One can use an oversimplified picture of an atom with its electrons arranged in concentric *shells* that are identified by quantum numbers, n = 1, 2, 3, . . . , or by letters, K, L, M, N, . . . , beginning with the innermost shell outward, each shell subdivided and each subdivision having a fixed quota of electrons. The arrangement of electrons is summarized in Table 4-2. The shells are often shown as circles with the electrons neatly arranged around the circles and described as *orbiting* about the nucleus (Fig. 4-1).

Although this is convenient, it may give the false impression that atoms are

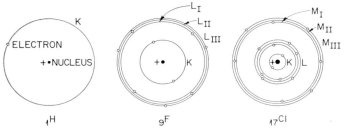

FIGURE 4-1. An illustration of the subshell arrangement and the relative sizes of atoms. Hydrogen, fluorine, and chlorine are given as examples. Open circles represent the electrons that occupy each subshell.

TABLE 4-2.   THE OCCUPATION CAPACITIES OF THE
ELECTRON SHELLS OF THE ATOM

n	PRIMARY SHELL LETTER DESIGNATION	SUBSHELL DESIGNATION							TOTAL CAPACITY
		I	II	III	IV	V	VI	VII	
1	K	2	—	—	—	—	—	—	2
2	L	2	2	4	—	—	—	—	8
3	M	2	2	4	4	6	—	—	18
4	N	2	2	4	4	6	6	8	32
5	O	2	2	4	4	6	6	8	32
6	P	2	2	4	4	x*	x	x	32
7	Q	2	x	x	x	x	x	x	32

*The subshells marked x are available to electrons but they are not needed by atoms in their ground states to accommodate the maximum of 103 electrons which corresponds to the 103 elements.

flat and that all electrons move in circles, never approaching the nucleus, and rotating with angular momentum. Many atomic physicists prefer to think that electrons may rotate about and oscillate toward and away from the nucleus, even passing through it at times, in a continuous motion so complex that the physicists avoid trying to predict the exact position of any electron at any time. Instead, they try to determine the *probability* of finding the electron at some given position in the coordinate system of the atom. It is known, for example, that electrons in subshell I described in Table 4-2 have no angular momentum and have a significant probability of passing through the nucleus. It is also known that the probability that an electron will be at some particular radial distance from the nucleus is the greatest at the distance represented by the radius of the shell in the simpler model. This fact is used to relate the *Bohr model*, which we will discuss later, to this more sophisticated *probability model*. Figure 4-2 is presented to give an idea of the probability model concept. Rather than showing discrete shells for the electrons to occupy, we show a "probability cloud" whose density represents the probability of finding the electron at a given position in the atom.

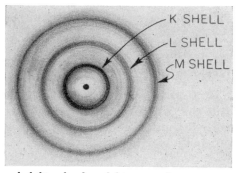

FIGURE 4-2.   The probability cloud model is somewhat nearer to a true picture of the atom than the orbital model shown in Figure 4-1. The blurred image represents a "time exposure" of electrons in motion. The reader should visualize the atom as having a spherical shape. The regions of high electron density appear dark and are located at radii corresponding to the orbital radii given in equation 10.

CLASSIFICATION OF ATOMS

Atoms are classified according to the number of protons, Z, the number of neutrons, N, and the number of nucleons, A, in their nuclei. Each different combination of Z and A identifies a distinct species of *nuclide.* (You need only two numbers, Z and A, because $N = A - Z$.) All nuclides that have the same proton number are *isotopes* of a specific chemical element. Atoms with the same proton number have the same number of electrons, and the number of electrons in the atom determines that atom's chemical characteristics. The different nuclides of one element are *isotopes* of that element. The isotopes have the same proton number, Z, but different mass numbers, A; hence they have different neutron numbers, N. Nuclides that have the same mass number, A, but different proton numbers, Z, are classed as *isobars.* Nuclides that have the same neutron number, N, but different proton numbers, Z, are classed as *isotones.* If the nuclei of one specific nuclide (same Z and same N numbers) differ from one atom to another in the manner in which the protons and neutrons are arranged within the nucleus, the different nuclei are called *isomers,* a term used by organic chemists to describe molecules that have the same atoms in different configurations. The number and arrangement of protons and neutrons in the nucleus determine whether the nucleus is stable or unstable. The stability of the nucleus determines the stability of the atom as a whole. Unstable nuclei will, at some time, spontaneously change to a more stable form, emitting radiation in the process. The atoms built around such unstable nuclei are said to be *radioactive* and such species are called *radionuclides.*

To identify nuclides we use the conventional chemical symbol with the mass number as a superscript and, when it is helpful, the proton number as a subscript. For example:

Isotopes of carbon are $^{11}_{6}C$, $^{12}_{6}C$, $^{13}_{6}C$, $^{14}_{6}C$.
Isobars of the mass number 12 are $^{12}_{5}B$ $^{12}_{6}C$ $^{12}_{7}N$.
Isotones of the neutron number 6 are $^{9}_{3}Li$, $^{1}_{4}Be$, $^{11}_{5}B$, $^{12}_{6}C$, $^{13}_{7}N$, $^{14}_{8}O$.

In these examples ^{11}B, ^{12}C, and ^{13}C are stable; the others are *radionuclides.* Some of these are illustrated in Figure 4-3.

An inventory of the nuclides in 1964 listed 80 stable elements, 259 stable nuclides, and 1130 radionuclides (Goldman, 1964). Twenty-three of the 103 different chemical elements that have been discovered or created artificially have no stable atomic forms.

REVIEW OF CONCEPTS OF ENERGY

Dynamic properties of atoms, of their nuclei, and of their radiations are described in terms of mechanical and atomic energy. Before we go further in the description of atoms, we must review the basic physics of energy.

A particle or a system of particles is said to have energy when it has the ability to do *work.* In physical terms, work is performed when something is moved a distance D against an opposing force F. The amount of work done in such a process is computed by multiplying the displacement by the opposing force:

$$Work = F \times D \tag{3}$$

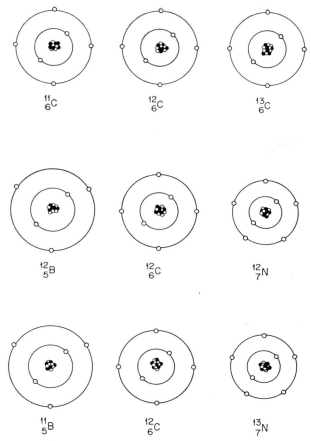

FIGURE 4-3.   Examples of *isotopes* (top row), *isobars* (center row), and *isotones* (bottom row). Protons in the nuclei are represented by black circles. The subdivision of the L-shells is not shown in this figure.

For example, work is done on an object when it is lifted up against the force of gravity, on a nail when it is driven into a board against the resisting force of friction, on a bullet when it is accelerated down a gun barrel against the resistance of the bullet's inertia, and on a space capsule when it is fired into outer space against gravitational, inertial, and frictional forces. On the atomic scale, work is done when an electron is accelerated or ejected from an atom against the electrical force of attraction of the nuclear charge and when a charged particle is slowed down as it penetrates a material medium that resists its advance.

When work is done, energy is transferred from the acting system to the system that is acted upon. Energy may take on a number of different forms. Stored energy is called *potential energy,* energy due to motion is called *kinetic energy,* and energy that appears as heat is *thermal energy.* Work done in lifting a weight to some height above its original position in a gravitational field gives that weight potential energy. Work done in driving a nail generates thermal energy and noise, or sound energy. Work done in accelerating a particle gives that particle kinetic energy.

A system containing potential, thermal, sound, or kinetic energy is capable of doing work. A weight on a grandfather's clock does work in driving the clock-work, a heated boiler can drive a steam engine, a sound wave can produce vibrations in an eardrum, and a moving bullet can produce heat in a target.

Energy stored in the atom is potential energy. Energy radiated from an atom is kinetic energy. When high-speed quanta of radiation are slowed down in an absorbing medium, they transfer kinetic energy into other forms, such as heat, atomic excitation, and, in the case of the scintillation crystal, visible light.

Potential energy is sometimes described as negative. If work has to be done in order to bring a system to a desired state, we can say that in its original state, its potential energy is negative relative to its desired state. For example, consider the lifting of a 20 pound bucket of water from a well 40 feet deep. The work required is 800 foot-pounds. When the bucket is at the bottom of the well, it has a potential energy of —800 foot-pounds relative to the surface of the ground and zero potential energy relative to the bottom of the well. If it were lifted to a height of 30 feet above the bottom of the well, the bucket would have a potential energy of 600 foot-pounds relative to the bottom of the well and a potential energy of —200 foot-pounds relative to the ground level (Fig. 4-4).

Kinetic energy is always positive. When an object gains speed, its mass increases because of its velocity. The increase in the kinetic energy of an object is related to its increase in mass through the Einstein equation

$$\Delta E = c^2 \cdot \Delta m \tag{4}$$

where c is a constant, m represents mass, and the symbol Δ is read "a change of . . ." If mass is expressed in atomic mass units (a.m.u.), the factor c^2 has the value 931.4 Mev. per a.m.u. By manipulating physical units, one can show that the value of c may be reduced to 3×10^{10} cm./sec., which is the speed with which light, x-rays, and gamma-rays move through a vacuum. The increase in energy, E, as a result of the motion, is equal to the kinetic energy that an object gains; therefore, one may write

$$\text{Kinetic energy} = (m - m_o)c^2 \tag{5}$$

where m is the observed mass of the object in motion and m_o is the observed mass of the object at rest. If the velocity of the object is given as v and is much less than the speed of light (the case that holds for most things in our civilization), equation 6 transforms into the form

$$\text{Kinetic energy} = \tfrac{1}{2} m_o v^2 \tag{6}$$

The relation between a change of mass and a change of energy given in equation 4 holds for potential forms of energy as well as for kinetic forms. When there is a gain or a loss of stored or potential energy in a nuclear or even in a chemical reaction, there will be a corresponding loss or gain of mass. In chemical reactions, energy changes per atom are too small to cause measurable changes in mass; therefore chemists do not observe the apparent failure of the "law" of conservation of mass. But in nuclear reactions and in radioactive decay processes, energy changes in each atom are sufficient to result in clearly evident mass changes.

ENERGY UNITS

Energy can be expressed in units of *ergs* (dyne-centimeters), *joules* (watt-

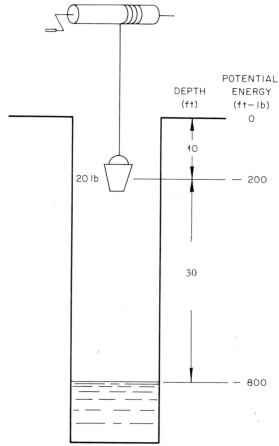

FIGURE 4-4. Energy levels associated with a 20 pound bucket in a well in the earth's gravitational field. The operator stands on the earth's surface, and considers this to be a good reference level. He arbitrarily assigns a value of zero to the potential energy of the bucket at the ground level. Here the bucket is shown at a −200 foot-pound energy level. If it were lifted to a height of 10 feet above the ground level, it would have an energy of +200 foot-pounds.

seconds), or *foot-pounds* for mechanical problems. Chemists generally use the *kilocalorie,* the amount of energy required to raise the temperature of 1 kg. of water from 14.5° to 15.5° C. Nuclear physicists use a unit called the *electron volt,* abbreviated e.v., the *kilo* electron volt, kev., and the *million* electron volt, Mev. The electron-volt is the amount of energy required to push an electron or a proton or anything else carrying the electron charge, e, through a region where there is a change of one volt of electrical potential. One kilocalorie is the equivalent of 2.62×10^{22} e.v. When a chemist delivers 1 kilocalorie of energy to a mole of material, he delivers to that material an average energy of 0.0435 e.v. per molecule.

ENERGY LEVELS OF ELECTRONS IN ATOMS

Electrons are held within the atom by electrical forces. The energy that is required to pull an electron away from an atom is referred to as *binding energy.*

The electron in the hydrogen atom exists only in states with well defined energies given by the expression:

$$E_{e-} = -\frac{13.6}{n^2} \text{ e.v.} \tag{7}$$

where n is a whole number with values of 1, 2, 3, 4, 5, 6 . . . Normally hydrogen atoms are in the "ground state" described by n = 1. Excited states are designated by higher values of n. Using the concept that electrons might orbit about the nucleus at a fixed distance, Niels Bohr found the orbit radius could be expressed:

$$R_{e-} = 0.53 \times 10^{-8} \text{ } n^2 \text{ cm.} \tag{8}$$

If Bohr's model is extended to larger atoms, it is found that electrons exert repulsive forces on one another and simple expressions are not easily derived for the electron energy and the orbital radii. Still there are approximate expressions

$$E_{e-} = -\frac{13}{n^2} (Z')^2 \text{ e.v.} \tag{9}$$

and

$$R_{e-} = 0.53 \times 10^{-8} \text{ } n^2/Z' \text{ cm.} \tag{10}$$

that can be used. Here Z' represents the average number of nuclear protons that influence an electron through a "fog" of intervening electrons. In lead, for example, with 82 protons, an electron in the innermost orbit (n = 1) will be affected by only 81 protons. The outermost electron in the orbit (n = 6) behaves as if there were only 0.74 protons in the nucleus as a result of interference caused by the other 81 electrons. This leads to an outer orbit radius of 1.6×10^{-8} cm., in agreement with the size of the lead atom given on page 78.

A diagram showing energy states in hydrogen is given in Figure 4-5. To separate the electron from the nucleus requires 13.58 e.v. of energy. In the figure, this is represented as the energy required to lift the electron from the bottom to the top of the well. Any additional energy that the electron might receive goes into that kinetic energy required to give it a velocity to use in roaming about in space free of its atom. If by some process 13.04 e.v. is delivered to the atom, the electron may be lifted from the lowest level, n = 1, to the −0.54 e.v. level, n = 5. An atom with one or more of its normal complement of electrons raised to energy levels higher than the lowest levels available to them is said to be "excited." A hydrogen atom with its only electron excited to the n = 5 level, where the binding energy is 0.54 e.v., can lose its excess energy by one or more transitions, in the course of which energy is radiated from the atom. The transitions allowed are those represented by a model of the electron "falling" from a higher energy level to a lower one. For each drop, a discrete quantity of radiated energy is emitted. Each quantity must correspond to the energy lost by the electron as it drops from one level to the next. In Figure 4-5, 10 different transitions are shown to be possible for the deexcitation of the hydrogen atom we have been discussing. If one observes the radiation emitted from a sample containing a large number of hydrogen atoms that were excited to the n = 5 state, he should expect to find the energy radiated in the form of quanta having the 10 discrete energies 13.04, 12.73, 12.07, 10.19, 2.85, 2.54, 1.88, 0.97, 0.66, and 0.31 e.v.

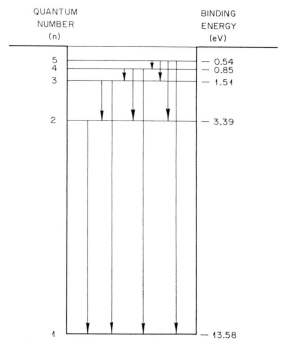

FIGURE 4-5. A well model showing the lowest five energy levels assigned to the electron in the hydrogen atom. The energies are given by equation 7. Normally, the electron would be found in the lowest energy state at the bottom of the well. Excitation may raise it to any of the higher energy states or even completely out of the well. The latter case would correspond with the removal of the electron from the atom. Arrows indicate 10 possible deexcitation transitions that are possible for an atom whose electron was initially excited to the n = 5 level.

In contrast with hydrogen, the lightest atom, tungsten is used as a typical example of a heavy atom. Figure 4-6 shows the 17 different energy levels occupied by the 74 electrons in this element in its normal unexcited state. The binding energies are greater in tungsten than in hydrogen because the 74 protons in the tungsten nucleus pull against the orbiting electrons with greater force than the single proton of the hydrogen nucleus can. The tungsten atom can be excited by delivery to it of sufficient energy to remove an electron from any of the levels shown in the figure and place it at an energy greater that that of the uppermost bound state that is shown. Such a removal is followed by a cascading of electrons from high level into the vacancies that exist in the lower levels. As is the case for all atoms, quanta of radiation are emitted for each transition. Because the binding energies in tungsten are so great, they are stated in thousands of electron volts, kev.

The radiation quanta emitted in the deexcitation of an atom are of the electromagnetic form called "photons." This name is used because some of them—those with energies ranging from 1.7 to 3.0 e.v.—are the carriers of visible light. Of the ten different photon groups given for the case of the deexcitation of the hydrogen atom, only three are visible: those with 1.88, 2.54, and 2.85 e.v. of energy. High-energy photons such as those that would be emitted following the removal of one electron from a low level in tungsten are called "characteristic" x-rays. These will be discussed in more detail later in this chapter, under the heading Atomic Radiation Processes.

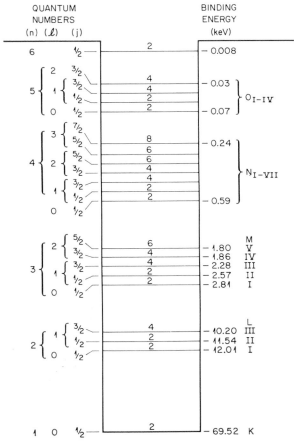

FIGURE 4-6. Energy levels of the occupied electron shells in the tungsten atom ($Z = 74$). The energy scale is distorted in order to show each level. Spectroscopic shell identification is shown on the right. The number of electrons that normally occupy each level is given by the numeral above that level. The quantum numbers in the three columns to the left of the well are: n, the *principle quantum number*, which is most important in determining the level energy as given in equation 9; ℓ, the *orbital angular momentum* quantum number describing the motion of the electron in its orbit; and j, the *total angular momentum* quantum number giving the amount of angular momentum due to both the orbital and spin motions of the electron. Electrons may drop from a higher level to a lower level provided that (1) there is an electron vacancy in the lower level, and (2) the quantum number ℓ changes by one unit, and the quantum number j does not change by any number greater than 1. Other transitions are forbidden. For each transition one photon or one Auger electron will be emitted from the atom.

ENERGY LEVELS IN THE NUCLEUS

The nucleons also occupy definite energy levels in the nucleus, but there are some differences. Only two nucleons of the same type, neutron or proton, may occupy one energy level. For each nuclide, there is one set of energy levels available to protrons and another set available to neutrons.

A nucleus is in its "ground state" when its lowest energy levels are filled. Figure 4-7 shows the energy levels of a nucleus of $Z = 7$, $N = 8$ in its unexcited state. Excitation may be accomplished by raising either a proton or a neutron to an unoccupied energy level, as indicated by the arrows in the figure. The energies involved in nuclear transitions are much greater than the atomic level

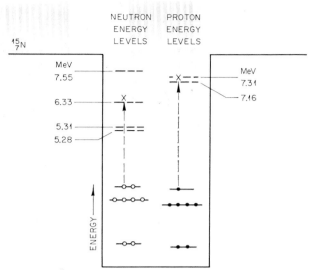

Figure 4-7. Energy levels of the nucleus of nitrogen-15. Occupied levels of the nucleus in its normal state are shown as solid lines. Dashed lines represent available levels for nuclear excitation. In nuclear wells, energy of excitation is positive relative to the energy of the highest occupied state. We are not willing to assign quantum numbers to the levels, but the excitation energies are well known. Nuclei can be excited from their normal conditions by bombardment with photons or high-energy charged particles.

energies, and the very energetic photons that are emitted when nuclei return to their ground state are identified as gamma-ray photons.

Two nuclei having the same value for Z and the same value for N but different nucleon configurations, which is expected when one is excited to a different state from the other, are called "isomers." Thus nitrogen-15 in an excited state is an isomer of nitrogen-15 in the ground state. Nuclear transitions that result in deexcitation by the emission of photons are often called "isomeric transitions."

Take care to distinguish between nuclear and atomic excitation. The former is associated with the configuration and energy of particles in the nucleus only; the latter is associated with the electrons that cavort about the nucleus.

RADIOACTIVITY

THE NATURE OF RADIOACTIVITY

When Becquerel and the Curies discovered radioactivity, the radiations from uranium and radium samples seemed to be continuous and inexhaustible. Between 1899 and 1902 Owens, Rutherford, and Soddy discovered that some elements lost their radioactive properties in a consistent fashion that varied from one element to another. The loss of radioactivity was called "decay." Rutherford also recognized that the source of some radioactive elements lay in samples of *other* radioactive elements and he reasoned that some radioactive atoms were *"disintegrating"* and producing other radioactive atoms, electrons, alpha particles, and gamma radiations. Thus, Rutherford coined the terms "decay" and "disintegration" in the early 1900's.

The nature of radioactivity is well understood today. Rutherford did not have as clear a picture of radioactive decay because until 1911 he did not visualize the atom as having a nucleus. Yet he correctly described the equation of radioactive decay.

Let N_t represent the number of radioactive atoms in a given sample at any time t. There is some degree of uncertainty about when any unstable nucleus will disintegrate, but the probability that a radioactive atom will disintegrate into another atomic form in a period of time, dt, is given by the expression

$$dP = \lambda dt \tag{11}$$

where λ is the symbol expressing the expectation that an atom will disintegrate in a unit of time. It is most often called the *decay constant*.

If we consider the population of atoms, $N_t{}^1$, and the number dN(t) that disintegrate in the period dt, we can derive the equation:

$$\frac{-dN_t}{N_t} = \lambda dt \tag{12}$$

This expresses that the fractional change of the population, $-dN_t/N_t$, in the time interval dt, is negative, signifying a decreasing number of atoms.

We can rewrite equation 12 in the form

$$R_t = -\frac{dN_t}{dt} = \lambda N_t \tag{13}$$

where R_t and dN_t/dt both express the rate of disintegration of the radioactive atoms in the sample under observation. There are two popular ways of expressing disintegration rates: in (1) disintegrations per second (or per minute), or in (2) curies, millicuries, or microcuries. The curie, abbreviated c. or Ci, is a practical unit for expressing the activity of a quantity of radioactive material. It is accepted that:

  1 curie (c) = 37,000,000,000 disintegrations/sec.
  1 millicurie (mc) = 37,000,000 disintegrations/sec.
  1 microcurie (μc.) = 37,000 disintegrations/sec.

This unit was adopted because it once was believed that 1 gram of radium underwent 37×10^9 disintegrations per second. We have better values for the disintegration rate of 1 gram of radium now, but the curie is officially established as 37×10^9 disintegrations per second.

The expression for N_t that satisfies equation 13 is

$$N_t = N_0 e^{-\lambda t} \tag{14}$$

where N_0 is the number of radioactive atoms in a sample at some arbitrary starting time when t = 0. Because equation 14 holds true at any time,

$$R_t = \lambda N_t = \lambda N_0 e^{-\lambda t} = R_0 e^{-\lambda t} \tag{15}$$

---

[1] In our notation, N_t and R_t are to be read "N (or R) at the time t." We mean by this that the population N_t and the disintegration rate R_t vary as functions of time. If we wish to specify some definite time such as t = 0 (when the counting might have started) or another time, t_1, we shall print it N_0 or N_{t_1}.

R is expressed in units of disintegrations per second or as "radioactivity" in curies.

The symbol e represents the number 2.71828, which is the base of the natural system of logarithms. Since

$$e = 10^{0.43429} \tag{16}$$

we can rewrite the solutions of equations 13 and 14.

$$N_t = N_0 \times 10^{-0.434\lambda t} \tag{17}$$

$$R_t = R_0 \times 10^{-0.434\lambda t} \tag{18}$$

HALF-LIFE AND THE COMPUTATION OF RADIOACTIVITY

The behavior of the functions given in equations 14, 15, 17, and 18 is shown in Figures 4-8 and 4-9. In Figure 4-8, the coordinates are linear. In Figure 4-9, logarithmic coordinates are used for the ordinates. The time coordinates are given in units of half-life rather than in one of the more familiar units of time. *Half-life,* $T_{\frac{1}{2}}$, is that period in which half of a population of atoms disintegrates. Because of the relation expressed in equation 13, it is also that period in which the dis-integration rate drops to one half of its initial value. It can be shown that

$$e^{-0.693} = \frac{1}{2} \tag{19}$$

and therefore the fraction $\dfrac{N_t}{N_0}$ is equal to one half when the product λt in the equations 14, 15, and 18 is given by

$$\lambda t = \lambda T_{\frac{1}{2}} = 0.693 \tag{20}$$

When this expression is used, λ and $T_{\frac{1}{2}}$ must be expressed in reciprocal units of time; that is, if λ is the disintegration expectation per second, $T_{\frac{1}{2}}$ must be ex-pressed in seconds. Often half-lives are given in units of hours, days, or years, but disintegration rates are expressed in terms of the number of events per

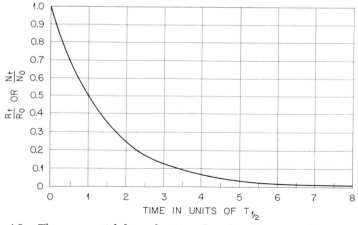

FIGURE 4-8. The exponential decay function plotted on linear coordinates. For each half-life time interval the value of this function is reduced by one half. The value of this function will never reach zero.

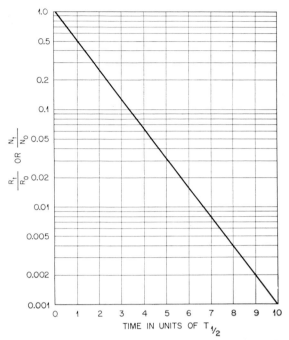

FIGURE 4-9. The exponential decay function plotted on semilogarithmic coordinates. The apparent distortion of the ordinate scale allows one to plot this function as a straight line.

second. We shall show in the following examples the steps that must be followed in order to express λ in the proper units.

From equation 20 the value of λ is found to be

$$\lambda = \frac{0.693}{T_{\frac{1}{2}}} \tag{21}$$

If we substitute this into equations 14 and 17, we have a simple form of the radioactivity decay equation:

$$\frac{R_t}{R_0} = \frac{N_t}{N_0} = e^{-0.693\frac{t}{T_{\frac{1}{2}}}} \tag{22a}$$

$$\frac{R_t}{R_0} = \frac{N_t}{N_0} = 10^{-0.301\frac{t}{T_{\frac{1}{2}}}} \tag{22b}$$

The fraction $\frac{t}{T_{\frac{1}{2}}}$ may be recognized as the number of half-lives involved in the decay of the material. For those more familiar with the logarithms expressed to the base 10 that are available on ordinary slide rules, equation 22b may be expressed in a more useful form:

$$\log_{10}\frac{R_0}{R_t} = \log_{10}\frac{N_0}{N_t} = 0.301\frac{t}{T_{\frac{1}{2}}} \tag{23}$$

Consider several examples:

Example 1. Iodine-131 decays with a half-life of 8.05 days. Find the probability of the disintegration of one atom of ^{131}I in 1 second.

COMPUTATION.

$$T_{\frac{1}{2}} = 8.05 \text{ days} \times 24 \frac{\text{hr.}}{\text{day}} \times 3600 \frac{\text{sec.}}{\text{hr.}} = 6.93 \times 10^5 \text{ sec.}$$

Using equation 21, $\lambda = \dfrac{0.693}{T_{\frac{1}{2}}} = \dfrac{0.693}{6.93 \times 10^5} = 10^{-6} \text{ sec.}^{-1}$. This means that if we could single out one atom and watch it for 1 second, the chances of its decaying in that second are only one in a million.

Example 2. Determine the number of radioactive ^{131}I atoms in a 30 μc. sample.

COMPUTATION. Use equation 13 and your knowledge that 1 μc. equals 37,000 disintegrations per second. Then $R = 30 \times 37,000 = 1,110,000$ disintegrations per second. But $R = \lambda N$, so $N = \dfrac{R}{\lambda} = \dfrac{1,110,000}{10^{-6}} = 1.11 \times 10^{12}$ atoms. At this point we should mention that 10^{12} atoms of iodine is not a very large quantity. One microgram of iodine contains 4.75×10^{15} atoms. The 30 μc. sample weighs about 1/4000 of a microgram. Stated another way, ^{131}I weighs about 8 *micrograms per curie.*

Example 3. Suppose we have 30 μc. of phosphorus-32 today. What will its activity be 30 days from now?

COMPUTATION. In this case, we use either the graph in Figure 4-9 or equation 23. The half-life of ^{32}P is 14.3 days; the ratio $\dfrac{t}{T_{\frac{1}{2}}} = \dfrac{30}{14.3} = 2.1$. Using equation 23, $\log \dfrac{R_0}{R_{20}} = 0.301 \times 2.1 = 0.633$. From the log tables, $0.633 = \log 4.296$, so $\dfrac{R_0}{R_{30}} = 4.296$ or $R_{30} = \dfrac{30 \ \mu\text{c.}}{4.296} = 7 \ \mu\text{c.}$

MEAN LIFE, EFFECTIVE LIFE

The *mean life* of a radioisotope is different from the half-life. The half-life is the period in which the activity (or population) of a radioactive material will decrease to one-half its initial value. Take a sample decaying at the rate of 1 mc. We know that this rate will decrease with time, but if we assume that it *will not* decrease, but will continue at the initial rate until all the radioactive atoms disintegrate, the time required for this to happen is the *mean life* of the atom. Since the initial decay rate is given as $R_0 = \lambda N_0$, the number of atoms initially present can be expressed $N_0 = \dfrac{R_0}{\lambda}$, but in light of the preceding discussion, $N_0 = R_0 \overline{T}$, where $\overline{T}$ is our symbol for mean life. Comparison of the last two relations for N_0 lead us to the conclusion that the expression for *mean life* is

$$\overline{T} = \frac{1}{\lambda} \tag{24}$$

Now, because $T_{\frac{1}{2}} = \dfrac{0.693}{\lambda}$, it follows that

$$\overline{T} = 1.44 T_{\frac{1}{2}} \tag{25}$$

Mean life is useful for computing the dose due to "infinite exposure" because the product of the mean life and the initially observed disintegration rate is equal to the total number of atoms that will eventually disintegrate.

In biological systems, the physical half-lives and mean lives of radioisotopes tell only a part of the story. Since living systems have their own way of eliminating materials, this too must be taken into consideration. This biological removal can be expressed as a *biological half-life* provided it approximates an exponential rate. The biological half-life of a given material in a given location in the body is related to an excretion probability, λ_b, just as half-life of a sample of a radioisotope is related to the disintegration probability λ. If a radioactive material with a physical disintegration probability λ were incorporated in a compound that disappears from a specified organ with a biological excretion probability λ_b, then the radioactivity has an even greater probability of disappearing from the site of interest. The *effective disappearance probability* can be expressed

$$\lambda_{eff} = \lambda_b + \lambda \tag{26}$$

and the *effective* half-life can be given by

$$T_{\frac{1}{2}eff} = \frac{0.693}{\lambda_b + \lambda} = \frac{T_{\frac{1}{2}b} \times T_{\frac{1}{2}}}{T_{\frac{1}{2}b} + T_{\frac{1}{2}}} \tag{27}$$

For example, if the physical half-life of an element x is 8 days and biological half-life in the liver of the compound that incorporates x is 2 days, the effective half-life of the radioactivity in the liver can be computed as follows:

$$T_{\frac{1}{2}eff} = \frac{(2) \times (8)}{2 + 8} = 1.6 \text{ days}$$

One should not rely upon the simple exponential function—equation 14—to describe the clearance of radioactive materials from all living systems. Often the mechanisms involved lead to a complicated clearance curve. When this is the case, the simple relations given in equations 26 and 27 do not hold because the terms λ_b and $T_{\frac{1}{2}b}$ are not constants and it is misleading to use the term "biological half-life."

SPECIFIC ACTIVITY

The concentration of activity in a sample containing radioactive material is called *specific activity*. This can be expressed by any combination of units of activity and of quantity that is appropriate to the occasion, e.g., millicuries per gram, microcuries per liter, or curies per cubic foot.

TABLE 4-3.   QUANTA OF ATOMIC RADIATION

NAME	SYMBOL	MASS (a.m.u.)	CHARGE	COMMENTS
Alpha	α	4.0015	$+2e$	Nucleus of ^{4}He atom
Electron	e^-	0.000549	$-e$	One of the atomic constituents
Positron	e^+	0.000549	$+e$	The anti-electron (we will explain later)
Neutrino	ν	0	0	Appears whenever an electron is absorbed by or emitted by a nucleus
Photon	γ	0	0	A quantized carrier of electromagnetic energy

TABLE 4-4. NUCLEAR DISINTEGRATION PROCESSES

NAME	SYMBOL	RADIATION EMITTED *	CHANGE IN THE NUCLEUS Z	A
1. *Isomeric Transitions*				
Gamma-ray decay	γ	γ	0	0
Internal converson	c, e	$e^- (\gamma_x, e_A^-)(\gamma_b)$	0	0
2. *Isobaric Transitions*				
Beta decay	β^-	$e^-, \nu, (\gamma_b)$	+1	0
Positron decay	β^+	$e^+, \nu, (\gamma_a), (\gamma_b)$	-1	0
Electron capture	e.c.	$\nu, (\gamma_x, e_A^-)$	-1	0
3. *Alpha Decay*	α	α	-2	-4

* (γ_x, e_A^-), characteristic x-rays and Auger electrons resulting from the filling of an electron vacancy; (γ_b), bremsstrahlung photons produced by electrons and positrons; ν, neutrino; (γ_a), annihilation photons produced by positrons.

The number of radioactive atoms in a radiopharmaceutical is surprisingly small compared with the number of molecules of solvent. Using the results of the second example in this chapter, together with the information that 1 ml. of water contains approximately 3×10^{22} molecules, we find that a solution of radioactive sodium iodide (^{131}I) with a specific activity of 30 $\mu c.$ per milliliter will have in it one ^{131}I atom for approximately 3×10^{10} molecules of water. The term specific activity is also used to designate the weight of radioactive atoms relative to the total weight of the element, but this use is less common.

ATOMIC RADIATION PROCESSES

Radionuclides disintegrate by six distinctly different nuclear processes. In each case the atom loses a discrete amount of energy that must be carried off by one or more atomic particles or quanta. Some characteristics of the five important particles emitted from radioactive materials are summarized in Table 4-3. The first three of these particles have observable "rest mass" and charge. When one of these leaves an atom it will carry with it kinetic energy due to its motion, and the atom will lose both charge and mass. The last two do not have a "rest mass." They have never been observed at rest and one may assume that they never exist in a motionless state. Both move with the velocity of light and carry small discrete quantities of energy. The distinct difference between photons and neutrinos is that the photon has electromagnetic properties and the neutrino does not. The photon is generated in a region of high electric and magnetic fields such as those existing in the atom, and interacts strongly with particles or systems of particles that have associated electromagnetic fields. The neutrino, on the other hand, has nothing to do with electricity or magnetism, and, having no mass, is not very reactive. Its existence was postulated in 1931 to explain the apparent failure of the principle of conservation of energy in beta decay processes, but it was not observed until 1954.

Table 4-4 presents the characteristics of the six disintegration processes.

Each type of disintegration can be indicated by a *decay scheme,* a diagram that is designed to give a full picture of the pattern of disintegration of the atom. Figures 4-14 to 4-20 include typical examples. A decay scheme is a combination of a graph and an energy level diagram. The vertical scale represents the energy involved in the disintegration process. The horizontal scale represents the atomic number of the nuclides. Isomeric states of a nuclide are indicated by horizontal lines (energy levels). Transitions are indicated by arrows drawn from an initial state to a following state. In the case of an isomeric transition, in which the atomic number does not change, arrows are drawn vertically downward.

In the case of beta decay, an electron-neutrino pair is emitted from the nucleus which loses one unit of negative charge. As a result, the proton number, Z, increases by one. The transition is indicated by an arrow drawn downward to the right. In the case of positron decay or of nuclear electron capture, the charge of the nucleus decreases by one unit, and the transition is indicated by an arrow drawn downward to the left.

The characteristics of a specific type of radiation are determined not only by the nature of the particles or quanta that carry off the radiant energy, but also by the process in the atom that leads to the emission. Because of this, the "rays" are classified by their mode of origin rather than by their constituents. For example, visible light, characteristic x-rays, bremsstrahlung, and gamma-rays are forms of electromagnetic radiation and consist of streams of photons; and beta-rays, conversion electrons, and Auger electrons are radiations consisting of electrons. The particles are similar; only the places of origin are different.

THE ISOMERIC TRANSITIONS

Gamma-ray decay occurs when an atomic nucleus falls to a state of lower energy by simply rearranging its internal structure. There are certain well defined

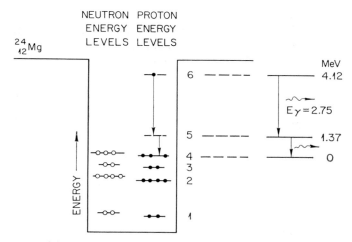

(*a*) NUCLEAR ENERGY LEVELS   (*b*) DECAY SCHEME

FIGURE 4-10.   Hypothetical energy levels in the nucleus of magnesium-24 and the scheme of the isomeric decay. This nuclide in the 4.12 Mev. excited state is the daughter product of beta decay of sodium-24. The two gamma-rays are associated with sodium-24 radioactivity. The numerals used to designate the proton energy levels are not nuclear quantum numbers.

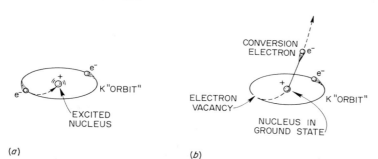

FIGURE 4-11. The process involved in internal conversion. (*a*) One of the K-shell electrons passes into the excited nucleus. (*b*) The excitation energy of the nucleus is transferred to that electron leaving a vacancy in the K-shell. Electrons from other shells have relatively smaller probabilities of coming into the nucleus and receiving the excitation energy.

ways in which neutrons and protons may be arranged within the nucleus. For each configuration, there is a different amount of energy stored in the nucleus. We can imagine vertically stacked shelves in the nucleus on which there are the nucleons, each shelf or "level" able to accommodate no more than two nucleons of the same kind, and each successively higher shelf representing a successively higher energy level. In Figure 4-10, we have illustrated hypothetical energy levels in the nucleus of magnesium-24. Its eleventh proton is sitting on the sixth proton level and the fifth and fourth levels are not filled. Imagine the proton as dropping first to level 5 and then to level 4, which is as far as it can go because all lower levels are filled.

In the case of a can of beans falling from a pantry shelf to the floor, potential energy is converted into heat and sound. In the case of a nucleon, potential energy lost in a transition is radiated as a photon. Suppose we assume that in magnesium, proton level 5 is 1.37 Mev. (in energy) higher than level 4 and that level 6 is 4.12 Mev. higher than level 4. The energy lost by the proton in the first drop from level 6 to level 5 would result in the release of 2.75 Mev. of energy. This energy would all go toward creating one photon. The second transition, from level 5 to level 4, would result in the generation of a 1.37 Mev. photon.

If we had a very large number of atoms of ^{24}Mg in the state of excitation illustrated in Figure 4-10, photons of 2.75 Mev. and 1.37 Mev. would radiate from the sample in all directions as these atoms decay to their ground states.

This scheme of transitions could be shown in the potential well representation of Figure 4-10 (a), but to save space, only the unfilled levels are shown in the decay scheme in Figure 4-10 (b).

METASTABLE STATES AND INTERNAL CONVERSION

Transitions of the type just described are very probable; that is, the excited states have high probabilities of decaying to lower energy states and their λ's have large values such as 10^{12} per second. But there are some excited states that take much longer to dissipate. They act as if there were some block to their decaying by the process of photon emission. These are the *metastable states*. They have half-lives that are very long in comparison to their companion states and decay probabilities that are very low. While a nucleus is in a metastable state, it is under constant bombardment of the s-electrons of the K-shell and the first subshells of the other major electronic shells. When an electron comes in contact with the nucleus on one of these "passes," it is possible for the nucleus to transfer its energy of excitation to the electron. If this happens, all the energy of excitation that the nucleus wishes to lose in the isomeric transition is carried away from the nucleus by the electron. The electron will then break free of the atom and travel away with a kinetic energy equal to the difference between the energy lost by the nucleus and the binding energy holding the electron in the atom. This gives the nucleus an alternative means of losing energy. It may emit a photon, or, if conditions are right, it may transfer its excitation energy to an electron belonging to its own atom. The electron that receives this energy is called a *conversion electron.*

The ratio of internal conversion events to photon emission events associated with the decay of one metastable state is the ratio $\frac{e}{\gamma}$ or α, the *conversion coefficient.* Its value may range from zero (no conversion) to infinity (complete conversion).

Following electron conversion, the atom is left with one of its orbital electrons missing. The vacancy will be filled by an electron from a higher energy level, and other cascading electron transitions will follow until all vacancies from the nucleus outward are filled. The last vacancy will be filled by a "free electron" picked up by the atom to complete its full complement of electrons. Each time one of these electron transitions takes place, the atom loses energy which can be carried away by two means: (1) by generation of a photon (known as a *characteristic x-ray*), or (2) by freeing additional electrons from the atom through the Auger process. The fraction of these transitions in which the energy is carried away by photons is called the *fluorescent yield, ω.* The Auger process in the orbital electron shells is analogous to the internal conversion process at the nucleus.[2]

An example of isomeric transitions is the decay of technetium-99m. The decay scheme and the electron energy levels appear in Figure 4-12. There are two routes by which the metastable state can decay—0.68 per cent of the transitions are directly to the ground state and the other 99.32 per cent take place by a two-stage process. Both transitions from the metastable state are highly converted in a manner typical of the decay of a metastable state of long half-life. The decay of the 140 kev. state is mostly by photon emission because its inherent decay probability is much higher than the decay probability of the metastable state. But even in that transition, there is a measurable internal conversion; 116 conversion electrons will be emitted for every 1000 gamma-ray photons. This is to say that of every 1116 transitions from the 140 kev. state to the ground state, 116 will involve internal conversion. The electrons that carry off the nuclear energy come from the K-, L-, M-, and N-shells. The data presented in Figure 4-12 indicate that the ratio of conversion of electrons from these shells occurs in the ratio K:L:(M+N) = 790:100:30. The binding energies of electrons in the shells of the technetium atom are given on the electron energy level diagram in Figure 4-12. K-shell electrons that are ejected from the atoms as a result of the 140 kev. transition will leave the atom with the kinetic energy

---

[2] More about this subject is given by Slack and Way (1959), pages 64–70, and by Wapstra et al. (1959), Chapter 7.

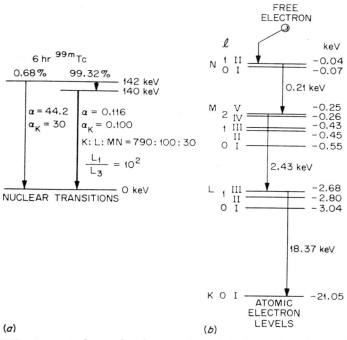

FIGURE 4-12.   Isomeric decay of technetium-99m. (a) The nuclear decay scheme giving the conversion coefficients and the relative numbers of conversions of electrons from the K-, L-, and M-shells associated with the 140 kev. transition. (b) Electron energy levels similar to those shown in Figure 4-6 for tungsten. One of many possible cascade schemes to fill a K-shell vacancy is shown.

$$E_{e_K} = 140 - 21 = 119 \text{ kev.}$$

L-shell electrons will leave with the energy

$$E_{e_L} = 140 - 3 = 137 \text{ kev.}$$

The M-shell and N-shell electrons will carry off almost the full value of the 140 kev. because they are bound by such small forces. Following the conversion of a K-shell electron in one atom, there will be a succession of electronic transitions as first the K-shell vacancy, and then other resulting vacancies, are filled. It is possible that one atom might follow the scheme shown at the right in Figure 4-12 and that characteristic x-ray photons having energies of 18.37, 2.43, and 0.21 kev. will leave the atom. Other atoms might decay in a different manner. Those that follow the same scheme of filling vacancies may emit Auger electrons instead of photons. This is more likely for transitions having smaller jumps in energy, as from an N-shell to an M-shell, than for jumps of greater energy difference (L to K), in which the fluorescent yield, ω, is larger. Other atoms follow different schemes for filling vacancies. The simplest transition that can follow the conversion of a K-shell electron is for an electron from outside the atom to fall directly into the K-shell vacancy. Other more complicated schemes can be followed. The only rules are that energy must be lost by the atom in each transition and that transitions are permitted only between levels with orbital quantum numbers, i, that differ by 1. The principle of the conservation of energy applies—the sum of the energy of all the x-ray photons and Auger electrons that leave an atom after the removal of a K-shell electron will be 21 kev. This energy, added to the energy carried off by the conversion electron (119 kev.), results in a sum of 140 kev. that is lost by the nucleus in the transition. Similar rules apply if the conversion electron comes from the L-, M-, or N-shell.

A feature characteristic of internal conversion can be illustrated by considering the 2 kev. transition. In this transition, the nucleus can lose only 2 kev. Only electrons that require less than 2 kev. to break away from the atom can serve to carry off this energy. Electrons in the K-shell and L-shell of technetium require from 2.68 to 3.04 kev. Although the K- and L-shell electrons come in contact with the nucleus, they do not serve as nuclear energy carriers. That role is left to M- and N-shell electrons. Available data indicate that M-shell electrons are much more likely to carry off this energy than are N-shell electrons; the ratio in favor of the M-shell electrons is 70:9. A situation somewhat similar to this exists in the radioactive decay of mercury-197.

We do not observe low-energy photons in the emission spectrum resulting from the 2 kev. nuclear transition. There are practically no nuclear gamma-ray photons emitted, and the fluorescent yield of the transitions between the N- and M-shell energy levels is very low. Almost all the radiated energy is carried off by electrons and these are not easily detected because of their low energies. They will contribute to ionization and radiation dose, however, and therefore are not inconsequential.

The distribution of energy among the photons and the electrons that are emitted from a radioactive source is called the spectrum of radiation. Photons that are produced by nuclear and atomic transitions from one energy level to a lower one carry away discrete quantities of energy and their spectra are called "line spectra." Conversion electrons also carry off discrete quantities of energy and yield line spectra. An example of the spectra of the electrons and photons from isomeric transitions is shown in Figure 4-13. Later, we shall show examples of continuous spectra of both photons and electrons.

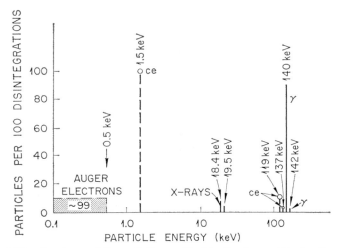

FIGURE 4-13.   Spectrum of the radiation emitted in the decay of technetium-99m. Electron lines are dashed and capped with open circles. Photon lines are solid. The height of each line represents the number of quanta emitted per 100 disintegrations. Many x-ray lines have been omitted for the sake of clarity. Auger electrons have line spectra that are crowded closely in the low-energy region of the spectrum.

THE ISOBARIC TRANSITIONS

Atoms that are produced by bombarding stable atoms with neutrons, protons, deuterons, and alpha particles, and atoms that are created in the chains of the decay of such naturally radioactive elements as uranium and thorium, may be formed with an imbalance in the number of protons and neutrons in their nuclei. Such nuclei possess excessive energies and are unstable. If the excess energy in the nucleus of an atom exceeds the binding energy of an unwanted nucleon (about 8 Mev.), the offending nucleon will promptly break free of the nucleus. This happens often in the course of the production of radioisotopes in a nuclear reactor. But if the internal energy associated with the imbalance is less than the binding energy of a nucleon, escape is out of the question. The nucleus may reach a state of satisfaction with the ratio of protons and neutrons, however, by changing one of its neutrons into a proton or vice versa. In that case, the number of nucleons, A, will not change but the number of protons, Z, will increase or decrease by one. Such a transfiguration is called an "isobaric transition." Of course, if the number of protons in the nucleus changes, the nuclear charge must change correspondingly. Nature calls upon its lightest charge carriers, electrons and positrons, to effect the change. Neither of these particles can exist as residents of the nucleus; therefore an electron must be destroyed at the nuclear surface or either an electron or positron (leptons) must be generated at the nucleus much as the photon is generated in an isomeric transition. In any of these cases, a neutrino appears as a by-product and competes with the charged particles for some of the energy liberated when the nucleus decays. Isobaric processes fall into three categories: beta decay, positron decay, and electron capture.

BETA DECAY, β^-

Beta decay is the isobaric transition that leads to the emission of the electron-neutrino pair.[3] This occurs when a neutron disappears and a proton appears in its place within the nucleus. With this change, the proton number, Z, of the nucleus increases by one, but the mass number does not change. One of the simplest examples of beta decay is the case of the ^{32}P atom. The nuclide $^{32}_{15}P$ is made by adding a neutron to the stable nuclide $^{31}_{15}P$ in an exothermic irreversible process. There is only one stable nuclide of the element phophorus, since all other isotopic forms have either too many or too few neutrons to be stable. Phosphorous-32, for example, contains an odd number of protons (15) and an odd number of neutrons (17). This is a very unsatisfactory configuration. Only five nuclides with odd numbers of both neutrons and protons are stable (hydrogen-2, lithium-6, boron-10, nitrogen-14, and tantalum-180). The unstable nucleus can become a nucleus of stable $^{32}_{16}S$ (sulfur) when one neutron changes into a proton. This is possible because the unstable nucleus has sufficient internal energy to generate an electron and a neutrino, and then to give the pair 1.71 Mev. of kinetic energy and settle down to the stable nucleus of the ^{32}S atom. The decay scheme is shown in Figure 4-14. It is a simple jump from the ^{32}P

---

[3] Not everyone agrees with this nomenclature. There are many who prefer to call *all* isobaric transitions "beta decay" and to classify this form as *negatron emission*. Because the first beta-rays were identified as rays of electrons, we prefer to maintain the initial meaning. This is consistent with the concept that a "beta particle" is an electron.

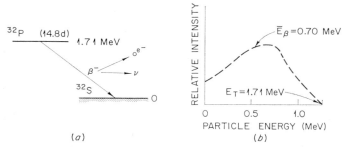

(a)   (b)

FIGURE 4-14. Beta decay of phosphorus-32. (a) The nuclear decay scheme showing the energy of the transition and the particles emitted in the course of the decay. The 1.71 Mev. is shared by the electron and the neutrino. (b) The spectrum of the electrons (beta particles) emitted. The maximum energy of the electrons is 1.71 Mev. The average energy is 0.70 Mev. A linear energy scale is used in this beta spectrum.

nucleus to the ^{32}S nucleus in its ground state. The difference in the energies of the two levels represents the energy shared by the electron and the neutrino. The distribution of energy, E_β, of electrons (beta particles) is illustrated as the continuous spectrum in Figure 4-14 (b). The greatest energy that any of the electrons have is equal to the transition energy E_T. The laws that govern the distribution of the electron energies are known but are too complex to be reviewed here. The average energy of the electrons is always less than the energy of the transition, E_T. In the case of the decay of ^{32}P it is given as $\bar{E}_\beta = 0.70$ Mev., which is about 40 per cent of E_T. Although the energies of the electrons emitted from the nucleus vary from zero to E_T Mev., the same amount of energy, 1.71 Mev., is always carried away by the electron and the neutrino together. We can state this relation:

$$E_\beta + E_\nu = E_T \tag{28}$$

The nature of the spectra of "beta emitters" must be understood when these materials are applied to clinical uses. Some tests require the use of pure beta emitters such as carbon-14 and sulfur-35 which have decay schemes similar to that of ^{32}P. When the radioactivity of the samples is measured, the wide variation in the energies of the emitted electrons can cause counting errors because transmission of electrons through sample material and through detector windows is strongly dependent upon the energy of the electron and absorption is significant at all energies. One must also take into account the distribution of the electron energies in computing the radiation dose delivered to organs of the body as a result of beta decay. Only the electrons deliver radiation dose to tissue. Neutrinos have no mass and no charge. They have only an extremely small chance of interacting with tissue—so small that one can ignore it completely. To compute the radiation dose delivered to tissue from beta emitters, we usually rely on the values of the average electron energy, $\bar{E}_\beta$, that are obtained by nuclear radiation spectroscopists.

There are about 23 cases of simple beta decay similar to the example that we have given. The major differences among them are the transition energy, E_T, and the shape of the electron spectrum. But there are many more beta-emitting radionuclides. One route of decay is to an excited isomeric state of the daughter nuclide. Some follow alternative routes. When isomeric decay is associated with beta decay, the radiation emitted from a sample contains electrons, neutrinos, and gamma-ray photons. In some cases there may also be conversion electrons, x-ray photons, and Auger electrons. Examples are given in Figures 4-15 and 4-16. The decay scheme of ^{131}I is shown in Figure 4-15. Seven different modes of beta decay have been confirmed. Each leads to the formation of xenon-131 atoms in excited states. Ninety per cent of the beta transitions of ^{131}I involve the transfer of 606 kev. to an electron-neutrino pair and leave the daughter xenon nucleus in the 365 kev. excited state. In an 806 kev. transition, 0.8 per cent of the ^{131}I atoms decay to a metastable state of ^{131}Xe that has a half-life of 12 days. The latter has a high probability of electron conversion decay to the ground state. In considering such a decay scheme, we must remember that each atom of ^{131}I can decay only once, by one of the processes shown in the decay scheme. The percentages stated in the diagram are the "branching ratios" and give the odds on which route is likely to be followed. In Figure 4-15, you can see that the predominant beta particle spectrum must have a maximum electron energy of 0.608 Mev., and that the greatest number of gamma-ray photons will have an energy of 0.365 Mev.

Positron decay, β^+

Positron decay, β^+, is one of two ways in which an unstable atom can convert a nucleon from a proton to a neutron. The transmutation of the nucleon is accomplished as a positron and a neutrino are formed at the nucleus. The energy that the nucleus loses in the transition goes into generating the two particles and in giving them both kinetic energy. The positive charge lost by

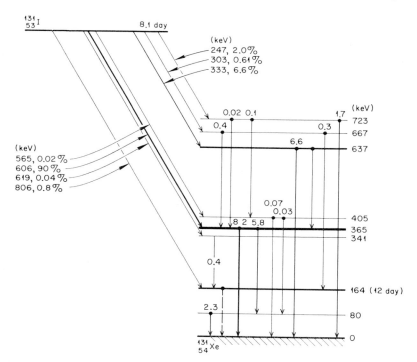

Figure 4-15. The decay scheme of iodine-131, after Graeffe and Walters (1967). The predominant transitions are shown as bold lines. The dashed arrow represents the transition from the 164 kev. isomeric state of xenon-131 which occurs by internal conversion.

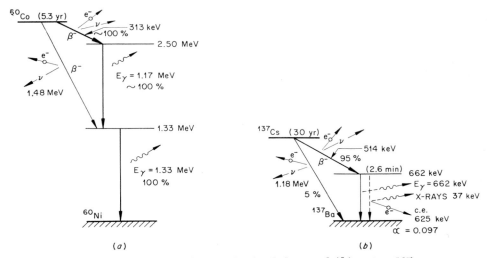

FIGURE 4-16. Decay schemes of (*a*) cobalt-60 and (*b*) cesium-137.

the nucleus is carried off by the positron. As in beta decay, the charged particle and the neutrino share the kinetic energy. The energy spectrum of positrons emitted from a sample of a positron-decaying nuclide is continuous and of similar shape as the beta decay spectrum.

Few positron-decaying radioisotopes have lives long enough to be useful in nuclear medicine. Sodium-22, whose decay scheme and spectra are shown in Figure 4-17, is a good example. The nucleus of this atom contains 11 protons and 11 neutrons. This arrangement of odd numbers of both types of nucleons is unstable and results in the change of a proton to a neutron. The end product is a nucleus of 10 protons and 12 neutrons containing less energy than the original.

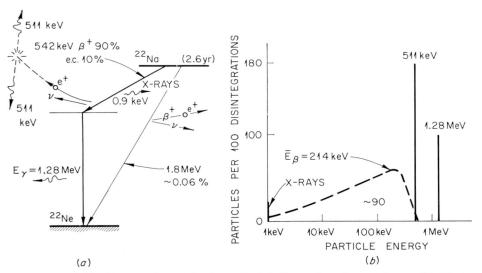

FIGURE 4-17. Positron decay of sodium-22. (*a*) The nuclear decay scheme. (*b*) Electron and photon spectra using logarithmic coordinates for the energy of the particles. The positron spectrum is continuous, as is the electron spectrum in beta decay (see Fig. 4-14).

The energy difference between the two nuclei is sufficient to allow the generation of the positron and the neutrino, plus an additional 1.82 Mev. Sodium-22 achieves positron emission in one of two ways. One is to deliver 0.542 Mev. to the positron-neutrino pair; the other is to give all 1.82 Mev. to the pair. More than 99 per cent of ^{22}Na atoms decay by the first route. After the positron and neutrino have been ejected, the residual nucleus is that of neon-22 in an excited state, which immediately decays to the ground state by an isomeric transition that produces a 1.276 Mev. photon. Only 6 of 10,000 ^{22}Na atoms decay by the transition that leads directly to the ground state of ^{22}Ne.

The radiation spectra that result from the positron decay transitions in ^{22}Na consist of a continuum with positron and neutrino energies ranging from 0 to 0.542 Mev., a strong gamma-ray component of 1.276 Mev. photons, and a very weak positron-neutrino spectrum ranging from 0 to 1.82 Mev. In addition to the radiations given off by the ^{22}Na atoms, there is a gamma-like 0.511 Mev. annihilation radiation that originates from material in intimate contact with a positron emitter. This radiation is associated with the mutual destruction of positrons and electrons and will be described in our consideration of the interaction of radiation and matter.

ELECTRON CAPTURE, e.c.

The second way that an unstable atom can convert a proton to a neutron is by the electron capture process. The change within the nucleus is the same whether positron emission or electron capture is the mode of decay, and for this reason the two processes compete with each other. The emitted radiations resulting from the two processes and the energy transfer mechanisms, however, are quite different. Because of these differences, one or the other of the two decay processes—positron decay or electron capture—will be favored.

Some unstable, proton-rich nuclei never decay to a lower-energy isobar by positron emission, because there is not enough difference in energy between the unstable nucleus and the prospective daughter nucleus to create a positron. That process requires that the atom lose at least two electron masses or that it lose an energy of at least 1.022 Mev., which atoms do not have. The atoms are unstable, but cannot get into a more stable condition by changing one of their protons into a neutron because of the lack of sufficient transition energy. In such cases, the nucleus makes use of the deeply penetrating orbital s-electrons as in the process of internal conversion, but it uses it for a different purpose.

If an orbital electron passes through one of these unstable nuclei, there is some degree of probability that it will be captured by the nucleus and its charge will neutralize the charge of one proton. To capture the electron the nucleus must manufacture a neutrino, which is necessary for the interaction between the nucleus and the electron (or positron). The nucleus creates a neutrino while the electron is passing through, captures the electron, and ejects the neutrino. The neutrino carries away the energy that the nucleus loses in the internal transmutation process.

As an example, let us consider the decay of iron-55. The decay scheme is shown in Figure 4-18. In this case, the energy that the nucleus of the iron atom has available for the transition to manganese-55 is 0.217 Mev.—not enough to produce a positron. The average waiting period for the time when conditions

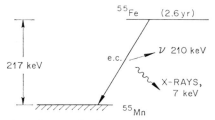

FIGURE 4-18. The simple electron-capture decay of iron-55.

become right for the capture of the electron is roughly 3.9 years. When an electron orbiting in the K-shell is captured, the ^{55}Fe nucleus is transformed to a ^{55}Mn nucleus and a neutrino is ejected which carries away the 0.210 Mev. of energy. This particle is the only radiation emitted from the nucleus. It is capable of penetrating a lead shield as thick as from the earth to the moon, so that it will not interact with the human body.

Since the neutrino is given 0.210 kev. of the nuclear transition energy of 0.217 kev., what about the difference of 7 kev.? The K-shell electron that was captured was bound in its shell by the 7 kev. energy. After the electron is captured by the nucleus and removed from its normal place in the K-shell, the atom is in a state of excitation of 7 kev. What follows is the usual series of electronic x-ray and Auger electron producing events described in the earlier discussion of internal conversion. At the end of the decay process, the nucleus has emitted only the single neutrino, but the atom has radiated a series of x-ray photons or Auger electrons whose total energy amount to 7 kev. Therefore, we should not expect to get much useful radiation from ^{55}Fe unless radiation with less than 7 kev. of energy is desired.

Some nuclides that decay by electron capture, however, are important in nuclear medicine. Tungsten 181 is an example. Its decay scheme is shown in Figure 4-19. Of the electron-capture transitions, 60 per cent are to the ground state of ^{181}Ta. The x-rays emitted from tantalum as a result of the capture of K-shell electrons have energies of 56 kev. and less. It is conceivable that there might be some scanning or tracer applications for such low-energy photon radiations.

Electron-capture nuclides that decay from the parent nucleus to a daughter in an excited state which, in turn, produces a desirable single-energy gamma-ray

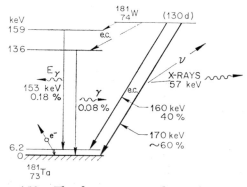

FIGURE 4-19. The electron-capture decay of tungsten-181.

are particularly attractive in nuclear medicine because the radiation is almost all in the form of photon and neutrino energy with very little high-energy electron energy; yet the half-life is of a reasonable duration. Electron-capture nuclides are becoming increasingly popular because of the absence of the positron and beta particle radiation.

ALPHA DECAY

Alpha radiation is not clinically useful, but some radionuclides that undergo alpha decay are. Radium-226 and radon-222 are examples. These are long-lived parents that produce a chain of short-lived gamma-ray emitters used in brachytherapy. Radon-222 is a typical alpha emitter. This gas emanates from radium and is encapsulated in gold seeds or in glass needles for surgical implantation in tumors. The modes of decay are shown in Figure 4-20. There are two branches in the decay scheme. The 5.59 Mev. transition directly to the ground state of radioactive polonium-218 accounts for more than 99 per cent of the disintegrations. The transition energy is shared by the emitted alpha particle and the recoiling daughter nucleus, but because only two bodies are involved in alpha decay, whereas three are involved in beta decay (the electron, the neutrino, and the recoiling nucleus), the principle of conservation of momentum dictates that all alpha particles from one transition shall have the same energy. When a 5.59 Mev. transition in ^{222}Rn occurs, the alpha particle will receive 5.48 Mev. of kinetic energy and the recoiling nucleus will receive 0.11 Mev. This same sort of thing happens in all alpha decay processes, so that alpha particles exhibit line spectra similar to gamma-ray photons, electron-capture x-ray photons, and conversion electrons. The other type of decay occurs in only 7 of 10,000 disintegrations. In these rare cases, radon atoms lose 5.08 Mev. in ejecting the alpha particle and the residual polonium atoms recoil with an energy of 510 kev., which they lose almost immediately by emission of a photon.

THE INTERACTIONS OF RADIATION WITH MATTER[4]

In general terms, radiation is an outward flow of energy from a source of energy, and is often pictured as *rays* fanning out from the source; when the radiation is collimated, it is pictured as well defined cones or *beams*. There was a time when all radiations were thought of as wavelike disturbances moving away from their sources. Now, we assign wavelike behavior to radiation beams when it suits our purposes, but we find at times that the wave concept cannot adequately describe the processes involved in nuclear and atomic radiations or the manner in which radiations interact with matter.

All particles of radiation carry with them discrete quantities of energy. The presence of a beam of radiation can make itself known only if some of the energy carried by the particles is transferred into an absorbing medium by

---

[4] Comprehensive treatments of this subject are given by Evans (1955), Chapters 18–25, and by Johns and Laughlin (1956).

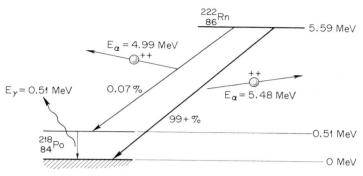

FIGURE 4-20.   Alpha decay of radon-222.

means of some interaction. Radiation that passes through a detector without loss of energy cannot be detected. Radiation that passes through tissue without transferring energy to the tissue delivers no radiation dose to the tissue.

The target material with which particles of radiation interact consists of tiny, dense, widely spaced, and positively charged atomic nuclei in a space sparsely populated by negatively charged electrons. In solids the nuclei can be considered to be motionless and spaced at distances that range from 14,000 nuclear diameters (in osmium) to 50,000 nuclear diameters (in lithium). The electrons are bound to their atoms by electrical forces, and their motion creates strong magnetic fields within the atoms. The atoms are usually bound together to form molecules, but the radiation particles generally do not interact with molecules as entities because of their size. Radiation particles may interact with nuclei, electrons, or atoms through many reaction mechanisms, and their energy may be transferred in part or *in toto* to nuclei, electrons, atoms, or molecules.

INTERACTIONS OF CHARGED PARTICLES WITH MATTER

The charged particles of radiation include the electron, positron, proton, deuteron, and alpha particle. The first two are known as light particles, the rest as heavy particles. The electron, positron, and alpha particle are present in radiations from radioactive materials. High-speed protons and deuterons are produced in accelerators, as well as high-speed electrons and alpha particles. Electrons and positrons moving at high velocities are often found as secondary forms of radiation that receive their high kinetic energies from photons. These charged "secondaries" are important forms of radiation because they are the basis upon which gamma and x-ray photons produce tissue damage, ionization of gases, and scintillations in crystal detectors.

The forces that interact between charged particles and matter are the electrical (Coulomb) forces that exist between charged bodies. If we let q_1 and q_2 represent the charge (in e.s.u.) on body 1 and body 2 and let d represent the distance between them (in centimeters), the mutual force between the two charged bodies is given by Coulomb's law:

$$F = \frac{q_1 q_2}{d^2}$$

(29)

If the charges are alike in polarity (both + or both −), the force between them is repulsive. If the charges have unlike polarities (one + and the other −), then the force is attractive. The negatively charged electron will experience both a repulsive force in encounters with electrons and an attractive force in encounters with atomic nuclei. The positively charged positron, proton, deuteron, and alpha particles have the opposite interaction forces.

As a charged particle passes among the atoms of an absorbing material, it may (1) dislodge electrons from atoms to form positive and negative ions, (2) excite electrons to higher energy levels in atoms, (3) set up vibrations of molecules in the vicinity of its path, (4) break a molecular chain, or (5) produce electromagnetic radiation in the form of photons from sites along its path when it is forced to suddenly change its course or slow down. The first process, *ionization,* is useful because the free ions in gases can be used for the detection of radiation. The production of photons by deacceleration and deflection of particles is important only for high-energy electrons and positrons and is identified with two processes—*bremsstrahlung* and *Cerenkov radiation production.* Each of these processes depletes a charged particle of some of its energy. Each time an electron is removed from an atom, the energy required to remove it (the binding energy) plus the kinetic energy that it has after leaving the atom must be supplied by the particle. About 1 or 2 e.v. is required to remove an electron from the outer shell of the atom; more energy is required to dislodge electrons from deeper shells. Energy is required of fast particles in the excitation of atomic electrons to higher energy levels in an atom. The excitation of molecular vibrations and the production of electromagnetic photons also require some of the particle's energy. As a charged particle moves through air, it will generate one ion pair[5] for every 35 e.v. that it loses. Only 16 per cent of this 35 e.v. goes into the production of the ions. The remaining 84 per cent of the energy goes into the other dissipative processes.

The energy that a particle loses to its surrounding medium for each unit of its path length is called the *linear energy transfer,* abbreviated *LET.* It is often expressed in such units as electron volts per micron. As a charged particle loses energy in one process or another, it will eventually lose all of its kinetic energy and almost come to a stop. It will not stop completely because when it reaches a very slow speed, it loses its ability to cause further damage along its path and becomes an extraneous wanderer among other molecules of the absorbing material. The alpha particle picks up free electrons and becomes a neutral helium atom. The proton and deuteron each pick up one electron and become neutral hydrogen atoms. The electron joins a large group of "free electrons" that seem to be omnipresent. The positron does things that we shall consider as a separate topic.

The number of ion pairs produced along each unit of length of the trajectory of the particle is called *specific ionization.* It differs from one charged particle to another, from one material to another, and from one particle energy to another. In air, an 8 Mev. alpha particle will have a specific ionization of about 2000 ion pairs per millimeter at the beginning of its path. As it slows, this figure increases to a maximum of about 7000 ion pairs per millimeter before the alpha particle begins to pick up electrons that will neutralize its charge.

---

[5] One ionizing event produces a negative electron and a positively charged atom. These two constitute an *ion pair.*

TABLE 4-5. RANGES OF 8 MEV. AND 1 MEV. CHARGED
PARTICLES IN AIR AND IN WATER*

ENERGY (Mev.)	PARTICLE	RANGE IN AIR (cm.)	RANGE IN WATER (mm.)
8	Alpha	7.3	0.1
	Proton	77	1.1
	Electron (Positron)	3440	41
1	Alpha	0.5	0.007
	Proton	2.3	0.03
	Electron (Positron)	350	4.2

* Computed from expressions and graphs that appear in Chapters 18 and 21 of Evan (1955).

The distance that a charged particle travels through a material from the point of its origin to the place where it no longer acts as a destructive radiation particle is called its *range*. The ranges of some typical examples are given in Table 4-5. Ranges represent the farthest distance that particles penetrate into a material. This may be less than the actual path length traveled. The paths of the heavy particles are essentially straight lines with very few drastic deflections. For heavy particles, the range is almost the same as the average path length. The paths of the light particles, however, are very tortuous, and the average path length is about twice as great as the range of these particles. This difference in the behavior of the heavy and light high-speed particles as they travel through matter is understandable when we take into account the masses of the high-speed particles and the electrons and nuclei with which they must interact. The heavy particles will penetrate the sea of electrons in the absorbing material without much change in direction. The atomic electrons are pulled out of their normal orbits by the attractive force of the heavy particle as it passes by. The fast electrons and positrons, on the other hand, have the same mass as the atomic electrons (and considerably less mass than the nuclei). They are easily deflected from their original paths on each encounter with electrons and undergo marked changes in course when they pass close to nuclei. Thus, they travel through mat-

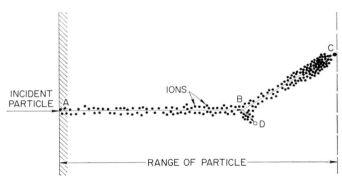

FIGURE 4-21. The course of a heavy charged particle through matter. In this example a glancing nuclear collision is indicated at *B*. Ions are formed along the track left by the recoiling ionized atom *D*. The primary particle comes to rest at *C*. The density of ions is greatest just before the particle comes to rest. It is here that the linear energy transfer is greatest.

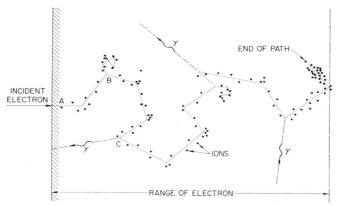

FIGURE 4-22. The path of an electron undergoing multiple scattering. The density of ions formed along the track is less than that seen for the heavier particles. At *B* some of the electron's energy is transferred to another electron. The path of the secondary electron is sometimes called a delta ray. At *C* a photon is formed due to the bremsstrahlung process. Other delta rays and bremsstrahlung photons are generated in subsequent scattering encounters. Near the end of the path, the ion density increases.

ter with frequent changes in direction. Great differences in the LETs of the heavy and light particles are explained in a similar manner. As the heavy particles move straight through an atom, they dislodge electrons from their atomic orbits and lose energy rapidly. Electrons, on the other hand, move about and do not give up their energy so quickly. In water, the linear energy transfers of a 1 Mev. alpha particle and a 1 Mev. electron are approximately 260 kev./micron and 0.2 kev./micron, respectively, a quite striking difference.

The bremsstrahlung[6] process deserves particular attention. When a charged particle is either deflected from its path or has its velocity changed (both changes are *accelerations*) it radiates electromagnetic energy in the form of photons. For each acceleration process, one photon will be generated and will carry away all the energy lost in the process.

Charged particles undergo significant accelerations only when they come under the influence of the charge of the nucleus as they pass very close to it. The intensity of radiation from a deflected or decelerated particle is proportional to the square of the acceleration that it undergoes. For particles of a given energy. the acceleration due to the passage near a nucleus varies directly with the Z number of the nucleus, and z, the number of unit charges on the particle; and inversely with M, the mass of the particle. The intensity of bremsstrahlung varies between materials and particles as Z^2z^2/M^2. Particles of small mass, M (electrons and positrons), are much better producers of bremsstrahlung than the heavier protons and alpha particles. Materials of high atomic number (tungsten, lead, and so forth) are better bremsstrahlung-producing targets than water, tissue, aluminum, or plastics. Bremsstrahlung are the primary component of the x-rays used in radiology. In x-ray tubes, electrons are accelerated relatively slowly to energies of several hundred kilo electron volts and then suddenly stopped as they hit the tungsten ($Z = 74$) target. Bremsstrahlung are also produced when electrons (or positrons) pass through bone, tissues, walls of glass sample holders, windows of detectors, and scanner collimators.

---

[6] This is a compound German word formed of *Bremse,* brakes, and *Strahlung,* radiation. We might translate it as "retardation radiation."

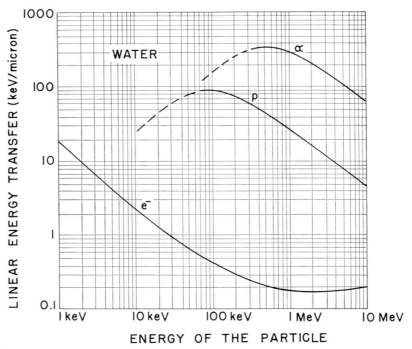

FIGURE 4-23.   Linear energy transfer of the electron, the proton, and the alpha particle in water as a function of the energy of the particle. As particles lose energy, the rate of transfer of energy to surrounding materials increases. The peaks of the curves occur at energies at which the particle velocities are too slow to effect energy transfer. The curves were obtained from theoretical expressions and experimental data given by Fano (1963), Northcliffe (1963), and Janni (1966).

For electrons of a given energy, E (million electron volts), the fraction of energy that appears as bremsstrahlung is given by the expression[7]

$$f = \frac{ZE}{1400} \tag{30a}$$

The bremsstrahlung spectrum of photons is continuous even though all the elec-

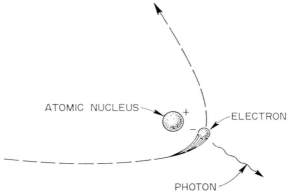

FIGURE 4-24.   The bremsstrahlung process.

[7] Taken from Evans (1955), pages 617 and 619.

trons that strike a target carry and lose the same energy in the target. The reason is that different amounts of energy are lost on each bremsstrahlung-producing encounter. The maximum energy that a photon can have, however, is the energy that the electron carries into the target.

For electrons or positrons in a beta-ray beam having its own continuous spectrum, the fraction of energy in the incoming beam that is radiated as bremsstrahlung is given by

$$f = \frac{ZE_T}{3000} \tag{30b}$$

where E_T is the energy of the transition producing the beta radiation (the maximum energy of the beta particles) (Evans, 1955).

Although bremsstrahlung are not emitted from radioactive atoms, they constitute a sort of "extraneous gamma radiation" that the unwary clinician might neglect to take into account in interpreting his gamma-ray counts or scans. Bremsstrahlung also provide a way to use pure beta-emitting radioisotopes as sources of gamma-like radiation in high-Z materials such as bone.

Another gamma-like radiation is associated with positron radiation. Positrons are like electrons in producing ionization, excitation, and bremsstrahlung.

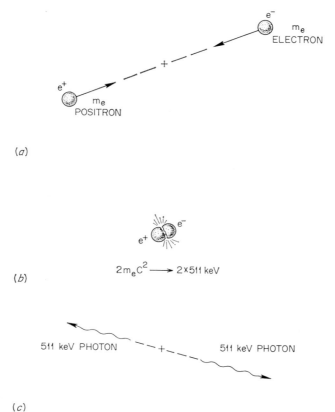

FIGURE 4-25. The annihilation of a positron, e+, and an electron, e-. (a) The two anti-particles are pulled toward their common center of mass by the electrical force of their opposite charges. (b) They meet at X and annihilation takes place. (c) All that is left of the two particles is two 511 kev. photons that carry off the energy that once was in the form of the masses of the two particles.

Their positive charges require no modifications of the laws describing their inter-actions. Fast positrons can transfer energy to electrons in atoms without crashing into them. But near the ends of their paths they are slowed down to such low energies that they may be pulled into contact with an electron. When a positron and an electron come together, their opposite charges add to zero and the masses of both disappear or are *annihilated*. The annihilation of the two masses leads to a creation in their places of two *annihilation* photons, each having an energy of 511 kev. (We mentioned previously that the energy equivalent ($E = mc^2$) of the electron and the positron is 511 kev.) Annihilation photons always have an energy of 511 kev. and cannot be distinguished from gamma-ray photons of the same energy, except for one added feature. The two annihilation photons always leave the site of the collision in diametrically *opposite directions*. Two detectors can be connected in *coincidence circuits* that respond only if each receives 511 kev. photons simultaneously. Under such circumstances, the detectors record counts only if the site of the annihilation lies on a straight line between them. Because the range of positrons in tissues is only a few millimeters, the site of the annihilation is always very close to the location of the positron-emitting radio-active material. This feature is used in positron scanning and for the operation of the positron camera. It can be used to give an excellent "fix" on the location of tagged chemicals emitting positrons without the use of collimators.

---

[8] "Intensity" is the flow of energy across a surface.

THE PASSAGE OF UNCHARGED PARTICLES THROUGH MATTER

Photons, neutrons, and neutrinos carry no charge, and react with matter in a very different fashion than the charged particles. They do not experience long-range Coulomb-law forces, and interact only in direct collision "one-hit" processes. Therefore, the large-scale behavior of beams of the neutral particles differs from the behavior of beams of charged particles.

The measure of the *intensity* of a beam of radiation is the amount of radiated energy per unit of time crossing a unit area perpendicular to the direction of motion of the particles in the beam. It is convenient to express this intensity in terms of the number of kilo electron volts of energy crossing a square centimeter per second. If we consider a beam in which each particle has an energy E, we can express the beam intensity[8]

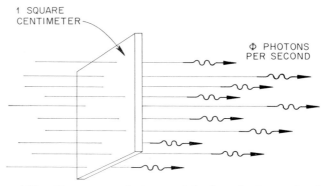

1 SQUARE CENTIMETER

Φ PHOTONS PER SECOND

FIGURE 4-26. The conceptual picture of the flux of a beam of radiation.

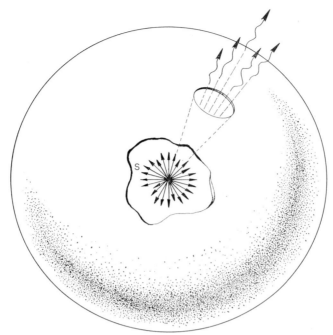

Figure 4-27. The relation between the intensity of radiation and the rate of particle emission from a point source, showing five photons per second leaving an opening of 1 sq. cm. in a sphere with a radius of 10 cm.

$$I = \Phi E \tag{31}$$

where Φ represents the *particle flux*, that is, the number of particles crossing a square centimeter per second. Suppose, for example, that 50 photons per second cross a square centimeter, each carrying 100 kev. The intensity of this beam would be 5000 kev./cm.²/sec.

The intensity and flux of a beam of radiation from a small source (often called a "point source") vary inversely with the square of the distance from the source to the point of the measurement provided that there is no absorption or scattering of the radiation between the source and the point of measurement (Fig. 4-27).

Suppose that we wanted to know the flux and intensity that we might expect to measure at a distance $r = 10$ cm. from a source, S, that radiates 144 kev. photons at the rate of 6282 per second. Normally each photon has an equal opportunity of radiating in any direction; that is, the same number of photons can be expected to pass through any chosen square centimeter of the surface of a sphere of radius r whose center is located at the position of the source. With no absorption or scattering, we expect all photons that leave the source to cross through the surface of the sphere. The area of the surface of any sphere is given as $4\pi r^2$ cm.²; therefore we would expect the particle flux to be given by

$$\Phi = \frac{R}{4\pi r^2} = \frac{6282 \text{ photons/sec.}}{4\pi(10)^2 \text{ cm.}^2} = 5 \text{ photons/cm.}^2\text{/sec.}$$

Since each photon carries 144 kev., the intensity of the radiation at 10 cm. would be

$$I = \Phi E_\gamma = 720 \text{ kev./cm.}^2/\text{sec.}$$

The *inverse-square law* holds for all radiation from a point source that is not attenuated by absorption or scattering, whether it be collimated in a narrow beam or radiated in all directions.

The removal of particles from a radiation flux due to scattering or absorption is called *attenuation*. The expression for the attenuation of a radiation flux is similar to the expression for radioactive decay

$$\frac{\Phi_x}{\Phi_0} = e^{-\mu x} \tag{32}$$

where μ represents the *linear attenuation coefficient*, x represents the thickness of material attenuating the beam, Φ_0 is the flux that would be measured without the attenuating material in the beam, and Φ_x is the flux that is measured with the attenuating material in the beam. This is illustrated in Figure 4-28.

The product μx is the probability that a neutral particle will be absorbed or scattered by a very thin absorber x cm. thick. In the earlier section on radioactive decay, the product λt was described as the probability that an atom would disintegrate in t seconds. The products μx and λt, then, both represent probabilities and may be treated mathematically in the same manner. The expressions for half-life, equations 20 and 21, work equally well in defining a half-value layer (HVL), so that one can say

$$\text{HVL} = \frac{0.693}{\mu} \tag{33}$$

This is the thickness of material that will reduce the intensity of radiation by one half. In shielding and radiation dosimetry discussions the thickness of material that will reduce radiation intensity to one tenth of its unattenuated value is often referred to as the tenth-value-layer (TVL). This is given by

$$\text{TVL} = \frac{2.3}{\mu} \tag{34}$$

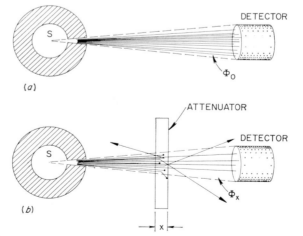

FIGURE 4-28. Attenuation of a radiation flux. (*a*) Without an attenuator in the beam, the flux of particles reaching the detector is Φ_0. (*b*) The attenuator of thickness x reduces the particle flux at the detector to Φ_x.

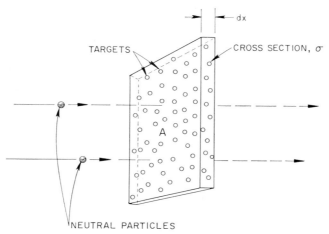

FIGURE 4-29. The concept of "cross section" of target atoms (electrons or nuclei will do just as well). The area A is partially blocked by the target atoms each having an area σ. The larger σ, the less likely it is that the incident particles could get through the thin section of material without suffering a collision.

The exponential law that is followed in the attenuation of neutral particles predicts that you can never achieve a barrier so thick that all particles will be removed from the beam. This is not the case with charged particles, which appear to have a finite range in all materials.

For a better understanding of the meaning of the coefficient μ, consider the microscopic nature of the one-hit interaction of a neutral particle and a target. Figure 4-29 shows a thin section of attenuating material having a face of area A, a thickness dx, and N interaction targets per unit of volume, each offering to the beam of incoming particles a *cross section* area of σ cm.^{2}. If the material is so thin that no target is behind another, the total area blocking the transmission of particles in the beam will be σ N Adx cm.^{2} and the fraction of the area A that is blocked is

$$f = \frac{\sigma \, N \, A dx}{A} = \sigma \, N \, dx \qquad (35)$$

If a beam having a particle flux of Φ_0 were incident on the area A, the fraction of particles removed from the beam per square centimeter per second could be expressed in terms of the fraction of the area that is blocked:

$$\frac{-d\Phi}{\Phi} = \sigma \, N \, dx$$

or we can write

$$d\Phi = -\Phi \, \sigma \, N \, dx. \qquad (36)$$

We use the minus sign because the flux is *depleted* as it travels through the thickness dx.

Equation 36 and its solution are similar to equation 12. The expression for the flux that passes through a sheet of material x cm. thick is given as

$$\Phi_x = \Phi_0 \, e^{-\sigma \, Nx} \qquad (37)$$

If we compare equation 37 with equation 32, we see that μ is equal to σ N; that is, μ is the product of the cross section of each interaction center and the number of interaction centers per unit volume of the target material. Linear attenuation coefficients for photons of different energies passing through water, sodium iodide, and lead are shown later in Figure 4-36.

There is another approach to the problem of beam attenuation. A number of authors prefer to use a *mass attenuation coefficient*, μ_m. This is simply the linear attenuation coefficient, μ, divided by the mass density ρ of the target material. It is expressed

$$\mu_m = \frac{\mu}{\rho} = \sigma_a x \text{ (atoms per gram)} = \sigma_a \frac{N_a}{A} \tag{38}$$

where N_a is the Avogadro number (6.025×10^{23} atoms per gram-atomic weight) and A is the gram-atomic weight (also the nuclear mass number) of the material.

When the mass attenuation coefficient is used, the attenuation equation is written

$$\Phi_x = \Phi_0 e^{-\mu_m \rho x} \tag{39}$$

and the product ρx is expressed in the units grams per square centimeter. This is the mass that lies behind each square centimeter of target material. When foils or windows are very thin, this is easier to measure than the linear thickness, x. We cut out a sample having an area of 1 cm.² and weigh it.

Let us consider some examples. Suppose we have a material such as lead that has a mass absorption coefficient of 5 cm.²/g. for 100 kev. photons. Lead has a mass density $\rho = 11.35$ g./cm.² and a gram-atomic weight of 207.19.

Example 1. What is the cross section that a lead atom presents to a 100 kev. photon? From equation 38,

$$\sigma = \mu_m \frac{A}{N_a} = (5 \text{ cm.}^2/\text{g.}) \frac{207.19 \text{ g.}}{6.025 \times 10^{23} \text{ atoms}}$$

$$\sigma = 1.72 \times 10^{-21} \text{ cm.}^2/\text{atom}$$

Cross sections for these processes are such small areas that we sometimes use a special unit of area called the *barn*, which equals 10^{-24} cm.². With this unit, the cross section of the lead atom to 100 kev. photons is 1720 barns.

Example 2. What is the tenth-value layer (TVL) of lead in a beam of 100 kev. photons? Since the TVL is attained when the exponent $\mu x = 2.3$,

$$\text{TVL} = \frac{2.3}{\mu} \text{ in cm.}$$

But $\mu = \mu_m \rho = (5 \text{ cm.}^2/\text{g.})(11.35 \text{ g./cm.}^3) = 56.75 \text{ cm.}^{-1}$; therefore the TVL $= \frac{2.3}{56.75} = 0.04$ cm.

Example 3. A sheet of lead foil 5 cm. by 10 cm. weighs 10 g. If a flux of 400 photons per square centimeter per second enters a detector in a beam of 100 kev. photons, what will be the flux if this sheet of lead is placed in the beam?

The foil has a mass per unit of area of $\rho x = \frac{10 \text{ g.}}{50 \text{ cm.}^2} = 0.2$ g./cm.²

The mass attenuation coefficient is $\mu_m = 5$ cm.²/g.

The transmitted beam is given by

$$\Phi_x = \Phi_0 e^{-\mu_m \rho x}$$

$$\Phi_x = 400 \times e^{-5 \times 0.2} = 400 \times e^{-1} = 400 \times \frac{1}{e}$$

but e = 2.718, so

$$\Phi_x = 400/2.718 = 147 \text{ photons/cm.}^2/\text{sec.}$$

If the counting rate were 400 counts/min. without the lead foil in the beam, we would expect it to drop to 147 counts/min. with the foil placed between the source and the detector.

Example 4. Patients have mass attenuation coefficients similar to water (when there are no bones in the way). Let us calculate what might happen to 27.5 kev. x-ray photons that are the predominant radiation from ^{125}I. For present purposes, we shall ignore some practical considerations that are not accounted for by the attenuation coefficient, and we shall calculate only the number of photons of 27.5 kev. that will pass directly from a point source, through the tissue, and into the window of a detector. Let us assume our source emits 3700 photons/sec. at the specified energy and that it is located 2 cm. deep in tissue and 4 cm. from the window of a detector that offers an acceptance area of 5 cm.^{2}.

If there is no absorbing tissue between the source and the detector, the flux of photons arriving at the detector as calculated from the inverse-square law will be

$$\Phi_0 = \frac{R}{4\pi r^2} = \frac{3700}{4\pi(4)^2} = 73.5 \text{ photons/cm.}^2/\text{sec.}$$

The attenuation due to 2 cm. of tissue (we use water as tissue-equivalent) is 0.38 cm.^{2}/g. for 27.5 kev. photons. Since water has a mass density $\rho = 1$, the linear attenuation coefficient is $\mu = 0.38$ cm.$^{-1}$. Thus

$$\mu x = 0.38 \text{ cm.}^{-1} \times 2 \text{ cm.} = 0.76$$

and

$$e^{-\mu x} = e^{-0.76} = 0.466$$

so that the flux that reaches the detector after penetrating the tissue should be

$$\Phi_x = \Phi_0 e^{-\mu x} = (73.5 \text{ photons/cm.}^2/\text{sec.})(0.466)$$

$$\Phi_x = 34.2 \text{ photons/cm.}^2/\text{sec.}$$

Since the detector window offers an acceptance area of 5 cm.^{2}, we expect the number of photons that impinge on the window each second to be

$$(5 \text{ cm.}^2) \times (34.2/\text{cm.}^2/\text{sec.}) = 171/\text{sec.}$$

Whether the detector will count at the rate of 171/sec. is another matter. This depends on the efficiency of the detector and the settings of the electronic pulse-height discriminators that follow it—problems to be considered in the chapter on the measurement of radiation.

We have considered so far only the process of *removal* of neutral particles from a beam of radiation. It is very important to take into account processes that *add* radiation flux to the original beam. These include *broad-beam scattering*, *multiple scattering* in thick materials, *fluorescence*, and *bremsstrahlung*. Each

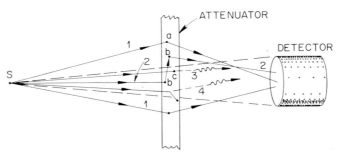

Figure 4-30. Processes occurring in attenuating materials that cause increases in counting rates at detectors. Those illustrated are *1,* broad-beam scattering; *2,* multiple scattering; *3,* fluorescence following photoelectric capture; and *4,* bremsstrahlung due to electrons being stopped in the attenuator.

process is illustrated in Figure 4-30. Broad-beam scattering is the process of scattering radiation initially not directed toward the detector into the detector. The effect of this scattering is to make the source seem to be more extended than it really is and to increase the apparent flux. When a neutral particle is scattered it *may* lose energy to its scattering target. If the energy of the scattered radiation is less than the energy of the initial radiation, we identify it as "degraded" scattered radiation. Almost all scattered radiation of interest to us undergoes degrading scattering. In thick attenuators some radiation might first be deflected from the path leading toward the detector, only to be scattered back toward the field of view of the detector. Fluorescence is characteristic x-radiation from atoms that may have been ionized or excited by either charged particles or photons. These characteristic x-rays have energies that are limited by the energy differences in the binding energies of the electron shells. Only materials with high atomic numbers present a problem in this regard. The highest energy of fluorescent radiation that we encounter is the 87 kev. x-ray from lead. The energy of such radiation from bone (calcium) is about 4 kev., which we would not expect to detect outside a patient. Bremsstrahlung may be generated in patients, in counting samples, or in collimators by high-speed electrons of any origin, nuclear, atomic, or photon-accelerated. The energies extend to the energy of the high-speed electron and the photon spectrum may overlap a gamma-ray or x-ray line that a scintillation counter is measuring. The clinician should be aware of these effects, since techniques have been developed specifically to minimize artifacts that may be caused by them.

PHOTON INTERACTIONS WITH MATTER

Photons are the workhorses of diagnostic nuclear medicine, since they make possible external counting, such as scanning. Photons have the greatest penetrating power of the detectable atomic radiations, whereas alpha particles, electrons, and positrons cannot be detected by an external detector.

Over the past several centuries, there has been disagreement about the nature of electromagnetic radiation. Newton (1642–1727) believed that light had a corpuscular nature. A scientist of that period, Huygens, explained many optical phenomena by assuming that light is wavelike, but until early in the 1800's most scientists supported Newton's ideas. New experiments in the nineteenth century seemed to "prove" that light had to be wavelike; after Hertz in 1887 generated microwaves that reflected and refracted as did light, physicists were convinced that the corpuscular concepts of Newton were incorrect. Further experimentation with light and x-rays in the period between 1900 and 1930, however, have shown that we must consider electromagnetic radiations as consisting of "corpuscular" photons when we describe their origination and interaction with matter, but as waves when we consider their reflection, refraction, and interference. We have learned to live with this "duality" in understanding light and the other electromagnetic radiations by accepting the idea that these radiations are truly corpuscular and that the "waves" are artificial concepts that give us a statistical foundation for predicting where the particles will go.

It is not easy to envision photons—entities that carry discrete quantities of kinetic energy, E_γ, and travel through space as particles. They travel at only one speed, the speed of light, c. They carry momentum given by the expression

$$p_\gamma, \text{ the momentum of a photon } = \frac{E_\gamma}{c} \tag{40}$$

and they can exert forces on impact with certain objects. Because they are electromagnetic and have no real mass, they interact only with things that have electrical and magnetic properties, such as electrons, positrons, electromagnetic fields in atoms, and electromagnetic fields in nuclei.

When we use the concept of waves in describing the propagation of x-ray beams or gamma-ray beams, we find the wavelength from the expression

$$\lambda = \frac{h}{p_\gamma} = \frac{12.39}{E_\gamma} \tag{41}$$

where h is Planck's constant; the wavelength, λ, is given in Angstrom units (10^{-8} cm.); and E_γ is expressed in kev. Equation 41 is useful in translating wavelength language to photon-energy language.

Photons are known to interact with matter by more than 10 different processes. In nuclear medicine the three most important ones are *Compton scattering, photoelectric absorption,* and *pair production.*[9]

COMPTON SCATTERING

This is the interaction that causes degraded scattering of photons, an interaction between photons and electrons in direct collision. A photon of energy E_γ strikes an electron. As a result of the collision, the electron will pick up energy from the photon and leave the site of the collision with a high velocity. We shall call the energy of the electron E_e, and designate the angle between the path of the incoming photon and the departing electron by θ. Following simple laws of motion, the incident photon scatters away from the site of the collision with less energy and at another angle from its original path, ϕ.

Because the kinetic energy of the system is conserved, we can write

$$E_\gamma = E'_\gamma + E_e \tag{42}$$

---

[9] An excellent detailed treatment of these topics is given by Evans (1955), Chapters 23–25.

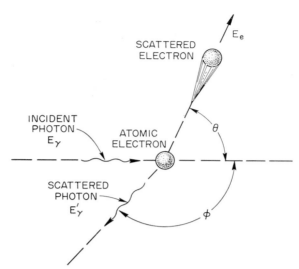

FIGURE 4-31. The Compton scattering interaction.

The amount of energy that the scattered photon has left after the collision depends upon the energy that the incident photon had and the angle of the scattering of the photon:

$$E'_\gamma = \frac{E_\gamma}{1 + \dfrac{E_\gamma}{511}(1 - \cos \phi)} \tag{43}$$

In these equations, energy is expressed in kilo electron volts. In Table 4-6 are given values of the energies of scattered photons and recoil electrons at scattering angles of 45, 90, 135, and 180 degrees for several photon energies that are of interest in nuclear medicine. The degradation of photon energy at these different scattering angles can be compared from one incident photon energy to another. Low-energy photons do not lose much energy upon scattering. The 27.5 kev.

TABLE 4-6. SOME INTERESTING X-RAYS AND GAMMA-RAYS AND THE ENERGIES OF
THEIR COMPTON-SCATTERED PHOTONS AND ELECTRONS
AT $\phi = 45$, 90, 135, AND 180 DEGREES

		ϕ, ANGLE PHOTON IS SCATTERED							
		45°		90°		135°		180°	
SOURCE RADIO- NUCLIDE	PHOTON ENERGY E_γ (kev.)	E'_γ (kev.)	E_e (kev.)	E'_γ (kev.)	E_e (kev.)	E'_γ (kev.)	E_e (kev.)	E'_γ (kev.)	E_e (kev.)
^{125}I	27.5	27.1	0.4	26.1	1.4	25.2	2.3	24.8	3.3
^{197}Hg	77	73.7	3.3	66.9	10.1	61.3	15.7	59.2	17.8
^{99m}Tc	141	130.5	10.5	110.5	30.5	95.9	45.1	90.9	50.1
^{203}Hg	279	240.5	38.5	180.5	98.5	144.1	134.9	133.7	145.3
^{131}I	364	301.1	62.9	212.6	151.4	164.3	199.7	150.1	213.9
^{85}Sr	513	396.4	116.6	256	257	189	324	170.5	342.5
^{60}Co	1330	754	576	369	961	244	1086	214	1116
—	∞	1740	—	511	—	299	—	256	—

x-ray from ^{125}I loses up to only 3.3 kev. On the other hand, high-energy photons may lose an appreciable fraction of their energy upon being scattered. The 1330 kev. photon from cobalt-60, for example, retains only 214 kev. upon 180 degree scattering (a complete reversal of direction). If $E\gamma$ in equation 43 is extended to infinity, an *upper limit* to the energy of the scattered photon at each different scattering angle will be found. For example, the highest energy that a photon scattered 180 degrees can possibly have is 256 kev.

The energy that a photon loses upon being scattered is transferred to the target electron. We can see in Table 4-6 that in the case of the higher-energy incident photons, the scattered electrons receive very large kinetic energies. These electrons are "swift charged particles" that pass through matter ionizing atoms, exciting molecules, generating bremsstrahlung, and otherwise causing disturbances. Photons that react with electrons in Compton scattering deliver radiation dose to tissue as the result of these high-speed electrons. At most, in one such event, a photon can create only one ion directly, an ion formed from the atom that lost the scattered electron. The scattered "recoil" electron, on the other hand, can create one pair of ions for every 35 e.v. of energy that it receives from the photon. After the high-speed recoil electron leaves the site of the collision, it will follow a tortuous path through the surrounding material, which might be tissue, lead in a scanner collimator, or sodium iodide in a scintillation crystal. In the latter material the high-speed electron, *not the photon,* will excite molecules to such energy levels that they emit very low-energy (about 3 e.v.) visible blue photons as they decay to a ground state. The light appears to come from the "track" of the swift electron. This light flash is the "scintillation"—our most useful tool for the detection of photons in nuclear medicine. The intensity of the scintillation is proportional to the amount of energy that the electron loses in the crystal and is related to the energy of the incoming photon by equation 43.

Because the Compton interaction is one between photons and electrons, the collision cross section, σ_c can be expressed in terms of a target area per *electron*. In Figure 4-32 the area is expressed in barns. Since each atom has Z electrons, equation 38 might be used to convert the values given in Figure 4-32 into the dimensions useful for expressing the scattering probability in terms of a mass absorption coefficient by letting σ_a equal $\sigma_c Z$. Thus, the expression for the Compton scattering mass attenuation coefficient would be

$$\sigma_c' = \sigma_c \frac{Z}{A} N_a \text{ cm.}^2/\text{g.} \tag{44}$$

For photons with energies much greater than the binding energies of the electrons in the target atoms, the attenuation coefficients obtained from equation 44 should not vary greatly from one material to another, because all electrons have the same cross section for interacting with a photon of a given energy and because the ratio Z/A does not vary greatly over the full range of the periodic table of the elements. The fraction of an incident flux of photons that can pass through material x cm. thick without undergoing Compton scattering can be found by using σ_c' in place of μ_m in equation 39.

In addition to the curve labeled σ_c giving the probability of a photon being scattered from each electron, two other cross sections, σ_s and σ_a, are shown in Figure 4-32. These are the energy-scattering and the energy absorption cross sections. The fraction of the incident photon energy which is scattered in the average

Compton collision is given by the fraction σ_s/σ_c. On the other hand, the fraction of the incident photon energy absorbed in the average Compton collision is given by the fraction σ_a/σ_c. This latter fraction is used in determining the radiation dose to patients and the energy transfer to absorbers due to Compton collisions. Some authors choose to call σ_a the "real absorption cross section."[10]

In Figure 4-36 we have compared the attenuation coefficients for the three primary photon interactions in water, which is representative of body tissues. Compton scattering predominates over the others for photon energies ranging from 25 kev. to 10 Mev. As the atomic number of the material increases, this range becomes smaller. For example, in lead the Compton scattering process is the most important one only from 800 kev. to 3 Mev.

PHOTOELECTRIC ABSORPTION

In this interaction, a photon enters an atom and is completely absorbed. Its energy is used to eject an electron with a kinetic energy that is equal to the photon energy less the binding energy that holds the electron in the atom:

$$E_e = E_\gamma - E_{en} \tag{45}$$

where E_{en} represents the binding energy of an electron in the nth shell. After such an event has taken place, the atom is left in an ionized state with one electron missing. A readjustment is made by electrons falling into vacancies producing x-rays and Auger electrons, and the atom emits a total energy that is equal to E_{en}. The shell-filling process is the same as that following internal conversion (Fig. 4-12).

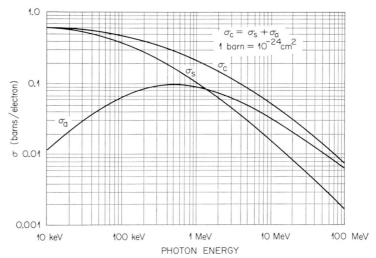

FIGURE 4-32. The Compton scattering cross sections in units of barns per electron. The collision cross section is given by the top curve labeled σ_c. The two lower curves are useful in determining the fraction of incident photon energy scattered and absorbed from the beam.

---

[10] An excellent set of examples using these scattering and absorption fractions is presented by Johns (1955), pages 174–177.

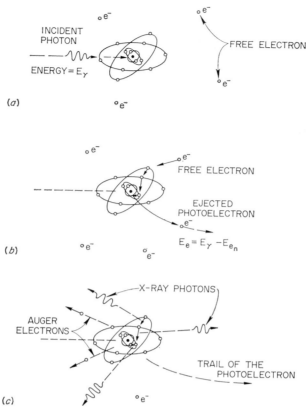

FIGURE 4-33.   The photoelectric absorption process. (*a*) The incident photon with an energy E_γ approaches an atom in absorbing material. (*b*) The photon interacts with the electric and magnetic fields inside the atom and in the process transfers all of its energy to an electron that occupies an inner shell. The electron then leaves the atom. In escaping from the pull of the nucleus, it loses the energy E_{e_n}. The atom is left in an excited state and electrons from other shells begin a cascading process. (*c*) As the cascading process continues, x-rays and Auger electrons are emitted from the atom. These particles carry off the energy E_{e_n} among them. Thus the atom finally returns to its original state, replacing the ejected electron with a free electron that drifts in from outer space.

There appears to be an interaction between the photon and the electromagnetic fields that exist inside the atom between the electrons and the nucleus. The closer an electron is to the nucleus, the stronger these electromagnetic fields and the more likely it is that a photon will transfer its energy to an electron. If a photon brings into the atom enough energy to liberate a K-shell electron, it will transfer its energy to that electron rather than to one farther from the nucleus, giving the K-shell electron an 80 to 20 preference over the others. If the energy of the incident photon does not exceed the binding energy of the K-shell, the photon will, if it interacts at all, transfer its energy to a less tightly bound electron, always preferring the inner- to the outer-shell electrons.

The electrical charge of the nucleus has a strong effect on the cross section for this reaction. (We call the cross section for the photoelectric interaction τ_a.) The cross section will increase with the proton number, Z, *roughly* as Z^4. The exponent seems to vary from 4.0 to 4.6 as the photon energy increases from 100 kev. to 3000 kev.

The energy of the photon has an "adverse" effect on the photoelectric cross section. As the photon energy, $E\gamma$, increases, the cross section decreases. We can approximate the interaction cross section with K-shell electrons[11]

$$\tau_a \cong \text{constant } \frac{Z^4}{E_\gamma^3} \qquad (46)$$

In Figure 4-34 we have plotted the photoelectric cross section for tungsten and for tin. The most outstanding features of these plots are the discontinuities that we call the *absorption edges*. They illustrate dramatically the fact that photons prefer to interact with inner-shell electrons but that they cannot do so unless they have sufficient energy to break the electrostatic bonds between the electrons and the nuclei. These edges are often considered in matching the radiation from a radiopharmaceutical to the sodium iodide scintillation detector and its surrounding shield and collimator. In Figure 4-35 we have illustrated this by comparing the attenuation coefficients of lead (used in collimators) and water (tissue

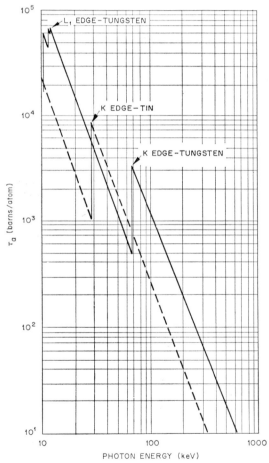

FIGURE 4-34. The photoelectric cross section in tungsten and tin. The effects of the atomic number, Z, and the photon energy, $E\gamma$, expressed in equation 46 are clearly shown here.

---

[11] See Evans (1955), page 698.

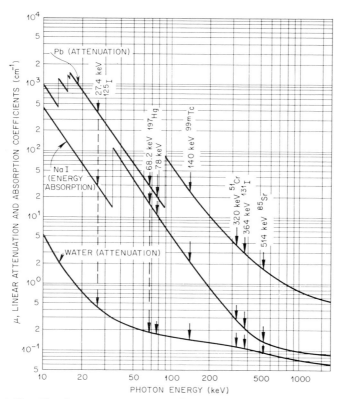

FIGURE 4-35. The linear attenuation coefficients for lead and water and the energy absorption coefficient for sodium iodide for photon energies of interest in nuclear medicine. Photon groups associated with the radiation of some radiopharmaceuticals are indicated in the figure so that the penetrability of water and lead can be compared with the energy absorption capability of the scintillation crystal for these particular radionuclides.

equivalent) with the energy absorption coefficient of sodium iodide for photon energies that are currently used in nuclear medicine. For scanning or for body counting, we prefer to use a radionuclide emitting photons that are not strongly absorbed in tissue, that *are* strongly absorbed in the sodium iodide crystal, and that can be collimated by a strong attenuation in the lead shielding. The energy of the photons that best meet these requirements appears to be in the neighborhood of 90 to 100 kev.

The photoelectric interaction predominates over Compton scattering for photons of low energy and for absorbing materials of high atomic number. Although an atom completely absorbs the photon in one of these events, the energy of the photon is converted largely into charged particle radiation which, in turn, rapidly transfers this energy into the absorbing medium and produces radiation effects in tissue or generates scintillations in a crystal detector. Those x-rays that leave the target atom after each interaction may have sufficient energy to leave the absorbing body. These constitute the fluorescent radiation illustrated in Figure 4-30. X-rays originating from photoelectric interactions in scintillation crystals are one way in which some of the energy brought into the crystal by an incoming photon is removed and results in a so-called *escape peak* that appears as an artifact in the pulse spectra in some scintillation counting systems. Examples appear in Figure 5-18.

PAIR PRODUCTION

The third interaction is possible only if the incident photon has an energy exceeding 1.022 Mev. If a high-energy photon comes very close to the atomic nucleus, it can interact with the very intense electromagnetic fields within and near the nucleus in such a way that all of its energy goes into the production of two electron masses of opposite charge (an electron and a positron) which possess kinetic energy. This effect illustrates the Einstein principle that there is an equivalence between energy and mass. An equation relating the energies of the components of this interaction is

$$E_\gamma = c^2 m_{e^-} + c^2 m_{e^+} + E_{e^-} + E_{e^+} \tag{47}$$

where we use the subscripts e^- and e^+ to designate the electron and the positron. The masses of the two particles are the same (Table 4-3) and the energy $m_e c^2$ is 511 kev. (0.511 Mev.). A total of 1.022 Mev. of the energy of the incoming photon is required to create the two masses. The remaining energy, if there is any, is divided between the positron and the electron but not necessarily equally. For example, if a 1.33 Mev. gamma-ray photon from ^{60}Co decay were to undergo this reaction near a nucleus (of *any* atom), the electron and the positron would share 0.31 Mev. (310 kev.) in any number of different ratios. The resulting charged particle spectrum would be a continuum for the electrons and a continuum for the positrons, but each pair that appears in conjunction with the disappearance of the 1.33 Mev. photon will have energies that add to 310 kev. Because electromagnetic fields are required for this interaction, it is more likely to occur if the nuclear charge is high, i.e., for materials of high atomic number.

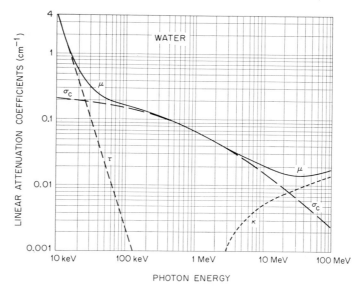

FIGURE 4-36. The behavior of the linear attenuation coefficient for photons interacting with water. The contributions to the total coefficient of the photoelectric effect, τ, the Compton process, σ_c, and the pair production process κ are shown. The data are from Grodstein (1957).

For photons of a given energy, the cross section per atom, κ_a, appears to vary as Z^2. Also, the cross section increases as the energy of the incident photon increases. The typical behavior of the attenuation coefficient is shown in Figure 4-36.

For most of the radionuclides in nuclear medicine, pair production does not take place, but occasionally we use gamma-rays having photon energies exceeding 1.02 Mev. The electron-positron "pair" behave as separate ionizing charged particles as they move through matter and it is they, not the photon, that produce the radiation effects in the surrounding material. The positron produced in pair production is no different from the positron produced in radioactive decay. At the end of its trail it will undergo an annihilation with an electron, and the annihilation photons, both having energies of 0.511 Mev., will appear. Thus energy is conserved. The 1.022 Mev. that the incident photon lost in producing the electron-positron mass will reappear later in the form of the two annihilation quanta.

SUMMARY OF PHOTON INTERACTIONS

Each of the three interactions we have reviewed employs different mechanisms and behaves differently from one target element to another and from one photon energy to another. All three, however, are explained as one-hit photon interactions in which the photon interacts with a target of a given cross section. The total cross section for a photon interaction is expressed as the sum of the three separate interaction cross sections. We have presented some of these in units of barns per atom. More often in the literature each cross section is expressed as mass attenuation coefficients in units of square centimeters per gram or as linear attenuation coefficients in units of 1/cm. Conversion from one set of units to another is not difficult.

We have shown some of the attenuation cross section curves in Figures 4-32, 4-34, 4-35, and 4-36. Ross and Harris in Chapter 5 show others in Figure 5-12. Tables of these for a large number of different attenuating materials are presented by Johns (1961) and in Grodstein, NBS Circular 583 (1957).

Although the three processes are distinctly different, they have two characteristics in common. They all follow the exponential absorption law, equation 37, and they all act as mechanisms whereby energy is transferred from the photon to charged particles. Without this feature photons could not be detected nor could they deliver radiation doses to tissues. The development of instruments, choices of radionuclides, and effective use of gamma-ray and x-ray sources in nuclear medicine depend upon our understanding of the behavior of these three interactions.

REFERENCES

Evans, R. D.: The Atomic Nucleus. McGraw-Hill Book Co., New York, 1955.
Fano, U.: Penetration of Protons, Alpha Particles and Mesons. *Ann Rev. Nucl. Sci.* 13:1, 1963.
Goldman, D. T.: Nuclides and Isotopes. Ed. 7. Publ. APD-35G, General Electric Company, Schenectady, N. Y., 1964.

Graeffe, G., and Walters, W. B.: Decay of [129]Cs and ^{131}I to the Levels in [129]Xe and [131]Xe. *Phys. Rev.* 153:1321, 1967.

Grodstein, G. W.: X-Ray Attenuation Coefficients from 10 keV to 100 MeV. NBS Circular 583, U. S. Department of Commerce, National Bureau of Standards, Washington D. C., 1957.

Ianni, J. F.: Calculations of Energy Loss, Range, Pathlength, Straggling, Multiple Scattering, and the Probability of Inelastic Nuclear Collisions for 0.1- to 1000-MeV Protons. AFWL-TR-65-150, Air Force Weapons Laboratory, Kirtland Air Force Base, New Mexico, 1966.

Johns, H. E.: The Physics of Radiology. Ed. 2. Charles C Thomas, Springfield, Ill., 1961.

Johns, H. E., and Laughlin, J. S.: Interaction of Radiation With Matter. *In* Hine, G. J., and Brownell, G. L. (eds.): Radiation Dosimetry. Academic Press, New York, 1956.

Northcliffe, L. C.: Passage of Heavy Ions Through Matter. *Ann. Rev. Nucl. Sci.* 13:67, 1963.

Slack, L., and Way, K.: Radiations from Radioactive Atoms in Frequent Use. U.S. Atomic Energy Commission, Washington, D. C., 1956.

Wapstra, A. H., Nijgh, G. J., and Van Lieshout, R.: Nuclear Spectroscopy Tables. North Holland Publishing Company, Amsterdam, 1959.

CHAPTER V

MEASUREMENT OF RADIOACTIVITY. PHYSICAL PRINCIPLES OF RADIONUCLIDE SCANNING. WHOLE-BODY COUNTING. LIQUID SCINTILLATION COUNTING

D. A. ROSS

C. C. HARRIS

DAVID E. KUHL

RICHARD C. REBA

HENRY N. WAGNER, Jr.

ARTHUR KARMEN

129

MEASUREMENT OF RADIOACTIVITY[1]

D. A. Ross
C. C. Harris

MEASURING RADIATION FROM A PATIENT

Radionuclides can be administered harmlessly to patients if the dose is kept small. New radiopharmaceuticals are coming into use more and more widely in medical research and diagnosis. Their major advantage is that the emitted radiation can be detected even when the amount of the radionuclide present, by actual weight, is almost nothing. For example, ^{131}I weighs about 8 *millionths* of a gram per *curie*, and we need only a few millionths of a curie (μc.) for a thyroid test. We could administer as much as 100 μc. of carrier-free ^{131}I—an amount that emits 3 million useful gamma rays every second—with the assurance that we would be adding less than a billionth of a gram (10^{-9} g.) to the body iodine "pool," and that the dose will therefore diffuse into the prevailing iodine without disturbing it in the least.

Ordinarily it is no trick to *detect* the emitted radiation, but it may be difficult to *measure* it quantitatively, for there are pitfalls lying in wait for the unwary, the naïve, and the wishful. The measurement of the radiation coming from a small sample is fairly easy, but if the source is buried in a patient, the problem of obtaining an accurate measurement may tax our resources.

When we measure a nuclide through its radiation we are making the tacit assumption that the number of rays emitted per second is proportional to the amount of the radionuclide present. According to the law of radioactive decay, during any second the same fraction of whatever is there will decay. In mathematical terms:

$$\text{disintegration rate,} \quad \frac{dN}{dt} = -N\lambda$$

where N is the number of radioactive atoms present, and λ is the "decay constant," which has a characteristic value for each radionuclide. Thus if we can measure the disintegration rate, and can obtain λ from tables,[2] we will have a measure of quantity. Each radionuclide has a characteristic number of rays emitted per disintegration (it is 1:1 only exceptionally); therefore if we measure rays emitted per second it will give us disintegrations per second, which in turn will give us the amount.

The catch is that when we use a detector, we do not count all the rays emitted per second, for they leave the disintegrating atoms in all directions and many of them miss the detector entirely. Moreover, a gamma photon will not necessarily be counted if it does reach the detector. Consequently *count rate* repre-

---

[1] Research sponsored by the U.S. Atomic Energy Commission under contract with the Union Carbide Corporation.

[2] If the table gives half-life instead of λ there is an easy conversion:

$$\lambda = \frac{0.693}{\text{half-life in seconds}}$$

sents only a fraction of the *disintegration rate,* and unless additional information is available the count rate tells us little.

To avoid this difficulty, we measure by comparison, counting first the unknown and then a standard containing a known number of microcuries of the same nuclide. Then, since the instrument is presumably seeing the same fraction of the generated rays each time, we can set up a proportion:

$$\frac{\text{unknown } \mu\text{c.}}{\text{standard } \mu\text{c.}} = \frac{\text{counts/sec. from unknown}}{\text{counts/sec. from standard}}$$

and therefore:[3]

$$\text{unknown } \mu\text{c.} = \text{standard } \mu\text{c.} \times \frac{\text{count rate from unknown}}{\text{count rate from standard}}$$

With this comparative approach we do not have to know what percentage of the emitted rays the system is counting, but *it must be the same percentage for the standard as for the unknown!* This may be difficult to achieve when the unknown is located inside a patient, for the number of rays reaching a detector depends not only on the position of the source but on what surrounds the source, namely, the patient's tissues, through which the outgoing rays must pass. It is very important for an operator to understand why this is so, for the validity of his work hinges on how successfully he can cope with this problem.

INTERACTION, ABSORPTION, AND DEFLECTION

The fundamental problem is that gamma rays, or gamma photons as they are more commonly called, interact with matter as they pass through it. They collide with the atoms and displace some of the electrons from their orbits— hence the name "ionizing radiation." The denser the material, the more of these collisions there will be; thus there are many in lead, fewer in a patient's tissues, very few in air, and none in a perfect vacuum. Whenever a collision occurs the photon is either *deflected* or *destroyed.*

When a photon collides with an electron the latter acquires some of the photon's energy, and leaves its atom with a velocity that depends on the amount of energy received. If the photon energy was not very high (say, 50 kev. or less for patient-like media) the electron is likely to absorb all of it, in which case we call the process a *photoelectric interaction.* Here the photon vanishes and a high-speed *photoelectron* emerges. If the energy of the photon is higher, on the other hand, the electron is not likely to absorb all of it; in this case there will be two products of the interaction: (1) a high-speed electron, and (2) a secondary photon carrying less energy than its parent primary. This process is called *Compton scattering;* the dislodged electron is a *Compton electron* and the secondary photon is a scattered or *degraded photon.* The high-speed electrons produced in both types of interaction collide repeatedly with other atoms and produce ionizations of their own, thus dissipating the kinetic energy. Simi-

---

[3] In situations in which a knowledge of the actual number of microcuries is not necessary, the standard can be merely a known fraction of the dose given the patient, in which case the unknown is rated as a percentage of the administered dose:

$$\% \text{ of dose in unknown} = \% \text{ of dose in standard} \times \frac{\text{counts/sec. from unknown}}{\text{counts/sec. from standard}}$$

larly, the scattered photons may undergo further interaction and produce more ions. If the absorbing material is thick enough it will absorb substantially all of the liberated electrons and scattered photons, in which case all the energy contained in the primary photon is expended in ionizing the absorber. The greater the primary energy, the more ionized atoms there will be.

The photoelectric process involves *bound electrons,* especially those in the inner electron shells (K, L, and so forth), and the interaction is most probable when the energy of the approaching gamma ray approximately matches the binding energy of the electron in its path. The binding energy depends on the nuclear charge (proton or Z number) and accordingly the probability of interaction, called the photoelectric cross section, is heavily dependent on the element involved. This is much less true for a Compton interaction, which involves *"free" electrons,* namely, those actually unattached, or so weakly bound that the binding energy is negligible. Compton cross section, therefore, depends mainly on the density of free electrons that the photon sees in its path, and apart from this it depends very little on the nature of the absorbing material.

There is another important difference between the two processes. Immediately after a photoelectric interaction the atom finds itself with one of its inner electron orbits vacant, and an x-ray is generated as this vacancy is filled in from the outer shells. The x-ray will have approximately the energy of the electron shell where the vacancy occurred,[4] and thus will be characteristic of the atom. After a Compton interaction, on the other hand, there will be no x-ray, for the dislodged electron had no binding energy worth mentioning.

Another important side effect in a Compton collision is that the photon must bounce off at an angle if it is to transmit any of its energy to an electron.[5] Thus in a scattering medium some of the photons will appear to go around corners, and only in a vacuum will they all travel in straight lines.

A third way in which a photon can interact with an absorbing medium is by the process of *pair production.* Part of the photon's energy is converted into matter, creating an electron-positron pair.[6] This takes 511 kev. for each member of the pair, this energy being Einstein's equivalent for an electron's resting mass. Pair production can never occur, therefore, unless the incident energy exceeds $2 \times 511 = 1022$ kev., and the process remains quantitatively unimportant until the energy reaches 2 Mev. or more, which is infrequent in nuclear medicine. In pair production, a positron and an electron are created, and the energy greater than 1022 kev. is carried away by the two particles in the form of energy of motion.

The electron then produces ions in the usual manner. The positron, however, is short-lived; its ionizing collisions quickly slow it down, whereupon it attracts an unattached electron in the neighborhood and the phenomenon of *annihilation* occurs. The two particles neutralize each other electrically and

---

[4] More properly: for a K vacancy the x-ray's energy will be mainly K − L, and so on.

[5] Compton (1923) worked out the relationships in detail. He found that if E represents the primary energy (in kev.), E' the energy of the scattered photon, and ϕ the angle through which it is deflected off course, then:

$$E' = \frac{E}{1 + \dfrac{E}{511}(1 - \cos \phi)}$$

[6] A positron is a particle having the same mass as an electron, but the charge is positive instead of negative.

vanish, and in their place appear two new photons, which are emitted in opposite directions. Each has an energy of 511 kev., which just matches the resting-mass energies of the annihilated positron and electron. Accordingly, when a high-energy photon is absorbed by pair production, the end products are a number of ionized atoms, and two 511 kev. gamma photons, called *annihilation radiation*, that leave the scene of their generation in opposite directions. In some of the scanning instruments ingenious use is made of this 180 degree relationship.

The original photon and the resulting annihilation radiation will almost always have different directions.

Interactions within the Patient. When some organ in a patient contains radioactive material, the radiation coming out of the body (the only radiation available to an external detector) will differ both in quality and in quantity from that emitted by the disintegrating atoms. Many of the emerging photons will be degraded in energy, and will not be traveling in their original directions. Some photons will not come out at all, having undergone a series of Compton collisions followed by a final photoelectric interaction in which the photon disappears. Some photons will come out undegraded, having failed to collide with anything. It is important to recognize that only these last can provide a reliable guide to (a) the position of the source, and (b) the energies characteristic of its decay process. If you need to find out *where* the radioactivity is, or *what* radionuclide it is, you must try to look only at the undegraded photons. If you also need to know *how much* radioactivity is there, you have a more difficult problem on your hands, one that will be made easier if you can establish the energies of the photons being counted. These are some of the reasons why spectrometry is important in nuclear medical work.

The changes in the character of the radiation will vary with the nature and thickness of the tissues through which the radiation passes. Thus they will differ from one patient to another, from one part of a patient to another part of the same patient, and from one direction of exit to some other direction. People who like their technical problems easy will do well to stick to the counting of liquid samples and give patients a wide berth.

Detector geometry

For our purposes it will be preferable to think of gamma rays not as waves but as particles: electrically neutral, submicroscopic particles emerging from metastable nuclei, traveling with the speed of light (1000 feet per microsecond *in vacuo*), and each carrying a tiny parcel of energy.[7] The quantity of energy is very important, for it determines (a) what kind of response the photon will produce in a sodium iodide crystal, and (b) what modifications the photon may undergo before it reaches the detector.

For the moment, however, let us consider a small, radioactive source surrounded only by air. Figure 5-1 shows such a source, pictured at the center of

---

[7] The amounts of energy are so small that the usual CGS unit, the dyne-centimeter or *erg*, is much too big to be practical. The unit for gamma photons is the *electron volt*, which is 1.6 million-millionths of an erg. A thousand e.v. ($= 1$ kev.) is therefore 1.6 billionths of an erg, and a million e.v. ($= 1$ Mev.) is 1.6 millionths. Ordinary x-rays, and many of the gamma rays, fall in the range of 1 to 300 kev.; other gamma rays, and the more penetrating or "super-voltage" x-rays, have higher energies—e.g., the ^{60}Co radiation at 1.17 and 1.33 Mev. In sharp contrast with these are the puny little photons that transmit visible light—e.g., orange light (600 mμ) at 2 e.v.

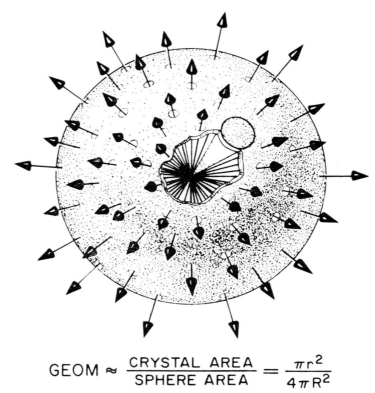

$$\text{GEOM} \approx \frac{\text{CRYSTAL AREA}}{\text{SPHERE AREA}} = \frac{\pi r^2}{4\pi R^2}$$

FIGURE 5-1. *Detector geometry* (= geometrical efficiency = extrinsic detector efficiency). The source is imagined at the center of a spherical shell (radius R), with the crystal (radius r) resting on the surface of the sphere. The photons are emitted in all directions, and the fraction reaching the crystal will be:

$$\text{Geometry} = \frac{\text{spherical surface covered by crystal}}{\text{total spherical surface}} = \frac{\pi r^2}{4\pi R^2}$$

It is easy to lose 99 per cent of the emitted radiation. (Redrawn after Ross et al., 1965.)

a spherical shell, with the detecting crystal on the surface. The photons come out in all directions, and clearly many will miss the detector completely. For convenience let us classify them into "sheep" and "goats," the sheep being accepted whereas the goats are cast out. There will be a *cone of entry*, with its apex at the source and its base at the crystal; this cone will contain the sheep. In the illustration the sheep are heavily outnumbered by the goats, so we say that "the detector geometry is poor."

It is not hard to estimate just how poor it will be, for the ratio of the sheep to all the emitted rays will be $\dfrac{\text{area of front face of crystal}}{\text{total area of spherical shell}}$; namely, $\dfrac{\pi r^2}{4\pi R^2}$ where r is the radius of the crystal and R that of the sphere. Suppose the source is suspended in the air, 5 in. in front of a 2 in. by 2 in. cylindrical crystal (Fig. 5–2A). The calculation shows that only 1 per cent of the rays will find the detector—99 goats for every sheep.

What will happen if we back the detector off to 10 in.? To catch the same cone of sheep the crystal would have to be twice as big as before, making its presenting area four times as large (Fig. 5–2A). So if we back the crystal away without making it any bigger it will catch only one quarter of the former 1 per cent. This is the basis of the *inverse-square law*, which states that the count rate varies inversely as the square of the source-to-detector distance. Double the distance, it says, and you divide the count rate by four.

This inverse-square argument is valid only if the angle of the cone is small,[8] so that for short distances or large crystals the inverse-square law gets into

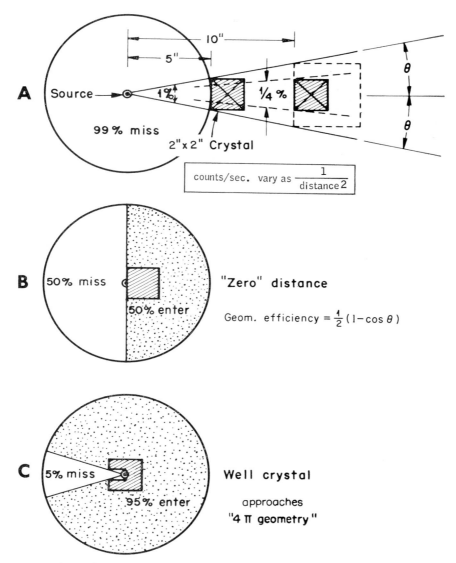

FIGURE 5-2. Three stages of detector geometry. *A,* With the source 2½ crystal diameters away, the geometry is down to 1 per cent. Double the distance and it becomes 0.25 per cent—*inverse-square law. B,* With the source against the crystal the geometry will be 50 per cent—*cosine law* (see text). *C,* With a well crystal the geometry approaches 100 per cent (4π), but the sample must be small.

---

[8] Otherwise πr^2, the area of the *flat* face of the crystal, will not be a fair equivalent for the corresponding, *curved* area on the surface of the sphere.

trouble. For example, if the distance is reduced to zero (Fig. 5–2B) the count rate will certainly not become infinite, as the law says it should; in fact the crystal will still let half of the radiation get away. A more reliable law, which holds true even when the angle of the cone is large, says that the geometrical efficiency will be $\frac{1}{2}$ $(1 - \cos \theta)$, where θ is the "angle of generation" of the cone, namely, half the angle of the apex as seen from one side (Fig. 5–2A). At zero distance θ becomes 90 degrees and its cosine is therefore zero; this law, accordingly, says that at zero distance the geometry will be 50 per cent, which is correct. The *cosine law* is less convenient than the other,[9] but is more widely applicable. It holds whenever the detector presents a circular outline to the source, and that is the only restriction.

We can improve the geometry of Figure 5–2B further by using the "well" principle, inserting the sample into a hole drilled part way into the crystal (Fig. 5–2C). Here there might be 95 per cent sheep and 5 per cent goats, so that a switch from Figure 5–2A to 5–2C would improve the geometry nearly one hundred fold. This helps to give a well counter its high sensitivity, in terms of counts/sec./μc. The drawback is that an ordinary well crystal can admit only small samples. The number of escaping photons will depend on how far down in the well the source is placed; thus the volume of the sample will have a bearing on the geometry, and for comparisons to be valid the volumes must be the same. Unless, of course, a correction factor is applied.

We can take almost any counting situation involving a small source and a cylindrical crystal, and calculate the fraction of the total emitted radiation that will reach the crystal—so long as the source is in the air. When it is surrounded by a scattering medium, however, the pretty, straight-line pictures of Figure 5–2 lose some of their value. Any photon that incurs a Compton collision will be deflected from its original course, and thus what should have been a sheep may become a goat, as shown in Figure 5–3. Alternatively a goat may become a sheep, and one must remember that there are enough goats to make this a very real possibility. Furthermore, a photon that starts off as a sheep may get killed in a photoelectric crash. In short, *absorption and scattering modify the percentage of the generated photons that will reach the crystal.* Thus, although the tidy diagrams of Figure 5–2 are valuable in orienting our thinking about detectors in general, they cannot be trusted in the patient-counting situation. Counts/sec./μc. can be one thing in one patient and something else in another. Or—which is not only worse but more probable—counts/sec./μc. may be one thing when you count a patient and something else when you count the standard representing a known fraction of the administered dose. Yet similar geometry is essential if a quantitative comparison is to be valid, for the counter must register the same fraction of all disintegrations both times.

Patient Phantoms. The usual way out of this difficulty is to construct a phantom in which the standard of comparison will be counted, the phantom's job being to duplicate the patient's geometry. When making thyroid measurements, for example, we use a neck phantom so contrived that the absorption

---

[9] In ordinary practice, θ is specified by its tangent rather than its cosine, where $\tan \theta = r/R$, the ratio of detector radius to source distance. The cosine is readily obtainable from this ratio, since

$$\cos \theta = \frac{1}{\sqrt{1 + \tan^2 \theta}}$$

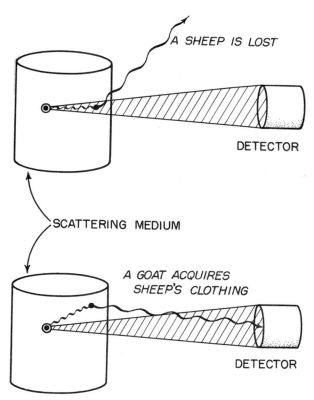

FIGURE 5-3. If the source is contained in a patient, the detector geometry becomes disturbed. The sheep should stay within the cone subtended by the detector while the goats depart into outer darkness, but scattering can deflect a sheep out of the cone (above), or a goat into it (below).

and scattering in the phantom will closely imitate what happens in a human neck containing a radionuclide-loaded thyroid gland in the usual position. But the problem is a difficult one. The phantom might be able to imitate *one* particular neck with reasonable success, but in the clinic the test will involve many necks in all sizes and shapes. Moreover, the gland itself is likely to vary in size, shape, and position, especially if it is diseased. A neck phantom, therefore, cannot provide a perfect solution to the difficulty. If we could decide not to count scattered radiation, the phantom would need to mimic only photoelectric absorption, and thus one source of error would be removed. The geometry in which the standard is counted would then be a better match for the disturbed geometry caused by the patient's tissues.

Energy-Selective Counting. A gamma-ray spectrometer is an instrument that will count gamma rays with due regard to their energies, and can therefore be made accept only those energies selected by the operator. It behaves, in effect, like the tuning circuit in a radio, which can let in a desired signal and suppress all others. This feature permits a spectrometer operator, in many cases, to reject the degraded photons and count only the undeflected, primary photons. We say "in many cases" rather than "always," because when the primary energy is low (20 to 130 kev.) the energy change accompanying a Compton collision may be so small that the spectrometer cannot distinguish between the primary and the degraded radiation.[10] Given a higher primary energy, however, a spectrometer can reject much of the scatter, thus greatly enhancing the reliability of a comparison between a patient count and the standard count, when the latter is made with a sample of the same radionuclide, counted outside the patient in a realistic phantom. If the phantom could be an accurate facsimile there would be no geometry problem, but human beings differ and a phantom cannot simulate everybody.

Any measuring process depends on the collaboration of three ingredients: (1) the method, (2) the instrument, and (3) the operator. An operator will do a much better job if he understands what is going on in his instrument; therefore let us inquire into its mechanism.

THE PULSE-HEIGHT SPECTROMETER

BASIC PRINCIPLE: PULSE HEIGHT MEASURES GAMMA ENERGY

The end result that we are striving for is an answer to the question, "How many gamma rays per second?" This will be obtained with a device that counts electrical pulses, namely, a scaler or a rate meter. Accordingly we must change an incoming gamma ray into an electrical pulse. If we are to count the rays with due consideration for their energies ("How many photons per second in the energy band between p and q kev.?"), the pulse must carry some kind of energy characterization or tag all the way from the detector to the point at which the energy discrimination is made. The energy tag is the pulse's height, or voltage. All through the following discussion of the spectrometer's mechanism, therefore, we will find the requirement that *pulse height be proportional to gamma energy.*

OVERALL COUNTING SYSTEM

A gamma-ray spectrometer consists of several components, each of which contributes to counting a selected fraction of the photons that interact in the detector. The system has two main subdivisions: the *detector* and the *processing unit.* The detector is a "transducer": it accepts the incoming photons and produces their electrical analog, a stream of output pulses, much as a microphone accepts incoming sound waves and changes them into electrical waves. The processing unit is the analyzer: it measures and counts the pulses, and condenses their information into a rational, overall picture.

The components and their functions are as follows:

Detector

SCINTILLATION CRYSTAL. Generates a flash of light, the *scintillation,* for each absorbed photon, the intensity of the flash being proportional to the amount of gamma energy absorbed. The crystal has a *shield* to keep out background

---

[10] Compton's formula (footnote 5) shows that the maximum energy a 30 kev. photon can lose in a Compton collision is only 3 kev., and this presents the spectrometer with an impossible assignment. For a fuller discussion of this problem consult Ross et al., 1965.

radiation, and a *collimator* that permits it to detect radioactivity coming only from the desired direction.

PHOTOMULTIPLIER (or multiplying phototube, or simply phototube). In response to each scintillation, the photomultiplier produces a burst of electrons whose number is proportional to the intensity of the flash. An important accessory for the phototube is the *high-voltage supply*, which provides suitable potentials for the electrodes of the tube.

Processing Unit

INTEGRATOR. Adds up the number of electrons delivered by the phototube, producing a pulse whose voltage is proportional to this charge. Integration is accomplished most simply by a capacitor (Fig. 5–4), but often a feedback amplifier is used.

PULSE SHAPER (or differentiator, or clipper). A device that cuts off the tails on the pulses derived from the integrator, so that a new pulse cannot look deceptively tall as a result of standing on its predecessor's tail.

VOLTAGE AMPLIFIER. Amplifies the shaped pulses from millivolts to volts,

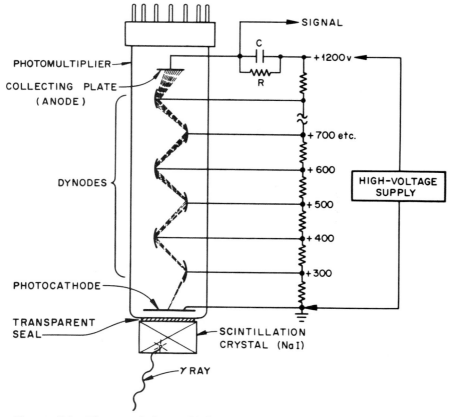

FIGURE 5-4. The crystal-photomultiplier unit develops an electrical pulse for each interacting gamma ray. The blue-violet light of the scintillation liberates electrons from the *photocathode*. These are multiplied enormously while they cascade through a series of *dynodes* to the final collecting plate, or *anode*. The electrodes receive their potentials from a *resistor string* powered from the system's *high-voltage supply*. Voltages shown are approximate only.

so that they can be sorted effectively. A *gain control* provides manual adjustment of the amplification, or voltage gain, so that pulse height may be related to gamma-ray energy by a convenient ratio. A *preamplifier* may contribute to the gain, but its main function is to provide enough power so that the pulses can be transmitted from the detector unit to the main chassis without incurring heavy losses in the connecting cable. The preamplifier may also provide the integrating function. Throughout the amplifying system, *linearity* between input and output is important; so also is *rapid recovery* from the effects of a large input pulse.

Pulse-height selector (or differential discriminator). Provides an electronic window analogous to the slit in an optical spectroscope. This component generates an output pulse for each input pulse whose tip falls within the window, and ignores all others. Sill height and window opening are adjustable: the *E dial* (or base) controls the sill height; the *ΔE dial* (window width) controls the spacing between sill and top. For special purposes the sill and top may be independently adjustable.

Scaler. Counts the pulses that come through the analyzer. Together with a *timing clock* this gives the number per second or minute. Alternatively, the counting rate can be indicated directly by rate meter. The newer "digital rate meters," used for dynamic studies, give the effect of a succession of scalers. A multichannel analyzer can also perform this function (see p. 160).

Recorder. Although not an essential part of a spectrometer, recorders are used in many applications to record the count rate continuously as a function of time.

Of the foregoing components, those in the detector need most careful consideration, because the transformation of gamma photons into electrical pulses is not a perfect process, and unless the operator understands the detector he can seriously misinterpret the data being recorded.

The scintillation crystal

As we have seen (p. 133), ionizations occurring in the patient are a nuisance: they deposit potentially injurious energy, they steal this energy from the photon, and often they steal the whole photon. Ionizations produced in the detector, on the other hand, are a necessity, for we have no way of measuring or even detecting a gamma ray except through the ions that are produced. We do our best, therefore, to enhance ion production in the detector. We would like each photon to expend *all* its energy in the detector; any that escapes in the form of a scattered photon will cause the spectrometer to underestimate the energy of the incoming photon.

Light Production. Certain substances have the property of emitting a flash of light when ions are produced within them. The photoelectric and Compton processes release high-speed electrons, and these interact with nearby material and knock other electrons out of their orbits. The orbital vacancies attract unbound or loosely bound electrons, and as each of these falls into a vacant orbit, thus losing potential energy, a photon of equivalent energy is released. The resulting multitude of practically simultaneous, tiny flashes of light is the *scintillation*.

Most of the detecting crystals used in medicine are made of sodium iodide, activated with a trace of thallium [NaI(Tl)]. Sodium iodide is dense (3.67 g./cc.), and most incoming photons of reasonable energy interact in some manner. In addition to the advantage of high stopping power, the crystal has a good light output; its blue-violet emission is well suited to good phototubes, and—most important—the crystal is transparent to its own light. NaI(Tl) is a medium-speed scintillator:[11] although it is fast enough to permit high counting rates, it does not unduly complicate the design of the processing circuitry.

One of the most valuable properties of sodium iodide is that the total light in the scintillation is nearly proportional to the energy deposited in the crystal by the photon. The higher the incoming energy, the more ions are produced, and the more numerous the flashes of light as the atoms deionize. Therefore more total light is emitted in the scintillation. If the entering photon deposits all its energy in the crystal, the amount of light in the scintillation will then provide a measure of the photon's energy.

Intrinsic Crystal Efficiency. Usually only a fraction of the photons leaving the source will reach the detector, and of those that do only some will produce ions. Others go straight through, leaving the detector unaffected. If we know the thickness of the crystal and the absorption coefficient of sodium iodide for the energy concerned, we can calculate the percentage of the incident rays that will be lost in this way. A measured figure is better, however, because the rays arriving near the outer edge of a cylindrical crystal may cut through the corner, thereby encountering a reduced thickness of sodium iodide. From measurements we can derive an efficiency figure, defined as follows:

$$\text{intrinsic total efficiency} = \frac{\text{photons that cause scintillations}}{\text{all incident photons}}$$

This figure will, of course, depend on the energy of the incoming radiation.

PHOTOMULTIPLIER TUBE

Light Conversion. The next step is to convert the scintillation into an electrical pulse. If we allow light (especially violet light) to strike a substance whose outer orbital electrons are very weakly bound, some of the electrons will be knocked loose. This is the photoelectric process in the usual sense, referring to visible or near-visible light. The detached electrons can be captured by the electrostatic attraction of a positively charged conductor located nearby, and a current is produced. Figure 5–4 shows how this principle works in a spectrometer. A photomultiplier tube—a vacuum tube with a glass envelope that permits the light to enter—is used. Deposited on the inside of the entering window is the photocathode, a very thin layer of a compound (e.g., cesium and antimony) whose electrons are easily dislodged. Near it is a structure called a dynode, charged about 300 v. positive to the photocathode. Electrons liberated from the photocathode are therefore pulled toward the dynode, and the result is an electron current. If the illumination is very brief, as with a sodium iodide

---

[11] In sodium iodide, the light starts to come forth as the gamma ray interacts. A quarter microsecond later, 63 per cent of the total light, on the average, has emerged. At the end of 1 μsec., substantially all the light has been emitted (see Fig. 5–6*B*).

scintillation, a burst of electrons will leave the photocathode and the tube will then become quiescent again.[12] Understandably, the more intense the scintillation, the more electrons the burst will contain.

Electron Multiplication. If the gamma photon is low in energy, so that the scintillation is weak, there might be no more than a dozen or so electrons freed from the photocathode. The system will therefore need great amplification before a scintillation becomes usable. The first stage of amplification is carried out inside the multiplier tube; a series of 10 or more dynodes, each about 100 v. more positive than the one before it, are used (Fig. 5–4). The structure of the first dynode, and the voltage it carries, are so designed that the liberated electrons are accelerated toward it at high speed, and they interact with its specially prepared surface so that other electrons are knocked loose. The augmented cloud of electrons then is attracted by the second dynode; they again interact and multiply their number. At each dynode the number of emitted electrons is three to five times the number that arrived; thus the amplification achieved by a series of (say) 10 dynodes can be enormous, e.g., $4^{10} \cong 1$ million.

Beyond the last dynode there is the positive collecting plate, the anode; the arrival of the cloud of electrons causes the anode's potential to jump a few millivolts in the negative direction, thus providing a pulse that can be amplified and counted.

These are the processes of light sensing and electron multiplication that give these tubes the name of "photomultiplier." We loosely call them "phototubes" or "multiplier tubes" for short, though clearly neither term is accurate.

High-Voltage Supply. The number of emitted electrons at the surface of a dynode depends upon how fast the incident electrons are traveling when they strike the dynode; this depends in turn on the strength of the electrostatic field accelerating them. The electron multiplication or gain is therefore dependent on the voltage difference between dynodes, and in fact the gain is roughly proportional to the voltage difference. The dynodes derive their potentials from a series of voltage-dividing resistors whose high end is connected to a d.c. voltage supply (Fig. 5–4). If the high voltage should increase by 1 per cent, the voltage on each dynode will increase by 1 per cent, and therefore the electron gain at each stage will also increase by about 1 per cent. This means that the overall gain will increase by about 10 per cent (since $1.01^{10} \cong 1.10$); this is why the high-voltage supply for a scintillation dectector must be very carefully stabilized if constant gain is to be maintained. Constant gain is important because the pulses are subsequently to be accepted or rejected on the basis of pulse height. In spectrometers, then, the demands on the high-voltage supply are particularly exacting, and special care must be taken in designing the regulating circuits. A warm-up time of an hour or more may be needed to allow the stabilizing circuits to reach equilibrium.

The crystal and phototube must operate in a coordinated fashion. For example, the photocathode must be sensitive to the light produced by the scintillator; if the scintillator is of the type that produces less light than sodium iodide (for example, some of the organic scintillators), the phototube must have an especially low noise level. A recent trend has been to manufacture the crystal and phototube as an integral unit.

---

[12] Actually there is a low-grade *dark current,* but this need not concern us here.

Reflector and Optical Coupling. Figure 5–5 shows how the components of a typical detector are arranged. The crystal is optically coupled to the sensitive end of the photomultiplier tube, using a cement that readily transmits ultraviolet light. There must be an approximate match of refractive index between the cement and the surfaces to minimize the reflection of light back into the crystal. Care must be taken to exclude all air bubbles, since they would provide reflecting surfaces. The exit surface of the crystal, however, is the only one that should transmit light; at all other surfaces the light should be reflected in order to increase the collecting efficiency. Current practice is to have only the exit surface highly polished; the other surfaces are rough-ground, and between these surfaces and the protective can there is a brilliantly white reflecting powder, such as alpha-alumina (aluminum oxide).

Canning and Magnetic Shielding. The crystal and the reflecting powder are usually enclosed in a thin, aluminum can that lets gamma rays in easily but excludes room light (Fig. 5–5). In a low-energy detector, the can must be particularly thin. The purpose of the can is to keep water vapor away from the sodium iodide, which is hygroscopic. A magnetic shield is often incorporated into the can, since stray magnetic fields influence the electron paths between the various elements inside the photomultiplier tube and thus may change the electron gain. Alternating-current transformers also produce 60 cycle magnetic flux—particularly transformers of the voltage-regulating type. Phototubes without magnetic shielding must be kept well away from this kind of transformer, preferably at a distance of at least 5 feet. Furthermore, a magnetically unshielded

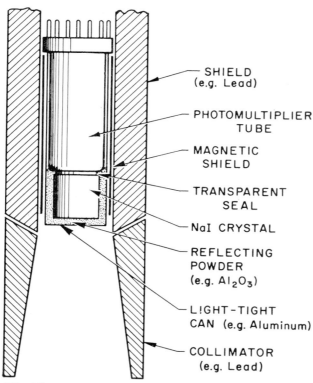

FIGURE 5-5. The principal components of a typical sodium iodide detector.

phototube may change its amplification if it is merely switched from a vertical to a horizontal orientation, or otherwise moved about, owing to the earth's magnetic field.

PHOTOTUBE OUTPUT CIRCUIT

The intensity of the scintillation determines how many electrons leave the photocathode, and for each of these electrons there will be perhaps 500,000 arriving at the anode. If we could count these we would be measuring the scintillation.

Each electron carries a minute electrical charge: 6.24×10^{18} make up 1 coulomb. When we measure an electrical charge, therefore, we are really counting electrons.

If we connect the anode directly to the high-voltage supply, the arriving electrons will quickly disappear, leaving us with no useful signal. We can make them generate a voltage by placing a resistance in the circuit, but this tells us only the rate of flow (current), not the total number of electrons.

Integration. On the other hand, if we make the electrons charge up a capacitor (condenser), we can obtain their total number by measuring the voltage developed between the capacitor's plates. Capacitors follow the law: $Q = CV$, where Q is the charge (number of electrons), C is the capacity, and V is the voltage between the plates. It follows that voltage and charge are proportional, since C is a constant. Taking advantage of this, we place a condenser in the phototube's anode lead (Fig. 5–4), and lead off the voltage surge to the amplifying system. Each time a collection of electrons arrives, the voltage decreases a few millivolts and the size of this decrease is a measure of the number of electrons. Thus through a series of proportionalities the voltage change measures gamma energy.

PULSE SHAPING

A stream of incoming photons could be made to cause a series of negative voltage steps at the phototube's anode, the voltage getting lower each time. If we allowed this to happen, the tube would soon stop functioning; therefore we let the anode's electrons pass into the high-voltage supply through a resistance placed in parallel with the integrating capacitor (Fig. 5–4). This run-off must not be too fast or it will hamper the development of the step voltage, which takes 1 or 2 μsec. to reach completion (Fig. 5–6B). We therefore proportion the resistance and capacity in such a way that the step will be followed by a long "tail" that returns the system to equilibrium, as shown in Figure 5–6A.

All the information we want is contained in the step voltage; the tail is a handicap, for if another pulse comes along soon enough it could be superimposed on its predecessor's tail and thus look larger than it is. To eliminate the tail, leaving a zero baseline ready for the next pulse, a circuit called a differentiator (or clipper) is used. It may be built from resistors and capacitors, but if large pulses are anticipated (e.g., from cosmic rays hitting a large crystal) it is better to use a device called a *delay line* (Fig. 5–7). The step-and-tail pulse is applied to the open end of the line, whose far end is carefully short-circuited. The pulse travels down the line, reflects from the shorted end with reverse

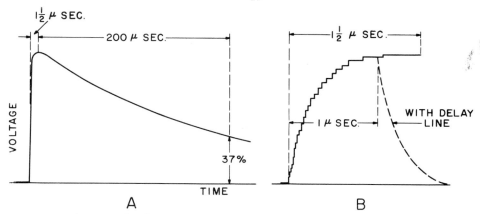

FIGURE 5-6. *A,* The electrical pulse delivered by the phototube has a steeply rising *step* followed by a more slowly declining *tail.* We eliminate the tail, since it carries no information and can deceive the analyzing circuits (see *delay line,* p. 144). Normally this pulse is negative in sign. *B,* The step, viewed with expanded time scale. The numerous subflashes that make up the scintillation are over in a microsecond or so. The dashed curve shows what happens when the delay line cancels out the tail—see the insert in Figure 5-7. (Redrawn from Ross, 1959.)

polarity, and returns to the input end about a microsecond after it entered. During the delay, the original step is free to drive the amplifier, but after 1 μsec. the reflected pulse cancels out the tail. The result is a brief pulse whose leading edge is the original step and whose trailing edge is a mirror-image step that restores a clean baseline (Figs. 5–6B and 5–7).

Double Differentiation. It is almost always desirable to differentiate the integrator's output twice instead of once. This produces a double-sided pulse with approximately equal areas above and below the baseline. Such pulse shaping helps the following amplifier cope with overloads and sudden changes in pulse rate. In addition, it improves the performance of pulse-sorting circuits by eliminating shifts due to high counting rates. Single differentiation is used primarily for simplicity and economy; the problems mentioned must then be dealt with in other ways.

PREAMPLIFIER

Since a movable detector is desirable, there will usually be several feet of electrical cable between the detector and the main electronic unit. The capacities in a long cable can attenuate a phototube's output pulse considerably, and the preamplifier's chief function is to prevent this by putting adequate current into the pulse at the detector end of the cable. The preamplifier may or may not increase the pulse's *voltage,* depending on design requirements. Sometimes it also performs the integrating function, in which case it is called a *charge-sensitive preamplifier.*

The preamplifier and the main amplifier should be properly matched together; it is best to procure both from the same manufacturer.[13]

---

[13] The integrator, clipper, and voltage amplifier comprise a specific system known in the language of nuclear instrumentation as a *linear amplifier.* This system has the definite requirement that it produce a voltage pulse whose height is proportional to the total charge in an input pulse. Any preamplifier used must fit properly in this arrangement of functions. This system is not the same as "linear amplifiers" used in other applications.

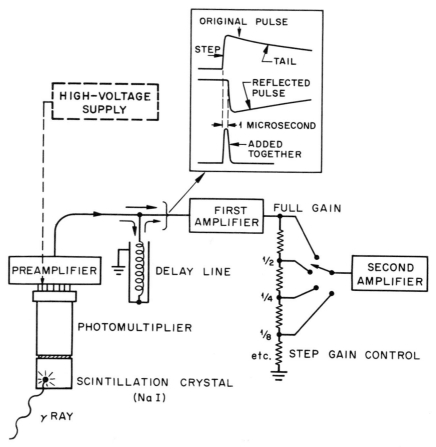

FIGURE 5-7. Detecting, pulse-shaping, and amplifying components of a typical pulse-height spectrometer. (Redrawn from Ross, 1959.)

A typical system is shown in Figure 5–7. In this configuration, integration is done by a capacitor at the input of the preamplifier, and differentiation (by delay-line clipping) at the input of the main amplifier.

The high-voltage supply is not a functional part of the preamplifier, but often it is most practical to feed the high voltage through the preamplifier to the string of voltage-dividing resistors (Fig. 5–4) mounted on or near the photo-tube's socket.

With the arrangement of Figure 5–7, the preamplifier's output characteristics influence the operation of the delay-line clipper. If another preamplifier with different properties is substituted for the proper one, the clipper may only distort, rather than eliminate, the tail of the pulse. An improperly clipped pulse, when further amplified, can cause errors.

VOLTAGE AMPLIFIER

The pulses delivered by a detector, after integration and clipping and even some preamplification, are usually only a few millivolts in height. Further amplification is necessary, and the amplifier must preserve the proportionality between the input and output pulses over a wide range of input heights.

Voltage amplification is usually provided by two or more sections. The amplification, or gain, in each of these sections is stabilized by negative feedback. Though it requires the use of more vacuum tubes or transistors, feedback helps to linearize the system and keep the amplification constant from day to day.

In vacuum-tube systems, the circuits that sort the pulses according to voltage are likely to operate on pulses up to 100 v. in height; in transistorized circuits the pulse-height analyzer can be designed to operate on pulses up to 10 v. Since the pulses available from the clipper are of the order of millivolts, vacuum-tube amplifiers will generally provide gains of the order of 3000 to 10,000, and transistorized systems about a tenth of this.

The voltage amplifier must be designed in such a way that it recovers quickly after overload—that is, after receiving an input pulse too large to be amplified linearly. In addition, it must put out no false pulses during the recovery. This overload precaution is necessary because cosmic rays carry extremely high energies and therefore make bright scintillations, especially in a large crystal. General-purpose pulse amplifiers, not designed to cope with the overload hazard, are frequently unsatisfactory.

Gain Control. The system's voltage gain (= amplification) can be controlled by adjusting the phototube's voltage (p. 142), but it is often more convenient to control the gain at the amplifier. This can be done by placing a voltage divider between two amplifier sections, as shown in Figure 5–7. The control usually works in steps, each of which decreases the gain by half; thus a four step control would provide full gain, and one half, one fourth, and one eighth of full gain. The 1:2 ratios are not intended to be precise, and the divider is usually made of low-cost, 5 per cent resistors. The gain is adjusted by using a gamma source of known energy; the method is described in the section on operation, page 163.

PULSE-HEIGHT SELECTOR OR ANALYZER

This is the device that determines which pulses are to be counted and which are not. We have indicated that the peak height of each pulse is a measure of the energy deposited in the crystal by the incoming photon. Therefore, when we sort these pulses by height, it is the equivalent of sorting the gamma rays according to their energies. We can select a given band of energy and count only the photons within that band. If we want the complete spectrum, we select a narrow band and sweep it through the whole range of energies, recording the count rates as the sweep proceeds.

A pulse-height selector operates on this principle. If we want to count all pulses whose maximum heights are between 60 and 70 v., we use an electronic window with controls by which we can set the window sill at 60 v. and the window itself for a 10 v. opening. This window, according to our "instructions," will ignore all pulses whose maximum heights are higher than 70 v. or lower than 60. This 10 v. band of pulse heights will correspond, of course, to a certain energy band among the incoming gamma rays, and by selecting a window sill level and a window opening we can select any group of gamma energies in which we may be interested.

To look at an entire spectrum, one may use the continuous-recording method already mentioned, sweeping a narrow window slowly over the entire range of pulse heights. The spectra shown in Figures 5–9, 5–20 to 5–22, and 5–24 to 5–28 were made in this way. Alternatively one may use a point-by-point approach, setting a narrow window at a succession of adjacent locations and taking a count each time, until the whole spectrum has been analyzed (see Figs. 5–11, 5–13, and 5–16). Figures 5–17, 5–18, and 5–19 were made with multichannel analyzers (p. 160), in which a couple of hundred windows can accumulate counts concurrently.

Circuit Operation. The fundamental element is a "trigger" circuit, called a discriminator, which will fire only if the voltage delivered to its input exceeds a certain critical level, or "threshold;" below that level it remains quiescent. The discriminator circuit ignores any incoming pulse that is too small, but will fire completely, with no in-between states permitted, if the incoming pulse reaches or exceeds the threshold.

We use two threshold-type discriminators, one set above the other, with their outputs subject to a veto, or "anticoincidence," circuit. The veto circuit passes the output of the lower discriminator only if there is no simultaneous output from the upper discriminator. In this way any scaler or rate meter connected to the output of the veto circuit counts only those pulses whose heights fall in between the thresholds of the upper and lower discriminators, that is, "fall within the window" (Fig. 5–8).

Pulse-Height Selector Controls. The window width is controlled in two ways on most modern equipment. In one system when the window-sill control is altered, the window sill and window top move up or down together, maintaining the same spacing between them. The spacing between window sill and window top is called the "window;" its width is set by an appropriate control.

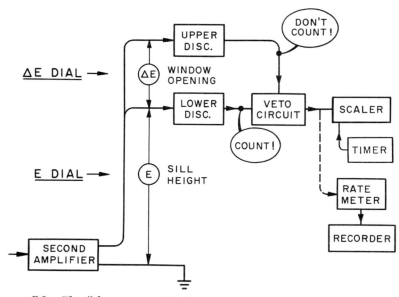

Figure 5-8. The "electronic window" and the pulse-counting components of a pulse-height spectrometer. (Redrawn from Ross, 1959.)

The other system sets the window top with an independent control (upper discriminator threshold). The former system is useful when searching for the narrow regions of maximum counting rate that indicate peaks in a spectrum, and in actually plotting spectra. The constant window width ensures that we measure the same amount of the energy spectrum no matter where the window sill is set. The second method is useful when it is desired to set both window sill and window top precisely to certain energy equivalents.

PULSE COUNTING

The information from the pulse-height analyzer is in the form of a stream of pulses with random time intervals between them. The anticoincidence circuit makes these pulses all about the same size, for we have already made the energy selection, and the proportional relationship between pulse height and energy is no longer needed. The remaining problem is to count the pulses over a known time to obtain the average rate per second or per minute. This is usually done by an ordinary scaler and timer (Fig. 5–8).

One can also obtain the count rate by means of a rate meter. If a changing count rate is to be studied, and a continuous record of the rate is needed, the relatively low-cost, conventional rate meter can be used if the changes are not too rapid. Harris et al. (1966) comment upon several methods of recording a changing counting rate.

THE PULSE-HEIGHT SPECTRUM

A gamma-ray spectrum is a photon spectrum, similar to a light spectrum except that the energies are thousands of times higher. Each gamma-emitting nuclide has a characteristic spectrum: a graph that answers the question, "Of all the gamma photons emitted by these disintegrating atoms, what percentage have such-and-such an energy, what percentage have another, . . .?" and so on until all the emitted rays are accounted for. A few radionuclides emit only one kind of gamma photon; many more emit several kinds. Two familiar examples are shown at the top of Figure 5–9. Practically 100 per cent of the gammas emitted by ^{51}Cr have a single energy: 322 kev. Iodine-131 emits five principal energies and some less important ones. In contrast to beta emission, it is characteristic of gamma emission that the energies are discrete and discontinuous; thus the true emission spectrum is a series of lines with nothing in between, not a continuous graph as in a beta spectrum.

Below the line spectra in Figure 5–9 are pulse-height spectra for the same two nuclides. Each gamma ray is represented by a hump instead of a line, and there may be a broad hump, or even a plateau, that has no counterpart at all in the line spectrum. We must find out why this distortion occurs.

BASIC NATURE OF A PULSE-HEIGHT SPECTRUM

We try to design the detector in such a way that the height (voltage) of the phototube's output pulse will be proportional to the energy of the gamma photon that caused the scintillation. If we succeed, we can sort the pulses in

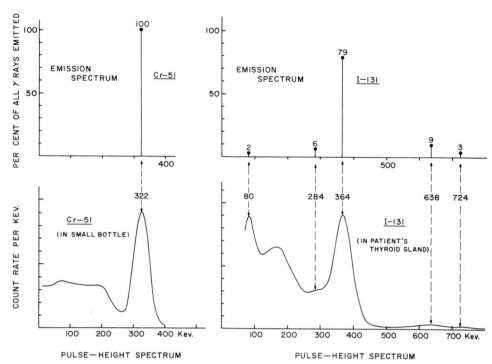

Figure 5-9. *Top,* Emission spectra for Cr-51 (left) and I-131 (right). Abscissae show the energies of the photons emitted; the figure over each line shows the percentage of the total gamma emission. Note that this is *not* percentage of disintegrations: in Cr-51, for example, only one disintegration in 10 emits the 322 kev. ray. But 100 per cent of the rays have this energy. *Bottom,* Pulse-height spectra for same nuclides. NaI crystal, 2 inches by 2 inches; scattering materials near source as noted. (Redrawn from Ross, 1959.)

terms of height, and this will be equivalent to sorting the photons in terms of energy. The original question, "What percentage of the incoming photons have an energy of (say) 100 kev.?" will then become the analogous question, "What percentage of the pulses have a height of (for example) 10 v.?"

Gamma-ray spectra are intended to indicate the distribution of energies in the photons arriving at the detector; actually they show the distribution of heights in the detector's output pulses. A spectrum can be plotted in terms of percentage of the incoming photons per kev. energy interval, with the actual interval used—e.g., 5 kev.—being stated.

DISTORTIONS LOSS OF RESOLUTION

Let us now consider why a line (Fig. 5–9, *top*) becomes a hump (Fig. 5–9, *bottom*).

Imagine a stream of photons, all of the same energy, entering the detecting crystal. Some go right through it, leaving no ions; some are completely stopped in the sodium iodide, depositing all of their energy; and some give part of their energy to an electron in a Compton collision, but the deflected photon escapes from the crystal, taking the rest of the energy with it. Let us consider first the second group, the photons that undergo *total absorption.* Since these all bring the same energy into the crystal, and all of it is absorbed, the electrical pulses should all have the same height.

But not all of the photon's energy appears in the flash of the scintillation: a small and somewhat variable fraction is turned into heat. The scintillations produced by the incident, "monoenergetic" photons have nearly the same intensities, but not quite. Moreover, not all of the light of a scintillation enters the phototube.

The phototube adds to the dispersion. The photocathode is not completely uniform in sensitivity throughout its area; therefore the number of photoelectrons released will depend on the part of the cathode that is closest to the scintillation. The nonuniformity is likely to be more prominent in tubes of large diameter. If the scintillation is weak, as when the incident energy is low, the photocathode may release so few electrons that they will be subject to statistical variations. We must expect, therefore, that the spectrometer's resolving power will be poor at the lower energies. Statistical variations also occur in the paths that the electrons take from dynode to dynode. The high-voltage supply for the phototube may not be adequately filtered; this will impose a 60 or 120 cycle fluctuation in the electron gain. Finally, if either the phototube or the amplifier is noisy, one pulse may stand on the crest of a noise wave while another stands in a trough; this causes random variations in the heights of the pulses.

For these and other reasons, monoenergetic gamma radiation does not produce pulses that are all the same height. With a well made detector most of them will have nearly the same size, but on either side of this *mode* there will be other pulses, some taller and some shorter than they should be. The more nearly alike they are, for a given incoming energy, the better is the *resolution* of the detector.

MEASUREMENT OF RESOLUTION

The various sources of dispersion just mentioned spread a spectral line out into a hump or peak. This is called the *total-absorption peak,* since the pulses constituting this group all come from scintillations caused by total absorption of the incoming gamma energy. The total-absorption peak approximates the familiar, bell-shaped "normal distribution." If it is narrow and sharp, we know that all the total-absorption pulses have very nearly the same height, and that the resolution is good. The sharpness of the peak, therefore, is an index of resolution. Use is made frequently of a horizontal line through the peak at a level half the peak height; the width of the peak along this line is called "full width at half maximum," or F.W.H.M. (see Fig. 5–22). The resolution is this width (kev.) expressed as a percentage of the peak energy (also kev.). Since the resolution is energy-sensitive, deteriorating as the energy goes down, it is understood to be measured at 662 kev. (^{137}Cs) unless otherwise specified. A low figure indicates good resolution. Eight per cent is a typical value of resolution of a sodium iodide crystal.

FURTHER DISTORTION: ENERGY ESCAPE FROM THE CRYSTAL

Let us consider other sources of distortion in the pulse-height spectra of Figure 5–9. The ^{51}Cr spectrum is not a single, bell-shaped peak, centered on 322 kev. with some 10 per cent of spread. There is also a broad plateau extending downward from about 200 kev., with a prominent trough between the plateau and the main peak.

This part of the spectrum is largely the result of Compton scattering, and is referred to as the *Compton plateau*. In sodium iodide the photoelectric process is highly probable only at rather low energies; therefore when a medium-energy ray enters the crystal, the most likely event is a Compton collision. Usually this is followed by another, and perhaps others, until the energy is reduced to a level at which a photoelectric interaction occurs, and absorption is total (Fig. 5–10, *left*). But anywhere in the prephotoelectric stage—particularly after the first collision, when the energy is still fairly high—the scattered photon may escape from the crystal (Fig. 5–10, *right*). The result is a weaker scintillation, a smaller electrical pulse, and a count in the spectrum somewhere to the left of the total-absorption peak.

The trough just to the left of the main peak indicates that *nearly*-total absorption is infrequent: either absorption will be total or it will fall short of total by a considerable margin. Compton's equation (page 132) predicts this phenomenon. A colliding photon can give all, or only some, of its energy to the electron in its path, but it cannot give *nearly* all. E'/E is the fraction of the original energy that the scattered photon carries away; therefore $1 - \dfrac{E'}{E}$ is the fraction that the electron receives. This quantity approaches a maximum as the angle of deflection nears 180 degrees, where cosine $\phi = -1$. At that point the electron's fraction reaches $\dfrac{E}{E + 256}$, and cannot get any larger (Fig. 5–20B).

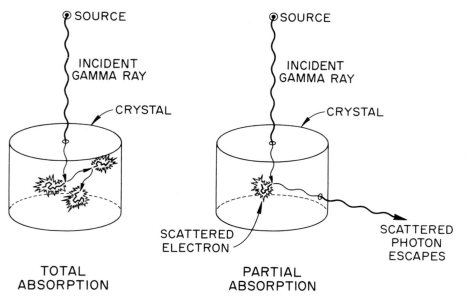

FIGURE 5-10. If a pulse-height spectrum is to be reliable, all the energy of the incoming photon must be absorbed in the crystal, the final event being a photoelectric one (left). If the crystal is small, or the energy high, some photon energy may escape (right). (Redrawn from Harris et al., 1959.)

Consequently, unless the scattered ray collides again, the fraction of energy delivered to the crystal cannot lie in the gap between $\dfrac{E}{E + 256}$ and 1. This results in a trough, whose theoretically sharp edges (see Fig. 5–11) have been rounded off by (1) multiple Compton collisions, and (2) imperfect resolution.

Figure 5–11 illustrates a pulse-height spectrum for ^{137}Cs, plotted in counts per second per 20 kev. (the interval used), versus energy. The vertical axis is a logarithmic scale, which is a convenient way of making the small details look larger, so that they can be studied more effectively. Cesium-137 decays to a ^{137m}Ba daughter that emits monoenergetically at 662 kev.; this photon is 11 per cent converted, and produces a 32 kev. barium x-ray. (We have removed this component from the spectrum to avoid complicating the discussion.) The detecting crystal was small ($1\frac{1}{2}$ in. diameter by 1 in.), permitting considerable loss of scatter produced in the crystal.

This spectrum consists of a total-absorption peak and a Compton distribution. The total count rate is about 700 per second. If there were no distortion in the spectrum, therefore, it would consist of a single line at 662 kev., reading 700 counts/sec. on the vertical scale. If all the reacting photons had been totally absorbed, imperfect resolution would simply have spread the ideal line out into a narrow peak, bell-shaped if plotted with linear coordinates. This peak would

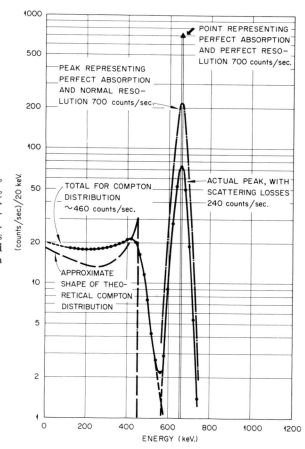

FIGURE 5-11. Solid curve, Pulse-height spectrum from ^{137}Cs, adjusted to take out the barium K x-ray (32 kev.) and predetector scatter. NaI crystal, $1\frac{1}{2}$ inch by 1 inch. Total count rate about 700 counts per sec. Other curves, Theoretical data, as indicated. (Redrawn from Harris et al., 1959.)

contain a total of 700 counts/sec., since it would represent all the reacting photons. In Figure 5–11 we have drawn the imaginary peak as the dot-dashed curve. But the total-absorption peak actually obtained contains only 240 counts/ sec., the other 460 counts/sec. were in the Compton continuum as a result of partial absorption.

FURTHER DISTORTION: PREDETECTOR SCATTERING

Usually by the time the radiation reaches the detector some scattering has occurred, so that many of the photons are already degraded in energy. They have interacted with other atoms in the source, or in the material surrounding the source, or in the air between the source and the detector, or in the walls of the detector's collimator or shield, or in the can or the alumina reflector surrounding the crystal (Fig. 5–5). In the pulse-height spectrum for ^{51}Cr (Fig. 5–9) some of the substandard pulses were due to predetector scattering rather than to energy loss from the crystal. This process is still more prominent in the ^{131}I pulse-height spectrum at lower right in Figure 5–9, for there the radioactivity was contained in a thyroid gland in a human subject. The hump between 100 and 200 kev. is one of the consequences.

It is important to recognize differences between predetector and intra-detector scattering, i.e., scattering within the patient and within the crystal. The energy resulting in the scintillation is electron energy: energy transferred to the crystal's electrons by any or all of the three modes of interaction between a photon and matter. In a succession of scattering interactions in the crystal, each collision increases the probability that the absorption will become total, since the photon energy decreases each time. We therefore prefer a large crystal in order to enhance the number of Compton interactions leading up to a final photoelectric absorption. In the patient, on the other hand, these same processes become drawbacks, for the only kind of energy we can detect coming from the patient is *photon* energy; the electron energy is not emitted. Each Compton collision in the patient, therefore, *decreases* the experimenter's chances of learn-ing something useful: it changes the photon's direction (important in the patient though not in the crystal) and increases the probability that not even a lower-energy photon will be emitted. Moreover, it increases the radiation to the patient. Scattering within the patient, therefore, is particularly bothersome.

Since the information remaining after predetector scattering will reside in photons rather than in electrons, the trough-and-plateau relationships described for the crystal will be precisely reversed in predetector scattering: the trough will be near zero and the plateau to its right. Each may, and probably will, be masked by other, concomitant processes.

In summary, when a spectrum of a monoenergetic emitter is obtained from a patient, its Compton region will be registering both good and bad photons. The bad ones are scatter produced in the patient, goats masquerading in sheep's clothing (Fig. 5–3), with their change of direction compromising the detector's geometry. The good photons in the Compton region reached the detector unde-graded by going straight, but they then suffered the misfortune of producing substandard pulses because some of their energy escaped from the crystal. A large crystal helps to separate the sheep from the goats. It provides most of the sheep with total absorption, thus placing them in the primary peak where they belong, and where they can be counted by a pulse-height selector.

MINIMIZING SCATTERING EFFECTS

To reduce the distortions that we have been discussing, we should like to minimize both Compton and photoelectric processes in the patient, and maximize photoelectric absorption in the crystal. There is little that one can do about a patient, who will resist any attempt to modify his architecture, but there is much that can be done about the detector. The most important thing is to use as large a crystal as one can tolerate, physically and fiscally. Let us see why.

For a given distance, a large-diameter crystal improves the detector geometry (= *extrinsic* efficiency), thus increasing the fraction of the emitted radiation that reaches the crystal. If the crystal is thick, it will reduce the chance that a photon might go all the way through without interacting; thickness improves the total *intrinsic* efficiency. Whenever the incident radiation is plentiful, a lost count does less harm than a count registered through partial interaction; in other words, no information is sometimes better than false information. But if the emission rate is low, we cannot afford to lose counts; therefore we make the crystal with as large a solid angle as we can, and make it thick enough to reduce the straight-through "leakage." Four half-thicknesses will reduce leakage to around 6 per cent. This requires about 5 cm. (2 in.) of sodium iodide at 300 kev.; the higher energies will need more.

A large crystal has an additional and still more important virtue. Just as it reduces straight-through leakage, it also reduces outward leakage of scattered photons; thus it encourages the multiple interactions that are the predominant means of obtaining total absorption (Fig. 5–10, *left*). Even in a small crystal multiple interactions are important. The curves in Figure 5–12 show that at 662 kev. a Compton interaction is *nine times* more likely than a photoelectric one. It follows that if there were no multiple interactions, and the photoelectric process provided the only total absorption, the full-energy peak in Figure 5–11 would contain only one tenth of the pulses, the rest being derived from single-scattered Compton events, with a maximum absorbed energy of 477 kev. (p. 120). Yet in the actual spectrum more than a third of the pulses are in the total-absorption peak, even with a crystal only 1½ in. by 1 in.

Figure 5–13 shows two spectra obtained from ^{51}Cr—322 kev. Here we have used two sodium iodide crystals, one twice the diameter of the other, the larger three times as thick as the smaller. They were set up with the same geometry, the larger being twice as far from the source. When the readings are totaled, the 3 in. by 3 in. crystal gives 43 per cent more total counts. But, more important, it provides 69 per cent more *peak* counts. This is because the larger crystal offers more material for multiple interactions, so that over 80 per cent of all counts appear in the total-absorption peak. If the gamma energy chosen for this illustration had been higher, the difference between the crystals would have been greater. A 3 in. diameter, 2 in. thick crystal provides nearly all of the advantage of the 3 in. thick crystal at this medium energy; this accounts for the current popularity of the 3 in. by 2 in. crystal.

CRYSTAL EFFICIENCY

It is clear from the foregoing discussion that not every incident gamma ray will produce a scintillation, and that of all scintillations produced, some will be

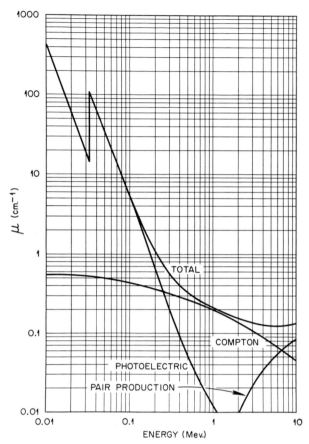

FIGURE 5-12. How the stopping power of sodium iodide changes with energy. The top curve is the total linear attenuation coeffcient (μ), excluding undegraded (coherent) scattering; the curves below show its three components. (Graphs by Harshaw Chemical Co., from data by White-Grodstein, NBS Circular No. 583.)

"good" (i.e., will report faithfully on the incoming energy) and others less faithful. Let us now define several indices.

$$\text{Extrinsic efficiency} = \text{geometrical efficiency}$$

$$= \frac{\text{gamma photons reaching crystal}}{\text{all gamma photons emitted from radioactive source}}$$

$$\text{Intrinsic total efficiency} = \frac{\text{all scintillations}}{\text{total incident photons}}$$

$$\text{Intrinsic peak efficiency} = \frac{\text{total-absorption scintillations only}}{\text{total incident photons}}$$

$$\text{Peak-to-total ratio (P/T)} = \frac{\text{total-absorption scintillations}}{\text{scintillations of any kind}}$$

The intrinsic peak efficiency is the product of intrinsic total and P/T. These quantities depend on the entering energy, and on the size and shape of the crystal. They are also dependent on the position of the source, and thus are not purely intrinsic. The reason for this lies in the process of "corner cutting." The escape of a scattered photon from the crystal is more probable if the Compton collision occurs near one edge; it will be still more probable if the photon enters the front face near the edge and at an angle, tending to cut through the corner. Corner cutting will be minimal if the source is either close to the crystal or far away; it will be prominent when the source is one crystal-radius away from the front face. Large crystals not only reduce leakage, but also decrease corner cutting; the large, front face presents proportionately more interior and less edge to a source in the unfavorable, middle-distance position. At times the middle-distance position cannot be avoided (e.g., with a honeycomb collimator). A practical solution in such a case is to bevel the front edge of the crystal, and decrease the corner cutting that would otherwise occur.

In summary, if the crystal is large: (1) there will be more incident rays, for the same source distance; (2) more of the incident rays will interact; (3) a larger fraction will interact totally.

Figure 5–14 shows the relation between crystal efficiency and energy; the left set of curves describes intrinsic total efficiency and the right set shows intrinsic peak efficiency. The crystal size (in inches) and the source-to-crystal distance (in centimeters) are indicated in each case. The total-efficiency curves illustrate the effects of corner cutting. All the curves emphasize that efficiency improves—sometimes quite rapidly—as the photon energy decreases.

When scattering occurs within the source (i.e., the patient), the crystal can

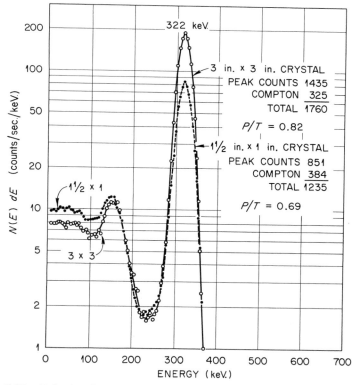

FIGURE 5-13. Pulse-height spectra from a ^{51}Cr source, using two NaI (Tl) crystals at the same geometry: 20 cm. distance for the 3 inch by 3 inch crystal and 10 cm. for the 1½ inch by 1 inch. The larger crystal, in spite of the greater source-to-crystal distance, gives 43 per cent more total counts than the smaller crystal, and 69 per cent more peak counts.

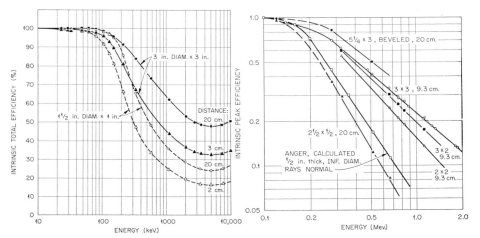

FIGURE 5-14. Intrinsic efficiency, as a function of energy, for a variety of sodium iodide crystals. *Left,* Intrinsic total efficiency for 3 inch by 3 inch and 1½ inch by 1 inch crystals, with two source distances for each. Corner cutting is severe (efficiency reduced) when the source is about half a crystal diameter away. (Redrawn from Harris et al., 1959.) *Right,* Intrinsic peak efficiency for crystals with dimensions indicated (in inches), for source-to-crystal distances shown. See text for discussion. (From Harris et al., 1965.)

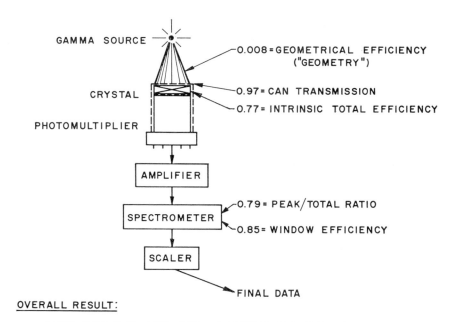

OVERALL RESULT:

0.008 x 0.97 x 0.77 x 0.79 x 0.85 = <u>4 COUNTS</u> PER <u>1000 RAYS</u> EMITTED.

FIGURE 5-15. The emission rate of a source is usually much higher than the recorded count rate. Unless a well crystal is used, the detector geometry is responsible for most of the waste. The figures given are typical, but they vary widely with geometry, crystal dimensions, energy, and so forth.

detect the scattered rays more easily than the primary ones; moreover, the smaller the crystal, the more prominent this selective effect will be, for the curves slope upward and to the left more steeply when the crystal is small. We have seen (p. 136) that scattering within the patient makes it difficult to compare the patient count and the standard, and that one way to circumvent this is to make use of a phantom so constructed that it imitates the patient. If the counting system accepts all energies, the phantom must be realistic in terms of both absorption and scattering, which is practically impossible because of variability in size and shape of different patients. A properly operated spectrometer can disregard much of the scatter; this scatter-rejecting function is all the more important if the crystal is small, since the small crystal emphasizes the scatter.

OTHER PHOTON ESCAPE PHENOMENA

We have been discussing nonspecific escape of photon energy from the crystal, which results in partial absorption of the original photon energy. There

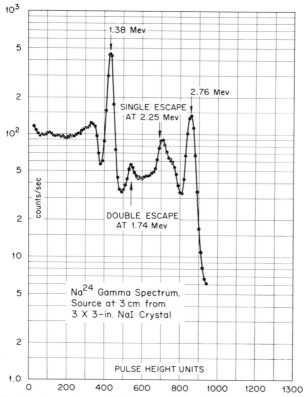

FIGURE 5-16. Spectrum from a Na²⁴ source, placed 3 cm. from a 3 inch by 3 inch NaI crystal. Each pulse-height unit corresponds to 32.5 kev. The primary spectral peaks at 2.76 and 1.38 Mev. are easily recognized. Since pair production will occur at these energies, escape of some of the resulting annihilation radiation causes lesser peaks to appear: for single escape, at 2.25 Mev. (= 2.76 − 0.511); and for double escape, a still smaller peak at 1.74 Mev. (= 2.76 − 2 × 0.511). Similar escape peaks are not found below the 1.38 Mev. peak because this energy is only a little more than the minimum required for pair production, namely, 2 × 511 = 1022 kev. This photon therefore produces many Compton electrons but few positron-electron pairs (see Fig. 5-12). (From Harris et al., 1959.)

are, in addition, two special kinds of escape. One occurs when the incoming energy is high enough to make pair production frequent. The two 511 kev. photons of the annihilation radiation are highly penetrating ($X_{1/2} \cong 2$ cm.), and one or both of them may leave the crystal without contributing to the scintillation. In such a case the intensity of the flash is diminished by a definite amount, namely, by 511 kev. if one ray escapes, or twice that if both escape. Thus in a spectrum of ^{24}Na (Fig. 5–16) there is a prominent, primary peak at 2760 kev.; a small, single-escape peak at 2250 kev. ($= 2760 - 511$), and still smaller, double-escape peak at 1740 kev. ($= 2760 - 2 \times 511$).

In the other special kind of escape, what would have been a total absorption scintillation is substandard by about 28 kev., the energy of an iodine ($K - L$) x-ray. This happens when the energy of the incoming gamma ray is fairly low, in which case (a) the gamma-ray will interact close to the entrance surface, and (b) photoelectric interaction is probable. In this interaction, a photoelectron is ejected from the K shell of an iodine atom; this causes a scintillation. For complete absorption of the photon's energy, however, the K x-ray produced by the filling of the K-shell vacancy must also be absorbed within the crystal. This x-ray may come off in any direction, of course, but if the interaction was only 1 or 2 mm. deep, and the x-ray goes back toward the surface, it will have a chance to escape from the crystal. Whenever that happens, the scintillation will represent the energy of the incoming ray minus the 28 kev. lost in the escaping x-ray. For this reason, a pulse-height spectrum showing a total-absorption peak below 150 kev. often shows, in addition, a smaller peak placed 28 kev. to the left of the primary peak. Several examples of these *escape peaks* may be seen in Figure 5–18.

MULTICHANNEL ANALYZERS

Spectrometers of the kind we have been discussing are called *single-channel* analyzers because they determine the count rate for a single band of energies. All other energies are discarded; this lowers the count rate and impairs statistical precision. Instead of having a single scaler, counting pulses in a narrow energy band, we can use a whole series of scalers representing a series of adjoining energy bands; we can measure the voltage of each pulse and direct it into the scaler whose band covers that voltage. We need a multichannel *memory*, preceded by an *addressing unit* that looks at the voltage of each pulse and then routes it into the correct memory channel. After an appropriate counting time we can determine for each channel how many counts have accumulated, and the answers will enable us to plot the spectrum. With this approach none of the pulses are thrown away, and it becomes possible to obtain low-level, gamma-ray spectra without an inordinate counting time.

The memory of a multichannel analyzer is usually made up of tiny magnetic rings ($\frac{1}{16}$ in. diameter), each of which can store either 0 or 1 in a binary code. A collection of these rings can provide 500 memory channels in a space no bigger than a lunch box, each channel being capable of storing up to a million counts. A standing spectrum can be made to appear on the face of a cathode-ray tube. The multichannel memory also prints out its numbers through a printer or typewriter; it can also plot out the spectrum on a chart.

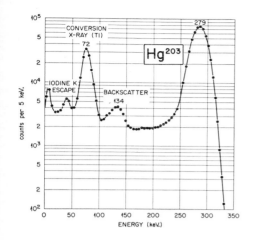

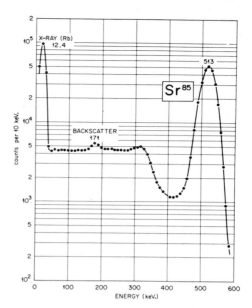

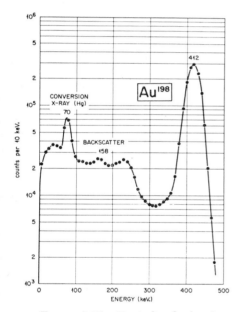

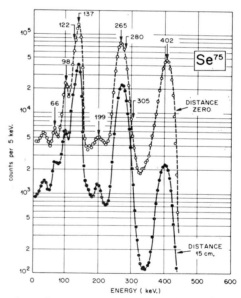

FIGURE 5-17. Typical pulse-height spectra from four gamma emitters in the medium-energy range. Hg²⁰³, Sr⁸⁵ and Au¹⁹⁸ are plotted from data by Heath (1964); all used a 3 inch by 3 inch NaI crystal at 10 cm.; energy bandwidths are as shown on the ordinate. Se⁷⁵ was run in our laboratory using a 3 inch by 3 inch NaI crystal. Two source distances were used to show how summing effects can alter the configuration of the spectrum. The 402 kev. state of the excited As⁷⁵ daughter undergoes transition to ground state by (at least) two routes: (1) directly, with the emission of a 402 kev. gamma ray, and (2) in a two-stage cascade, emitting photons at 137 and 265 kev. The two are very nearly coincident in time, since the half-life of the intermediary state is less than 10 micromicroseconds. With a typical source-to-crystal distance—that is, with poor geometry—only one member of a synchronous pair is likely to enter the crystal, but if both of them should happen to do so the scintillation will look like a 402 kev. one. Accordingly if the geometry is improved (upper curve), the 402 kev. peak increases considerably in relative strength. To avoid overload problems, a weaker source was used for this curve.

Summing phenomena are particularly prominent in a well counter, owing to the excellent geometry. They must be carefully considered whenever spectral data are to be used for a quantitative assay.

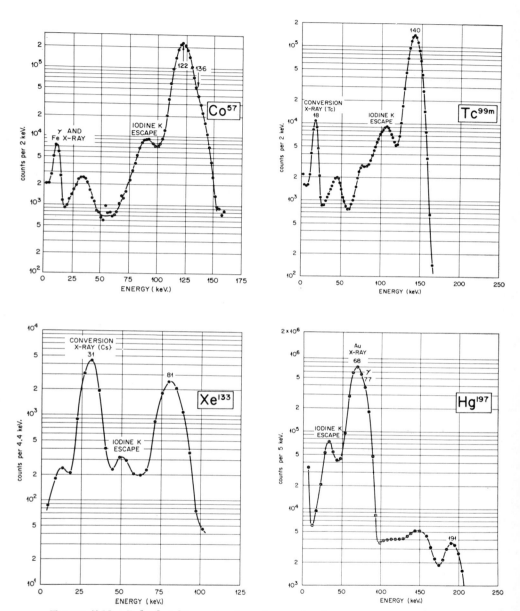

Figure 5-18. Pulse-height spectra from four rather low-energy gamma emitters. Xe^{133} and Hg^{197} are from Heath's data (1964), with a 3 inch by 3 inch crystal at 10 cm. Co^{57} is ours, run at 20 cm. from a 3 inch by 3 inch crystal suspended up in the laboratory air, some 8 feet above the floor and well away from walls; backscatter is therefore minimal. Tc^{99m} is also ours, run at 23 cm. from a 3 inch by 3 inch crystal in a 4 inch lead box. All spectra are net.

Exercise. For each of these nuclides, calculate the energy of the backscatter peak, $256E/(256 + E)$. Note how it crowds toward the primary when the energy is low, so that all the single-collision scatter is contained in a narrow band. Look for the Compton edge at $E^2/(256 + E)$.

The device that measures the height of each pulse is called an *analog-to-digital converter* (A.D.C.) The pulse height—the analog of energy—is converted into a number; the taller the pulse, the larger the number. With modern circuitry, the A.D.C. works so fast that it can process a pulse in 100 μsec. or less, after which it is ready for a new pulse.

The multichannel analyzer enormously reduces the time and labor required to obtain a gamma-ray spectrum.

THE MULTISCALER

A multichannel analyzer has an important accessory capability; most of these instruments provide for operation in what is called the "multiscaler mode." To do this the A.D.C. is disconnected, and the memory system counts pulses without regard for their heights. (Normally the multiscaler is preceded by a separate, single-channel spectrometer.) A timing device opens one channel after another to the oncoming pulses, and each channel accumulates counts for a selected, short time interval. With this manner of operation, the plotted-out contents of the memory will show the course of a changing count rate as a function of time. The advantage of this system over a conventional recording rate meter is that the memory has no inherent lag, as the storing circuit of a rate meter has (Harris et al., 1966). The multiscaler is therefore particularly valuable in studying rapidly changing count rates, the only limitation being that enough counts must accumulate in each channel. The duration of the time intervals is chosen with this in mind.

OPERATING POLICIES

A pulse-height spectrometer can be made to count gamma radiation *selectively*, according to the adjustment of its controls. Although this is a substantial advantage, it bestows on the operator the responsibility of operating the instrument properly.

GAIN ADJUSTMENT

If only a limited portion of the spectrum is to be counted, the instrument's controls must be adjusted in such a way that it will count only the correct spectral band. We therefore need to establish the relationship between *dial divisions* and *gamma energy*. The relationship will depend on the overall electrical gain (including phototube multiplication): a scintillation of given intensity will be counted by a high window if the amplification is high, or by a lower one if the gain is turned down.

The panel control that adjusts the window sill is often called the *E-dial*; it is usually a 10 turn potentiometer with 1000 scale divisions. The window opening is adjusted by a ΔE-*dial*, and the circuits are often arranged so that the E and ΔE divisions are equivalent. In such a case the position of the center of the window, which is what we require for calibrating purposes, is $E + \frac{1}{2}\Delta E$ divisions. Since 1000 kev. spans most of the energies used in medical work, the gain adjustment most often preferred is one that gives 1 kev. per E-dial division.

The method of calibration is as follows. (1) Select a convenient, mono-energetic source whose energy is known, (2) set up the E and ΔE dials so that the *center* of a narrow window falls at the number of divisions corresponding to the source energy, and (3) adjust the gain until the pulses come into this window. A window opening of 20 divisions is usually suitable for this purpose, and the half-window then has the convenient value of 10 divisions.

Cesium-137 is a favorite calibrating source: the 662 kev. photon from the ^{137m}Ba daughter is adequate, and the 30 year half-life permits a small permanent standard to be kept. Cesium-137 also provides a 32 kev. barium x-ray, which is useful for zero-adjusting purposes. For the medium-energy range, ^{203}Hg provides a gamma ray at 279 kev. and an x-ray at 72. Its half-life of 47 days, however, means that it will have to be renewed fairly often. For the range below 100 kev., 1.3 year ^{109}Cd emits a gamma of 88 kev. and an x-ray at 22. Whatever source is to be used, it should be small, and set up in the air in front of the detector with a minimum of scattering material around it. With ^{137}Cs, 1 to 20 μc. is usually suitable for use with an external detector; for a well crystal, with perhaps 100 times the efficiency, much less activity can be used.

To calibrate with ^{137}Cs the window is set so that E = 652 and ΔE = 20, making E + $\frac{1}{2}\Delta$E = 662. The primary pulses coming from the amplifier need to be adjusted in height so that they will pass into the window. If we start with the gain low and slowly increase it, the pulses will at first lie below the window sill, and as the amplification is increased and pulses begin entering the window, the count rate will rise. In terms of the pulse-height spectrum of Figure 5–20B, the primary peak will move to the right as the gain is increased, and as the peak passes into the region of the window, the count rate increases. If the gain becomes too high, the pulses will reach up above the window and the count rate will fall again. When the gain has been adjusted for maximum count rate, 1 E division = 1 kev.

The means of controlling the gain will vary from instrument to instrument. The amplifier often has a stepwise, coarse gain control and also a continuously variable, fine control. Gain can also be adjusted through the high voltage supplied to the multiplier tube in the detector, and sometimes this high-voltage knob is the only continuous gain control that the system has. It is important to remember that though the calibrating source may be monoenergetic, its spectrum is likely to contain more than one peak (for example a backscatter peak or an x-ray) and it is important not to standardize the wrong peak. The way to avoid this mistake is to bring the primary peak into the window *from below*, starting with a gain that is low. If this is done, the first peak to come into the window will be the primary one.

Some indicator for count rate must be used for this adjustment; a "howler" provides an audible signal, and leaves the operator's eyes free to watch the dials. The howler produces a note whose pitch rises as the count rate rises; when the spectral peak matches the window the pitch will be highest. The desired end point is not sharp, however, for small changes in the position of the peak cause little change in count rate. For this reason, check the gain adjustment by offsetting the E-dial 30 divisions, first below, and then above, its calibrating position. The two off-center count rates should be about equal.

If a howler is not available, any other suitable count-rate indicator can be used. A rate meter can be used, or the rate of flashing of the neon lights in a scaler, or the rate of rotation of the pattern in a dekatron tube. These are usually adequate to signal approximate equality between the two off-center count rates, and it should be possible to locate the primary peak within two or three divisions of the E dial.

Two sources of error may occur in the E-dial calibration. These are: (1) amplifier nonlinearity, and (2) E-zero offset.

Amplifier Nonlinearity. This can destroy the proportional relationship between gamma energy and pulse height. If the E-dial and the amplifier are both working correctly, one should be able to calibrate with ^{137}Cs and then find that ^{51}Cr (for example) comes to a peak with the window at the expected setting. If the amplifier is nonlinear this will not be possible.

E-Zero Offset. A low-energy standard should be kept so that the E-zero can be checked. Cadmium-109 is a good one: it has a half-life of 1.3 years; its metastable daughter (^{109m}Ag) emits a transitional gamma photon at 88 kev.,[14] and a silver x-ray at 22 kev. A straight line drawn through two or more calibrating points should pass through the origin when extended, and if it does not, there is usually an adjustment that can correct the zero as needed.

Because these two troubles may be present, it is good general policy to *use the ^{137}Cs standard only to achieve an approximate calibration.* Unless the peak in the sample is markedly asymmetrical, (e.g., ^{133}Ba) one should make the final gain adjustment with the actual sample material. This, coupled with the practice of comparing with a known standard in a good phantom, minimizes the hazards due to nonlinearity and zero misadjustment.

WINDOW OPERATION

One must next decide which energy band will be most effective: where the band should be centered (window position) and how wide it should be (window opening). A spectrometer can be helpful in four principal ways: (1) in achieving a good "signal-to-noise ratio" (S/N); (2) in minimizing statistical uncertainty; (3) in providing stable (i.e., drift-free) operation; and (4) in producing a gamma-ray spectrum.

Signal and Noise: the S/N Ratio. The window's basic function is to *reject;* it counts only a fraction of the incoming pulses. The window should be set to accept counts that bring in reliable information, while rejecting data that will not provide information. In the parlance of engineering, the window's job is to reject as much of the noise as possible, so that the signal stands out prominently.

The signal *usually* corresponds to the net count rate—the gross rate minus the background. But there are other kinds of noise besides the ordinary background.

We must distinguish two basically different kinds of noise because each requires separate treatment. In one situation the noise is severe but constant in quantity; here one tries to measure the noise carefully and subtract it. In the other situation the noise is variable in amount, although its average value may be low; one cannot measure it accurately, and the only hope is to make it small in comparison with the signal. If there is a high signal-to-noise ratio, or S/N, the

---

[14] Because of the 91 per cent conversion, procure 10 times as much as would be suggested by the disintegration rate.

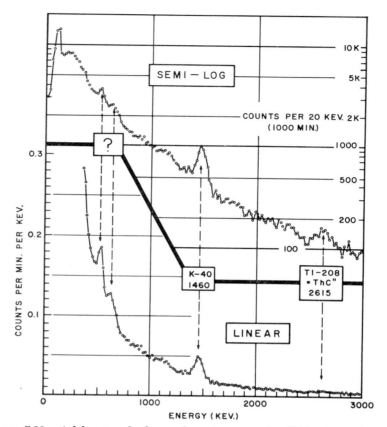

FIGURE 5-19.   A laboratory background spectrum, run for 1000 minutes (overnight) to bring out its weak structure. NaI crystal, 3 inch by 2 inch, inside a 4 inch lead box; multichannel analyzer at 20 kev. per channel; semilog and linear plotting. Note very low count rates (scale at left). In the spectra we can recognize K-40 (probably in the detector), Tl-208 (a thorium daughter), and small peaks near 500 and 600 kev., perhaps due partly to pair production (511 kev.), and partly to fallout contamination: e.g., Ru-106 → Rh-106 (513 and 625 kev.), Sr-85 (513 kev.), and so forth.

In ordinary backgrounds, where the shielding is much thinner, this structure is usually diluted out of sight.

variations in the noise component are likely to be insignificant and the average noise level can be subtracted.

Noise can be of several kinds. The first is the ordinary and ever-present *room background,* arising from cosmic-ray degradation products and from the minute quantities of radionuclides that are always present in building materials, the detector itself, its shield, and some of the electronic components located within the shield. These nuclides include ^{40}K, the various members of the ^{238}U and ^{232}Th families, and perhaps some of the fallout elements. Room background has the virtue that it is usually constant, but it can become variable because of improperly shielded sources (including spilled radioactive material), because of patients harboring radioactivity who may walk about in nearby rooms (a wall is often very poor protection), because of x-ray or therapy machines that get turned on and off, and so forth.

Ordinarily background is nearly *structureless*—that is, it has no prominent peaks in it. The low-energy end of the spectrum will rise because of the prevalence of scattered radiation. In the middle range it presents a reasonably smooth curve, representing degradation products more than primary rays. With exceptional shielding and a long counting time, some signs of structure will often appear. This is illustrated in Figure 5–19, in which a count was continued all night with a 3 in. by 2 in. crystal inside a 4-in.-thick lead box. The peak at 1460 kev. is undoubtedly due to ^{40}K, which occurs in one atom in every 8500 of natural potassium. Because this element is distributed so widely in nature, and because of its high solubility, a manufacturer must exercise extreme care to keep ^{40}K out of the crystal, the phototube, and the electrical components mounted on the phototube's socket, all of which will be inside the shield. Indications of the radium or thorium daughters may also be seen in a background spectrum; in Figure 5–19 there is little or no evidence of radium, but the thorium family produces a weak ^{208}Tl peak at 2615 kev.

The peak near 500 kev. might be due partly to annihilation radiation, resulting from pair production by any high-energy gamma ray (p. 126), but contamination from fallout is a more likely possibility. Ruthenium-106, for example, produces a ^{106}Rh daughter emitting at 513 and 624 kev. Strontium-85 (513 kev.) might possibly have been present as a laboratory contaminant, although this would not explain the peak in the low 600's. In any case it must be emphasized that these features are seen here only because of the good shielding and the long count; ordinarily they would be buried, unseen, in a statistically poor, unstructured, "background continuum" (Fig. 5–22, lower curve). When a spectrum is unstructured, the count rate is *approximately proportional to the window opening.*

When an organ in a patient is being studied, there will be not only the room background but also a *body background* from the parts of the patient that one does not wish to include in the count—that is, from the so-called *nontarget* areas. This kind of background will not be structureless, for it is derived largely from the administered radionuclide. It is important to realize, however, that the *body-background spectrum may not match that of the target organ,* because there will be different degrees of absorption and scattering in the various tissues concerned. Thus the thyroid spectrum will differ from that of the nonthyroid neck background; the latter is likely to differ from a thigh spectrum; and so on. It is unwise therefore to subtract a nontarget count from a target count without considering the spectra.

Another kind of noise occurs when two radionuclides are present. The photons from the higher-energy nuclide produce a *"cross-talk" background* as a result of Compton scattering that complicates the measurement of the lower-energy nuclide. This problem is discussed subsequently.

Scattered radiation is usually noise, particularly when the unknown sample and the standard for comparison cannot be counted under the same geometric conditions. In a well counter, on the other hand, the dimensions and position of the standard can duplicate accurately those of the unknown; so that both the primary and the scattered rays are proportional to the radionuclide content, and the inclusion of the scatter-counts will add to the count rate and improve the statistical reliability.

Inclusion of some of the scattered radiation has been found helpful in the counting of whole patients and other large samples (Gibbs, 1962, 1963). With a properly chosen energy band, the increased scatter from a large source can help to compensate for the increased losses by absorption, so that the results depend little on the size of the source and the distribution of the nuclide within it.

Scattered radiation is a problem when a position-sensitive detector is trying to locate a source within a patient. A scattered ray, by definition, has been deflected out of its original course and therefore looks as if it were coming from a location other than the true one. We speak of the *target* region, at which the collimator is aimed, and everywhere else is *nontarget;* we wish to keep T/NT, the *target-to-nontarget ratio*, high. Thus T/NT in scanning is the counterpart of S/N elsewhere, for the nontarget counts are not wanted and are therefore classed as noise.

Noise can also be electrical in origin. No amplifier is completely free of noise, and there will be small amounts of "hissing," a.c. hum, power-line static, and so forth. A resting phototube also puts out small amounts of *dark noise*. A signal pulse that happens to occur on the crest of a noise wave will look taller than an identical pulse standing in a trough; thus electronic noise impairs resolution. When the signal pulses are small, the noise pulses will be proportionately larger; this is why quiet amplifiers and phototubes are particularly important when low-energy counting is to be done. Not all electrical noise is of low voltage, however; spike pulses can get into the amplifier through improperly shielded leads or through the power lines. Any device with sparking contacts can cause this kind of trouble: a commutator-type motor, the reversing d.c. motor on a scanner, the relays in an electric typewriter, and so on. It is sound policy to keep such devices off the power line that supplies the amplifier and high-voltage unit.

From the foregoing classes of noise—backgrounds and other unwanted counts —the reader can pick out the two kinds: the *constant* and the *unpredictable*. The latter are particularly troublesome, because they can be dealt with only in terms of average and individual values that may fluctuate widely. The only hope, as mentioned earlier, is to keep the S/N ratio high, by any means at your disposal.[15] One way is to operate the spectrometer window effectively, because both the location and the opening of the window have an important effect on the S/N ratio.

Count Rate and "Enclosed Area." An important basic principle is that if one represents the window on a linear pulse-height spectrum as in Figure 5–20B, with its sill to the left and top to the right, the count rate will be proportional to the *area* lying under the window: the area bounded on each side by the window sill and top, and lying between the curve of the spectrum and the baseline.[16] We often label the vertical axis "count rate," but what we really mean is "count rate per kev. of window opening;" for if we widen the window it will accept more pulses and accordingly we must specify the window opening if the count rate is to mean anything. Let us suppose that the spectrum was

---

[15] If a neighboring x-ray installation is the source of the trouble you may have to consider moving your laboratory to a distant location. X-ray equipment not only makes photons, it also throws brief, heavy loads on the power lines, making the line voltage dip from time to time, perhaps beyond the compensating capacity of the regulating circuits in your instruments. Therapy for line-voltage variations is discussed on page 142.

[16] Whenever we speak of an area under a spectral curve, we are referring to a plot in which both axes have linear scales. In a semilog spectrum the "area under the curve" becomes infinite ($\log 0 = -\infty$).

constructed by taking counts with a 1 kev. window, placed successively at the various energy levels along the horizontal scale. If we need to know the count rate for a window spanning the range from 300 to 301 kev., we imagine a narrow, vertical strip standing with its lower end on the baseline between 300 and 301 kev., and reaching up until it comes to the curve. The height of the strip is, of course, an index of the count rate, which can be read off against a vertical scale at the left.

Suppose that for the 300 to 301 strip the reading is 2000 counts/min., and that for 301 to 302 kev. is 2100. If we place a 2 kev. window so that it spans from 300 to 302, it will count all the pulses passed by the two 1 kev. windows; accordingly its rate will be 2000 + 2100 = 4100 counts/min. For a 40 kev. window we would be adding up 40 vertical strips instead of two, and a consideration of the figure will show that the sum of all these strips will be the area lying under the curve, enclosed between the lower and upper limits of the window at 300 and 340 kev.

The conclusion is that no matter where we place a window on a spectrum plotted with linear coordinates, no matter how large we make its opening, the count rate will be proportional to the area bracketed by the window.

Window Opening and Count Rate. Let us apply the area concept to window opening, taking a simple case first. Referring to Figure 5–20B, suppose we place a 40 kev. window with its center at 140 kev.; it will be looking at the heavily shaded area 40 kev. wide. If one doubles the opening, and keeps the window centered at 140 kev., the count rate will double, since the area doubles. In a region where the spectrum is straight, the count rate will be proportional to window opening to a reasonably good approximation. This will hold for the

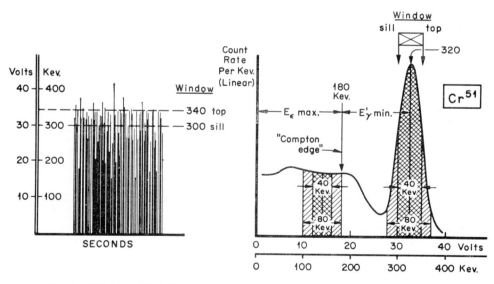

A. ACTUAL PULSES   B. PULSE - HEIGHT SPECTRUM

FIGURE 5-20.   The electrical pulses (A) can be sorted out according to pulse voltage, and thus according to gamma energy. The count rate per kev. can then be plotted into the spectrum (B). The shaded areas relate to the discussion of the effects of window opening on count rate. For discussion of the plateau, trough, and Compton edge see page 152. (Spectrum from Ross, 1959.)

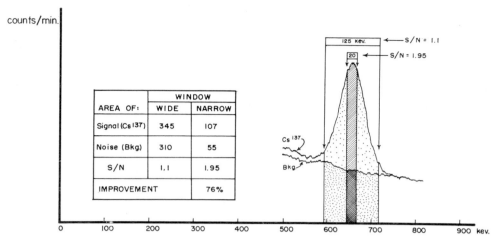

AREA OF:	WINDOW	
	WIDE	NARROW
Signal (Cs 137)	345	107
Noise (Bkg)	310	55
S/N	1.1	1.95
IMPROVEMENT		76%

FIGURE 5-21.   The signal-to-noise ratio (S/N) improves when a wide window is narrowed. The cost is high, however, in terms of lost counts. The coordinates are linear. (From Ross, 1959.)

Compton plateau or for a background spectrum and it will be nearly true for narrow windows almost anywhere.

Consider now what happens if we move the 40 kev. window to the primary peak, and repeat the procedure. If you start with a 40 kev. opening centered on the peak, and then widen 20 kev. on each side, you will not double the area, for the lightly shaded strips added on are not as tall as the dark, central pair. In this case, therefore, the doubled opening will see less than twice the area of the narrower one; count rate will *increase with* window opening, but it will *not be proportional to* it. Flatness or insignificant curvature in the spectrum makes for the proportional relationship, whereas "structure" destroys it. Over a peak in the spectrum, the count rate will increase more slowly, proportionately, than the window opening; over a trough the opposite will be true.

Window Opening and S/N Ratio.   Figure 5–21 illustrates the operation of the foregoing theory in an actual case: the counting of a weak ^{137}Cs source in the presence of an unstructured background. The areas concerned were measured with a planimeter, and the results are given, in arbitrary units, in the small table at the left of the figure. We see that when a narrow window was opened up to six times its width, the background increased to about six times its former level; the signal count, on the other hand, increased only threefold, so that the S/N ratio was cut nearly in half. The lesson is clear: *if the counting problem calls for maximizing the S/N ratio, and the background is unstructured, center the window over a high, primary peak and keep it reasonably narrow.* This will throw away counts, of course, but it throws away background faster than signal. One must procure plenty of signal counts, however, if this method is to be used.[17]

Window Opening and Statistics: S^2/B.   Let us now consider the other situation in which noise is a problem: when it is measurable, and constant in

---

[17] This is a good reason for not carrying the narrowing process too far. When the edges of the window are riding up at 70 per cent of the peak value, the S/N has reached 90 per cent of its maximum. There is little to be gained, therefore, by narrowing further, and much to be lost in terms of impaired statistics.

quantity, but at a high level, so that it threatens to obscure the signal. Here the gross count is only a little greater than the background, and the net count (signal) is small. The problem is to measure, with acceptable accuracy, a small difference between two quantities, each of which is subject to random fluctuations that threaten the small difference with very large percentage errors. Suppose we can measure two quantities with unusually good reliability (standard deviation 1 per cent of average), and that one of them is 105 units and the other is 100. If the variations are random, statistical theory says that:[18]

$$(105 \pm 1\%) - (100 \pm 1\%) = 5 \pm 29\%$$

Clearly the error can become great when the difference is small.

The S.D. is a measure of variability, and is derived, properly speaking, by considering the fluctuations in a number of measurements of the same thing. A more meaningful measure of variation is the *fractional standard deviation* (F.S.D.), which is simply the S.D. expressed as a fraction of the average. The statisticians call it the *coefficient of variation*.

What about the increased count rate delivered by a wide window? We remember that opening the window will reduce the S/N ratio, but perhaps the increasing count rate could more than offset this. There is an optimum window opening for use when the gross count is only a little larger than background, a compromise between rising count rate and falling S/N.

We would like to have a relationship between gross count (G) and background (B) in order to make the small net sample count, $S = G - B$, of greatest statistical validity.[19] The S.D. for S can be calculated if we know those for G and B; we cannot measure the latter two with single counts but we can estimate them by using the square-root rule. Applying statistical theory we write:

$$(\text{S.D. for net count})^2 = (\text{S.D. for gross count})^2 + (\text{S.D. for background})^2$$

$$\cong \sqrt{G}^2 + \sqrt{B}^2 = G + B = (S + B) + B$$

$$\cong S + 2B$$

$$\therefore \text{expected S.D.} \cong \sqrt{S + 2B}$$

and expected F.S.D. $\cong \dfrac{\sqrt{S + 2B}}{S}$ where S and B are *total counts* (not count rates), and the sample and background are counted for equal times.

In those situations in which the signal is weak and background is a problem, S will be considerably smaller than 2B, and the expected F.S.D. then approximates $\dfrac{\sqrt{2B}}{S}$. If we want this quantity to be small we must make its reciprocal large. To obtain a simple "figure of merit," for use in comparing one counting arrangement with some alternative one, we can eliminate the 2. On this basis,

---

[18] S.D. for a sum or difference:

$$(\text{S.D.}_{a \pm b})^2 = (\text{S.D.}_a)^2 + (\text{S.D.}_b)^2$$

[19] Note that we are still dealing with accumulated counts, not count rates, and that $S = G - B$ only if the sample and background have the same counting time.

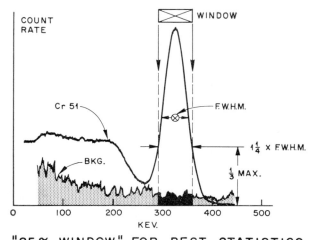

"85% WINDOW" FOR BEST STATISTICS

FIGURE 5-22.   For a statistically optimum window, make the top and sill cut the peak at about one third of the peak height. The precision deteriorates, though not much, if you try to include the remaining 15 per cent of the total-absorption pulses (see Fig. 5-23). (Spectra courtesy of ORINS Medical Division, from Ross et al., 1965.)

$\dfrac{S}{\sqrt{B}}$ should be large; its square should also be large, and thus we can use the "S^2/B rule," which says that for the most reliable measurement of a weak sample, the ratio (net sample)^2/background should be made as large as possible.

The sample spectrum will contain prominent peaks, but the background usually will not; consequently S and B will vary differently with respect to window opening. When we were trying to correct for a moderate but variable background, we selected the window opening that would maximize S/N; when a feeble signal is almost lost in a steady background, we select the opening that will maximize S^2/B. Or, better, we select the window that will minimize $\sqrt{S + 2B}$ /S.

We can solve this problem with the help of two assumptions. One is that the background count rate will be approximately proportional to the window opening, for reasons that we have already discussed (p. 169). The other assumption is that the shape of a total-absorption peak will approximate that of the bell-shaped "normal curve of error," whose mathematical properties are well known. This assumption will hold fairly well for the upper half of the peak, and will also hold fairly well for the lower half unless escape phenomena or scattering markedly distorts the left side slope. We can calculate S and B for a series of window openings, determine the F.S.D. in each case, and find out where it goes through a minimum.

An example of a statistically optimum window is shown in Figure 5-22, which shows a ^{51}Cr peak. The window sill and top of the window cut the primary peak at the two points where the count rate is about *one third of maximum;* this makes the opening some 25 per cent greater than F.W.H.M., the full width at half maximum. This window will detect only 85 per cent of the counts in the total-absorption peak; if you attempt to count the other 15 per cent, the small increase in signal is counterbalanced by the more rapidly mounting background, and the precision gets worse. When the signal is very weak, then, 85 per cent *window efficiency* provides the best solution.

Frequently the optimum window setting is not necessary: the opening can be made somewhat narrower or wider without greatly changing the reliability. This is shown in the curves of Figure 5–23, in which the estimated F.S.D. (per cent), representing the uncertainty of a count, is plotted as a function of window opening. The uncertainty is greatest when the window is narrow, and decreases as the window opening increases. The uncertainty reaches a broad minimum, however, where the opening is between 1 and 1½ times F.W.H.M.; anywhere in this range the window will be operating near its best. We shall see in the following section that wider openings may be preferred if stability is a problem.

The curves of Figure 5–23 are plotted for three values of S/N (as measured at maximum, with a narrow window) and the conclusion regarding the optimum opening is the same for all three. In deriving these curves the relationship F.S.D. $\cong \sqrt{S + 2B}/S$ was modified because it presupposes equal counting time for sample and background. A simple extension of the F.S.D. formula

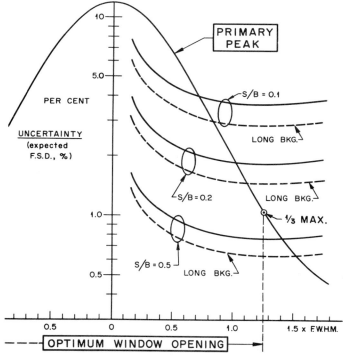

FIGURE 5-23. Statistical uncertainty, as gauged by the expected fractional standard deviation (per cent), is plotted against window opening, expressed in terms of the full width at half maximum (F.W.H.M.). Three pairs of curves are shown, each assuming an arbitrary signal-to-background ratio, as indicated. Solid lines assume equal sample and background times; dashed curves show the 20 per cent or so improvement that is obtainable if background is counted five times as long as the sample. The primary peak is the normal curve of error, on linear coordinates; the F.S.D. curves are semilog.

permits the use of count rates instead of total counts, thus providing for different sample and background counting times:

$$\text{Expected F.S.D.} \cong \frac{1}{\sqrt{R_s t_s}} \sqrt{1 + \frac{R_b}{R_s}\left[1 + \frac{t_s}{t_b}\right]}$$

where R_s and R_b are the counts/min. for the sample (net) and background, and t_s and t_b are the two counting times, also in minutes.

The curves of Figure 5–23 were derived from this formula. Optimum window opening is about the same for all. The solid curves assume equal counting times; the dashed ones show that a fivefold background counting time can reduce the uncertainty to 80 per cent of what it was. There is, however, a law of diminishing return: a tenfold background time would not be more than 4 per cent better than a fivefold one. In practice, therefore, a "long background" counting time should last five times as long as the sample time, unless additional background time costs nothing. Another consideration is that the longer the background counting time, the greater the chance that something may happen to make the result unrepresentative of the background present while the sample was being counted. If the background is variable, the best thing to do is to find out why it varies and correct it. Failing that, all that can be done (when the sample is very weak) is to use equal sample and background counting times, taking half of the background count just before the sample, and the other half just afterward.

Window Opening and Count-Rate Stability. Count rate will depend on window position, but it should not be *critically* dependent. Either the gain or the window position may drift, since no electronic instrument can hold its adjustment indefinitely. Line-voltage changes may exceed the compensating capacity of the instrument; a photomultiplier tube may be temperature-sensitive; someone may move a magnetized screwdriver (many tools are magnetized these days) close to an unprotected phototube, thus changing its gain; and so on. Consequently an unanticipated change in gain is a very real possibility, and we should design operating policies to minimize the harm that might result.

Let us consider first a drift in window position in terms of the area principle (p. 169). If we keep the window centered over a primary spectral peak, and widen the opening, strips of area will be added on at each side, and the count rate will rise. If, on the other hand, the opening stays the same but the position shifts, area is gained at one side but lost at the other, and the effect on count rate will depend on whether or not the gain exceeds the loss. Count-rate stability will be best if we can make gain and loss about equal. Figure 5–24 shows a ^{131}I spectrum with a window centered, initially, on the main primary peak. As the window drifts upward, area is gained on the right and lost on the left. The unhatched rectangle designated "net loss" represents the change in area, for the other area components approximately cancel each other. Our concern is to keep the net-loss rectangle small.

The width of this rectangle represents the amount of drift. For a given amount of drift the height of the net-loss rectangle depends on how steep the sides of the peak are at the points where the curve is cut by the vertical lines representing the window top and sill. Clearly we should keep away from the steep places in the spectrum, and place the window top and sill where the curve slopes only gently—namely, either near the top of the peak or near the bottom. Either should keep the rectangle small.

A narrow window has two obvious faults. It is poor statistically, since the F.S.D. rises when the window is narrowed (Fig. 5–23). Secondly, to get good stability the net-loss rectangle should not only be small, it should be a small *percentage* of the total area seen by the window. If this area is small, as when the window is narrow, even a small rectangle could represent a sizable fraction of the total. In contrast, the much larger area under a wide window makes a small rectangle still less important. There is little doubt, therefore, that the wide window is better.

Fortunately there is no great difference between a window designed for stability and one giving best statistics; the broad minima in the F.S.D. curves (Fig. 5–23) give us a generous amount of leeway, and there will not be much statistical loss if the window is made somewhat wider than the ideal "85 per cent." Moreover, the statistics will be of major concern only if the signal is weak, so in most situations maximum window efficiency is unnecessary. If there is a stability problem, the window limits should be set fairly near the baseline. The system will then be less affected by drift, the window efficiency will be high, and the statistics will still be close to the best obtainable.

For a given window and peak, the maximum count rate will occur when the window top and sill intersect the sides of the peak at equal heights above the baseline; with such a window a net-loss rectangle will appear no matter which way the window is shifted. Unless the peak is symmetrical, therefore, the center line of a wide window, adjusted for maximum count rate, will not pass through the tip of the peak. Stability is best, of course, when the window is adjusted for maximum rate, for that is the point where an imaginary spectrum, run with this wide window, will have near-zero slope.

Now let us turn from the problem of a drifting window to that of drifting amplification. In the former case, illustrated in Figure 5–24, the window moves

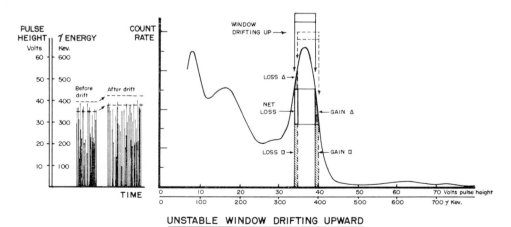

UNSTABLE WINDOW DRIFTING UPWARD

FIGURE 5-24. When a properly placed window drifts upward, area is gained at the right but lost at the left. Two triangular areas for gain and loss balance each other; so do the gain and loss rectangles. Net loss is therefore the clear rectangle. I-131 spectrum from a patient's neck. (From Ross, 1959.)

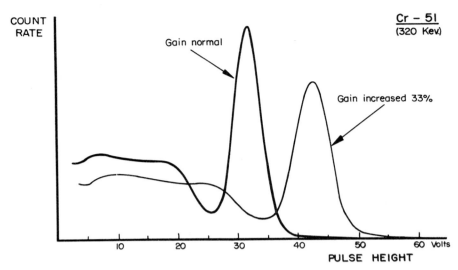

Figure 5-25. Effect of increased amplification on a Cr-51 spectrum. The peak moves to the right in direct proportion to the gain, but because the underlying areas must remain constant, the peak height varies inversely as the gain. Measures designed to protect against drifting gain should take this into account. (From Ross, 1959.)

relative to the spectral peak, whereas when the gain changes, the peak creeps out from under a stationary window. These two kinds of drift are not strictly comparable, although in most instances they are approximately so. If a drifting peak could move to one side without changing its size, we could apply the same argument that we have used for the drifting window; but the peak *does* change its size as it moves. If it shifts to the right it becomes shorter and fatter; to the left it grows taller and thinner.

Figure 5–25 shows how the spectrum of ^{51}Cr changes when the gain is increased 33 per cent: the 320 kev. peak, originally at 32 v., moves out to 43 v., and its height is reduced at the same time. This is because the total area under the curve must remain the same, since it represents the total number of scintillations occurring in the crystal per minute, irrespective of how tall or short the resulting electrical pulses may be. These scintillations depend only on the incoming radiation, and not on how the operator chooses to process the pulses. Although the gain may change, then, the area under the spectrum does not. Consequently if the peak moves to the right in the ratio of 4:3, its height must shrink in the ratio of 3:4.

This circumstance permits the gain-change problem to be explored mathematically. For protection against drifting gain the window sill and top should *not* cut the peak at equal heights above the baseline: the sill should cross the curve at a higher level than the top, in such a way that the ratio between the higher and lower count rates is that of the window-top voltage to window-sill voltage (Fig. 5–26, bottom). This ratio will be near unity if the window opening is not large compared to the sill height, and in such a case an adjustment designed to protect against gain change will also correct for window drift. As the lower energies are approached, however, the resolution of the spectrometer becomes poorer and the total-absorption peak becomes proportionately broader.

The ratio of V_2 to V_1 (Fig. 5–26) then becomes considerably greater than 1; when this happens a single window placement will not be ideal for both kinds of drift. In such cases it is usually best to protect against gain change, since this is more likely to occur. To this end, maximum count rate should be found by adjusting the gain, instead of searching it out with the E-dial. It is important to bear this in mind during beta scintillation counting, in which a broad, low-voltage peak is the rule rather than the exception.

Prevention of Drift. From what has been said it will be clear that preventing drift is far better than learning to live with it. Apart from competent instrument design, steady a.c. power is the most important preventive. A voltage-regulating transformer will often be needed. To deliver a constant output voltage, the transformer requires a constant load, so it should not be loaded with devices that are turned on and off. If necessary, isolate the spectrometer and its high-voltage supply, and operate these instruments only from the regulating transformer, using the raw a.c. line for less vulnerable, intermittently operating components such as a strip-chart recorder, printout typewriter, X-Y plotter, tape punch and reader, and so on. Also, procure a transformer with the proper volt-ampere capacity: for effective performance the transformer should be loaded to between 67 and 97 per cent of its full rating.

If the line-voltage variations are too great to be coped with in this way,

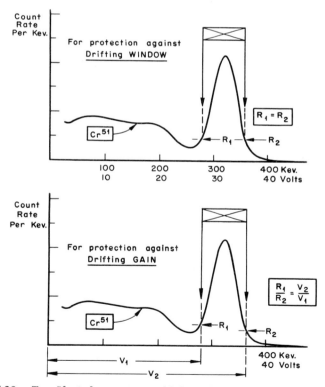

FIGURE 5-26.   *Top,* If window position is likely to drift, the top and bottom of the window should cut the peak at equal heights above the baseline ($R_1 = R_2$). *Bottom,* If the gain is likely to drift, the relationship shown in the lower figure should be used. This becomes important when the peak is broad, e.g., at the lower energies, or in beta counting.

try to connect the counting instruments to a private power line whose use is under your control, because then you can prevent its being subjected to heavy, intermittent loads—e.g., from electric ovens, refrigerators, air conditioners, x-ray equipment, elevator motors, air compressors, floor buffers,[20] and so on. Make the connection for this line as far back toward the power station as possible, for there the wiring will be heavy, and other people's intermittent loads will be a smaller percentage of the total wattage available at the point where your line is connected. It may be difficult to obtain such a line, for it will be a rare administrator who understands why it is necessary, and a rare electrician who will not hold out for a conveniently short connection.[21]

Constant temperature in the counting room is also important, but *do not* operate either a heater or an air conditioner from the instrument line!

Instability of Window Opening. We have been discussing unwanted changes in window position, relative to the primary peak of interest. What about spontaneous changes in window *opening?* These are much harder to detect; can we correct for them?

Two measures can be taken. The first is to use a *wide window,* which we have already decided is best for most quantitative counting. When the window is wide, the enclosed area is large, and the top and sill intersect the spectrum at low level. Consequently an uncompensated area change produced by a change in window opening (a) will be small, because the rectangle involved is not tall, and (b) will be a small fraction of the total enclosed area.

The second measure is to count *by comparison,* which is a good idea for several reasons. The net count rate from an unknown sample is compared with that obtained from a known quantity of the same nuclide, counted under the same or equivalent conditions. If conditions are equivalent the spectra will be similar, in which case a minor shift in either the window or the peak will have substantially the same effect on sample and standard alike, and the ratio between the counts will remain unaltered. It is easy to understand, on the basis of the area concept, why the two spectra must be similar. Sometimes, of course, it is difficult to obtain comparable counting conditions.

Whenever two counts are to be compared, the smaller the time lapse between them, the less important any drifting problem will be.

Asymmetrical Window Settings. Sometimes special circumstances make it advisable to set the window somewhat higher than the normal, stability-oriented position in which the sill and top intersect the primary peak at equal heights above the baseline. The asymmetrical variant should be considered (a) if scattered radiation is highly objectionable, and (b) if the energy is sufficiently low to make it difficult for the spectrometer to reject the scatter (Ross et al., 1965). We have pointed out (p. 120) that a spectrometer's resolution deteriorates as

---

[20] Buffers are an intolerable abomination. They not only throw heavy loads on and off the power lines, making life miserable for any laboratory that needs a steady line voltage, but they scatter spore-bearing dust throughout the hospital, they vastly increase the slippery-when-wet hazard, and they make a floor merely look clean instead of being clean. They have no business in any hospital, and an outright ban is long overdue.

[21] With annoying stubbornness, one of us insisted on a restricted instrument line for the low-background, whole-body counting installation at Oak Ridge Institute of Nuclear Studies Medical Division, and this provision has paid off handsomely in terms of improved voltage stability. The 120 v., single-phase power is derived from a small, step-down transformer fed directly from one of the high-voltage distribution lines outside the building.

the energy decreases, and to make matters worse, the energy band into which a photon may be scattered in a single Compton collision becomes narrower as the primary energy gets lower, so that the scatter band is close to the primary line (Ross et al., 1965: Fig. 3, p. 112). Differentiation between a primary and a scattered ray requires greater precision at the time when the spectrometer's precision is becoming worse. The rejection of scattered energies lying close to the primary will be more effective if the window is shifted a little to the right, so that its sill rides well up on the left-hand limb of the peak. The price paid for the improved S/N ratio is a somewhat reduced count rate, plus increased vulnerability to drifting; consequently this expedient should not be used unless needed. By the same token, the primary energy should not be any farther below 130 kev. or so than is necessary; the possible drawbacks should be borne in mind whenever a switch to a low-energy gamma emitter appears desirable for other reasons.

Scans illustrating the clean-up value of the asymmetrical window are shown in Ross et al. (1965). Conventional and asymmetrical window settings have been tabulated for several nuclides of clinical interest (Harris, 1964).

Plotting a Pulse-Height Spectrum. The way to approach any new or difficult counting problem is to see first of all what the sample and background spectra are like in the actual counting situation that you wish to use—and to take remedial measures if they are unfavorable. The spectra are even more important if you are trying to count more than one nuclide. A spectrum may be needed to check the radiochemical purity of supplied material, or to establish the identity of an unknown nuclide when evidence of contamination appears. It is a good plan to start with a sample containing a generous amount of activity,[22] and to take all practicable measures to assure constant room temperature, adequate warm-up time, well stabilized a.c. power, and so forth. If appreciable background is present, it must be determined and subtracted for each window position.

If spectral information in the low-energy range is needed, it is well not to trust the window at low E-dial settings. Use more amplifier gain, so that the pulses of interest can be seen at E-dial settings above 50 divisions (on a 1000 division scale). It is also possible to use more high voltage on the phototube, but *first look up the maximum voltage* that the tube will tolerate. High gain, of course, can precipitate noise problems, and it may become necessary to find a quieter amplifier or phototube. Analyzers vary considerably in regard to noise, and also to the E-dial reading below which the window will become unreliable.

Multiple-Nuclide Counting. When two radionuclides are present in the same sample, there is need for careful use of the spectrometer window. Corresponding to the two primary peaks selected for counting, there will be an *upper window* for the "upper nuclide" and a *lower window* for the "lower" one. For illustration we might take ^{59}Fe and ^{51}Cr, two nuclides that are frequently used in blood studies (Fig. 5–27). The high-energy photons from the iron component produce many substandard pulses, some due to escape from the crystal and

---

[22] Like many other things, generous source activity can be overdone. A high-activity source can be impairing the function of the phototube and amplifier, while at the same time the pulse rate coming through the window may be low because of a narrow opening. Remember that the window can protect the rate meter from overload, but it does not protect the detector or amplifier (Fig. 5–8).

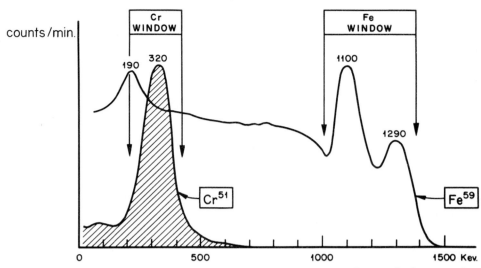

FIGURE 5-27. Double-nuclide counting is illustrated by Fe[59] and Cr[51]. The lower window will see room background as usual, and this should be constant in quantity. In addition, however, there will be a *cross-talk background* thrown into the lower window by the upper nuclide; the cross-talk will therefore be proportional to the amount of upper nuclide present. (Spectra from Ross, 1959.)

others due to predetector degradation. It is against these iron-derived pulses, scattered into the lower window from above, that the radiation from the ^{51}Cr must be counted. We may call this added noise the *cross-talk background,* to distinguish it from the ordinary, room background that will also contribute to the gross, lower-window count.

The cross-talk background will have the virtue of being steady, and in being proportional to the amount of upper nuclide present. The way to deal with it, therefore, is to procure a pure sample of the upper nuclide and count it with both windows, subtracting out the upper and lower room backgrounds to get net counts. The measurements must be made using the same detector and geometry (e.g., a well counter) that will be used later in the actual experi- ment, for otherwise the spectra are likely to change. This determination tells the operator that every time he has 100 net counts in the upper window it will produce a certain number of counts of cross-talk background in the lower window. Once this ratio has been established, the net, upper-window count in an unknown mixture can be used to correct for the cross-talk. The percentage of cross-talk will depend, of course, on the spectrum of the upper nuclide and on the positions and openings for the two windows. The latter must be selected with considerable care, perhaps after one or two pilot experiments. The windows will be different for each pair of nuclides.

Much of the success of a double-nuclide determination hinges on whether one can, by careful planning, arrange for a reasonable sample-to-background ratio in the lower window. The problem becomes additionally complicated if the selected peaks are so close together that the lower nuclide also cross-talks into the upper window, as ^{51}Cr might well do into a conventional ^{131}I window. This creates a situation in which one may choose to measure ^{131}I by its topmost two gamma rays (Fig. 5–9), which are normally shunned because their abundance is low. Double counting is discussed in greater detail in Ross (1959).

Large Windows and High Energies. Many spectrometers have ΔE dials that give a maximum window opening equal to 100 E-dial divisions, and sometimes a need arises for a pass band greater than 100 kev. This is easily obtained by reducing the amplifier gain, so that each E division becomes equal to 2 kev. instead of the usual 1—or, for that matter, any other calibration ratio that the operator finds convenient. These reduced gain settings also permit operation of a window in the regions above 1000 kev., which is the top of the range in many spectrometers if one uses the ordinary 1:1 calibration. The only precaution to bear in mind is that usually the ratios on the panel control are not intended to be mathematically precise, and one should always restandardize a new gain using a single gamma peak of known energy. Again, as recommended earlier, the final adjustment of the gain is carried out on the actual peak that one wishes to count.

THRESHOLD OR "INTEGRAL" COUNTING

Some spectrometers are provided with a switch that disconnects the window-top mechanism but not the window sill; this permits an operator to count all gamma rays having energies greater than a chosen threshold value. This feature is not used often, for the window type of operation is usually preferable. It may be helpful, however, to include a discussion of the threshold mode of counting, since many commercial scintillation counters are not spectrometers and will operate only on the threshold basis. In many situations these instruments are capable of doing a creditable job, provided they are operated with intelligence and understanding.

Figure 5–28 shows the differential (i.e., window) and integral (threshold) spectra for a small source, suspended in air in a plastic container 3 mm. thick. The nuclide is ^{133}Ba, which emits several gamma rays plus a 31 kev. x-ray from the cesium daughter. For the differential spectrum the count rate was recorded continuously with a rate meter while the window, 5 kev. wide, was swept slowly to the left at a constant speed of 300 kev. per hour. When the differential spectrum was finished, the window-top circuit was inactivated and the window sill, now the threshold, was again swept downward at the same speed, thus providing the integral spectrum shown in the same figure. For the latter the sensitivity was decreased to about 1/16 of its former value in order to keep the curve on the chart, for removal of the window top always makes the count rate higher, especially when the threshold is low.

It is not difficult to visualize the nature of a threshold spectrum. Imagine that we have located a 5 kev. window at the top of the 363 kev. peak in the differential spectrum. It will be counting a tall, narrow strip of area between this peak and the baseline. If the sill is kept where it is and the window top is moved to the right, the area will increase and the count rate will go up, leveling off at a maximum when the window top is well over to the right. There is then little difference between such a count rate and one taken with the threshold at 360 kev. and no window top. Both systems are seeing all of the area lying under the differential curve and to the right of the threshold line.

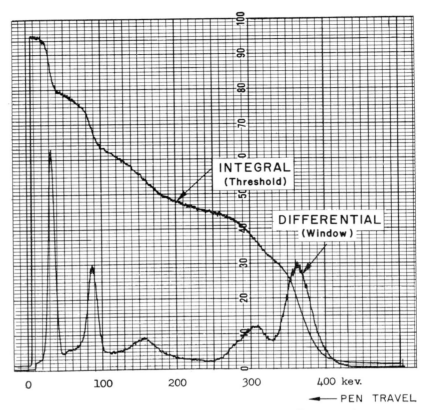

FIGURE 5-28. Differential and integral spectra for a small source of [133]Ba, in air. Note that the integral curve rises more steeply wherever the differential spectrum shows a maximum. Because the integral spectrum is not flat anywhere there may be stability problems. It was recorded at about 1/16 sensitivity to keep it on the chart. (Spectra courtesy of ORINS Medical Division, from Ross et al., 1965.)

If we now move the threshold toward the left, the area increases, rapidly where the differential curve is high above the baseline (because there the strips of area being added on are tall), and slowly where it is lower. As the threshold moves to the left, the area always grows, and therefore the integral curve is always rising. There are no peaks in the integral spectrum.

The positions of the peaks in the differential spectrum are indicated in the integral spectrum by places where the curve rises steeply. It is opposite the peaks that area is being added most rapidly by the moving threshold. Thus the integral curve is steep near 363 and 85 kev., where the differential spectrum is well above the baseline; in fact, the integral curve is equally steep at these two places because the two peaks in the differential spectrum are about the same height. The integral curve is still steeper in the 31 kev. region, where the peak is higher. Conversely, it slopes only gently at 450, 240, and 10 kev., where the differential spectrum is low.

It is the absence of spectral peaks that makes the calibration of a threshold instrument's E dial awkward. In a spectrometer all one has to do is search out a dial setting for a maximum count rate, whereas in a threshold instrument one has to find a setting where the rate is rising most steeply. This is a much greater chore.

Operating Policies. In some threshold instruments, the only way to set the threshold is by means of a potentiometer located inside the cabinet; some instruments have a control on the panel. How do you decide where to set it?

As in the case of the spectrometer, it depends on the problem. For *scatter rejection* a threshold system can be nearly as effective as a window: the threshold is placed in the trough just to the left of the primary peak, since nearly all the scatter will fall below this level. For dealing with *background* this same location will probably be adequate, although the only way to be sure is to test several threshold positions, determine S^2/B for each (p. 171), and then select the best. Background may be more of a hazard in a threshold instrument than in a spectrometer because the absence of a window top allows a wide band of high-energy gamma rays to contribute to background; one can only hope that they will not be too numerous. *Stability* is likely to be the most urgent problem, for the continually climbing integral curve (Fig. 5–28) provides no plateau anywhere, and stability is therefore never as good as in a properly operated spectrometer. One should select the place where the *per cent change in count rate*, per kev. of threshold shift, *is lowest*. Anything that can be done to prevent threshold shift or gain change will be highly desirable.

In many commercial threshold counters there is no panel E dial, but only an internal threshold, which is left at a constant setting, and a continuously variable high-voltage control. Since the high voltage controls the phototube gain, the higher the gain, the more pulses will exceed the threshold and be counted. A plot of count rate versus high voltage is approximately the mirror image of the integral spectrum shown in Figure 5–28; the high count rates will be toward the right, since the higher the voltage, the more the counts. The relationship between count rate and high voltage is not linear (it is a power function—see p. 142) so the curve will be compressed at the right-hand end. Control over effective threshold by the high voltage is better than nothing, although it is important to remember that the gain changes *very rapidly* with high voltage.

Virtues and Vices. We can summarize the advantages and disadvantages of threshold counters. They are electrically simpler than spectrometers, are cheaper, and fail less frequently. The count rates with threshold machines are higher, other things being equal, since a wide band of energies is accepted. The background rates are also higher, so the increased count rate is helpful only if the S^2/B has actually increased. As in the spectrometer, a characteristic threshold position is needed for each nuclide. Dial calibration is quick and easy with a spectrometer, but is a time-consuming nuisance in the threshold instrument. Stability is inferior in threshold operation, for the integral spectrum has no flat regions.

CONCLUSION

The virtues of the spectrometer in nuclear medicine, and its vices, may be summarized. The spectrometer offers the operator:

(1) A means of determining which gamma energies the instrument is

counting, and the ability to adjust the energy pass band to the counting problem at hand;

(2) Relative freedom from errors due to scattered radiation;

(3) A greatly improved signal-to-background ratio, since most of the background is not recorded;

(4) Improved stability, when the instrument is operated correctly;

(5) Greater freedom in using two nuclides together, since the instrument can, within limits, select the characteristic radiations individually;

(6) A powerful analytical tool that can check the radiochemical purity of supplied material, or establish the identity of an unknown nuclide, through the plotting out of the gamma-ray spectrum.

These advantages become available only at a price. A spectrometer is somewhat more expensive than an ordinary "threshold" scaler, which, in effect, has a window sill but no window top. There are more components in a spectrometer and some of these may fail. It requires careful and informed operation.

PHYSICAL PRINCIPLES OF RADIONUCLIDE SCANNING[23]

David E. Kuhl

Radionuclide scanning provides pictures of the body distribution of radiopharmaceuticals that have been administered to the patient, for the purpose of medical diagnosis. At the turn of the century, radiographic examination revolutionized medicine by making possible inspection of internal organs without incision. The recent introduction of radionuclide scanning has been another major advance in the search for better ways to evaluate the structure and function of internal organs without injury to the patient.

The important advantages of scanning depend on characteristics peculiar to the technique. A typical advantage of any study using a radioactive label is that extremely small amounts of material can be measured very precisely. Initially this measurement was possible only when a sample of urine, feces, blood, or tissue was separated from the patient. It was soon recognized that gamma-rays penetrate body tissues and can be detected externally. Scanning extends this detection to picture formation and gives information concerning the spatial distribution and the amount of radioactive material within a living patient.

Usually scanning is a search for structural information, and answers questions about the presence or absence of a lesion, or about position, size, boundaries, and relationships of normal and diseased structures. More recently, scanning has been applied to quantitative measurement of organ function as well. Both kinds of information depend on a prior knowledge that specific differences can

[23] Supported by USAEC Contract No. AT (30-1)-3175(USPHS Research Grant No. C-4456, and USPHS Research Career Program Award CA-14,020 from the National Cancer Institute. NYO-3175-34.

exist between normal and abnormal tissues in the selective accumulation of radioactivity.

At first, scanning appears to be the simplest of procedures, but closer examination shows that the overall detection system is a complex one. Too often a potential application fails when the administered radioactivity is restricted by the radiation dose to the patient, or the differential concentration between the structure and its surroundings is small and transient, or the detector makes poor use of the emitted radiation, and the final picture is unintelligible. For success, each part of this complex diagnostic system must be chosen for optimal efficiency. If the physician is to be effective in supervising and interpreting the results of the procedure, he must understand these complexities, especially if he hopes to contribute to the advance of this rapidly developing field.

The fundamental problems in scanning concern the biological and physical properties of the labeled compound, the configuration and location of the structure to be visualized, and the performance of the detection instrument.

THE LABELED COMPOUND

The suitability of a labeled compound in scanning depends on the physical properties of the label and the biological properties of the compound.

The radionuclide should emit gamma-rays that are sufficiently energetic to penetrate tissue and get out of the body, but not so energetic that they easily penetrate the shielding of the detecting device. These requirements usually limit the choice of photons for scanning to those in the energy range of 20 to 600 kev.

Ideally the radionuclide should emit no alpha particles, beta particles, conversion electrons, or very low-energy photons since these have an extremely limited range in tissue and contribute to the radiation dose without providing useful information. The radiation dose from these useless emissions is important since it limits the amount of radioactive material that can be given to the patient.

The biological properties of the compound should permit selective partitioning of its distribution between structures of interest. A variety of physiologic mechanisms have been employed to obtain this differential: active transport of iodine into the thyroid gland, phagocytosis of colloids by liver cells, red cell sequestration in the spleen, capillary blockade with macromolecules in the lungs, diffusion of small molecules into brain tumors, and localization of large molecules in blood compartments (Wagner, 1964). The most favorable situation is that in which there is a large quantity of radioactivity in the structure to be visualized and little or none in the surrounding areas.

The time course of the labeled compound in the structure is determined by biological mechanisms as well as the physical half-life of the label. This time course influences the choice of the time of study as well as the amount of radioactive material given. Any radioactivity remaining after completion of the study provides no more information but contributes radiation dose to the patient and limits the amount of radioactive material that can be used. The optimal effective half-life is slightly less than the amount of time between injection and the study (Wagner and Emmons, 1965). For a detailed discussion of radiopharmaceuticals, the reader is referred to Chapter VI.

THE STRUCTURE TO BE SEEN

The anatomical features of the internal organs also influence the radiation pattern projected from the body. These are the least controllable parameters of the study system. Even in an idealized system, the cross-sectional area and thickness of the structure determine the intensity of the emitted photons. The signal is reduced with increasing distance of the structure from the detector (divergence) and with thickness of overlying tissues (attenuation). Surrounding tissues can add scattered radiation to the signal. In a real system, there are additional anatomical complexities. The configuration of the structure's edge and the presence of neighboring structures may be crucial factors which determine whether or not the information of interest can be obtained. Respiration or other types of motion may further blur the data. Overlying ribs and arms may shield the region of interest and peculiar deformities of posture may add additional challenges.

THE IMAGING DEVICE

The imaging device portrays the three-dimensional distribution of radioactivity as a two-dimensional picture. A lens system would suffice if gamma-rays could be focused, but they cannot. An autoradiograph would suffice if the patient were a thin sheet of radioactivity, but he is not. Other means must be used to reconstruct the image of radioactivity deep within the body.

There are two types of imaging instruments. The first is the *moving detector device,* or scanner, with which the distribution of radioactivity is recorded by establishing a relative motion between the detector and the subject over the entire region of interest. The second is the *stationary detector device,* or camera, which is not moved, but views the entire field of interest and records the distribution from all points simultaneously.

Both types of instruments have two major parts, a *detection system* and a *display* (Fig. 5-29). The detection system also has two parts, a *collimator* and an *image converter.* The collimator forms an image of the distribution of radioactivity by passing only gamma-rays coming from selected directions. The image converter, a combination of a *detector component* and a *data transfer component,* responds to the radiation image passed by the collimator and converts it to a pattern of signals to which the display unit responds. The display unit reproduces this pattern of signals as a visible picture representing the original spatial distribution of radioactivity.

There is no completely satisfactory imaging system; moving detector devices are better for some applications, and stationary detector devices are better for others. A perfect imaging device would effectively use every incident photon to form a signal which would be positioned in exactly the same pattern as that from which the photons originated. All real instruments distort and obscure this information to some extent. Even if a perfect imaging device existed, it would not be possible to distinguish images of radioactive structures if too few photons arrived at the detector. The common limitations of all scanning procedures at present are that the number of photons emerging from the patient is small and our efficiency in using these photons to form images is poor. Regardless of the imaging system used, the best picture results when there is a maximal differential in recorded photons between a structure and its surroundings, and when enough photons have been recorded to make the statistical reliability of this difference high. Sensitivity and spatial resolution are two concepts that are useful in characterizing how well an imaging system can accomplish this.

Sensitivity, as a general term, describes how many counts a detection system will record from a known distribution of radioactivity. Sensitivity is usually expressed as the ratio of the number of counts measured to the number of photons emitted from a source under specified conditions. *Spatial resolution,* as a general term, describes the maximal capability of a detection system to distinguish fine spatial detail in a distribution of radioactivity, in the idealized circumstance when a sufficiently large number of counts are available so that random fluctuations are negligible and background counts need not be considered. Several different expressions of spatial resolution are in use. Usually an improvement in either sensitivity or spatial resolution is at the expense of the other and a compromise must be effected for best results. For example, if the spatial resolution of a detection system is too fine, sensitivity may be too low and statistical fluctuations may obscure real differences in the distribution of radioactivity. However, if spatial resolution is too poor, although sensitivity will be high, important spatial details such as boundaries and interfaces will be obscured. To show more clearly this compromise between sensitivity and spatial resolution we will describe these concepts more specifically.

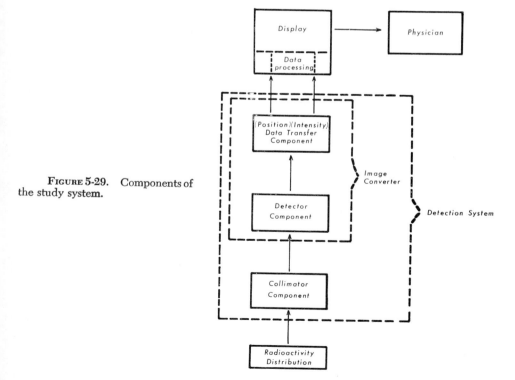

FIGURE 5-29.   Components of the study system.

CHARACTERIZING THE RESPONSE OF A DETECTION SYSTEM: SENSITIVITY AND SPATIAL RESOLUTION[24]

TOTAL RESPONSE

The *response,* or output, of the detection system is the spatial distribution of counts representing the spatial distribution of radioactivity in the source. This representation is a distortion of the original pattern because of absorption and scatter processes within the source and distortions introduced by each component of the detection system. The total counting rate, C_t, corresponding to a small part of the distribution, is due to collimated primary radiation, C_{coll}, scattered radiation, C_{scat}, and primary radiation that has penetrated the collimator septa or shielding of the detection system, C_{penet}, or:

$$C_t = C_{coll} + C_{scat} + C_{penet} \tag{1}$$

The scatter fraction (f_s) and penetration fraction (f_t) designate the relative contribution to the total counting rate of scattered radiation and primary radiation that penetrates the septa or shielding (Beck, 1966).

These two fractions are defined as:

$$f_s = \text{scatter fraction} = \frac{C_{scat}}{C_{coll}}$$

$$f_p = \text{penetration fraction} = \frac{C_{penet}}{C_{coll}}$$

Then
$$C_t = C_{coll} (1 + f_s + f_p) \tag{2}$$

First we will consider the ideal case when there is negligible penetrating and scattered radiation ($C_t = C_{coll}$), and no attenuation in the source.

RESPONSE TO COLLIMATED PRIMARY RADIATION

EFFICIENCY

In an ideal system in which penetrating radiation, scatter, and attenuation in the source are negligible, the only significant distortions of the response occur within components of the detection system. A common distortion is a smaller number of output signals from a component than input signals to the component. This loss of counting data is specified by the term *efficiency,* ϵ, for each component and is defined as the ratio of the number of output events to the number of input events for the component. This fraction expresses the performance of the component with respect to its theoretical maximal performance, when the efficiency should equal one.

The efficiency of the entire detection system, ϵ_{syst}, is equal to the product of the efficiencies of its component parts (Fig. 5-29). Therefore the efficiencies of

---

[24] This formulation of sensitivity and spatial resolution evolved from discussion among the following people in the period from 1963 to 1967: W. J. MacIntyre, Chairman; S. O. Fedoruk; C. C. Harris; D. E. Kuhl; and J. R. Mallard.

the entire detection system, ϵ_{syst}, the collimator, ϵ_g, the image converter, ϵ_i, the detector component, ϵ_d, and the data transfer component, ϵ_{dt}, are related as:

$$\epsilon_{syst} = \epsilon_g \, \epsilon_i = \epsilon_g \, \epsilon_d \, \epsilon_{dt} \qquad (3)$$

Collimator efficiency, ϵ_g, is the ratio of the number of photons passing through the open space of the collimator to the number of photons emitted by the source. This fraction is independent of photon energy and is dependent only on geometrical considerations of collimator construction (scatter, attenuation, and septum penetration are neglected).

Image converter efficiency, ϵ_i, is the ratio of the number of recorded counts to the number of primary photons incident on the detector. This fraction is dependent on the energy of the primary photons incident on the detector. Image converter efficiency is equal to the product of the efficiencies of its parts, the detector component and the data transfer component. The detector efficiency, ϵ_d, is the ratio of the number of ionizing events that take place in the detector to the number of primary photons incident on the detector. The data transfer efficiency, ϵ_{dt}, is the ratio of the number of counts recorded to the number of ionizing events in the detector.

SENSITIVITY

The *point sensitivity*, S_p, of the detection system is defined as the fraction of photons per unit time detected from a point source in air at any position in space. If C_p is the counting rate measured for a source emitting ρ_p photons per unit time,

$$C_p = \rho_p \, \epsilon_{syst} \qquad (4)$$

and

$$S_p = \frac{C_p}{\rho_p} = \epsilon_{syst} = \epsilon_i \, \epsilon_g = \epsilon_i \, \Omega \qquad (5)$$

where Ω represents the geometrical fractional solid angle of view of the detector seen through the collimator by the point source.

(The point sensitivity, S_p, and the efficiency, ϵ_{syst}, are equal only in the ideal case considered here in which penetrating radiation, scatter, and attenuation in the source are negligible.)

If a point source is moved linearly across the aperture of a collimator in a direction perpendicular to the length, L, of the collimator such that the emission rate is ρ photons per unit length, the integrated response would be the same as the counting rate from a line source emitting ρ_L photons per unit time per unit length and occupying the same position as the path traversed by the point.

$$C_L = \int_y \rho_L \, S_p \, dy \qquad (6)$$

and

$$S_L = \frac{C_L}{\rho_L} = \int_y S_p \, dy \qquad (7)$$

where C_L is the counting rate measured from a line source emitting ρ_L photons per unit time per unit length, and *line sensitivity*, S_L, is the sensitivity of the detector to a line source of concentration ρ_L photons per unit time per unit length.

The variation of the line sensitivity, S_L, with transverse displacement of the line source at a distance Z from the collimator face is defined as the *line-spread function*, $S_L(x)$, and is illustrated in Figure 5-30.

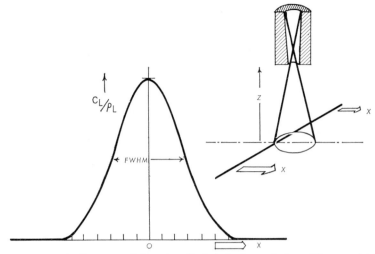

Figure 5-30. The line-spread function, S_L (x), is the variation of line sensitivity, S_L (i.e., the counts recorded per photon emitted per unit length), as a line source is moved across the axis of the collimator at the distance Z. The full width at half maximum (F.W.H.M.) is the distance in centimeters between half-maximum values on this profile.

The *plane sensitivity*, S_a, is defined as the ratio of the number of photons recorded by the detection system to the number of photons emitted per unit area from an extended plane source perpendicular to the collimator axis containing a uniform concentration of radioactive material which emits ρ_a photons per unit time per unit area. If C_a is the counting rate for a plane source at any distance, Z, from the collimator face,

$$C_a = \int_x \int_y \rho_a S_p \, dx \, dy \qquad (8)$$

and

$$S_a = \frac{C_a}{\rho_a} = \int_x \int_y S_p \, dx \, dy \qquad (9)$$

where the integral is taken at the distance Z.

The integration of the line-spread function over the entire field of interest is identical with the measurement of S_a provided that the line source is sufficiently long to cover fully the field of view at all distances of the source to the collimator face. Thus, for an extended line source of concentration ρ_L photons per unit time per unit length, plane sensitivity is given by

$$S_a = \frac{\int_x C_L \, dx}{\rho_L} = \int_x S_L \, dx \qquad (10)$$

Plane sensitivity is of special importance in the comparison of detection systems. This is because the response to a plane source is independent of the distance from the detector, provided the plane source covers the field of view uniformly and attenuation, penetration, and scatter are negligible (Mayneord, 1950; Beck, 1961). On the other hand, point sensitivity and line sensitivity do not possess this property and must be spatially localized before the measured sensitivities can be used for system comparisons.

SPATIAL RESOLUTION

Spatial resolution refers to the capability to distinguish the fine details in a spatial distribution of radioactivity. Various attempts have been made to characterize spatial resolution. For example, some investigators have measured spatial resolution in terms of the minimal distance by which two point sources could be separated and still be distinguished. This method is imprecise and depends on the criteria of detecting the separation. Other investigators have used the width of the counting rate profile from a single line source or point source at an arbitrary level. The most common index of this type is the full width at half maximum (F.W.H.M.), the distance in centimeters between the half-maximum value response of the counting rate profile recorded at a specific distance Z between the source and collimator face (Fig. 5-30). This single value is too simple to describe fully the ability of the detection system to respond to fine spatial detail. The *modulation transfer function* (M.T.F.) is a more complete description of spatial resolution.

The M.T.F. was developed to analyze the performance of imaging systems in several other fields (Perrin, 1960; Morgan, 1962). Beck (1964a, b, 1966) and others (Cradduck et al., 1966; Frey, 1966; Gopalo Rao and Wagner, 1967) have recently applied this concept to describe the spatial resolution of scanning.

The *object modulation,* m_o, or object contrast, for a plane sinusoidal distribution of radioactivity is the ratio of the difference to the sum of the maximum and minimum concentrations of radioactivity. The object modulation may be expressed by the equation:

$$m_o = \frac{\rho_{max} - \rho_{min}}{\rho_{max} + \rho_{min}} \tag{11}$$

where ρ_{max} and ρ_{min} are the maximum and minimum concentrations of activity of the plane sinusoidal distributions (Fig. 5-31).

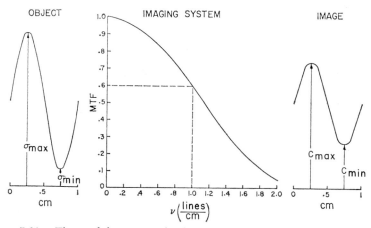

FIGURE 5-31. The modulation transfer function, M.T.F., is the efficiency of transferring the object modulation to the image modulation for a spatial frequency component of a radioactive distribution. In this example, the object modulation of a one-line-per-centimeter structure is $m_o = \dfrac{\rho_{max} - \rho_{min}}{\rho_{max} + \rho_{min}} = \dfrac{0.9 - 0.1}{0.9 + 0.1} = 0.8$, and is transferred by the detection system with an efficiency (M.T.F.) of 0.6 to an image modulation given by $m_e = m_o \times$ M.T.F. $= (0.8)(0.6)$ $= 0.48$. (Adapted from Beck et al., 1967.)

The *image modulation,* m_c, or the image contrast, is the ratio of the difference to the sum of the corresponding observed counting rates. The image modulation may be expressed by the equation:

$$m_c = \frac{C_{max} - C_{min}}{C_{max} + C_{min}} \tag{12}$$

where C_{max} and C_{min} are the maximum and minimum observed counting rates over the plane sinusoidal distribution (Fig. 5-31).

The *M.T.F.* is the efficiency of transfering the object modulation, or object contrast, of a radioactive distribution to an observed counting rate modulation, or image contrast, and is stated for each separation distance between the objects. It is given by the expression:

$$\text{M.T.F.} = \frac{m_c}{m_o} = \frac{\text{image modulation}}{\text{object modulation}} \tag{13}$$

To describe completely the spatial resolution of the detection system for plane sinusoidal distributions at a specific distance Z from the collimator, the M.T.F. must be obtained for an entire range of separation of the two concentrations (Fig. 5-31). This could be accomplished by measuring radioactive models, but that would be tedious. All the required data are contained in the line-spread function (Fig. 5-30) from which the M.T.F. can be calculated for all values of spatial frequency.

The M.T.F. is the Fourier transform of the line-spread function and can be calculated for all values of separation (expressed as spatial frequency in terms of lines per centimeter) by measurement of the line spread function alone (Perrin, 1960).

$$\text{M.T.F.} = \frac{\int_{-\infty}^{+\infty} S_L \cos 2\pi\nu x \, dx}{\int_{-\infty}^{+\infty} S_L \, dx} \tag{14}$$

In theory, all radiation images may be resolved into a spectrum of spatial frequencies. The M.T.F. predicts the response of the detection system to the included spatial frequencies. The M.T.F. may be determined in several ways, but the most convenient is to determine the line-spread function and compute the Fourier transform of it. The M.T.F. reflects the maximum capability of the system for transferring spatial information. For validity, the detection system must be operated within its region of linear amplitude (output proportional to input) and sufficient counts must be available to make random fluctuation negligible when the line-spread function is determined.

Indices such as the F.W.H.M. of the line-spread function can be useful, but the M.T.F. is a much more rigorous and versatile characterization of spatial resolution. For example, broadening of the line-spread function due to penetrating radiation occurs primarily below the half-maximum point. The degradation of spatial resolution will be shown by an attenuation of the M.T.F., but may not be reflected when F.W.H.M. is cited.

The M.T.F. is of special use in analysis of the entire detection system, since the composite M.T.F. of the entire system may be determined by multiplying the M.T.F. of the component parts, frequency by frequency, across the range of spatial frequencies.

CONCLUSIONS

1. The most useful expressions for characterizing the response of a detection system in terms of sensitivity and spatial resolution are the plane sensitivity, S_a, and the modulation transfer function, M.T.F. Plane sensitivity has only one value for sources in air at all distances, when penetration and scatter are negligible, and therefore does not require an arbitrary choice of source position or source dimension. The M.T.F. is a complete description of spatial resolution at a specific distance Z from the collimator.

2. The line-spread function can be easily measured and accurately reproduced in different laboratories (Hine and Vetter, 1965; Hine, in press), and contains all the data required for calculation of both the plane sensitivity and the M.T.F. Plane sensitivity, S_a, can be determined by integrating the line-spread function. The M.T.F. can be computed as the Fourier tranform of the line-spread function.

IMAGING DEVICES

MOVING DETECTOR DEVICES (SCANNERS)

In the moving detector device, or scanner, systematic relative motion is established between the detector and the distribution of radioactivity, counting

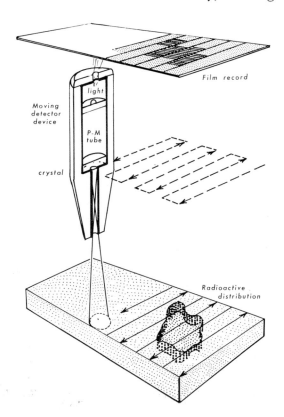

FIGURE 5-32. Moving detector device. A collimated detector device is moved in a rectilinear raster over the distribution of radioactivity which is reproduced as a photorecording.

data are collected sequentially, and the distribution is finally reproduced as a two-dimensional picture (Fig. 5-32). This was the first type of imaging device to be introduced in nuclear medicine (Cassen et al., 1951; Mayneord and Newberry, 1952) and is still the most commonly used.

The collimator is usually a radiation-opaque shield that restricts the field of view to radiation coming through one or more holes from a small volume of the radioactive object at any one time. Alternatively, time-coincident detection can be used for collimation of photons that possess inherent directional properties, that is, positron annihilation radiation (Wrenn et al., 1951; Brownell and Sweet, 1953).

The image converter (see page 186) has two parts: the detector, usually a scintillation phosphor, and the data transfer component (see Fig. 5-29).

The scintillation phosphor is usually a sodium iodide (Tl) crystal measuring ½ to 8 in. in diameter and from ½ to 2 in. in thickness. The larger crystals increase the sensitivity of the detection system, but also require more heavy shielding and introduce additional problems.

The data transfer component consists of the intensity unit and the positional unit.

The intensity unit is usually a photomultiplier tube, a linear amplifier, and a discriminator. Upper and lower discriminators are adjusted to pass only those pulses from the photomultiplier tube that are associated with primary radiation and to reject a large number of those pulses associated with scattered radiation (Allen et al., 1954, 1955; Francis et al., 1955). The interrelation of phosphor, photomultiplier tube, and discriminator has already been described in this chapter.

The positional unit is a system of motors that move the detector over the patient's body in a systematic and preset pattern. The most common scanning pattern is a rectilinear raster, that is, alternate back and forth motion on successive lines until the entire field of study is systematically scanned.[25] The limits of the field of study are chosen to include the structures of interest. The line spacing and scan speed are preset so that enough counts for a good picture will be recorded in a tolerable period of examination time. Usually this examination time is 15 minutes to 1 hour in duration.

The most common display for moving detector devices is *photorecording* on film (Kuhl et al., 1956; Bender and Blau, 1959; Herring, 1960). As counts are detected, a light is caused to flash as it is moved mechanically back and forth over film with a motion synchronous to the detector; a photographic picture of the distribution of radioactivity is produced (Fig. 5-33A).

THE COLLIMATOR COMPONENT[26]

The response of an ideal detection system (i.e., when $C_t == C_{coll}$ and $\epsilon_1 = 1$; see equations 2 and 5) can theoretically be calculated in terms of the collimator efficiency, ϵ_g, which depends only on the collimator dimensions and configuration. These calculations are limited in applicability, but have been used by many

---

[25] The early Greeks called the rectilinear raster *Boustrophedon* (as the ox turns) in describing their ancient form of writing in which the lines run, as in plowing, alternately left to right and right to left.

[26] This formulation of sensitivity and spatial resolution evolved from discussion among the following people in the period from 1963 to 1967: W. J. MacIntyre, Chairman; S. O. Fodoruk; C. C. Harris; D. E. Kuhl; and J. R. Mallard.

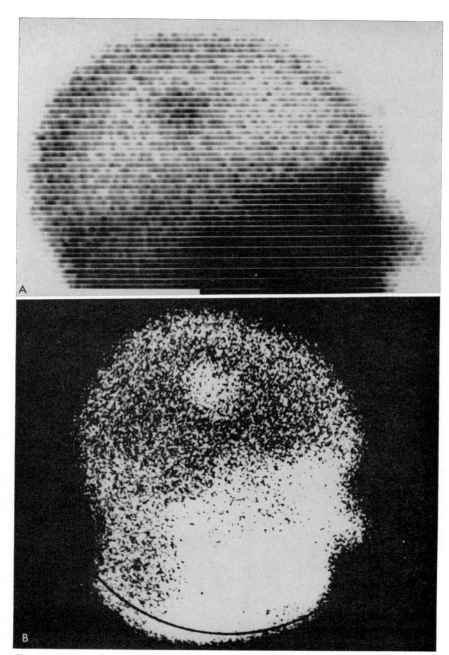

FIGURE 5-33. Photorecordings of brain metastasis in right parietal lobe made using 10 mc. of ^{99m}Tc pertechnetate. A, Scanner view at 40 minutes after injection. Three-inch diameter crystal with focused collimator. Twelve-minute study time. B, Camera view at 3 hours after injection. Eleven-inch crystal with multihole collimator. Two-minute study time.

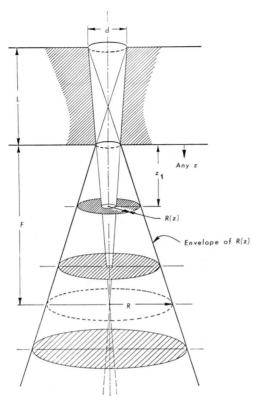

FIGURE 5-34. Single-hole collimator with tapered walls. The field of view enlarges as the distance, z, increases. (From MacIntyre et al., to be published.)

investigators in order to better understand what the real system is measuring (Beck, 1961, 1964b; Brownell, 1958, 1959, 1962; Courtial and Gandy, 1964; Cradduck and Fedoruk, 1962; Dewey and Sinclair, 1961; Ephraim, 1964; Francis et al., 1962; Harris et al., 1963a, 1964; Myers and Mallard, 1964; Myhill, 1961; Newell et al., 1952; Rotenberg and Johns, 1965; Simons, 1962, 1964; Van der Does de Bye, 1956).

The simplest collimator has a single hole in a lead shield (Fig. 5-34). The hole may have straight or tapered walls. The field of view defined by a single-hole collimator enlarges as the distance, Z, from the collimator increases. The geometric radius of view at any distance, Z, is called R. At the focal distance, F, of a tapered hole, the geometrical radius of view is given by the expression:

$$R_F = \frac{F}{L} d \qquad (15)$$

where d is the hole diameter at the large end and L is the collimator length. It has been shown (Harris et al., 1964) that the radius, R_F, is approximately the same as the F.W.H.M. of the response for collimators with no septum penetration.

The single-hole collimator has largely been replaced by the multihole focused collimator (Newell et al., 1952) in which many tapered holes are used with a single large detector (Fig. 5-35). This arrangement increases the number of photons passing through the collimator by N, the number of holes, while keeping the radius of the field of view in the focal plane, R_F, approximately the same as that of a single-hole collimator. The multihole focused collimator with a large crystal is an improvement over the single-hole collimator with a small crystal because sensitivity is improved while spatial resolution is preserved in the focal plane.

The point-spread function, or the rise and fall of counting rate as a point source is moved across the field of view, can be calculated in the focal plane and is approximately triangular in shape. Point-spread functions at other distances from the collimator are more difficult to calculate and exhibit other shapes, ranging from an approximately rectangular shape at the collimator face to a nearly Gaussian configuration at distances beyond the focal plane. These calculations are valuable in the design of collimators; in practice, system performance is evaluated using experimental data.

To characterize the response of the entire detection system to sources in air, in terms of sensitivity and spatial resolution, we need only make simple experimental measurements of a line source. Line-spread functions may be obtained by plotting counting rate versus distance as a capillary tube filled with a radioactive solution is moved in a straight line perpendicular to the central axis of the collimator.

Plane sensitivity, S_a, the response to a uniform plane source, is obtained by integrating the line-spread function over one dimension (equation 10). This term is useful in comparing the response of different detection systems under similar conditions. Conditions of measurement, such as source dimensions, source material, photon energy, and discriminator setting must be specified.

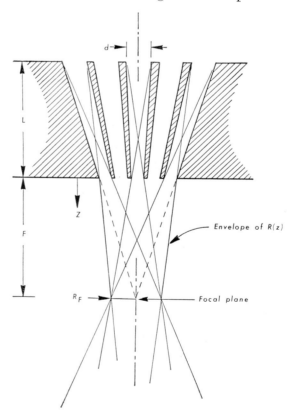

FIGURE 5-35.   Multihole focused collimator. The field of view is smallest in the focal plane. (From MacIntyre et al., to be published.)

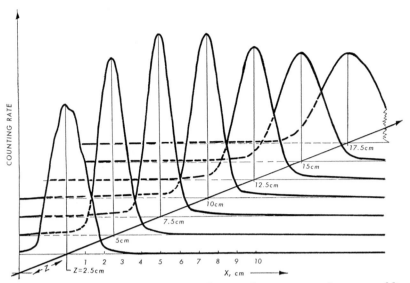

FIGURE 5-36. The response of a moving detector device expressed as a set of line-spread functions measured at different distances, Z, from a multihole focused collimator with a 7.5 cm. focal distance. (Adapted from Hine, in press.)

Plane sensitivity, S_a, for an air medium is approximately the same at all distances Z from the collimator, provided penetrating radiation, C_{penet}, is an insignificant part of the total response.

A set of line-spread functions measured at different distances from the collimator (Fig. 5-36) contains the information necessary to describe completely the spatial resolution of the detection system. The F.W.H.M. may be obtained directly from the plotted data. The M.T.F. (Fig. 5-37) is a more complete expression of the spatial resolution and can be computed by taking the Fourier transform of each line-spread function (p. 192).

The total response of the detection system includes primary collimated radiation, scattered radiation, and penetrating radiation (equations 1 and 2). The scatter fraction, f_s, depends chiefly on the source medium, source dimensions, photon energy, and discriminator settings. Attenuation in a volume distribution of radioactivity decreases the quantity of primary radiation, but may increase the quantity of scattered radiation reaching the detector. The penetration fraction, f_p, depends chiefly on the photon energy, collimator material, and collimator design and construction. Since attenuation in the collimator material is exponential, penetrating radiation can never be completely eliminated, but will be insignificant when low-energy photons are used with a properly designed and constructed collimator of high-density material.

When the contribution of scattered radiation and penetrating radiation is appreciable, the line-spread function is changed as shown in Figure 5-38A. Detection of this radiation that originates outside the geometrical field of view results in a broadening of the line-spread function, degradation of the M.T.F. (Fig. 5-38B), and increase in plane sensitivity, S_a, by the factor $(f_s + f_p)$. The factor $(f_s + f_p)$ is equal to the difference between the integrals of the line-spread functions measured with and without scatter and penetration.

The total response of a moving detector device can be measured to test

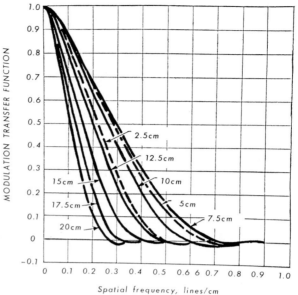

FIGURE 5-37. Modulation transfer functions computed by taking the Fourier transform of each line-spread function in Figure 5-36. (From MacIntyre et al., to be published.)

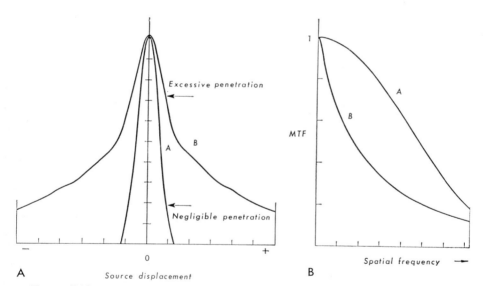

FIGURE 5-38. Detection of septum-penetrating radiation broadens the line-spread function (A) and degrades the M.T.F. (B). (From MacIntyre et al., to be published.)

whether it is performing as expected with a specific radionuclide. The response to a given radionuclide can be characterized in terms of sensitivity by measuring the plane sensitivity, S_a, and spatial resolution can be described in terms of the modulation transfer function using data contained in a set of measured line-spread functions made at different distances, Z, from the collimator in air. These data can be compared with a second set of measurements of a low-energy photon emitter which approximate the response to collimated primary radiation. Unless the two sets of data are identical, there is an appreciable contribution of scattered or penetrating radiation in the original response. Scattered and penetrating radiation broaden the line-spread function, which increases the plane sensitivity, S_a, by the factor $(f_s + f_p)$, and which degrades the M.T.F.

SCANNERS

The most commonly used scanner today has a single sodium iodide (Tl) crystal 3 in. in diameter and 2 in. thick. The most frequently used collimator for this scanner has a focal length of approximately 3 in. and a geometrical radius of view in the focal plane of approximately ½ in. The duration of a scanning study is usually 15 minutes to one hour for each view.

One approach to increasing the speed of the examination is to enlarge the area of the detector. Assuming that the focal distance and geometrical radius of view in the focal plane are the same as with the 3-in. diameter detector, this change should increase the plane sensitivity, S_a, in proportion to the square of the radius of the detector. The threefold gain in sensitivity with a 5-in. diameter detector and the sevenfold increase in sensitivity with an 8-in. diameter detector are considerable improvements over the sensitivity of the ordinary 3-in. diameter crystal, but not without a price. McAfee et al. (1966) have reported the advantages and disadvantages of an 8-in. diameter detector system. The improved sensitivity permits scans to be completed in a fraction of the time required with a 3-in. diameter detector system, but this advantage is at the expense of spatial resolution. A 3-in. diameter detector subtends a solid angle of 25° at the focal point, a 5-in. diameter detector subtends 40°, and an 8-in. diameter detector subtends 45° to 60°. The 3-in. diameter detector maintains spatial resolution approximately constant over a considerable distance on either side of the focal plane; the larger detectors do not. The deterioration of spatial resolution on either side of the focal plane could be reduced if the larger detector were equipped with a collimator of longer focal length, but the sensitivity would fall.

An 8-in. diameter detector with focused collimator is satisfactory for rapid scanning of relatively thin structures that can be positioned in the focal plane, such as kidneys, thyroid, or bone. With a large organ such as the liver, spatial resolution will be poor with this device.

An alternative way to reduce examination time is to use multiple detectors of moderate size. Beck et al. (1967) have constructed a brain scanner with four detectors especially designed for use with lower-energy photons. Although each of the four crystals is only 2 in. in diameter, the overall performance of the four units, each with a very efficient collimator, makes it possible to obtain paired images of superior quality in less than 10 minutes.

Hindel and Gilson (1967) described a high-speed scanning system that includes a 10-channel detector which moves over the patient at speeds from 0.2 to 4 cm./sec. (Fig. 5-39). The lead-shielded detector consists of 10 adjacent, parallel, sodium iodide (Tl) crystals; each is 6 in. long, 2 in. thick, and ⅜ in. wide. Each crystal has its own collimator, photomultiplier tube, amplifier, and pulse-height analyzer. Each operates as a separate detector. On each path along the x-axis, the detector assembly views 10 lines whose widths are determined by the spatial resolution of the collimator. At the end of a pass, the detector assembly steps a selected distance (0.15, 0.3, or 0.6 cm.) and scans the patient again. Since the distance between adjacent channels is 1 in., a complete picture can be obtained in 16, 8, or 4 passes.

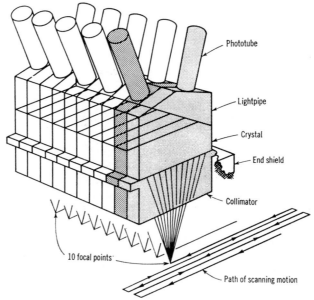

Phototube

Lightpipe

Crystal

End shield

Collimator

10 focal points

Path of scanning motion

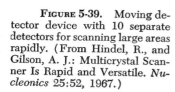

FIGURE 5-39. Moving detector device with 10 separate detectors for scanning large areas rapidly. (From Hindel, R., and Gilson, A. J.: Multicrystal Scanner Is Rapid and Versatile. *Nucleonics* 25:52, 1967.)

This configuration of multiple detectors permits high-speed recording of relatively thick structures without the penalty of poor spatial resolution in positions outside of the focal plane. In addition, this system is readily applied to the scanning of large areas, such as the lungs. The study field is not limited by the size of the detector, as is the case with stationary detector devices.

STATIONARY DETECTOR DEVICES (CAMERAS)

In stationary detector devices, sometimes referred to as cameras, the emission pattern is determined without motion of the detector or the patient. The stationary detector device is of special advantage when all parts of the study field must be examined simultaneously. The stationary detector device is a more recent development than the moving detector device for radionuclide imaging (Anger et al., 1956), but its basic principle is much older. Röntgen (1895) reported using a pin-hole aperture and photographic film to make images of the anode of his x-ray tube. Both the moving and stationary detector devices are essentially a combination of a collimator for producing the radiation image and an image converter for changing this radiation image into a picture (see Fig. 5-29). But in a moving detector device, intensity information and positional information are transferred in separate processes. The data transfer component of the stationary detector device performs both these functions simultaneously.

MEASURING THE RESPONSE[27]

Calculation of the response of the stationary detector device is more difficult than for a moving detector device. Even in an idealized system in which

[27] This formulation of sensitivity and spatial resolution evolved from discussion among the following people in the period from 1963 to 1967: W. J. MacIntyre, Chairman; S. O. Fedoruk; C. C. Harris; D. E. Kuhl; and J. R. Mallard.

scattered and penetrating radiation are negligible and the image converter is assumed to have maximal performance, it is difficult to calculate the expected spatial resolution from a pin-hole collimator, which projects a point source as a coma, or a multihole collimator, which can project a point source as a cluster of images on the detector.

The response of a stationary detector device can be characterized in terms of sensitivity and spatial resolution by using the same principles applied to the moving detector device (pp. 197–199). For each component of both the moving and the stationary detector systems, there is degradation of information. In the moving detector device, the degradation is best described from measurements of the system as a whole. In the stationary detector device, it is more useful to consider separately the geometrical degradation introduced by the collimator and the additional degradation introduced by the image converter. In all practical systems now in use, the most significant distortion of the original image signal occurs in the collimator component.

The total response of a stationary detector system can be characterized in terms of plane sensitivity, S_a, and spatial resolution, as described by the M.T.F., by using a set of measured line-spread functions obtained by moving an uncollimated line source across the face of the collimator at different distances, Z, from the collimator in air. The efficiency and spatial resolution of the image converter can be characterized in terms of efficiency, ϵ_i, and the M.T.F., by using a set of measured line-spread functions obtained by moving a slit-collimated line source across the face of the detector with the collimator removed (Cradduck et al., 1966).

If the response of the image converter is not uniform over the whole area of the detector, the line-spread function and ϵ_i will vary from point to point. The overall variations in efficiencies of the image converter may be expressed as the ratio of the change in ϵ_i to the value of ϵ_i at the center of the detector.

The degradation and the distortion of the response introduced by scattered and penetrating radiation may be treated in a manner similar to that described on p. 199. The line-spread function of the image converter at the point of measurement is the pattern of variation of count rate at that test point as a slit-collimated beam of radiation from a line source is moved across the detector face.

The plane sensitivity, S_a, is the integral of all line-spread functions obtained by moving an uncollimated line source across the field of view. When the area of the object is less than the field of view of the detector, A_v, it is more meaningful to express sensitivity in terms of plane sensitivity per unit area of the field of view, or $\dfrac{S_a}{A_v}$.

All investigators do not yet use common expressions for sensitivity and spatial resolution. If they did, it would be less difficult to compare the performances of different stationary detector devices than it is now.

THE COLLIMATOR COMPONENT

The three types of collimation for a stationary detector system are pin-hole collimation, multihole collimation, and positron-coincidence collimation. Positron-coincidence collimation will be described on p. 208.

Pin-Hole Collimation. The pin-hole collimator (Fig. 5-40) is a shallow aperture at the end of a conical lead shield that projects an inverted radiation image onto the detector (Röntgen, 1895; Anger, 1958, 1963, 1966; Mallard and Myers, 1963a and b; Jammett et al., 1964; Cradduck and Fedoruk, 1965). The aperture is usually lined with tungsten, platinum, or other high-density materials and has a diameter measuring approximately 1/16 to 3/8 in. The diameter of the pin-hole defines the solid angle of radiation accepted by the collimator for each point of the source and, therefore, influences both the spatial resolution and sensitivity of the detection system.

The line-spread function for a test point on the detector can be obtained by moving a line source across the pin-hole at distance Z and plotting the variation in counting rate at the test point with respect to the distance. Enlarging the aperture widens the line-spread function and degrades the spatial resolution, but increases the plane sensitivity, S_a.

When the distances L and Z are increased, but the diameter, D, is kept the same, spatial resolution will be improved and will be reflected in narrowing of the line-spread function. But the plane sensitivity, S_a, will decrease, since the angular field of view is decreased.

When the diameter of the detector, D, is increased, both plane sensitivity, S_a, and spatial resolution are improved. A larger object can be viewed at a shorter distance (angular field of view is increased) and there is a corresponding improvement in plane sensitivity, S_a. At the same time, spatial resolution is improved, since the line-spread function is narrowed as the distance, Z, is reduced.

Although sensitivity and spatial resolution can be improved by increasing the diameter of the detector, this change exaggerates other problems of magni-

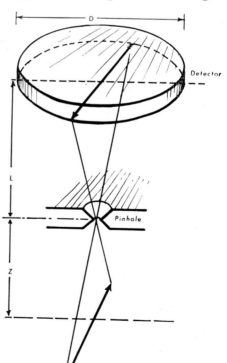

FIGURE 5-40. Pin-hole collimator projects inverted radiation image on detector.

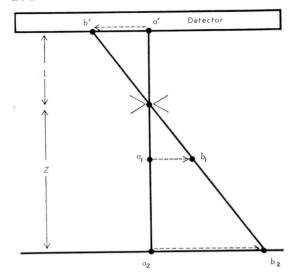

FIGURE 5-41. Pin-hole collimator distortion. The short line source, a_2-b_2, and the shorter line source, a_1-b_1, project the same radiation image, $a'-b'$, on the detector. The geometrical shape of the radiation image and that of the radioactive object do not coincide when pin-hole collimation is used.

fication and distortion (Mallard and Myers, 1963a and b). The angular field of view of the pin-hole collimator makes impossible a true plane view (orthogonal projection) of the distribution. One consequence of this inherent distortion is illustrated in Figure 5-41. The radiation image of point b_2 will coincide with the radiation image of point b_1 on the detector. The length of the radiation image of the short line source a_2-b_2 will be the same on the detector as the length of the shorter line source a_1-b_1. The radiation image enlarges as the distance, Z, decreases and the geometrical shape of the radiation image will not coincide with that of the radioactive object.

Other distortions are inherent in the pin-hole design. At the periphery of the detector a point source is imaged as a coma (commatic aberration), and a unit distance on the detector represents a greater distance on the object than at the center (pin-cushion distortion).

The magnification distortion of the pin-hole collimator is usually a disadvantage, but it can be used to advantage to accommodate subjects of different sizes by placing them close to or far from the aperture. Pin-hole collimation gives the best combination of sensitivity and resolution and the fewest adverse effects of distortion when used for small objects, such as the thyroid gland, which can be positioned a few inches from the aperture (Anger, 1966b). With an administered dose of 15 to 25 μc. of iodine-131, pictures can be obtained with an Anger camera (p. 206) in 3 to 9 minutes (Anger and Rosenthal, 1959).

Although the pin-hole collimator is well adapted for the study of small objects, the most commonly used collimator for the stationary detector device is the multihole collimator, which is better adapted for the study of larger objects.

The multihole collimator (Fig. 5-42) is an array of straight or tapered holes in an absorbing material that covers the entire area of the detector. The multihole collimator avoids many of the distortion problems encountered with the pin-hole collimator and projects a radiation image on the detector very close in size to that of the object. The field of view is approximately the same regardless of distance.

The spatial resolution is best closest to the multihole collimator and is degraded with increasing distance. The resolution of the focused collimator of a moving detector device is best on the geometric focal plane, which is some distance from the collimator. With both types of collimator, the sensitivity to an extended source is independent of distance, provided attenuation in the object is neglected. Analysis of the spatial resolution of the multihole collimator is complicated by the multiple radiation images produced on the detector by a point source. Photons from a point source pass through more than one hole of the collimator to reach the detector (Fig. 5-42). In this instance, an index of spatial resolution such as the F.W.H.M. of the counting rate profile is not an adequate description of the spatial resolution of the multihole collimator. But M.T.F.s can be obtained from line-spread functions measured as described previously and will adequately describe the degradation in spatial resolution caused by the satellite responses.

The properties of a single-hole collimator, already discussed, also apply to each hole of the multihole collimator. Thus, the performance of the multihole collimator is determined by the number of holes, hole diameter, length of hole, septum thickness, and collimator material. A more efficient collimator can be designed for use with low-energy gamma-rays, since the septa can be thinner and more holes of smaller diameter can be used for a given size crystal. Collimator efficiencies can be improved if multihole collimators are made of tungsten alloy rather than lead because the septa can be thinner and more holes of the same diameter can be used per unit area. An increase in sensitivity of from 21 per cent for collimators designed for 280 kev. to 30 per cent for those designed for 410 kev. is possible (Anger, 1964).

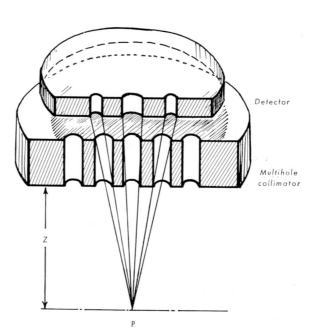

FIGURE 5-42. Multihole collimator with straight-parallel holes. Photons from a point source can pass through more than one hole and produce satellite radiation images on the detector. (Adapted from MacIntyre et al., to be published.)

Detector

Multihole collimator

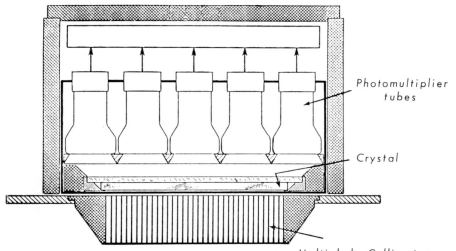

FIGURE 5-43.   Stationary detector device with single phosphor and position-sensing photomultiplier array. (Adapted from Anger, 1966.)

THE IMAGE CONVERTER

The image converter in the stationary detector device is a combination of a large-area detector component and a component for transferring both intensity and positional information. The large-area detector converts the radiation pattern projected by the collimator into a corresponding pattern of interactions which are, in turn, converted by the data transfer device into intensity and positional signals which serve as the input to a picture display. Sensitivity and spatial resolution are limited by the collimator, even before the radiation pattern is presented to the image converter. Further degradation of this information by the image converter can be measured as described on p. 202.

There are three principal kinds of image converters: the phosphor-photomultiplier, the phosphor-image intensifier, and the gas-filled chamber.

Phosphor-Photomultiplier. SINGLE PHOSPHOR WITH POSITION-SENSING PHOTOMULTIPLIER ARRAY.   In 1956, Anger introduced an image converter that became the first practical stationary detector device for clinical diagnostic use. This device is illustrated in Figure 5-43. The collimator projects the radiation image onto an 11-in. diameter sodium iodide (Tl) crystal that is ½ in. thick. The crystal is viewed through a 1½-in.-thick transparent light guide by a hexagonal array of 19 photomultiplier tubes. The position of scintillations in the crystal determines the proportionate division of light among the tubes. A computing circuit senses the tube outputs as they are activated by scintillations in the crystal, determines the position of each scintillation in the crystal, and sends position signals to an oscilloscope that reproduces the scintillations as point flashes of light on the screen. A substantial number of those scintillations produced by scattered radiation are rejected by processing the summed output signals from the photomultiplier tubes by means of a pulse-height analyzer. A camera makes a time exposure of the screen as the flashes are integrated into an image of the radiation pattern (see Fig. 5-33B).

The spatial resolution of the image converter corresponding to a point on the detector is limited by the statistical factors that determine the light division among the photomultiplier tubes, and by the scattering of gamma-rays in the crystal. The loss of resolution is inversely proportional to the square root of the brightness of the scintillation, and for this reason this specific type of image converter cannot be used for very low-energy gamma-rays. The loss of spatial resolution in the image converter is mainly due to statistical fluctuations inherent in the operation of photomultiplier tubes. The error in correct localization of a scintillation in a ½-in.-thick crystal due to scattering is very slight (Cradduck and Fedoruk, 1965) and little distortion of the signal is introduced in the final display. A thick crystal would increase the loss of spatial resolution due to scatter. Using a window of the pulse-height analyzer equal to 1.5 times the F.W.H.M. of the photopeak, with the collimator removed, the separation of a barely distinguishable double line in the final picture is approximately 0.38 in. at 150 kev., 0.28 in. at 279 kev., and 0.25 in. at 264 kev. (Anger, 1966b). The experimentally measured photopeak detection efficiencies, ϵ_d, with the pulse-height analyzer set to accept nearly all of the photopeak, are 0.75 for 169 kev., 0.34 for 279 kev., 0.22 for 364 kev., 0.13 for 510 kev., and 0.10 for 662 kev. (Anger, 1966b).

The spatial resolution of this type of image converter with a ½-in.-thick crystal is good at energies greater than 70 kev. and the performance of the collimator is the more important limitation of the spatial resolution of the entire detection system (Anger, 1966b; Anger and Davis, 1964; Cradduck and Fedoruk,

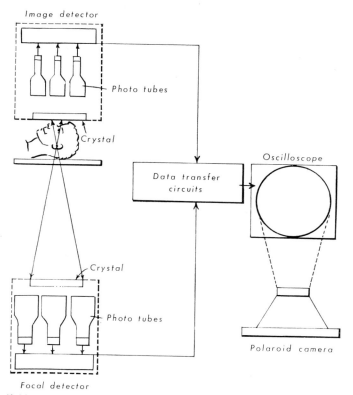

FIGURE 5-44. Positron camera. Only scintillations time-coincident in image detector and focal detector are displayed. (Adapted from Anger, 1966.)

1965; Mallard, 1966; Myers et al., 1966). With the ½-in. thick crystal, however, high detection efficiency can be obtained only at the lower energies. The upper limit of photon energy is approximately 700 kev. This is due to problems with gamma-ray penetration of the lead collimator septa and is common to all detection devices.

Several investigators have used two-dimensional multichannel analyzers with the Anger camera when they required quantitative (numerical) data (Mallard and Myers, 1963b; Cradduck and Fedoruk, 1965; Myers et al., 1966; Wilks and Mallard, 1966). Adam et al. (1967) processed these digital data further in a computer to correct for differences in response over the crystal area.

POSITRON-COINCIDENCE OPERATION. In 1963, Anger introduced the positron camera, a modification of his earlier stationary detector device (Fig. 5-44). In its present form, the patient is placed between two image converters. One image converter, called the image detector, is identical to that described on p. 206. The other, called the focal detector, is similar in operation, but has a 9-in.-diameter by 1½-in. crystal. No metal collimator is used in the system.

When a positron is emitted, it combines with a negative electron and produces two 0.51 mev. annihilation gamma-rays that travel away from the point of origin in exactly opposite directions. When this gamma-ray pair causes coincident scintillations in the two detectors, the scintillation in the image detector is displayed on the oscilloscope screen. Any scintillations occurring in the image detector that are not in time coincidence with gamma-rays detected by the focal detector are not displayed. Since scintillations from a point source of positrons occur over a wide area on the image-detector crystal, correction signals from a computing unit are used to shift the positions of the flashes on the oscilloscope screen so that data corresponding to points lying on the same plane are superimposed. As a consequence, there is a plane of best focus that can be adjusted at the time of the study. With the positron-coincidence operation, deep-lying structures are demonstrated just as well as those on the surface. This is because the total path of two gamma-rays through tissue is always the same. This feature is advantageous when midline structures are to be visualized or when it is necessary to correct for absorption; the absorption correction in a positron system depends only on the total thickness of the tissue and not on the tissue between the primary detector and the source alone, a distance that is difficult to determine.

A disadvantage of the positron camera is that it overloads easily and its use is limited to activities of less than 50 μc. or so. With these activities, exposure times are usually 1 to 5 minutes. On the other hand, the positron camera has an extremely low background (a few counts per hour) so that long exposures can be made of objects containing very little radioactivity. For very low activities of positron emitters, the positron camera has a high sensitivity combined with good resolution for structures deep within the object.

MULTIPLE PHOSPHORS IN RANK AND FILE ARRAY. In some stationary detector devices, the image converter is a fixed array of many individual detectors (Fuchs and Knipping, 1955; Gross et al., 1964). Here, position information is limited to discrete addresses, one for each detector, instead of being continuously distributed across a large-area detector.

In 1962, Bender and Blau reported construction of a stationary detector device that contains a mosaic of 294 individual phosphors arranged in a 14 by

21 rectangular array, 6 by 6 in. in size. Each phosphor is a 2-in.-thick, ⅞-in.-diameter, sodium iodide (Tl) crystal. In front of the phosphor array there is a multihole collimator containing 294 tapered holes, one corresponding to each phosphor (Fig. 5-45A). Originally, data transfer was achieved with the same position-sensing photomultiplier tube arrangement as used in the Anger camera. Later, a rank and file coincidence method was evolved for the data transfer component (Fig. 5-45B) for determining which phosphor in the array had detected a gamma-ray (Bender and Blau, 1962, 1963, 1964).

Each of the 294 phosphors in the array is optically coupled by two plastic light pipes to one of 14 rank photomultiplier tubes (horizontal position) and one of 21 file photomultiplier tubes (vertical position). A pulse occurring simultaneously in one rank photomultiplier tube and in one file photomultiplier tube uniquely identifies the phosphor in which a scintillation has occurred. These data are stored in a magnetic core memory. If scintillations have occurred in more than one crystal as a result of scattered radiation, an anticoincidence system prevents the event from being stored. In addition, the summed signal from the 14 rank photomultiplier tubes is introduced to a pulse-height analyzer, which selects for storage only those events associated with the total-absorption photopeak, thereby rejecting most of the counts representing scattered radiation. At the end of the study, data can be extracted from the magnetic core memory, displayed on an oscilloscope screen, manipulated by a digital data processor, or transferred to magnetic tape for subsequent analysis. There are two complete magnetic core memories, each of which has a core position corresponding to each of the 294 phosphors. To correct for differences in response between phosphors, data from a uniform plane source can be stored in memory 1, data from the patient's distribution of the same radionuclide can be stored in memory 2, and the final picture data can be normalized by displaying the ratio of the data in the two memories.

This stationary detector device is well adapted to the collection of rapidly

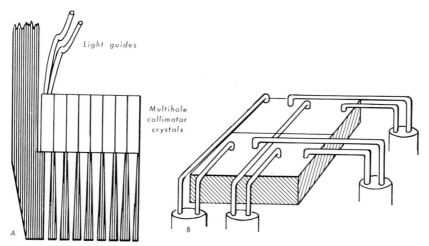

FIGURE 5-45. Stationary detector device with multiple phosphers in rank and file array. Each of the 294 phosphors is optically coupled by two plastic light pipes (A) to one of 14 rank photomultiplier tubes and one of 21 file photomultiplier tubes (B) which uniquely identify the phosphor position. (Adapted from Tech. Report ALF5, Baird Atomic Inc.)

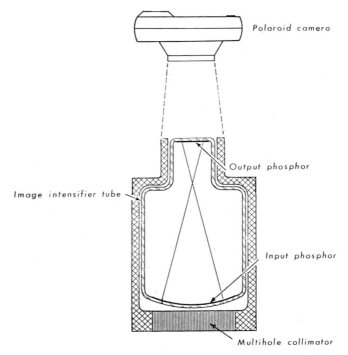

FIGURE 5-46.   Stationary detector device with image intensifier tube.

changing counting data that must be spatially oriented. For example, the instrument has been used to record the flow of iodine-131 Hippuran through the different parts of the kidney and to record the passage of barium-137m through heart chambers. Numerical data from individual parts of organs can be recorded as a function of time by integrating selected areas from a sequence of pictures.

This device is not well adapted to studies that require fine structural detail since the maximal number of picture elements possible is limited to 294, the number of phosphors in the device.

Phosphor Image Intensifier. In 1955, Kellershohn and Pellerin suggested that an x-ray image intensifier could be used for imaging the distribution of radioactive tracers in patients.

In 1963, Ter-Pogossian et al. demonstrated an ^{125}I distribution in the thyroid gland using an x-ray image intensifier fitted with a multihole collimator and a Polaroid camera. The image converter of this instrument is an 8-in.-diameter image-intensifier tube that has a thin input phosphor inside a glass envelope (Fig. 5-46). A multihole collimator projects a radiation pattern upon the input phosphor and produces a corresponding light pattern. The input phosphor is in contact with a photocathode which converts the optical image into an electron image. The electrons are electrostatically focused and accelerated in the image-intensifier tube to form a small image on the fluorescent output screen. A light gain of approximately 6000 can be obtained with this apparatus. The final optical image can be further processed by an image orthicon television system, or can be photographed directly.

The input phosphor is thin and has a poor detection efficiency for gamma-rays higher in energy than 150 kev. With ^{125}I (27 kev.) 26 per cent of the photons striking the glass envelope interact and are recorded as detectable events.

Because of its poor efficiency for any but low-energy photons, this image-intensifier device can be considered a special-purpose instrument for use with radionuclides having energies of less than 150 kev. (iodine-125, mercury-197, xenon-133, cobalt-57, and technetium-99m). It has no provision for reducing the detection of scattered radiation with pulse-height analysis. This is not a serious deficiency when the instrument is applied to the imaging of low-energy photons since, even with sodium iodide (Tl) crystal detectors, it is not possible to separate efficiently the scattered radiation of low-energy gamma emitters (Ross et al., 1965; Eichling et al., 1966). Compton scatter of photons with energies lower than approximately 100 kev. takes place with little loss of photon energy and therefore it is difficult to exclude these scattered photons when pulse-height analysis is used.

The image-intensifier device is capable of transferring position information with very little distortion. Spatial separations on the order of a few millimeters can be distinguished by using this image converter, provided that there are sufficient counts. The practical spatial resolution of the whole detection system is determined by the collimator, as is the case with the other stationary detector devices already described.

Gas-Filled Chamber. In 1964, Kellershohn et al. introduced a stationary detector device for use with low-energy gamma-rays in which a self-triggering spark chamber was the image converter (Fig. 5-47). This chamber measures 20 cm. in diameter and is filled with argon or xenon gas. A potential difference of several kilovolts, somewhat lower than the breakdown voltage, is maintained between a parallel aluminum cathode and glass anode. A fine-mesh grid at intermediate potential provides some discrimination against detection of undesired events. When low-energy gamma-rays produce recoil electrons in the gap between the cathode and the first grid, the voltage difference causes additional electrons to be produced by collisions and an avalanche follows. A columnar discharge, or spark, is produced in the second part of the chamber and then is

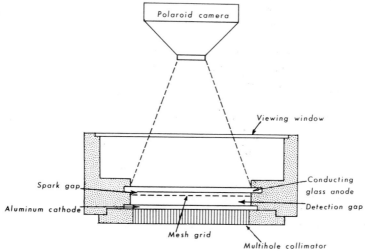

FIGURE 5-47. Stationary detector device with spark chamber.

rapidly extinguished. The sparks can be photographed through the glass end of the chamber as discrete luminous dots. The detection efficiency of this spark chamber for ^{197}Hg (70 kev.) is only about 0.10 and the counting rate is limited to about 100 counts per second (Lansiart and Kellershohn, 1966).

Horwitz et al. (1965) have constructed a spark chamber of slightly different design that uses a silver-plated glass cathode and a transparent anode of electrically conducting glass.

Use of a gas-filled chamber as an image converter for a stationary detector device has attracted interest because of its apparent simplicity. The potential application of the spark chamber for radionuclide imaging is limited, however, by its low detection efficiency as well as its restriction to use with very low-energy photons.

HYBRID DETECTOR DEVICE

GENERAL DESCRIPTION

Hybrid detector devices combine features of both the moving and stationary detector devices. There are several types of hybrid devices, but usually a stationary detector views the distribution of radioactivity in one dimension and then is moved across the patient so that the distribution of radioactivity is determined in two dimensions.

Multiple-Detector Array for x-Axis Viewing; y-Axis Translation. The first hybrid detector device of this class was described by Anger in 1953. A later version of this instrument has 64 scintillation detectors, each with a 1-in.-diameter by 1-in.-thick sodium iodide crystal, arranged in four rows 30 in. long (Anger, 1966). Each detector has a single-hole collimator. As the detector array examines the width of the body, the patient is moved slowly in a longitudinal direction. For each count detected, a flash of light appears on the oscilloscope screen in a position corresponding to that of the counter. A sheet of photographic film is moved in front of the oscilloscope screen synchronous with the patient's movement and a picture of the radioactive distribution is recorded on the film.

A typical total-body scan requires only 6 minutes. The detection efficiency is good for high-energy gamma-rays such as the 1.1 and 1.3 mev. emissions from iron-59. The instrument is particularly suited for bone marrow scanning with iron-59 and bone scanning with fluorine-18 (0.51 mev.) in which large areas must be covered, but fine spatial resolution is not required.

Single Phosphor with Position-Sensing and Photomultiplier Tubes for x-Axis Viewing; y-Axis Translation. In 1966, Davis and Martone described a hybrid detector device with which a large area was examined by a moving "line" detector. In this instrument, a solid rod of sodium iodide (Tl), 2 in. in diameter and 8 in. long, is viewed by a pair of photomultiplier tubes, one bonded to each end. A radiation image is projected on the side of the crystal rod by a multihole collimator. The position of a scintillation along the axis of the rod is directly proportional to the logarithm of the ratio of the fluorescent radiation fluxes measured by the end-viewing photomultiplier tubes. The position of the scintillation is sensed electronically and is represented as a flash of light in a corresponding position on an oscilloscope screen. The summed signal is subjected to pulse-height analysis to reduce detection of scattered radiation. The patient is moved past the detector. The position of the light spot on the oscilloscope screen depends on both the position along the length of rod at which the scintillation occurred and the position of the rod with respect to the longitudinal travel of the patient.

Davis has reported a liver scan made with this instrument using 300 μc. of gold-198 with a scanning time of 2 minutes and 36 seconds. The instrument has the advantage of being relatively simple. Its sensitivity is probably intermediate between commonly available moving and stationary detector devices, but the resolution is rather poor, especially for lower-energy photons such as ^{99m}Tc (140 kev.).

Camera for Simultaneous x-Axis and y-Axis Viewing; Rectilinear Translation of both Camera and Recording Film. In 1966, Harper et al. reported using a hybrid instrument in which an Anger camera is moved so that its field of view sweeps across the region to be examined. At the same time, the oscilloscope camera film is moved to keep in register the image moving on the oscilloscope screen. The field of view of the Anger camera is equal to the crystal area when a multihole collimator is used. But, by moving the camera, a much larger area of the patient can be examined.

This approach combines some of the best features of the moving detector device (large and adjustable study field) and the stationary detector device (speed), and could be of particular value in those studies in which the area is large and good spatial resolution is required.

COMPARISON OF IMAGING DEVICES

It is valid to compare the performance of a moving detector device and a stationary detector device in terms of the time required to accumulate a given total count from equal areas when spatial resolution is the same for both devices. On this basis, a moving detector device with a single small phosphor is not as good as a stationary detector device with a large phosphor. This is not surprising, but one should not conclude that stationary detector devices are always better than moving detector devices. Each of the two types has special advantages and special disadvantages, but the similarities of the two techniques are more striking than their differences.

In principle, the moving detector device is superior because it is efficient for a wide range of photon energies, the study field can be adjusted to accommodate large structures, and the response is uniform over the entire study field. But there are stationary detector devices that are efficient for all but the most energetic photons (image intensifier for low energies, phosphor-photomultiplier for moderate energies); the study field of a moving camera is not limited by the size of its detector (hybrid techniques); and data processing can be used to equalize the response across the field of view of the stationary detector device.

In principle, the stationary detector device is superior to the moving detector device because the time of study is shorter and all parts of the field of interest can be viewed at once. But the time of study with a moving detector device may be equal if it is provided with a detector area equivalent to the stationary devices (Harris et al., 1967). (Of course, there are practical limitations to increasing the size of detector used with a focused collimator in a moving detector device. Too large a detector produces a large solid angle of view that can give very poor resolution on either side of the focal plane.) Alternatively, study time with the moving detector device can be reduced by using multiple individual detectors of moderate size.

No imaging device is ideal for all applications. The present trend is to choose a special-purpose instrument that is most suitable for solution of the problem. For example, when the distribution of a moderate-energy emitter must be determined in less than 30 seconds, a stationary detector device of the phosphor-photomultiplier type can be used. One could choose a stationary detector device of the phosphor-image intensifier type to demonstrate a rapidly changing, high-intensity distribution of low-energy photons (^{133}Xe, 81 kev.). A moving detector device shielded with very high-density material can be used to determine distribution of high-energy photon emitters (^{59}Fe, 1.1, 1.3 mev.). With other applications that impose less stringent requirements for performance, there is a wider latitude for choice among the different types of imaging devices.

SPECIAL-PURPOSE TECHNIQUES

TOMOGRAPHIC SCANNING

Tomographic, or section, scanning is used to obtain information that might otherwise be lost because of image overlap (Kuhl, 1963, 1964; Kuhl and Edwards, 1963, 1964, 1966a; Kuhl et al., 1966b; Cassen, 1964; Hisada et al., 1967). Image overlap is inherent in rectilinear scanning, since the record is a summation of images of radioactivity from many different depths in the body. In section radionuclide scanning, principles of roentgen tomography are applied to separate these images of radioactivity according to their depths. Specific levels of interest can be examined without significant interference from structures at other levels.

In roentgen tomography, both the x-ray tube and the film are moved in opposite directions during exposure. At the same time, the inclination of the tube is changed uniformly to generate a region of beam convergence in the body plane to be studied. Images of structures at this level are reinforced continuously as the film is exposed; images of structures above or below this level are spread over a wider area of film. As a consequence, only the structures in a section of the body at the specified level are well defined in the tomograph. For images of other levels, the process must be repeated.

This same principle can be extended to radionuclide scanning in several ways. For example, a rectilinear scan can be made using a focused collimator with a very wide solid-angle field of view on either side of the focal plane. In this instance, photon emissions divergent *from* a body plane simulate the x-rays convergent *to* a body plane in roentgen tomography. Only those radionuclide distributions at the level of the focal plane are sharply defined. However, for successful suppression of images on other planes, the solid angle of view must be much larger than is usually found with conventional focused collimators. Cassen (1964) has successfully applied this method of section scanning using a focused collimator that has a very large solid angle of π steradians. This collimator has a spherical cap configuration, an 18 cm. radius to focus, and 2200 holes; it is backed by a 23-kg. crystal aggregate. As in conventional roentgen tomography, this method requires preselection of the level of interest and a separate study to obtain each section image.

Hisada et al. (1967) perform section scanning with a four detector system. Two detectors are opposed with the patient in between. Each of the remaining detectors is positioned oblique to one of the opposed detectors. Signals from the detectors are mixed in three combinations. Sections parallel to the long axis of the body have been helpful in disclosing small lesions in large organs.

Kuhl et al. (1963, 1964, 1966) use transverse section scanning to demonstrate the radioactivity in a cross section of the brain approximately 1 or 2 cm. thick. A section image results when a pair of detectors completes a sequential series of 24 tangential scan lines (at 7.5° angular intervals) around the complete circumference of the patient's head. All counting data are recorded on perforated tape. Each complete section requires 10 to 20 minutes of scanning time. In its original form, the record was made by exposing the film of an oscilloscope camera with a thin line of light that was given motion and orientation matched to the detector's line of view. Twenty-four separate exposures of the film integrated the data into an image of the distribution of radioactivity in the section. This method has been improved by using computer summation.

The transverse section data are reorganized by a digital process. Overlapping bands of film exposure are replaced in the section image by an orderly rectilinear matrix of picture elements, each element representing the sum of counts detected over that address in each of 24 paths of the detectors. The original scan data from each detector are first transferred from perforated paper tape to a magnetic storage drum. A program tape controls all subsequent sequences of the translation operation. For each picture element of the final display, counts from 24 corresponding elements of original data—one per scan tangent—are extracted from the drum, added, divided by 24, and punched into another tape. This processed tape is then used to generate the final section image. Twelve minutes are required to perform the 181,000 operations necessary to translate the transverse section image into a rectilinear raster of 10,000 picture elements.

The transverse section of the brain improves the examination of the base of the cranial vault and gives additional information about tumor boundaries.

TRANSMISSION SCANNING

Transmission scanning is used to improve the spatial orientation within the body of the radionuclide emission scan (Kuhl et al., 1966a). Accurate evaluation of a radionuclide distribution in the body requires that the spatial relationships of emission scan data be oriented to the anatomy of the patient. Usually, data on the scan record are keyed to anatomy either by using reference marks to represent external features of the body or by superimposing the scan image over a roentgenogram of the region (Kuhl et al., 1956). These methods may introduce inaccuracy due to geometrical distortions; also, if the patient moves during the scan, counting data and anatomical reference may no longer correspond.

Transmission scanning can be employed to reduce these inaccuracies. During a conventional emission scan, a small radioactive source of either americium-241 or iodine-125 is made to move under the patient to follow the motion of the detector. The photons from this source are collimated and directed through the patient to the detector. Pulse-height analysis is used to separate the emission and transmission counting data which are then recorded separately. As the scan progresses, the point-to-point variation of counting rate from the transmitted beam depends on attenuation by anatomical structures. The transmission scan image that is reconstructed from these data is similar to a roentgenogram of the scanned part and can be oriented to the corresponding emission scan image with negligible geometrical distortion. Any patient movement during the study is apparent in both records.

DETECTABILITY

Optimizing the Performance of the Imaging System

In choosing the radiopharmaceutical, the time for study, and the combination of components that make up the detection system, the problem is always that of maximizing the information available to construct the image, while reducing the cost in terms of time and radiation dosage to the patient. There are always statistical fluctuations imposed by the relatively few photons available. The problem is that of effecting a suitable compromise between sensitivity and spatial resolution. There is not yet general agreement as to how this can best be achieved. It is agreed that a method of systems analysis would be useful if it aided in specifying which detection system should be used to perform a given task, in designing a system to meet these specifications, in giving us knowledge of the lower limits of detectability of lesions, in proving or disproving the feasibility of new scanning studies, and in allowing workers in different laboratories to compare their results.

It is easy to compare systems that have the same resolution or the same sensitivity, but this is not the usual case. Most often it is necessary to make a compromise between sensitivity and resolution. If the spatial resolution is very fine, sensitivity may be too low and it may not be possible to distinguish adjacent regions because of poor statistics. But if spatial resolution is very poor, there may be insufficient spatial information to distinguish differences in the distribution of radioactivity even though the corresponding high sensitivity is associated with negligible statistical variation (Brownell, 1964).

To evaluate the necessary compromise between spatial resolution and sensitivity, some investigators have used the information capacity of the scan image as a criterion for comparison (Beck, 1964a; Brownell, 1964; Cederlund, 1964; Gregg, 1965). These studies suggest that there is probably an optimal number of counts that should be recorded for each "resolution area" making up the picture in order to maximize the information content of the picture. This number is independent of the detection system. As a consequence, if the activity level, study time, or detector sensitivity is increased, the spatial resolution should be narrowed to maintain the number of counts per "resolution area" constant at this optimal value for the best possible picture. Brownell (1964) conducted experiments in which observers evaluated a family of simulated scan images produced with a digital computer; he concluded that the optimal number of counts per resolution element is independent of activity, but may vary with the detail of the pattern being observed.

Another approach is to compare imaging systems on the basis of a figure of merit that is proportional to the time required to distinguish statistically a difference in activity between two samples, one representing the radioactive object and the other representing adjacent radioactivity (Dewey and Sinclair, 1961; Beck, 1961, 1964a, b, 1966; Matthews, 1964; Wagner and Emmons, 1965; Kuhl, 1965; Simons and Bailey, 1967). At present, this formulation has been more widely applied to evaluating practical scanning problems.

Beck (1961, 1964a, b, 1966) has used a figure of merit, Q, that is proportional to the reciprocal of the time required to distinguish a statistically significant difference between counting rates corresponding to adjacent regions. If C_1 and C_2 are the true mean counting rates over two adjacent regions, the counting time over these regions required to obtain enough counts to distinguish the difference between C_1 and C_2 with a given statistical reliability is inversely proportional to the figure of merit, Q, which is given by:

$$Q = \frac{(C_1 - C_2)^2}{(C_1 + C_2)} \tag{16}$$

Figures of merit may be compared between different detection systems. A system with a figure of merit half that of another system will require twice as long a counting time for detection of the difference between C_1 and C_2.

The figure of merit is maximal when the diameter of the field of view of the collimator equals the diameter of the radioactive object (Newell et al., 1952; Dewey and Sinclair, 1961; Simons and Bailey, 1967). Such figures of merit are insufficient to enable a choice to be made of the collimating systems that will give the best spatial resolution of the structure (Simons and Bailey, 1967), but detection systems may be compared on the basis of their figures of merit if they have the same resolution.

Although it has not yet been demonstrated that maximizing this figure of merit corresponds to maximizing the likelihood of diagnosis, analyses on the basis of figures of merit have already increased our understanding of certain physical relationships:

1. The optimal effective half-life of a labeled compound is 0.69 times the elapsed time between administration and measurement when radiation dose is a consideration (Wagner and Emmons, 1965).

2. The optimal energy range for gamma-rays used in brain scanning with a moving detector device and a focused collimator is 100 to 200 kev. when the physical characteristics of the source and the design parameters of the collimated detector are considered (Beck, 1961).

3. The optimal energy range for gamma-rays used in liver scanning with a moving detector device and a focused collimator is the same as for brain scanning, 100 to 200 kev. (Kuhl, 1965), but it is even more important that the radiopharmaceutical have suitable physical and biological characteristics that result in the production of large numbers of photons per unit radiation dose (Beck, 1966; Kuhl, 1965).

4. Focused collimation gives a higher probability for detection of brain tumors than positron-coincidence collimation (Beck, 1961; Matthews, 1964), but the preference for focused collimation need not necessarily apply when high-energy photons are used (Matthews, 1964).

Eventually it may be practical to make an optimal choice of each component of the detection system completely on the basis of a calculated analysis of the specific detection problem, but this has not yet been accomplished.

DISPLAY AND PROCESSING

The first scan images were rows of black marks made on paper by a *mechanical printer* that was activated each time a preset number of counts had accumulated from a moving detector (Cassen et al., 1951). Regions of higher counting rate were represented as regions of higher mark density. Differences in mark density between regions could be distinguished when they were greater than four or five times the standard deviation of the differences (Matthews, 1964). Later, color coding was introduced to improve the contrast of mark recordings (Mallard and Peachey, 1959; Mallard et al., 1964). Now, mark recording has largely been supplanted by *photorecording* (Kuhl et al., 1956; Bender, 1957; Herring, 1960). The contrast of images on film is more easily varied to improve perception of lesions, and the character of the display is more readily understood by persons accustomed to radiographic images.

In most photorecorders for moving detector devices, film is exposed by a light source coupled mechanically to the moving detector; oscilloscope cameras have also been used as photographic recorders with moving and stationary devices (Mayneord and Newberry, 1952; Anger et al., 1956; MacIntyre et al., 1958; Kuhl, 1964; Kuhl and Edwards, 1964, 1966a, b). The intensity of the light source is controlled by the counting rate and the illuminated region of the film corresponds to the scanning raster. In this way, the spatial variation of detector response is represented on the film as variation in photographic density.

The distortions introduced by the photorecorder are added to those introduced by each successive prior component in the detection system. The most important distortions produced by the photorecorder are:

1. The latitude, or range, of a direct photorecording on film is limited to about two magnitudes (Laughlin et al., 1964); it is less when high contrast is used. The activity distribution must be prejudged and the recorder must be carefully adjusted before the study. Even then counting data may be lost in the very low and very high film densities.

2. If the diameter of the light spot is large, spatial resolution can be degraded.

3. A nonlinear relationship between film density and counting rate can distort the edge and interface gradients in the picture.

4. A long rate meter time constant in the photorecorder of a moving detector device can degrade spatial resolution due to the lag imposed on the photorecorder response (Gopalo Rao and Wagner, 1967).

The present trend in scanning is to store the data intact during the study procedure and to perform any special operations on the data at a later time. For example, closed-circuit television viewing (Bender and Blau, 1959) and rescanning densitometry (Harris et al., 1963b, 1964) have been used for analysis of the photographic record after scanning. Other approaches to optimizing image contrast have included magnetic tape recording of scan data followed by time-compression replay with oscilloscope-camera film recording (Berne and Jonsson, 1959) or storage tube display (Bonte et al., 1963). Numerical printout has been used when the quantitative counting data were of more importance than picture quality (Beattie and Bradt, 1961). Recently, magnetic or perforated paper tape recording of the original counting data has been employed by some workers as a prelude to digital data processing (Kawin et al., 1964; Schepers and Winkler, 1964; Brown, 1964; Weber et al., 1965; Sprau et al., 1966; Kuhl and Edwards, 1966b, 1967).

Considerable attention is now being given to computer processing of scan data and it is likely that the results of these studies will extend the usefulness of the scanning technique. At present computer processing of scan data is limited to very few centers. However, two optical processing devices are readily available and should be more widely applied. These are the glass diffusion filter and the diminishing lens.

The glass diffusion filter (Anger et al., 1965) is useful for smoothing random fluctuations in density in the image. In accordance with the statistics of detection, a random variation in the number of counts in each picture element is superimposed on the ordered variation, which constitutes the real emission image. When the number of counts in each element is low, the random fluctuations between elements make perception more difficult. The spottiness of the picture can be diminished by integrating counts over areas wider than one picture element. This can be accomplished by spatial averaging using digital computation (Schepers and Winkler, 1964; Charleston et al., 1964; Sprau et al., 1966; Kuhl and Edwards, 1967) or by printing the picture with a light spot larger than each individual element (MacIntyre et al., 1958; Charleston et al., 1964; MacIntyre and Christie, 1966). Almost the same results can be accomplished by viewing sharply printed scan images through a diffusion filter (framing glass) held from 1 to 5 in. above the image. The amount of diffusion obtained with the filter is directly proportional to the distance between the glass and the picture, and can be controlled by the physician. The diffusion filter is most useful for distinguishing low-contrast images with unsharp edges.

The diminishing lens also aids in the perception of the unsharp border of an ill defined image, but for different reasons. The perception of an image depends on the spatial gradient of retinal illumination by the image (Tuddenham, 1957). The spatial gradient of brightness on the film recording has been determined by all of the parameters of the detection system and display discussed so far. But the spatial gradient of retinal illumination depends also on viewing conditions. Minification of the picture, increase in viewing distance, and use of a diminishing lens all cause the projection of the brightness difference representing the image border to cover fewer retinal receptor cells. This increases their differential illumination and improves perception of the image border.

SUMMARY

The best picture will result from a scanning study when there is a maximal differential in recorded photons between a structure and its surroundings and when enough photons have been recorded to make the statistical reliability of this difference high. These conditions depend on the biological and physical properties of the labeled compound, the configuration and location of the structure to be visualized, and the performance of the detection system.

The maximal performance of a detection system is characterized in terms of sensitivity (plane sensitivity, S_a) and spatial resolution (M.T.F.). In a particular detection system, an improvement in either sensitivity or spatial resolution is usually at the expense of the other. There is agreement that a compromise must be effected for best results. It is not yet clearly understood how this can best be accomplished.

Each component of the detection system causes some loss in both sensitivity and spatial resolution, but the principal restriction occurs in the first component, the collimator.

In the moving detector device, or scanner, the multihole focused collimator is preferred to a single-hole collimator since a crystal of larger area can be used. Sensitivity is thus improved while spatial resolution is preserved in the focal plane. But if the detector area is too great, spatial resolution of the focused collimator will be poor in positions other than in the focal plane. Alternatively, one may use multiple detectors of moderate size, each with a focused collimator, to improve sensitivity of a moving detector device.

In the stationary detector device, or camera, the pin-hole collimator is preferred for viewing small objects placed close to the aperture, and the multihole collimator is preferred for larger objects.

The advantages of a scanner over a camera are: it is efficient for a wider range of photon energies, the study field can be adjusted to accommodate large structures, and the response is uniform over the study field. The advantages of a camera over a scanner are that the time of study is shorter and all parts of the field of interest can be viewed at once. Hybrid techniques can be used to combine the advantages of each method, but no imaging device is ideal for all applications.

The best display system for any imaging device is one in which data destruction is negligible, yet there is provision for modifying the data to satisfy the psychophysiological requirements of perception.

WHOLE-BODY COUNTING

Richard C. Reba
Henry N. Wagner, Jr.

A whole-body counter is used to measure the radioactivity within the entire human body. It is an external detection system with the lowest possible spatial resolution, as opposed to scanning devices that portray the distribution of radioactivity within the body with a high degree of spatial resolution.

Whole-body counters were first developed to measure the radioactivity within the bodies of persons who had ingested radium-containing paint. Since then, they have been used for a variety of other purposes, which are listed in Table 5-1.

Many uses of whole-body counters require a high degree of sensitivity, which greatly increases their cost. Large numbers of carefully balanced photomultiplier tubes, heavy shielding, and high maintenance requirements all contribute to the cost. Fortunately, for many clinical studies, such as measurement of gastrointestinal absorption, relatively insensitive systems can be used. Even systems designed for biomedical research can be relatively simple and inexpensive. An example is a portable unit used to measure the cesium-137 content of people living in remote parts of Alaska (Palmer, 1966). It consists of an unshielded detector with a battery-operated single-channel analyzer. Another system uses a minimal amount of lead shielding to decrease background radiation by arranging lead bricks in a configuration referred to as "shadow shielding," which eliminates the background radiation in the direct field of view of the crystal detector. Using this principle, it is possible to obtain a whole-body counter of low cost, small size, and adequate sensitivity that is completely transportable. If a single 3 by 3 in. crystal detector and a single-channel spectrometer are used, the cost can be less than \$10,000. The sensitivity of such a system is in the nanocurie range for many tracers, such as iron-59 and cobalt-58. The background in such a system, for photon energies above 500 kev., is as low as that in a large iron room with only slightly less sensitivity. There is little variation in sensitivity for people of different size.

TABLE 5-1.   USES OF WHOLE-BODY COUNTERS

Public Health
> Monitoring personnel of reactors, cyclotrons, and nuclear laboratories
> Monitoring fallout (primarily ^{137}Cs and ^{131}I)
> Evaluation of patient exposures in medical utilization of radioactive tracer materials
> Evaluation of accidental exposure to radiation

Medical Diagnosis and Research
> Intestinal absorption of various elements and compounds
> Metabolism of elements, drugs, hormones, proteins, vitamins, and nutrients
>> Special studies utilizing very short-lived radionuclides
>>> Studies utilizing isotopes with short physical half-lives, such as $^{13,16}N$, $^{15,18}O$, ^{11}C, and ^{28}Mg
>>> Studies using isotopes with short biological half-lives such as the rare gases, xenon and krypton
> Measurement of body content
>> Potassium deficiency
>> Lean body mass and fat content
>> Whole-body sodium (^{24}Na), calcium (^{49}Ca), nitrogen (^{16}N), and chlorine (^{38}Cl) by whole-body activation analysis
> Detection of genetic abnormalities
>> Muscular dystrophy (^{40}K content)
>> Hemachromatosis (^{59}Fe absorption)

Other
> Large animal whole-body counter
> Large-volume sample counter, e.g., counting meteorites and foodstuffs

A whole-body counter designed to measure relatively large quantities of activity has been built at the Oak Ridge Institute of Nuclear Studies (Morris et al., 1964). It consists of a 2 by 2 in. sodium iodide crystal mounted 9 feet above the subject in an unshielded room. Although designed for measurement of therapeutic quantities of radioactive tracers, it can measure precisely 10 μc. of ^{131}I within a patient during a 10 minute counting period. Recently Morris (1965) described the use of four 3 by 3 in. crystals for a diagnostic whole-body counter.

OUTLINE OF THE HISTORY OF TOTAL-BODY COUNTING

An outline of the development of total-body counting is given in Table 5-2. Soon after the discovery of radioactivity by Becquerel in 1896, it was learned that exposure to ionizing radiation could be harmful or even fatal. Ingestion, as in the case of luminous dial painters, inhalation, as in the case of uranium

TABLE 5-2. DEVELOPMENT OF WHOLE-BODY COUNTING*

DATE	EXPERIMENTER AND APPARATUS	SUBJECT OBSERVA-TION TIME	APPROXIMATE LIMIT OF DETECTION (STANDARD ERROR)	
			AS μg. ^{226}Ra EQUIVA-LENT	AS A PERCENTAGE OF TOTAL BODY POTASSIUM
1929	Schlundt et al. Ion chamber at 1 atm.		5	
1933	Schlundt et al. Ion chamber at 1 atm.		0.2	
1937	Evans Geiger-Müller tube		0.1	
1947	Hess and McNiff Ion chamber at 1 atm.		0.03	
1951	Sievert High-pressure ion chamber	2 hr.	0.005	50
1953	Burch and Spiers Differential high-pressure ion chambers	2 hr.	0.003	30
1956	Sievert High-pressure ion chambers underground	3–4 hr.	0.001	10
1956	Los Alamos 4π liquid scintillator (Anderson, 1956)	15 min.	0.0001	1
to	Argonne National Laboratory NaI scintillator (Marinelli, 1956)	15 min.	0.0003	3.5
1960	Leeds Plastic scintillator apparatus (Bird and Burch, 1958)	15 min.	0.0001	1.5

* From Vennart, J.: Use of Whole-Body Counters in Radiological Protection. *Nature* 204:1041, 1964.

miners, or injection, as in the case of Thorotrast administration for radiographic studies, may be the means of entry of radioactive material.

To determine the amount of radium within the bodies of the dial painters, Schlundt (1929) used small ionization chambers directed toward the backs of the subjects from a distance of 30 cm. Evans (1937) measured whole-body radioactivity with Geiger-Müller tubes, and outlined the principles and problems involved in the techniques of whole-body counting.

Among the problems that Evans discussed were those resulting from variations in the configuration of the body of one person compared to another and the geometrical relation between the detector and the subject. How to account for changes in detection efficiency due to the effects of tissue absorption and

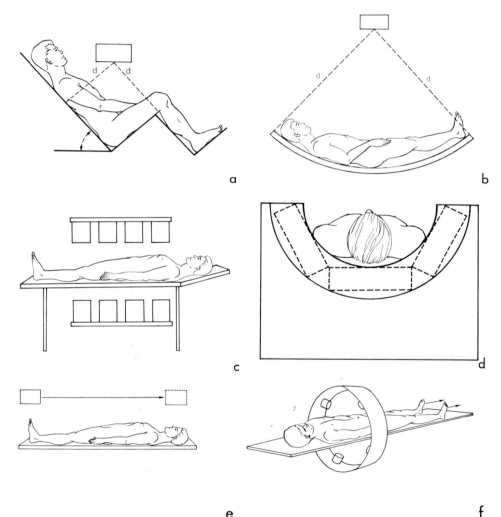

FIGURE 5-48.   Detector-patient configuration in whole-body counters: e shows a system in which the detector moves; f shows a system in which the patient is moved; the others are stationary systems. In a, the standard chair position, d usually equals 42 cm. In b, the arc position, d usually equals 1.00 to 1.74 meters. c, Multiple detectors used to achieve uniformity of response and to increase sensitivity. d, a 2π system; either a solid or a liquid scintillator can be used.

TABLE 5-3. CHARACTERISTICS OF SEVERAL TYPES OF WHOLE-BODY COUNTERS

Detectors

High sensitivity: Adult ^{40}K estimate requires 100–200 sec. for 98% precision
    4π liquid scintillation
    Massive shielding and highest cost
    Independent of isotope distribution
Medium sensitivity: 2π liquid scintillation or multiple crystals
Low sensitivity: Adult ^{40}K estimate requires 1000–3000 sec. for 98% precision
    Single large crystal or shadow shield type
    Minimal shielding and moderate cost
    Suitable for most clinical studies
Very low sensitivity: Ionization chambers or Geiger-Müller tubes

Shielding

Steel, lead, water, gypsum, cement, concrete, chalk, plaster, talc, dunnite, marble, serpentine aggregate, rock

Electronics

Single- or double-channel analyzer
Multichannel analyzer

Data Presentation

Visual: oscilloscope
Manual: scaler, x-y plot, typewriter
Automatic data processing: punch cards, digital punch or magnetic tape

---

scattering were also outlined. Some of the most common detector-patient configurations that have been used are illustrated in Figure 5-48. These were developed to achieve uniform sensitivity regardless of the distribution of radioactivity within the body.

The type of detector has also changed considerably as whole-body counters have evolved. During the 1940's, ionization chambers sensitive enough to detect the gamma-ray equivalent of 0.03 μg. of radium with a 1 hour counting period were developed. Schlundt and Evans had been able to detect only 5 to 100 μg. Sievert (1951) first used four large-volume high-pressure ionization chambers surrounding the subject. Using water as a shield and placing his counter in a cave under 55 meters of rock, he reduced the minimal detectable activity to 0.002 μg. of radium if the counting times were as long as 8 hours.

Sievert (1956) was the first to measure natural radioactivity in living man. He measured the natural potassium-40 of the body as a function of age, sex, and body weight. During the early 1950's, the development of methods for producing large scintillation detectors led to great technical improvements (Marinelli, 1957; Anderson, 1957). Plastic scintillators were used by Bird and Burch (1958), although the energy resolution is less with organic scintillators than with sodium iodide. However, ^{137}Cs can be separated from the photopeak area of ^{40}K and the ^{40}K content of an adult can be measured within 1000 seconds with a 2 per cent counting error.

Burch and Spiers (1953) and Reines et al. (1953) carried out the first quantitative measurements of total-body potassium from measurement of ^{40}K. Their results were comparable to those based on the use of ^{42}K to estimate total exchangeable potassium and on chemical measurements of cadavers.

In 1957 Anderson described further improvements in the 4π liquid detector, and in 1959 Anderson and Laugham reported the results of ^{40}K body potassium measurements of 1590 persons, analyzed according to age and sex. They confirmed earlier reports of the linear relationship between body potassium and lean body mass. Using a 2 minute counting period, they could detect the naturally occurring ^{40}K (15 mg. or about 10^{-8} curies) in an adult man with 95 per cent precision.

TYPES OF WHOLE-BODY COUNTERS

Table 5-3 lists the characteristics of various components of whole-body counters; Table 5-4 outlines their general advantages and disadvantages. Overall sensitivity is related to the type of detector. The most sensitive are the liquid or plastic scintillation counters, which are useful for studies of low levels of radioactivity, the identity of which is known. Because of their limited size, crystal detectors are less sensitive and therefore require longer counting times than liquid detectors. For example, a detector with a single 8 by 4 in. crystal requires a counting period up to 1 hour to determine the ^{40}K content of the human body with acceptable precision, whereas this can be done in a 4π liquid scintillation counter in 3 to 4 minutes.

Thallium-activated sodium iodide crystals are used in most whole-body counters. Gamma-ray spectrometry makes possible simultaneous study of two or more radionuclides. Identification of unknown radionuclides requires the use of inorganic crystals, such as sodium iodide, to permit resolution of gamma-ray energy.

Multiple crystals not only increase sensitivity but also permit localization of radioactivity within specific parts of the body. With liquid scintillators, usually only two nuclides can be measured simultaneously (Fig. 5-49). An advantage of liquid scintillators is that they can be put in containers that completely surround the body. Spectral resolution of liquid detectors can be improved by increasing the thickness of the scintillator (to 12 in.) and by using very large photomultiplier tubes (Van Dilla and Anderson, 1962).

Usually a sodium iodide crystal detector system is best for clinical purposes, and the liquid scintillator systems are best for measurement of large numbers of

TABLE 5-4. GENERAL ADVANTAGES AND DISADVANTAGES OF WHOLE-BODY COUNTERS

Advantages

Total metabolic balance studies may be performed with ease, with precise measurements of the rate of tracer loss from the body without the inconvenient and at times unreliable collection of urine, feces, sweat, or respired air. Large numbers of normal and hospital outpatients may be conveniently studied.

Studies may be performed resulting in a *very low* radiation dose enabling the safe study of normal children and pregnant women.

Studies may be performed resulting in *no* radiation dose to the subject. By measurement of natural ^{40}K, evaluation of lean body mass, fat, and nutrition are possible.

Disadvantages

Complex equipment, which is expensive to obtain and maintain, is required.

Absolute calibration is difficult to achieve.

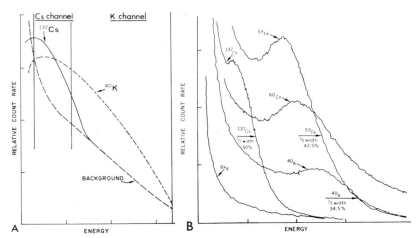

FIGURE 5-49. A, Gamma spectra from a liquid scintillation counter with coincidence counting. B, Gamma spectra from a liquid scintillation counter.

persons to determine the body content of known radionuclides, such as ^{137}Cs and ^{40}K.

In both types of systems it is important to keep the background low and to avoid fluctuations in background from thermionic emission as well as cosmic and other radiation. Steel is the most commonly used shielding material. Five to seven inches of steel, four inches of lead, or three and a half feet of water is effective. At times other materials are chosen on the basis of local availability. In the construction of whole-body counters, it is important to check the building materials to be sure that they are free of radioactive contaminants. Cobalt-60 and ruthenium-103 have been found in steel, and in the vicinity of nuclear reactors or cyclotrons, argon-41 and nitrogen-11 may be present as contaminants of air. Air-borne particles of dust contaminated with radon can become a problem if air filters are not used. In addition to the use of shielded rooms, the crystal detectors themselves are often encased in lead together with their photomultiplier tubes.

A common type of whole-body counter consists of a single large crystal or multiple small crystals mounted inside a room constructed of thick steel walls. The patient enters the room and is positioned in a special chair or other support. Room air is continuously cooled, filtered, and circulated. Closed-circuit television permits observation of the patient, and music is often used to prevent boredom and reassure the patient during long counting periods.

A useful system for clinical studies is that in which the patient moves in relation to the detector. One detector is above and the other below the patient; this increases the sensitivity and obviates the need for having the patient in both prone and supine positions.

When liquid scintillators are used, an arrangement of the type illustrated in Figure 5-50 is often used. It consists of a horizontal tank and well, a cylindrical shield, organic scintillators and solvents, and the litter on which the patient lies (Reba et al., 1968b). The detector consists of a double-walled stainless steel cylindrical tank, the inner wall of which surrounds the patient and

Schematic drawing of whole body counter

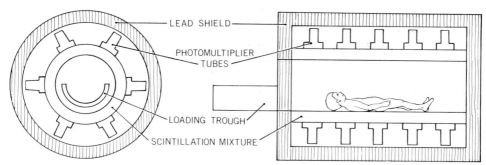

Figure 5-50. 4π liquid scintillation counter. (From Reba, R. C., et al.: Determination of Total Body Potassium by Measurement of K-40. *In* Cheek, D. B. (ed.): Human Growth: Body Composition, Cytology, Energy and Intelligence. Lea & Febiger, Philadelphia, 1968.)

also forms the inner wall of the tank containing the liquid scintillator. Around the outer wall of the tank is a steel shield. Multiple photomultiplier tubes are connected in parallel so that all scintillations are viewed by at least two photo-tubes. Coincidence counting is often used with liquid scintillation systems to reduce background.

CALIBRATION OF WHOLE-BODY COUNTERS

In most measurements of radioactivity, exact knowledge of detector efficiency is unnecessary since the unknown is usually compared to a standard. The best way to calibrate whole-body counters is to inject a known activity of the radionuclide of interest into the patients to be studied. In some cases this is impractical because of the long half-life of the radionuclide. In such cases, another nuclide distributed in the same manner but with a shorter half-life and similar energy can be used. For example, ^{42}K, which emits monoenergetic 1.52 Mev. photons and has a 12.5 hour half-life, can simulate ^{40}K, which emits 1.46 Mev. photons; ^{132}Cs, with a 6.5 day half-life and 0.67 Mev. gamma photons, can simulate ^{137}Cs (0.662 Mev.; half-life, 30 years). Overall detection efficiency varies from patient to patient because of individual geometrical differences. When each test patient cannot be calibrated individually, the calibration can be performed on a group of patients similar to the test patients and is usually expressed on a weight basis.

In 4π liquid scintillation whole-body counters, sensitivity is a simple linear function of weight between 30 and 180 pounds. For patients less than 30 pounds, counting efficiency is nonlinear and requires a multiple order polynomial to describe the relation of count rate to weight. The linear portion of the calibration curve is adequate for most clinical studies including those involving children. In some whole-body counters, height must also be considered in efficiency calibrations. Other methods of calibration involve the use of a hollow plastic manikin, or body configurations made of sugar, rice, or other materials of suitable specific gravity that are free of radioactivity. Bottles containing known amounts of radioactivity are also used. Correction must be made daily for changes in sensitivity. Additional corrections must be made with liquid detectors, since the mass of the sample or subject may suppress background.

The efficiency of the instrument for a given person can be estimated from his weight, using experimentally determined calibration curves as a basis. For many clinical problems, exact knowledge of counting efficiency is not necessary since the determination is a direct comparison between an initial value determined shortly after administration of the dose and a value obtained at some later time.

DATA PROCESSING

Modern data processing techniques can be applied to whole-body counting and serve several useful functions: integration of photopeak activity, evaluation of counting errors, reduction of noise by smoothing processes, normalization of spectra, spectral stripping, and efficiency calculations.

APPLICATIONS

RADIUM DIAL PAINTERS

The first studies based on whole-body counting are not only of historical interest but also are the basis of estimates of permissible body burdens of radioactive substances.

Evans (1967) has recently reviewed the data concerning radium dial painters. He points out that the selection of 0.1 μg. of radium as the maximal permissible body burden was based on the study of 30 patients and that today after the thorough study of about 700 additional persons, this figure remains a safe and conservative guide for evaluating skeletal deposition of radioactivity. The gamma-ray spectrum of a person who ingested radium is shown in Figure 5-51.

The symptoms and sequelae of radium poisoning are related to dose. With a residual body burden of less than 0.5 μg. of radium, there is no shortening of life and no clinically significant signs or symptoms. With doses greater than 0.5 μg., the life span is shortened and there is a high incidence of malignant tumors (about 40 per cent). Osteoporosis, osteomyeletis, spontaneous fractures, osteogenic sarcomas (after 7 to 43 years), and carcinomas of the paranasal sinuses or mastoids (after 19 to 41 years) are also common. Leukemia does not appear to have an increased incidence.

THOROTRAST TOXICITY

Thorotrast, colloidal thorium dioxide, unlike radium, which goes to the bone, is accumulated and retained by the reticuloendothelial cells, which are primarily in the liver, spleen, and bone marrow. Patients who received diagnostic doses of thorotrast have subsequently devoloped hepatic tumors, leukemia, and various other hematological disorders.

Uranium toxicity

The inhalation hazard from the occupational exposure of uranium miners is well established. Comparison of uranium miners and a group of other persons matched for age and smoking habits has revealed a significant increase in the incidence of lung cancer among the miners (Wagoner et al., 1965; Saccomanno et al., 1964), which was related to inhalation of ^{222}Rn and its daughters. The number of oat cell, round cell, and polygonal cell cancers was increased, whereas epidermoid cancer was decreased. The cancers were highly malignant and the miners died within a few months of diagnosis.

Radioactive fallout

The major long-lived atmospheric contaminants liberated during testing of nuclear weapons are cesium-137 and strontium-90. Cesium-137 decays to barium-137m, which emits a 0.662 Mev. gamma-ray and has been observed in the gamma spectra of normal persons since 1956 (Miller and Marinelli). Monitoring by various laboratories throughout the world has provided data on the level of radioactive fallout from nuclear weapons tests. Iodine-131, zirconium-95/

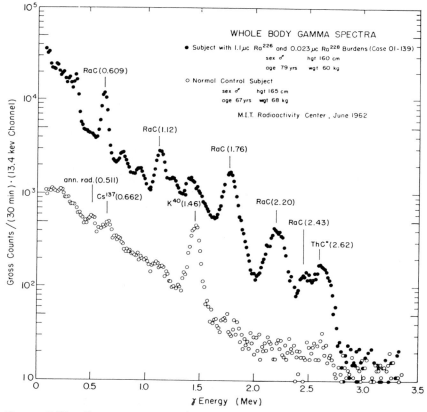

Figure 5-51. Gamma spectrum of a radium dial painter. (From Evans, R. D.: The Radium Standard for Boneseekers—Evaluation of the Data in Radium Patients and Dial Painters. *Health Phys.* 13:267, 1967.)

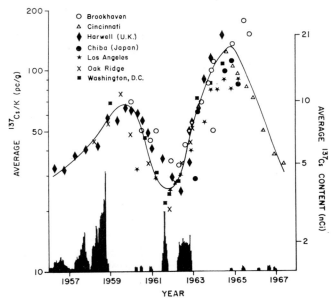

FIGURE 5-52. Cesium-137 body burdens from 1956 to 1967 related to nuclear weapons testing (indicated by black bars at the bottom).

niobium-95, ruthenium-103, -106, and sodium-22 have been identified by low-level whole-body counting.

There is a delay of 8 to 12 months between the time of atmospheric contamination and the appearance of ^{137}Cs in human beings. Particles can be detected in rain and air samples halfway around the world from the site of detonation as early as 1 week after a bomb test. The atmospheric contaminants are incorporated into food products and then ingested. Other radioisotopes of cesium have been detected in man or his environment; ^{134}Cs has been found in Alaskan Eskimos, and ^{136}Cs has been detected in cow's milk.

The cesium content of the body is usually reported as the cesium-potassium ratio, which has been found to be a convenient index. Cesium content is affected by both age and sex, increasing in both sexes to about age 20 and then decreasing slightly thereafter, with less in the adult female. Although most investigators have assumed a Gaussian distribution for total-body ^{137}Cs/^{40}K ratios, Leitnaker and associates (1965) and Ellett and Brownell (1965) observed their data to be skewed and believe ^{137}Cs concentrations best fit a log-normal or gamma distribution. The average biological half-life of ^{137}Cs in adults is quite variable and averages about 100 days; in infants up to 37 days of age, the biological turnover is 7 to 10 days (Vennart, 1964).

Figure 5-52 illustrates the body content of ^{137}Cs obtained from reports in the literature (Rundo and Newton, 1964; Scott, 1964; Leitnaker et al., 1965; Cohn et al., 1965; MacDonald et al., 1965; Iluma et al., 1967; Kolde, 1967; *Radiological Health Data*, 1962). The shaded area represents the relative frequency of atmospheric nuclear weapons testing over the same period. There is a delay of 8 to 12 months before the radioactive cesium appears in man. Although the levels are nearly the same in persons throughout the world, adults in northern areas—Alaskan Eskimos and Finnish, Swedish, and Norwegian Laplanders (not included in this figure)—have body burdens of ^{137}Cs about 50 to 100 times those of people living in temperate zones. Ecological studies have established the lichen → caribou → man cycle as the route taken by the ^{137}Cs in those groups with high levels (Hanson, 1967). The highest levels reported during 1964-1965 (about 150 picocuries of cesium per gram of potassium) contributed about ⅐ of the background dose rate from all natural sources of radiation.

The ^{131}I content in the thyroid gland of normal children as a result of fallout has been monitored and illustrates the use of low-level detectors to assay the radioactivity of people and foodstuffs. Such data provide the basis for determining whether or not the maximal permissible concentrations of radioactivity in food and water have been exceeded.

INDUSTRIAL MONITORING

Whole-body counters have also been useful for monitoring industrial workers exposed to environments containing unusual amounts of radioactivity. Zinc-65 has been detected in some cyclotron workers, as well as in the local population. Certain persons working with nuclear reactors have also been found to be contaminated with various radionuclides. Among the identified radionuclides are chromium-51, cobalt-58, cobalt-60, zinc-65, zirconium-95/niobium-95, silver-110m, iodine-131, and cerium-141.

Whole body counters have been used to estimate the absorbed thermal neutron dose resulting from reactor accidents (Hurst et al., 1959). Measurements were made of the amount of ^{24}Na produced by the exposure. They have also been used to allay the fear of contamination and obviate unnecessary treatment. The absorbed dose can be estimated without having to await the results of excreta collection and analysis.

RADIOPHARMACEUTICAL STUDIES

Whole-body counting is useful in the development of radiopharmaceuticals. Even with the use of short-lived isotopes, long-term retention data are required to make possible estimation of permissible doses (see Chapter XVII). An isotope with more suitable physical characteristics is often used to study the element of interest. For example, indium-114 has been used to study the metabolism of indium, even though the short-lived indium, ^{113m}In, was of primary interest. Beasley and his associates (1966) used technetium-95m (half-life, 60 days) and technetium-96 (half-life, 4.3 days) to determine the physiological behavior of technetium-99 (half-life, 2×10^5 years) and technetium-99m (half-life, 6 hours).

CLINICAL APPLICATIONS

The major differences between clinical and public health studies based on whole-body counting is that in clinical studies the radionuclide of interest is known and the levels of activity are usually much higher. In studies of intestinal absorption, elimination, and whole-body turnover rates, absolute calibration is not necessary, since after a gamma-emitting radionuclide is administered, we compare the initial measurement with measurements made at some later time. A major advantage is that one need not collect excreta. Some metabolic studies require data on "pool" size, and the administered dose must be high enough to permit a precise count of plasma, urine, or other body fluid samples. Studies can be extended for months or even years, or reliable short-term data can be obtained with a reduction of radiation dose to the patient because of the great sensitivity of the method.

One of the major problems associated with clinical uses of whole-body counting is a change in detection efficiency due to translocation of radioactivity within the body. For example, immediately after ingestion of ^{59}Fe, the radioactivity is primarily distributed within the gastrointestinal tract (stomach, upper small intestine, and portal circulation); the ^{59}Fe is eventually transported to the bone marrow and after about a week is released back into the circulation in red blood cells. These changes of location of the tracer often change the count rate.

Another example of uneven distribution is radium, which is accumulated selectively in specific parts of the skeleton, such as the skull. Vitamin B_{12}, cesium, calcium, and iodide are also distributed unevenly.

POTASSIUM METABOLISM

One of the most frequent uses of whole-body counting has been measurement of the ^{40}K content of the body. This nuclide occurs naturally, and comprises 0.0118 per cent of the naturally occurring element. Because of the constant abundance of ^{40}K, measurement of the nuclide provides an indirect measurement of the quantity of potassium in the body. The accuracy of serial whole-body counting of ^{40}K as a means of studying potassium metabolism is as accurate as the alternate method of measuring the exchangeable potassium space with ^{42}K. The latter requires repeated administration of radioactive material.

Clinical studies of potassium balance using whole-body counters are not as sensitive as the classic balance studies because the coefficient of variation of an individual determination is large (10 to 15 per cent). Therefore, the method is best suited for studies of groups of patients, in which the random errors are smaller and differences in mean values are more significant.

Measurement of ^{40}K can be used to estimate lean body mass (Anderson and Langham, 1959). Since the potassium content of extracellular fluid and fat is low, most of the potassium of the body is contained within the other cellular elements of the body, referred to as *lean body mass.*

Forbes and Hursh (1963) and Forbes (1965), using a single large crystal, found a sex difference in the ^{40}K content of the body that began at about 16 years of age, but they did not find a correlation with weight. Using a 4π liquid scintillation detector, Reba and his associates (1968a) found that with separation of the sexes, total-body water and total-body potassium could be related in a linear fashion in the growing child. In young girls, height and body potassium were linearly related but in boys there was a sharp break in the relation of total potassium to height. This is believed to be related to the increased muscle growth at the time of adolescence in the male (Fig. 5-53).

Measurement of lean body mass is helpful in studies of obesity. Benoit and his associates (1965) found that during total starvation 65 per cent of the weight loss of obese persons was due to loss of lean body mass; only 35 per cent was due to loss of adipose tissue. When the same persons were on a low-calorie, high-fat diet, only 3 per cent of their weight loss was due to loss of lean body mass, and the loss of fat was greater than during absolute deprivation of food. Christian et al. (1964) found that obese young adults on dietary weight reduction lost only fat, and lean body mass remained the same.

Forbes (1964) defined two types of obesity in children. In one type, both

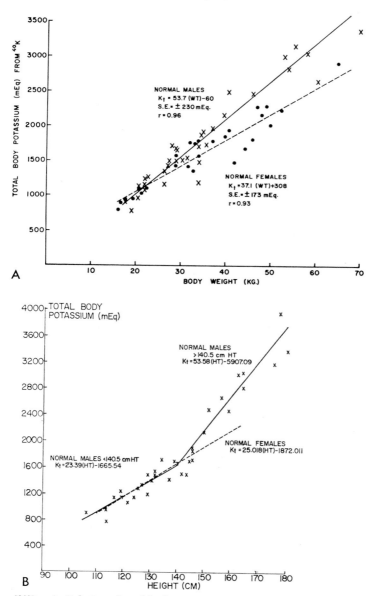

FIGURE 5-53. A, Relation of total body potassium to body weight in children. B, Relation of total body potassium to height in children. (From Reba, R. C., et al.: Body Potassium and Lean Body Mass. In Cheek, D. B. (ed.): Human Growth: Body Composition, Cytology, Energy and Intelligence. Lea & Febiger, Philadelphia, 1968.)

lean body mass and body fat was increased; in the other, only the fat content was increased.

Hypokalemia is a complication of a wide variety of medical and surgical disorders, and may progress to a severe degree before being diagnosed. A significant decrease in body potassium can be present with normal serum potassium. Metabolic balance studies, 24 hour urinary potassium excretion, 48 hour exchangeable space, and muscle biopsy are alternative methods for measuring body potassium, but whole-body counting is rapid, simple, and effective. For example, patients with primary muscle diseases, such as muscular dystrophy, have been found to have significantly decreased body potassium. The degree of potassium deficit correlates with the severity of the disease. Healthy family members, parents and siblings, of these patients also have significant decreases in body potassium allowing the ready identification of this genetic trait (Blahd et al., 1964).

Iron

Iron deficiency is a common nutritional deficiency. The early studies of iron absorption and excretion were obtained from balance studies of stable iron, and later by measurements of ^{55}Fe and ^{59}Fe incorporation into red cells, together with the fecal excretion of unabsorbed radioiron. The whole-body counter can be used to measure directly the body retention of orally administered iron, to establish dietary iron requirements, to quantify loss of iron and of labeled red cells, and to determine the metabolic turnover of radioiron.

The percentage absorption of iron is related to the age of the patient and to the administered dose (up to 5 mg.). In the absorption test, 0.1 to 10 μc. of ^{59}Fe and 0.25 to 5.00 mg. of a ferrous salt are administered and the first whole-body measurement is obtained 4 to 10 hours later. The percentage of the dose absorbed is estimated from a single measurement 14 to 21 days later. With a 0.25 mg. dose of carrier iron, normal absorption after 2 to 3 weeks is 5 to 25 percent in normal adults. Because of problems resulting from the variable anatomical distribution of radioactivity, random errors of the order of 10 to 20 per cent or greater are common, yet the precision is sufficient for most clinical purposes.

The chemical form of the administered iron is a significant factor in determining the amount absorbed; equivalent amounts of ferric ion or iron incorporated into food are less efficiently absorbed than the ferrous ion (Chapter IX). Ionic iron ingested with meals is less efficiently absorbed than that administered on an empty stomach. Patients with dumping syndrome due to Billroth II type operations have normal absorption of free ferrous iron but not the iron incorporated in food (Reizenstein and Höglund, 1966).

The most sensitive indication of iron deficiency is the finding of increased absorption of radioiron. Increased iron absorption is often found in advanced pregnancy, hemolytic anemia (despite increased iron stores), iron overload anemia, polycythemia, chronic pancreatitis, and liver disease. Increased iron absorption is found in accelerated erythropoiesis from any cause. Premenopausal adult women normally have a greater iron absorption than adult men because of decreased iron stores. Patients with hemochromatosis have increased absorption of iron, as do some of their relatives apparently free of the disease. Whole-body counting makes possible their detection.

Decreased iron absorption may occur in chronic illnesses, such as rheumatoid arthritis, steatorrhea, and aplastic anemia, and in obese adolescent females. Patients with uremia have been found to have normal absorption of iron, although incorporation of iron into hemoglobin is depressed. Increased dietary intake of phosphates and phytates and gastric achylia may also lead to decreased intestinal absorption of iron. Depressed absorption is often seen in patients with decreased erythropoiesis.

The average rate of daily loss of iron as determined by whole-body counting varied from 0.05 to 0.193 per cent per day in normal adults. These values are somewhat higher than those based on measurement of fecal excretion since iron loss in skin desquamations and other routes is reflected in the whole-body count. Iron loss (and absorption) is two to three times higher in menstruating women; in postmenopausal women, the values are very close to those of adult men. Iron deficiency results in a decreased rate of iron loss from the body (Reizenstein and Höglund, 1966).

Vitamin B_{12}

In studies of vitamin B_{12} metabolism, whole-body counting offers several advantages. It avoids the necessity of collection of urine or feces; it is not necessary to administer a flushing dose of the stable vitamin; and long-term studies can be carried out easily. Usually the initial value is obtained 4 to 6 hours after administration of the oral dose of vitamin B_{12} and body retention is measured after 7 to 10 days.

Using whole-body counting after a 0.5 μg. dose, Heyssel (1966) found absorption of up to 17 per cent of the dose even in patients with pernicious anemia.

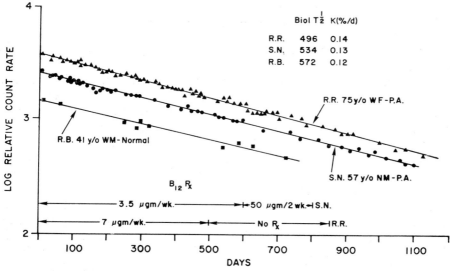

FIGURE 5-54. Body content of ^{60}Co vitamin B_{12} as a function of time in a normal person and two patients with pernicious anemia. Administration of stable vitamin B_{12} had no demonstrable effect on the turnover rate. (From Heyssel, 1967.)

Others have noted absorption as high as 20 to 30 per cent in some patients with pernicious anemia. This was not affected by simultaneous administration of intrinsic factor. Intestinal absorption as determined by this method is usually between 45 and 80 per cent. A second dose of labeled vitamin B_{12} administered 5 hours after the first is absorbed to the same degree as the first. This makes possible simultaneous measurement of vitamin B_{12} absorption with and without intrinsic factor (Reizenstein et al., 1961). Two different nuclides of cobalt (e. g., [58]Co and ^{60}Co) are used as labels.

Long-term studies have demonstrated that the metabolism of administered radiolabeled vitamin B_{12} is the same in normal persons and persons with pernicious anemia (Fig. 5-54) (Heyssel et al., 1965; Heyssel, 1967). The loss of vitamin B_{12} from the body is 1.5 to 5.0 µg. per day; the higher values agree closely with the observations of the time required to develop vitamin B_{12} deficiency after absorption of the vitamin stops, e.g., 3 to 8 years after total gastrectomy.

Cobalt-57 is not used in whole-body counting because of the low energy of the emitted gamma photons; [58]Co and ^{60}Co are more commonly used.

CALCIUM AND STRONTIUM

Calcium deficiency is usually the result of inadequate dietary intake or malabsorption. Most studies of calcium metabolism have been based on balance techniques or on measurements of blood and urine following intravenous administration of stable or radioactive calcium.

Cederquist (1964) and Sargent et al. (1966) have reviewed the studies of calcium and strontium using whole-body counting in the investigation of bone metabolism and disease. The intestinal absorption of calcium has been measured 7 days after the oral administration of 0.5 to 10 µc of [47]Ca in a manner identical to that employed for iron and vitamin B_{12}. There is a graded decrease in the percentage absorption of calcium with increasing doses of carrier in the range of 0.1 µg. to 2000 mg. When [47]Ca is given with 200 mg. of calcium lactate, normal adults retain an average of 39 per cent (range 28 to 54 per cent). Absorption of [47]Ca given with milk is less than when given with an equivalent amount of inorganic calcium, particularly in patients with gastric or pancreatic disease (Deller et al., 1965).

The results with whole-body counters have correlated well with other data. A correction can be made for the amount of endogenous calcium excreted during a previous or subsequent oral test by whole-body counting following intravenous administration of [47]Ca. Patients who have undergone gastric surgery or are suffering from intestinal malabsorption, conditions that are known to be associated with calcium deficiency, have decreased absorption. Patients with sarcoidosis, those receiving vitamin D therapy or anabolic hormones, and those with active acromegaly have normal or increased absorption.

Strontium-85 has been used to study bone metabolism, since strontium and calcium behave similarly in bone metabolism. Once [85]Sr is incorporated into bone, it is handled physiologically like calcium; the long-term retention within the body is related to the rate of resorption of bone. Because of the short physical half-life of [47]Ca (4.7 days) the longer-lived [85]Sr (64 day half-life) is used for longer-term studies. Both calcium and strontium must be used if one is to obtain a complete picture of calcium metabolism by whole-body counting (Sargent et al., 1966). Although ^{45}Ca is now available for long-term studies, whole-body counting with ^{85}Sr provides the only practical means of measuring the turnover of calcium analogs in bone. The metabolism of intravenously injected calcium in metabolic bone disease, such as osteoporosis, or in metastatic breast cancer, can be studied with a whole-body counter.

PROTEIN METABOLISM

Various plasma protein fractions labeled with gamma-emitting radionuclides have been used to measure rates of degradation of plasma proteins. In these studies, one assumes that the rate of elimination of radioactive tracer from the body reflects the rate of protein catabolism. Whole-body counting provides more accurate and more precise data than measurement of the rate of loss of label from the plasma or measurement of urinary radioactivity. The most frequently used label in these studies has been radioactive iodine.

The disappearance of ^{131}I protein from the body appears to be a single exponential function of time from day 3 to 4 to at least day 45 to 50. The usual half-time of albumin in the body is about 20 days (17 to 22 days) in adult males (Lippincott et al., 1961b). Carbon-14-labeled albumin and globulin are not metabolized in the same way as the ^{131}I-labeled proteins, even when more recent methods of iodinating proteins are used.

The half-times of ^{131}I-labeled human gamma globulin range from 5.5 to 19 days (Lippincott et al., 1961a). There is no significant difference in the turnover

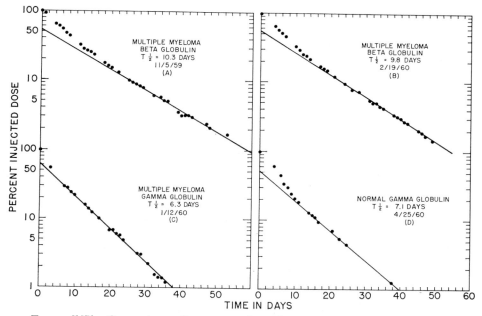

FIGURE 5-55. Comparisons of turnovers of ^{131}I-labeled proteins in a hypergammaglobulinemic patient with multiple myeloma. (From Lippincott, S. W., et al.: Determination of Radioactively Labeled Globulin Turnover by the Direct Whole-Body Counting Technique. *J. Clin. Invest.* 40:697, 1961.)

rates of labeled normal gamma globulin, myeloma gamma globulin, and myeloma beta globulin when studied in the same patient (Fig. 5-55).

The increased levels of globulin in plasma of patients with multiple myeloma appear to be caused by increased synthesis at a rate greater than the increased catabolism of these proteins. On the other hand, the slower rate of gamma globulin catabolism in some patients, together with a decrease in plasma globulin concentration, indicates a decreased rate of synthesis of gamma globulin. Albumin and gamma globulin metabolism have also been studied in the nephrotic syndrome and in various malignancies (Cohn et al., 1966). Natural progression of the disease and the effects of various therapeutic measures can be quantified by the effect on the rate of decrease in whole-body radioactivity.

IODINE METABOLISM

Extrathyroidal metabolism of both thyroxine and triiodothyronine has been determined using whole-body counting (Fisher and Oddie, 1964; Oddie et al., 1964). Thyroxine turnover is about 10 per cent per day in normal persons and somewhat higher in patients with hyperthyroidism. Triiodothyronine has a faster turnover rate, about 50 per cent per day.

About 85 per cent of an orally administered dose of both thyroxine and triiodothyronine was absorbed from the gastrointestinal tract. Degradation rates of both were similar after intravenous and oral doses, but there was a time delay in the degradation of triiodothyronine thought to be due to transient sequestration in the liver. The degradation rate of triiodothyronine was 0.53 per cent per day and of thyroxine 0.11 per cent per day. The apparent volume of distribution of triiodothyronine was 31 liters and of thyroxine 10 liters.

Whole-body counting has also been used in the follow-up of patients with metastatic thyroid carcinoma, for example, to assay whether any functioning metastatic tissue remains after ablative therapy (Oberhausen, 1966). Whole-body retention of more than 3 per cent of the dose of radioiodine 3 days after administration is presumptive evidence of functioning thyroid metastases.

REGIONAL BLOOD VOLUMES

Regional blood volumes can be determined by the use of whole-body counting. After the total blood volume is determined by the indicator dilution method, the patient is placed in the whole-body counter. After the total counts are recorded, the regional blood pool of interest is completely shielded and a repeat count is taken. The fractional decrease times the total blood volume is the volume of the region of interest (Sevelius et al., 1965).

BLOOD LOSS

Serial whole-body counting of patients after intravenous injection of labeled red blood cells can be used to monitor blood loss, for example, during surgical procedures. Measurements can be made immediately before and after operation. Calibration can be achieved by comparing the results of whole-body counting with the indicator dilution technique performed immediately before surgery.

Electrolytes (other than potassium)

Whole-body counting has been used to simplify measurements of exchangeable body pools of electrolytes, e.g., sodium, potassium, and bromine. Jagger and his associates (1963) used this method to measure [22]Na retention for long periods and found the method superior to usual balance techniques for the study of sodium metabolism. Patients have been assayed for up to 4 years after a single 25 μc. administration of [22]Na. A small component, 0.35 per cent of the injected dose, has a biological turnover of about 1000 days, believed to represent a bone "compartment." Such data could have been obtained only with a whole-body counter.

Veall used a simple whole-body counter to measure sodium retention for a period of up to 1 month after the administration of 20 μc. of [22]Na (Veall, 1962). Dahl and his associates (1962) found a prolonged biological half-life of [22]Na in patients with essential hypertension. Recently, however, Dahl et al. (1966) were unable to find a significant difference in the long-term whole-body turnover of sodium in patients with essential hypertension.

Miscellaneous uses

Activation Analysis. A new application of whole-body counting is to measure the radioactivity induced in the body by intentional exposure to high-energy or thermal neutrons for the purpose of determining the body content of elements such as sodium, chlorine, and calcium. Anderson and associates (1964) exposed two human patients to neutrons and then performed whole-body gamma-ray spectroscopy. Sodium-24, chlorine-38, and calcium-49 were readily identified. The values obtained for total-body sodium were almost identical to those estimated from the 24 hour [24]Na exchangeable space. Chlorine and calcium measurements were also attempted and although the correlation was not as good as for sodium, the values were reasonable. Total-body radiation dose was 0.1 rad.

The alpha beam from a cyclotron used for pituitary irradiation has induced ^{11}C activity in patients. Total-body disappearance was measured by whole-body counting and breath analysis (Sargent, 1962).

Bremsstrahlung Detection. Although whole-body counting is usually based on measurement of emitted gamma photons, the method has also been applied to radionuclides that decay only by emission of beta particles. For example, phosphorus-32, strontium-89, and strontium-90 have been measured in the body when present in amounts of 0.01 to 0.02 μc. (Bengtsson, 1964).

Trace Element Analysis. Copper (in Wilson's disease), zinc, trivalent chromium, and manganese (in extrapyramidal disease) have all been studied with whole-body counting. Cotzias (1963) has shown that body turnover of manganese is related to the level of dietary manganese and that the excretion of radiomanganese can be increased by oral administration of the stable element. Such experiments have led Cotzias and his co-workers to believe that manganese, like zinc, is under homeostatic control. Whole-body turnover studies have been used to predict the effect of chelation therapy in subjects suffering from chronic manganese poisoning (Mena et al., 1967).

Trivalent chromium has been difficult to study because of its poor intestinal

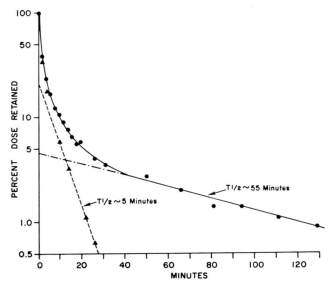

Figure 5-56. Body content of ^{85}Kr after intravenous administration. Less than 1 per cent of the dose was present in urine voided after the last body count.

absorption and immediate binding to serum proteins after intravenous administration. This latter property has allowed the evaluation of protein loss from the body after injection of ^{51}CrCl$_3$. In the absence of protein loss, there is little variation in the whole-body turnover of trivalent chromium.

Using four species, mice, rats, dog, and man, Richmond et al. (1962) have related the whole-body retention of zinc (^{65}ZnCl$_2$) to body weight, basal metabolism, and energy expended (calories per gram per day). In all instances smooth curves were obtained, implying that when properly defined, data from smaller mammalian species can be extrapolated to man. The best estimate of the long-term biological half-life of zinc is 300 to 450 days (Spencer et al., 1965).

Radiation Dosimetry. As discussed in Chapter XVII, whole-body counters have been useful in providing the biological data necessary for the calculation of radiation dose. In these studies, it is imperative that the entire injected dose of the radiopharmaceutical be accounted for, even when we are uncertain of its localization. The whole-body counter is particularly useful under these circumstances. For example, the total-body content of Krypton-85 was measured after it had been administered by intravenous injection. It could be demonstrated that less than 1 per cent of the dose remained after 2 hours (Fig. 5-56). This ruled out sequestration of the radionuclide in unsuspected areas.

LIQUID SCINTILLATION COUNTING

Arthur Karmen

Solutions of certain fluorescent compounds emit light when ionizing radiation deposits energy in them. Liquid scintillation counting is based on detecting and measuring this light. Although it can be used to detect many types of ionizing radiation, liquid scintillation counting is particularly useful for counting low-energy alpha or beta particles.

Since the sample can usually be incorporated directly into the solution of the scintillator, there are no losses of counts from absorption of the radiation in a counter window or from self-absorption of the radiation in the sample. The efficiency of counting is higher than in solid sample counting. Even beta particles of very low energy, such as those from tritium, can be counted with high efficiency. Compared to gas counting methods, larger quantities of sample can be counted and preparation of the sample for counting is simpler. Since the light output is proportional to the energy deposited in the scintillator, several isotopes that emit particles of different energies can be counted simultaneously.

THE SCINTILLATION PROCESS

The liquid scintillator consists of a dilute solution of one or more fluorescent compounds dissolved in a solvent. The radioactive particle or photon deposits energy in the solvent, causing excitation of the fluorescent solutes, which release the energy as a burst of light. This light interacts with the photocathode of a photomultiplier tube and gives rise to an electrical pulse which is amplified, analyzed, sorted according to its size, and counted.

THE SOLVENT

The solvent serves two functions: it dissolves the fluorescent solutes and the sample, and it absorbs and transfers the energy of the radioactive particle. Since not all liquids transfer electronic excitation with equal efficiency, the choice of solvents is limited. Commonly used solvents include toluene, xylene, dioxane, and several other alkyl benzenes. Fortunately, many organic compounds are quite soluble in these solvents. Other compounds can be solubilized by the addition of small quantities of other solvents that do not interfere with either the generation or emission of the scintillations.

THE PRIMARY SOLUTE

PPO (2,5 diphenyloxazole), PPD (phenyldiphenyloxadiazole), and *p*-terphenyl are examples of fluorescent compounds used as primary solutes. They receive the excitation energy from the solvent and emit it as a burst of light. Since concentrations of 5 to 10 g. per liter are required for maximal light output, poor solubility in toluene can limit the usefulness of a compound as a primary solute. *p*-Terphenyl, for example, was one of the earliest primary solutes and is still one of the least expensive. But, because *p*-terphenyl is not very soluble in cold toluene, PPO, which is more soluble, is now more commonly used.

THE SECONDARY SOLUTE

The wavelength of the light emitted by most primary solutes is shorter than that to which the photomultiplier is most sensitive. A secondary fluorescent solute such as POPOP (1,4-bis-2-[5-phenyloxazolyl]-benzene) is added to the solution to absorb the photons emitted by the primary solute and to emit photons of a longer wavelength. The photomultiplier then detects more of the emitted light photons and the efficiency of counting is improved. Because of its more ideal emission spectrum, POPOP would be an ideal primary solute were it not for its low solubility in toluene. It is an effective secondary solute or wavelength shifter even at concentrations one tenth that of the primary solute, i.e., about 0.5 g. per liter.

DETECTING THE SCINTILLATIONS

Interaction of a low-energy radioactive particle with the liquid scintillator gives rise to only a small number of photons. Sensitive photomultiplier tubes are required for their detection. Unfortunately, the photocathodes of sensitive photo-multiplier tubes tend to emit electrons even in the absence of light that are indistinguishable from those emitted when light photons interact with the photocathode. Three measures are employed to reduce the resulting noise or background counting rate. First, the photomultiplier tubes are refrigerated to reduce this thermionic emission. Second, since interaction of a burst of light photons with the photocathode generally gives rise to a number of electrons simultaneously, the electrical pulses are usually larger than those that follow single thermionic electrons. Pulse-height analysis is therefore often helpful in distinguishing signal from noise pulses. The third and most effective measure is coincidence counting. When the scintillator absorbs a beta particle, it emits a number of light photons simultaneously. Two photomultiplier tubes view the scintillator. Their outputs are so arranged that only pulses that appear in both tubes simultaneously are counted. This is effective in reducing background be-cause the probability of simultaneous thermionic emission of electrons from both photomultiplier tubes is small. Through the use of refrigerated photomultiplier tubes, coincidence counting, and pulse-height analysis, typical background count-ing rates, under conditions suitable for carbon-14 assay at 80 per cent efficiency, are frequently less than 10 counts/min.

INSTRUMENTATION

The unknown sample is usually counted in 10 to 15 ml. of scintillator solution in a 20 ml. glass or polyethylene counting vial which is coupled by a light pipe to the photosensitive surfaces of two selected photomultiplier tubes. The pulses in the outputs of both tubes are fed to the coincidence network and also are electrically summed to reflect more closely the total number of photons detected. This sum pulse is amplified, subjected to pulse-height analysis, and sorted into one or more scalers according to its size.

Several factors in addition to the energy deposited by the radioactive event determine the size of the electrical pulse. These include the chemistry of the scintillator, the voltage on the photomultiplier tube, and the gain of the amplifier. To achieve comparable efficiencies of counting for each sample in a series, we generally attempt to keep the chemistry of the scintillator as constant as possible and to compensate electrically for small changes in that chemistry. We then choose instrument settings for counting each isotope that yield the highest efficiency-to-background ratios. One method of selecting these settings is as follows: An unquenched sample of liquid scintillator containing tritium is placed in the sample well. Each scaler channel is defined by an upper and lower pulse-height discriminator; i.e., the pulse must exceed the lower but not the upper discriminator to be registered in the channel. The lower discriminator of one channel is set just high enough to exclude amplifier noise and the upper discriminator is set at its maximum, thus defining a "wide window." With the amplifier gain set at midscale, the high voltage is adjusted until the counting rate in that window is maximal. These settings will be close to optimal for counting tritium in an unquenched sample since most of the tritium pulses will be counted and most of the larger pulses that originate from background radiation will be excluded. Then a known quantity of tritium dissolved in the same scintillation solution as the unknown sample is placed in the well. The amplifier gain is increased until the counting rate in the window is again maximal. These settings are close to optimal for tritium in the actual samples to be counted, for the same reasons.

Amplifier gain settings are adjusted for each isotope in the same way. For example, since the beta of ^{14}C is more energetic than that of the tritium, it gives rise to larger pulses. At settings optimized for tritium, many of these pulses will exceed the levels of the upper discriminator. Since the optimal settings for a given isotope are those that yield the maximal number of counts in a wide window, the amplifier gain must therefore be decreased for ^{14}C counting.

Liquid scintillation counters that can count as many as 400 samples automatically are available. These instruments sort pulses into as many as five separate scalers. The versatility of this equipment makes possible a number of different approaches to counting.

COUNTING OF SAMPLES THAT CONTAIN DIFFERENT ISOTOPES

If the amplifier gain and the window settings are chosen properly, each channel can be set to count only one of several different isotopes. A series of samples, each of which contains only one isotope, can then be counted automatically during the same time period. This ability to count different isotopes in the same series of samples can greatly increase the counting capability of a laboratory.

AUTOMATIC MONITORING FOR QUENCHING

Although self-absorption is not a significant problem in liquid scintillation counting, as it is when samples are counted on planchets, a comparable problem that is often encountered is that certain samples contain compounds that quench; i.e., interfere with the generation or the emission of the light pulses. Two mechanisms of quenching are generally distinguished: "chemical quenching" and "color quenching." Thus compounds such as carbon tetrachloride interfere with the transfer of energy from solvent to solute or with the emission of light by the solute. Colored compounds, particularly those that are yellow in solution, interfere primarily by absorbing the emitted light. Since most samples cause some degree of quenching, particularly when present in high concentrations, the efficiency of counting may vary from one sample to the next. It is generally important to estimate the efficiency of counting in each sample. There are several methods for doing this. One of these, known as the "channels ratio" method, is based almost entirely on pulse-height analysis. Window and gain settings for one channel are optimized for an unquenched sample of the isotope to be counted. A second channel is set to record only a fraction of those pulses, generally those above the average pulse height. As long as the chemistry of the scintillator remains constant, the pulse-height spectrum remains constant and the ratio of the counts in the two channels remains the same. If a chemical or color-quenching agent diminishes the number of photons emitted, some of the large pulses are converted into smaller pulses and the ratio shifts downward. Once the relationship between this ratio and the efficiency of counting is determined by counting samples containing known quantities of isotope and graded quantities of quenching agent, the counting efficiency for each isotope can be estimated from the shift in the ratio.

DETERMINATION OF EFFICIENCY WITH INTERNAL STANDARDS

When a more accurate estimate of efficiency is required, it is helpful to determine the efficiency of counting of *each* isotope in *each* sample in *each* channel by first counting the mixtures and then repeating the count, first after the addition of a known quantity of ^3H and then again after the addition of a known quantity of ^{14}C. Standard solutions of ^3H- and ^{14}C-labeled toluene, which do not themselves quench, are used for this purpose.

DETERMINATION OF EFFICIENCY WITH EXTERNAL STANDARDS

Another approach to monitoring for quenching is to count each sample as usual and then to expose it to a high-energy gamma source and to count it again. When the sample is exposed to the gamma source, the spectrum of pulses will include many that are much larger than those emitted when ^{14}C or ^3H alone is present. The discriminator and gain settings for one or more channels are set up to record portions of the spectrum containing the largest pulses. If the sample is quenched and the amplitude of all pulses is decreased, the counting rate in these channels will decrease or the ratio of pulses will change. A series of samples that each contain a constant, known quantity of either ^{14}C or ^3H and graded quantities of a quenching agent are counted to determine the relationship between the efficiency of counting ^{14}C and ^3H in their respective channels and the counting rates of the external standard in its respective channels. Once this relationship is known, the efficiency of counting of each isotope in the unknown sample in each of the channels can be estimated directly from the counting rate of the external standard in its own channels.

BALANCE-POINT COUNTING

We can optimize the setting of the amplifier for a given isotope and then reduce the upper discriminator setting so that a small fraction of the largest pulses is excluded from the window. Then, if a quenching agent is added, the amplitude of some of these pulses will be reduced so that they are counted in the window. At the same time, a number of smaller pulses will be reduced in size below the threshold of the lower discriminator. If the window settings are chosen properly, the number of pulses decreased in size so that they are counted in the window will be equal to the number decreased below the level of the lower discriminator, and the counts within the window will be relatively insensitive to quenching. This mode of operation, called "balance-point counting," is often the optimal method.

SIMULTANEOUS COUNTING OF TWO ISOTOPES

Two isotopes emitting beta particles of different energies, such as ^{14}C and ^3H, can be assayed simultaneously in the same sample by means of pulse-height analysis. Since the energy of the beta particles of each isotope extends continuously from very low levels up to a maximal energy characteristic of the isotope, the beta spectra of all different isotopes overlap to some degree. Some of the pulses from the more energetic isotope always appear in the channel optimized for the isotope with the lower energy. The spectrometer is set for simultaneous ^{14}C and ^3H counting as follows. One channel is optimized for each isotope. The efficiency of counting of each isotope in each channel is determined by counting known samples of each isotope separately. When a sample containing a mixture of both is counted, the quantity of each can be calculated from the counting rates in each window by the use of two simultaneous equations. Usually, in ^{14}C–^3H simultaneous counting, the lower level discriminator for the upper or ^{14}C channel is raised somewhat above the optimal level so that all the pulses of the ^3H are excluded. The counts in this channel will then be due only to ^{14}C. The quantity of ^3H present is calculated after the contribution of ^{14}C is subtracted from the counting rate in the lower channel.

Automatic equipment is now available that offers automatic background subtraction, automatic external standardization, and built-in special-purpose computers for calculating and printing out the number of disintegrations per minute for each isotope in each sample.

SAMPLE PREPARATION

A sample can be dissolved in the scintillator, suspended in the scintillator, or coated on the surface of the scintillator, or, alternatively, the scintillator can be dissolved or suspended in the sample. Each method offers advantages for specific applications.

COUNTING OF SOLUTIONS

The simplest method for preparing a sample for liquid scintillation counting is to dissolve the sample in the scintillation solution. Toluene, which is one of the best scintillation solvents, is also a good solvent for lipids, hydrocarbons, and other such relatively nonpolar, fat-soluble compounds. Appreciable quantities of many of these compounds can be dissolved in the scintillator solution without decreasing its counting efficiency. Others cause quenching and can be counted efficiently only in dilute solution.

More polar compounds that are not very soluble in toluene can often be counted in toluene solutions containing small quantities of solvents such as ethanol. The counting efficiency of these solutions is usually appreciably less than that of toluene alone. However, as much as 1 ml. of water can be incorporated into a toluene:ethanol (70:30) mixture and counted with fairly high efficiency. Other similar additives are used for other specific compounds.

COUNTING OF SUSPENSIONS

Many materials can best be counted by suspending rather than dissolving them in the liquid scintillator. For example, carbon dioxide can be precipitated as barium carbonate and then suspended in the liquid scintillator with the help of a thixotropic gelling agent such as Thixcin or Cab-o-sil. Silica gel from thin-layer chromatography plates can be counted in the same way. Samples deposited on filter paper—such as sections of paper chromatograms—can be counted by depositing the entire strip of paper in the liquid scintillator. The efficiency with which these suspended materials are counted is surprisingly good. Light scattering in the sample is not as great a problem in liquid scintillation counting as it is in most other optical systems. Many samples that appear quite opaque because of light scattering can be counted with high efficiency.

COUNTING OF AQUEOUS SOLUTIONS BY PLACING THEM IN
CONTACT WITH FINELY DIVIDED CRYSTALLINE SCINTILLATORS

Another method for counting aqueous solutions is to suspend finely divided crystals of organic scintillator within them. Steinberg (1959) simply poured the solution to be counted over a weighed amount of crystalline anthracene in a conventional counting vial. The efficiency for ^{14}C was quite high (50 per cent or more). The system was also useful for tritium counting even though the efficiency was only about 1 per cent, because a relatively large sample could be counted. This work was the basis of the use of finely divided anthracene crystals for detecting the radioactivity in flowing liquids effluents of ion exchange and other columns such as are used for amino acid analysis.

High-boiling organic materials can be collected from the gas phase and counted on crystalline scintillators coated with a thin film of silicone oil (Karmen and Tritch, 1960). The counting efficiency is high because the radioactive material is in close contact with the scintillator. This technique is particularly useful for collecting and counting high-boiling materials in the effluent of gas chromatography columns.

We can usually choose from a number of alternative methods for counting a given type of sample. In choosing, one considers the specific radioactivity as well as the total radioactivity of the sample. When the specific radioactivity is low, we choose a method that permits counting of a large sample even if its efficiency is low. When the quantity of radioactivity is small, the method that offers higher efficiency may be more useful. Whatever method is chosen, it is best to count samples that contain both large and small quantities of material with the same sensitivity. Since solutions and suspensions are counted with different efficiencies, the radioactive material should be either completely in solution or completely in suspension rather than distributed between the two phases.

APPLICATIONS

The compositions of some useful scintillation solutions are given in Table 5-5.

COMPOUNDS SOLUBLE IN TOLUENE

Solutions of toluene-soluble lipids, hydrocarbons, steroids, and other similar organic compounds can be counted by pipetting an aliquot into PPO-toluene-POPOP. If the sample is dissolved in a solvent that quenches, such as chloroform, the solvent should be evaporated and the sample redissolved in benzene or toluene before the scintillator solution is added. The efficiency of counting can be determined by either the internal standard or the easier external standard method.

COMPOUNDS NOT SOLUBLE IN TOLUENE

Dilute solutions of many water-soluble compounds can be incorporated into one of the toluene-ethanol scintillation mixtures or into Bray's solution (Table 5-5). Care should be taken not to exceed the solubility of the compound in cold scintillation solution, or there may be a continual decrease in the counting rate as more and more of the radioactive material precipitates and is counted with lower efficiency. In assays in which the solubility is doubtful, it is often better either to prepare toluene-soluble derivatives of the radioactive compound or to precipitate it completely and count it as a suspension. Compounds such as Hyamine hydroxide form toluene-soluble derivatives with carbon dioxide, many hydroxy acids, and amino acids. Peptides, proteins, whole tissue, and tissue extracts can be solubilized by heating with a Hyamine solution. Unfortunately, chemiluminescence is sometimes encountered in these solutions. The occurrence of this phenomenon can be recognized if nonradioactive "blank" samples of the tissue are counted. It may be decreased by neutralizing the sample before counting.

Many inorganic cations such as barium, calcium, cadmium, potassium, rubidium, and cesium can be counted as salts of organic acids. They can also be counted as derivatives of di(2)-ethylhexyl phosphoric acid and other similar organic complexing agents.

TABLE 5-5. TYPICAL SCINTILLATION SOLUTIONS

SOLVENT (ml.)	PRIMARY SOLUTE (g./l.)		SECONDARY SOLUTE (g./l.)	
For toluene-soluble materials				
Toluene 1000	PPO	5	POPOP	0.1
Xylene 1000	PPO	4	POPOP	0.05
For carbon dioxide				
Toluene 1000	PPO	4	POPOP	0.05
(Add 1 ml. hydroxide of Hyamine, 1 N in methanol, to each 15 ml. of solution)				
For aqueous solution				
Toluene 500	PPO	4	POPOP	0.01
Ethanol 500				
Naphthalene 60 g.	PPO	4	Dimethyl POPOP	0.02
Ethylene glycol 20 ml.				
Methanol 100 ml.				
Dioxane to 1 liter (Bray, 1960)				

BIOLOGICAL MATERIAL

Several methods have been described for assaying whole blood, urine, and tissue for ^{14}C and ^3H by liquid scintillation counting. Usually there is little problem if only small quantities are to be assayed. The entire sample is dissolved in toluene with the aid of an agent such as Hyamine hydroxide. However, if the specific activity of the sample is low and it becomes necessary to count somewhat larger quantities, problems may arise. For example, if radioactivity is present in a variety of chemical compounds, some may tend to precipitate while others remain in solution. Knowledge of the chemical nature of the radioactive compounds is very useful in these instances. When larger quantities of tissue are to be counted, more accurate results may be obtained if the sample is subjected to combustion to carbon dioxide and water before counting. Combustion also eliminates problems involved in counting compounds that are difficult to dissolve, or that form colored solutions, or that act as chemical quenching agents. One of the most convenient methods is oxygen flask combustion.

LIQUID SCINTILLATION COUNTING OF CARBON DIOXIDE

Carbon dioxide can be trapped and counted in a solution of an organic base such as phenylethyl amine, ethanolamine, or hydroxide of Hyamine, all of which form toluene-soluble carbonates. These may be counted in the usual PPO-POPOP-toluene mixtures. Since the light output is generally diminished by the presence of these bases, the efficiency is somewhat less than with unquenched solutions, even with amplifier gain set somewhat higher than usual. This technique is most useful for counting samples of about 1 mM. of CO_2. When smaller quantities are to be counted, as, for example, in studies of the release of CO_2 from an incubated tissue specimen, it may be more convenient to trap the CO_2 on filter paper soaked with a solution of inorganic base, and then to dry the paper and put it directly into the PPO-toluene. For counting larger quantities, CO_2 can be collected in a solution of sodium or potassium hydroxide and then precipitated as barium carbonate by the addition of barium hydroxide. The barium carbonate is suspended in PPO-toluene with the help of Cab-o-sil or a similar gelling agent.

A convenient method for determining the specific radioactivity of CO_2 in expired air is to blow it through a drying agent and then over the surface of a measured quantity, usually 1 mM., of Hyamine hydroxide solution containing phenolphthalein as a pH indicator (von Schuching and Abt, 1965). When the indicator is decolorized, signaling that the carbon dioxide has neutralized the Hyamine, PPO-toluene is added and the sample is counted as usual. The specific radioactivity is calculated directly from the counting rate. This method circumvents the many problems associated with measuring the $^{14}CO_2$ and $^{12}CO_2$ concentrations in the expired air separately.

SCINTILLATION COUNTING OF GASES

Carbon dioxide-14 and tritium-labeled hydrogen in the gas phase can also be counted by passing them through a tube filled with small anthracene crystals. The scintillations are approximately the same size as those produced by ^{14}C

and ^3H in a liquid scintillator and the same equipment can be used to measure them. A useful application of this detector is in measuring ^{14}C and ^3H in the effluent of a gas chromatography column. The column effluent is passed through a combustion train which converts organic compounds to $^{14}CO_2$ and $^3H_2$ and then through the detector. The sensitivity of the anthracene crystal scintillation counter for ^{14}C is comparable to that of an ionization chamber or proportional counter. It is less sensitive to changes in the composition of the gas; this is helpful if the sample contains compounds of different specific activities. In addition, ^{14}C and ^3H can be assayed simultaneously through the use of pulse-height analysis.

INTERPRETATION OF RESULTS

In all metabolic studies with labeled compounds, we cannot assume that the radioactivity in a particular tissue or body fluid is in the same chemical form as the original compound administered. This is particularly true for ^{14}C- and ^3H-labeled compounds, most of which are readily metabolized and are useful primarily because they are metabolized. A correct interpretation of the results of an experiment frequently hinges on the accuracy with which the radioactive compounds are identified. This, in turn, depends directly on the adequacy of the chemical methods used to isolate and purify the sample before counting. For example, following its intravenous administration, ^{14}C-labeled palmitate disappears from the blood with a half-time of about 2 minutes and almost immediately thereafter, ^{14}C-labeled bicarbonate appears. The total ^{14}C in the blood soon after the injection reflects both palmitate and bicarbonate radioactivity which must be separated if the clearance of palmitate from the blood is to be determined. Several simple extraction procedures can be used to accomplish this separation. After several more minutes have passed, esters of palmitic acid and other metabolites appear in the blood, and a more elaborate extraction or chromatographic separation is necessary.

Another instance in which chemical separation is of great importance is in the simultaneous measurement of ^{14}C and ^3H in double-isotope derivative assays, as, for example, in the assay of testosterone. This assay is usually performed as follows: a small quantity of high-specific-activity ^3H-testosterone is added to the sample. The testosterone is extracted and then reacted with a ^{14}C-labeled reagent such as ^{14}C-acetic anhydride. The labeled testosterone acetate is then extracted, isolated, and counted for ^3H and ^{14}C. The total quantity of testosterone in the final sample is calculated from the ^{14}C and the specific radioactivity of the ^{14}C-anhydride, and the recovery of the testosterone in the original sample is estimated from the ^3H level. The total quantity of testosterone in the original mixture is then calculated. The accuracy of this method depends on the separation of testosterone from the other compounds in the sample that can react with acetic anhydride and on the separation of the testosterone acetate from the acetates of these other compounds. To insure the purity of the final product, the labeled acetate is usually chromatographed in several different systems until the ratio of ^{14}C to ^3H no longer decreases with succeeding separations. The accuracy of the final result depends directly on how well this purification is carried out.

The value of the results in a biological study involving ^{14}C- and ^3H-labeled compounds may depend as much on the resolution of the chemical methods used to separate the radioactive compounds as on the method of counting. One of the most useful features of liquid scintillation counting techniques, among which we may include the counting methods based on the use of finely divided solid scintillators, is that they are readily adaptable for use with many kinds of chromatographic methods.

Although liquid scintillation counting is useful in biological studies primarily because of its high sensitivity for ^{14}C and ^{3}H, a significant factor that determines its utility is the convenience with which a large number of samples can be counted in a given day. This convenience is partly attributable to the ease with which samples may be prepared for counting and partly to the automatic counting equipment that is available. Because of this convenience, liquid scintillation counting is the method of choice for most ^{3}H and ^{14}C assay. A variety of methods have been developed to apply it to the assay of many other radionuclides as well.

REFERENCES

MEASUREMENT OF RADIOACTIVITY

Compton, A. H.: A Quantum Theory of the Scattering of X-rays by Light Elements. *Physical Rev.* 21:483, 1923.

Gibbs, W. D.: The "Hot-Patient Counter." ORINS-42. Clearing House for Federal Scientific and Technical Information, National Bureau of Standards, Springfield, Va., 1962, p. 45; A New Large-Volume Radioactive Sample Counter. ORINS-43. Clearing House for Federal Scientific and Technical Information, National Bureau of Standards, Springfield, Va., 1963, p. 88.

Harris, C. C.: Certain Fundamental Physical Considerations in Scanning. *In* Quinn, J. L., Ed.: Scintillation Scanning in Clinical Medicine. W. B. Saunders Co., Philadelphia, 1964, p. 13.

Harris, C. C., Hamblen, D. P., and Francis, J. E., Jr.: Basic Principles of Scintillation Counting for Medical Investigators. ORNL-2808. Clearing House for Federal Scientific and Technical Information, National Bureau of Standards, Springfield, Va., 1959.

Harris, C. C., Satterfield, M. M., Bell, P. R., and Ross, D. A.: A Comparison of Various Methods of Rate Recording. *In* Croll, M. N., and Brady, L. W., Eds.: Recent Advances in Nuclear Medicine. Appleton-Century-Crofts, New York, 1966.

Harris, C. C., Satterfield, M. M., Ross, D. A., and Bell, P. R.: Rectilinear vs. Stationary Scanners. Presented at A Symposium on Fundamental Problems in Scanning, Chicago, May 8–9, 1965. Charles C Thomas, Springfield, Ill., 1966.

Heath, R. L.: Scintillation Spectrometry: Gamma-Ray Spectrum Catalogue. TID-4500. Ed. 2. Vols. 1 and 2. Clearing House for Federal Scientific and Technical Information, National Bureau of Standards, Springfield, Va., 1964.

Ross, D. A.: Medical Gamma-Ray Spectometry. ORINS-30. Clearing House for Federal Scientific and Technical Information, National Bureau of Standards, Springfield, Va., 1959.

Ross, D. A., Harris, C. C., Satterfield, M. M., and Bell, P. R.: New Challenges in Clinical Counting. *Jap. J. Nuclear Med.* 2:81, 1965.

Ross, D. A., Harris, C. C., Satterfield, M. M., Bell, P. R., and Jordan, J. C.: Low-Energy Gamma-Emitters in Scanning and Other Clinical Applications. *Radioaktive Isotope in Klinik und Forschung* 6:108 (*Strahlentherapie* Supplement vol. 60) Urban & Schwarzenberg, München-Berlin, 1965.

General References

Crouthamel, C. E.: Applied Gamma-Ray Spectrometry. International Series of Monographs on Analytical Chemistry, Pergamon Press, New York, 1960.

Neiler, J. H., and Bell, P. R.: The Scintillation Method. *In* Siegbahn, K., Ed.: Alpha, Beta, and Gamma-Ray Spectroscopy. Vol. I. North-Holland Publishing Co., Amsterdam, 1965, p. 245.

Physical principles of radionuclide scanning

Adam, W. E., Loreny, W. J., and Scheer, K. E.: Quantitative Untersuchungen mit der Szintillationskamera. *In* Hoffman, G., and Scheer, K. E. (eds.): Radioisotope in der Lokalisationsdiagnostik. F. K. Schattauer-Verlag, Stuttgart, 1967.

Allen, H. C., Jr., and Risser, J. R.: Simplified Apparatus for Brain Tumor Surveys. *Nucleonics* 13:28, 1955.

Allen, H. C., Jr., Risser, J. R., and Greene, J. A.: Improvements in Outlining of Thyroid and Localization of Brain Tumors by the Application of Sodium Iodide Gamma-Ray Spectrometry Techniques. *In* Proceedings of the Second Oxford Radioisotope Conference, Oxford, July 19-23, 1954. Vol. I. Academic Press, New York, 1954, pp. 76-96.

Anger, H. O.: A Multiple Scintillation Counter In-vivo Scanner. *Amer. J. Roentgen.* 70:605, 1953.

Anger, H. O.: Scintillation Camera. *Rev. Sci. Instr.* 29:27, 1958.

Anger, H. O.: Gamma-Ray and Positron Scintillation Camera. *Nucleonics* 21:56, 1963.

Anger, H. O.: Scintillation Camera with Multichannel Collimators. *J. Nucl. Med.* 5:515, 1964.

Anger, H. O.: Whole Body Scanner Mark II. *J. Nucl. Med.* 7:331, 1966a.

Anger, H. O.: Survey of Radioisotope Cameras. *ISA Trans.* 5:311, 1966b.

Anger, H. O., and Davis, D. H.: Gamma-Ray-Detection Efficiency and Image Resolution in Sodium Iodide. *Rev. Sci. Instr.* 35:693, 1964.

Anger, H. O., Mortimer, R. K., and Tobias, C. A.: Visualization of Gamma-Ray Emitting Isotopes in the Human Body. *In* Proceedings of the International Conference on the Peaceful Uses of Atomic Energy 14:204, 1956.

Anger, H. O., and Rosenthal, D. J.: Scintillation Camera and Positron Camera. *In* Medical Radioisotope Scanning. International Atomic Energy Agency, Vienna, 1959, p. 59.

Anger, H. O., Van Dyke, D. C., Gottschalk, A., Yano, Y., and Schaer, L. R.: The Scintillation Camera in Diagnosis and Research. *Nucleonics* 23:57, 1965.

Beattie, J. W., and Bradt, G.: Digital Printout System for Whole Body Scanner. *IRE Trans. Biomed. Electronics* 8:24, 1961.

Beck, R. N.: A Theoretical Evaluation of Brain Scanning Systems. *J. Nucl. Med.* 2:314, 1961.

Beck, R. N.: A Theory of Radioisotope Scanning Systems. *In* Medical Radioisotope Scanning. Vol. I. Proceedings of the Symposium on Medical Radioisotope Scanning Held by the International Atomic Energy Agency in Athens, April 20-24, 1964. IAEA, Vienna, 1964a, p. 35.

Beck, R. N.: Collimators for Radioisotope Scanning Systems. *In* Medical Radioisotope Scanning. Vol. I. Proceedings of Symposium on Medical Radioisotope Scanning Held by the International Atomic Energy Agency in Athens, April 20–24, 1964. IAEA, Vienna, 1964b, p. 211.

Beck, R. N.: Radioisotope Scanning Systems. *ISA Trans.* 5:335, 1966.

Beck, R. N., Charleston, D. B., Eidelberg, P., and Harper, P. V.: The ACRH Brain Scanning System. *J. Nucl. Med.* 8:1, 1967.

Bender, M. A.: Photoscanning Detection of Radioactive Tracers "in vivo." *Science* 125:443, 1957.

Bender, M. A.: The Digital Autofluoroscope. *In* Medical Radioisotope Scanning. Vol. I. Proceedings of the Symposium on Medical Radioisotope Scanning Held by the International Atomic Energy Agency at Athens, April 20-24, 1964. IAEA, Vienna, 1964, p. 391.

Bender, M. A., and Blau, M.: Photoscanning. *In* Medical Radioisotope Scanning. International Atomic Energy Agency, Vienna, 1959, p. 31.

Bender, M. A., and Blau, M.: The Autofluoroscope. *In* Kniseley, R. M., et al. (eds.): Progress in Medical Radioisotope Scanning. Oak Ridge Institute of Nuclear Studies, Oak Ridge, Tenn., 1962a, p. 151.

Bender, M. A., and Blau, M.: The Clinical Use of the Autofluoroscope. *J. Nucl. Med.* 3:202, 1962b (Abstr.).

Bender, M. A., and Blau, M.: The Autofluoroscope. *Nucleonics* 21:52, 1963.

Berne, E., and Jonsson, U.: Einmagnetischer Analysator für die quantitative Auswertung von Scintigrammen. *Nuclear Med.* 1:80, 1959.

Bonte, F. J., Krohmer, J. S., and Romans, W. C.: Magnetic Tape Recording of Scintillation Scan Data. *Int. J. Appl. Radiat.* 14:273, 1963.

Brown, D. W.: Digital Computer Analysis and Display of the Radioisotope Scan. *J. Nucl. Med.* 5:802, 1964.

Brownell, G. L.: Theory of Radioisotope Scanning. *Int. J. Appl. Radiat.* 3:181, 1958.

Brownell, G. L.: Theory of Isotope Scanning. *In* Medical Radioisotope Scanning. Proceedings of a Seminar Organized by the International Atomic Energy Agency and World Health Organization, Vienna, February, 1959. IAEA, Vienna, 1959, p. 1.

Brownell, G. L.: Problems in Radioisotope Visualization. *In* Kniseley, R. M., et al. (eds.):

Progress in Medical Radioisotope Scanning. Oak Ridge Institute of Nuclear Studies, Oak Ridge, Tenn., 1962, p. 158.

Brownell, G. L.: Theory of Radioisotope Scanning. In Medical Radioisotope Scanning. Vol. I. Proceedings of the Symposium on Medical Radioisotope Scanning Held by the International Atomic Energy Agency in Athens, April 20-24, 1964. IAEA, Vienna, 1964, p. 3.

Brownell, G. L., and Sweet, W. H.: Localization of Brain Tumors with Positron Emitters. Nucleonics 11:40, 1953.

Cassen, B.: Theory of Scanning and Imaging of Radioisotope Distributions. In Medical Radioisotope Scanning. Vol. I. Proceedings of the Symposium on Medical Radioisotope Scanning Held by the International Atomic Energy Agency in Athens, April 20-24, 1964. IAEA, Vienna, 1964, p. 77.

Cassen, B., Curtis, L., Reed, C., and Libby, R.: Instrumentation of I^{131} Used in Medical Studies. Nucleonics 9:46, 1951.

Cederlund, J.: Information Theory and Radioisotope Scanning. In Medical Radioisotope Scanning. Vol. I. Proceedings of the Symposium on Medical Radioisotope Scanning Held by the International Atomic Energy Agency in Athens, April 20-24, 1964. IAEA, Vienna, 1964, p. 57.

Charleston, D. B., Beck, R. N., Eidelberg, P., and Schuh, M. W.: Techniques Which Aid in Quantitative Interpretation of Scan Data. In Medical Radioisotope Scanning. Vol. I. Proceedings of the Symposium on Medical Radioisotope Scanning Held by the International Atomic Energy Agency in Athens, April 20-24, 1964. IAEA, Vienna, 1964, p. 509.

Courtial, J., and Gandy, A.: Note sur la sensibilité et le pouvoir de resolution en scintigraphie. In Medical Radioisotope Scanning. Vol. I. Proceedings of the Symposium on Medical Radioisotope Scanning Held by the International Atomic Energy Agency at Athens, April 20-24, 1964. IAEA, Vienna, 1964, p. 91.

Cradduck, T. D., and Fedoruk, S. O. J.: A Study of Collimators for Use in Radioisotope Scanning Techniques. J. Canad. Ass. Radiol. 13:9, 1962.

Cradduck, T. D., and Fedoruk, S. O.: An Experimental Determination of the Overall Spatial Resolution of a Scintillation Camera. Phys. Med. Biol. 10:67, 1965.

Cradduck, T. D., Fedoruk, S. O., and Reid, W. B.: A New Method of Assessing the Performance of Scintillation Cameras and Scanners. Phys. Med. Biol. 11:423, 1966.

Davis, T. P., and Martone, R. J.: The Hybrid Radioisotope Scanner. J. Nucl. Med. 7:114, 1966.

Dewey, W. C., and Sinclair, W. K.: Criteria for Evaluating Collimators Used in In Vivo Distribution Studies with Radioisotopes. Inst. J. Appl. Radiat. 10:1, 1961.

Eichling, J. O., Ter-Pogossian, M. M., and Rhoton, A. L.: Analysis of the Scattered Radiation Encountered in Diagnostic Scanning. Radiology, 86:142, 1966.

Ephraim, K. H.: Clinical Photoscintillography: Technique and Applications. In Medical Radioisotope Scanning. Vol. I. Proceedings of a Symposium Held by the International Atomic Energy Agency in Athens, April 20-24, 1964. IAEA, Vienna, 1964, p. 291.

Francis, J. E., Jr., Bell, P. R., and Harris, C. C.: Medical Scintillation Spectrometry. Nucleonics 13:82, 1955.

Francis, J. E., Jr., Harris, C. C., and Bell, P. R.: A Focusing Collimator for Research in Scanning. J. Nucl. Med. 3:10, 1962.

Frey, H. S.: Evaluation of Photoscanner. Invest. Radiol. 1:314, 1966.

Fuchs, W., and Knipping, H. W.: Eine gamma-Retina. Naturwissenschaften, 42:493, 1955.

Gopalo Rao, U. V., and Wagner, H. N.: Effect of an Analog Ratemeter on the Modulation Transfer Function in Radioisotope Scanning. Radiology 88:504, 1967.

Gregg, E. C.: Information Capacity of Scintiscans. J. Nucl. Med. 6:441, 1965.

Gross, W., Schlesinger, E. B., and de Boves, S.: A Scintillation Camera for Kinetic Studies of Radioactive Nuclides in the Brain. In Medical Radioisotope Scanning. Vol. I. Proceedings of a Symposium Held by the International Atomic Energy Agency in Athens, April 20-24, 1964. IAEA, Vienna, 1964, p. 401.

Harper, P. V., Gottschalk, A., Charleston, D. B., and Yasillo, N.: Area Scanning with the Anger Camera. J. Nucl. Med. 7:373, 1966 (Abstr.).

Harris, C. C., Bell, P. R., Francis, J. E., Jordan, J. C., and Satterfield, M. M.: Collimators for Radioisotope Scanning. In Progress in Medical Radioisotope Scanning. Oak Ridge Institute of Nuclear Studies, Oak Ridge, Tenn., 1963a, p. 25.

Harris, C. C., Bell, P. R., Francis, J. E., Jordan, J. C., and Satterfield, M. M.: Data Recording for Radioisotope Scanning. In Progress in Medical Radioisotope Scanning. Oak Ridge Institute of Nuclear Studies, Oak Ridge, Tenn., 1963b, p. 66.

Harris, C. C., Bell, P. R., Satterfield, M. M., Ross, D. A., and Jordan, J. C.: The Design and Performance of a Large High-Resolution Focusing Collimator. In Medical Radioisotope Scanning. Vol. I. Proceedings of a Symposium Held by the International Atomic Energy Agency in Athens, April 20-24, 1964. IAEA, Vienna, 1964, p. 193.

Harris, C. C., Satterfield, M. M., Ross, D. A., and Bell, P. R.: Rectilinear vs. Stationary Scanners. *In* Gottschalk, A., and Beck, R. (eds.): Fundamental Problems in Radioisotope Scanning. Proceedings of a Symposium Held in Chicago, May 8-9, 1965. Charles C Thomas, Springfield, Ill., 1967.

Herring, C. E.: A Universal Photo-Recording System for Radioisotope Area Scanners. *J. Nucl. Med.* 1:83, 1960.

Hindel, R., and Gilson, A. J.: Multicrystal Scanner Is Rapid and Versatile. *Nucleonics* 25:52, 1967.

Hine, G. J.: *Nucleonics* (in press).

Hine, G. J., and Vetter, H.: Evaluation of Focusing Collimator Performance. *Nucl. Med.* 4:333, 1965.

Hisada, K. I., Hiraki, T., Ohba, S., and Matsudaira, M.: Simultaneous Performance of Isosensitive Scanning and Bilamicroscanning. *Radiology* 88:129, 1967.

Horwitz, N. H., Lofstrom, J. E., and Forsaith, A. L.: The Spinthericon: A New Approach to Radiation Imaging. *J. Nucl. Med.* 6:724, 1965.

Jammet, H., Gorgora, R., Morichére, J., and Desneiges, P.: "Étude d'une caméra à scintillations: Description et applications cliniques. *In Medical* Radioisotope Scanning. Vol. I. Proceedings of a Symposium Held by the International Atomic Energy Agency in Athens, April 20-24, 1964. IAEA, Vienna, 1964, p. 355.

Kawin, B., Huston, F. V., and Cope, C. B.: Digital Processing Display System for Radioisotope Scanning. *J. Nucl. Med.* 5:500, 1964.

Kellershohn, C., Lansiart, A., and Desgrez, A.: Sur deux nouveaux types de detecteur pour caméra à rayons X ou Y. *In* Medical Radioisotope Scanning. Vol. I. Proceedings of a Symposium Held by the International Atomic Energy Agency in Athens, April 20-24, 1964. IAEA, Vienna, 1964, p. 333.

Kellershohn, C., and Pellerin, P.: Sur la possibilité d'utiliser un tube amplificateur d'image pour mettre en évidence la localisation et la distribution d'un corps radioactif. *C. R. Soc. Biol.* 149:533, 1955.

Kuhl, D. E.: Section Scanning for Image Separation. *In* Progress in Medical Radioisotope Scanning. Proceedings of a Symposium at the Medical Division of the Oak Ridge Institute for Nuclear Studies, Oct. 22-26, 1962. U.S. Atomic Energy Commission, Oak Ridge, Tenn., 1963, p. 171.

Kuhl, D. E.: A Clinical Radioisotope Scanner for Cylindrical and Section Scanning. *In* Medical Radioisotope Scanning. Vol. I. Proceedings of a Symposium on Medical Radioisotope Scanning Held by the International Atomic Energy Agency in Athens, April 20-24, 1964. IAEA, Vienna, 1964, p. 273.

Kuhl, D. E.: Influence of Collimator Design, Photon Energy and Radiation Dose on Detection Effectiveness in Liver Scanning. *Phys. Med. Biol.* 10:93, 1965.

Kuhl, D. E., Chamberlain, R. H., Hale, J., and Gorson, R. O.: A High-Contrast Photographic Recorder for Scintillation Counter Scanning. *Radiology* 66:730, 1956.

Kuhl, D. E., and Edwards, R. Q.: Image Separation Radioisotope Scanning. *Radiology* 80:653, 1963.

Kuhl, D. E., and Edwards, R. Q.: Cylindrical and Section Radioisotope Scanning of the Liver and Brain. *Radiology* 83:926, 1964.

Kuhl, D. E., and Edwards, R. Q.: Reorganizing Transverse Section Scan Data as a Rectilinear Matrix Using Digital Processing. *J. Nucl. Med.* 7:332, 1966a.

Kuhl, D. E., and Edwards, R. Q.: Perforated Tape Recorder for Digital Scan Data Store with Grey Shade and Numeric Readout. *J. Nucl. Med.* 7:269, 1966b.

Kuhl, D. E., and Edwards, R. Q.: Digital Techniques for On-Site Scan Data Processing. *In* Gottschalk, A., and Beck, R. (eds.): Fundamental Problems in Radioisotope Scanning. Proceedings of a Symposium Held in Chicago, May 8-9, 1965. Charles C Thomas, Springfield, Ill., 1967.

Kuhl, D. E., Hale, J., and Eaton, W. L.: Transmission Scanning: A Useful Adjunct to Conventional Emission Scanning for Accurately Keying Isotope Deposition to Radiographic Anatomy. *Radiology* 87:278, 1966a.

Kuhl, D. E., Pitts, F. W., Sanders, T. P., and Mishkin, M. M.: Transverse Section and Rectilinear Brain Scanning with ^{99m}Te Pertechnetate. *Radiology* 86:822, 1966b.

Lansiart, A. J., and Kellershohn, C.: Spark Chambers in Nuclear Medicine. *Nucleonics* 24:56, 1966.

Laughlin, J. S., Kenny, P. J., Corey, K. R., Greenberg, E., and Weber, D. A.: Localization and Total Body High-Energy Gamma-Ray Scanning Studies in Cancer Patients. *In* Medical Radioisotope Scanning. Vol. I. Proceedings of a Symposium Held by the International Atomic Energy Agency in Athens, April 20-24, 1964. IAEA, Vienna, 1964, p. 253.

Mallard, J. R.: Medical Radioisotope Visualization (A Review of Scanning). *Int. J. Appl. Radiat.* 17:205, 1966.

Mallard, J. R., Duggan, M. H., Myers, M. J., and Wilks, R. J.: An Analysis of Quantitative Colour Display for Scanning. In Medical Radioisotope Scanning. Vol. I. Proceedings of the Symposium on Medical Radioisotope Scanning Held by the International Atomic Energy Agency in Athens, April 20-24, 1964. IAEA, Vienna, 1964, p. 423.

Mallard, J. R., and Myers, M. J.: The Performance of a Gamma Camera for the Visualization of Radioactive Isotopes In Vivo. Phys. Med. Biol. 8:165, 1963a.

Mallard, J. R., and Myers, M. J.: Clinical Applications of a Gamma Camera. Phys. Med. Biol. 8:183, 1963b.

Mallard, J. R., and Peachey, C. J.: A Quantitative Automatic Body Scanner for the Localization of Radioisotopes In Vivo. Brit. J. Radiol. 32:652, 1959.

MacIntyre, W. J., and Christie, J. H.: The Use of Data Blending to Reduce Statistical Fluctuations in Radioisotope Scanning. Radiology 86:141, 1966.

MacIntyre, W. J., Christie, J. H., and Tatsuno, I.: The Evaluation of Straight-Bore, Tapered, and Focusing Collimators as a Function of Gamma-ray Energy. In Medical Radioisotope Scanning. Vol. I. Proceedings of the Symposium on Medical Radioisotope Scanning Held by the International Atomic Energy Agency in Athens, April 20-24, 1964. IAEA, Vienna, 1964, p. 153.

MacIntyre, W. J., Fedoruk, S. O. J., Harris, C. C., Kuhl, D. E., and Mallard, J. R.: Sensitivity and Resolution in Radioisotope Scanning. A report to the ICRU. (To be published.)

MacIntyre, W. J., Rejali, A. M., Christie, J. H., Gott, F. S., and Houser, T. S.: Techniques for the Visualization of Internal Organs by an Automatic Radioisotope Scanning System. Int. J. Appl. Radiat. 3:193, 1958.

Matthews, C. M. E.: Comparison of Coincidence Counting and Focusing Collimators with Various Isotopes in Brain Tumor Detection. Brit. J. Radiol. 37:531, 1964.

Mayneord, W. V.: Some Applications of Nuclear Physics to Medicine. Brit. J. Radiol. Suppl. 2, 1950.

Mayneord, W. V., and Newberry, S. P.: An Automatic Method of Studying the Distribution of Activity in a Source of Ionizing Radiation. Brit. J. Radiol. N.S. 25:589, 1952.

McAfee, J. G., Mozley, J. M., Natarajan, T. K., Fueger, G. F., and Wagner, H. N., Jr.: Scintillation Scanning with an Eight-Inch Diameter Sodium Iodide (Tl) Crystal. J. Nucl. Med. 7:521, 1966.

Morgan, R. H.: The Frequency Response Function. A Valuable Means of Expressing the Informational Recording Capability of Diagnostic X-Ray Systems. Amer. J. Roentgen. 88:175, 1962.

Mortimer, R. K., Anger, H. O., and Tobias, C. A.: The Gamma-Ray Pinhole Camera with Image Amplifier. In University of California Radiation Laboratory Report UCRL-2524, 1954.

Myers, M. J., Kenny, P. J., Laughlin, J. S., and Lundy, P.: Quantitative Analysis of Data from Scintillation Cameras. Nucleonics 24:58, 1966.

Myers, M. J., and Mallard, J. R.: Some "Depth-Independent" Collimators for In Vivo Radioisotope Scanning. Int. J. Appl. Radiat. 15:725, 1964.

Myhill, J.: Theory of Multichannel Collimated Scintillation Detectors. Int. J. Appl. Radiat. 12:10, 1961.

Newell, R. R., Saunders, W., and Miller, E.: Multichannel Collimator for Gamma-Ray Scanning with Scintillation Counters. Nucleonics 10:36, 1952.

Perrin, F. H.: Methods of Appraising Photographic Systems. J. Soc. Motion Picture Television Engrs. 69:151, 239, 1960.

Röntgen, W. C.: On a New Kind of Rays. Preliminary Communication to the Würzburg Physico-Medical Society. Sitzberger. Physik-Med. Ges. Würzburg 137:132, 1895.

Ross, D. A., Satterfield, M. M., Jordan, J. C., Harris, C. C., and Bell, P. R.: Low Energy Gamma Emitters in Scanning and Other Clinical Applications. In Radioaktive Isotope in Klinik und Forschung. Proceedings of the Fifth International Symposium in Vad Gastein, Austria, January 1964. Urban & Schwarzenberg, Munich, 1965, p. 108.

Rotenberg, A. D., and Johns, H. E.: Collimator Efficiency and Design. Phys. Med. Biol. 10:51, 1965.

Schepers, H., and Winkler, C.: An Automatic Scanning System, Using a Tape Perforator and Computer Techniques. In Medical Radioisotope Scanning. Vol. I. Proceedings of a Symposium Held by the International Atomic Energy Agency in Athens, April 20-24, 1964. IAEA, Vienna, 1964, p. 321-329.

Simons, H. A. B.: The Calculation of Gamma Ray Penetration of the Walls of Cylindrical and Conical Collimating Holes. Phys. Med. Biol. 6:561, 1962.

Simons, H. A. B.: The Comparison Between Collimator Theory, Extended to Allow for the Effect of Wall Penetration, and Experiment. In Medical Radioisotope Scanning. Vol. I. Proceedings of a Symposium Held by the International Atomic Energy Agency in Athens, April 20-24, 1964. IAEA, Vienna, 1964, p. 115.

Simons, H. A. B., and Bailey, J. M.: An Investigation into the Usefulness of "Figure-of-Merit" as a Criterion of a Collimating System. *Phys. Med. Biol.* 12:29, 1967.

Sprau, A. C., Tauxe, W. N., and Schaapel, D. W.: A Computerized Radioisotope-Scan-Data Filter Based on a System Response to a Point Source. *Mayo Clin. Proc.* 41:585, 1966.

Ter-Pogossian, M., Kastner, J., and Vest, T. B.: Autofluorography of the Thyroid Gland by Means of Image Amplification. *Radiology* 81:984, 1963.

Tuddenham, W. J.: The Visual Physiology of Roentgen Diagnosis. *Amer. J. Roentgen.* 78:116, 1957.

Van der Does de Bye, R. N.: Analysis of the Scintiscanning Problem. *Nucleonics* 14:128, 1956.

Wagner, H. N., Jr.: Pharmacological Principles in the Development of Radiopharmaceuticals for Radioisotope Scanning. *In* Quinn, J. L. (ed.): Scintillation Scanning in Clinical Medicine. Based on a Symposium Held at Bowman-Gray School of Medicine. W. B. Saunders Co., Philadelphia, 1964, p. 16.

Wagner, H. N., and Emmons, H.: Characteristics of an Ideal Radiopharmaceutical. *In* Radioactive Pharmaceuticals. Oak Ridge Institute of Nuclear Studies, Oak Ridge, Tenn., 1965, p. 1.

Weber, D. A., Kenny, P., Pochaczevsky, R., Corey, K. R., and Laughlin, J. S.: Liver Scans With Digital Readout. *J. Nucl. Med.* 6:528, 1965.

Wilks, R. J., and Mallard, J. R.: A Small Gamma Camera—Improvements in the Resolution, a Setting-Up Procedure and a Digital Print-Out. *Int. J. Appl. Radiat.* 17:113, 1966.

Wrenn, F. R., Jr., Good, M. L., and Handler, P.: The Use of Positron-Emitting Radioisotopes for the Localization of Brain Tumors. *Science* 113:525, 1951.

WHOLE-BODY COUNTING

Anderson, E. C.: The Los Alamos Human Counter. *Brit. J. Radiol.* Suppl. 7:27, 1956.

Anderson, E. C., and Langham, W. H.: Average Potassium Concentration of the Human Body as a Function of Age. *Science* 130:713, 1959.

Anderson, E. C., Osborn, S. B., Tomlinson, R. W. S., Newton, D., Rundo, J., Salmon, L., and Smith, J. W.: Neutron-Activation Analysis in Man In Vivo. *Lancet* 2:1201, 1964.

Beasley, T. M., Palmer, H. E., and Nelp, W. B.: Distribution and Excretion of Technetium in Humans. *Health Phys.* 12:1425, 1966.

Bengtsson, L. G.: Human Beta Bremsstrahlung Detection by Means of Thin and Thick Sodium Iodide Crystals. *In* Assessment of Radioactivity in Man. Proceedings of the Symposium. International Atomic Energy Agency, Vienna, 1964, p. 91.

Benoit, F. L., Martin, R. L., and Watten, R. H.: Changes in Body Composition during Weight Reduction and Obesity. *Ann. Intern. Med.* 63:604, 1965.

Bird, P. M., and Burch, P. R. J.: The Relative Performance of Large Volume Plastic and Liquid Scintillators. *Phys. Med. Biol.* 2:217, 1958.

Blahd, W. H., Cassen, B., and Lederer, M.: Decreased Body Potassium in Nondystrophic Relatives of Patients with Muscular Dystrophy. A Biochemical Trait. *New Eng. J. Med.* 270:197, 1964.

Burch, P. R. J., and Spiers, F. W.: Measurement of the Gamma Radiation from the Human Body. *Nature* 172:519, 1953.

Cederquist, E. S.: Clinical Application of Whole-Body Counting of ^{85}Sr and ^{47}Ca in Patients with and without Widespread Malignant Skeletal Disease. *Acta Radiol.* Suppl. 232:34, 1964.

Christian, J. E., Combs, L. W., and Kessler, W. V.: The Body Composition of Obese Subjects. *Amer. J. Clin. Nutr.* 15:20, 1964.

Cohn, S. H., Gusmano, E. A., and Love, R. A.: Recent Trends in the Level of Fall-Out Caesium-137 in Man. *Nature* 205:537, 1965.

Cohn, S. H., Lippincott, S. W., and Korman, S.: Protein Metabolism in Neoplastic Diseases Using the Whole Body Counting Technique. *In* Clinical Uses of Whole-Body Counting. Proceedings of a Panel. International Atomic Energy Agency, Vienna, 1966, p. 212.

Cotzias, G. C.: Trace Metals: Essential or Detrimental to Life. Brookhaven Lecture Series, Number 26 (BNL 828), April 10, 1963, pp. 1-14.

Dahl, L. K., Lax, L. C., Young, C. R., Shackow, E., and Knudson, K.: Failure to Confirm a Prolongation of the Biological Half-Life of ^{22}Na in Hypertensive Patients. *Circulation Res.* 19:750, 1966.

Dahl, L. K., Smilay, M. G., Silver, L., and Spraragen, S.: Evidence for a Prolonged Biological Half-Life of Na^{22} in Patients with Hypertension. *Circulation Res.* 10:313, 1962.

Deller, D. J., Worthley, R. W., and Martin, H.: Measurement of Ca-47 Absorption by Whole-Body Gamma Spectrometry. *Aust. Ann. Med.* 14:223, 1965.

Ellett, W. H., and Brownell, G. H.: Statistical Study of the Distribution of [137]Cs Fallout Between Individual Members of a Large Population. In Meneely, G. R., and Linde, S. M. (eds.): Radioactivity in Man. Second Symposium. Charles C Thomas, Springfield, Ill., 1965, p. 540.

Evans, R. D.: Radium Poisoning: II. The Quantitative Determination of the Radium Content and Radium Elimination Rate of Living Persons. Amer. J. Roentgen. 37:368, 1937.

Evans, R. D.: The Radium Standard for Boneseekers—Evaluation of the Data in Radium Patients and Dial Painters. Health Phys. 13:267, 1967.

Fisher, D. A., and Oddie, T. H.: Whole-Body Counting of ^{131}I-Labeled Triiodothyronine. J. Clin. Endocr. 24:733, 1964.

Forbes, G. B.: Lean Body Mass and Fat in Obese Children. Pediatrics 34:308, 1964.

Forbes, G. B.: Toward a New Dimension in Human Growth. Pediatrics 36:825, 1965.

Forbes, G. B., and Hursh, J. B.: Age and Sex Trends in Lean Body Mass Calculated from [40]K Measurements: With a Note on the Theoretical Basis for the Procedure. Ann. N.Y. Acad. Sci. 110:255, 1963.

Hanson, W. C.: Cesium-137 in Alaskan Lichens, Caribou and Eskimos. Health Phys. 13:383, 1967.

Heyssel, R. M.: Absorption and Excretion of Vitamin B_{12} Measured by Whole Body Counting. In Clinical Uses of Whole-Body Counting. Proceedings of a Panel. International Atomic Energy Agency, Vienna, 1966, p. 241.

Heyssel, R. M.: Unpublished Data, 1967.

Heyssel, R. M., Bozian, R. C., Darby, W. J., and Meneely, G. R.: Turnover of Co[60]-Labeled Vitamin B_{12} in Patients with Pernicious Anemia. In Meneely, G. R., and Linde, S. M. (eds.): Radioactivity in Man. Second Symposium. Charles C Thomas, Springfield, Ill., 1965, p. 331.

Hurst, G. S., Ritchie, R. H., and Emerson, L. C.: Accidental Radiation Excursion at the Oak Ridge Y-12 Plant—III. Determination of Radiation Doses. Health Phys. 2:121, 1959.

Iluma, T. A., Uchiyama, M., Nagai, T., Ishihara, T., Saiki, M., and Yamagata, N.: Body Burdens of Cesium-137 in Japan. Nature 214:133, 1967.

Jagger, P. I., Hine, G. J., Cardarelli, J. A., and Burrows, B. A.: Influence of Sodium Intake on Exchangeable Sodium in Normal Human Subjects. J. Clin. Invest. 42:1459, 1963.

Kolde, H. E.: Cesium-137 Burdens of Cincinnati Residents. Radiol. Health Data 8:559, 1967.

Leitnaker, F. C., Reba, R. C., and Woodward, K. T.: Cesium-137 Burdens in Man. Radiol. Health Data 6:227, 1965.

Lidén, K.: The Metabolism of Cesium in Man. In Assessment of Radioactivity in Man. Proceedings of the Symposium. International Atomic Energy Agency, Vienna, 1964, p. 33.

Lippincott, S. W., Cohn, S. H., Hamel, H., Fine, S., and Korman, S.: Determination of Radioactively Labeled Globulin Turnover by the Direct Whole-Body Counting Technique. J. Clin. Invest. 40:697, 1961a.

Lippincott, S. W., Cohn, S. H., Robertson, J. S., and Farr, L. E.: In Vivo Measurement by the Whole-Body Gamma Spectrometer of the Degradation Rate of I[131] Labeled Normal Albumin. Lab. Invest. 10:481, 1961b.

MacDonald, N. S., Hepler, M., James, E., Hamel, R., Dernell, T., and Stern, A. J.: Changes in Human Body Burdens of Gamma-Radioactivities, 1960-64. Nature 206:1127, 1965.

Marinelli, L. D.: The Use of NaI-Tl Crystal Spectrometer in the Study of Gamma-Ray Activity In Vivo: A Summary of Developments at the Argonne National Laboratory. Brit. J. Radiol. Suppl. 7:38, 1956.

Mena, I., Marin, O., Fuenzalida, S., and Cotzias, G. C.: Chronic Manganese Poisoning. Clinical Picture and Manganese Turnover. Neurology 17:128, 1967.

Miller, C. E., and Marinelli, L. D.: Gamma Ray Activity of Contemporary Man. Science 124:122, 1956.

Morris, A. C.: A Diagnostic-Level Whole-Body Counter. J. Nucl. Med. 6:481, 1965.

Morris, A. C., Ross, D. A., and Travis, J. C.: A High-Level Whole-Body Counter. Int. J. Appl. Radiat. 15:391, 1964.

Oberhausen, E.: Liquid Scintillation Whole-Body Counting. In Clinical Uses of Whole-Body Counting. Proceedings of a Panel. International Atomic Energy Agency, Vienna, 1966, p. 3.

Oddie, T. H., Fisher, D. A., and Rogers, C.: Whole-Body Counting of ^{131}I-Labeled Thyroxine. J. Clin. Endocr. 24:628, 1964.

Palmer, H. E.: Simplified Whole Body Counting. Health Phys. 11:95, 1966.

Reba, R. C., Cheek, D. B., and Leitnaker, F. C.: Body Potassium and Lean Body Mass. In Cheek, D. B. (ed.): Human Growth: Body Composition, Cytology, Energy and Intelligence. Lea & Febiger, Philadelphia, 1968a.

Reba, R. C., Leitnaker, F. C., and Woodward, K. T.: Determination of Total Body Potassium by Measurement of K-40. In Cheek, D. B. (ed.): Human Growth: Body Composition, Cytology, Energy and Intelligence. Lea & Febiger, Philadelphia, 1968b.

Reines, F., Schuch, R. C., Cowen, C. C., Jr., Harrison, F. B., Anderson, E. C., and Hayes, F. N.: Determination of Total Body Radioactivity Using Liquid Scintillation Detectors. *Nature* 172:521, 1953.

Reizenstein, P., Cronkite, E. P., and Cohn, S. H.: Measurement of Absorption of Vitamin B_{12} by Whole Body Spectrometry. *Blood* 18:95, 1961.

Reizenstein, P., and Höglund, S.: Absorption and Excretion of Iron Measured by Whole-Body Counting. *In* Clinical Uses of Whole-Body Counting. Proceedings of a Panel. International Atomic Energy Agency, Vienna, 1966, p. 255.

Richmond, C. R., Furchner, J. F., Trafton, G. A., and Langham, W. H.: Comparative Metabolism of Radionuclides in Mammals. I. Uptake and Retention of Orally Administered Zn^{65} by Four Mammalian Species. *Health Phys.* 8:481, 1962.

Rundo, J., and Newton, D.: Increase in the Caesium-137 Content of Men Due to Radioactive Fall-Out. *Nature* 203:537, 1964.

Saccomanno, G., Archer, V. E., Saunders, R. P., James, L. A., and Beckler, P. A.: Lung Cancer of Uranium Miners on the Colorado Plateau. *Health Phys.* 10:1195, 1964.

Sargent, T.: Metabolic Studies with Fe^{59}, Ca^{47} and C^{11} in Various Diseases. *In* Whole-Body Counting. Proceedings of the Symposium. International Atomic Energy Agency, Vienna, 1962, p. 447.

Sargent, T., Linfoot, J. A., and Issac, E. L.: Whole Body Counting of ^{47}Ca and ^{85}Sr in the Study of Bone Diseases. *In* Clinical Uses of Whole-Body Counting. Proceedings of a Panel. International Atomic Energy Agency, Vienna, 1966, p. 187.

Schlundt, H., Barker, H. H., and Flinn, F. B.: The Detection of Radium and Mesothorium in Living Persons. *Amer. J. Roentgen.* 21:345, 1929.

Scott, L. M.: An Analysis of Cesium Body Burdens. *Health Phys.* 10:415, 1964.

Sevelius, G., Patrick, D. R., O'Connor, B., Patrick, E., and Coleman, B.: Determination of Blood Volume Distribution by Whole Body Counting. *In* Meneely, G. R., and Linde, S. M. (eds.): Radioactivity in Man. Second Symposium. Charles C Thomas, Springfield, Ill., 1965, p. 48.

Sievert, R. M.: Measurement of Gamma Radiation from the Human Body. *Arkiv. für Fysik.* 3:337, 1951.

Sievert, R. M.: Measurements of Low Level Radioactivity, Particularly the Gamma Radiation from Living Subjects. Proceedings of the International Conference on Peaceful Uses of Atomic Energy 13:187, 1956; *Strahlentherapie* 99:185, 1956.

Spencer, H., Rosoff, B., Feldstein, A., Cohn, S. H., and Gusmano, F.: Metabolism of Zinc-65 in Man. *Radiation Res.* 24:432, 1965.

Van Dilla, M. A., and Anderson, E. C.: Human Counters Using Liquid Scintillators. *In* Whole-Body Counting. Proceedings of the Symposium. International Atomic Energy Agency, Vienna, 1962, p. 41.

Veall, N.: Clinical Whole-Body Counting with Simple Detection Systems. *In* Whole-Body Counting. Proceedings of the Symposium. International Atomic Energy Agency, Vienna, 1962, p. 397.

Vennart, J.: Use of Whole-Body Counters in Radiological Protection. *Nature* 204:1041, 1964.

Wagoner, J. K., Archer, V. E., Lundin, F. E., Holaday, D. A., and Lloyd, J. W.: Radiation as the Cause of Lung Cancer among Uranium Miners. *New Eng. J. Med.* 273:181, 1965.

General References

Allsopp, C. B. (ed.): The Measurement of Body Radioactivity. Proceedings of a Conference. *Brit. J. Radiol.* Suppl. 7, 1957.

Assessment of Radioactivity in Man. Proceedings of the Symposium. Vols. I and II. International Atomic Energy Agency, Vienna, 1964.

Clinical Uses of Whole-Body Counting. Proceedings of a Panel. International Atomic Energy Agency, Vienna, 1966.

Cohn, S. H.: The Whole-Body Counter in Medical Research and Diagnosis. *In* Lawrence, J. H. (ed.): Progress in Atomic Medicine. Grune & Stratton, New York, 1965.

Mehl, J. G.: Single and Multiple Detector Systems for Whole-Body Counting. *In* Hine, G. J. (ed.): Instrumentation in Nuclear Medicine. Vol. I. Academic Press, New York, 1967.

Meneely, G. R. (ed.): Radioactivity in Man, a Symposium. Charles C Thomas, Springfield, Ill., 1961.

Meneely, G. R., and Linde, S. M. (eds.): Radioactivity in Man. Second Symposium. Charles C Thomas, Springfield, Ill., 1965.

Van Dilla, M. A., Anderson, E. A., Richmond, C. R., and Schuch, R. L.: Large Organic Scintilla-

tion Detectors. *In* Hine, G. J. (ed.): Instrumentation in Nuclear Medicine. Vol. 1. Academic
Press, New York, 1967.

Whole-Body Counting. Proceedings of the Symposium. International Atomic Energy Agency,
Vienna, 1962.

LIQUID SCINTILLATION COUNTING

Bray, G. A.: A Simple Efficient Liquid Scintillator for Counting Aqueous Solutions in a Liquid
Scintillation Counter. *Anal. Biochem.* 1:279, 1960.

Karmen, A., and Tritch, H. R.: Radioassay by Gas Chromatography of Compounds Labeled
with Carbon-14. *Nature* 186:150, 1960.

Olivera, V. T., Denham, C., and Davidson, J. D.: Oxygen Flask Combustion in Determination
of ^{14}C and ^{3}H in Biological Materials. *Anal. Biochem.* 4:188, 1962.

Steinberg, D.: Radioassay of Aqueous Solutions Mixed with Solid Crystalline Fluors. *Nature*
183:1253, 1959.

von Schuching, S. L., and Abt, A. F.: Carbon-14 Fat Oxidation Test: A New Method for Measuring Fat Absorption in the Human. *In* Rothchild, S. (ed.): Advances in Tracer Methodology.
Vol. 2. Plenum Press, New York, 1965.

CHAPTER VI

THE
RADIOPHARMACEUTICAL

HENRY N. WAGNER, Jr.
BUCK A. RHODES

Radioactive drugs differ from other drugs in that they are usually given to provide information rather than to elicit a pharmacological response. Thus, we cannot simply apply pharmacological principles, such as dose-response relationships, directly to radioactive drugs, although problems such as sterility, pyrogenicity, and chemical stability apply to all drugs whether radioactive or not.

Radioactive pharmaceuticals are divided into two major categories: in the first group are those drugs that will eventually be used in nonradioactive form. In such cases, the labeled drug is used as a tracer, to provide fundamental information about the biochemistry or pharmacology of the stable drug. In the second group, the radionuclide remains an essential part of the drug, which will always be given in radioactive form, either to gain information or to suppress a biological function, such as the function of the thyroid gland in hyperthyroidism.

LABELED PHARMACEUTICALS

Labeled pharmaceuticals have been used to study drug localization, mechanisms of catabolism, rates of excretion, absorption from the intestinal tract or injection sites, metabolic products, homogeneity of preparations, and rates of disintegration and release. They are also used to identify products (using techniques such as activation analysis), to determine the age of a product, to sort tablets according to activity, and to provide control of a production line operation.

For example, the search for useful new pharmacological agents is often advanced by the application of tracer techniques to help identify pharmacologically active metabolites. Zins, Ursprung, and Weeks (1965) observed that an experimental compound, diallylmelamine, was a vasodilator as well as an antisecretory drug. Although the antisecretory effect was immediate, the hypotensive effect did not appear for several hours. There was no correlation between the blood or tissue levels of the administered compound and the hypotensive effect, suggesting that the latter might be due to the formation of an active metabolite. Therefore, diallylmelamine was labeled with ^{14}C, and chromatographic systems were developed for the separation of the metabolites of diallylmelamine from blood and urine. Seven were found. Administration of inhibitors of the metabolism of the parent compound prolonged the duration of the hypotensive action and increased blood levels of the metabolites. After rats were given ^{14}C-labeled diallylmelamine, pooled urine samples were concentrated, and three major metabolites were separated by countercurrent distribution. The isolated labeled metabolites were then reinjected, and their hypotensive activity was tested. Two failed to show hypotensive activity, but the third produced significant lowering of blood pressure. Subsequent synthesis of unlabeled metabolites made possible more extensive pharmacological testing and confirmed the finding that an active metabolite of diallylmelamine, formerly believed to be only an antisecretory drug, could be itself classified as a hypotensive drug. This is one of many examples of experiments that would have been virtually impossible without the use of radioactive tracer techniques.

TABLE 6-1. "WELL ESTABLISHED" RADIOPHARMACEUTICALS*

ISOTOPE	CHEMICAL FORM	USE
^{131}I ^{125}I	Iodide	Diagnosis of thyroid function
^{131}I ^{125}I	Iodinated human serum albumin	Blood volume determinations; pericardial effusions; cardiac scans; circulatory studies; and placenta previa
^{131}I	Iodinated human serum albumin macroaggregates	Lung scans
^{131}I ^{125}I	Rose bengal	Liver function studies
^{131}I	Cholografin (iodipamide)	Cardiac scans for pericardial effusions
	Labeled renal function compounds	Kidney function studies
^{131}I	Labeled fats or fatty acids	Fat absorption studies
^{51}Cr	Chromate Chloride	Spleen scans (labeled red cells); red cell tagging and survival studies; placenta previa; and plasma and blood volume determinations
^{59}Fe	Chloride or citrate	Iron turnover studies
^{57}Co or ^{60}Co	Labeled vitamin B$_{12}$	Diagnosis of pernicious anemia
^{131}I ^{125}I	Iodide	Thyroid scans
^{131}I ^{125}I	Iodinated human serum albumin	Brain-tumor localization
^{131}I ^{125}I	Rose bengal	Liver scans

TABLE 6-1   (CONTINUED)

ISOTOPE	CHEMICAL FORM	USE
^{131}I ^{125}I	Labeled renal function compounds	Kidney scans
^{198}Au	Colloidal	Liver scans
^{203}Hg or ^{197}Hg	Chlormerodrin (Neohydrin)	Brain scans and kidney scans
^{131}I	Iodide	Treatment of hyperthyroidism or cardiac dysfunction
^{32}P	Soluble phosphate	Treatment of polycythemia vera and bone metastases
^{32}P	Soluble phosphate	Treatment of leukemia
^{131}I	Iodide	Treatment of thyroid carcinoma
^{198}Au	Colloidal	Intracavitary treatment of pleural and peritoneal effusions or ascites
^{198}Au	Colloidal	Interstitial treatment of cancer
^{32}P	Colloidal chromic phosphate	Intracavitary treatment of pleural and peritoneal effusions
^{32}P	Colloidal chromic phosphate	Interstitial treatment of cancer
^{85}Sr	Nitrate or chloride	Bone scans on patients with diagnosed cancer
^{51}Cr	Human serum albumin	Diagnosis of gastrointestinal protein loss

* From Cunningham, R. E.: Discussion. *In* Andrews, G. A., et al.: Radioactive Pharmaceuticals. U. S. Atomic Energy Commission, 1966.

RADIOACTIVE PHARMACEUTICALS

Radioactive pharmaceuticals are often used to evaluate the function of a biological unit, for example, to determine whether a tumor actively concentrates iodine, or to measure differences in regional blood flow. At other times, radioactive pharmaceuticals are used to obtain an image of an organ or lesion, for example, to visualize space-occupying lesions of the kidneys. Some substances provide both functional and structural information. Certain other agents are used to deliver therapeutic radiation to a particular biological site, for example, to the thyroid.

The usefulness of radiopharmaceuticals depends on the physical characteristics of the radionuclide as well as upon the chemical and biological behavior of the labeled material. The substances can be characterized by four major parameters: (1) biological behavior; (2) type and rate of radioactive decay; (3) detection characteristics; and (4) production factors.

Table 6-1, modified from Cunningham (1966), summarizes the radiopharmaceuticals that are considered by the Atomic Energy Commission to be "well established." As we shall see, many others are widely used, even though their use is still officially considered to be investigational.

DESIGN OF A RADIOPHARMACEUTICAL

A radiopharmaceutical may be chosen because of chemical properties that result in its tendency to accumulate in a particular organ or region of the body.

TABLE 6-2. MECHANISMS OF LOCALIZATION*

ACTIVE TRANSPORT	CAPILLARY BLOCKADE
Thyroid scanning with iodide	Lung scanning with macroaggregated albumin (MAA) or indium particles
Renal scanning with chlormerodrin	Renal scanning with particles
Liver scanning with rose bengal	Brain scanning with particles

PHAGOCYTOSIS	SIMPLE OR EXCHANGE DIFFUSION
Liver scanning with colloidal particles	Bone scanning with ^{18}F, ^{85}Sr, ^{87m}Sr or ^{47}Ca
Spleen scanning with the same materials	Brain tumor scanning
Bone marrow scanning with colloidal particles	

CELL SEQUESTRATION	COMPARTMENTAL LOCALIZATION
Spleen scanning with heat-damaged red blood cells	Cardiac scanning for pericardial effusion
Spleen scanning with mercurihydroxypropane (MHP)	Mediastinal scanning for aneurysms
	Placental scanning for placenta previa

* From Wagner, H. N., Jr.: Nuclear Medicine: Present and Future. *Radiology* 86:601, 1966.

Examples of some localization mechanisms are listed in Table 6-2. Most of these processes occur quite rapidly so that measurements can be made shortly after administration of the radiopharmaceutical. In most cases, the radionuclide must emit gamma radiation of a type that can be detected with a high degree of spatial localization. At other times, samples of breath, blood, or urine may be studied, and these methods require different physical characteristics of the radionuclide.

Much of the current interest in the medical applications of tracer techniques has resulted from our ability to detect and measure radioactivity within the body by means of radiation detectors directed toward the body. External counting techniques greatly extend the information obtainable by examination of bodily materials—such as urine, blood, and feces, or of bits of tissues taken surgically—despite the fact that spatial resolution is still quite low. We need only compare a conventional radiograph with a current scanning image of an organ to see how much the resolution of the latter must be improved. However, if we look at a series of scans, we can see the value of radioisotope methods: we obtain information on both structure and function.

The resolution of scanning procedures, which is about $\frac{1}{25}$ that of radiography, is low because of the statistical limitation associated with the use of small quantities of radioactivity. The number of photons emitted by the radiopharmaceutical within the body is several orders of magnitude less than the number passing through a person in a conventional x-ray examination. Therefore, in the design of radiopharmaceuticals, we strive constantly to increase the number of emitted photons, always keeping in mind the total cost in terms of radiation dose and expense.

The steps in the design or selection of a radiopharmaceutical can be outlined as follows: (1) establish that the diagnostic problem to be solved or the physiological parameter to be measured requires one of several possible radiopharmaceuticals; (2) establish the maximum permissible radiation dose (in rads) that can reasonably be given to obtain the desired information; (3) determine the time course of each radiopharmaceutical in the organ or target of interest as well as in other parts of the body, particularly in the region surrounding the target; (4) determine the optimum time when the measurements should be made for each radiopharmaceutical under consideration; (5) determine the dose of each radiopharmaceutical (in microcuries) that can be administered up to the maximum permissible dose (in rads) or to the level that provides adequate information; (6) calculate a figure of merit or ranking for each radiopharmaceutical, based on an ideal detection system; (7) correct the figures of merit for the type of radioactive decay, the detection parameters, and the production factors for each radiopharmaceutical; and (8) choose the radiopharmaceutical that best meets all criteria. Let us now consider these steps in more detail.

Determination of the maximum permissible dose (MPD) for a given patient or for a given physiological experiment in man is an exceedingly complicated problem, but the criteria recommended by the International Commission on Radiological Units and Measurements (ICRU) and the International Commission on Radiological Protection (ICRP) can be used as guidelines. To obtain the necessary information, it will not be necessary in most cases to give radiation doses as great as the maximum permissible dose. In some cases, however, the gains associated with the procedure will require doses equal to or (rarely) even greater than the MPD.

In each case, we must keep in mind that the overall effectiveness of the study should be judged by the value of the information in relation to the cost of the procedure. The value of the new information can be measured in terms of how it alters our knowledge of the probabilities that the patient has certain diseases—and by the precision, accuracy, and value of this information. The total cost of the radiopharmaceutical includes the actual and potential risk to the patient in terms of mortality and morbidity, as well as financial cost in terms of personnel, time, space, equipment, and materials.

From the standpoint of radiation dose, many of the physiological processes under study in medicine today occur at sufficiently rapid rates that measurements can be made shortly after administration of the radiopharmaceutical. It is therefore possible to use radionuclides that disappear rapidly by radioactive decay so that large doses can be given safely. In this way, the number of emitted photons can be increased and spatial resolution improved.

In all measurements of radioactivity, we must be able to distinguish *significant* changes in counting rate from those caused by statistical fluctuations in the rate of radioactive decay. Although it is true that by increasing our observation time sufficiently we can, in theory, obtain a large enough counting rate to reduce the variance to insignificant levels, in practice we must limit both the radiation dosage and the counting period to values that frequently result in low counts and correspondingly high variances.

For example, an important consideration in scanning is the time course of the radioactivity in the target organ compared to that in the surrounding nontarget area. A number of criteria can be used to aid in the solution of the problem of selecting the optimum time to carry out the scan. The *target-to-nontarget* activity ratio would be a useful criterion if the measurements were precise and undistorted by statistical fluctuation. We could afford to allow both target and nontarget activity to be small if the ratio of the two were high. It would then be possible to amplify the results to bring the target activity up to any predetermined level. But when we deal with low counts that have a large random variability, we must be concerned with the absolute levels of activity as well as the target-to-nontarget ratios. Thus, we might prefer a smaller ratio if we could obtain greater amounts of radioactivity in both the target and nontarget areas, and thereby make more precise measurements.

Another simple criterion that could be used is to maximize the arithmetical difference between the target and nontarget radioactivity; but this has the same basic fault as the first criterion: it takes no account of the absolute values and the variances.

A criterion that has been used in various forms by Beck (1961), Dewey and Sinclair (1961), and Matthews (1964), consists of defining a figure of merit (m) for the target (T) and nontarget (NT) activities, according to the equation

$$m = \frac{T - NT}{\sqrt{T + NT}}$$

The denominator is an index of the combined error of the difference, T — NT. The figure of merit that we use at present is similar, but differs in that we consider the *relative* standard deviation of the difference. Thus

$$m = \frac{T - NT}{(T + NT)^{\frac{1}{2}}/(T - NT)} \quad \text{or} \quad \frac{(T - NT)^2}{(T + NT)^{\frac{1}{2}}}$$

This maximization of the difference between target and nontarget radioactivity, while minimizing the error of difference, is somewhat analogous to the term *contrast* as used in radiographic procedures. It has the advantage of taking into account both the absolute and relative counting rates in the target and nontarget areas.

The next factor in the design or selection of a radiopharmaceutical is the type of radioactive decay. In external detection systems, only x-ray, gamma, and annihilation radiations provide detectable photons at the surface of the body. Beta particles, conversion electrons, and low-energy photons are absorbed within the tissues of the body and contribute to the radiation dose without providing information.

Certain generalizations can be made: the total radiation dose from a single beta particle or positron is usually an order of magnitude greater than that from a gamma ray. Consequently, differences in gamma-photon energy are generally less important from the standpoint of radiation dose than whether or not the nuclide emits beta particles or positrons. Differences in half-life are also often outweighed by whether or not the nuclide decays with beta or positron emissions, particularly if the energy is high.

The effect of the gamma-photon energy on the design of the detection system is usually of greater importance than the effect of different gamma energies on radiation dose. For example, low-energy x-rays and gamma-rays of energy 20 to 150 kev. are easily absorbed by elements having intermediate values of atomic number. On the other hand, hard gamma-rays in the range of 250 kev. to 2 mev. are not stopped by thicknesses of any materials other than the heaviest and most dense elements, such as lead, gold, and thallium. Most scanning and camera detectors designed for spatial localization depend upon the use of gamma radiation with energy of less than 500 kev. Higher energy radiations have the advantage of being less degraded by tissue absorption; but the hard gamma radiation increases the required size of the detector crystal and the amount of shielding material, thereby limiting the sensitivity and ultimately the resolution by requiring thick collimator septa. A gamma-photon energy of greater than 600 kev. is usually a compelling reason *not* to use a nuclide if spatial localization is required.

Charlton (1966) has outlined the practical aspects of the *development* of a radiopharmaceutical—from the time the radionuclide is selected through the steps of its production, its synthesis into suitable chemical form, and its being tested for quality and purity.

PRODUCTION OF A RADIONUCLIDE

The use of high-flux nuclear reactors makes possible the production of nuclides of high specific activity, the economical use of targets, reduction in the masses of the target material to be processed, and the use of multistage nuclear reactions. An example of the latter is the production of ^{28}Mg by the sequential nuclear reactions:

$$^6\text{Li}(n,\alpha)^3\text{H}; \quad ^{26}\text{Mg}(^3\text{H},p)^{28}\text{Mg}$$

Enriched stable isotopes are used when feasible in the production of radionuclides because a higher specific activity is obtained and the product has less radionuclidic impurities. For example, native iron contains a natural abundance of only 0.33 per cent ^{58}Fe. If ^{59}Fe is prepared by irradiating iron two hundred fold enriched in ^{58}Fe, the specific activity of the product is proportionally increased.

The cyclotron is used in nuclear medicine to produce nuclides of two principal types. First, those nuclides whose decay characteristics are preferable to other nuclides of the same element that are available from nuclear reactors; and, second, isotopes of elements of obvious biological importance (such as carbon, nitrogen, and oxygen) for which no reactor-produced nuclides exist. Examples of the first category are: ^{123}I, ^{52}Fe, ^{199m}Hg, ^{49}Cr, ^{61}Cu, and ^{73}Se; examples of the second are ^{11}C, ^{13}N, and ^{15}O.

Baker (1966) has outlined the main steps in the production of radionuclides in a reactor:

1. A suitable target is prepared and irradiated with neutrons.

2. The irradiated target is processed by simple dissolution or by more complicated separations—including ion exchange, precipitation, and distillation—to remove undesirable impurities or to concentrate the product nuclide.

3. The radionuclides are placed in inventory, dispensed, and packaged for shipment.

The most important reaction used for radionuclide production is the (n,γ) reaction, in which "thermal" neutrons are captured with coincident formation of a gamma-ray. Other common reactions use fast neutrons that are of sufficiently high energy to remove other particles as they penetrate the target nuclei. In general, the more energetic the impinging neutron, the more extensive the "damage" to the nucleus, i.e., the greater the mass knocked out. The (n, fission) reaction is used to produce relatively large quantities of nuclides, such as ^{131}I, ^{137}Cs, ^{144}Ce, ^{90}Sr, ^{99}Tc, and ^{133}Xe. The (n,p) reaction is used to produce ^{58}Co, ^{32}P, and ^{35}S.

If we examine the list of the known nuclides, we see that the most common half-life is about 1 hour. About 24 per cent of the nuclides have a half-life of 1 hour to 1 day, and 20 per cent have a half-life of 1 day to 1 year. (About 290 radionuclides have a half-life of 1 hour to 1 day, 240 have a half-life of 1 day to 1 year, and 83 have a half-life greater than 1 year.) About half of each group belong to the group of neutron-excess nuclides, and the other half are neutron-deficient. In general, neutron-excess nuclides are produced in nuclear reactors, and the neutron-deficient are produced in cyclotrons.

One advantage of cyclotron-produced radionuclides is that they are generally carrier-free. They are often positron-emitters or they emit useful characteristic x-rays as the result of electron capture. Frequently, the only practicable radionuclide of an element is one made in a cyclotron. An example of the use of nuclides of high specific activity is the study of trace elements, when one does not wish to disturb the system under investigation by administering reactor-produced nuclides that are often of low specific activity.

The need for large numbers of photons for precise temporal and spatial localization (without undue radiation dosage) makes short-lived nuclides particularly attractive in biomedical studies. To use these effectively, it is necessary to be near a source of production of short-lived nuclides, or to use what is called a *nuclide generator*. These devices make short-lived nuclides available at long distances from the source of production. They consist of a longer-lived parent nuclide that produces a short-lived daughter nuclide as it decays. Usually the daughter nuclide is separated by chemical means at intervals and the parent is left to generate a fresh daughter. A classic example is the separation of the 3.8 day ^{222}Rn from the 1620 year ^{226}Ra in the preparation of radon seeds.

The first widespread application of a generator system in nuclear medicine was the ^{132}Te-^{132}I system developed by Brookhaven National Laboratory in 1954. Although the 2.3 hour ^{132}I generator has found only moderate use in the United States, ^{132}I has been widely used in Europe. Other systems have subsequently been devised at Brookhaven and elsewhere to supply radionuclides with half-lives varying from a few minutes to several days.

A generator is based on the principle that a daughter nuclide can be separated readily and repeatedly from its longer-lived parent nuclide. Differences in chemical behavior are used to achieve the separation. The general relationship between parent and daughter radioactivity can be derived from the interaction of the decay constants of the two radionuclides. After the daughter nuclide has been removed from the parent, the daughter activity increases progressively as the parent decays until the two activities become equal; the maximum activity of the daughter always occurs at this point. Thereafter, the daughter activity exceeds the activity of the parent until they reach a state of "transient equilibrium," at which point the ratio of the two activities remains constant and both appear to decay with the half-life of the parent (Figure 6–1).

After separation from the parent, the daughter, of course, decays with its own characteristic half-life.

We can predict the amount of daughter activity that can be separated at any time after a previous separation. As the frequency of removal of the daughter nuclide is increased, the total daughter activity separable in a given time period (or over the whole lifetime of a generator) increases until it reaches a maximum (steady continuous separation).

Typical generators used for ^{132}I, ^{99m}Tc, ^{68}Ga, and ^{87m}Sr consist of a small glass column containing aluminum oxide on which the parent activity is firmly adsorbed. The alumina is retained in the tube by a porous glass disk. An outer housing made of plastic protects the column against breakage during shipment and handling. The daughter activity is eluted from the generator by pouring the proper reagent through the column and collecting the eluate in a suitable vessel. The entire operation may be shielded or even automated. The lead shipping container is frequently used in shielding the generator during elution.

Richards (1966a) has recently outlined numerous parent-daughter relationships potentially suitable for generator systems. Eight have been developed to the point of commercial availability. Of the eight parent-daughter generator systems listed, six were developed at Brookhaven National Laboratory. Although

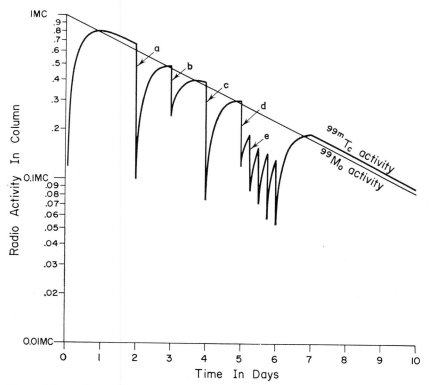

Figure 6-1. Relative activities of ^{99}Mo (parent) and ^{99m}Tc (daughter) showing ingrowth of ^{99m}Tc after elution: *a*, 85 per cent elution after 48 hours of ingrowth; *b*, 50 per cent elution after 24 hours; *c*, 80 per cent elution after 24 hours; *d*, 60 per cent elution after 24 hours; *e*, repeated 60 per cent elutions after 6 hours.

TABLE 6-3. NUCLIDE GENERATORS*

DECAY SCHEME PARENT ⟶ DAUGHTER ⟶ DECAY PRODUCT	PRINCIPAL PHOTON ENERGY Mev.	USES OR POTENTIAL USES
$^{28}\text{Mg} \xrightarrow[21.3h]{\beta^-,\gamma} {}^{28}\text{Al} \xrightarrow[2.3m]{\beta^-,\gamma} {}^{28}\text{Si}$	1.780	Aluminum tracer
$^{38}\text{S} \xrightarrow[2.9h]{\beta^-,\gamma} {}^{38}\text{Cl} \xrightarrow[38m]{\beta^-,\gamma} {}^{38}\text{Ar}$	2.150	Chlorine tracer
$^{42}\text{Ar} \xrightarrow[3.5y]{\beta^-} {}^{42}\text{K} \xrightarrow[12.4h]{\beta^-,\gamma} {}^{42}\text{Ca}$	1.530	Potassium tracer
$^{68}\text{Ge} \xrightarrow[280d]{EC} {}^{68}\text{Ga} \xrightarrow[68m]{\beta^+, EC} {}^{68}\text{Zn}$	0.511	Positron scanning and bone studies
$^{72}\text{Se} \xrightarrow[8.4d]{EC,\gamma} {}^{72}\text{As} \xrightarrow[26h]{EC, \beta^+} {}^{72}\text{Ge}$	0.835	Arsenic tracer and positron scanning
$^{82}\text{Sr} \xrightarrow[26d]{EC} {}^{82m}\text{Rb} \xrightarrow[6.3h]{EC, \beta^+, \gamma} {}^{82}\text{Kr}$	0.770	
$^{83}\text{Rb} \xrightarrow[83d]{EC,\gamma} {}^{83m}\text{Kr} \xrightarrow[1.9h]{\gamma} {}^{83}\text{Kr}$	0.032	Lung scanning and blood flow measurements
$^{87}\text{Y} \xrightarrow[80h]{EC,\gamma} {}^{87m}\text{Sr} \xrightarrow[2.8h]{\gamma} {}^{87}\text{Sr}$	0.388	Bone scanning
$^{90}\text{Sr} \xrightarrow[28y]{\beta^-} {}^{90}\text{Y} \xrightarrow[64h]{\beta^-} {}^{90}\text{Zn}$	1.730	Therapy
$^{99}\text{Mo} \xrightarrow[67h]{\beta^-,\gamma} {}^{99m}\text{Tc} \xrightarrow[6h]{\gamma} {}^{99}\text{Tc} \longrightarrow$	0.140	Scanning: brain, thyroid, etc. Albumin tagging
$^{111}\text{Ag} \xrightarrow[7.5d]{\beta^-,\gamma} {}^{111m}\text{Cd} \xrightarrow[49m]{\gamma} {}^{111}\text{Cd}$	0.150	Scanning
$^{113}\text{Sn} \xrightarrow[118d]{EC} {}^{113m}\text{In} \xrightarrow[1.7h]{\gamma} {}^{113}\text{In}$	0.392	Scanning
$^{115}\text{Cd} \xrightarrow[2.2d]{\beta^-,\gamma} {}^{115m}\text{In} \xrightarrow[4.5h]{\gamma} {}^{115}\text{In}$	0.335	Scanning
$^{125}\text{Sb} \xrightarrow[2.7y]{\beta^-,\gamma} {}^{125m}\text{Te} \xrightarrow[58d]{\gamma} {}^{125}\text{Te}$	0.110	Scanning
$^{131}\text{Ba} \xrightarrow[11.6d]{EC,\gamma} {}^{131}\text{Cs} \xrightarrow[9.7d]{EC} {}^{131}\text{Xe}$	0.029	
$^{132}\text{Te} \xrightarrow[3.2d]{\beta^-,\gamma} {}^{132}\text{I} \xrightarrow[2.3h]{\beta^-, \gamma} {}^{132}\text{Xe}$	0.670	Thyroid studies and double tagging
$^{137}\text{Cs} \xrightarrow[30y]{\beta^-,\gamma} {}^{137m}\text{Ba} \xrightarrow[2.6m]{\gamma} {}^{137}\text{Ba}$	0.662	Dynamic studies
$^{189}\text{Ir} \xrightarrow[11d]{EC,\gamma} {}^{189m}\text{Os} \xrightarrow[5.7h]{\gamma} {}^{189}\text{Os}$	0.030	Scanning
$^{194}\text{Hg} \xrightarrow[130d]{EC} {}^{194}\text{Au} \xrightarrow[1.7d]{EC, \beta^+} {}^{194}\text{Pt}$	0.327	Scanning
$^{226}\text{Ra} \xrightarrow[1622y]{\alpha} {}^{222}\text{Rn} \xrightarrow[3.8d]{\alpha} {}^{218}\text{Po} \longrightarrow$	0.352 (of RaB and many others)	Therapy, myelography

*This list of generators includes those that have been used (Richards, 1966a) and several additional generators that look promising because of physiological importance of the element, the desirable physical half-life of the parent and daughter, or the energy and abundance of the photons emitted. For a more extensive listing of generators, see Brucer, M.: 118 Medical Radioisotope Cows. *Isotop. Radiat. Technol.* 3:1, 1965.

the list is not long, a variety of biomedical applications has been made: [137]Ba with an extremely short half-life is useful for rapid dynamic studies; ^{68}Ga is useful as a positron-emitter for studies of bone; [132]I is useful for short-term or repetitive thyroid studies and double-labeling experiments; [87m]Sr is useful for bone scanning; and ^{99m}Tc, because of its desirable physical properties, has a growing list of tracer and scanning applications. Generator systems that have been used, along with some potentially useful generators, are listed in Table 6–3.

RADIONUCLIDIC PURITY

Charlton (1966) has defined radionuclidic purity as *the proportion of the total activity present as the stated radionuclide.* Daughter radionuclides are often excluded. Primary considerations are the nature of the impurities and the intended use of the product. Usually it is possible to predict the radionuclidic impurities that will be present, and frequently they can be eliminated with little trouble. At times, the impurities may be of no consequence—for example, [199]Au in [198]Au—which results from the sequential reactions:

$$^{197}\text{Au}(n,\gamma)^{198}\text{Au}; \quad ^{198}\text{Au}(n,\gamma)^{199}\text{Au}$$

Since [199]Au has a low-energy beta radiation and a half-life similar to [198]Au, for many purposes (such as liver scanning) the presence of [199]Au does not create a problem.

On the other hand, [126]I, with its beta emission and high-energy gamma emission, is an objectionable impurity in [125]I. It arises from the nuclear reactions:

$$^{124}\text{Xe}(n,\gamma)^{125}\text{Xe} \xrightarrow{\text{EC}} {}^{125}\text{I}; \quad ^{125}\text{I}(n,\gamma)^{126}\text{I}$$

To solve this problem, the [126]I is allowed to decay to about 1 per cent of the ^{125}I activity; the [126]I can be allowed to decay to even lower levels if desired. Long-lived impurities in shorter-lived radionuclides are particularly objectionable, since the degree of impurity increases with time. Mercury is an example. Until recently, enriched [196]Hg was not readily available and [197]Hg was prepared from natural mercury. This led to contamination of [197]Hg with [203]Hg at a level of about 4 per cent of the total activity at the time of delivery. By the end of a week, however, the contamination had risen to 21 per cent of the [197]Hg content. Fortunately, enriched [196]Hg has become readily available and the problem no longer exists.

In many cases, radionuclidic purity can be determined by gamma spectrometry; but this is not possible in the case of beta-emitters, or in the case of impurities that have gamma-photon energies similar to that of the major nuclide. In such cases, chemical separations must be used.

PRODUCTION OF A RADIOCHEMICAL

As yet, few biologically significant organic compounds are widely used in nuclear medicine. Thyroid hormones and cyanocobalamin (vitamin B_{12}) are among the few. One reason for the paucity is that most biologically important compounds do not contain elements other than carbon, hydrogen, oxygen, nitrogen, phosphorus, and sulfur—elements for which it has thus far been difficult to obtain gamma-emitting nuclides. We have had to resort to "foreign labeling," in which a radionuclide of an element not present in the natural compound is introduced. Examples of foreign-labeled compounds include iodinated proteins, iodinated fats, and ^{99m}Tc-labeled albumin. Whether such a foreign-labeled molecule is suitable depends upon the stability of the labeled compound before and after administration, the extent to which the properties of the original molecule are altered, and the specific information that is sought. For example, if we wish only to delineate the cardiac blood pool for the purpose of detecting a pericardial effusion, it is of no consequence that ^{99m}Tc-labeled albumin is not handled metabolically in a manner similar to natural albumin; it is only necessary that it remain in the vascular compartment during the time required for the imaging procedure.

A word of caution: *a radiopharmaceutical designed for and satisfactory for one purpose should not be used for a different purpose without due care.*

At times, we can use chemical analogs—such as selenium as a substitute for sulfur, rubidium and cesium for potassium, and pertechnetate for iodide —provided we keep our purposes clearly in mind.

Bayly (1966) has pointed out that thus far the development of radiopharmaceuticals has been based to a large extent on the physical characteristics of the radionuclides. Various physical factors—such as half-life, type of radiation, nuclear reactions involved in production, and daughter nuclides—have been carefully considered, but biochemical considerations have been subordinate. Usually, when a given substance is labeled with a foreign nuclide, the chemical properties are found to have been significantly altered by the procedure. Inulin is a good example, as we will show. For a compound to be used for measurement of glomerular filtration rate, it must:

1. Be physiologically inert
2. Exist in the blood in a form that is completely filterable at the glomerulus
3. Not be synthesized or broken down by the tubules
4. Not be reabsorbed by the tubules
5. Be conveniently estimated in blood (and urine)
6. Be conveniently available and stable on storage

These requirements are fulfilled by inulin, and many studies have been done with this substance; its main fault is that its chemical measurement is difficult and time-consuming. Therefore, the idea occurred of using a labeled compound to facilitate the chemical determinations. Although biosynthetic labeling with ^{14}C was possible, it would have been excessively expensive. Therefore, three other methods of labeling inulin were tried: it was iodinated after the introduction of a number of allyl groups; an inulin carboxylic acid ^{14}C was prepared by condensation of inulin with cyanide ^{14}C; and a tritiated derivative was prepared by partial methylation of inulin with methyl-T sulfate. Since none of these compounds was chemically the same as inulin, their behavior *in vivo* had to be compared with that of inulin. Although claims that they had the same behavior have been made, more recent work has shown that their behavior is not identical with that of inulin—a result that is hardly surprising in view of the chemical alterations.

Because of the previous experience with the use of stable inulin to measure glomerular filtration rate, the attempt to synthesize labeled inulin was worthwhile, but one always had to return to the primary requirements and to consider whether the labeled compound met them. Nelp, Wagner, and Reba (1964) successfully used the readily available cyanocobalamin [57]Co. More recently, ^{51}Cr ethylenediamine tetraacetate (EDTA) and [125]I- or ^{131}I-iodothalamate have also been used. Sigman et al. (1965) have determined that the renal clearance of sodium iothalamate in man closely approximates that of inulin. In a subsequent study (Sigman et al., 1966), these results were extended and confirmed. The major advantage of these agents is that radioactivity can be measured instead of using complex colorimetric procedures. Furthermore, the determinations are not affected by those substances that may alter chemical techniques.

RADIOCHEMICAL PURITY

As defined by Charlton (1966), radiochemical purity is *the fraction of the stated radionuclide present in the stated chemical form*. If we say that a preparation of l-triiodothyronine labeled with ^{131}I is 99 per cent radiochemically pure, we mean that 99 per cent of the ^{131}I is in the chemical form of l-triiodothyronine. Radiochemical impurities might be iodide ion ^{131}I, or l-thyroxine [131]I.

Radiochemical impurities can be detected by a variety of analytical techniques; but paper, thin-layer, and gas chromatography are used most often. Radiochemical impurities may arise during the manufacture of the labeled compound or during its subsequent storage. Decomposition from self-irradiation is a specific problem of radiopharmaceuticals, particularly in the case of high specific activities. Examples in which decomposition has been a problem include cyanocobalamin (^{60}Co), diisopropylfluorophosphonate (^{32}P), and l-triiodothyronine (^{131}I). Specific activity, physical form, nature of the solvent, concentration of the solution, pH, presence of trace metals, presence of light, and temperature are all important factors affecting decomposition.

In addition to radiation decomposition, chemical decomposition may take place—for example, during sterilization by autoclaving. In such cases, sterilization is achieved by passing the final solution through a bacterial filter.

Whether or not a particular radiochemical impurity is tolerable depends upon the circumstances. For example, chromic ion (^{51}Cr) is formed in solutions of sodium chromate (^{51}Cr) by radiation decomposition. Although chromic ion does not label red blood cells, neither has it any adverse effect in the procedure.

Rose bengal ^{131}I often contains a certain amount of incompletely iodinated tetrachlorofluoresceins, but these behave similarly to rose bengal and therefore do not interfere with the usefulness of the product for the study of liver function.

Iodinated triolein presents a much more complex problem. At times in the past, the labeled material has consisted almost entirely of labeled impurities. Most preparations of triolein have contained labeled diglycerides and monoglycerides, which are metabolized differently from triolein and have resulted in the poor reputation of procedures designed to detect steatorrhea.

Inorganic iodine contaminating some early commercial preparations of ^{131}I iodohippurate interfered with the use of this compound in the study of renal function. These are a few examples of the pitfalls awaiting the unwary.

QUALITY CONTROL

Licensure by the U.S. Atomic Energy Commission requires that by-product material shall not be used in human beings until its pharmaceutical quality and assay have been established. It is necessary to establish and record the identity, quality, and quantity of all ingredients in the product and to demonstrate that the techniques used in its formulation will yield a dosage form of the highest possible safety, reliability, and effectiveness.

Ahrens (1966) has pointed out the need to include quality control procedures in the routine use of radioactive substances. The importance of this type of control is illustrated by the requirement of the Journal of Lipid Research that authors specify what they have done to investigate and insure the purity of radioactive compounds used in their studies. Another example is the Atomic Energy Commission's requirements for license for medical use of ^{99m}Tc generators. The user must show that the ^{99}Mo contamination does not exceed 1 μc. per millicurie of ^{99m}Tc. Also the ^{99m}Tc must be tested to show that ^{103}Ru, ^{132}Te, and ^{131}I are less than 0.1 μc. and that the aluminum content is less than 0.05 mg. per millicurie of ^{99m}Tc. A radioassay of overall accuracy of 10 per cent is required.

STERILIZATION AND STERILITY TESTING

Two methods are used. The first uses saturated steam under pressure in an autoclave and is preferred for solutions whose constituents will withstand the physical conditions of 121° C. at 18 p.s.i. Autoclaving is not suitable for oils because water must be present in the product for steam to be generated within the sealed container. The second method consists of passing the product through a sterilizing filter of proper type, and is useful for true solutions as well as for small colloidal products. Because of the small chemical quantities involved with many radiopharmaceuticals, we avoid the use of filtration media that are adsorptive, such as asbestos-filter or Seitz filters. A membrane filter made of cellulose esters is useful in sterilizing many radiopharmaceutical products, including those in alcoholic, hydroalcoholic, aqueous, or oil vehicles.

In addition to their sterilizing properties, these filters can be used to clarify suspensions and to sort particles according to size. Briner (1960) recommends a filter with 0.45 micron pores in the sterile filtration of materials that are not blood products or blood derivatives. For the latter, he recommends a filter with 0.22 micron pores to remove certain aberrant or mutant microorganisms, believed to be of the family *Pseudomonadaceae*.

The *United States Pharmacopeia* specifies that two media should be used to test for sterility of radiopharmaceutical products: fluid thioglycollate and fluid Sabouraud medium. After inoculation, the thioglycollate tubes are incubated at 30 to 32° C. for at least 7 days and those containing Sabouraud medium at 22 to 25° C. for at least 10 days.

PYROGENS AND PYROGEN TESTING

Most febrile reactions associated with pharmaceutical agents are due to pyrogenic substances of microbiological origin, but some are not. The latter include reactions to lysergic acid diethylamide, 5-hydroxytryptophan, intravenous fat emulsions, and other colloids. The term *pyrogen* is usually restricted to heat-stable substances that result from contamination by bacteria, viruses, yeasts, or molds and produce any or all of the following symptoms: monophasic or biphasic fever, chills, malaise, mild to moderate pain in joints, leukopenia, and other less well defined clinical signs, such as apprehension, pallor, and substernal oppression. Viable or even killed organisms need not be present in an injectable product for the material to be pyrogenic. Bacterial products, called endotoxins, are the major cause of pyrogenic reactions. Thus, sterility is not an indicator of lack of pyrogenicity, nor is sterilization a procedure intended to inactivate pyrogens in injectable products. Pyrogens are inactivated by autoclaving at 160° C. for 10 hours.

The *United States Pharmacopeia* specifies the procedures used in pyrogen testing. The test animals must be healthy mature rabbits, each weighing not less than 1.5 kg. The control temperature is determined in each of three animals; no animal can be used with a control temperature exceeding 39.8° C.

An appropriate amount of the product to be tested is injected into a marginal ear vein of each of three rabbits within 30 minutes of the time the control temperature is obtained. The temperature of each rabbit is recorded at hourly intervals for 3 hours. The volume injected into each animal must be at least an equivalent human dose, on a weight basis. In actual practice, from three to ten times the equivalent human dose is usually used to provide a greater safety factor.

If none of the animals shows an individual temperature rise of 0.6° C., or more above its control temperature, and if the sum of the temperature rises in all three animals does not exceed 1.4° C., the test material meets the requirements for the absence of pyrogens. If one or two rabbits exhibit a rise in temperature of 0.6° C. or more, or if the sum of the temperature rises in the three rabbits exceeds 1.4° C., the test must be repeated with five more rabbits. If not more than three of the eight rabbits show temperature rises of 0.6° C. or more, and if the sum of the eight temperature rises does not exceed 3.7° C., the product meets the requirements for the absence of pyrogens.

EXAMPLES OF SOME RADIOPHARMACEUTICALS

RADIOACTIVE IODINE

Brucer (1966) pointed out that radioactive iodine was responsible for the growth of the field of nuclear medicine from its infancy to its present adolescence. The value of radioactive drugs was recognized when it was demonstrated that an "atomic cocktail" could "cure" cancer of the thyroid. In Brucer's words:

> Of course, it was only a small portion of cancers that were cured, and the definition of "cure" had to be considerably stretched. But even after the radiotherapist despaired, and with metastases the surgeon couldn't touch, radioiodine "cured" the disease. The treatment of carcinoma of the thyroid seems to be the decisive single event that put the word *medicine* in *nuclear medicine*.

TABLE 6-4. ISOTOPES OF IODINE[*]

MASS NUMBER	HALF-LIFE	RADIATIONS Mev.	PRINCIPAL PHOTON Mev.	ESTABLISHED BIOMEDICAL USEFULNESS
117	6.5m		0.34, 0.51	
118	13.9m		0.51, 1.15	
119	19.5m	β^+	0.26, 0.73	
120	1.3h	$4.0\beta^+$	0.51, 0.62, 1.52	
121	2.1h	EC, $1.1\beta^+$	0.028, 0.21	*
121m	80 μsec.	I.T.	0.028, 0.06, 0.19	
122	3.5m	EC, $3.1\beta^+$	0.028, 0.51, 0.56, 3.1	
123	13.3h	100% EC	0.028, 0.16	*
124	4.2d	EC, $2.2\beta^+$	0.028, 0.51, 1.69	*
125	60.0d	100% EC	0.028, 0.035	*
126	13.3d	EC, $0.87\beta^-$	0.028, 0.39, 0.67	*
126m	2.6h	I.T.		
127	stable			*
128	25.0m	$2.12\beta^-$	0.45, 0.54	*
129	16 x 10⁶y	$0.15\beta^-$	0.029	*
130	12.5h	$1.02\beta^-$	0.74, 1.15	*
131	8.0d	$0.61\beta^-$	0.36, 0.64	*
132	2.3h	$1.60\beta^-$	0.76, 1.41	*
133	21h	1.3 β^-	0.53, 0.85	
134	53m	2.5 β^-	0.85, 1.8	
135	6.7h	1.4 β^-	1.28, 1.69	
136	86 sec.	5.6 β^-	1.32, 3.2	
137	24 sec.	β^-(n)		
138	6.3 sec.	β^-(n)		
139	2.0 sec.	β^-(n)		

[*] After Myers, W. G.: Radioisotopes of Iodine. In Andrews, G. A., et al.: Radioactive Pharmaceuticals. U. S. Atomic Energy Commission, 1966.

Iodine is unique among the elements that compose the human body in that iodine has two dozen radioactive isotopes—almost double that of any other "physiological" element (Myers, 1966). Some of the most important isotopes are listed in Table 6-4. Table 6-5 is a summary of the properties of an "ideal" gamma-emitting isotope, against which we can judge the relative merits of the various available isotopes (Myers, 1966).

In 1938, [128]I became the first of the iodine radionuclides to be applied in the life sciences (Hertz et al. 1938; Hamilton, 1938). Despite the 25 minute half-life of this nuclide, Hertz, Roberts, and Evans (1938), using a Geiger-Müller tube, clearly demonstrated the rapid accumulation of radioiodine in the thyroid gland after intravenous injection of labeled iodine into rabbits. These studies came only 4 years after the discovery of artificially produced radioactivity by Joliot and Curie (1934).

Iodine-129 has a specific activity of only 0.16 μc. per milligram because of its very long half-life; in essence, it can be considered a stable isotope; and it has been used in studies in animals to improve the sensitivity of the chemical detection of iodide and iodinated amino acids of biological significance (Rhodes and Wagner, 1966). Experimental animals were fed enriched [129]I as the sole source of iodine until equilibration of the entire iodine content of the body had been replaced by the 87 per cent enriched [129]I. Neutron activation analysis of [129]I

TABLE 6-5. PROPERTIES OF AN "IDEAL" GAMMA-EMITTING ISOTOPE
THAT MINIMIZE RADIATION EXPOSURE*

1. The energy of the gamma rays should assure:
   a. Adequate tissue penetration with minimum scatter
   b. Maximum photoelectric interactions in readily manipulatable detectors that have minimum background sensitivities
   c. Maximum directionality for highest resolution
   d. Minimum collimator penetration to maximize the umbra
2. It should have the shortest practicable physical half-life that is compatible with the physiological half-period of the phenomenon under study
3. It should give a minimum of useless radiation from beta particles, Auger or conversion electrons, or both, and low-energy photons following electron capture or internal conversion or both
4. It should have the maximum "gamma-ray merit ratio" (usable gamma-ray signal/useless energy absorbed locally)

* From Myers, W. G.: Radioisotopes of Iodine. In Andrews, G. A., et al.: Radioactive Pharmaceuticals. U. S. Atomic Energy Commission, 1966.

gives an increase in the analytical sensitivity of iodine analyses by a factor of approximately 1000 compared to other methods of measuring iodine.

The development of various isotopes of iodine has been outlined by Brucer (1966).

At first, the California group (Hamilton and Soley) was using 25-minute iodine-128. Sometime around 1938, Hamilton complained that this was not very good (for logistic, not metabolic, reasons). Seaborg (now AEC chairman; then Professor of Chemistry at the University of California) and Livingston synthesized and identified iodine-131 with an 8-day half-life. Although this was satisfactory scientifically, a reasonable production method had not been worked out, but another substitute did become available, the 12.5 hour iodine-130. This longer 12.5 hour half-life was sufficient to allow clinical work.

In 1941, Irving Ariel and a group at the University of Rochester described in detail a method for making both 25-minute iodine-128 and 12.5 hour iodine-130 from bombardment of tellurium in the cyclotron. The 25-minute activity died away and the 12.5 hour iodine was then used in animal physiology studies. In 1946, Earl Chapman (a physician at the Massachusetts General Hospital) and Robley Evans (a physicist at the Massachusetts Institute of Technology) described in detail a method for producing the 8-day iodine-131, also with cyclotron bombardment of tellurium, but this time with deuterons rather than protons.

After the nuclear reactor was developed during World War II, a new method for producing the 8-day iodine-131 became available. Iodine-131 was one of the many radioisotopes resulting from fission. All that was needed was a little chemical engineering to make very large volumes of very pure, very high specific activity eight-day radioiodine. The original AEC saw to it that this was done. By the time a big new fission-product separation plant was built in Oak Ridge, a newer AEC had so irritated the pharmaceutical houses (just beginning distribution during the 1950's) that they went back to the tellurium irradiation method, but now with neutrons in a reactor . . . a Canadian reactor at that.

The principal emissions of ^{131}I are listed in Table 6-6 (Myers, 1966). Its half-life of 8 days unnecessarily increases the radiation exposure for most tracer studies, as does the high-energy beta emission. The 364 kev. gamma-ray most commonly used in such measurements is emitted in only 80 per cent of the

TABLE 6-6. EMISSION OF 8.05 DAY ^{131}I[*]

| BETA PARTICLES | | GAMMA-RAYS | | CALCULATED NARROW-BEAM |
| ENERGY | ABUNDANCE | ENERGY | ABUNDANCE | HALF-THICKNESS IN WATER |
kev.	%	kev.	%	cm.
815	0.7	722	3.0	8.5
608	87.2	637	9.0	8.0
335	9.3	364	80.0	6.3
250	2.8	284	5.3	5.7
		163	0.7	4.7
		80	2.2	3.8

* From Myers, W. G.: Radioisotopes of Iodine. *In* Andrews, G. A., et al.: Radioactive Pharmaceuticals. U. S. Atomic Energy Commission, 1966.

disintegrations. Calculated narrow-beam half-thicknesses for ^{131}I are 1.5 cm. in sodium iodide and 0.24 cm. in lead. Moreover, the 637 and 722 kev. gamma-rays emitted in about 12 per cent of the disintegrations create problems in directionalized detectors designed for optimum collimation of the 364 kev. gamma-ray. In almost all respects, ^{131}I fails to fulfill the criteria for an ideal gamma-isotope of iodine for *in vivo* diagnostic applications.

Iodine-132 is available as the decay product of the 3.2 day ^{132}Te parent. The emission of high-energy gamma-rays and beta particles makes this nuclide unsuitable for scanning.

Myers (1966) pioneered the use of ^{125}I in medicine and has emphasized its numerous advantages. Reid and Keston (1946) discovered this nuclide in a solution containing radioiodine isotopes separated from tellurium after bombardment with deuterons in the Massachusetts Institute of Technology cyclotron 6 months previously. They wrote, "Upon injection into rats, large fractions of the carrier-free material injected could be found in the excised thyroid glands . . ."

This was the only published report of an application of ^{125}I in biology until 1959, when one of Myers' students described in his master's thesis the initial animal study designed to utilize some of the desirable physical properties of 27 to 35 kev. ^{125}I photons (Vanderleeden, 1959; Myers and Vanderleeden, 1960). Chief emissions from ^{125}I, with their approximate energies and abundances, are listed in Table 6-7. The radiations from ^{125}I of principal interest for external detection are given in detail in Table 6-8, with the approximate abundances of each. Calculated narrow-beam half-thicknesses in water, aluminum, sodium iodide, copper, and lead of the characteristic x-rays from ^{125}I are given in Table 6-9.

The half-thicknesses of about 0.2 mm. in sodium iodide make possible the use of scintillation crystals about 1 to 2 mm. thick. Moreover, the interactions in sodium iodide occur almost entirely by the photoelectric process. The half-thickness in aluminum of about 1.8 mm. assures adequate penetration through a thin aluminum window of an aluminum-canned NaI(Tl) scintillation detector.

The half-thicknesses of about 0.02 mm. in lead and about 0.06 mm. in copper simplify construction of highly efficient collimators with almost no septal penetration. No beta particles are emitted to give rise to useless radiation. The radiation exposure from ^{125}I is less than that from ^{131}I, even though the half-life of the former is 7.5 times as long, because of the much higher gamma-ray merit ratio.

TABLE 6-7. CHIEF EMISSIONS FROM 60 DAY ^{125}I*

ENERGY AND TYPE	NUMBER/100 DISINTEGRATIONS
Photons	
28 kev. K x-rays	137
35 kev. gamma-rays	7
4 kev. L x-rays	7
Monoenergetic Electrons	
34 kev. conversion	2
31 kev. conversion	11
23 kev. Auger	23
4 kev. conversion	80
3 kev. Auger	48

* From Myers, W. G.: Radioisotopes of Iodine. *In* Andrews, G. A., et al.: Radioactive Pharmaceuticals. U. S. Atomic Energy Commission, 1966.

TABLE 6-8. ^{125}I 27.2 TO 35.4 KEV. PHOTONS*

TYPE	ENERGY kev.	NUMBER EMITTED PER 100 DISINTEGRATIONS†	PER CENT OF TOTAL
Kα_1 x-ray	27.5	74.4	51.6
Kα_2 x-ray	27.2	38.2	26.5
Kβ_1 x-ray	31.0	20.2	14.0
Kβ_2 x-ray	31.7	4.0	2.8
Gamma-ray	35.4	7 ± 2	5.0

* From Myers, W. G.: Radioisotopes of Iodine. *In* Andrews, G. A., et al.: Radioactive Pharmaceuticals. U. S. Atomic Energy Commission, 1966.
† The total number of 27.2 to 35.4 kev. photons in each 100 disintegrations is 144 ± 6.

TABLE 6-9. CALCULATED NARROW-BEAM HALF-THICKNESSES OF 27.4 KEV. PHOTONS*

ABSORBER	DENSITY	cm.²/g.	HALF-THICKNESS cm.
Water	1.000	0.425	1.65
Al	2.717	1.44	0.177
NaI	3.667	10.2	0.0185
Cu	8.927	14.0	0.00555
Pb	11.290	40.5	0.00152

* From Myers, W. G., and Vanderleeden, J. C.: Radioiodine-125. *J. Nucl. Med.* 1:149, 1960.

The 60 day half-life provides a shelf life that is convenient for synthesis, shipping, and storage.

Iodine-123 emits 159 kev. gamma-rays in about 84 per cent of the disintegrations (Table 6-10). These have a calculated narrow-beam half-thickness in water of 4.7 cm., which provides adequate penetration for most applications in nuclear

TABLE 6-10.   [123]I GAMMA-RAYS AND X-RAYS USABLE IN DIAGNOSIS*

PHOTONS	ENERGY kev.	NUMBER EMITTED PER 100 DISINTEGRATIONS
Gamma-rays	159	84
X-rays	28 (av.)	92

X-RAY TYPE	ENERGY kev.	PER CENT OF X-RAYS	NUMBER EMITTED PER 100 DISINTEGRATIONS
$K\alpha_1$	27.5	54.4	50.0
$K\alpha_2$	27.2	27.9	25.6
$K\beta_1$	31.0	14.7	13.5
$K\beta_2$	31.7	3.0	2.8

* From Myers, W. G.: Radioisotopes of Iodine. *In* Andrews, G. A., et al.: Radioactive Pharmaceuticals. U. S. Atomic Energy Commission, 1966.

medicine, and compares favorably with the corresponding value of 6.3 cm. for the 364 kev. gamma-ray emitted in 80 per cent of the disintegrations of [131]I. The calculated narrow-beam half-thickness of the 159 kev. gamma-rays in NaI is 0.36 cm.; that in lead is only 0.037 cm. Highly efficient detectors for these gamma-rays can be small and light in weight. The high directionality of the detectors optimally designed to match the 159 kev. gamma-ray should make ^{123}I human serum albumin especially useful for scanning brain tumors, as pointed out by Matthews (1964).

Characteristic tellurium K x-rays of 27.2 to 31.7 kev. are emitted from ^{123}I atoms in about 92 per cent of the disintegrations (Table 6-10). The energies of these x-rays are identical to those that accompany the decay of [125]I (Table 6-8). Consequently they have the same calculated narrow-beam half-thickness ($\sim$ 1.7 cm.) (Table 6-9) and experimental broad-beam half-thickness ($\sim$ 2.3 cm.) in water described previously for [125]I. The 159 kev. gamma-rays and the 28 kev. (average) x-rays emitted by ^{123}I are easily separable by pulse-height discrimination circuitry or by differences in absorption by metals.

The mass absorption coefficient in water of 28 kev. x-rays is 0.405 cm.^{2}/g. and of 159 kev. gamma-rays is 0.148 cm.^{2}/g. This large difference in absorption coefficients makes feasible the estimation of the depth of point sources of ^{123}I in water phantoms. The possibility of developing this method of determining depth has been discussed briefly (Myers, 1964).

The 13.3 hour half-life of ^{123}I is conveniently long for most of the determinations now being carried out with [131]I. The half-life of ^{123}I is sufficiently long to permit the labeling of thyroxine and other amino acids. It is adequate also for the labeling of compounds such as 2,6-diiodosulfanilate, rose bengal, and iodohippurate as well as for the tagging of iodinated insulin and other iodinated proteins and fatty acid derivatives. The high specific activity of about 70 billion disintegrations per second per microgram (1900 curies per milligram) may prove to be advantageous, or even essential, for some studies.

Iodine-123 decays solely by electron capture. Therefore it emits no useless and undesirable beta particles in diagnostic procedures. This advantage, plus the 14.5 fold shorter half-life, ensures that radiation exposures will not exceed a few per cent of ^{131}I in studies such as the 24 hour uptake of labeled iodide by the thyroid (Table 6-11).

The half-life (13.3 hours) of ^{123}I permits serial administrations to be made at intervals of about 3 days or longer without significant residual ^{123}I from a previous dose. Thus one may readily follow the dynamics of disease processes or treatment.

The differences in photon energies and half-lives of different radioisotopes of iodine will permit multiple labeling. For example, the iodine atoms in each of the three positions in a triiodothyronine molecule might be labeled separately with ^{123}I, ^{125}I, and ^{126}I or ^{131}I to study their metabolic fates. Similarly, serial studies may be made by giving ^{125}I for the first measurement, ^{123}I for the second, and finally ^{126}I or ^{131}I, while successively rejecting the photons of lower energy with a spectrometer or by differential absorption in metals.

Protection by shielding from ^{123}I photons during syntheses, handling, transportation, and storage is simplified by effective absorption in lead. Spills of ^{123}I and contamination of glassware and instruments are rapidly self-scavenging because of the 13.3 hour half-life.

In all respects, then, ^{123}I fulfills our criteria for ideal gamma-isotopes for *in situ* and *in vivo* diagnostic procedures more closely than any other radio-nuclide of iodine (Table 6-12) (Rhodes, et al., 1967).

Iodine-121 decays with a 2.1 hour half-life by electron capture in 91 per cent of the disintegrations and by emitting 1.13 Mev. positron particles in 91 per

TABLE 6-11. RELATIVE MERIT OF ISOTOPES OF IODINE
FOR A 24 HOUR THYROID UPTAKE TEST*

IODINE ISOTOPE	DIFFERENTIAL COUNTING		INTEGRAL COUNTING
	PHOTON ENERGY (Mev.)†	RELATIVE NO. OF DETECTABLE PHOTONS/- MINUTE/RAD‡	RELATIVE NO. OF DETECTABLE PHOTONS/- MINUTE/RAD‡
123	.159	25.03	26.91
124	.511	.54	1.64
125	.028	3.11	—
126	.386	.44	1.24
128	Half-life too short for 24 hour uptake measurement		
129	Specific activity too low for accurate 24 hour uptake measurement with ordinary external counting equipment		
130	.54	2.00	5.98
131	.364	1.00	1.0ᶜ
132	.67	.03	.08
133	.53	1.52	1.44

* From Buddemeyer and Rhodes, 1966.
    † When more than one photon is emitted, the one giving the highest number of detectable photons per disintegration was used.
    ‡ Relative to ^{131}I. "Detectable photons" are those that escape the thyroid and its overlying tissue and which would be detected by a 3 x 3 in. NaI crystal 10 cm. from the source. For differential counting, photons escaping without attenuation were assumed to be detected with the intrinsic photopeak efficiency of the crystal; for integral counting, any photons not fully absorbed were assumed to be detected with the total intrinsic efficiency of the crystal. The figure was computed for measurements made 24 hours after administration of the isotope. Dose in rads is the cumulative thyroid self-dose including that during the period of biological uptake and continuing until biological and/or physical decay was complete.

TABLE 6-12. ADVANTAGES AND DISADVANTAGES
BASED ON THE PHYSICAL HALF-LIFE

SHORT HALF-LIFE

Advantages	Disadvantages
1. Reduced radiation to patients	1. High levels of radiation during preparation
2. Repeatable at frequent intervals	2. Short shelf life
3. Improved counting statistics	3. Decay during period of measurement
4. Rapidly self-scavenging	4. Production and quality control more difficult

LONG HALF-LIFE

Advantages	Disadvantages
1. Simpler production and testing	1. Higher dose to patient
2. Longer shelf life	2. Radiation self-decomposition
3. Long-term studies possible	3. Contamination more serious
4. Activity constant during measurement	4. Progressive increase in background radiation during serial studies

TABLE 6-13. EMISSIONS OF 2.1 HOUR ^{121}I*

CHIEF DECAY MODES	ENERGY Mev.	ABUNDANCE	GAMMA-RAYS		CALCULATED NARROW-BEAM HALF-THICKNESS IN WATER cm.
			ENERGY kev.	ABUNDANCE %	
Electron capture		91 ± 1	~28	~85†	1.7
		9 ± 1	511	~18	7.2
β^+	1.13				
Excited state of ^{121}Te		100	214	~91 ± 1‡	5.1

* From Myers, W. G.: Radioisotopes of Iodine. *In* Andrews, G. A., et al.: Radioactive Pharmaceuticals. U. S. Atomic Energy Commission, 1966.
† Calculated value based on the assumption that electron capture is solely K-capture, there is about 8 ± 1 K-conversion of the 214 kev. gamma-ray, and the radiative yield is 0.855.
‡ About 9% conversion (K = 8 ± 1, L = about 1) is assumed.

cent. After either mode of decay, a 214 kev. gamma-ray is emitted in less than 5 nanoseconds by an excited state of 17 day ^{121}Te. The 17 day ^{121}Te decays by electron capture, followed by emission chiefly of 575 kev. gamma-rays.

Iodine-121 has many properties of an ideal gamma-isotope for certain diagnostic applications. The 2.1 hour half-life of ^{121}I is close to that of 2.3 hour ^{132}I. When a high degree of directionality is essential, the lower energies of the ^{121}I photons (Table 6-13) will be more advantageous than the ^{132}I gamma-rays, most of which are emitted with much higher energies.

The positron particles emitted in about 9 per cent of the disintegrations, plus the approximately 2.1 hour half-life, permits the use of ^{121}I in conjunction with the positron scintillation camera.

IODINATION

Iodination has long been used as a convenient means of labeling compounds of biomedical interest. One iodination procedure is substitution of iodine for hydrogen according to the reaction:

$$R\text{—}H + I_2 \rightleftarrows R\text{—}I + HI$$

All methods of direct iodination involve the iodine in the $+1$ oxidation state, and in free molecular iodine, the structure $I^-\text{—}I^+$ is presumed. The iodine may be in the form $KI \cdot I_2$ or it may be prepared nascent *in situ* or just before use by oxidation of (radio)iodide with such agents as iodate, nitrite, persulfate, or hydrogen peroxide.

This type of iodination is mild, it causes little degradation, and its activity (concentration) can be buffered by controlling the pH and the concentration of iodide. It has been used for iodinating albumin and other proteins in mildly alkaline solutions. Amino acids and proteins have also been radioiodinated by the electrolysis of a mixed solution of the radioiodide and the substance to be iodinated. This technique has been used for radioiodination of tyrosine, tyrosine-cystein mixtures, serum albumin, fibrinogen, and gamma globulins.

Another form of iodination is reaction with ICl. Iodine monochloride is a vigorous iodinating agent for many types of compounds (Tubis, 1966). Iodine monochloride as such may be added to the reaction or may be formed from KI or KIO_3, or by the use of *p*-toluenesulfone-dichloramide (dichloramine-T), which in the presence of ^{131}I forms ^{131}ICl (Murray and Williams, 1958).

Radioiodine can be introduced by the Sandmeyer reaction into ring compounds containing primary amino groups such as benzine amine (Tubis, 1966). In this reaction the primary amino group is diazotized and treated with radio-iodine. The diazonium group is replaced by the iodine. This method can serve as a general one and has been used to prepare ^{131}I iodotrypan blue (Bloch and Ray, 1946).

Exchange reactions with radioiodine occur with free I_2, radioiodide or other forms, and are related to molar ratios and times of interaction, the influence of daylight or ultraviolet, the various solvents, and the temperatures (Tubis, 1966). The degree of exchange varies from a trace to 100 per cent (Murray and Williams, 1958).

A specific example will demonstrate the principle of exchange. Iodine-131 can be exchanged for ^{127}I in sodium iodohippurate at a slightly acid pH of 6 at $100°$ C. for 2 hours (Tubis, Posnick, and Nordyke, 1960). Various modifications of this procedure have been proposed; and in another method a trace of ICl is used, which seems to facilitate exchange (Anghileri, 1964).

Thus far, we have considered ^{131}I-labeled protein preparations in which only a small fraction of the protein molecules contain the radioactive label. For example, in turnover studies of serum albumin in man, observations on the fate of the labeled protein can be carried out for 5 to 6 weeks with the use of an amount of albumin less than 1/25,000 the human body albumin content and with less than one molecule in 25,000 bearing a substituted atom of ^{131}I (Yalow and Berson, 1966).

Certain protein hormones are present in concentrations several million fold less than that of serum albumin. Yet, as a result of the methods devised by Hunter and Greenwood (1962), Greenwood, Hunter, and Glover (1963), and Berson and Yalow (1963), a turnover study with ^{131}I-labeled insulin can be carried out with a "tracer dose" that contains 100 μc. at a specific activity of about 40 to 50 mc. per milligram and that does not exceed 10 per cent of the extra-pancreatic insulin content of the body in the fasting state.

> Criteria for suitability of labeled hormone in immunoassay are simply that the labeled material should retain the ability to bind completely to specific antibody and should not bind non-specifically to other serum proteins. It is not essential that the labeled compound retain the identical immuno-chemical behavior as the unlabeled hormone, but only that the hormone used as standard and endogenous hormone compete identically against the binding of labeled hormone. Indeed, if the radioactive label is attached to the hor-mone near an antigenic site, alteration of immunochemical reactivity can be anticipated. In insulin, HGH (human growth hormone) and parathyroid hormone, it appears that the labeled and unlabeled hormones show similar binding to antibody in most antisera, but there is evidence that this is not necessarily true for ACTH (adrenocorticotrophic hormone). (Yalow and Berson, 1966.)

The first use of ^{131}I-labeled proteins of high specific activity was in the radio-immunoassay of insulin. To meet this need, Berson and Yalow (1966) prepared ^{131}I-labeled insulin at specific activities up to 300 mc. per milligram by a modification of the nitrous acid oxidation method of Pressman and Eisen (1950). This was replaced by the method used for iodination of human growth hormone by Hunter and Greenwood, which Berson and Yalow and co-workers have sub-sequently applied to insulin (1963), ACTH (1964), parathyroid hormone (1963), and other proteins as well as human growth hormone (Roth et al., 1963).

TECHNETIUM-99M

Technetium-99m illustrates certain other general principles. This nuclide was initially considered for medical applications because of its favorable nuclear characteristics. The 6 hour half-life is sufficiently long for many applications. The energy of the gamma radiation (140 kev.) has satisfactory tissue penetration and yet is readily collimated. The short half-life and the absence of beta radiation make feasible the administration of millicurie amounts, yielding high counting rates and improved spatial resolution. As the pertechnetate ion (TcO_4^-), which is the most stable form in aqueous solutions, technetium resembles iodide. The most useful application of pertechnetate thus far has been in brain scanning—not because of any increased tumor specificity of this agent but primarily because of reduced scanning times and improved precision resulting from the ability to administer large doses.

The parent nuclide, ^{99}Mo, is produced in a nuclear reactor as a fission product from the neutron irradiation of uranium, or by the thermal-neutron bombardment of molybdenum. The fission-product process has the advantage of yielding a carrier-free product, thereby allowing the adsorption of large amounts of the radionuclide on an ion exchange generator system without danger of leakage of the parent molybdenum activity. Molybdenum-99 produced by the neutron irradiation of molybdenum requires less elaborate equipment for process-ing and entails substantially fewer problems of waste disposal.

The ^{99m}Tc generator, developed at the Brookhaven National Laboratory in 1957, is based on the adsorption of carrier-free ^{99}Mo on an alumina column. The technetium is eluted by pouring 0.9 per cent sodium chloride solution through the column; 90 to 95 per cent of the ^{99m}Tc activity is eluted in a form requiring little further processing before clinical use. Generators of this type can be prepared containing more than 500 mc. of molybdenum and yield a technetium product having less than 0.1 μc. of total radioactive contaminants per millicurie of ^{99m}Tc. The product is often eluted into a plastic syringe to which is attached a presterilized microfilter holder. The solution is filtered into a sterile evacuated bottle. If the solution is to be autoclaved, the product can be allowed to flow directly from the syringe through the needle into the bottle without filtering. A second needle is used for venting the bottle (Richards, 1966b).

Radioassay can be carried out in a well-type ionization chamber that has been calibrated against a ^{57}Co standard. This method avoids the necessity of diluting the doses before counting in a well-type scintillation counter.

After separation from the parent ^{99}Mo, ^{99m}Tc grows back and reaches a maximum in about 23 hours (see Fig. 6-1). Thus, daily milkings yield large batches of product. However, more frequent milkings yield still more total activity within a given period of time, although the amount per milking is reduced. The growth of technetium reaches 50 per cent of maximum in about 6 hours; thus it is possible to elute several times a day.

Technetium-99m can be supplied directly to the user separated from the parent ^{99}Mo, which is retained by the supplier. However, because of the relatively short half-life of ^{99m}Tc, the problems of scheduling and shipping are great, but have been overcome by several commerical manufacturers.

After intravenous injection as the pertechnetate solution, ^{99m}Tc is concentrated in the stomach, colon, urinary bladder, thyroid, mucous, and salivary glands. Similar distribution is observed after intraperitoneal, oral, or intravenous administration (Harper et al., 1966).

The effectiveness of pertechnetate for brain scanning depends on its exclusion from normal brain tissue. Since pertechnetate is one of the ions actively trapped by the thyroid, good images of the gland are obtained with 1 mc. of ^{99m}Tc. The advantage over ^{131}I is that the gland receives about 1/1000 the radiation dose (Harper et al., 1966). The scan can be carried out within minutes of administration of the dose, thus avoiding the necessity of having the patient return after 24 hours (the usual time for scanning when using iodide). Scanning with ^{99m}Tc pertechnetate has occasionally been helpful in patients with reduced accumulation of radioactive iodine, because the larger doses of ^{99m}Tc have provided better visualization of thyroid tissue. Ordinarily, however, a nuclide of iodine would seem preferable to technetium for thyroid scanning, since the ratio of target-to-nontarget activity is much higher with iodide when the thyroid uptake is normal. Iodide is retained in the thyroid gland, but pertechnetate decays; hence in iodine scanning one can wait for the extrathyroidal level to fall to very low values.

Intravenously administered ^{99m}Tc sulfur colloid is rapidly removed by the reticuloendothelial system and may be utilized for visualization of the liver, spleen, and bone marrow (Harper et al., 1966).

When ^{99m}Tc pertechnetate in 2.5 N hydrochloric acid is reduced by treatment with ascorbic acid, the radionuclide combines with iron to form a substance a large part of which is promptly excreted in the urine after intravenous injection; the remaining ^{99m}Tc becomes fixed in the kidney and may be utilized for renal scanning (Harper et al., 1966).

Technetium-99m can be bound to albumin by several methods to yield a radiopharmaceutical useful for blood-pool scanning (Stern, McAfee, and Zolle, 1966). Unlike ^{99m}Tc pertechnetate, ^{99m}Tc albumin does not concentrate in the thyroid, salivary, and gastric glands, nor is it excreted in the urine and feces. After intravenous injection, the blood clearance of ^{99m}Tc albumin almost parallels that of ^{131}I-labeled albumin, which has also been used for cardiac blood-pool scanning and for placental scanning. The ^{99m}Tc-labeled albumin may also be prepared in the form of large aggregates that are useful for lung scanning.

Indium-113m

This radionuclide, recently introduced into nuclear medicine (Stern et al., 1966, 1967; Goodwin et al., 1966) is another example of the value of short-lived nuclides that decay by isomeric transition. Indium-113m can be eluted from its parent nuclide, tin-113, which has a half-life of 118 days and thus need be obtained at much less frequent intervals than the molybdenum-technetium generator. The latter must be obtained weekly because of the 67 hour half-life of ^{99}Mo. The higher gamma photon energy of ^{113m}In (390 kev.), compared to 140 kev. for ^{99m}Tc, is more easily resolved by gamma-ray spectrometry, which makes easier the precise delineation of the size and shape of certain lesions.

The ^{113}Sn-^{113m}In generator system was first described by Pinajian of the Oak Ridge National Laboratory. The tin nuclide is produced by thermal neutron activation, and is adsorbed on ion exchange resins or other media. Hydrochloric acid is used as an eluent. Indium-113m compounds have been developed for lung, brain, liver, spleen, bone marrow, and blood-pool scanning.

We prepared and screened several complexes of indium and found that indium chelates, such as diethyltriamine-pentaacetic acid (DTPA), give tumor-brain concentration ratios in experimental tumors in mice comparable to those found with pertechnetate. Indium chelates (EDTA and DTPA) readily diffuse into the extracellular fluid and are rapidly excreted by the kidney. The blood clearance half-time of indium chelates in man is about 70 minutes, with over 50 per cent of the administered dose appearing in the urine in approximately 2 hours. The physical characteristics of ^{113m}In (1.7 hour half-life, no beta emission) allow millicurie doses to be given without danger of excessive patient radiation.

The higher energy of ^{113m}In (390 kev.) requires collimators with thicker septa than those used with ^{99m}Tc. To achieve equal sensitivity, it is necessary to use collimators with less spatial resolution. We compared ^{99m}Tc pertechnetate and ^{113m}In DTPA in paired studies of a series of patients with a variety of brain tumors and other mass lesions. Accumulation of radioactivity in the mucous glands of the face, the frontal sinuses, the salivary glands, and the choroid plexus noted with ^{99m}Tc pertechnetate was not seen with ^{113m}In DTPA. Consequently, it was not necessary to administer atropine and perchlorate (as we do in the case of pertechnetate) to remove these normal areas of concentration that occasionally lead to problems in interpretation. Tumors and other lesions were visualized equally well with both agents. At this time, it appears that [113mIn] DTPA is as good as [99mTc]-pertechnetate as a brain scanning agent.

The measurement of regional pulmonary arterial blood flow by radioisotope scanning after the injection of radioactive particles is useful in the diagnosis of several pulmonary diseases and in physiological studies of the pulmonary circulation. Indium-labeled iron hydroxide particles offer certain advantages over [131I]-labeled macroaggregated albumin (MAA). Carrier-free [113mIn] can be easily incorporated into iron hydroxide particles of relatively uniform size (20 to 40 micra), which can be sterilized by autoclaving. The final specific activity of the particles is not less than 20 μc. per μg. After intravenous injection of a 2 mc. dose, approximately 90 per cent of the particles are trapped in the lungs. Although the radioactivity decays with a physical half-life of 1.7 hours, the particles of iron hydroxide leave the lung with a half-time of about 12 hours. Both indium and iron hydroxide are not toxic to animals with doses of at least 10,000 times higher than those used for lung scanning in man.

The new agent provides higher photon yields than are permissible with [131I]-MAA. No toxic, hemodynamic, or pyrogenic reactions have been observed to date. With the usual 300 μc. dose of [131I]-MAA, the absorbed radiation dose to the lungs is about 4.5 rad per millicurie, compared to about 0.75 rad per millicurie with the [113mIn] particles. The high count rates obtained with [113mIn] make it possible to obtain better images in less time than with the [131I]-MAA. The indium particles are much less expensive, and it is not necessary to administer thyroid-blocking agents, such as Lugol's solution, as in the case of [131I]-MAA.

Liver, spleen, and bone marrow scanning may be performed with a variety of radiocolloids, which are phagocytized in the reticuloendothelial system after intravenous injection. Carrier-free [113mIn] can be easily made into a colloid which is taken up by the RES. Gelatin (U.S.P.) is added to a column eluate of [113mIn] and the solution adjusted to pH 7 to 8 with dilute sodium hydroxide. The final gelatin concentration approaches 2 per cent (20 μg./ml.). In mice, after intravenous administration, the liver concentration approaches 80 per cent and the spleen 10 per cent; the rest is in the bone marrow (4 per cent per gram) and other RES sites.

Preliminary calculations indicate an approximate radiation dose to the liver of 0.5 rad per millicurie, with a lesser amount to the spleen and bone marrow. For liver, spleen, and bone marrow scanning we have used 1 to 2, 3, and 5 to 8 millicuries, respectively. Visualization of these tissues is excellent and comparable to scans obtained with [99mTc]-sulfur colloid. One distinct advantage of [113mIn] colloid—in addition to decreased scattering because of the 390 kev. photon—is the absence of radioactivity in the gastrointestinal tract and bladder. The latter problem has been associated with preparations of [99mTc]-sulfur colloid containing free pertechnetate ([99mTcO_4]) ion and in those patients receiving [99mTc]-pertechnetate for a brain scan 24 hours before the liver, spleen, or bone marrow scan.

Indium-113m can also be made into a chemical form suitable for blood-pool scanning. In contrast to [99mTc] albumin, which takes approximately 1 hour to prepare and requires many steps including Millipore filtration for sterilization, carrier-free [113m]In eluted from a [113]Sn-[113m]In generator can be stabilized with gelatin, adjusted to pH 3.5 to 4.0, sterilized by autoclaving, and ready for use in approximately 30 minutes. Observations of immunoelectrophoretic patterns obtained from *in vitro* incubation of the preparation with whole blood reveal that the [113m]In, in this form, is bound to plasma transferrin.

The blood levels of the [113m]In-protein complex remain high (half-time approximately 3 hours) and, unlike ^{99m}Tc pertechnetate, which may accumulate in the bladder, thereby interfering with the interpretation of the placenta scan, urinary excretion of [113m]In is of the order of 0.06 to 0.1 per cent of the administered dose. The usual dose for satisfactory placental and cardiac scanning is 1 and 2 mc., respectively.

RADIOACTIVE ORGANIC COMPOUNDS OF MERCURY

Since 1949, radioactive mercury has been used as a tracer for mercurial diuretics. Threefoot, Ray, Burch, et al. (1949) studied the plasma regression of [203]Hg meralluride (Mercuhydrin) following its intravenous injection in man. In 1956, Borghgraef and his associates provided basic pharmacologic data on the mercurial diuretic [203]Hg chlormerodrin. In dogs, the kidneys bind 100 to 150 μg. of chlormerodrin per gram of tissue; the liver and spleen bind the material to a lesser degree. In experiments on both rats and dogs, Greif and his colleagues (1956) found the concentration of radioactivity after the administration of [203]Hg chlormerodrin to be highest in the outer renal cortex, decreased in the medulla, and lowest in renal papillary tissue. The mercury was found bound to the soluble fraction of the renal tubular cells and to a lesser extent in the mitochondrial fraction. Of 13 labeled mercurials studied by Kessler, Lozano, and Pitts (1957), the one with highest concentration in the kidney was [203]Hg chlormerodrin. When administered shortly after the administration of the diuretic, dimercaprol (British anti-lewisite) causes a rapid discharge of chlormerodrin into both urine and renal venous blood. Diuretic doses of chlormerodrin are 95 per cent protein-bound in plasma, despite the fact that radioactivity is rapidly accumulated in the kidneys and liver.

The first use of [203]Hg chlormerodrin in nuclear medicine was in 1959, when Blau and Bender used it in the detection of brain tumors. Shortly thereafter, McAfee and Wagner (1960) reported its use in kidney scanning. Subsequently, other groups have also successfully used [203]Hg chlormerodrin in brain and renal scanning, using it in the latter case as an aid in detecting unilateral renal disease in hypertensive patients and in detecting space-occupying kidney lesions.

Renal scanning after administration of radioactive chlormerodrin provides structural information. If the rate of accumulation of radioactivity is monitored with paired external radiation detectors directed toward the kidneys, additional information about the relative function of the two kidneys can be obtained (Reba et al., 1963). Functional data can also be obtained by serial kidney scanning.

An important difference between radioisotope scanning and contrast radiography of the kidneys is that the scanning technique does not require the high urinary concentration of material necessary to achieve opacity to x-rays. The relative concentration of the radionuclide with respect to its surroundings is the important factor, rather than the absolute concentration. Therefore, even in mild renal disease, chlormerodrin may be concentrated to a sufficient degree to provide interpretable scanning images. Scanning patients who have frank uremia confirms the fact that hepatic accumulation of mercurial diuretics increases in the presence of renal disease. If the blood urea nitrogen exceeds 60 to 80 mg. per 100 ml., very little information can be obtained with ^{203}Hg or ^{197}Hg chlormerodrin.

Cysteine inhibits the binding of organic mercurials by the liver more than it inhibits renal binding; ^{197}Hg chlormerodrin-cysteine complex has been used in renal scanning of patients with renal insufficiency. By inhibiting the binding of the chlormerodrin by tissues other than renal, the renal concentration is increased and delineation of the kidneys is improved.

The replacement of the radionuclide ^{203}Hg by ^{197}Hg is another radio-pharmaceutical advance that exemplifies the continual interaction of such factors as the radiation detection instruments, the chemical structure of the basic drug, and its radioactive label. Because of the short half-life of ^{197}Hg, the radiation to the patient is much less than with ^{203}Hg, thus solving the problem of excessive radiation produced by the prolonged retention by the kidneys of about 10 per cent of a chlormerodrin dose.

An intravenous dose of 100 to 150 μc. of ^{203}Hg-labeled chlormerodrin results in a rather high radiation dose to the kidneys. On the basis of studies of normal persons for as long as 20 weeks, the dose to the kidneys is calculated to be 23 rads; the dose received by the blood, other organs, and total body is only 0.13 rads. Although 50 per cent of the injected radiomercurial is recovered in the urine in 8 hours, and 66 per cent in 24 hours, 9 per cent is retained in each kidney after the first 48 hours, with a relatively long effective half-life of 28 days. Other authors have estimated the radiation dose to the kidneys by 150 μc. to be from 7 to 15 rads—even as much as 30 rads.

To reduce the renal radiation dose, several workers have recommended use of ^{203}Hg-labeled Salyrgan instead of labeled chlormerodrin. The concentration of Salyrgan in the kidneys begins to fall within 15 minutes of injection because of its more prompt urinary excretion. Unfortunately, however, the peak renal concentrations are considerably lower than those obtained with chlormerodrin.

The ^{197}Hg nuclide has many characteristics ideal for external scintillation counting and scanning: its physical half-life is 2.7 days, it has no beta emission, and it is available in high specific activity. Its principal gamma energy of 77 kev., plus the characteristic x-radiation of 69 kev., permit high-resolution scintillation scanning. A dose of 150 μc. of ^{197}Hg-labeled chlormerodrin results in a renal radiation dose of only 1.5 rads, and a total body dose of only 0.012 rads. Because of the marked reduction in renal radiation, the ^{197}Hg material is preferable to that labeled with ^{203}Hg.

In addition to brain and renal scanning, a third area of usefulness of radioactive organic compounds of mercury in nuclear medicine is spleen scanning. The pharmacological basis of spleen scanning is that the spleen is the most efficient organ in the body at removing moderately damaged red blood cells from the circulation. This ability is utilized to achieve a concentration of radioactivity in the spleen sufficiently high to permit its visualization by scanning. Originally we labeled several milliliters of the patient's red cells with ^{51}Cr and then heat-damaged the cells just enough so that the spleen would remove them from the circulation (Wagner et al., 1962).

More recently we have developed a new radiopharmaceutical, 1-mercuri-2-hydroxypropane (MHP), labeled with either ^{203}Hg or (preferably) ^{197}Hg, which offers significant advantages over the ^{51}Cr heat-treatment method (Wagner et al., 1962, 1964). The technique consists of withdrawing several milliliters of blood from the patient, adding the organic mercurial MHP labeled with ^{197}Hg or ^{203}Hg, and reinjecting the labeled red cells intravenously. The MHP-induced damage to the red cells results in their accumulation in the spleen, which can then be delineated by scanning techniques.

The compound 1-iodomercuri-2-hydroxypropane (IMHP) was first synthesized by Sand and Hofmann in 1900. In 1957, while studying the relationship between structure and diuretic activity of a series of mercurial compounds, Kessler, Lozano, and Pitts included this substance. Since the material had no diuretic effect, the attention of those investigators was not particularly directed toward their finding of an unusually high concentration of the IMHP in the spleen; but fortunately they included the data on organ distribution in their report. Because of our interest in physiological concentrating mechanisms, such as those related to the spleen, we synthesized a related compound, 1-bromo-mercuri-2-hydroxypropane.

Mercuric nitrate, labeled either with ^{197}Hg or ^{203}Hg and diluted with mercuric acetate solution, was used as the starting material. Propane gas was bubbled through the solution while potassium hydroxide was being added very slowly. Enough potassium hydroxide was added to increase the pH to between 9 and 10, and the propane bubbling was continued for another hour. The resultant solution containing 1-acetomercuri-2-hydroxypropane was then treated with sodium bromide saturated with carbon dioxide; and the resultant precipitate, 1-bromomercuri-2-hydroxypropane, was purified by recrystallization.

To obtain material of higher specific activity, the reaction was carried out on a micro scale, without adding carrier mercuric acetate. The bromide precipitation step was also omitted. A total of 95 per cent of the radioactivity in solution after the alkalinization of the mercuric acetate (or nitrate) in the presence of propane was tightly bound by human erythrocytes when incubated in heparinized whole blood. The specific activity of the resultant material ranged between 10 μc. and 2000 μc. per milligram Hg, depending on the specific activity of the starting material. Prior to use in human subjects the material was sterilized by filtration through a millipore (Swinney) filter and tested for sterility and pyrogenicity. A dose of 1 mg. per kilogram was found to be without toxicity in dogs. The human dose never exceeded 0.1 mg. per kilogram.

Initially, MHP was injected intravenously. Although this procedure delineated the spleen satisfactorily in some persons, in others the accumulation of the material in the kidneys, as well as in the spleen, led us to discard this procedure.

The technique finally selected was as follows: 0.5 to 15 ml. of whole blood was withdrawn from the patient, and the needle was left in the antecubital vein. The blood was added to a sterile Vacutainer containing 100 μc. of ^{203}Hg-labeled or 300 μc. of ^{197}Hg-labeled MHP, plus 1 mg. of stable MHP per milliliter of packed red cells. After several inversions of the tube to insure mixing, the blood was withdrawn into the same syringe and immediately injected again into the patient. The scanning procedure was routinely carried out at 1 to 2 hours after injection, but scanning could be delayed for a period of 4 to 5 hours.

Both inorganic mercuric ion (Hg^{++}) and organic mercurial ions ($R—Hg^+$) have a high affinity for sulfhydryl groups. Presumably, MHP reacts with the protein sulfhydryl groups of the red cell, forming R—Hg—S protein compounds. Most organic mercurials react to some extent with red blood cells. For example, about 20 per cent of injected chlormerodrin is bound by red blood cells, although most of it is bound by the renal tubular cells. The important characteristic of MHP is that, of all organic mercurials tested, it is the most tightly bound by human red blood cells. When MHP was incubated at room temperature with heparinized whole blood in the proportion of 1 to 2 mg. per milliliter of red blood cells, approximately 98 per cent of the radioactive mercury was bound to the red cells. Also, serial washing in tenfold volumes of 0.9 per cent saline did not reduce the amount of bound MPH to the extent observed with the other organic mercurials.

The accumulation of MHP in the spleen could be explained by chemical damage to the red blood cells, which then became sequestered in the spleen. This mechanism was confirmed by the following experiment. Human red blood cells were labeled with ^{51}Cr sodium chromate by a method that resulted in a normal red cell survival (half-time of cell removal, 25 to 35 days). When similarly labeled red cells were incubated with 1 to 2 mg. of stable MPH and then injected into the patient, the ^{51}Cr radioactivity over the spleen increased progressively.

Additional evidence that MHP resulted in splenic sequestration of red blood cells was obtained by histological examination of the spleen tissue of rabbits. These animals were sacrificed serially after injection of rabbit red cells that had been treated with MHP. Myriads of red cells could be seen in the splenic pulp, especially in the sinusoids.

In extensive studies of diuretic and nondiuretic mercurial compounds in dogs, it has been established that chemical doses of 1 mg. of mercury per kilogram body weight are safe. With labeled MHP, one should always keep the dose of mercury below 0.1 mg. per kilogram body weight. At this low level, toxic reactions should never occur.

What of the radiation hazard? Since the labeled red cells are promptly cleared from the blood, the total body radiation is slight. Nor is splenic radiation significant, since the radioactivity remains in the spleen for only a few hours. The limiting organ from the standpoint of radiation is the kidney. After the initial breakdown of the red blood cells in the spleen, the urinary excretion of the radioactivity is at a nearly constant rate of about 0.5 per cent of the dose per day. Fortunately, at least one fourth of the radioactivity appears in the stool, presumably from biliary excretion. The radiation to a 150 g. kidney from a dose of 100 μc. of MHP ^{203}Hg is about 70 rads. The use of ^{197}Hg is preferable, since the radiation dose will thus be not more than 7 rads.

SELENIUM-SUBSTITUTED SULFUR COMPOUNDS

The lack of suitable gamma-emitting isotopes of carbon, hydrogen, nitrogen, oxygen, sulfur, and phosphorus has severely limited the choice of compounds for studies requiring *in vivo* counting. Sometimes it is possible to label a molecule by substitution of a side group, for example, to substitute an iodine for a hydrogen, without seriously affecting the biological behavior of the molecule. As a general rule, however, molecules labeled in this way are prevented from taking part in normal biochemical processes because of the change in molecular structure. Other times it is possible to label a molecule by substitution in the skeleton of a molecule, for example, to replace a carbon atom with a silicon atom in an organic molecule, without altering the molecular structure to the degree that the biological behavior is changed. An example of this approach has been the preparation of gamma-emitting analogues of sulfur-containing compounds by substituting ^{75}Se for sulfur. Selenium-75 has a half-life of 127 days and decays by electron capture with the emission of several gamma-rays of which the 265 and 280 kev. gammas are most commonly used. The atomic radii and solvating abilities of sulfur and selenium analogues are sufficiently similar so that only minor differences in chemical behavior are usually found.

Selenocystine and selenomethionine were first synthesized several years ago and since then numerous other amino acids, as well as nucleic acid constituents, coenzymes, and hormones, have been prepared. These include selenopurines and selenopyrimidines, selenopantethine, selenocoenzyme A, selenoctic acid, Se-adenosylselenomethionine, selenoglutathione, and selenoxytocin. More recently these compounds have been used as reagents for the synthesis of peptides (Mautner, 1966).

An illustration of this category of radiopharmaceutical is ^{75}Se selenomethionine. Its biological behavior was found (Blau and Manske, 1961; Spencer and Blau, 1962) to parallel that of methionine, including participation in protein synthesis. One to two hours after administration of the compound, approximately 6 per cent of the dose was found in the pancreas of dogs, a concentration eight to nine times that in liver, which is the area of second highest concentration. Thus ^{75}Se selenomethionine was evaluated as a pancreatic scanning agent. Subsequent studies have revealed other uses. Selenomethionine parallels methionine in the synthesis of blood proteins and in transport across the intestinal wall (Blau and Holland, 1966). On the other hand, selenomethionine appears to be metabolized quite differently from methionine in protein metabolism. Hence when selenomethionine is used as a substitute for methionine in any experiment, the equivalence of the two compounds must first be established. This is usually accomplished by comparing its metabolism to that of ^{35}S methionine in experimental animals (Hansson and Blau, 1963).

Radioactive selenomethionine can be prepared by chemical synthesis from ^{75}Se or it can be produced by biosynthesis using yeast grown on a low sulfur medium containing selenium (Blau, 1961). The usual dose in patient studies, 250 μc., contains approximately 50 μg. of selenium which is the same amount of selenium ingested in a usual diet and a thousand fold below the toxic levels of selenium (Sollman, 1957). The estimated radiation dose to the patient from pancreas scanning with this agent is 0.6 rad, total body dose, delivered over a period of several months (Blau and Bender, 1962).

Mautner (1966) has summarized the important role of sulfur-containing compounds in biological processes. High-energy sulfur compounds occupy a central position in group- and energy-transfer reactions. Disulfide bonds play an important role in the maintenance of the tertiary configuration of proteins. Amino acids containing sulfur have been implicated in catalytic sites of several enzymes. Sulfur compounds are of major importance in chemotherapy. There is even a role for the simple inorganic isologs, for example ^{75}Se-selenate has been used as a substitute for sulfate in the measurement of extracellular fluid volume (Albert et al., 1966). It is predictable that future uses of ^{75}Se in nuclear medicine will exceed those of the past.

LABELED PARTICLES

To gain insight into the mechanism by which bacteria are removed from the circulation, Drinker and Shaw (1921) and Lund et al. (1921) observed the fate of colloidal manganese injected into the circulation of animals and found, as had Voigt in 1914, that the foreign particles accumulated in the liver, lung, and spleen, as the result of phagocytosis by the reticuloendothelial system. Large particles were found to accumulate in the lung by the process of capillary blockade.

The distribution of injected particles depends to a great extent on their size and the site of injection. Smaller particles (less than 1 micron in diameter) are removed with great efficiency by the liver and spleen, and have been used to estimate liver blood flow and phagocytic function of the Kupffer cells of the liver (Taplin et al., 1966). They are also useful in liver, spleen, and bone marrow scanning.

Larger particles (greater than 10 microns in diameter) are used for estimating regional blood flow. It can be shown that the accumulation of particles greater in size than the pulmonary capillary bed is directly proportional to regional pulmonary arterial blood flow (Tow et al., 1966). The particles must be uniformly mixed in the blood, must be removed in the initial circulation through the capillary bed, and must not be appreciably metabolized or otherwise removed during the period of observation.

Taplin et al. (1966) have described how labeled particles came to be used as lung scanning agents. In 1952, Dobson and Jones observed that particles of chromic phosphate larger than 1 micron were retained in the lungs after intravenous injection. Temporary pulmonary retention of intravenously injected colloidal gold and colloidal albumin suspensions of much smaller size (10 to 200 millimicrons) was also observed during studies of reticuloendothelial function. As a result of the work of Halpern and his group (1956), human serum albumin could be prepared in the form of colloidal particles of different sizes, labeled with a variety of radionuclides.

Large aggregates that fulfill the criteria for measuring regional blood flow in man were first prepared from high specific activity human serum albumin. A 0.1 per cent solution was adjusted to pH 5.5, the isoelectric point of the albumin, and heated for 4 to 15 minutes in an oscillatory water bath at 100°C. (Wagner et al., 1964).

Labeled particles are being put to an increasing number of new uses. For example, colloidal [198]Au has been adapted by Baker, Migita, and Wagner

(1967) to the measurement of liver regeneration rates. After maximum liver uptake of colloidal gold, part of the liver is removed surgically and the specific activity of the removed tissue is determined. Once this colloid becomes localized in the liver, it remains there at least for a period of weeks; hence as liver tissue regenerates, the specific activity of the liver decreases in proportion to the rate of regeneration and can be used for its measurement.

Hydrous ferric oxide is another example of a colloidal radiopharmaceutical. During the formation of the iron particles, coprecipitation and occlusion of trace substances occurs and has been used for many years in water treatment and radiochemistry. If we form the *floc* in the presence of carrier-free radio-nuclides, especially metal ions, a suspension of particles can be prepared that has the chemical properties of colloidal iron oxide together with useful radio-nuclidic properties of the tracer. Since a large variety of nuclides can be incorporated into the iron colloid, the physical properties of the nuclide, i.e., the half-life and the gamma-ray energy, can be made optimum. Iron particles have not been found to be toxic in amounts necessary for biomedical studies, and the biochemistry of colloidal iron is extensive. An example of this type of particulate radiopharmaceutical is ^{113m}In-labeled hydrous iron oxide, a lung scanning agent (Stern et al., 1966).

Four types of toxicity must be considered with colloidal radiopharmaceuticals: (1) albumin aggregates might be antigenic; (2) particles can block a significant fraction of a capillary bed or overload the phagocytic cells; (3) on dissolution of the particles, certain colloids can release toxic chemicals into the circulation; and (4) the physical and chemical characteristics of the particles might become altered during storage and lead to any of the first three. It is usually possible, however, to prepare colloids of high specific activity and obtain useful results with physiologically insignificant numbers of particles. Sols can be prepared that are stable for long periods of time.

CARBON COMPOUNDS

The usefulness of carbon-labeled compounds in biomedical research is apparent from their widespread applications, but they have not been widely used in nuclear medicine. Of the two available radioisotopes of carbon, ^{11}C has a half-life of 20.3 minutes and ^{14}C a half-life of 5760 years. Neither emits gamma-rays although annihilation radiation allows ^{11}C to be detected externally. Other carbon isotopes have less desirable physical characteristics; for example, ^{10}C has a half-life of only 19.1 seconds.

Cyclotron-produced ^{11}C carbon dioxide has been used in metabolic and respiratory studies, as has ^{11}C carbon monoxide (Matthews et al., 1966) Carbon-11 is produced by bombarding boron (a molten boric oxide target) with 15 Mev. deuterons. The reactions are ^{10}B(d,n)^{11}C and ^{11}B(d,2n)^{11}C. Five per cent carbon monoxide or carbon dioxide carrier gas mixed with argon is passed through silica gel absorbers into a target box. Both ^{11}CO and ^{11}CO$_2$ are formed in the target box. If ^{11}C-labeled carbon monoxide is required, the ^{11}CO$_2$ is absorbed in soda lime. If ^{11}C carbon dioxide is required, the ^{11}CO is oxidized by cupric oxide at 850° C. In production of CO$_2$, 5 per cent CO$_2$ in helium is used instead of argon to eliminate the ^{41}Ar contamination. Matthews et al. (1966) estimate that the absorbed tissue dose per breath of 5 mc. of ^{11}CO is 0.128 rad to the lungs and 0.211 rad to the blood. For $^{11}CO_2$, the lung dose is 0.220 rad and the blood dose 0.055 rad. The use of more complex carbon compounds labeled with ^{11}C requires rapid chemical synthesis followed by immediate use.

Uses of ^{14}C-labeled compounds are described in the chapter on metabolic diseases (Chapter 14). Compounds of short biological half-life are usually employed to decrease the radiation exposure. Substances that might result in the incorporation of ^{14}C into molecules of genetic importance are also avoided. Because of the absence of gamma radiation, we can only sample body fluids; for example, glucose metabolism can be evaluated by measuring the radioactivity of expired CO_2 following the administration of ^{14}C-labeled glucose.

Carbon-14 has been quite useful in many *in vitro* clinical tests. For example, a simple screening test for congenital galactosemia consists of incubating galactose-1-^{14}C with blood cells from newborn infants. Carbon-14 CO_2 production is measured. The blood cells of the galactosemic child do not produce labeled CO_2, whereas the normal blood cells release considerable quantities of CO_2 during the galactose incubation (Weinberg, 1961).

RADIOACTIVE GASES

In 1955, Knipping et al. introduced the use of radioactive ^{133}Xe for studying lung function. The following year $^{15}O_2$ was first used in biological investigations (Ter-Pogossian and Powers, 1958) and was soon developed as an agent for the study of lung function (Dyson et al., 1958). Nitrogen-13 and ^{11}C-labeled

TABLE 6-14. RADIOACTIVE GASES OF BIOMEDICAL INTEREST

GAS	HALF-LIFE	RADIATIONS	PRINCIPAL PHOTON ENERGY
^{11}CO, $^{11}CO_2$	20.4m	β^+	0.511
$^{13}N_2$	10.05m	β^+	0.511
$C^{15}O$, $C^{15}O_2$	2.07m	β^+	0.511
^{77}Kr	1.2h	β^+, E, γ	0.108
^{79}Kr	34h	E, β^+, γ	0.044
^{83m}Kr	1.9h	γ	0.012
^{85m}Kr	4.4h	β^-, γ	0.150
^{85}Kr	10.76y	β^-, γ	0.52
^{87}Kr	76m	β^-, γ	0.40
^{123}Xe	1.85h	E, β^+, γ	0.15
^{125}Xe	18h	E, γ	0.187
^{127}Xe	36.4d	E, γ	0.20
^{129m}Xe	8d	γ	0.040
^{131m}Xe	12d	γ	0.164
^{133m}Xe	2.3d	γ	0.233
^{133}Xe	5.27d	β^-, γ	0.081
^{135}Xe	9.2d	β^-, γ	0.25
^{222}Rn	3.8d	α	0.51

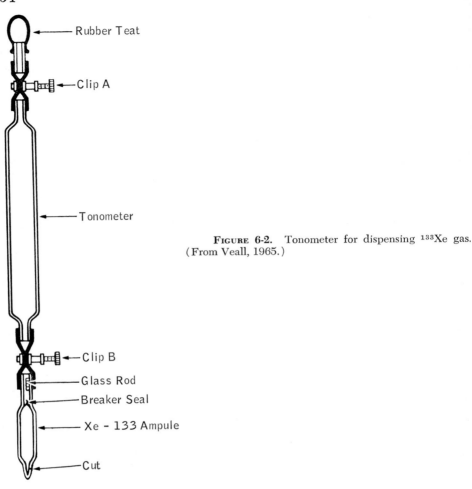

Rubber Teat

Clip A

Tonometer

FIGURE 6-2.   Tonometer for dispensing ^{133}Xe gas. (From Veall, 1965.)

Clip B

Glass Rod

Breaker Seal

Xe - 133 Ampule

Cut

carbon dioxide and carbon monoxide have also been useful in this type of study. Except at institutions located very near cyclotrons, only the noble gases have been generally available. In addition to 5.27 day ^{133}Xe, 9.2 hour ^{135}Xe and 10.3 year ^{85}Kr have been used. Because the noble gases are excreted rapidly in the breath, high levels of activity can be used without excessive radiation hazard, and the radiation dose is nearly independent of physical half-life. Table 6-14 enumerates some of the physical properties of the useful or potentially useful radioactive gases.

Matthews et al. (1966) have outlined the uptake, distribution, and fate of radioactive gases in the body.

There are five stages in the fate of radioactive gases in the body. First, the initial uptake of the gas in a region of lung after a single breath will depend on the ventilation to that region of the lung. Next, during a subsequent breath-hold period, the radioactivity will be removed from the alveolar air by the blood. The extent to which this occurs may be limited by diffusion or by solubility and blood flow. Third, the radioactivity is removed from the lungs by the blood flow. Fourth, it may exchange with tissue pools in the systemic capillaries. Finally, radioactivity returns to the lungs in the venous blood and may be expired.

The principal uses of the radioactive noble gases in nuclear medicine are the assessment of regions of decreased ventilation and perfusion in the lungs and the regional blood flow in other areas. The radiopharmaceutical is prepared either as a labeled gas which the patient inhales or it can be injected as a solution containing the dissolved gas. Preparation methods, developed by Veall (1965), are illustrated in Figures 6-2 and 6-3. Figure 6-4 shows injection sites and detector placements for measuring regional blood flow. Figures 6-5 and 6-6 are examples of the clearance curves obtained in this type of study.

Lassen and Munck (1955) measured cerebral blood flow using [85]Kr, a method that illustrates the use of inert radioactive gases to measure organ perfusion rates according to the principles developed by Kety and Schmidt (1948) using nitrous oxide. Because the radioactive gas can be quantified by external counting, the need for collection and analysis of multiple blood samples is avoided. The procedure is not only simpler and faster than the nitrous oxide method, but more exact measurements are obtained with less discomfort to the patient. A technical simplification in the measurement of cerebral blood flow has been proposed by Mallett and Veall (1965). Three millicuries of ^{133}Xe diluted with air to a concentration of approximately 2 mc. per milliliter is withdrawn from the rubber teat at the top of the tonometer with a grease-free, water-lubricated syringe and is injected into a rubber tube connecting an oxygen

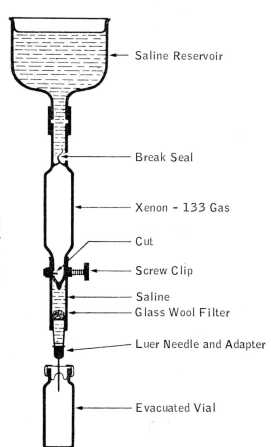

FIGURE 6-3. Method for preparing saline solution of [133]Xe. (From Veall, 1965.)

Saline Reservoir

Break Seal

Xenon - 133 Gas

Cut

Screw Clip

Saline

Glass Wool Filter

Luer Needle and Adapter

Evacuated Vial

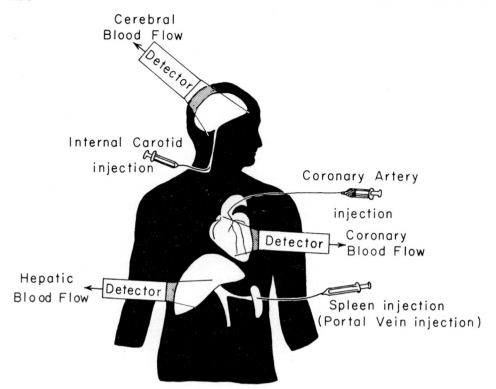

FIGURE 6-4. Measurement of regional blood flow with ^{85}Kr and ^{133}Xe. (From Wagner 1964.)

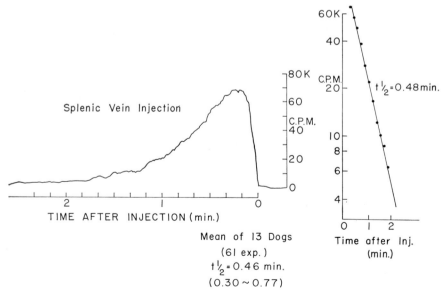

FIGURE 6-5. Clearance of ^{133}Xe from the liver of the dog after splenic vein injection. (From Wagner, 1964.)

cylinder to a 6 liter spirometer. The xenon is then blown into the spirometer with a short puff of oxygen. The apparatus initially contains air, and oxygen is added during the course of the experiment at a rate sufficient to replace that consumed by the patient. The CO_2 produced is absorbed with Calsoda. A pilot's mask connects the spirometer to the patient and the spent radioactive gas is vented to the outdoors. The patient breathes ^{133}Xe-labeled air on closed circuit for 5 minutes and then is allowed to breathe room air. The measurement of desaturation curves and hence tissue clearance rates are obtained by means of extracranial counters. The curves can be analyzed to give fast and slow exponential components with half-periods of about 1.5 minutes and 10 minutes. This technique is a simple atraumatic method for semiquantitative clinical studies of cerebral blood flow, but has not yet been widely accepted.

Krypton-85 and xenon-133 were used by Holzman et al. (1964) to measure blood flow in the human forearm. Following an injection of a solution of physiological saline containing the dissolved gas into the volar surface of the forearm, an external detector placed over the site of injection was used to obtain the half-time of disappearance of radioactivity. Muscle blood flow measured with ^{133}Xe after a histamine injection has been used as a diagnostic method in peripheral arterial disease (Lindbjerg, 1965).

The radioactive noble gases have been used in the study of circulation to other organs. For example, Singleton et al. (1965) used [85]Kr in the detection of intracardiac shunts and concluded that the increase in sensitivity of this method permitted detection of small shunts not demonstrated by oxygen saturation. Arborelius (1965) used [85]Kr in the study of pulmonary circulation during bronchospirometry. He found that the [85]Kr technique is more precise than the conventional oxygen uptake technique.

Another application of radioactive gases is the use of radiolabeled bubbles or foams. Russian neurosurgeons have used intrathecal injections of radon and xenon for isotope myelography. In the presence of a spinal canal block, the radioactive bubble would stop at that level in its ascent and produce a sharp

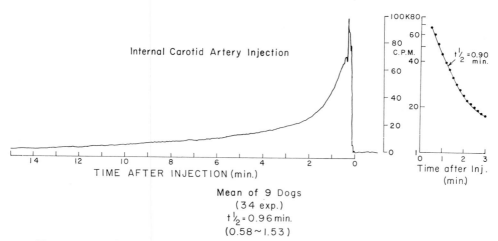

Internal Carotid Artery Injection

$t_{\frac{1}{2}} = 0.90$ min.

Time after Inj. (min.)

TIME AFTER INJECTION (min.)

Mean of 9 Dogs
(34 exp.)
$t_{\frac{1}{2}} = 0.96$ min.
(0.58 ~ 1.53)

FIGURE 6-6.   Clearance of ^{133}Xe from the brain of the dog after internal carotid artery injection. (From Wagner, 1964.)

spike in the record as the detector probe was passed along the spinal column (Hübner and Brown, 1965).

WHEN SHOULD A RADIOPHARMACEUTICAL BE USED?

A radiopharmaceutical should be used in patients when the value of the information gained or effect produced outweighs the risks involved. Whenever the use of a radiopharmaceutical is considered, the decision for use should not be made unless the user can say with some certainty that the information gained will be sufficient for the diagnosis or that the effect achieved will be useful in treatment. With radiopharmaceuticals, both underdosing and over-dosing are serious errors. If too few microcuries are administered and insufficient information is gained, the patient has been exposed to needless radiation.

In normal persons radiopharmaceuticals may be used when these volunteers or their legal guardians have been adequately informed of the potential risks as well as of the benefits.

Two international policies serve as general guides in deciding when to use radioactivity in human studies: the Declaration of Helsinki ("In the purely scientific application of clinical research . . . it is the duty of the doctor to remain the protector of the life and health of that person on whom clinical research is being carried out"); and the International Code of Medical Ethics ("Any act or advice which could weaken physical or mental resistance of a human being may be used only in his interest") (LeRoy, 1966).

REFERENCES

Albert, S. N., Albert, C. A., Hirsch, E. F., Brecker, I. N., and Numerof, P.: Selenate as a Substitute for Sulfate in the Measurement of Extracellular Fluid Volume. *J. Nucl. Med.* 7:290, 1966.

Anghileri, L. J.: A Simplified Method for Preparing High Specific Activity ^{131}I-Labeled Hippuran. *Int. J. Appl. Radiat.* 15:95, 1964.

Arborelius, M., Jr.: Krypton-85 in Study of Pulmonary Circulation during Bronchospirometry. *Scand. J. Clin. & Lab. Invest.* 17:253, 1965.

Baker, P. S.: Reactor-Produced Radionuclides. *In* Andrews, G. A., Kniseley, J. W., and Wagner, H. N., Jr.: Radioactive Pharmaceuticals. U.S. Atomic Energy Commission, 1966.

Baker, R. R., Migita, T., and Wagner, H. N., Jr.: Parenchymal and Reticuloendothelial Cell Function after Subtotal Hepatectomy in the Dog—a Correlation with Quantitative Measurements of the Rate of Regeneration. Unpublished data.

Bayly, R. J.: A Biochemical View of Radiopharmaceutical Development. *In* Andrews, G. A., Kniseley, J. W., and Wagner, H. N., Jr.: Radioactive Pharmaceuticals. U.S. Atomic Energy Commission, 1966.

Beardsley, R. E.: Radiation Control. *In* Gershenson, D., and Greenberg, D.: The Natural Philosopher. Vol. 1. Blaisdell Publishing Co., New York, 1963.

Beck, R. N.: A Theoretical Evaluation of Brain Scanning Systems. *J. Nucl. Med.* 2:314, 1961.

Berson, S. A., and Yalow, R. S.: Antigens in Insulin Determinants of Specificity of Porcine Insulin in Man. *Science* 139:844, 1963.

Berson, S. A., Yalow, R. S., Aurbach, G. D., and Potts, J. T., Jr.: Immunoassay of Bovine and Human Parathyroid Hormone. *Proc. Nat. Acad. Sci.* 49:613, 1963.

Blau, M.: Biosynthesis of (^{75}Se) Selenomethionine and (^{75}Se) Selenocystine. *Biochim. Biophys. Acta* 49:389, 1961.

Blau, M., and Bender, M. A.: ^{75}Se-Selenomethionine for Visualization of the Pancreas by Isotope Scanning. *Radiology* 78:974, 1962.

Blau, M., and Bender, M. A.: Radiomercury ([203]Hg) Labeled Neohydrin: A New Agent for Brain Tumor Localization. *J. Nucl. Med.* 3:83, 1962.

Blau, M., and Holland, J. F.: Metabolism of Selenium-75 L-Selenomethionine. *In* Andrews, G. A., Kniseley, J. W., and Wagner, H. N., Jr.: Radioactive Pharmaceuticals. U.S. Atomic Energy Commission, 1966.

Blau, M., and Manske, R. F.: The Pancreas Specificity of ^{75}Se-Selenomethionine. *J. Nucl. Med.* 2:102, 1961.

Bloch, H. S., and Ray, F. E.: Organic Radioiodo Compounds for Cancer Research. *J. Nat. Cancer Inst.* 7:61, 1946.

Borghgraef, R. R. M., Kessler, R. H., and Pitts, R. F.: Plasma Regression Distribution and Excretion of Radiomercury in Relation to Diuresis Following the Intravenous Administration of [203]Hg Labeled Chlormerodrin to the Dog. *J. Clin. Invest.* 35:1055, 1956.

Briner, W. H.: Quality Control, Pyrogen Testing, and Sterilization of Radioactive Pharmaceuticals. *In* Andrews, G. A., Kniseley, J. W., and Wagner, H. N., Jr.: Radioactive Pharmaceuticals. U.S. Atomic Energy Commission, 1966.

Brucer, M.: Vignettes in Nuclear Medicine. No. 2. Nuclear Consultants, St. Louis, 1966.

Buddemeyer, E. U., and Rhodes, B. A.: Personal Communication. 1966.

Charlton, J. C.: Problems Characteristic of Radioactive Pharmaceuticals. *In* Andrews, G. A., Kniseley, J. W., and Wagner, H. N., Jr.: Radioactive Pharmaceuticals. U.S. Atomic Energy Commission, 1966.

Cunningham, R. E.: Discussion. *In* Andrews, G. A., Kniseley, J. W., and Wagner, H. N., Jr.: Radioactive Pharmaceuticals. U.S. Atomic Energy Commission, 1966, p. 687.

Dewey, W. C., and Sinclair, W. K.: Criteria for Evaluating Collimators Used in In Vivo Distribution Studies with Radioisotopes. *Int. J. Appl. Radiat.* 10:1, 1961.

Dobson, E. L., and Jones, H. B.: The Behavior of Intravenously Injected Particulate Material: Its Rate of Disappearance from the Blood Stream as a Measure of Liver Blood Flow. *Acta Med. Scand.* 144(Suppl. 273):1, 1952.

Drinker, C. K., and Shaw, L. A.: Quantitative Distribution of Particulate Material (Manganese Dioxide) Administered Intravenously to Cats. *J. Exp. Med.* 33:77, 1921.

Dyson, N. A., Hugh-Jones, P., Newbery, G. R., and West, J. B.: The Preparation and Use of Oxygen-15 with Particular Reference to its Value in the Study of Pulmonary Malfunction. Proceedings of the Second United Nations International Conference on the Peaceful Uses of Atomic Energy, Geneva, 1958. 26:103, 1958.

Goodwin, D. A., Scheffel, U., Wagner, H. N., Jr., and Kramer, H. H.: Indium-113m Colloid: A New Radiopharmaceutical for Liver Scanning. *Nucleonics* 24:65, 1966.

Greenwood, F. C., Hunter, N. M., and Glover, J. S.: The Preparation of 131-I-labeled Human Growth Hormone of High Specific Radioactivity. *Biochem. J.* 89:114, 1963.

Greif, R. L., Sullivan, W. J., Jacobs, G. S., and Pitts R. F.: Distribution of Radiomercury Administered as Labeled Chlormerodrin (Neohydrin) in the Kidneys of Rats and Dogs. *J. Clin. Invest.* 35:38, 1956.

Halpern, B. N., Biozzi, G., Benacerraf, B., Stiffel, C., and Hillemand, B.: Cinétique de la phagocytose d'une sérumalbumine humaine spécialement traitée et radiomarquée et son application à l'étude de la circulation hépatique chez l'homme. *C.R. Soc. Biol. (Paris)* 150:1307, 1956.

Hamilton, J. G.: The Rates of Absorption of the Radioactive Isotopes of Sodium, Potassium, Chlorine, Bromine and Iodine in Normal Human Subjects. *Amer. J. Physiol.* 124:667, 1938.

Hansson, E., and Blau, M.: Incorporation of ^{75}Se-Selenomethionine into Pancreatic Juice Proteins In Vivo. *Biochem. Biophys. Res. Comm.* 13:71, 1963.

Harper, P. V., Lathrop, K. A., and Gottschalk, A.: *In* Andrews, G. A., Kniseley, J. W., and Wagner, H. N., Jr.: Radioactive Pharmaceuticals. U.S. Atomic Energy Commission, 1966.

Herrera, N. F., Gonzalez, R., Schwartz, R. D., Diggs, A. M., and Belsky, J.: [75]Se Methionine as a Diagnostic Agent in Malignant Lymphoma. *J. Nucl. Med.* 6:792, 1965.

Hertz, S., Roberts, A., and Evans, R. D.: Radioactive Iodine as an Indicator in the Study of Thyroid Physiology. *Proc. Soc. Exp. Biol. Med.* 38:510, 1938.

Holzman, G. B., Wagner, H. N., Jr., Iio, M., Rabinowitz, D., and Zierler, K. L.: Measurement of Muscle Blood Flow in the Human Forearm with Radioactive Krypton and Xenon. *Circulation* 30:27, 1964.

Hübner, K. F., and Brown, D. W.: Scanning of the Spinal Subarachnoid Space after Intrathecal Injection of [131]I Labeled Human Serum Albumin. *J. Nucl. Med.* 6:465, 1965.

Hunter, W. M., and Greenwood, F. C.: Preparation of Iodine-131 Labeled Human Growth Hormone of High Specific Activity. *Nature* 194:495, 1962.

Joliot, F., and Curie, I.: Artificial Production of a New Kind of Radioelement. *Nature* 133:201, 1934.

Kessler, R. H., Lozano, R., and Pitts, R. F.: Studies on Structure—Diuretic Activity Relationships of Organic Compounds of Mercury. *J. Clin. Invest.* 36:656, 1957.

Kety, S. S., and Schmidt, C. F.: The Nitrous Oxide Method for the Quantitative Determination of Cerebral Blood Flow in Man: Theory, Procedure and Normal Values. *J. Clin. Invest.* 27:476, 1948.

Knipping, H. W., Bolt, W., Valentin, H., and Endler, P.: Regionale Funktionsanalyse in der Dreislauf -und Lungen-Klinik mit Hilfe der Isotopenthorakographie und der skeletiven Angiographie der Lungengefäbe; Beitrag zur präoperativen Funktionsanalyse in der Thoraxchirurgie. *München. Med Wschr.* 99:46, 1957.

Lassen, N. A., and Munck, O.: The Cerebral Blood Flow in Man Determined by the Use of Radioactive Krypton. *Acta Physiol. Scand.* 33:30, 1955.

LeRoy, G. V.: Guidelines for Safe Use of Radiopharmaceuticals. *In* Andrews, G. A., Kniseley, J. W., and Wagner, H. N., Jr.: Radioactive Pharmaceuticals. U.S. Atomic Energy Commission, 1966.

Lindbjerg, I. F.: Measurement of Muscle Blood Flow with ^{133}Xe after Histamine Injection as Diagnostic Method in Peripheral Arterial Disease. *Scand. J. Clin. & Lab. Invest.* 17:371, 1965.

Lund, C. C., Shaw, L. A., and Drinker, C. K.: Quantitative Distribution of Particulate Material (Manganese Dioxide) Administered to the Dog, Rabbits, Guinea Pig, Rat, Chicken, and Turtle. *J. Exp. Med.* 33:231, 1921.

Mallett, B. L., and Veall, N.: The Measurement of Regional Cerebral Clearance Rates in Man Using Xenon-133 Inhalation and Extracranial Recording. *Clin. Sci.* 29:179, 1965.

Matthews, C. M. E.: Comparison of Isotopes for Scanning. *J. Nucl. Med.* 6:155, 1965.

Matthews, C. M. E., Dollery, C. T., Clark, J. C., and West, J. B.: Radioactive Gases. *In* Andrews, G. A. Kniseley, J. W., and Wagner, H. N., Jr.: Radioactive Pharmaceuticals U.S. Atomic Energy Commission, 1966.

Mautner, H. G.: The Synthesis and Reactions of Sulfur and Selenium Compounds. *In* Andrews, G. A., Kniseley, J. W., and Wagner, H. N., Jr.: Radioactive Pharmaceuticals. U. S. Atomic Energy Commission, 1966.

McAfee, J. G., and Wagner, H. N., Jr.: Visualization of Renal Parenchyma by Scintiscanning with [203]Hg Neohydrin. *Radiology* 75:820, 1960.

Murray, A., III, and Williams, D. L.: Organic Synthesis with Isotopes. Part 2. Interscience Publishers, New York, 1958.

Myers, W. G.: Discussion. *In* Kniseley, R. M., and Tauxe, W. N. (eds.): Dynamic Clinical Studies with Radioisotopes. U.S. Atomic Energy Commission (TID-7678), Oak Ridge, Tenn., 1964, p. 211.

Myers, W. G.: Radioisotopes of Iodine. *In* Andrews, G. A., Kniseley, J. W., and Wagner, H. N., Jr.: Radioactive Pharmaceuticals. U.S. Atomic Energy Commission, 1966.

Myers, W. G., and Vanderleeden, J. C.: Radioiodine-125. *J. Nucl. Med.* 1:149, 1960.

National Bureau of Standards. Handbook 92, Safe Handling of Radioactive Materials. Superintendent of Documents, U.S. Government Printing Office, Washington, D.C. 1964.

Nelp, W. B., Wagner, H. N., Jr., and Reba, R. C.: Renal Excretion of Vitamin B-12 and its Use in Measurement of Glomerular Filtration Rate in Man. *J. Lab. Clin. Med.* 63:480, 1964.

Pressman, D., and Eisen, H. N.: The Zone of Localization of Antibodies. V. An Attempt to Saturate Antibody-Binding Sites in Mouse Kidney. *J. Immun.* 64:273, 1950.

Reba, R. C., McAfee, J. G., and Wagner, H. N., Jr.: Radiomercury-Labeled Chlormerodrin for In Vivo Uptake Studies and Scintillation Scanning of Unilateral Renal Lesions Associated with Hypertension. *Medicine* 42:269, 1963.

Reid, A. F., and Keston, A. S.: Long-Life Radioiodine. *Phys. Rev.* 70:987, 1946.

Rhodes, B. A., and Wagner, H. N., Jr.: Are Iodotyrosines Normal Constituents of Plasma? *Nature* 210:647, 1966.

Rhodes, B. A., Wagner, H. N., Jr., and Gerrard: Iodine-123: Development and usefulness of a new radiopharmaceutical. *Isotopes Radiation Technology* 4:275, 1967.

Richards, P.: Nuclide Generators. *In* Andrews, G. A., Kniseley, J. W., and Wagner, H. N., Jr.: Radioactive Pharmaceuticals. U.S. Atomic Energy Commission, 1966a.

Richards, P.: The Technetium-99m Generator. *In* Andrews, G. A., Kniseley, J. W., and Wagner, H. N., Jr.: Radioactive Pharmaceuticals. U.S. Atomic Energy Commission, 1966b.

Roth, J., Glick, S. M., Yalow, R. S., and Berson, S. A.: Hypoglycemia: A Potent Stimulus to Secretion of Growth Hormone. *Science* 140:987, 1963.

Sand, J., and Hofmann, K. A.: Einwirkung von Propylen und Butylen auf Mercurisalze. *Berichte Deutsch. Chem. Ges.*, 33:1353, 1900.

Sigman, E. M., Elwood, C. M., and Knox, F.: The Measurement of Glomerular Filtration Rate in Man with Sodium Iothalamate [131]I (Conray). *J. Nucl. Med.* 7:60, 1966.

Sigman, E. M., Elwood, C. M., Reagan, M. E., Morris, A. M., and Catanzaro, A.: The Renal Clearance of I[131] Labelled Sodium Iothalamate in Man. *Invest. Urol.* 2:432, 1965.

Singleton, R. T., Dembo, D. H., and Scherlis, L.: Krypton-85 in Detection of Intracardiac Left-to-Right Shunts. *Circulation* 32:134, 1965.

Sollmann, T.: A Manual of Pharmacology. Ed. 8. W. B. Saunders Co., Philadelphia, 1957, p. 1230.

Spencer, R. P., and Blau, M.: Intestinal Transport of Selenium-75-Selenomethionine. *Science* 136:155, 1962.

Stern, H. S., Goodwin, D. A., Scheffel, U., Wagner, H. N., Jr., and Kramer, H. H.: In-113m for Blood-Pool and Brain Scanning. *Nucleonics* 25:62, 1967.

Stern, H. S., Goodwin, D. A., Wagner, H. N., Jr., and Kramer, H. H.: In-113m—A Short-Lived Radioisotope for Lung Scanning. *Nucleonics* 24:57, 1966.

Stern, H. S., Goodwin, D., Wagner, H. N., Jr., and Kramer, H. H.: Iron (^{113m}In) Hydroxide: A New Radiopharmaceutical for Lung Scanning. *Nucleonics* 24:10, 1966.

Stern, H. S., McAfee, J. G., and Zolle, I.: Technetium-99m-Albumin. *In* Andrews, G. A., Kniseley, J. W., and Wagner, H. N., Jr.: Radioactive Pharmaceuticals. U.S. Atomic Energy Commission, 1966.

Taplin, G. V., Johnson, D. E., Kennady, J. C., Dore, E. K., Poe, N. D., Swanson, L. A., and Greenberg, A.: *In* Andrews, G. A., Kniseley, J. W., and Wagner, H. N., Jr.: Radioactive Pharmaceuticals. U.S. Atomic Energy Commission, 1966.

Ter-Pogossian, M., and Powers, W. E.: The Use of Radioactive Oxygen-15 in the Determination of Oxygen Content in Malignant Neoplasms. Proceedings of the First UNESCO International Conference of Radioisotopes in Scientific Research, Paris, 1957. 3:625, Pergamon Press, New York, 1958.

Threefoot, S. A., Ray, C. T., Burch, G. E., Cronvich, J. A., Milnor, J. P., Overman, W., and Gordon, W.: Concentration-Time Course in the Plasma of Man of Radiomercury Introduced as a Mercurial Diuretic. *J. Clin. Invest.* 28:661, 1949.

Tow, D. E., Wagner, H. N., Jr., Lopez-Majano, V., Smith, E. M., and Migita, T.: Validity of Measuring Regional Pulmonary Arterial Blood Flow with Macroaggregates of Human Serum Albumin. *Amer. J. Roentgen.* 46:664, 1966.

Tubis, M.: Special Iodinated Compounds for Biology and Medicine. *In* Andrews, G. A., Kniseley, J. W., and Wagner, H. N., Jr.: Radioactive Pharmaceuticals. U.S. Atomic Energy Commission, 1966.

Tubis, M., Posnick, E., and Nordyke, R. A.: Preparation and Use of ^{131}I Labeled Sodium Iodohippurate in Kidney Function Tests. *Proc. Soc. Exp. Biol. Med.* 103:497, 1960.

Vanderleeden, J. C.: The Development of Counting Techniques for Low Energy Gamma Radiation for Applications in Biology. M.S. Thesis. The Ohio State University, 1959.

Veall, N.: The Handling and Dispensing of ^{133}Xe Gas Shipments for Clinical Use. *Int. J. Appl. Radiat.* 16:385, 1965.

Voigt, J.: Untersuchungen über die Verteilung und das Schicksal des Kolloiden Silbers im Säugertierkörper. I. Zur Kenntnis des kolloidalen Silbers. *Biochem. Z.* 62:280, 1914.

Voigt, J.: Über die Verteilung und das Schicksal des kolloidalen Silbers im Säugetierkörper. II. Was erfahren wir aus quantitativen analysen über die Verteilung? *Biochem. Z.* 63:409, 1914.

Voigt, J.: Über die Verteilung und das Schicksal des kolloiden Silbers im Säugetierkörper. III. *Biochem. Z.* 68:477, 1915.

Voigt, J.: Über die Verteilung des Kolloiden Jodsilbers im Säugetierkörper nach intravenöser Injektion. *Biochem. Z.* 89:220, 1918.

Wagner, H. N., Jr.: Radiopharmaceuticals—Their Use in Nuclear Medicine. *Nucleonics* 24:62, 1966.

Wagner, H. N., Jr., McAfee, J. G., and Winkelman, J. W.: Splenic Disease Diagnosis by Radioisotope Scanning. *Arch. Intern. Med.* 109:673, 1962.

Wagner, H. N., Jr., Weiner, I. M., McAfee, J. G., and Martinez, J.: 1-Mercuri-2-hydroxypropane (MHP): A New Radiopharmaceutical for Visualization of the Spleen by Radioisotope Scanning. *Arch. Intern. Med.* 113:696, 1964.

Weinberg, A. N.: Detection of Congenital Galactosemia and the Carrier State Using Galactose C-14 and Blood Cells. *Metabolism* 10:728, 1961.

Yalow, R. S., and Berson, S. A.: Preparation of High Specific Activity Iodine-131 Labeled Hormones: Use in Radioimmunoassay of Hormones in Plasma. *In* Andrews, G. A., Kniseley, J. W., and Wagner, H. N., Jr.: Radioactive Pharmaceuticals. U.S. Atomic Energy Commission, 1966.

Yalow, R. S., Glick, S. M., Roth, J., and Berson, S. A.: Radioimmunoassay of Human Plasma ACTH. *J. Clin. Endocr.* 24:1219, 1964.

Zins, G. R., Ursprung, J. J., and Weeks, J. R.: The Discovery and the Sequential Metabolism of a Long-Acting Hypotensive Agent. *In* Roth, L. J. (ed.): Isotopes in Experimental Pharmacology. The University of Chicago Press, Chicago, 1965, p. 361.

VII

THE THYROID GLAND

WILLIAM H. BEIERWALTES

HENRY N. WAGNER, Jr.

R. L. VOUGHT

A. T. MASI

OUTLINE OF THE HISTORY OF IODINE AND ITS RELATION TO THE THYROID GLAND

H. N. Wagner, Jr.

The first milestone along the road to an understanding of the importance of iodine in thyroid physiology occurred when Courtois, a saltpeter manufacturer in France, told a chemist named Clement about a new gas that he had discovered.[1] Desormes and Clement announced Courtois' discovery at the Institut Impérial de France in 1813. Two months later, the following was recorded in the *Proceedings of the Royal Society* in London:

> Sir Humphrey Davy communicated, in a letter to the President, a long paper from Paris, on a new gas discovered in that city by M. Courtois, a manufacturer of saltpeter. It appears that this gas was discovered about two years ago, but such is the deplorable state of scientific men in France that no account of it was published till the arrival of our English philosopher there. . . . M. Gay-Lussac has devoted his attention to an examination of its history and properties. Meantime, Sir Humphrey has made a great number of experiments on it, and would have made several more had he not wanted the necessary apparatus in Paris.

Thus began a dispute over priority between two great scientists, Davy and Gay-Lussac, that lasted for years. Chattaway (1909) writes:

---

[1] The discovery was first announced in the newspaper *Le Moniteur Universal,* No. 336, Dec. 2, 1813, p. 1344, col. 1; later reported in *Annales de chimie* 88:304, 1813.

> Courtois discovered iodine and prepared it in a pure state; Gay-Lussac thoroughly investigated it, demonstrated its close relationship to chlorine, established its elementary nature and named it. Davy did little more than make these discoveries known in England.

Sharp (1913) has presented another viewpoint:

> Both Courtois and Clement failed to recognize that iodine was an element; this honour being reserved for Davy who gave it its name. Gay-Lussac laid claim to the title of this discovery and he certainly was the first—in 1813—actually to publish the fact that iodine was an element, but it appears that Davy had communicated the fact to Gay-Lussac during a conversation which took place between the two men while Davy was on a visit to Paris. Altogether the weight of evidence as to priority of discovery is in favor of Davy, but he failed to get it into print first.

A relationship between iodine and goiter was suggested by Coindet (1820), who reported the discovery of a "remedy against goiter." Only 8 years after the discovery of iodine, he guessed that iodine was the substance in burned sponge that had been found to be effective in the treatment of goiter for at least seven centuries. His idea may have been based on the work of Fyfe, an Edinburgh chemist, who reported in 1819 "some experiments made with a view of ascertaining the different substances from which iodine can be procured." Fyfe found high concentrations of iodine in marine products, including sponge. Coindet's discovery was described in an anonymous article in the *Edinburgh Medical and Surgical Journal* of 1824:

> We learn from the first memoir of Doctor Coindet, that in the year 1813, when searching for a formula in the work of Cadet, he found that Russell had recommended the ashes of *fucus vesiculosus*, or bladderwrack, under the name of A. *vegetabilis*, for the cure of bronchocele;[2] and he was led, from analogy between this substance and burnt sponge, so long famed, to suspect that iodine was the active principle of both. The great and unequaled success which resulted from its use in the treatment of bronchocele, at once indicated the power of iodine as a therapeutic agent, and encouraged Doctor Coindet to pursue his researches in rendering it an efficient article in the materia medica. . . .
>
> It is in medicine, as in other practical applications of human knowledge, that few innovations entitled to the name of discovery, few changes distinguished for sagacious conjecture, can be effected, without giving rise to dispute about the merits of the individual with whom the improvement was supposed to originate. It has been generally understood among the profession that the happy conjecture, which introduced iodine into medical treatment, originated with Doctor Coindet of Geneva; yet we find that his claim to this honour is disputed by one of his countrymen, Doctor J. C. Straub of Hofwyl, in the Canton of Berne. It is always difficult, and sometimes unsafe, to attempt to decide a question of this sort.

After iodine had been used for several years in the treatment of endemic goiter, the idea was presented that it was the *lack* of something, rather than the *presence* of something in drinking water that caused goiter, the latter idea going back at least to the first century A.D. In 1830, Prevost, a Swiss, stated that iodine deficiency might be responsible for goiter. The following year, Boussingault, a French chemist, recommended that domestic salt supplies be iodized to prevent goiter. The circumstances of this recommendation have been described by Kelly and Snedden (1958):

---

[2] In older literature, the term bronchocele was used for goiter.

In 1824, von Humboldt described the occurrence of goiter in the Andean plateau and referred to the striking fact that the inhabitants of goitrous localities recognized that salt from certain natural deposits was more beneficial than that from others. The following year, a young doctor named Roulin, who had recently come to Colombia from Paris full of information and ideas about Coindet's new iodine treatment of goiter, noted this and was instrumental in having samples of the salts analyzed by Boussingault. On analysis, Boussingault made the significant discovery that those salts instinctively preferred by the goitrous peoples contained most iodine.

This prompted his recommendation.

In 1852, Chatin, a professor of pharmacy in Paris, published a long series of papers on the natural occurrence of iodine. He demonstrated a lack of iodine in the air, soil, and water in districts of endemic goiter and recommended iodinization of the water supply. His experiments were severely criticized on technical grounds by a commission of the French Academy of Science, and his recommendations were ignored. Meanwhile, Boussingault's recommendation had resulted in the experimental use of iodized salt in several French districts. Large doses of iodine were given in the form of iodized salt and potassium iodide tablets and by inhalation. These measures resulted in toxic symptoms, and the studies were abandoned.

Over 50 years were to elapse before further study was made of the use of iodine in the prophylaxis of endemic goiter. The renewed emphasis resulted from the momentous work of Baumann, who in 1896 showed that the human thyroid gland contained iodine. Shortly thereafter, Marine carried out his classic experiments. We are fortunate to have a description by Marine (1954) of the evolution of his experiments:

> My first visit to Michigan was in March, 1907, when I made a horse-and-buggy visit to several farms between Ann Arbor and Pontiac to get a first-hand acquaintance with endemic goiter in sheep and to add to our collection of thyroids of cretin and goitrous dogs and calves the thyroids of cretin lambs which were at that time not easily obtained in northern Ohio. . . . The iodine content of a large series of dog, pig, cattle and also fish thyroids was found generally to vary inversely with the degree of hyperplasia. . . .
>
> When we tried to correlate these comparatively simple relations in animal thyroids with the morphology and iodine contents of a series of human thyroids, both autopsy and surgical, we encountered difficulties. . . . Most of the so-called colloid and nodular goiters were too variable in morphology and iodine content to be correlated with the animal series.
>
> On June 5, 1907, Lenhart and I removed one lobe [of the thyroid of an old dog] . . . which we classified as "colloid goiter."

Forty-six days later these investigators removed half of the remaining lobe and again the appearance was that of colloid goiter. When they subsequently removed portions of the remaining bit of thyroid, they found moderate hyperplasia and then, still later, marked hyperplasia.

> These and similar experiments established in our minds that compensatory hyperplasia in these longstanding and morphologically highly complex goiters was essentially identical with that observed by Halsted for normal thyroids of dogs. I think it was the most satisfying group of experiments we ever did. We now had a clue.

Thus the idea was introduced that goiter is an exaggeration of the normal physiological processes of hyperplasia with iodine deficiency and involution with iodine excess.

These studies led to widespread use of iodine to prevent goiter. In 1916, Kimball began an experiment on goiter prevention in 10,000 schoolgirls in Akron, Ohio. Not only did the administration of iodine prevent the development of goiters, but it was associated with the disappearance of thyroid enlargement in two thirds of the girls who had thyroid enlargement at the start of the study, far more than in the untreated control patients (Kimball, 1953). Elsewhere in the United States and throughout the world, similar programs were begun. Two years later, despite objections by many physicians who were convinced that an epidemic of hyperthyroidism would be precipitated, the general use of iodized salt was begun in Michigan. In 1924 the incidence of endemic goiter in Michigan was 39 per cent; by 1950 it had fallen to 1 per cent. In 1948, the Endemic Goiter Committee of the American Public Health Association said that endemic goiter should be classified as a deficiency disease and that federal legislation should be introduced to carry out goiter prophylaxis by the continuous use of iodized salt. This proposal failed to pass in the United States, but similar legislation was enacted in Canada and Colombia—an illustration of the successful integration of scientific knowledge and preventive medicine.

By 1915, Kendall had isolated an iodinated amino acid from the thyroid gland, demonstrated it physiological activity, and named the substance *thyroxine*. In 1926, Harington established the formula of this material and synthesized it. Sandell and Koltoff discovered the catalytic effect that exceedingly small amounts of iodine have on the reduction of ceric ions in the presence of arsenious acid. This finding became the basis for the determination of the protein-bound iodine (PBI) in plasma by Chaney (1940), and it provided an exceedingly important diagnostic tool. Modifications in the method included the widely used alkaline incineration method devised by Barker and his associates in 1951.

In the same year as the first determination of the plasma protein-bound iodine (1940), radioactive iodine was used for the first time by Hamilton and Soley at the University of California in Berkeley. The radionuclide ^{131}I was made by Glenn Seaborg and Ernest Lawrence, the inventor of the cyclotron in which it was produced. Hamilton and Soley measured the rate of urinary excretion of radioactive iodine in various human thyroid disorders. They suggested the use of an external Geiger counter over the thyroid gland to measure the rate and extent of accumulation of iodide. Following the introduction of radioactive isotopes of iodine, detailed knowledge of the synthesis, liberation, and peripheral utilization of thyroid hormones was developed.

ANATOMY OF THE THYROID GLAND AND NOMENCLATURE OF CERTAIN THYROID DISEASES

W. H. BEIERWALTES AND H. N. WAGNER, JR.

The thyroid gland has one lobe on each side of the trachea in front of and below the thyroid cartilage of the larynx. These lobes are joined by a connecting bridge, or isthmus, at their lower anterior portions. More commonly than not, a finger-like projection of thyroid tissue arises from the superior aspect of the left half of the isthmus of the thyroid and projects upward and toward the midline of the anterior surface of the neck for a distance of several centimeters. This "pyramidal" lobe is a thyroglossal tract remnant from the descent of the anlage of the thyroid gland from the region of the foramen caecum in the posterior portion of the tongue to the usual location of the adult thyroid. About 1 to 4 per cent of patients who have had total thyroidectomies later present evidence of functioning thyroid tissue in the midline, above the usual location of the thyroid.

Assessment of the physical size and weight of the thyroid gland by palpation depends not only on the intrinsic characteristics of the gland itself but also on its location in the neck and its texture, as well as on the distribution of tissues between the examiner's fingers and the subject's gland. Autopsy studies of unselected series of thyroid glands have shown that there is a continuous but skewed frequency distribution of gland weights, ranging from 5 to more than 100 g. The heavier glands (i.e., over 35 or 40 g.), which make up about 10 per cent of the frequency distribution, are usually considered to be goitrous. The modal frequency of gland weights in Harland's series of Jamaicans (1964) was 13 g., somewhat less than the 20 to 25 g. that was observed by Hazard and Kaufman in Cleveland, Ohio, in 1952. The difference may be related to the greater average total body weight of the North American compared to the Jamaican.

Mortensen, Woolner, and Bennett (1955) concluded from their autopsy series at the Mayo Clinic that mean thyroid weight increased with age, but this difference was not apparent after age 20 in Harland's study (1964). These three autopsy series included few patients under 20 years of age. Glands weighing over 40 g. were not encountered in young people. The upper limit of weight for a "normal" thyroid gland can be considered to be 40 g., which is two to three times the weight of the "modal" gland in these autopsy series. Since there is a positive correlation between body weight and thyroid weight in man and animals, a 40 g. gland in a 25 kg. child may be more than two or three times the weight of the modal gland among his peers; and, conversely, a 40 g. gland may be less than two or three times the weight of the modal gland of persons weighing 70 kg.

Usually an enlarged gland results in a "bulge," projecting anteriorly and laterally; the examiner must assess the weight on the basis of the size of the "bulge," a judgment that is quite subjective. However, the distribution of "bulge" size can be roughly correlated with gland weight. The physician can achieve more reproducible estimates of size if he adopts a standardized technique of inspection and palpation of the neck. One such technique, recently introduced by Crooks (1964), is as follows. The patient sits facing a light that gives diffuse, even illumination of the neck. The examiner observes the neck from three positions, directly in front, and obliquely from the patient's left and right. The patient is asked to swallow a sip of water while the examiner is in each of the three positions. Any swelling in the neck that appears to move upward on swallowing is recorded as "thyroid visible." High-intensity reading lamps are particularly useful for inspection of the neck, since they provide bright and uniform illumination of the neck and can be easily adjusted to patients of varying height. The gland is then palpated from behind the subject with the examiner's thumbs over the nape of the neck, which is slightly flexed. The patient is asked to swallow. A mass that moves upward is recorded as "thyroid palpable."

Since judgment of gland size is subjective, standardized diagnostic criteria must be used in epidemiologic surveys. Several such standards used in recent surveys are summarized in Table 7-1.

Most investigators agree that a gland that is visible and palpable is a goiter. Differences in judgment among observers arise because of differences in examination techniques. In some cases Crooks' method carried out by three observers has been used together with these criteria: a gland is goitrous if it is visible and palpable on swallowing to each of three observers when the observations and results of each observer are recorded independently of the other two.

The thyroid gland is composed primarily of cell-lined spheres that contain stored thyroid hormone in a form called colloid. Blood vessels and lymphatics course between the spheres. When the thyroid gland is abnormally active, as in exophthalmic goiter, it is very vascular and friable. The quantity and velocity of blood coursing through the arteriovenous anastomoses in such glands are frequently great enough to give the "bruit" or continuous murmur characteristic of arteriovenous aneurysms (Modell, 1933). A lymph node in the midline just above the thyroid isthmus is known as the Delphian node "because it is exposed first, and if diseased, will foretell the nature of the disease process to be found in the thyroid gland" (Means, 1948). The node may be enlarged in thyroiditis or in metastatic carcinoma of the thyroid gland. The more-lateral lymph nodes tend to follow the venous drainage of the thyroid, especially the jugular chains.

An enlargement of the thyroid gland from any cause is termed a goiter, or struma. An enlarged thyroid gland may be overactive without producing enough normally iodinated thyroid hormone to cause metabolic overactivity of the body cells. Thyroid overactivity may result from a subnormal intake of iodine as a result of deficient diet, puberty, or pregnancy, or as a result of deranged intrathyroidal metabolism of iodine. These goiters are classified as *endemic* (in a geographic region in which goiters are common) or *sporadic* (in a geographic region in which goiters are not common). A small goiter of this type is usually called *simple,* whereas the larger, more advanced goiters are usually called *colloid.*

A goiter may produce thyroid hormone at an excessive rate, and if there are no nodules visible or palpable on the surface of such a gland, the patient is said to have Graves' disease or exophthalmic goiter. A small percentage (2 to 5 per cent) of such patients do not have a clinically detectable goiter. Many do not have true exophthalmos (forward protrusion of the eyes) but only ap-

TABLE 7-1. DIAGNOSTIC CRITERIA FOR GOITER USED BY RECENT INVESTIGATORS

DATE	INVESTIGATOR, PLACE	MINIMAL CRITERIA FOR GOITER
1953	WHO	Palpable and 4 to 5 times normal size
1956	Sos, Szabo, and Raksanyi, Hungary	Visible enlargement
1959	Terpstra, Holland	> 2 or 3 times normal size
1963	Kilpatrick et al., England	> 40 g
1963	PAHO*	Palpable and "enlarged"
1964	Hadjidakis et al., Greece	Visible, head extended
1964	Crooks et al., Scotland	Visible, and palpable on swallowing
1965	London et al., Kentucky	> 40 g

*Recommendation of the First Conference on Research on Endemic Goitre. Caracas, Venezuela, April 1963. Sponsored by the Pan American Health Organization. Unpublished data.

parent exophthalmos, from upper lid retraction that exposes to view an increased surface area of the eyeball. If a hyperactive thyroid gland is nodular, the patient is generally said to suffer from Plummer's disease, or toxic nodular goiter, or toxic adenomatous goiter. Nodular goiters are usually benign but may be caused by malignant neoplasms, thyroiditis, or other pathological conditions. Inflammation of the thyroid (thyroiditis), either suppurative or nonsuppurative, can produce a goiter that is either smooth or nodular.

PHYSIOLOGY OF THE THYROID GLAND

FUNCTIONAL STATUS OF THE THYROID GLAND

When the thyroid gland is normally active, the patient is said to be *euthyroid*. When a patient is suffering from the effects of too much thyroxine, which causes generalized hyperactivity, he is said to be *hyperthyroid*. His thyroid gland produces thyroid hormone in "toxic" quantities, and he may be said to be suffering from *thyrotoxicosis*. The terms hyperthyroidism and thyrotoxicosis are now synonymous. In the older literature these were differentiated, since it was believed that in some patients there was a quantitative increase in the amount of normal thyroid hormone, whereas in others there was an abnormal or toxic kind of hormone.

A person will develop the same clinical picture, except for exophthalmos and lid retraction, if he is given large quantities of thyroid hormone either orally or parenterally. In such cases, the thyroid gland will actually become underactive because of the depression of thyroid-stimulating hormone (TSH) activity of the pituitary. The patient might be said to have induced thyrotoxicosis without hyperthyroidism.

The term *hypothyroidism* is used to describe the clinical state of a patient who suffers from too little stimulation of his bodily function by thyroid hormone. When there is a marked deficiency, or perhaps a total lack of circulating thyroid hormone, lasting for a long period of time, the hypothyroid patient develops the syndrome, *myxedema;* the term is used because of the infiltration of the skin, mucous membranes, and (to a lesser extent) all tissues of the body with a pseudomucinous substance. A patient suffering from severe and obvious lack of thyroid hormone is said to be myxedematous. This state may result from destruction of the thyroid gland or from loss or marked depression of its function. At times a gland may be quantitatively hyperactive and yet may fail to produce hormone that is metabolically active, with resultant hypothyroidism.

Hypothyroidism is the term used when the thyroid gland is underfunctioning because of abnormality in the thyroid gland itself. Secondary hypothyroidism refers to underfunction of the thyroid gland as a result of hypopituitarism.

METABOLISM OF IODINE

The functions of the thyroid gland can be considered under four headings:
1. Uptake of iodine by the thyroid

2. Organic binding of iodine
3. Storage of thyroid hormone
4. Release of thyroid hormone

Little information is available as to the chemical state of iodine in food-stuffs, but it appears that the digestive juices readily convert these compounds into metabolically useful forms that are promptly absorbed and appear in the serum as iodide.

Ingested iodine is absorbed from the gastrointestinal tract so rapidly that it can usually be detected in the thyroid gland within minutes. At least part of the absorption takes place in the stomach. Absorption has been found to be complete within an hour after ingestion (Hertz et al., 1938). Keating and Albert (1949) showed that the usual rate of absorption is 5 per cent per minute, although absorption may be delayed if the subject is not fasting. Normally, only trace quantities of ^{131}I can be found in the vomitus of patients who vomit 10 minutes or more after receiving an oral dose of ^{131}I. But if a patient has gastric retention from a peptic ulcer or gastric cancer, the absorption of ^{131}I may be sufficiently retarded to lower the usual results of the 2 hour measurement of ^{131}I uptake by the thyroid.

When fasting, the plasma inorganic iodide (PII) concentration in normal persons ranges from 0.1 to 1.0 μg./100 ml. (Wayne et al., 1964) and is directly proportional to the daily iodine intake (Vought and London, 1964). The thyroid, salivary, and gastric glands and the kidney remove iodine from the plasma exponentially; i.e., the rate of removal is proportional to the concentration of iodide in the plasma. Thus, the amount of plasma iodide cleared per unit of time depends on the plasma concentration of iodide, as well as on fractional uptake by the thyroid gland. The amount of plasma iodide taken up by the thyroid per unit of time, i.e., the absolute iodine uptake (AIU), is given by:

$$\text{AIU, } \mu\text{g./hr.} = \text{thyroidal clearance ml./hr.} \times \text{PII } \mu\text{g./ml.}$$

Thyroid clearance depends to a large extent on TSH stimulation and plasma inorganic iodine on dietary iodine intake. Usual values of the AIU are 0.5 to 6.0 μg./hr. in healthy nongoitrous persons.

The role of the *salivary* and *gastric glands* in iodine metabolism is not fully understood, but it cannot be ignored. Extrathyroidal iodine metabolism has recently been reviewed by Brown-Grant (1961). It appears that the salivary and gastric glands concentrate iodide about as efficiently as the iodide-trapping mechanisms of the thyroid, and that their concentrating mechanisms are inhibited by the same anions that inhibit thyroidal concentration of iodide. Salivary and gastric iodine concentrating mechanisms are *not* under TSH control. Recently, Vought and London (1964) measured the secretion rate of iodide in mixed saliva after paraffin-chewing stimulation and found that the rate was linearly dependent on dietary iodide intake at levels below 167 μg./day; the rate increased sharply at levels of high dietary iodine intake. Even at low levels of iodide intake, the salivary secretion rate, 3.0 to 3.6 μg./hr., was approximately equal to the AIU. Iodine in salivary and gastric secretions is not lost from the body since it is reabsorbed from the intestinal tract.

In the *kidney*, iodide is filtered by the glomeruli and about 73 per cent is normally reabsorbed by the tubules. As with the thyroid, the rate of renal excretion is proportioned to the PII, and the amount lost per unit of time depends on the renal iodide clearance and the PII concentration. Thus, the renal loss of iodide depends on the equilibrium among dietary iodine intake, the rate of glomerular filtration of iodide, and iodide reabsorption by the tubules.

At intake levels below 500 μg./day, the amount of iodine excreted per day in the urine of nongoitrous persons is usually equal to or slightly in excess of iodine intake (Vought and London, 1964).

In healthy subjects *fecal* iodine excretion usually amounts to 5 to 20 μg./day and is independent of iodine intake (Vought and London, 1964). Large amounts of iodine may appear in the feces after—in some cases, years after—the ingestion or injection of radiopaque dyes. Under normal circumstances, fecal iodine appears to be chiefly hormonal, i.e., as end products of thyroxine metabolism that are excreted via the liver and bile. Van Middlesworth (1965) has shown that in the rat there is a large enteric circulation of thyroxine.

In normal persons the *total* (urinary plus fecal) iodine excretion usually exceeds iodine intake at intake levels below 500 μg./day, according to studies over short periods of time. (Iodine excretion in the sweat is usually slight enough to be ignored.) The amount of iodine excreted over a period of time consists of two components, (a) a large fraction, 90 to 100 per cent of intake, plus (b) a relatively constant "obligatory" excretion of 30 to 50 μg./day, which is independent of intake. The obligatory iodine excretion is apparently both urinary and fecal, since the average total daily obligatory iodine excretion exceeds the average daily fecal iodine excretion (Vought and London, 1964).

Fifty-two to 84 per cent (average, 66 per cent) of tracer doses of ^{131}I were excreted in the urine by euthyroid subjects over a 48 hour period. Thyrotoxic subjects excreted only 6 to 32 per cent, with an average of 19 per cent. Myxedematous subjects excreted 72 to 91 per cent (Skanse, 1948).

Radioiodine in blood is found mainly in plasma and to a lesser extent in red blood cells. The thyroid clears ^{131}I from the plasma of hyperthyroid patients at the rate of 75 to 250 ml. per minute (Myant et al., 1950). This rate of clearance is dependent upon the diffusion space of ^{131}I and the rate of renal clearance, as well as on thyroid function.

IODIDE-CONCENTRATING MECHANISM OF THE THYROID

Along with certain other organs, such as the stomach and mammary and salivary glands, the thyroid gland is able to concentrate iodide to a high degree (Halmi, 1961). Almost one fifth of the iodide in the blood that perfuses the thyroid is extracted in a single passage through the gland. Iodide uptake and subsequent steps in the formation of thyroid hormone occur in rapid succession, although under abnormal conditions iodide uptake may be the only function of which the gland is capable. This may occur if organic binding of iodine is blocked with goitrogens or with large doses of iodine. Diseases may occur in which iodide may be concentrated without subsequent organic binding. Stanbury and Hedge (1950) first observed the familial occurrence of congenital goiter as a result of such defects.

Iodide trapping follows saturation kinetics, and may be inhibited (apparently competitively) by at least two types of anions, of which thiocyanate (SCN^-) and perchlorate (ClO_4^-) are representative. The energy source for iodide concentration appears to be high-energy phosphate bonds. Exact conditions of temperature, pH, and cationic composition are necessary.

A defect in iodide-concentrating ability has been found by Stanbury and Chapman (1960). A 15 year old boy with goiter and hypothyroidism was unable to concentrate iodide in his salivary glands and gastric mucosa and had a low thyroidal uptake of ^{131}I. The clinical picture was reversed completely and the goiter regressed after administration of large doses of iodide daily.

In the normal subject, the concentration gradient (expressed by the ratio of thyroid to serum iodide concentration, T/S) does not usually exceed 30:1. On the other hand, in Graves' disease, or in hyperplasia of the thyroid induced by drugs that block organification of iodine, the ratio may be as high as 500:1. In contrast to organically bound iodine, trapped iodide is readily discharged from the gland within a few minutes by thiocyanate, perchlorate, and certain other anions.

In normal persons and in patients with Graves' disease, trapped iodide is rapidly converted to monoiodotyrosine. The rapidity of this process is evidenced by the inability of thiocyanate to discharge significant amounts of ^{131}I that had been accumulated by the normal or toxic gland a few minutes earlier. Therefore, the rate of thyroidal clearance of plasma iodide may usually be taken as equivalent to the rate of organic binding of iodide.

OTHER IODIDE-CONCENTRATING MECHANISMS

Physiological sites of iodine concentration other than the thyroid, e.g., the bladder, stomach, and salivary glands, must be distinguished from functioning metastatic thyroid tissue in the evaluation of a patient with suspected carcinoma of the thyroid or in a patient being treated with radioactive iodine. Whenever turnover of iodine by the thyroid is rapid, as in hyperthyroid patients or in patients whose thyroid has been ablated by surgery or radioiodine, a high concentration of radioactivity may be found in the liver (Pochin, 1964). The radioactivity is in the form of thyroxine and possibly other metabolites of thyroxine. The radioactive thyroxine usually can be found within a few days of administration of the dose of radioactive iodine, and therefore can be distinguished from that due to the presence of functioning metastases, which usually have a maximum uptake at an earlier time (often at 6 to 12 hours).

ORGANIC BINDING OF IODINE

After iodide has been concentrated by the thyroid gland, presumably it is oxidized to hypoiodous acid and nascent iodine. The latter reacts immediately with tyrosine to form monoiodotyrosine and diiodotyrosine. Two molecules of diiodotyrosine are then coupled by an oxidative mechanism to yield the principal thyroid hormone, thyroxine. A second thyroid hormone, 3, 4, 3'-triiodothyronine, arises either from the coupling of monoiodotyrosine and diiodotyrosine or by deiodination of thyroxine. The latter reaction is believed by Pitt-Rivers to be unlikely, since thyroid tissue cannot be shown to deiodinate thyroxine (Pitt-Rivers, 1963).

It is generally believed that thyroid hormone synthesis occurs within the thyroglobulin molecule, but the exact site of iodination is not yet certain. Thyroglobulin is probably synthesized within the thyroid cell. Before thyroxine is secreted into the circulation the peptide linkage is broken, since normally thyroglobulin itself is not found in the blood.

At least two thirds of the thyroidal iodine is in the form of diiodotyrosine and monoiodotyrosine. An enzyme, dehalogenase, selectively removes the iodine from free iodotyrosines but spares free thyroxine and triiodothyronine, as well as the protein-bound iodotyrosines. Following deiodination of iodotyrosines within the thyroid, the iodide is reoxidized and recombined with thyroglobulin.

Stanbury and his associates have found goitrous patients who have defects in these metabolic pathways. Two sisters studied by Stanbury, Ohela, and Pitt-Rivers, (1955) were found to have iodotyrosines present in abundance but scarcely detectable amounts of thyroxine. Several families of goitrous subjects have been found who lack the enzyme dehalogenase (McGirr, 1960). In these patients monoiodotyrosine and diiodotyrosine leak from the thyroid in large amounts, and since the enzyme is also absent from peripheral tissues, the iodotyrosines are excreted unchanged in the urine.

Storage and release of thyroid hormone

The thyroid gland normally contains about 10,000 to 20,000 μg. of organic iodine, and secretes about 100 μg./day, mostly in the form of thyroxine. In thyrotoxicosis, this value may reach 1000 μg./day, or about 5 to 10 per cent of the total thyroidal iodine. After Graves' disease has been treated with ^{131}I, surgery, or antithyroid drugs, thyroidal iodine content may be reduced to values as low as 1200 μg. and yet normal quantities of thyroxine may be secreted. Since the normal thyroid gland secretes only 0.5 to 1 per cent of its iodine stores per day, even complete blockade of thyroxine production may require months to induce hypothyroidism.

By means of autoradiography it has been found that as organic binding of iodine occurs, thyroxine is secreted into the lumen of the thyroid follicles. This occurs within 20 to 30 minutes after the parenteral administration of a tracer dose of [131]I. The radioactivity is found at first as a ring at the periphery of the follicle. During the next 4 hours it becomes distributed throughout the colloid. There is evidence that ^{131}I thyroxine begins to leave the thyroid gland within 2 hours after a tracer dose of [131]I. Berson and Yalow (1963) have pointed out that since the specific activity of intrathyroidal thyroxine is at a peak within a day or so after ^{131}I administration, at least 50 per cent of thyroidal monoiodotyrosine and diiodotyrosine would have to be converted daily to thyroxine, unless there were a preferential short circuit for the conversion of newly accumulated thyroidal iodine into thyroxine. It is likely that there are at least two functionally distinct intrathyroidal iodine compartments with different turnover rates. Nadler et al. (1954) found that the turnover rate of iodine in the thyroid follicles of the rat was inversely related to the size of the follicles. Triantaphyllidis (1958) has also presented evidence that some thyroidal iodine has a faster turnover rate than others.

Transport and peripheral metabolism of thyroxine

Except under pathological conditions, such as dehalogenase deficiency, it is unlikely that iodotyrosines are secreted by the thyroid gland, although some evidence to the contrary has been put forward. In any case, the most important secretion by the thyroid is thyroxine, which binds immediately to a plasma protein (thyroxine-binding globulin or TBG) that is present in trace quantities and on electrophoresis migrates between alpha$_1$ and alpha$_2$ globulins. The reaction equilibrium is such that the normal ratio between free and protein-bound thyroxine is about 1:1000. Thyroxine-binding sites of secondary importance are also present in albumin and in a protein that on electrophoresis migrates in front of albumin (prealbumin). Triiodothyronine is also bound to the interalpha globulin, but less avidly than thyroxine.

Under various physiological and clinical conditions, the concentration of TBG varies; for example, it is increased in pregnancy or following the administration of estrogens, whereas in the nephrotic syndrome it is decreased. Binding of thyroxine by TBG may be an important regulator of the concentration of *free* thyroxine, which is believed to be the important physiological stimulant of metabolic activity. The rate of uptake of thyroxine by tissues may be controlled by competition between the binding capacities of plasma and cellular proteins.

If one injects labeled thyroxine intravenously in normal subjects, the half-time of clearance of radioactivity from the blood is about 6 or 7 days. Triiodothyronine has a shorter half-time, perhaps related to the decreased binding by plasma proteins. Iodine-131-labeled hormone produced by the thyroid gland is metabolized somewhat more rapidly than exogenous labeled thyroxine, possibly because the thyroid has incorporated radioactivity to a small degree into triiodothyronine. Metabolism of thyroxine is faster in hyperthyroidism and slower in hypothyroidism than in the euthyroid state.

Thyroxine is present in high concentrations in the liver and kidney, and in lower concentrations in the pituitary, intestine, adrenal, skin, and skeletal muscle. Because of its mass (about half the body weight) skeletal muscle accounts for most of the extravascular thyroxine.

In man, deiodination of thyroid hormones is the principal metabolic pathway (Pitt-Rivers, 1963). Over 80 per cent of the radioactivity is found as urinary iodide after injection of ^{131}I-labeled thyroxine. About 15 per cent is excreted in the feces.

PHYSIOLOGIC EFFECTS OF THYROID HORMONES

Thyroid hormone is essential for life in all mammals; it is involved in growth, maturation, and differentiation in the young, and in numerous metabolic processes in adults. It has an important function in the control of nitrogen, lipid, calcium, water, and electrolyte metabolism and in the regulation of the enzymes involved in protein synthesis; these processes are discussed in detail by Pitt-Rivers and Trotter (1965). The stimulation of these processes results in the overall effect on basal metabolic rate.

The administration of thyroxine to hypothyroid patients is not followed by an immediate response unless very large doses are given, in which case a response may occur within 6 to 12 hours. A latent period is also observed with triiodothyronine, but its duration is shorter, the onset being within a few days in contrast to about 2 weeks in the case of thyroxine. The duration of action of a single dose of triiodothyronine is also shorter than that of thyroxine.

DIAGNOSTIC TESTS OF THYROID FUNCTION

INTRODUCTION

A reasonable question concerning diagnostic tests of thyroid function is, why are there so many? At least two reasons may be cited. First, study of the function of the thyroid to detect specific abnormalities requires several procedures, each assessing a different aspect. One can no more evaluate total thyroid function by a single test than one can evaluate the entire cardiovascular system by measuring only the pulse rate, or the arterial or venous pressure alone.

A second reason is that each test has its own particular value, its strong and weak points—usually expressible in terms of specificity, sensitivity, reliability, or costs to the patient or physician. For example, one disadvantage of the radioiodine uptake test in the diagnosis of hypothyroidism is its lack of specificity, which may lead to misinterpretation if the patient has abnormal concentrations of iodine in the blood. The physician must have a basic knowledge of at least several diagnostic tests of thyroid function, must understand the role of each in the diagnostic process, and must be able to choose the most suitable ones according to the problem.

Many patients with increased thyroid function can be diagnosed by a careful medical history and physical examination. In other patients, laboratory tests of thyroid function, such as the serum protein-bound iodine (PBI) and the radioactive iodine uptake test, will be necessary to establish the correct diagnosis. The radioiodine tests of thyroid function indicate the rate of activity of the thyroid gland. The PBI measures the concentration of protein-bound iodine in plasma as an indication of the presence or absence of disease. None of these procedures measures the degree of clinical thyrotoxicosis. The basal metabolic rate correlates roughly with the degree of disease but is not specific, since in many clinical states, such as lung or heart disease, it may also be elevated. For this reason, radioiodine tests and PBI determinations have become the backbone of thyroid diagnostic procedures. Their main shortcoming results from the fact that many hospitalized patients receive organically bound iodine in the form of roentgenographic contrast media or as inorganic iodide in medications. Results may also be confusing when thyroid hormone has been taken surreptitiously (thyrotoxicosis factitia) or when the patient is producing metabolically inactive thyroid hormone (genetic hypothyroidism).

MEASUREMENT OF IODIDE ACCUMULATION

The most widely used test of thyroid function with radioiodine is direct measurement of the rate of accumulation of ^{131}I by the thyroid gland by means of an external radiation detector. A dose of ^{131}I is administered orally or intravenously. After standardized intervals, such as 1, 2, 6, or 24 hours, radioactivity in the thyroid is measured under standardized conditions and is compared to the amount present in a reference source containing a known quantity of ^{131}I. The amount of ^{131}I in the thyroid is usually expressed as a percentage of the administered tracer dose. The result measures the percentage of the extrathyroidal iodide pool that is being accumulated per unit time, sometimes referred to as the *fractional clearance* of iodide. Since the absolute quantity of iodide in the extrathyroidal iodide pool is usually not known, one cannot determine the absolute value of iodide accumulation in units of mass per unit time. Only the fractional clearance is used to indicate functional activity of the thyroid gland. The procedure is valid, since an overactive thyroid gland turns over the plasma iodide pool faster than a normally active gland, and an underactive gland turns over iodide more slowly, provided the body's iodide stores are within the usual range. Unfortunately, one may encounter patients whose extrathyroidal iodide stores are abnormally large, and the radioiodine accumulation is thereby depressed. Although at normal inorganic iodide levels the rate of accumulation of radioactive iodine by the thyroid is independent of the serum iodide concentration (Stanley, 1949), this is not true at higher levels of iodide. Childs and collaborators (1950) reported that in hyperthyroid subjects the iodide-trapping function was not altered by the administration of stable iodide in the range of 0.1 to 100 mg., but it was suppressed by 500 mg. or more. Stanley (1949) observed that the administration of 1.5 mg. of stable iodide daily for as long as a week did not change the radioiodine uptake.

Grayson (1960) has reviewed the factors that influence the radioiodine uptake test, such as the presence of certain drugs such as Lugol's solution, which contains about 5 to 8 mg. of iodine per drop, vitamin preparations, which may contain about 100 to 150 μg., and radiographic contrast media. Magalotti et al. (1959) and Wayne et al. (1964) have provided a convenient summary of the duration of action of various drugs that suppress iodine accumulation.

EARLY UPTAKE MEASUREMENTS

In the diagnosis of hyperthyroidism with radioiodine, it is frequently necessary to make an uptake measurement within 30 minutes to 6 hours after administering the dose. Some hyperthyroid patients incorporate tracer iodide into thyroxine and secrete labeled hormone so rapidly that the radioactivity in the thyroid may have returned to normal amounts within 24 hours. Errors will result in approximately 10 to 20 per cent of patients with hyperthyroidism if reliance is placed entirely on the 24 hour uptake value. If one measures radioiodine uptake within the first hour, it is better to use the intravenous route of administration to avoid variability resulting from differences in the rate of intestinal absorption. Oral doses have been employed successfully when the 2 hour uptake is measured (Pochin, 1960). It is usually possible to distinguish hyperthyroidism from normal thyroid function within a few minutes of the intravenous administration of the radioactive iodine. Therefore, if one wishes to reduce the radiation dose, after the early uptake measurement, one may administer sodium perchlorate to cause release of the trapped iodide (Mosier, 1963). This is particularly desirable in children.

LATE UPTAKE MEASUREMENTS

Although early uptake measurements (30 minutes to 6 hours) are useful in the diagnosis of increased thyroid function, it is not possible consistently to detect *decreased* thyroidal activity without waiting at least 6 hours, and preferably 24 hours, after administration of the dose before making measurements. The usual level of activity of the thyroid gland is not sufficiently great to permit differentiation between decreased and normal function within shorter periods of time. Another advantage of the late measurement is that the extrathyroidal iodine measured by the external radiation detector is less after 24 hours than within a few hours after administration of the dose.

In general, we prefer early uptake measurements to detect increased thyroid function, and late uptake measurements (either 24 or 48 hours) to detect decreased thyroid function.

THYROIDAL CLEARANCE OF PLASMA IODIDE

After intravenous injection or after ingestion and absorption of ^{131}I, the initial plasma level begins to fall as a result of several physiological processes, which include mixing of ^{131}I in the vascular compartment, diffusion into the extravascular space, thyroidal uptake, and renal excretion of radioactivity. The fall in the blood level of ^{131}I progressively decreases the rate of uptake of ^{131}I by the thyroid gland. Within 2 hours, secretion of ^{131}I in the form of labeled thyroxine begins. To control more of the numerous variables that influence the ^{131}I uptake measurement, clearance methods were applied by Myant, Pochin, and their associates (1949, 1950). These were needed, because in about 10 per cent of their patients, simple measurement of the thyroidal uptake or the urinary excretion of iodide gave equivocal results. For example, in the presence of severe renal disease, misleading values were obtained. Myant, Pochin, and Goldie (1949) and subsequently Berson and his associates (1952) found that measurement of the clearance of ^{131}I from the blood by the thyroid was the most reliable index of the thyroid's iodide-accumulating function. Goolden (1958) has summarized the advantages of measuring the rate of uptake of radioiodine by the thyroid at an early stage after an *intravenous* dose. Variability in absorption is avoided; the change in thyroidal radioactivity is greatest during the initial phase of accumulation; the rate of accumulation is not obscured by the simultaneous loss of labeled hormone from the gland; and plasma radioactivity can be measured with greater precision at this time. In addition, if one obtains a plasma sample and relates thyroidal accumulation to this value (thyroid clearance = rate of change of thyroidal ^{131}I $\div$ the plasma concentration of ^{131}I determined at the same time), a correction is made for extrathyroidal factors, such as renal iodide clearance rate and the rate of diffusion of iodide into the extravascular tissues. Finally, the result is not dependent on an exact knowledge of the administered dose.

Disadvantages of the clearance test are that it is more time-consuming than other tests, the dose must be given intravenously, and a blood sample must be obtained. Extrathyroidal radioactivity is proportionately higher at this time.

The thyroidal clearance method is usually reserved for diagnosing hyperthyroidism in patients who have been treated with radioiodine. The thyroid pool of organic iodine is often reduced in these patients (Berson and Yalow, 1954). This results in the early appearance of labeled hormone in the plasma, even though the total output of hormone may be within normal limits. The values for the thyroid uptake at 24 hours may therefore be spuriously low, whereas the values of the protein-bound ^{131}I at 48 hours may be spuriously high.

Although the results of Berson et al. (1952) as well as those of Coenegracht and Fraser (1955) indicate that early thyroid clearance measurements discriminate quite well between normal and increased thyroid function, they are less sensitive to reduced thyroid uptake, a weakness common to all tests performed within a few hours of administration of the dose. Therefore, decreased thyroid function must be assessed by other procedures such as the urinary excretion test or the 24 hour thyroidal uptake measurement.

URINARY EXCRETION OF IODIDE

Determination of the 24 or 48 hour excretion of radioiodine into the urine is a simple test and was among the first used to diagnose thyroid disease (Skanse, 1949). The principal disadvantage of these tests is their dependence upon the cooperation of the patient; if the collections are in error, the results will be misleading. In addition, in patients with renal disease or congestive heart failure the values may be the same as with increased thyroid function. For these reasons, urinary tests are used only infrequently.

McConahey et al. (1956) reported the results shown in Table 7-2.

TABLE 7-2. PERCENTAGE OF PATIENTS IN NORMAL RANGE IN DETERMINATION OF 24 HOUR EXCRETION OF ^{131}I (NORMAL RANGE = 37 TO 75 PER CENT OF DOSE)[*]

EXOPHTHALMIC GOITER	MYXEDEMA	NODULAR GOITER	
		Without hyperthyroidism	With hyperthyroidism
9	92	98	56

[*] Data from McConahey et al. (1956).

Fraser et al. (1953) measured urinary excretion between 0 and 8, 8 and 24, and 24 and 48 hours after administration of the dose and corrected for renal disease and errors in collection by determining an index consisting of the ratio of the *0 to 8 hour* to the product of the *8 to 24 hour* times the *0 to 48 hour* collection periods.

EFFECTS OF ANTITHYROID DRUGS ON RADIOIODINE TESTS

The uptake of ^{131}I by the thyroid of a hyperthyroid patient during the first few hours after administration of the radioiodine will not be slowed greatly by the administration of thiourea derivatives, unless they contain iodine—e.g., sodium iodothiouracil—because the trapping function of the thyroid is not altered appreciably. On the other hand, the 24 hour thyroidal ^{131}I uptake performed while the patient is taking antithyroid drugs will be suppressed (Schultz and Jacobson, 1952). The thiourea derivatives presumably depress the activity of the peroxidase enzyme system in the thyroid gland (DeRobertis and Grasso, 1946). Tolbutamide (Orinase) and carbutamide also possess antithyroid activity in the dose range used in the treatment of diabetes (Grayson, 1960). Para-aminosalicylic acid (PAS) and resorcinol are among the many drugs that inhibit iodine accumulation by the thyroid (Wayne et al., 1964).

IODINE DEFICIENCY AND RADIOIODINE TESTS

In most instances an avid uptake of radioiodine may be correctly assumed to be due to a high rate of uptake of stable iodide by the thyroid. Nevertheless measurement of the percentage of the administered radioiodine dose accumulated per unit time by the thyroid does not give a quantitative measurement of the accumulation of stable inorganic iodide. Occasionally an avidity for radioiodine may be attributable to an abnormally small extrathyroidal iodide pool, as in the case of certain patients with endemic goiter.

Ideally, one would like to be able to measure the concentration of inorganic iodide in plasma (Wayne et al., 1964). Unfortunately, this quantity is so small that it cannot be measured directly by methods available at present. In 1949, Stanley described a method for measuring the stable iodide accumulation by the thyroid gland using the radioiodine uptake of the thyroid and the specific activity of urine excreted simultaneously, i.e., the ratio of radioactive to stable iodide in the urine (Stanley, 1949). Koutras et al. (1961), Buchanan et al. (1961), and Alexander et al. (1962) have made extensive use of measurement of the urinary specific activity to study normal persons and patients with iodine-deficient goiters. Using these methods, the value of plasma inorganic iodide could be calculated and the normal range defined as 0.08 to 0.60 μg./100 ml. About half of the patients with nontoxic goiter examined by Wayne et al. (1964) had an increased uptake of radioiodine and a low value of plasma inorganic iodine (0.05 $\pm$ 0.01 [standard error] μg./100 ml.).

MEASUREMENT OF ORGANIC BINDING

An impaired ability of the thyroid to form monoiodotyrosine from iodide and tyrosine occurs during the administration of antithyroid drugs, such as the thioureas (Astwood, 1944) and in chronic thyroiditis (Hashimoto's disease) (Morgans and Trotter, 1957). Impaired organic binding has also been reported following radioiodine treatment of hyperthyroidism (Kirland, 1954), in certain patients with colloid nodular goiters, and in patients with recurrent colloid adenomatous goiter (Floyd et al., 1960).

Defective organification may be diagnosed by administering an oral dose of potassium thiocyanate (KSCN) or potassium perchlorate (KClO$_4$) 2 hours after the administration of a tracer dose of [131]I. In normal persons, radioiodine will be bound to tyrosine within this period of time, and no radioactivity will leave the gland. If a defect in organic binding of iodide is present, unbound ^{131}I is released from the thyroid gland shortly after the administration of these drugs.

MEASUREMENT OF STORAGE AND RELEASE OF THYROID HORMONE

Nodine et al. (1957) have described a method of estimating the "intrathyroidal exchangeable iodine," based on the increase in stable protein-bound iodine and protein-bound ^{131}I following the administration of TSH 9 days after a tracer dose of [131]I. Wayne et al. (1964) have also used this method, but it has not been

TABLE 7-3. RATES OF RELEASE OF LABELED THYROID HORMONE FROM THYROID GLAND

	RANGE	MEAN
Normal	7.0–164.0 days	30.5 days
Hyperthyroid	3.8–18.0 days	10.4 days

widely used clinically. The major limitation of the method is that it measures only the quantity of iodine with which the tracer dose has equilibrated in 9 days, and not the total quantity of iodine present in the thyroid. The method is of potential value in the diagnosis of iodine deficiency in which the total quantity of thyroidal iodine is decreased.

If an antithyroid drug is administered a day after the tracer dose, it creates a defect in organic binding and prevents recirculation of ^{131}I. The rate of decrease in daily thyroid counts may then be taken to represent the rate of release of labeled thyroid hormone from the thyroid gland. The secretion rate can be expressed as the biologic half-life of the radioactivity in the gland.

Values may also be expressed as the percentage of total ^{131}I in the thyroid gland released during a period of 24 hours (Greer and Shull, 1957).

Normal = 6.81 ± 0.75 per cent per day

Hypothyroid (suppression of normal pituitary function with triiodothyronine) = 1.05 ± 0.20 per cent per day

This technique has not been used clinically but has been useful in studies of the effect of TSH on hyperthyroid patients (Greer and Shull, 1957), as well as on the effect of triiodothyronine and thyroxine (Johnson et al., 1959) and iodide (Greer and DeGroot, 1956) on the activity of the thyroid gland.

Two simplified radioiodine tests have been valuable clinically for the measurement of the rate of release of thyroid hormone into the blood. The first measures the concentration of radioactive protein-bound iodine in the blood after administration of a tracer dose of ^{131}I (Clark et al., 1949). The second measures the PB ^{131}I concentration in the blood after a tracer dose of ^{131}I, as well as the level of ^{131}I in the saliva (Thode et al., 1954). In both tests, the amount of ^{131}I bound to plasma protein is higher than normal if the thyroid is overactive, and lower than normal if the thyroid gland is underactive. The "conversion ratio" of Clark et al. (1949) accentuates this difference by comparing the quantity of ^{131}I precipitated with plasma protein with the total ^{131}I in the unprecipitated blood. The quantity of ^{131}I excreted in saliva is less than normal in hyperthyroid patients.

The results obtained are shown in Table 7-4.

TABLE 7-4. RATE OF RELEASE OF THYROID HORMONE INTO THE BLOOD 48 HOURS AFTER THE DOSE

	PB^{131}I (% DOSE/LITER OF PLASMA)	CONVERSION RATIO
Euthyroid	0.13–0.05 at 48 hr.	13–42
Hyperthyroid	0.16	42
	(0.27 at 72 hr.)	

The major disadvantage of the use of the PB[131]I is that it may be elevated in a euthyroid individual who has a decreased thyroidal iodine pool. In this case the thyroid gland turns over ^{131}I at an elevated rate while maintaining a normal total concentration of thyroid hormone in the serum. The PB[131]I value may therefore be elevated even in the presence of myxedema (Bloom and Terpstra, 1953). The most common cause of a spuriously elevated PB[131]I is partial ablation of the thyroid by surgery or irradiation.

Plasma Levels of Thyroid Hormone

Thyroxine is readily bound by plasma proteins, primarily by a trace protein that migrates on electrophoresis between alpha$_1$ and alpha$_2$ globulins. Normally, these binding proteins are not fully saturated, and the ratio between free and protein-bound thyroxine is usually about 1:1000.

Hamolsky, Stein, and Freedberg (1957) described an *in vitro* test that provides an estimate of the number of unoccupied binding sites on thyroxine-binding plasma proteins. Triiodothyronine (T3) labeled with radioactive iodine is incubated with whole blood under standardized conditions, and subsequently the red blood cells are separated from plasma by serial washing. The amount of radioactive triiodothyronine bound by the red blood cells is inversely related to that bound by thyroid-hormone binding sites not previously occupied by thyroxine. An important advantage of the "T3 red cell uptake" test is that inorganic iodine or other iodine-containing compounds do not interfere. Therefore, even though the patient may be receiving iodine-containing medications or may have had a previous radiographic study with contrast media containing iodine, the test will still be valid. One disadvantage of the test is that the conditions of the incubation must be rigorously controlled, since pH, CO_2 partial pressure, number of washings, and other factors affect the results. A second disadvantage in the test is its relative nonspecificity.

In hyperthyroidism, as a result of an increased plasma level of free thyroxine, thyroxine-binding globulin (TBG) is nearly saturated. Since the binding of triiodothyronine by TBG is only one third to one fourth as strong as that of thyroxine, T3 will bind only to the unoccupied binding sites. Consequently, in hyperthyroidism, more T3 is bound by binding sites on red blood cells.

In hypothyroidism, since the amount of thyroxine bound by TBG is less, there are more unoccupied binding sites to which T3 can be bound. Consequently, less is bound by the red blood cells. There is no evidence that red blood cells themselves are different in hyperthyroid and hypothyroid patients.

In pregnancy, there is an increase in TBG without an associated increase in the level of free thyroxine. Although more thyroxine is bound per unit volume of plasma (evidenced by the elevated protein-bound iodine), the number of the unoccupied binding sites on TBG is also increased. Consequently T3 binding is increased, with a resultant decrease in the quantity bound by red blood cells. This test has been used as a pregnancy test, as well as an indication of abortion (Visscher, 1963).

Table 7-5 lists various clinical states influencing the results of the T3 red cell uptake test. In most cases, the abnormal values result from alterations in plasma proteins, either quantitative or qualitative.

TABLE 7-5. CLINICAL STATES INFLUENCING RESULTS OF THE T3
RED CELL OR RESIN UPTAKE TEST

Factors elevating the T3 red cell or resin uptake
    Anticoagulants—dicumarol, heparin
    Nephrotic syndrome
    Severe liver disease
    Severe metastatic malignancy
    Severe pulmonary insufficiency with CO_2 retention
    Paroxysmal atrial arrhythmias
    Uremia
    Leukemia
    Polycythemia vera
    Myelomatosis
    Severe chronic infectious diseases
    Salicylate therapy
    Testosterone therapy
    Prednisone therapy

Factors lowering the T3 red cell or resin uptake
    Pregnancy
    Estrogen therapy
    Propylthiouracil in hyperthyroid therapy
    Iodine in hyperthyroidism
    Ovulatory suppressants

Because red cells play only an indirect role in the T3 red cell uptake measurement, modifications have been made in the procedure to eliminate the errors arising from hematocrit differences, hemolysis, and red cell anomalies. Certain anion exchange resins have the ability to adsorb free T3 without affecting significantly the bound T3. Mitchell (1961) reported the use of an anion exchange resin to measure the degree of binding of thyroid hormones to plasma proteins. Initially he used Amberlite IRA-400 resin in the chloride or acetate form, but subsequently he changed to tris buffer at pH 5.0 to 5.2 in order to reduce variability in the results. Serum is equilibrated with thyroxine for 30 minutes. One milliliter samples of this mixture are added to tubes containing 1 ml. of resin and are shaken for 1.5 hours at 30°C. The tubes are then counted, the resin washed three or four times with distilled water, and counted again. The resin uptake is calculated by dividing the residual radioactivity by the initial radioactivity. Because of difficulties in reproducibility in repeated determinations, the results are compared to those obtained with simultaneous measurements of pooled normal serum. The use of a resin sponge improved the reproducibility, increased the simplicity of the test, and made differences more pronounced.

Sterling (1961) evaluated IRA-400 in the acetate, chloride, iodide, and hydroxyl cycles, as well as other resins, and found that IRA-400 in the formate cycle was the most satisfactory. His results were as shown in Table 7-6.

The resin methods offer greater simplicity and also decrease the time needed to perform the test. However, as in measurement of the red cell uptake of T3, these methods are not free from the possibility of technical errors and care must be taken to employ a well controlled technique. Essentially the same physiological factors that affect the T3 red cell uptake test affect the resin uptake of T3. Whether one uses the red cell method or a resin method, each laboratory must carefully establish its own normal and abnormal ranges before using the test clinically.

TABLE 7-6. MEASUREMENT OF THE DEGREE OF BINDING OF THYROID HORMONES
TO PLASMA PROTEINS USING IRA-400 IN THE FORMATE CYCLE*

THYROID STATUS	MEAN (%)	STANDARD DEVIATION	NUMBER OF PATIENTS
Normal	35	±2.2	35
Thyrotoxicosis	53	±7.8	44
Myxedema	27	±3.3	28
Pregnancy	25	±4.3	11

* Data from Sterling and Tabachnick (1961).

MEASUREMENT OF PERIPHERAL UTILIZATION OF THYROXINE

If ^{131}I-labeled thyroid hormone is injected intravenously and radioactivity in subsequent samples of blood is measured, the disappearance rate can be calculated. If the serum PBI is also measured, the extrathyroidal pool of thyroxine can be calculated by the isotope dilution principle. The absolute rate of organic iodine degradation (μg. of thyroxine metabolized per day) can be calculated as the product of the pool size and the fractional turnover.

The relatively rapid fall in the plasma radioactivity during the first day after injection is related to the diffusion of the tracer throughout the body's extrathyroidal organic iodine pool. A more gradual fall of the plasma radioactivity begins 2 days after injection and follows a straight line when plotted on semilog graph paper. This rate has been interpreted as being due to metabolic degradation of the administered radiothyroxine, and hence is a measure of the turnover rate of the hormone. The half-time of thyroxine clearance is obtained by extrapolating the linear component of the disappearance curve back to zero time. The turnover rate (k) is computed from the half-time ($t_{1/2}$) using the relation $k = \dfrac{0.693}{t_{1/2}}$, where $t_{1/2}$ = half-time in days and k = turnover rate, i.e., the fraction of the body's extrathyroidal organic iodine pool turned over per day.

Sterling and Chodos (1956) gave the following example from the data on a normal subject:

Half-time ($t_{1/2}$) = 6.7 days (obtained graphically)

$$\text{Turnover rate (k)} = \frac{\ln 2}{t_{1/2}} = \frac{0.693}{6.7} = 0.104 = 10.4\%/\text{day}$$

The extrathyroidal organic iodine (EOI) pool was estimated from the quotient

$$\frac{\text{total radioactivity injected}}{\text{radioactivity per microgram of PBI}}$$

The denominator is obtained from extrapolation to zero time, which represents plasma radioactivity if distribution had occurred immediately after injection.

If plasma PBI = 5.8 μg./100 ml.

Zero time plasma radioactivity = 1150 counts per min./ml.

$$\frac{1150}{5.8/100 \text{ ml.}} = 19{,}850 \text{ counts per min.}/\mu g. \text{ of PBI}$$

$$\frac{10{,}950{,}000 \text{ counts per min. injected}}{19{,}850 \text{ counts per min.}/\mu g. \text{ of PBI}} = 552 \text{ (EOI pool)}$$

The product of the EOI pool and the turnover rate (k) gives the degradation rate in micrograms of organic iodine per day.

$$552 \ \mu g. \text{ (EOI pool)} \times 10.4\%/\text{day (k)} = 58 \ \mu g. \text{ I/day}$$

This figure represents both the rates of formation and degradation, which are identical in a steady state with constant EOI pool. Sterling and Chodos (1956) reported the results shown in Table 7-7.

TABLE 7-7. RATES OF ORGANIC IODINE DEGRADATION IN VARIOUS CLINICAL STATES[*]

	NORMAL SUBJECTS	MYXEDEMA	THYROTOXICOSIS	HYPERMETABOLISM
[131]I thyroxine plasma t 1/2 (days)	6.6 ± 0.7	9.7 ± 1.4	4.4 ± 1.1	5.2 ± 0.8
thyroxine turnover rate (%/day)	10.5 ± 1.1	7.3 ± 1.1	16.9 ± 5.0	13.7 ± 2.5
extrathyroidal organic iodine pool (μg.)	548 ± 107	238 ± 60	1021 ± 173	753 ± 230
thyroxine degradation rate (μg./day)	57 ± 11	18 ± 4	197 ± 35	100 ± 18

[*] Data from Sterling and Chodos (1956).

An example of the use of these determinations in making a clinical diagnosis is reported by Beierwaltes and Robbins (1959). In a specific case the serum PBI and BEI indicated that a patient was hyperthyroid. The BMR and his symptoms indicated that he was hypothyroid. The patient's EOI was elevated to about the same amount as that found in thyrotoxicosis. The turnover rate was subnormal. The degradation rate in μg. of thyroxine iodine per day was within the normal range, indicating that he was euthyroid. The anomalies of the thyroid function tests were apparently the result of increased thyroxine binding by serum proteins.

THYROID SCANNING FOR VISUALIZATION OF THE LOCATION AND STRUCTURE OF THE THYROID

Thyroid scanning is an example of the use of a physiological mechanism to concentrate a radionuclide and make possible the visualization of the structure of an organ. The method usually is combined with measurement of the rate of accumulation of the tracer by the thyroid, thereby providing functional as well as anatomical information.

Among the principal uses of thyroid scanning are the identification of accessory thyroid tissue, which may be found anywhere in the midline from the

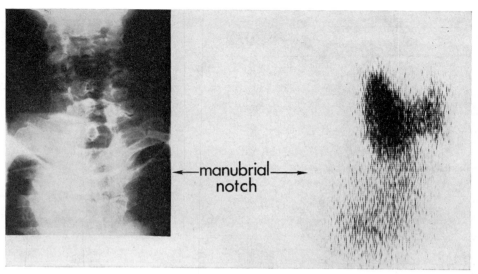

FIGURE 7-1.   Substernal extension of the thyroid in a euthyroid patient. Iodine-131 was the radionuclide used.

mouth to the diaphragm, and the localization of functioning metastatic neoplasms originating in the thyroid gland. A frequent diagnostic problem is defining the nature of superior mediastinal masses. An example is presented in Figure 7-1, which shows a large retrosternal goiter extending down into the mediastinum through the thoracic inlet. Many of these patients are middle-aged females who complain of shortness of breath or dysphagia. Some are believed initially to have asthma, whereas others have symptoms suggesting heart disease or increased thyroid function. In most cases, retrosternal goiters concentrate radioactive iodine sufficiently to permit definitive diagnosis by scanning. However, by improper use of contrast enhancement or background erase techniques, one may erroneously conclude that the mass does not concentrate iodine although it actually does, the false impression being created by the decreased concentration of iodine in the goiter relative to the normal thyroid tissue in its normal location. A small percentage of retrosternal goiters do not concentrate iodine to a significant degree. Therefore, failure of the lesion to accumulate iodine does not rule out the possibility that it is thyroidal tissue.

In most patients with thyrotoxicosis, it is possible to determine on clinical grounds whether the patient has *toxic nodular goiter* or *diffuse hyperplasia* of the thyroid gland, particularly if the patient has exophthalmos. Differentiation of these two diseases does not usually require scanning, but occasionally the ability to identify a functional nodule with suppression of the rest of the gland is of great value.

In the evaluation of thyroid nodules, scanning may reveal that what was believed to be a solitary nodule is in fact the largest nodule in a multinodular goiter, a distinction that is important in the management of the patient. Scanning is also of value in the differentiation of "hot" from "cold" nodules, i.e., those that concentrate radioactive iodine from those that do not. Another use of thyroid scanning is the evaluation of remnants of the thyroid gland following surgery. Postoperative scanning of patients who have had total thyroidectomy for thyroid carcinoma helps to define the nature of masses that appear in the region of the thyroid gland several years later. Superimposition of the scanning image on a radiograph of the region is of value because areas of increased or decreased radioactivity can be related to abnormalities in the tracheal air column.

An occasional diagnostic problem is differentiation of acute thyroiditis from hemorrhage into a thyroid nodule. Both conditions cause an acute febrile illness with swelling and tenderness in the thyroid and at times dysphagia. A diagnosis can be made if there is a decreased accumulation of radioiodine throughout the gland, a finding characteristic of diffuse inflammation of the gland, whereas in localized hemorrhage a filling defect may be observed within the contour of the thyroid gland. Confirmatory evidence of acute thyroiditis is provided by the finding of an elevation of the serum PB1, presumably the result of leakage of thyroxine from the inflamed thyroid cells.

Unfortunately, thyroid scanning is not very helpful in differentiating three diseases that are frequently confused clinically: Hashimoto's thyroiditis, multinodular goiter, and carcinoma of the thyroid. All may have the appearance of an enlarged thyroid gland with multiple filling defects.

In the interpretation of thyroid scans it is important to examine the patient. Only in this way can one determine whether an area of increased radioactivity corresponds to a palpable lesion in the thyroid gland.

Scanning has been used to obtain objective data concerning the size of the thyroid. Myhill and his associates (1965) found good correlation between the scanning image and the frontal view of the gland after surgical removal. Such data are useful since it is often difficult to obtain an accurate estimation of the true size of the gland by physical examination alone.

Renda and Wagner measured the frontal plane area of the thyroid in scans of normal persons and compared the results to patients with nodular goiters and hyperthyroidism (Fig. 7-2). Most normal persons had areas less than 20 sq. cm., whereas only about 17 per cent of the nodular and hyperthyroid group had thyroids smaller than 20 sq. cm. No normal person had a thyroid

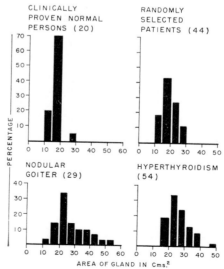

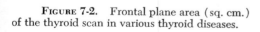

FIGURE 7-2.   Frontal plane area (sq. cm.) of the thyroid scan in various thyroid diseases.

whose frontal plane area measured greater than 30 sq. cm. Approximately 30 per cent of the "normal" persons had irregularities of the borders of the scan image suggesting a possible thyroid abnormality. Nine per cent had nonuniform distribution of the radioactivity within the gland. In the hyperthyroid group 11 per cent of the glands had irregular borders and 37 per cent showed nonuniform distribution within the gland. All of the clinically nodular glands had irregular margins and nonuniform distribution of the radioactivity.

STUDIES OF THE THYROID USING TECHNETIUM-99m

Following its administration to a human subject, technetium-99m pertechnetate accumulates in the thyroid gland. Because of the favorable physical characteristics of ^{99m}Tc, it has been suggested as a useful supplement to radioactive iodine for clinical assessment of both function and anatomical imaging of the thyroid gland (Harper et al., 1964; Degrossi et al., 1965). Unlike iodine, technetium is not organified within the gland. Figure 7-3 is the scan of a euthyroid patient who received 1 mc. of pertechnetate 30 minutes before the scan was obtained.

Technetium-99m is useful for patients with hypofunctional thyroids when statistical variations are pronounced because of the low concentrations. If the photon yield is increased by using pertechnetate, the image can be seen better on the scan (Fig. 7-4).

The chemical properties of pertechnetate allow for an estimation of the trapping mechanism of the thyroid gland. The measurements are difficult to

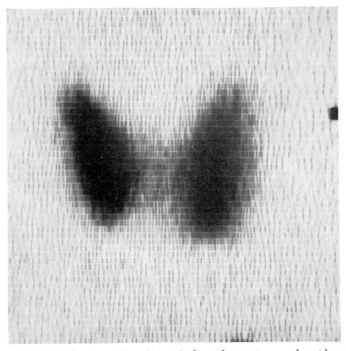

FIGURE 7-3. Technetium-99m (1 mc.) thyroid scan in a euthyroid person.

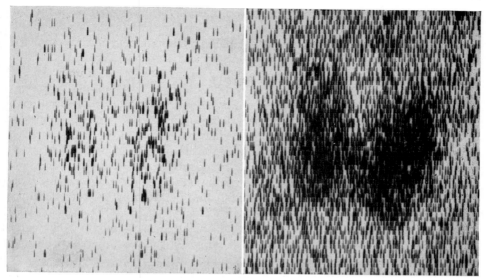

FIGURE 7-4.   *Left.* Iodine-131 (25 μc.) scan in a patient with a 2 hour uptake of 2 per cent, a 24 hour uptake of 2 per cent, and a history of exogenous iodide. *Right.* Technetium-99m pertechnetate (1 mc.) scan in the same patient on the same day.

interpret because of the rapidity of uptake and the generally high extrathyroidal activity. Andros et al. (1965) attempted to minimize these errors by determining the effect of perchlorate in bringing about release of ^{99m}Tc from the gland. They also limited the field of view with the focusing collimator. One to three per cent of the dose was found in euthyroid subjects with an eightfold to tenfold increase in hyperthyroidism and less than one per cent in hypothyroidism. Others have obtained similar values (Atkins and Richards, 1966).

STUDIES OF THYROID DISEASES WITH ^{14}C-LABELED COMPOUNDS

If the thyroid controls oxidative metabolism in general, disturbances of of function would be expected to occur with changes in the metabolism of ^{14}C-labeled compounds, both *in vivo* and *in vitro*. Although changes have been found, they cannot be interpreted as general increases or decreases in oxidative rate. Hyperthyroid patients form $^{14}CO_2$ from labeled glucose at an increased rate, but not from labeled palmitate or acetate (Gordon and Goldberg, 1964). In fact, according to these workers, and Johnson et al. (1963), $^{14}CO_2$ is produced from certain fatty acids faster in hypothyroid patients, and production becomes slower after treatment with thyroxine. In contrast, when labeled glucose is injected in hypothyroid patients, formation of $^{14}CO_2$ (particularly from glucose-1-^{14}C) is decreased, and an increase is produced by treatment.

These anomalous findings may be due to other differences in lipid metabolism, e.g., decreased intermediary pools of free fatty acids (FFA) or decreased incorporation of labeled FFA into other synthetic routes, both factors tending to increase the rate of appearance of $^{14}CO_2$. Lipsky et al. (1955) found in myxedematous patients a marked decrease in conversion of ^{14}C acetate into cholesterol and to a lesser extent into fatty acids. Normal results were restored by administration of triiodothyronine. Gould et al. (1955) reported a fourfold decrease in incorporation of ^{14}C acetate into plasma cholesterol.

The high rate of oxidation of ^{14}C-labeled palmitate and acetate in hypothyroidism may be on another basis. Goldberg and Gordon (1955) suggest that a high level of circulating thyroid-stimulating hormone of the pituitary (TSH) is at least partly responsible. Both euthyroid subjects and hypopituitary patients have an increased oxidation of labeled fatty acids following administration of pituitary TSH, but patients with primary hypothyroidism do not. The high rate of oxidation in these patients may be related to their high blood levels of endogenous TSH. Supportive evidence was the finding of an increase in oxidation produced in normal subjects by administration of propylthiouracil, presumably resulting in an increase of endogenous TSH. The changes in oxidation of labeled fatty acids caused by TSH (and the opposite effects of triiodothyronine) were not accompanied by significant changes in plasma levels of FFA.

It may be possible to use the rates of oxidation of palmitate-1-^{14}C before and after administration of exogenous TSH, to distinguish between primary hypothyroidism and that secondary to pituitary deficiency.

Gordon and Goldberg (1964) have also found a thyromimetic effect of the pyridine nucleotide coenzyme, DPN (NAD), when infused into hypothyroid patients. Oxidation of labeled palmitate and acetate fell sharply, but that of glucose-^{14}C and glucose-6-^{14}C rose. The DPN had no effect in euthyroid subjects.

In contrast to the increase in oxidation of glucose-1-^{14}C found *in vivo* as a result of increased thyroid hormone, Johnson and Redding (1963) reported that the blood of thyrotoxic rats and human patients, when incubated with methylene blue and glucose-1-^{14}C, shows only about half the rate of formation of $^{14}CO_2$ as normal blood. They suggest the use of this procedure as an *in vitro* method for estimating tissue levels of thyroid hormone activity. The reason for the paradoxical differences between *in vivo* and *in vitro* results with glucose-^{14}C is not yet clear, but such tests of thyroid functional activity may prove to be of great value.

In a study of the blood clearance of intravenously administered ^{14}C-tripalmitin, Kinsell et al. (1965) noted that a hyperthyroid subject metabolized secondarily formed lipoprotein twice as fast as other patients. This was indicated both by clearance from the blood stream and by formation of $^{14}CO_2$ over an 8 hour period. Conversely, Lipsky et al. (1955) described a slowing of the rate of removal of endogenously ^{14}C-labeled cholesterol from the blood of myxedematous patients. These studies suggest a future role of ^{14}C-labeled compounds in studies of thyroid diseases, fat metabolism, and obesity.

DISEASES OF THE THYROID GLAND

ACCESSORY THYROID TISSUE

Abnormalities may develop during the embryonic descent of the thyroid from the oropharynx to its usual position in the neck. A most common abnormality is the development of a pyramidal lobe projecting upward from the isthmus of the thyroid. Thyroid tissue may be found projecting from the back of the tongue or even within or beneath the tongue. When present, lingual thyroid tissue is usually the only functioning thyroid tissue. Occasionally, thyroid tissue is found in the mediastinum, even within the pericardial sac. Rarely, neoplastic thyroid tissue (teratoma) may be found in the ovary, where it is referred to as struma ovarii. Aberrant tissue may become apparent only after the normal thyroid has been removed surgically or by irradiation. Thyroid scanning can provide exact identification of the nature of these masses.

Intrathoracic goiters can be readily identified by scanning. Most are in the substernal region, although at times one may extend into the posterior thorax behind the superior vena cava. Usually these are acquired rather than congenital diseases.

CONGENITAL GOITER

An important cause of goiter is a genetic defect in one or more enzymes that control the synthesis of thyroxine. The diminished output of thyroxine results in compensatory hypertrophy and hyperplasia of the thyroid gland, forming a goiter. The mechanism is stimulation of the thyroid by thyroid-stimulating hormone (TSH) from the pituitary.

These congenital defects fall into five categories: (1) iodide-trapping defect, in which the thyroid, salivary glands, and gastric mucosa are unable to concentrate iodide; (2) iodide organification defect, in which iodide trapping occurs, but further conversion of iodide into monoiodotyrosine and diiodotyrosine does not occur, presumably because of absence of peroxidase enzymes; (3) iodo-tyrosyl-coupling defect, in which monoiodotyrosine and diiodotyrosine are not coupled to form thyroxine; (4) iodotyrosine dehalogenase defect, in which absence of a dehalogenase enzyme prevents deiodination of iodotyrosines not coupled to form thyroxine, with the result that iodotyrosines are lost in the urine and iodide deficiency develops; and (5) butanol-insoluble serum iodine states, in which abnormal unknown types of organic iodine compounds are found in the blood. Many of these patients have hypothyroidism. In others, hyperplasia of the thyroid may partially compensate for the defect and the patient remains euthyroid.

Other genetic defects, such as deafness and inability to taste phenylthiourea, may be found in a significant number. Although accurate diagnosis of the specific defect is possible only with radioisotope techniques described in other sections, the medical history and physical examination can provide valuable clues (Wayne et al., 1964). Goiter appearing in early childhood in a patient with a strong family history of goiter, especially if males are affected, is probably due to dyshormonogenesis; if the patient is hypothyroid, this is almost certainly the case. The differential diagnosis in patients with nontoxic goiter includes dyshormonogenesis, Hashimoto's disease, carcinoma of the thyroid, and iodine-deficient goiter. Any nontoxic goiter in a man, except in endemic areas, should arouse the suspicion of carcinoma or Hashimoto's disease, rather than a congenital lesion. The most common cause of goitrous hypothyroidism in adults is Hashimoto's disease.

Nontoxic Goiter

R. L. Vought

Nontoxic (simple) goiter is an important cause of enlargement of the thyroid gland and occurs sporadically or in endemics. Most investigators believe that simple goiter is the result of absolute or relative iodine deficiency, but other etiologic factors have been suggested. Many commonly used drugs have goitrogenic activity and must always be considered as a possible cause of goiter, particularly in patients with hypothyroidism. The prevalence of goiter remains high in recently developing countries, but many cases have been discovered in the rural areas of Western Europe and the United States. Diseases associated with goitrous populations include thyrotoxicosis, cretinism, deafness, and mental retardation; but the nature of the relationships to goiter and iodine metabolism is not completely understood.

The diagnosis of nontoxic goiter is based on: (a) an enlarged thyroid gland, (b) the presence of characteristic disturbances of iodine metabolism, and (c) the absence of hyperthyroidism. Meticulous inspection and careful palpation of the thyroidal region of the neck may be essential to recognition of an enlarged thyroid. Characteristic disturbances in iodine metabolism are: (a) increased radioiodine uptake by the thyroid, (b) low urinary iodine excretion, and (c) low plasma inorganic iodide. Isotopic studies of thyroidal hormonal synthesis are necessary if specific biochemical defects, such as those that occur in familial goiter, are to be identified. Most patients with simple goiter are clinically euthyroid and their BMR and PBI determinations are usually within normal limits; there is a general tendency, however, for the goitrous group to be hypermetabolic.

Since the studies of Stanbury, Brownell, and Riggs and their Argentinian collaborators, Perinetti, Itoiz, and Del Castillo (1954), it has been recognized that the goitrous thyroid gland differs from the nongoitrous gland in its avidity for iodine. The typical goitrous subject in an endemic goiter area has an increased radioiodine uptake, a low plasma inorganic iodine and decreased urinary excretion of stable and radioactive iodine. Koutras et al. (1960) found that sporadic goitrous patients, even when living in iodine-rich areas, had the same triad of findings.

The median [132]I uptake of goitrous and nongoitrous subjects in Kentucky was 22.9 per cent and 14.7 per cent of dose, respectively. Using the same technique in Scotland, the 2.5 hour [132]I uptakes for goitrous and normal persons were 39.9 per cent and 21.6 per cent, respectively. In Ecuador, Fierro found 24 hour ^{131}I uptakes of 34 per cent in nongoitrous subjects in Quito, and of 75 per cent and 68 per cent among the goitrous and nongoitrous subjects, respectively, in an endemic goiter area. The plasma inorganic iodine and urinary iodine excretion show similar variations and may also be within normal limits in goitrous subjects. A recent observation of goitrous subjects in Kentucky by London et al. (1965) indicates that the absolute uptake of inorganic iodide in goitrous subjects may be higher than in nongoitrous. Koutras et al. (1960) failed to find a significant difference between goitrous subjects and nongoitrous controls in Scotland.

The major differences in iodine metabolism between goitrous and non-goitrous may be summarized as follows:

1. The goitrous gland exhibits an extraordinary avidity for iodine, even after adequate iodine supplementation.

2. The goitrous gland usually contains as much iodine as the normal gland, but its concentration per unit mass is lower.

3. In healthy persons the urinary excretion of iodine is proportional to iodide intake, but in goitrous children no such correlation is found.

4. In healthy persons iodine excretion usually exceeds iodine intake, but in goitrous children iodine excretion is usually less than intake.

Three hypotheses have been proposed regarding the cause of simple goiter: (a) iodine deficiency, (b) infectious origin, and (c) goitrogens. Stanbury et al. (1954), Ermans et al. (1963), Beckers et al. (1964), and Wayne et al. (1964) support the argument that the high radioiodine uptake, low plasma inorganic iodine, and low urinary iodine excretion are evidence of concurrent or pre-existing dietary iodine deficiency. However, in these studies iodine balance was not examined. Also, dietary iodine deficiency has not been demonstrated by direct chemical measurement of the iodine content of diets.

The hypothesis of infectious origin apparently was well accepted before the turn of the century. McCarrison reported many experiments in which goiter was produced in man and animals by feeding polluted water and feces from goitrous subjects to previously nongoitrous animals. The epidemiological evidence (e.g., Costa and Montara, 1952) supporting an infectious hypothesis is inconclusive.

Goitrogens, substances that produce goiter, are of two types: (a) those that block the gland's iodine-trapping mechanisms, the perchlorate type, and (b) those that block the coupling of iodine and thyroxine, the thiouracil type. Some goitrogens occur naturally, e.g., those produced by plants of the *Brassica* family; others are pharmacological compounds that are used either because of their antithyroid activity, or despite it, their antithyroid activity being an unwanted side effect, e.g., thalidomide.

One of the most interesting observations of *Brassica*-induced goiter is that of Clements and Wishart in Tasmania (1956). In 1949 Clements was asked by Tasmanian health authorities to make a goiter survey of the island. As a result of the survey of some 8000 school children, iodine prophylaxis was recommended and carried out. However, rather than the expected decrease in goiter prevalence, 5 years later an *increase* in the condition was observed in nearly all age groups. The investigators were able to demonstrate that milk from cows fed kale fodder decreased the uptake of radioiodide in both man and experimental animals. They also demonstrated that milk from kale-fed cows induced active hyperplasia of the thyroid in the calves of these cows. In Finland as well, where narrow-stemmed kale is used extensively as cattle fodder, Virtanen (1961) and Peltola and Krusius (1960) have found goitrogenic substances in the milk of such animals. These substances include thiocyanate, presumably formed by enzymic action in the gut, and a thioxazolidine.

The medicinal goitrogens include many commonly used drugs, some sulfonamides and barbiturates, cortisone and hydrocortisone, progesterone, and phenylbutazone. A detailed history of drug usage is a necessity in the diagnostic evaluation of a patient with nontoxic goiter.

Prevalence and Health Significance of Nontoxic Goiter

R. L. Vought

The most recent and comprehensive survey of goiter prevalence is that of Kelly and Snedden, 1960. Endemics still exist in the classic mountainous areas, particularly the Himalayas, Andes, Carpathians, Caucasus, and in some areas of the Austrian, German, and Swiss Alps; in Switzerland the prevalence of goiter has decreased considerably since the introduction of iodine prophylaxis, but it still remains a problem in local areas; in the United States the current prevalence of goiter is apparently low in all regions, but exact figures are not available. Goiter is still prevalent in the Netherlands, Belgium, England, Scotland, and Wales.

The goiter endemias studied in recent years share common features. Endemic goiter is primarily a rural disease; the endemias are usually associated with poor sanitation, and sewage disposal is either absent or primitive. Although few careful studies of the association of goiter with polluted water supplies have been reported, it is possible that the water supplies of goitrous populations are predominantly either unprotected or poorly protected surface supplies or shallow wells. Careful studies show a clear association of endemic goiter with poverty, but not with starvation.

The medical and public health significance of goiter is increased by the associated diseases: cretinism, infantile myxedema, deaf mutism, and both hyperfunction and hypofunction of the thyroid gland. An association between goiter and mental retardation, stillbirths, and congenital deafness has also been suggested. Wayne et al. (1964) concluded that thyroid hormone in doses sufficient to suppress thyroid function is the treatment of choice in all forms of nontoxic goiter.

Suppurative Thyroiditis

H. N. Wagner, Jr., and W. H. Beierwaltes

Acute suppurative thyroiditis, at times resulting in the formation of abscesses within the thyroid, is a fulminating disease caused by pyogenic bacteria. The disease is characterized by fever, malaise, dysphagia, and pain and tenderness in the region of the thyroid. With radioisotope methodology, it is not possible to distinguish this disease from thyroid neoplasms, Riedel's struma, Hashimoto's disease, or hemorrhage into a preexisting adenoma or nodule. Suppurative thyroiditis is an exceedingly rare disease.

Acute Nonsuppurative Thyroiditis

This form of thyroiditis is infectious and is probably viral in origin. A characteristic finding is temporary failure of the thyroid to accumulate radioactive iodine (Werner, 1949), a manifestation of considerable diagnostic value. Restoration of thyroid function usually occurs before the patient develops symptoms of hypothyroidism. Some patients develop transient hyperthyroidism as a result of leakage of thyroxine from the inflamed gland. When this occurs, serum PBI is elevated, another characteristic manifestation.

The differential diagnosis must exclude pharyngitis, tonsillitis, and other infections of the throat; careful history taking and physical examination can usually establish whether the inflammation is in the neck or the throat. Some patients have fever of unknown origin, particularly if the thyroid is not conspicuously enlarged. Hemorrhage into a thyroid nodule may be confused with acute thyroiditis, although the former usually occurs in patients with a history of antecedent goiter, a significant clue to diagnosis.

The accumulation of radioiodine is usually normal in patients with hemorrhage into a nodule; an area of decreased radioactivity is sometimes found on the scan. Inflamed lymph nodes may be confused with thyroiditis, but can be distinguished by their lack of movement when the patient swallows. Differentiation of nonsuppurative from suppurative thyroiditis is essential, since the latter must be treated with antibiotics and occasionally by surgical drainage. Radioiodine uptake by the thyroid is usually normal in suppurative thyroiditis and the disease is clinically much more severe.

FACTITIOUS HYPERTHYROIDISM (THYROTOXICOSIS FACTITIA)

This syndrome should be suspected in a hyperthyroid patient with an elevated PBI and an abnormally low accumulation of radioactive iodine by the thyroid gland without evidence of thyroiditis. Iodine ingestion in an incorrectly treated patient with thyrotoxicosis may result in a similar syndrome, but the two can be differentiated by measurement of butanol-extractable iodine (BEI) as well as the total serum PBI. The latter is usually quite high, beyond the range found even in hyperthyroidism, whereas the BEI is much lower. If the patient ingests thyroxine or thyroid extract, the serum PBI will be much higher than if the patient is taking triiodothyronine, since the latter is more weakly bound by thyroxine-binding plasma proteins.

The absence of enlargement of the thyroid is an important manifestation in factitious hyperthyroidism, since nearly all patients with true thyrotoxicosis have palpable enlargement of the thyroid. The failure to find a palpable thyroid in the presence of hyperthyroidism and a low rate of accumulation of radioiodine should cause one to suspect thyrotoxicosis factitia, particularly in a neurotic person. The absence of exophthalmos is another important diagnostic clue, as is the usual finding of exacerbations and remissions of the factitious disease.

RADIATION EFFECTS

Radiation may decrease thyroidal uptake of radioiodine by producing a temporary thyroiditis, or even permanent injury to the thyroid gland. Werner (1955) reported that tracer doses of ^{131}I, totaling between 200 and 700 μc., had a significant therapeutic effect in some hyperthyroid patients. The euthyroid gland, on the other hand, is much less affected by such doses.

As will be discussed in detail subsequently, patients who have had thyroidectomy from either ^{131}I or surgery have little functional reserve in their thyroid glands; storage of thyroid hormone is slight or absent. Such patients may have an increased 2 hour uptake of ^{131}I and an elevated $PB^{131}I$.

HYPERTHYROIDISM

Diffuse hyperplasia of the thyroid gland results in an increased rate of turnover of radioactive iodine by the thyroid gland. Graves' disease is the term used to describe this condition, which is of unknown etiology; it is characteristically associated with exophthalmos. Administration of thyroid-stimulating hormone (TSH) to animals for prolonged periods can result in thyroid enlargement and increased thyroxine secretion but not exophthalmos. On the other hand, exophthalmos may be present in patients without thyrotoxicosis, although such patients often have an increased thyroidal uptake of radioactive iodine.

The diagnosis of Graves' disease is frequently quite easy on clinical grounds alone. Tracer studies may be useful in the following ways: (1) To confirm the diagnosis of Graves' disease, particularly if contaminating agents, such as radiographic contrast media, interfere with the serum PBI determination; (2) to differentiate thyrotoxicosis medicamentosa or thyrotoxicosis factitia from Graves' disease; (3) to distinguish anxiety states from thyrotoxicosis; (4) to distinguish nontoxic goiters from thyrotoxicosis, particularly when the PBI is elevated; and (5) to evaluate the degree of residual thyroid function in treated hyperthyroid patients.

Other diseases that may be confused with hyperthyroidism include anxiety states and neuroses, cardiac disease, gastrointestinal disease, myasthenia gravis, menopausal syndromes, and pheochromocytoma. For example, muscular weakness is common to both myasthenia gravis and thyrotoxic myopathy. Indeed, both diseases occur simultaneously with a greater incidence (about 5 per cent) than that expected on the basis of chance alone, a factor that increases the diagnostic problem. In patients with pheochromocytoma, transient thyroid enlargement may complicate diagnosis.

Differentiation between diffuse hyperthyroidism and toxic nodular goiter may be difficult; for example, if the patient has previously been operated upon for hyperthyroidism, regrowth of hyperplastic tissue in one or both lobes may result in the finding of nodular goiter. Usually, in cases of toxic nodular goiter, enlargement of the thyroid gland was present long before thyrotoxic manifestations developed; this is in contrast to the diffuse hyperplasia that usually occurs simultaneously with the manifestations of hyperthyroidism. The nodules of a toxic nodular goiter frequently cause mechanical disturbances such as encroachment upon the trachea, esophagus, or recurrent laryngeal nerve; in contrast, diffuse goiters usually do not. In Graves' disease, the size of the goiter only rarely parallels the severity of thyrotoxic manifestations; severe hyperfunction may be associated with goiters of moderate size, and large goiters may be only mildly hyperfunctioning.

The possibility of toxic nodular goiter should be considered if the 24 hour thyroid uptake of radioiodine is within normal limits in a hyperthyroid patient.

Whereas 10 to 25 per cent of patients with diffuse hyperplasia may have normal 24 hour uptake values, over half of the patients with toxic nodules have 24 hour values in the normal range, presumably because of the smaller mass of abnormal thyroid tissue (Skillern et al., 1962). Thyroid scanning can usually differentiate the two diseases with certainty. Exophthalmos is the most specific manifestation of Graves' disease; it is absent in patients with toxic nodular goiter.

Wayne (1960) found in a large series of patients that measurement of the radioiodine uptake and $PB^{131}I$ established the correct diagnosis in 98 per cent of the patients with hyperthyroidism, provided the patients were untreated and had not received iodine-containing compounds. In about 10 per cent of cases the two radioisotope tests gave discordant results; this led to the conclusion that both tests should be performed routinely. We usually measure both the radioiodine uptake and the PBI. If the results are discordant, and the radioiodine accumulation is above normal, the triiodothyronine suppression test may be of value. On the other hand, if hyperthyroidism is suspected and the radioiodine uptake is normal, estimations of plasma inorganic iodine or butanol-extractable iodine are most helpful, since they may indicate previous iodine administration. The T3 red-cell uptake test, or modifications using resins, may also be helpful, since iodine does not interfere with these determinations.

HYPOTHYROIDISM

The diagnosis of hypothyroidism is more difficult than that of hyperthyroidism. The condition may result from congenital defects, goitrogens, atrophy of the thyroid gland, thyroiditis, or hypopituitarism, or be the end result of hyperthyroidism of long duration. Myxedematous adults may manifest severe hearing impairment and initially go to an ear specialist, or they may be hospitalized in psychiatric institutions before the metabolic defect is recognized. Cardiovascular manifestations, such as bradycardia, serous effusions, angina pectoris, or congestive heart failure, may be prominent. A few patients are first diagnosed only after they suddenly lapse into coma. Hypothyroid patients frequently have the facial appearance of patients with renal diseases such as chronic glomerulonephritis or nephrotic syndrome. Anemia may be present and lead to the erroneous diagnosis of pernicious anemia.

Important manifestations of decreased thyroid function in children are mental retardation, delayed dentition, and impairment of growth and development. The thyroid gland may be completely absent, but usually minimal amounts of thyroid tissue can be found by scanning or at autopsy. Cretinism may be difficult to distinguish from nutritional deficiencies and mongolism.

A frequent diagnostic problem is the confirmation of the diagnosis of hypothyroidism in a patient who is taking thyroid medications on the basis of questionable or inadequate evidence. One course of action is to discontinue all treatment and observe the patient carefully for signs of clinical worsening. If the patient is hypothyroid, definite indications of physical and mental deterioration will usually appear within 60 to 90 days. Fortunately, this is usually not necessary. By giving thyroid-stimulating hormone (TSH), we can tell whether a patient taking thyroid replacement medication does in fact have decreased thyroid function. Suppression of thyroid function induced in normal persons by ingestion of thyroid hormone can usually be eliminated by administering 10 units of TSH daily for 1 to 5 days.

Because of the lack of specificity of a decreased rate of accumulation of radioactive iodine, it is usual to perform the radioiodine uptake test at 24 or 48 hours together with the protein-bound iodine (PBI) test.

HYPOTHYROIDISM SECONDARY TO HYPOPITUITARISM

To distinguish pituitary diseases, such as Simmonds-Sheehan disease, from primary disease of the thyroid, measurement of the response of the thyroid to TSH is helpful. After initial measurement of the plasma PBI and the rate of accumulation of radioiodine, the patient is given an intramuscular injection of TSH. The dosage schedule varies in different laboratories, but usually a minimum of two injections of 10 mg. each are given, followed by measurements of the ^{131}I uptake and PBI. In primary thyroid disease, neither rises significantly.

NEW GROWTHS

Cancer of the thyroid is among the diagnostic possibilities in a patient with either uniform enlargement of the thyroid or enlargement of one or more nodules in a normal-sized or goitrous gland. The differential diagnosis is most often between colloid nodular goiter and carcinoma of the thyroid.

The early stage of colloid nodular goiter consists of diffuse hypertrophy, hyperplasia, increased vascularity, and increased function. The second state includes diffuse enlargement with focal concentrations of ^{131}I on autoradiography. At later stages, the focal areas of increased activity disappear as a result of necrosis—which often results in hemorrhage and replacement by focal areas of fibrosis, calcification, or other retrogressive changes—but new foci of increased concentration of ^{131}I are present elsewhere in the gland. In the final stages, the grossly abnormal multinodular goiter results from a series of similar processes.

Although radioisotope scanning is less precise than autoradiography, scanning provides the same type of information concerning the evolution of colloid nodular goiter. Abnormality of the thyroid gland may be detected occasionally on scanning when it cannot be detected by inspection and palpation, particularly if the patient has symptoms that result from a mass in the thoracic inlet. Even with the thyroid in its normal position, if the patient has a short, thick neck, a goiter may not be detectable with certainty by physical examination.

If a nodule contains an increased concentration of radioactivity in comparison to the rest of the thyroid, it is called a "hot" nodule. Since thyroid cancer usually concentrates ^{131}I less avidly than normal thyroid tissue, a hot nodule is probably not cancerous. Hot nodules do not usually disappear after the administration of large doses of desiccated thyroid over periods of months or even years, presumably because they are autonomous and not dependent on TSH stimulation.

If little radioactivity accumulates in a nodule, it is termed "cold." One cause of a cold nodule is necrosis of a previously functional nodule; another is thyroid cancer. The finding of decreased concentration of ^{131}I in a clinically evident thyroid nodule increases slightly the likelihood of thyroid carcinoma. When the cold nodule is solitary and the remainder of the thyroid gland is relatively normal in size and has a relatively homogeneous distribution of ^{131}I, the statistical chance that the nodule is cancerous is nearly 50 per cent.

A fully developed multinodular goiter is usually easily recognized on the scan even though the clinician may see or feel only a solitary nodule. The diagnostic features of multinodular goiter are areas of increased ^{131}I concentration associated with multiple necrotic areas that register as cold. Areas of intermediate degrees of concentration of ^{131}I result from gradations between relatively normal thyroid tissue and retrogressive changes. In our experience, the incidence of carcinoma of the thyroid in multinodular goiters is low, probably less than 1 per cent. The scan may, therefore, be of considerable value in the judgment between surgical thyroidectomy and the risk of assuming that the gland is not cancerous.

Colloid nodular goiter is important because of its high incidence and the frequency of complications, which, in order of decreasing incidence, are: (1) tracheal deviation or compression; (2) thyrotoxicosis; (3) substernal extension; and (4) thyroid carcinoma.

Tracheal deviation or compression can be diagnosed by radioistope scanning and conventional radiography of the patient's trachea.

Thyrotoxicosis may develop as a result of autonomous hyperfunction of a single nodule or adenoma or it may be caused by the simultaneous occurrence of Graves' disease in a person with preexistent colloid nodular goiter.

In the scan of a patient with hyperthyroidism caused by autonomous hyperfunction of a solitary nodule, the nodule is usually the only area that concentrates ^{131}I, presumably because the increased output of thyroid hormone by the nodule depresses output of TSH by the pituitary gland. Delineation of the rest of the thyroid can sometimes be obtained by administering TSH and repeating the scan. TSH will stimulate the extranodular tissue and increase its uptake of radioactivity.

The finding of a hot nodule with suppression of uptake of the surrounding thyroid tissue does not furnish sufficient evidence for a diagnosis of thyrotoxicosis. An autonomously hyperfunctioning nodule may not secrete enough thyroid hormone to produce clinical thyrotoxicosis.

The incidence of substernal extension of multinodular goiters increases greatly with increasing age. The scan can demonstrate ^{131}I concentration in a a substernal mass and thereby establish with certainty that it is a goiter.

Thyroiditis may occasionally be confused with carcinoma of the thyroid. Hemorrhage into an adenoma or the presence of a rapidly growing anaplastic carcinoma of the thyroid may produce sudden swelling in the thyroid gland and simulate thyroiditis. As acute thyroiditis subsides, hard nodules may develop that simulate carcinoma. As mentioned previously, thyroid function is depressed by thyroiditis, so that the uptake of ^{131}I at 24 hours is usually less than 5 per cent of the administered dose, whereas the serum PBI may be elevated owing to release of stored thyroid hormone into the circulation through necrosis of follicular walls. These changes are usually present in the first week or two of the illness when there is extensive inflammation of the thyroid gland. The ^{131}I uptake and serum PBI are usually normal when there is hemorrhage into an adenoma. Rapidly growing undifferentiated carcinoma of the thyroid may cause complete replacement of the thyroid, resulting in a low radioactive uptake. In this instance serum PBI will be low rather than high.

If the diagnosis of thyroiditis is uncertain, the physician may begin a therapeutic trial of cortisone (Crile and Schneider, 1952). Cortisone administered to a patient with acute or subacute thyroiditis in dosage of 300 mg. per day for 1 day, then 200 mg. per day for 2 more days, usually results in complete subsidence of all symptoms or signs of thyroiditis. If this result does not occur, thyroidectomy should be considered. Hashimoto's and Riedel's struma may also be confused with carcinoma of the thyroid. One clue to the differential diagnosis is the fact that early in Hashimoto's thyroiditis the ^{131}I uptake may be elevated (Doniach et al., 1957); later the uptake may be decreased. Goitrous hypothyroidism developing in an otherwise normal adult is most commonly Hashimoto's disease. Release of radioactivity after administration of thiocyanate can be demonstrated in many patients with Hashimoto's disease. These patients are usually found to have decrease in size of the goiter after treatment with desiccated thyroid (Dodson et al., 1955)

CHRONIC THYROIDITIS (HASHIMOTO'S DISEASE)

A. T. MASI

In 1912, Hashimoto reported a disease of the thyroid in four Japanese women, for which he proposed the term "struma lymphomatosa" (Hashimoto, 1912). The disease is characterized by its histological features: (1) numerous lymphoid follicles; (2) striking changes of the acinar epithelium including its colloid content; (3) extensive connective tissue formation; and (4) diffuse round-cell infiltration. Other terms used subsequently to describe these lesions are lymphadenoid goiter, Hashimoto's struma, chronic thyroiditis, and lymphoid thyroiditis or struma.

The disease is not so rare as once was thought. In the United States, Hashimoto's disease is found in approximately 10 per cent of thyroidectomies (Masi et al., 1965). It is not known whether this represents an increase in the disease (McConahey et al., 1962; Macksood et al., 1961) or whether there has been an increase in frequency of thyroid surgery for nontoxic goiter. Geographic variables do not seem to play an important role in the frequency of this condition in the United States (Lindsay et al., 1952), and there is no special concentration in socioeconomic or sociocultural or religious groups (Masi, 1965).

Hashimoto's disease is most commonly found in middle-aged white females (Woolner et al., 1959) and has been reported to be rare in Negroes (Harland and Frantz, 1956) and in males (Marshall et al., 1948). However, such conclusions are based on the absolute numbers of cases diagnosed at thyroid operation without consideration of the selective aspect of patients undergoing thyroidectomy. Thyroid surgery is performed mainly on middle-aged white females, and Hashimoto's disease is usually diagnosed either at the operating table or on later examination of surgical pathology (Marshall et al., 1948; Danowski, 1962).

Autopsy data are a better indication of the distribution of Hashimoto's disease than are data based on clinical recognition. Such studies indicate that the histological changes of Hashimoto's disease, in both its focal (Goudie et al., 1959; Williams and Doniach, 1962) and diffuse (Mortensen et al., 1955) forms, increase continuously with age rather than peak in the middle years of life. Furthermore, the ratio of female to male prevalence appears from autopsy studies to be four to one, rather than approximately 20 to one as suggested by statistics derived only from cases found by thyroid surgery. The prevalence in whites compared to Negroes was found to be three to one in a large autopsy series (Masi, 1965). Studies such as these relate the distribution of this disease more closely to thyrotoxicosis and myxedema than was previously believed.

An adult patient with recent onset of a diffuse, firm goiter and hypothyroidism almost certainly has Hashimoto's disease. In approximately one fourth of the cases (Masi et al., 1965) the disease is found by a physician incidentally during a routine examination. Most often the diagnosis is first made at surgery (Harland and Frantz, 1956; Marshall et al., 1948), because the disorder is generally mild and the clinical findings nonspecific. The usual complaint of these patients before surgery is a goiter not associated with any physical discomfort (60 per cent). Fifteen per cent of patients with goiter complain of symptoms from mechanical pressure, such as dysphagia and dyspnea, especially when they lie down. A small proportion (5 per cent) complain of anterior neck pain or discomfort that may be suggestive of acute thyroiditis, although these symptoms are not as marked in Hashimoto's disease. Unlike persons with granulomatous thyroiditis, patients with Hashimoto's disease usually do not complain of fever or malaise.

Symptoms suggesting thyrotoxicosis, such as nervousness and weight loss, occur in a minority (5 per cent) of patients. The frequency of such symptoms has been sufficient, however, to suggest the bizarre name "Hashitoxicosis" to one group of workers (Means et al., 1963). A family history of thyrotoxicosis, on the other hand, is not rare in patients with diffuse thyroiditis.

Symptoms and signs of hypothyroidism tend to vary directly with the duration of the disease and with the diffuseness of the thyroiditis. In a large series of cases, probably 10 per cent or less have clinical myxedema at the time of their first examination. In 605 patients with Hashimoto's thyroiditis reviewed by Woolner, McConahey, and Beahrs, 8 per cent were myxedematous before surgery (Woolner et al., 1959). Among 188 patients with diffuse thyroiditis, 19 per cent were myxedematous, whereas among 417 patients with focal thyroiditis or thyroiditis with epithelial hyperplasia, only 3 per cent had myxedema.

Other complaints of patients before thyroid surgery are eye symptoms, exophthalmos, or concern about the cosmetic appearance of a full neck. Although virtually all patients with Hashimoto's disease who have a thyroid operation have a palpable abnormality of the gland, the same histological changes have been found at autopsy without any enlargement or nodularity (Mortensen et al., 1955).

Patients with Hashimoto's disease are most often operated upon to exclude the possibility of cancer or to treat the disease at its earliest possible stage. A minority of patients have mechanical pressure, anterior neck pain, or concern about appearance. The differentiation of chronic thyroiditis from cancer is difficult. Hashimoto's disease can present as a uninodular or multinodular goiter, although usually it causes diffuse enlargement. Palpable lymph nodes of the anterior cervical chain may suggest cancer rather than thyroiditis, but palpable enlargement of the midline Delphian node above the isthmus can occur with Hashimoto's disease (Means et al., 1963). The possibility of Hashimoto's disease should be considered whenever a presumptive diagnosis of nontoxic goiter or carcinoma is made. Ancillary tests can then be ordered to confirm or exclude this diagnosis. A definitive diagnosis, however, usually depends upon histological examination.

Although elevation of the serum gamma globulin (Fromm et al., 1950) and abnormalities of the colloidal gold test (Luxton and Cooke, 1956) have been reported, these results are found mainly in patients with advanced disease and myxedema. McConahey and his associates (1961) compared certain plasma protein measurements in patients with Hashimoto's thyroiditis and in euthyroid patients with adenomatous goiter. They found no significant differences in the sedimentation rate, thymol turbidity, or zinc turbidity tests. The patients with Hashimoto's disease had a higher frequency of abnormality of the serum albumin and the cephalin flocculation test, as well as a tendency to elevated gamma globulin levels, but these differences were small and the tests were not considered to have much value in the differential diagnosis of Hashimoto's disease.

An extensive literature exists on the various tests for serum antibodies to several thyroid antigens (Blizzard and Chandler, 1960; Doniach and Roitt, 1962). The more common tests are the tanned red-cell agglutination test for thyroglobulin antibody (Witebsky and Rose, 1956), the complement fixation test for a microsomal antigen of thyrotoxic glands (Trotter et al., 1957), and the Coons immunofluorescent technique on unfixed tissue sections for the microsomal antigen (Holborow, 1960).

These tests are positive in the highest proportion and in highest titer in patients with Hashimoto's disease (Roitt and Doniach, 1958), but they are also positive in most patients with nongoitrous myxedema and hyperthyroidism (Doniach et al., 1960), making differentiation from such conditions difficult on the basis of these tests alone. In euthyroid patients, strongly positive antithyroid antibody tests are good presumptive evidence of thyroiditis of the focal or diffuse variety; positive results would be less likely in cancer or adenomatous goiter, in which the results do not differ appreciably from those of normal persons (Doniach et al., 1960). Using the presence or absence of antithyroid antibodies as a criterion for classifying thyroiditis (e.g., "autoimmune" thyroiditis) is premature, however, because almost all evidence at present indicates that these humoral factors are a result rather than a cause of the disease process (Doniach and Roitt, 1962; Hall, 1962).

Certain tests of thyroid function have limited value in the diagnosis of Hashimoto's disease. The serum cholesterol is usually normal, although a minority of patients with clinical or other evidence of hypothyroidism may have values above 320 mg./100 ml. The basal metabolic rate also tends to be normal. The median value for the BMR among 120 white female patients with histologically diagnosed Hashimoto's disease discovered in a community-wide hospital survey was +3, with 15 per cent of patients having low values (less than or equal to −15) and 20 per cent of patients with high values (greater than or equal to +15) (Masi, 1965).

The PBI tends to be lower in persons with Hashimoto's disease than in the population at large. In a series of 53 white female patients, the *median* value of this test was 4.9 μgm./100 ml. (Masi, 1965), which is slightly lower than the value (*mean* 5.7 μgm./100 ml.) found by Lowrey and Starr (1959) in 1015 female employees of a general hospital. Because of the large amount of overlap, this laboratory procedure has only a slight chance of correlating with the histologic diagnosis of any given patient.

Patients with Hashimoto's disease have a relatively increased amount of nonthyroxine iodoprotein in their serum, which is measured in the PBI determination but not in the BEI test because it is butanol insoluble. McConahey and his colleagues (1961) emphasized the diagnostic value of the PBI-BEI difference as a clinical laboratory test to distinguish Hashimoto's disease from euthyroid adenomatous goiter. An abnormally high difference (above the normal upper limit of 1 μgm./100 ml.) was found in 47 per cent versus 10 per cent, respectively; and a strongly positive result (above 2 μgm./100 ml.) was found in 36 per cent versus 0 per cent, respectively. The BEI test is therefore a truer measure of active thyroid hormone, especially in Hashimoto's disease, than is the PBI measurement.

The plasma inorganic iodine level is normal (0.5 to 1.0 μgm./100 ml.) in Hashimoto's disease (Buchanan et al., 1961) and does not account for the discrepancy between PBI and BEI. In exceptional circumstances, however, an increased PBI-BEI difference might result from a markedly elevated serum iodide level, as in patients ingesting iodine-containing medications, because the BEI washing procedure removes free iodine to a greater degree than the PBI method.

A thyroid scan may be helpful if the patient has a nodule in the thyroid. In Hashimoto's disease, the nodule tends to concentrate the isotope more actively than the normal tissue, the opposite of the usual result in cancer. Usually, the thyroid is diffusely enlarged, with a diffuse distribution of the radioactivity.

The radioiodine uptake test is usually normal in Hashimoto's disease (Skillern et al., 1956), but it may be higher than one would suspect from the BEI or BMR. If the radioiodine uptake values for a group of patients with Hashimoto's disease are plotted on the ordinate and the BEI values on the abscissa, the points will tend to fall above the expected normal regression line. Uptake values may reach hyperthyroid levels, but unlike those in thyrotoxicosis, they are suppressible with exogenous thyroid hormone. Thus, the finding of a higher uptake value than one would expect from clinical examination or from a chemical test of thyroid function suggests Hashimoto's disease.

Buchanan and his co-workers (1961) have postulated that the thyroid in Hashimoto's disease has a diminished efficiency in the metabolism of iodine. This would explain the tendency for a rapid turnover of iodine in the thyroid, as evidenced by a relatively high iodine uptake compared to the output of physiologically active thyroid hormone, the increased amount of abnormal nonthyroxine iodoprotein found in Hashimoto's disease, and the elevated level of PB[131]I at 48 hours (Murray and McGirr, 1960). The latter is the single most discriminating tracer test in the diagnosis of chronic thyroiditis (Nilsson and Doniach, 1964). The finding that half of the patients have a rapid discharge of radioactivity after perchlorate administration suggests a defect in organic binding and transport of iodine. Subjects with chronic thyroiditis have an increased sensitivity to iodine, as in Graves' disease, which is aggravated by TSH administration (Dowling et al., 1963). The mechanisms of these abnormalities are not yet known.

Several studies that may have diagnostic value suggest that the thyroid in Hashimoto's disease is subject to increased TSH stimulation. When parenteral TSH is administered (4 to 10 USP units) to these patients, they do not respond adequately in terms of elevation of the radioiodine uptake (Skillern et al., 1956) or the PBI (Bowers et al., 1961), suggesting that the glands may be already under maximum TSH stimulation. El Kabir, Doniach, and Turner-Warwick measured the serum TSH levels in patients with various degrees of thyroiditis (El Kabir et al., 1963). Of 12 patients with normal or low radioiodine uptake, the TSH levels were abnormally elevated in 10. These preliminary studies, however, did not support the conclusion that Hashimoto's disease resulted from thyrotropic overstimulation because the TSH levels in patients with "mild thyroiditis" were normal or subnormal. Serial measurements of TSH levels must be carried out in the same patients and correlated with thyroid histology to test this theory.

DIFFERENTIAL DIAGNOSIS

A. T. MASI

An accurate diagnosis of Hashimoto's disease requires multiple laboratory tests. For example, a euthyroid female patient with a BEI of 4.0 and a radioiodine uptake of 55 per cent at 24 hours (which decreases to 25 per cent after 75 μgm. triiodothyronine per day for 1 week) has a 75 per cent probability of having Hashimoto's disease. If, in addition, the potassium perchlorate test is positive and the PB^{131}I is also elevated, the probability increases to 85 per cent. A definitive diagnosis requires histological examination. An unanswered question is whether confirmation of Hashimoto's disease is sufficient indication for a thyroid operation, particularly since no evidence has yet been found that Hashimoto's disease is associated with thyroid epithelial cancer or is a predisposing factor. Needle biopsy may be a useful diagnostic technique because of its negligible morbidity (Means et al., 1963).

Usually, Hashimoto's disease results in hypothyroidism; therefore, physiological doses of exogenous thyroid medication are often advisable as soon as the diagnosis is made. If the thyroid is enlarged before thyroid hormone therapy and regresses after therapy, this provides support for the diagnosis, and continuation of the medication is indicated. Administration of enough medication to maintain a euthyroid state and to prevent further thyroid enlargement is advisable.

If, on the other hand, a palpable thyroid abnormality or enlargement does not decrease in size after a 2 or 3 month trial of large dosage thyroid hormone, this is evidence against the diagnosis of Hashimoto's disease. In this case, thyroidectomy should be performed after evaluation of clinical variables such as sex, age, type of nodularity, and whether lymph nodes are palpable.

If Hashimoto's disease is diagnosed definitively after thyroid surgery, one must not hesitate to treat these patients with physiological doses of exogenous thyroid hormone. Hypothyroidism develops rapidly and to a severe degree after partial thyroidectomy (Woolner et al., 1959). Failure to give thyroid medication only postpones needed treatment; in the interim, the patient may risk the consequences of untreated hypothyroidsim. Although some patients with early Hashimoto's disease have a spontaneous regression of their goiter and do not require replacement therapy for a long time, this is unusual. An operative procedure may be necessary in those patients with symptoms arising from the mechanical pressure of an enlarged thyroid or in patients with a very firm thyroid of long duration that would not be expected to decrease in size with thyroid medication. If the gland is small, firm, and relatively fixed, an isthmectomy should suffice to relieve symptoms. If the gland is large, a bilateral subtotal thyroidectomy with or without isthmectomy should result in good symptomatic and cosmetic effects.

THERAPY OF THYROID DISEASES WITH RADIOIODINE

W. H. Beierwaltes and H. N. Wagner, Jr.

HYPERTHYROIDISM

Radioactive iodine was first used to treat thyrotoxicosis in 1941 (Hertz and Roberts, 1942; Hamilton and Lawrence, 1942). This form of treatment has been so satisfactory that one might ask, "Is ^{131}I the treatment of choice for all patients with thyrotoxicosis?" There are several reasons why this is not the case.

POSSIBLE CARCINOGENIC EFFECT

One reason why ^{131}I has not been used as the treatment of choice for hyperthyroidism at any age is that the radiation delivered to the thyroid gland might be carcinogenic after a period of years. Carcinoma of the thyroid has been observed in the thyroid glands of rats after ^{131}I (Goldberg and Chaikoff, 1952), although this work has not been confirmed. Thyroid cancer has been known to occur spontaneously with some frequency in the Long-Evans strain that was used in the original study (Frantz, 1956). To obtain a high incidence of cancer of the thyroid, both goitrogens and ^{131}I must be employed (Doniach, 1958). Maloof et al. (1952) found only one adenoma in the thyroids of 500 rats given doses of from 1 to 300 μc. of ^{131}I. Several reports of human thyroid cancers following external irradiation of the neck region in childhood have been published. In these patients the latent period for neoplasms has often been less than 10 years, and the association must now be regarded as well established.

On the other hand, it is doubtful whether irradiation in adult life predisposes to the development of thyroid carcinoma. In a survey of 100 patients with carcinoma of the thyroid, irradiation in adult life played no part in the pathogenesis of the disease (Kilpatrick et al., 1957). Between 100,000 and 200,000 thyrotoxic patients have been treated with ^{131}I during the past 20 years, yet the number of cases of carcinoma has not exceeded the usual incidence of thyroid carcinoma, 25 per 1,000,000 (Mustacchi and Cutler, 1956). If ^{131}I is carcinogenic in adults, the latent period must be much longer than that observed following external irradiation in childhood. The available evidence suggests that if ^{131}I therapy is restricted to adults the danger of subsequent development of carcinoma of the thyroid is remote.

RISK OF LEUKEMIA

The incidence of leukemia is definitely increased among patients treated with ^{131}I for thyroid cancer, but it has not proved to be a hazard in doses customarily used for hyperthyroidism. The usual dose of ^{131}I for this disease delivers from 5000 to 10,000 rads to the thyroid gland and five to eight rads to the whole body; this is evidently insufficient to increase the incidence of leukemia. Pochin (1960) was unable to show an incidence beyond that expected for the same number of people for the same period of observation.

CARCINOMA PRESENT IN THE THYROID

The presence of carcinoma should be suspected in any thyroid gland containing hard nodules. If it is possible that carcinoma may be present in the thyroid of a patient who has hyperthyroidism, ^{131}I treatment is contraindicated except as a possible method of preparing the patient for surgical thyroidectomy. The average dose of ^{131}I used to treat hyperthyroidism will not obliterate an area of carcinoma of the thyroid, particularly since such carcinoma concentrates iodine less avidly than does normal thyroid tissue (Fitzgerald and Foote, 1949), and far less avidly than hyperactive thyroid tissue. If the nodules of a goiter disappear after a dose of ^{131}I given as preoperative preparation for a patient with toxic nodular goiter, thyroidectomy need not be performed. If the nodules were a manifestation of carcinoma of the thyroid, they would not be destroyed by the small amount of ^{131}I used to treat exophthalmic goiter.

One type of nodular goiter rarely harbors carcinoma. When a patient develops recurrent exophthalmic goiter after a previous thyroidectomy, the goiter may consist of numerous firm or hard discrete nodules up to 3 to 5 cm. in size. In our experience these nodules have always shrunk satisfactorily after a dose of ^{131}I for hyperthyroidism. The radiation sensitivity provides evidence that these nodules represent postoperative remnants of hyperplastic tissue that have developed as a result of TSH stimulation.

LARGE MASS OF THYROID

Large toxic goiters (over 50 to 75 g.) are rarely shrunk to normal size by ^{131}I therapy; toxic nodular goiters shrink even less than diffuse hyperplastic goiters. Most substernal goiters do not shrink after ^{131}I therapy; in addition, such goiters may harbor unsuspected carcinoma. Therefore, nontoxic noncarcinomatous goiters should not be treated with [131]I. Since they concentrate ^{131}I even less well than toxic goiters, the dose necessary to shrink such goiters delivers an unnecessarily large amount of radiation to the patient.

PREGNANCY

One must avoid administering ^{131}I in treatment doses or even in tracer doses to any woman who might be pregnant. Transplacental diffusion of ^{131}I occurs, and the fetal thyroid has the ability to accumulate demonstrable amounts of ^{131}I by the twelfth week of gestation (Hodges et al., 1955).

SEVERE HYPERTHYROIDISM

In the treatment of severe hyperthyroidism one must be careful to avoid precipitating thyroid crisis or acute congestive heart failure as a result of rapid release of thyroid hormone into the blood stream by necrosis of follicular walls (Curran et al., 1958). Such patients should be treated initially with antithyroid drugs.

GENETIC DAMAGE

Genetic damage must be accepted as a risk to the individual patient, and to society in general, since mutations produced by ^{131}I are primarily recessive. The present rate of birth defects is thought to be of the order of 4 per 100 live births. About half of these occur on a genetic basis. If one estimates the effect on the mutation rate of the population as a whole, the increase produced by radioisotope therapy is small compared to the natural mutation rate, and impossible to detect. No existing data demonstrate that congenital abnormalities of any kind have been the result of radioiodine therapy.

The genetic effect of ^{131}I therapy to the total population of the Sheffield region in England was considered by Blomfield et al. (1959). They calculated, on the basis of 270 cases of thyrotoxicosis, a mean dose to plasma of 25 rads to women under 45 and men under 50, and a total genetically significant dose of 1516 rad-eq.[3] The investigators estimated that ^{131}I therapy for thyrotoxicosis had an effect equal to approximately 0.3 per cent of the natural background dosage. The effect of diagnostic radiology was estimated by Osborn and Smith (1956) to be 22 per cent of the natural background. These calculations suggest that the genetic hazard from ^{131}I treatment of hyperthyroidism, although present, is statistically small.

INDUCED HYPOTHYROIDISM

Stanbury and DeGroot (1964) have emphasized a major hazard of ^{131}I therapy. Since the introduction of radioiodine therapy, hypothyroidism has been accepted as a minor and easily remediable complication, occurring in 8 to 12 per cent of patients within the first few years of treatment (Chapman, 1955). Beling and Einhorn (1961) first recognized the more serious magnitude of the problem. In a virtually complete (99.4 per cent) follow-up of 791 patients, they found that hypothyroidism occurred in 7.5 per cent of patients within the first year, and thereafter at an annual increment of approximately 3 per cent per year for 7 years, by which time the incidence had reached 26.5 per cent. There was no evidence of any diminution of the annual increment of new cases. The general experience of others has been the same (Green, 1964). The mechanism of the phenomenon is suggested by the well accepted observation that although a cell may continue to function normally after relatively small doses of radiation, it may not reproduce itself normally. Consequently, function may cease at the time of first or subsequent cell replications.

Although the incidence of hypothyroidism after ^{131}I therapy increases progressively, the incidence after surgery is relatively stable. The findings of several

---

[3] rad equivalent genetic.

surgical series with long follow-up observations (Hurxthal et al., 1945; Bartels et al., 1956; Iversen et al., 1957) suggest that hypothyroidism is more common after ^{131}I therapy than after surgery.

We have followed a group of surgically treated patients for as long as 13 years together with a group of patients treated with ^{131}I. The cumulative incidence of hypothyroidism after ^{131}I was 2.7 per cent per year after treatment. The cumulative incidence in the surgically treated group was 1.7 per cent per year.

The incidence of hypothyroidism in the ^{131}I-treated patients without clinically detectable nodularity of the thyroid gland was higher than in the patients with nodular goiters. The incidence of hypothyroidism was particularly high in those patients who had had previous surgical therapy.

The use of smaller doses of radioiodine followed by antithyroid drugs has been proposed as a means of decreasing the incidence of subsequent hypothyroidism.

INDICATIONS FOR RADIOIODINE THERAPY IN HYPERTHYROIDISM

Previous Thyroidectomy for Hyperthyroidism. The risk of laryngeal palsy or parathyroid tetany is greater after a second thyroid operation than after the initial thyroidectomy. Major complications occur 20 times as frequently (Keating et al., 1958). Therefore, ^{131}I is the therapy of choice in patients of any age with goiter that recurs after thyroidectomy.

Exophthalmic Goiter in Persons Over 25 Years of Age. Radioiodine therapy is not usually given to hyperthyroid persons unless they are over 25 years of age, on the assumption that with older persons a normal life span will be completed before a possible carcinogenic effect of irradiation becomes manifest.

Impractically Long Preoperative Preparation. The longer a patient remains hyperthyroid, the more likely he is to develop complications such as progressive exophthalmos, thyrotoxic heart disease, thyroid crisis, or deleterious side effects of drug therapy (agranulocytosis, skin rash, or jaundice). For these reasons it is advisable to treat patients under 25 with ^{131}I if an unsuccessful attempt has been made over a period of 4 to 6 months to prepare the patient for thyroidectomy with antithyroid drugs.

Radioiodine is being used more widely in the preoperative preparation of patients with toxic nodular goiter (Crispell et al., 1955), since it is generally more difficult to treat such patients with antithyroid drugs than with ^{131}I. If the primary contraindication to ^{131}I therapy is the possibility that a nodular gland may harbor an unsuspected carcinoma, thyroidectomy can be carried out after the thyrotoxicosis has been relieved by ^{131}I.

Hyperthyroidism in the Presence of Contraindications for Surgery. Severe heart disease, or myocardial infarction of less than 1 year's duration, laryngeal palsy, severe emotional disturbance, severe hypertension, and severe disease of the lungs, liver, or kidneys are the most common surgical contraindications that make ^{131}I therapy preferable.

Hyperthyroidism with Malignant Exophthalmos. Malignant exophthalmos is progressive protrusion of the eyes, documented by increasing Hertel exophthalmometer measurements, plus one or more of the following physical signs:

lid or conjunctival swelling, extraocular muscle paresis, inability to close the eyes, and staining of the cornea with fluorescein dye (Beierwaltes, 1951, 1953). Thyroidectomy in a patient with these signs frequently results in an increase in the severity of the exophthalmos. Soley, Miller, and Foreman (1949) found a measured increase in exophthalmos in 30 per cent of patients treated with ^{131}I, in 26 per cent of those treated with roentgen irradiation of the thyroid gland, and in 40 to 50 per cent of those who had undergone subtotal thyroidectomy. Dobyns (1945) found an increase of more than 1 mm. in the exophthalmos in over 60 per cent of patients treated with thiouracil or surgery. Beierwaltes and Johnson (1956) found no significant change in measured exophthalmos in patients with toxic nodular or diffuse goiter when eye measurements were obtained at 3 and 6 month intervals after treatment of hyperthyroidism with [131]I. Further analysis showed that the Hertel exophthalmometer measurements at these time intervals after ^{131}I therapy were increased in one third of the patients, showed no change in one third, and showed a decrease in one third.

DOSAGE OF [131]I

Radioiodine therapy presents the same therapeutic dilemma as surgery. If one administers ^{131}I to a hyperthyroid patient with great care to avoid subsequent hypothyroidism, many patients will return with persistent or recurrent hyperthyroidism. With larger doses, the incidence of hypothyroidism will probably be at least 15 per cent. The physician may attempt to relieve thyrotoxicosis completely with one dose of ^{131}I, or he may repeat small doses at intervals over relatively long periods of time.

The size of the dose can be determined on the basis of four considerations. An average dose of 10 mc. of ^{131}I probably results in an equal incidence of subsequent hypothyroidism and persistent or recurrent hyperthyroidism. The usual patient with exophthalmic goiter requires a 10 mc. dose of [131]I. Variations from the average, including the percentage uptake of ^{131}I at 24 hours, or the effective half-life of ^{131}I in the thyroid gland, alter the dosage needed. If, by inspection and palpation, the weight of the gland is judged to be greater than the average of 35 to 50 g., 1 to 2 mc. is added to the average dose of 10 mc. If the 24 hour uptake value is markedly greater than the average of 65 to 75 per cent, the dose may be decreased by 1 to 2 mc. If the effective half-life of ^{131}I in the thyroid gland is likely to be less than the average of 13 days (Blomfield et al., 1959), the dose of ^{131}I may be correspondingly increased in an attempt to deliver the same amount of radiation during the shorter period of time. The effective half-life is usually decreased whenever there are decreased stores of ^{131}I in the thyroid. The radioiodine turnover is usually decreased in patients with recurrent hyperthyroidism after previous surgical or ^{131}I therapy or in the presence of Hashimoto's disease. The effective or biological half-life of ^{131}I may be determined by measuring the radioactivity in the thyroid gland daily after a tracer dose of [131]I.

Blomfield et al. (1959) have emphasized the importance of estimating the mass of the thyroid gland in determining the dose of [131]I. They found that with increasing mass of goiter, the percentage of patients who, after the first treatment, remain hyperthyroid increased, whereas the proportion becoming hypothyroid decreased.

Most physicians have discarded the use of a mathematical formula in calculating the dose of ^{131}I (Werner et al., 1949) because the weight of the thyroid gland cannot be estimated with sufficient accuracy. Physicians experienced with thyroid diseases (Soley et al., 1948) reported an error of from 42 per cent below to 31 per cent above the actual weight of the gland. Blomfield et al. (1959) compared the weight of the thyroid gland in six patients at autopsy with the estimates made by palpation before treatment with ^{131}I within 10 weeks previously. The weight of smaller glands was underestimated. When scanning techniques were used to study *in vitro* models to obtain an estimate of thyroid gland size (Blomfield et al., 1959), models less than 50 ml. in size led to an overestimation of size by as much as 50 per cent; above 50 ml. the accuracy was ± 25 per cent.

Variable factors render delivery of an optimal dosage of ^{131}I difficult. The biological half-life of a tracer dose varies and its determination requires an undesirably long time. The radiation sensitivity of the thyroid gland varies from one patient to the next. In 500 patients, Blomfield et al. (1959) found that despite an attempt to deliver a constant dose to the thyroid of 7000 rads, some patients received a dose to the thyroid of under 4000 rads and some over 10,000 rads, largely because of an unexpectedly shorter or longer effective half-life in the gland. The sensitivity of the thyroid to radiation varied so greatly from subject to subject that 10 per cent of those patients receiving 4000 rads became hypothyroid. Although the incidence of hypothyroidism in those receiving over 10,000 rads was slightly increased, additional treatment was required in a high percentage even in these patients.

To avoid hypothyroidism some physicians use doses as low as 2 to 4 mc. of ^{131}I. A few patients with exophthalmic goiter can be treated successfully with doses of ^{131}I as small as 4 mc. The principal disadvantage of this method of treatment is that most patients cannot be adequately treated with a single dose of this size. The maximum effect of each dose does not become evident for 3 months; therefore, if the patient requires several doses he may remain ill for an unnecessarily long period of time. Furthermore, the last dose, however small, may still induce hypothyroidism. In such instances, the patient has not only been allowed to remain ill for a long period of time, but he also has developed hypothyroidism. However, fractionation of the total dose is advisable when thyrotoxicosis is unusually severe, when the patient is elderly (either chronologically or physiologically), or when he has complicating illness. Nodular toxic goiter is almost always treated with multiple fractionated doses.

Individual doses should not be given more frequently than at 3 or 4 week intervals. When divided doses are given, a somewhat larger *total* dose of ^{131}I may have to be given, since one of the effects of the irradiation is to decrease the percentage taken up by the gland and increase the turnover rate (Freedberg et al., 1950). Thus, using equal doses, the amount of radiation delivered to the thyroid by each dose of ^{131}I is progressively less. Generally, the first dose is kept small to permit evaluation of the patient's response. If there is no worsening of the patient, manifest by cardiac complications or other untoward effects, each successive dose may be made slightly larger until the total calculated dose has been given. In seriously ill patients, 4 to 7 mc. has been found to be a safe initial dose. Successive doses may be 12 mc., then 17 mc., 29 mc., and so on.

The average total dose of ^{131}I necessary to relieve hyperthyroidism in patients with nodular toxic goiters has been about 34 mc. (McCullagh, 1952).

The maximum effect of a dose of ^{131}I in patients with hyperthyroidism usually does not become manifest for a period of 3 months (Beierwaltes and Johnson, 1956; Chapman et al., 1954). To shorten the period required to decide whether or not the patient will need a second dose of ^{131}I, a battery of tests has been designed to predict in advance the necessity for a second dose (Myant, 1953; Schultz and Zieve, 1955). These tests are based on the fact that after radioiodine administration, the first manifestations that change are the rate of uptake of radioiodine and the serum PBI. Later, as thyroid hormone stores are depleted, the patient's BMR falls, his serum cholesterol rises, and his clinical state improves. If ^{131}I uptake or serum PBI is still elevated 1 month after a therapeutic dose of ^{131}I, the patient should be given further treatment at that time. Normal values suggest that treatment has been adequate, even though the patient has not yet become clinically euthyroid. Although these tests may be helpful, they are more subject to error than observation of the patient's clinical status after 3 months.

POSSIBLE SEQUELAE OF ^{131}I THERAPY FOR HYPERTHYROIDISM

Thyroiditis. Thyroiditis develops within 1 to 2 days after treatment. This occurs in about 5 per cent of patients with toxic nodular or diffuse goiter, and is usually indicated by tenderness or pain in the region of the thyroid gland. Rarely there may be local heat, redness, and swelling. Symptoms of thyroiditis seldom last longer than 24 hours, but occasionally may persist as long as 3 to 7 days. If the patient is receiving anticoagulant drugs, the irradiation thyroiditis may lead to hemorrhage into the gland.

Worsening of Thyrotoxicosis. Patients with congestive heart failure may have worsening of their symptoms within 24 hours after the dose of [131]I. Symptoms of thyrotoxicosis may also become worse within a period of 24 to 48 hours and persist for 3 to 4 weeks. About 2 per cent of patients with diffuse toxic goiter and 10 per cent of patients with nodular toxic goiter had complications of this kind (Beierwaltes and Johnson, 1956). Seven per cent of the patients with nodular toxic goiter developed thyroid crisis. All were past 50 years of age and had heart disease or cerebral arteriosclerosis. They became more nervous and had increased pulse rate, increased congestive heart failure, anorexia, insomnia, and fever. None died, but two became psychotic for several weeks.

Hypothyroidism. Twenty per cent of patients with diffuse toxic goiter may develop temporary or permanent hypothyroidism (Beierwaltes and Johnson, 1956; Clark and Rule, 1955). This usually develops 3 months after the treatment dose, although it may not become apparent for years (Chapman et al., 1954) (see p. 345). Prominent early symptoms include muscle cramps, which occur whenever the patient sits or crosses his legs, and difficulty in opening and closing the hands. Because the hypothyroidism is usually of recent onset, large doses of thyroid can be started immediately, e.g., 1 grain (64 mg.) of desiccated thyroid, U.S.P., every day for 1 week, then 2 grains per day for 1 week, and then 3 grains per day thereafter. If the patient develops insomnia and increased nervousness on this dosage, his dosage should be reduced to 2 grains per day.

Persistent or Recurrent Hyperthyroidism After ^{131}I Therapy. In patients with malignant exophthalmos, it is advisable to tend to err on the side of high doses of ^{131}I. If the patient is left with persistent or recurrent hyperthyroidism after one dose of ^{131}I, his exophthalmos may progress after a second dose. If he is overtreated, no great harm is done, because the exophthalmos is usually treated with desiccated thyroid, even if the patient becomes euthyroid after ^{131}I treatment. If desiccated thyroid is administered while the patient is still hyperthyroid, the patient may develop worsening of the symptoms of thyrotoxicosis (Beierwaltes, 1953).

Only 10 per cent of our patients with nodular toxic goiter became hypothyroid after treatment with a single dose of ^{131}I. It is not surprising, then, that 36 per cent of the patients had persistent or recurrent thyrotoxicosis after one dose (Beierwaltes and Johnson, 1956). Twenty per cent of our patients with diffuse toxic goiter required more than one dose of ^{131}I, and 20 per cent became hypothyroid.

A higher percentage of patients with nodular goiter required multiple doses of ^{131}I than did patients with diffuse goiter, although no patient with nodular goiter required more than four doses. Repeated doses were usually given at 3 month intervals; therefore, some patients were not fully treated until an average of 1 year had elapsed.

What should be done if a patient returns 3 months or more after treatment with obvious residual or recurrent hyperthyroidism? Because of the danger of inducing hypothyroidism, we treat patients with persistent hyperthyroidism after therapy by administering antithyroid drugs of the thiourea type for a period of 6 months to a year. If there is persistence or recurrence of the symptoms of thyrotoxicosis after the antithyroid drugs are stopped, we re-treat them with radioiodine.

ANTITHYROID DRUGS AND ^{131}I THERAPY

Thiourea derivatives (thiouracil, propylthiouracil, Tapazole, and others) presumably exert their effect on the thyroid by depressing the rate of activity of the peroxidase enzyme system, thereby decreasing the formation of nascent iodine from iodide. The rate of formation of thyroxine is thereby retarded, whereas that present in the gland before the administration of the antithyroid drug is released into the blood and metabolized in the tissues of the body. Thus, the thyrotoxic state gradually abates. The decreased level of thyroxine in the blood stimulates the production of TSH by the anterior pituitary, resulting in increased hyperplasia, hypertrophy, and vascularity of the gland.

The aminobenzenes, such as para-aminobenzoic acid, and the sulfonamide drugs, such as sulfadiazine, act by competing with tyrosine for combination with free iodine, thereby blocking the production of thyroxine.

The mechanism of the antithyroid action of small doses of iodide is unknown; it may be that iodide decreases the action of TSH in stimulating thyroid cells. The thyroid reverts to a resting state and becomes involuted. Since thiouracil and iodine exert their effects in depressing thyroxine production by different mechanisms, simultaneous administration of the two agents causes a more rapid reduction in the basal metabolic rate than thiouracil alone. The action of iodine is of particular advantage to the surgeon. It is no longer necessary to discontinue thiouracil medication and administer iodine alone for 3 weeks to cause involution of the gland before surgery.

Use of Thiourea Derivatives in Preparation for [131]**I Therapy.** If a patient has been receiving a thiouracil derivative for treatment of hyperthyroidism, administration of the drug is usually stopped for at least 2 days before administration of a treatment dose of radioactive iodine. If he has severe untreated hyperthyroidism, he should not be treated with ^{131}I without preliminary preparation, since ^{131}I may cause necrosis of follicular walls and release stored hormones into the blood stream in quantities that can result in thyroid crisis. Signs of approaching thyroid crisis are poor appetite, insomnia, and fever. A hyperthyroid person past 40 years of age, who looks very ill and whose BMR is greater than + 50 per cent, should not be treated with ^{131}I without previous preparation even in the absence of more specific signs. These patients should be given sedation, bed rest, and thiouracil derivatives. When they have improved, are gaining weight, and have a drop in the BMR of 10 to 20 per cent or more, the thiouracil derivative can be stopped and a treatment dose of radioactive iodine given 2 days later.

GOITER IN RELATION TO ^{131}I THERAPY

What happens to the goiter after treatment of thyrotoxicosis with radioactive iodine? Decrease in the size of the goiter is the rule with diffuse goiter but is much less likely in nodular goiters, which are generally larger and require more radiation before they shrink to normal size. The radioactivity tends to concentrate in one or more hot nodular or paranodular tissue areas, in contrast to diffuse goiter, in which the radioiodine is more diffusely distributed. Many nodular goiters have relatively large areas of retrogressive change that do not concentrate radioiodine and therefore are not necrosed by [131]I.

Patients of ours who had roentgenographic evidence of substernal goiter showed no decrease in the degree of distortion of the trachea or esophagus after ^{131}I therapy, even when the part of the goiter in the neck decreased in size. Patients with a history of goiter and surgical thyroidectomy frequently have localized areas of functional hyperplasia, which are detected on physical examination as one or more firm or hard nodules near the thyroidectomy scar. The diagnosis of functional hyperplasia rather than carcinoma can be made if an abnormally high uptake of ^{131}I is found on scanning, with the total disappearance of the hot nodules 3 months after the administration of small doses of [131]I. Thyroid carcinoma does not concentrate ^{131}I as well as normal thyroid tissue, and consequently does not undergo necrosis after [131]I.

THYROIDECTOMY AFTER [131]I

Some patients with very large toxic goiters require thyroidectomy following treatment with [131]I. Radiation effects in the operative field after ^{131}I are less than after x-ray therapy, presumably because beta radiation from ^{131}I does not penetrate beyond the capsule of the thyroid gland. Therefore, little or no fibrosis is present around the thyroid. The irradiation decreases the vascularity and friability of the thyroid gland.

The surgeon should be aware that most thyroid cells remaining after ^{131}I therapy have been damaged by irradiation and therefore function subnormally. If he removes as much gland as he would from an unirradiated patient, a much higher percentage of his patients will develop hypothyroidism.

AURICULAR FIBRILLATION

What happens to auricular fibrillation after thyrotoxicosis is suppressed by [131]I? In our series, heart disease was present in 41 patients, or 50 per cent of those treated for toxic nodular goiter. Forty-four patients (18 per cent) with exophthalmic goiter had heart disease. Eighteen patients (22 per cent) with toxic nodular goiter and 21 patients (8 per cent) with exophthalmic goiter had auricular fibrillation. Only 39 per cent of the patients with toxic nodular goiter and auricular fibrillation reverted to normal sinus rhythm whereas 81 per cent of diffuse goiter patients with auricular fibrillation reverted to normal sinus rhythm at the time of disappearance of thyrotoxicosis. Andrus (1932) recorded that 33 per cent of patients with toxic nodular goiter and 15 per cent of patients with exophthalmic goiter have coexisting congestive heart failure. Lahey and Hurxthal (1934) reported a 71.5 per cent conversion after surgical thyroidec-tomy for toxic goiter. It is possible that many patients with auricular fibrillation who were cured of hyperthyroidism by ^{131}I but failed to convert to sinus rhythm had underlying heart disease.

WHAT DOES ONE TELL THE PATIENT?

Many patients, both men and women, are afraid that a dose of ^{131}I will cause sterility. The patient should be assured that this is an unwarranted fear. Women with hyperthyroidism have an increased incidence of menstrual irregu-larity, diminished fertility, and a higher than normal rate of fetal loss through miscarriage and stillbirth. These difficulties are decreased in frequency and severity by treatment of the thyrotoxicosis. However, excessive dosage of anti-thyroid drug, with resultant *hypothyroidism,* increases the risk of abortion in early pregnancy and can, in late pregnancy, cause hypothyroidism and goiter in the fetus. It is a rather common occurrence for thyrotoxic women with a history of reduced fertility and abnormalities of gestation to conceive within 2 or 3 months after a treatment dose of ^{131}I and proceed with a normal preg-nancy (Clark and Rule, 1955).

The typical patient knows little if anything about radioactivity and radio-active iodine. Therefore, the patient should be informed that he will drink a tasteless solution and will note no side effects. It should be explained that he will not feel the radioactivity and that no special precautions should be observed. He should be told that there is about a 5 per cent chance that he may develop tenderness over his thyroid gland for a few days after the treatment dose is given. Both patient and referring physician should understand that no improve-ment will occur for 1 or possibly 2 months. The patient should be warned to avoid iodides, antithyroid drugs, and desiccated thyroid because they may diminish the effect of the dose by blocking the recirculation of ^{131}I through the thyroid gland. It should be made clear to the patient and his referring physician that *other* drugs are not contraindicated. It is wise to give some sedative or reserpine during the first 2 months after treatment, to diminish hyperthyroid symptoms from withdrawal of antithyroid drugs and from leakage of stored thyroid hormone into the blood from necrosed thyroid cells.

We tell the patient that there is a 10 to 20 per cent chance that he may develop hypothyroidism, but that he can be kept in completely normal health by the administration of desiccated thyroid. He is also told that there is a 10 to 20 per cent chance that he may need more than one dose of ^{131}I. If it is planned to fractionate a patient's total dose, as explained earlier, the patient returns at monthly intervals for his fractional dose until the total estimated dose has been given. After that, he waits for 3 months before he returns for a complete thyroid reevaluation. All patients are asked to return 3 months after their total dose for a 2 hour uptake test and a brief medical history and physical examination. If the patient appears cured of his hyperthyroidism, we do not ask to see him again. If the patient appears well, but his ^{131}I uptake is still in the hyperthyroid range, we tell him that no further treatment is necessary but that it would be advisable to return for a repeat examination in 3 to 6 months. If goiter persists after disappearance of thyrotoxicosis, the patient is strongly urged to have thyroidectomy if there is no contraindication to surgery. Occasionally, a patient with thyrotoxicosis is allergic to iodides. He can still be given a treatment dose of ^{131}I because the treatment dose of ^{131}I for hyperthyroidism contains a total of only about 0.02 μg. of iodine. We have treated four patients who were severely sensitive to iodine, without reactions.

SUMMARY: INDICATIONS AND CONTRAINDICATIONS FOR THE USE OF ^{131}I IN THE TREATMENT OF HYPERTHYROIDISM

Radioiodine is *indicated* in the treatment of hyperthyroidism when a patient:

(1) has persistent or recurrent exophthalmic goiter following a previous surgical thyroidectomy;

(2) has exophthalmic goiter and is over 25 years of age;

(3) cannot be prepared for surgical thyroidectomy within a period of 6 months;

(4) refuses surgery or is believed unable to withstand surgery.

Radioiodine is *contraindicated* in the treatment of hyperthyroidism:

(1) in an exophthalmic goiter patient under 25 years of age, because of the possibility that ^{131}I irradiation might eventually cause cancer of the thyroid;

(2) as definitive treatment for a toxic nodular or larger goiter, because that goiter may harbor carcinoma;

(3) as definitive treatment for a large toxic goiter, because these goiters usually do not disappear after ^{131}I therapy;

(4) in a pregnant woman;

(5) while a patient is severely hyperthyroid.

CARCINOMA OF THE THYROID

GENERAL

Radioactive iodine is not the treatment of choice for carcinoma of the thyroid gland. The best available single therapeutic measure is surgery. No

TABLE 7-8. CUMULATIVE SURVIVAL IN PATIENTS WITH DIFFERENT TYPES OF
THYROID CARCINOMA AT MASSACHUSETTS GENERAL HOSPITAL

	5 YEARS	10 YEARS	20 YEARS
Papillary	73%	60%	45%
Follicular	71%	48%	24%
Undifferentiated	17%	17%	17%

patient should have ^{131}I treatment of thyroid carcinoma without total surgical thyroidectomy. The surgical treatment of this disease has become progressively more radical, despite the relative benignancy of thyroid carcinoma compared to carcinoma of other structures. A study at Massachusetts General Hospital (McDermott et al., 1954) reported the survival rates of patients with different morphologic types of thyroid carcinoma shown in Table 7-8.

The survival rate of papillary carcinoma, which constitutes over 60 per cent of all thyroid carcinomas, is excellent (Beahrs et al., 1951). A patient may have only local excision of a single carcinomatous nodule and remain asymptomatic for years.

Carcinoma of the thyroid tends to become more undifferentiated (McDermott et al., 1954; Sloan, 1954) and more invasive at ages 40 to 50 years, and consequently it should be treated in the same manner as other types of cancer. The procedure recommended at present is to excise the nodule in question and perform a bilateral subtotal thyroidectomy. One or more lymph nodes from each jugular chain, whether normal or abnormal in appearance, are excised at the same operation. All tissue removed is submitted for histological examination by frozen section. If no carcinoma is found, nothing further is done. If carcinoma is found only in the thyroid gland, a bilateral total thyroidectomy is performed. If one or more lymph nodes are found to contain carcinoma, a radical neck dissection is performed on that side of the neck, at the same time as the thyroidectomy.

A radical neck dissection should be done even if the patient has metastases *outside* the neck region. Total intracapsular thyroidectomy should be carried out before ^{131}I therapy, regardless of the extent or location of metastases, for these reasons: to prevent subsequent compression or invasion of the structures in the neck, such as the trachea, esophagus, and tributaries to the superior vena cava; to insure removal of an adequate biopsy specimen; to increase the radioiodine uptake of remaining cancerous tissue; and to decrease the level of circulating thyroid hormone so that TSH can stimulate increased accumulation of ^{131}I by metastases (Rawson et al., 1948; Wollman et al., 1953). Another reason for surgery before ^{131}I therapy is to provide a large specimen of the tumor, since some portions of tumor may concentrate ^{131}I and others may not. If only a small biopsy sample is removed, the material available for examination by the pathologist might erroneously indicate that the patient has only well differentiated metastases. More extensive resection, on the other hand, might reveal the presence of undifferentiated metastases and carcinoma as well.

EXTERNAL RADIATION THERAPY IN CARCINOMA OF THE THYROID

Although X-ray therapy has been disappointing in the treatment of carcinoma of the thyroid, we use it if the lesions remaining after surgery do not concentrate ^{131}I to a significant degree, as evidenced by scanning 6 weeks after surgery and cessation of thyroid medication. X-ray therapy rather than ^{131}I is also used in rapidly growing inoperable carcinoma of the thyroid, or in lymphosarcoma.

INDICATIONS FOR ^{131}I IN CARCINOMA OF THE THYROID

Patients should be treated with ^{131}I only if there is evidence of sufficient concentration of ^{131}I by the carcinoma to justify an attempt to destroy metastases with this nuclide. After the surgeon has attempted a total thyroidectomy, subsequent external counting over the thyroid region usually reveals persistent concentrations of ^{131}I, which are the result of residual normal thyroid tissue, functioning thyroid cancer, or a combination of both. Under such circumstances, ^{131}I is given to destroy all remaining normal and cancerous tissue.

When a patient with thyroid carcinoma is referred for possible radioiodine therapy, the examiner's first duty is to confirm the diagnosis. A patient should never be treated without confirmation of the diagnosis by pathological examination of tissue. Occasionally the diagnosis of thyroid carcinoma is made erroneously in patients with other diseases, such as thyroiditis.

The second step is to determine whether the carcinoma will concentrate ^{131}I to sufficiently high levels. Less than 50 per cent of carcinomas of the thyroid concentrate measurable amounts of radioiodine (Fitzgerald et al., 1949). Generally, when the histological section shows that the carcinoma contains colloid, the carcinoma will concentrate ^{131}I; if the neoplasm does not contain colloid, in most cases it will not concentrate ^{131}I significantly (Fitzgerald and Foote, 1949). Carcinoma containing colloid is designated as follicular or alveolar (Beierwaltes, 1952).

Follicular Carcinoma. Follicular (alveolar) carcinomas usually metastasize to bone via the blood stream. These tumors occur more commonly in young persons and tend to grow slowly and remain differentiated until the patient reaches age 40 to 50 years (Sloan, 1954).

Papillary Carcinoma. The papillary type of thyroid carcinoma comprises 50 to 60 per cent of all thyroid carcinomas (Fitzgerald and Foote, 1949; Beahrs et al., 1951). Less than one third concentrate radioiodine (Fitzgerald and Foote, 1949).

Papillary and Follicular Carcinomas. When papillary carcinoma of the thyroid concentrates ^{131}I, accumulation can usually be correlated with lakes of colloid that are present together with the papillary structures. A tumor is often designated by the pattern present in the majority of the histological sections. The term follicular has achieved general usage only recently, having been substituted for the term "papillary adenocarcinoma" or "papillary and alveolar carcinoma." The designations "adeno" or "alveolar" suggest glandular structure of any type, whereas "follicular" is more specific for the thyroid.

Papillary carcinomas may contain numerous small areas of calcification called calcospherites, which are most pronounced in papillary carcinoma of the ovary. Occasionally a patient may be referred for ^{131}I treatment because the pathologist cannot differentiate in cervical node biopsies between carcinoma from the ovary and carcinoma of the thyroid. In such cases, thyroidectomy will reveal no evidence of carcinoma.

More Undifferentiated Types. Other types of thyroid carcinoma may be grouped together as undifferentiated; none concentrates ^{131}I well enough for therapeutic purposes. It should again be emphasized that a thyroid carcinoma may show varied morphology in different parts of the same tumor. Biopsy of a single area may yield tissue that is not typical of most of the carcinomatous tissue. One patient had a biopsy of a single hard nodule that was found to be undifferentiated carcinoma. At postmortem examination all the other thyroid lesions and all metastases consisted of a well differentiated carcinoma that would readily have concentrated ^{131}I.

Primary and Metastatic Types. In addition to performing a total thyroidectomy, one of the metastases should be biopsied if possible. If these are functional, the patient can usually be cured by ^{131}I therapy. One should always consult with an experienced pathologist to decide whether or not carcinoma is present, and one should personally examine all thyroid sections to obtain the experience necessary for proper selection of candidates for ^{131}I therapy. The clinician has an almost unique opportunity to correlate functional studies with the histological appearance and clinical course.

DETERMINATION OF ^{131}I CONCENTRATION BY CARCINOMA

Thyroid cancer concentrates ^{131}I less avidly than normal thyroid tissue (Fitzgerald and Foote, 1949; Wollman, 1953). Unless a total thyroidectomy is performed, neither external counting over suspected metastases nor measurement of urinary excretion of ^{131}I will be of value in predicting the subsequent ability of the tumor to concentrate radioiodine. Definitive measurements of the uptake of ^{131}I by cervical, pulmonary, or bone metastases cannot be made before total thyroidectomy.

Radioiodine scanning and counting over suspected lesions with a stationary detector are useful techniques in the detection of concentrations of ^{131}I. At times, scanning may reveal areas of concentration too small to be detected by point counting, and scanning should be performed even if the 24 hour uptake of ^{131}I is quite low. The surgeon may also be unable to identify thyroid remnants at operation even though the scan clearly indicates their presence.

Originally it was hoped (Trunnell, 1949) that it would be possible to predict a good therapeutic response to ^{131}I if, after total thyroidectomy, the urine contained less than 30 per cent of a subsequent tracer or therapeutic dose of ^{131}I. Unfortunately, in practice, this did not prove to be the case. Urinary iodine excretion levels as great as 79 per cent in 72 hours have been observed in patients who subsequently had an unequivocal decrease in size of bone or lung metastases or disappearance of cervical nodes after a single treatment dose (Beierwaltes, 1952). A patient with a metastasis weighing only a few grams may accumulate a relatively small percentage of the total dose and yet achieve a high concentration of radioactivity per gram of tumor.

INDICES OF THYROID FUNCTION

In patients who have had a total thyroidectomy, a normal basal metabolic rate and serum protein-bound iodine indicate the presence of functioning thyroid carcinoma. However, after a total thyroidectomy in a normal person, the PBI falls first, and only after a period of 6 to 12 weeks (Means and Lerman, 1938) does the BMR fall to myxedematous levels. The serum PBI should therefore be used as the first indication of a lack of functioning thyroid tissue. Although a patient who becomes myxedematous after a total thyroidectomy clearly does not have enough functioning thyroid tissue, this is not an absolute indication of the absence of traceable carcinoma. The patient may have a small amount of functioning carcinoma that is not sufficient to maintain him in a euthyroid state. We have found concentrations of ^{131}I in residual thyroid tissue and in metastases in both jugular chains of lymph nodes in persons who became myxedematous after a surgical thyroidectomy.

ENHANCING UPTAKE OF ^{131}I BY THYROID METASTASES

When a patient with metastatic thyroid carcinoma has been evaluated and found to be a candidate for radioactive iodine treatment, can the uptake of ^{131}I be enhanced? Total thyroidectomy is the only certain way to increase ^{131}I uptake of metastases in patients with follicular carcinoma of the thyroid gland (Rawson et al., 1948). This operation not only increases TSH stimulation of the metastases, but also removes the chief competing site of uptake of radioiodine, i.e., the thyroid gland. Administration of exogenous TSH may increase ^{131}I uptake by metastatic carcinoma of the thyroid if the patient has been maintained in a euthyroid state by the administration of desiccated thyroid after thyroidectomy. Under these circumstances, endogenous TSH production will have been depressed.

GENERAL PROGRAM OF TREATMENT OF CARCINOMA OF THE THYROID

After the patient has had a total thyroidectomy and the degree of uptake of ^{131}I by metastases has been determined, he must be hospitalized for ^{131}I treatment. Only when his body content of ^{131}I is less than 50 mc. can he be discharged from the hospital. This is established by measurement of the amount excreted in the urine following the dose of ^{131}I. If functioning carcinoma is found 3 months after the first dose of ^{131}I, another dose is given, and it is repeated until the patient has become fully myxedematous and his carcinoma either has been completely ablated or fails to concentrate additional ^{131}I. The patient is then given desiccated thyroid at a dosage of 1 grain (64 mg.) a day for 1 week, then 2 grains (128 mg.) a day for 1 week, and then 3 grains (192 mg.) a day thereafter. He is asked to return once a year and to discontinue his thyroid medication 6 weeks before return. If no carcinoma is found, or if any carcinoma present does not concentrate ^{131}I, the patient resumes his thyroid medication and returns the subsequent year.

DOSAGE OF ^{131}I

The range of dosage of ^{131}I used in treating metastatic carcinoma of the thyroid has been determined largely on a trial-and-error basis. A large dose is necessary because carcinoma concentrates ^{131}I poorly. A hyperthyroid gland may be ablated with 15 or 20 mc. of ^{131}I, since it concentrates ^{131}I avidly. The euthyroid gland may be found to concentrate about 2 per cent of the administered dose per gram of thyroid tissue (Wollman, 1953). Yet investigators have found total regression of as much as 20 g. of metastases with as little as 200 mc. of ^{131}I (Beierwaltes and Johnson, 1956). Therefore, parameters other than the concentration of ^{131}I per gram of tumor tissue must be of importance. These include variations in radiation sensitivity of the tumor from patient to patient, variability of distribution of ^{131}I in metastases, the time course of radioactivity in the tumor, and perhaps other factors.

In children aged 3 to 12 years we usually limit the first dose of ^{131}I to 100 mc., and in adults, to 150 to 200 mc. Thyroid tissue in a critical location may undergo sudden swelling as a result of radiation thyroiditis or sudden necrosis and hemorrhage into a metastasis. Metastases may decrease dramatically in size after a treatment dose of as little as 60 mc. The largest single dose administered safely to a child under age 16, to our knowledge, was 315 mc. (Rawson et al., 1951). In some cases, metastases may be better treated by multiple doses of ^{131}I for this reason: a single metastasis may accumulate most of the dose of ^{131}I; the first dose may destroy this metastasis, and subsequent doses may then necrose the remaining metastases.

Generally, the greater the total weight of metastases, the larger the dose required to cause necrosis. Patients with the poorest concentration of ^{131}I in metastases require the highest blood level of ^{131}I to insure the maximum ^{131}I uptake in metastases, thereby increasing the radiation to hematopoietic tissue. The radiation delivered to hematopoietic tissue from a dose of ^{131}I is delivered during the iodide phase, before the ^{131}I has been taken up by the tumor, and after PB^{131}I has been released by the tumor. The latter causes more prolonged irradiation because of the continual release of the PB^{131}I from the tumor and the slow rate of breakdown of the ^{131}I-containing compounds in the blood. Radiation to blood is dependent upon a number of factors in addition to the quantity of the isotope administered and the retention during the first 48 hours (Stanbury et al., 1952). Rawson and his associates (1951) reported a fatality in a patient who had received 638 mc. of ^{131}I over a 14 month period, an amount that had a calculated radiation dosage of 1300 rep to the blood. The authors suggested that no dose calculated to deliver more than 500 rep to the blood be given. The generally accepted median lethal range of whole-body irradiation is about 500 roentgens. Five of Stanbury's patients, who received 200 mc. of ^{131}I in one dose for the treatment of thyroid carcinoma, received a total blood radiation dosage ranging from 76 to 232 rep during the first 9 days. One patient given 250 mc. received 112 rep; another patient given 300 mc. of ^{131}I received 103 rep. The Advisory Committee of the Atomic Energy Commission found no evidence that a single dose of larger than 200 mc. was more effective in treating thyroid cancer than a dose of 200 mc. or slightly less. They therefore strongly advise that single treatment doses larger than 200 mc. should not be used. Our usual dose for a patient with residual uptake only in the thyroid area is 150 to 165 mc. Our usual initial dose for patients with metastases outside the thyroid area is 200 mc.

Toxic effects of radioiodine therapy

Local Swelling. Local swelling from radiation thyroiditis, the first sign of toxicity after a treatment dose, is relatively rare, but may begin as soon as 6 to 10 hours after the dose, and rarely after 3 days. One boy 10 years of age developed massive swelling of the entire right side of the neck, extending from mandible to clavicle, about 8 hours after an oral dose of 60 mc. The swelling was not associated with infection, pain, tenderness, heat, leukocytosis, or fever, and disappeared in 24 to 36 hours. Another patient had had total thyroidectomy, with removal of superior mediastinal nodes and segmental resection of part of the left lung, for carcinoma. The first treatment dose of 180 mc. of ^{131}I was followed by sudden dyspnea and signs of left jugular and left subclavian venous obstruction; these complications began about 28 hours after therapy and were maximal at 36 hours.

Alarming toxic reactions such as these are entirely unpredictable and were not expected in either of these patients. A reaction was expected in five other patients with significant invasion of the trachea by the tumor, but it did not occur.

One patient had signs of spinal cord compression with pain, weakness, and early atrophy of the left arm. The scan indicated uptake in the region of the fourth cervical vertebra. The patient was given 180 mc. of ^{131}I and experienced no untoward effect. Three months after an additional dose of 180 mc. of ^{131}I, her fourth cervical vertebra was reossified. The patient was myxedematous, and no radioiodine uptake was detected over this area of the spine; all pain and signs of cord compression had disappeared.

A 13-year-old boy had extensive metastases in his lungs with clubbed fingers, cyanosis, and dyspnea. His scan demonstrated uptake of ^{131}I in the lung metastases. He was given 180 mc. of ^{131}I and experienced no detectable respiratory complications.

Irradiation Sickness. Other signs of toxicity are anorexia, nausea, or vomiting from irradiation sickness. In the doses commonly employed, these symptoms are usually mild, although some patients refuse breakfast the morning after a treatment dose.

Radiation Sialadenitis. Patients may complain of a metallic taste in their mouths within a few hours after the administration of a treatment dose of ^{131}I, which is excreted in part via the salivary glands. Schiff (1947) found that some euthyroid patients had saliva-to-serum ^{131}I ratios as high as 40:1 to 300:1. Schneyer (1953) reported that ^{131}I administered for treatment of thyroid cancer or hyperthyroidism may reversibly suppress salivary gland function.

Goolden et al. (1957) observed two patients who developed acute symptoms of radiation sialadenitis within 24 hours after a treatment dose of 100 mc. and 200 mc. It was calculated that the first patient received 707 rads and the second patient 680 rads to the salivary glands within the first 12 hours after the administration of the treatment dose. These authors point out that patients undergoing treatment for malignant disease of the mouth with x-rays or radium therapy almost invariably suffer from dryness of the mouth if both parotid glands are irradiated at dosage levels of the order of 500 to 1000 R.

We have observed mild tenderness of the submaxillary glands, but less commonly involvement of the parotid glands, after ^{131}I treatment. Swelling and tenderness of the submaxillary glands are more common after 3 months' treatment than in the first few days; they are usually associated with myxedema, and tend to disappear upon the administration of desiccated thyroid. In our experience, xerostomia after ^{131}I therapy is usually relieved when the induced myxedema is treated with thyroid medication.

Urinary Tract Effects. One of our patients with a large cystocele developed hematuria from cystitis after each treatment dose of 100 mc. Women should have a pelvic examination to check for the presence of this abnormality, since urine may be retained and produce an annoying cystitis. Although no other toxic effects have been noted in the urinary tract, renal insufficiency does result in retention of ^{131}I in the blood longer than usual. Therefore, the dose should be decreased to prevent excessive radiation. As small a dose as 50 mc. should be given initially, and after observation of its persistence in the blood and of its effect on the white blood cell count, one can determine whether a larger dose should be given subsequently.

Depression of Bone Marrow. Irradiation of bone marrow is increased by increased dosage of ^{131}I, poor uptake of ^{131}I in metastases, or decreased renal excretion of ^{131}I. Depression of bone marrow is increased by additional irradiation from x-ray sources, before, during, or after ^{131}I therapy. Resistance of bone marrow to irradiation is less in elderly persons, as well as persons with hypothyroidism (Kretchmar et al., 1952; Axelrod and Berman, 1951).

After large doses of ^{131}I, the lymphocyte count falls within a few hours, the leukocyte count within the first week, and the red cell and platelet counts within 1 or more weeks. The lymphocyte count is the last to recover (Kretchmar et al., 1952).

Of 57 patients treated with ^{131}I (Beierwaltes et al., 1956), 4 patients developed mild anemia and leukopenia; no depression of platelet count occurred. All had myxedema at the time of the blood changes; the latter returned to normal when a euthyroid state was produced by the administration of desiccated thyroid. The onset of myxedema in a woman of menstrual age may result in decompensation of hypoplastic marrow and in uterine hemorrhage (Goldsmith et al., 1952). Two patients, in whom myxedema was induced in the treatment of carcinoma of the thyroid, developed uterine hemorrhage so severe that they had to be hospitalized for transfusions.

In summary, a few practical suggestions can help to avoid severe depression of bone marrow function: (1) single doses larger than 200 mc. of ^{131}I should not be given; (2) smaller than usual doses should be given if uremia is present; (3) a patient should not be treated with doses at less than 3 month intervals, since the maximum effect from one dose will not become evident for at least that period of time (Maloof and Chapman, 1951); also, red blood cell and platelet counts may not fall to their lowest level within 2 to 3 months (Reinhard et al., 1946); (4) a patient who has leukopenia and is myxedematous should not be given additional doses, but should be given thyroid replacement therapy until his bone marrow has recovered; this usually occurs within 2 or 3 months, and thyroid medication is then stopped 6 weeks before retreatment; (5) a treatment dose of ^{131}I should not be given within 1 or 2 weeks of a course of x-ray irradiation to the neck nodes, lungs, or bones; (6) if depression of blood platelets occurs, further doses may result in the development of aplastic anemia.

Ovarian Function. A frequent question is whether exposure to ^{131}I will cause sterility. Studies of tissue concentration of ^{131}I at postmorten examination at varying periods after treatment doses of ^{131}I indicate low concentrations in gonads (Trunnell et al., 1950; Kurland and Freedberg, 1951). No patient under the age of 35 years is known to have ceased menstruating as a result of ^{131}I medication (Beierwaltes, 1952). Patients have also become pregnant despite therapeutic doses of 130 mc. of [131]I. One of our patients, a 19 year old girl, was given 362 mc. of ^{131}I in four divided doses over a period of 11 months for thyroid carcinoma that had metastasized to both lungs. She had had a total surgical thyroidectomy, and the carcinoma did not concentrate ^{131}I to a degree that prevented a relatively high plasma ^{131}I level; yet at no time did she experience disturbance of her menstrual cycle. She subsequently became pregnant and has had three normal children. Another 32 year old woman conceived despite induced myxedema and total amenorrhea. She delivered a normal boy 9.5 months after a 100 mc. treatment dose of [131]I. It must be emphasized, however, that *pregnancy is a contraindication to ^{131}I therapy.*

Each patient should be checked thoroughly for a thyroid tumor near the gonads before ^{131}I therapy is begun. If a patient has a teratoma of the ovary or testis, or a metastasis in pelvic bone that concentrates ^{131}I avidly, the gonads and other pelvic organs could receive high levels of radiation.

One instance of sterility following ^{131}I therapy has been reported (Kammer and Goodman, 1959) in a man who received 563 mc. in two doses; it is uncertain whether he was kept in a euthyroid state by replacement medication.

Radiation Pneumonitis and Fibrosis. Pulmonary insufficiency has resulted from irradiation with ^{131}I of thyroid carcinoma metastatic to the lungs (Rall et al., 1957). Two patients died, whereas four others showed x-ray evidence of pulmonary fibrosis. The authors concluded from their data that when a patient has diffuse metastasis in the lungs, a dose of 100 mc. of ^{131}I may deliver as much as 1000 to 2000 rads to the lungs. In such patients, an attempt should be made to keep the amount of ^{131}I in the lungs less than 125 mc.

URINARY EXCRETION OF ^{131}I AFTER TREATMENT DOSE

Patients are hospitalized for a treatment dose of ^{131}I for carcinoma of the thyroid so that they may be observed closely for local swelling of a strategically placed metastasis. In addition, the AEC requires hospitalization of any patient whose body contains 50 mc. or more of [131]I. When the total-body content of radiation drops below this figure, the patient may safely urinate into the usual sewerage system. We therefore measure the amount of radioactive iodine collected in each 24 hour urine sample and subtract this quantity of radioactivity from the amount initially administered to the patient, with suitable correction for decay, to determine when the patient may be discharged. It has been found necessary to carefully instruct the patient to collect the urine passed before having a bowel movement, to avoid losses of radioactivity.

Although we have observed wide variation from patient to patient in the rate of urinary excretion of ^{131}I, depending upon the functional capacity and total mass of the metastases, most patients given 100 mc. of ^{131}I will be ready for discharge after 3 days. Survey instruments may also be used to determine when a level of less than 7 milliroentgens per hour is emitted at the bedside near the patient's body. Thirty millicuries of ^{131}I produces a gamma ray exposure of roughly 9 mr. per hour 1 meter from the patient.

POST-TREATMENT HYPOTHYROIDISM

When the patient returns for the first follow-up examination, 3 months later, the classic clinical features of myxedema may not yet have become manifest. The serum PBI falls promptly after the source of thyroid hormone has been destroyed, and consequently the PBI is a good index of thyroid function under these circumstances. Since thyroid hormone continues to exert its effect on body cells for some time after the serum PBI falls (Lowenstein et al., 1945), the BMR and serum cholesterol have been found to be less reliable.

When the patient becomes totally myxedematous and no further uptake can be demonstrated in metastases, or all palpable and visible metastases are gone, no further ^{131}I treatment should be given.

TREATMENT WITH THYROID HORMONE

It has been stated that the myxedematous person is a happy "vegetable" with impaired intelligence and poor memory, who takes the ordinary troubles of life without the usual reaction to life's stresses. In our experience, this is not true. Housewives say that they are painfully aware of their myxedematous condition because they neglect their duties. One young physician had to stop practice because of ^{131}I-induced myxedema. Therefore, desiccated thyroid has been used to maintain the euthyroid state during treatment of thyroid carcinoma with ^{131}I, with TSH given just before treatment with ^{131}I to stimulate concentration of ^{131}I by metastases (Sturgeon et al., 1953). The regimen is as follows: (1) total thyroidectomy is followed by maintenance therapy with desiccated thyroid or l-thyroxine; (2) intramuscular or intravenous administration of 15 mg. of TSH is given twice a day for 5 or 6 days; (3) a tracer study is used to establish accumulation of radioactivity in the thyroid or other parts of the body, and the 72 hour urinary excretion of the tracer is measured; (4) if significant retention is found, a therapeutic dose of ^{131}I is given; (5) thyroid medication is continued, and TSH is again given during a repeat tracer test in 6 months.

We do not maintain the patient in a euthyroid state until he has been treated with ^{131}I to the point at which no further significant concentration of a tracer dose can be demonstrated. When TSH is stopped, the thyroid concentration of ^{131}I drops within a few days to lower levels than were present before TSH was administered. Furthermore, when thyroid medication is not administered, ^{131}I has been found in thyroid tissue 3 months after administration of a treatment dose of [131]I (Rawson et al., 1951). Daily administration of TSH for 3 months is not practical because of its expense. In addition, it may result in the formation of antibodies that nullify its effect.

RESULTS (HAYNIE, NOFAL, AND BEIERWALTES, 1963)

Two hundred patients with thyroid carcinoma received treatment at the University of Michigan between September 1947 and December 1960. During 1960 and 1961, follow-up examinations were performed on 76 per cent by means of thyroid function tests, x-rays, and radioiodine tests, with scans as the primary means of establishing freedom from disease. Twenty-two per cent of the patients died and 2 per cent were lost to follow-up. Sixty-seven per cent (52 of 82) of patients who proved to have had regional lymph node metastases that accumulated ^{131}I were apparently free of disease subsequently. Fifty-three per cent (30 of 82) of those patients with distant metastases that proved to accumulate ^{131}I were free of evidence of disease. In the other patients there had been no evidence of concentration of radioiodine in metastases.

The best results were obtained in young patients with well differentiated carcinoma. The usual total dose was about 150 mc., but those patients with distant metastases required about 350 mc. Although the mean follow-up interval was only about 5 years, the results are significant, since it was found that those patients who died of carcinoma did so within an average period of 2 years after treatment. No patient who was clinically free of disease for 3 years after completion of therapy was observed to have a subsequent recurrence of carcinoma.

REFERENCES

Alexander, W. D., Koutras, D. A., Crooks, J., Buchanan, W. W., MacDonald, E. M., Richmond, M. H., and Wayne, E. J.: Quantitative Studies of Iodine Metabolism in Thyroid Disease. Quart. J. Med. 31:281, 1962.

Andros, G., Harper, P. B., Lathrop, K. A., and McCardle, R. J.: Pertechnetate-99m Localization in Man with Applications to Thyroid Scanning and the Study of Thyroid Physiology. J. Endocrin. & Metabol. 25:1067, 1965.

Andrus, E. C.: Clinical and Experimental Observations Upon the Heart in Hyperthyroidism. Trans. Ass. Amer. Physicians 47:47, 1932.

Astwood, E. B.: Chemotherapy of Hyperthyroidism. Harvey Lect. 40:195, 1944–1945.

Atkins, H. L., and Richards, P.: Thyroid Trapping Function as Measured with Pertechnetate (Abstract). Read at 52nd Meeting of Radiological Society of North America, Chicago, November, 1966.

Axelrod, A. R., and Berman, L.: The Bone Marrow in Hyperthyroidism and Hypothyroidism. Blood 6:436, 1951.

Barker, S. B., Humphrey, M. J., and Soley, M. H.: The Clinical Determination of Protein-Bound Iodine. J. Clin. Invest. 30:55, 1951.

Beahrs, O. H., Pemberton, J., and Black, B. M.: Nodular Goiter and Malignant Lesions of the Thyroid Gland. J. Clin. Endocr. 11:1157, 1951.

Beckers, C., Crombrugghe, B., and de Visscher, M.: Dynamic Disturbances of Intrathyroid Iodine Metabolism in Sporadic Nontoxic Goiter. J. Clin. Endocr. 24:327, 1964.

Beierwaltes, W. H.: Irradiation of the Pituitary in the Treatment of Malignant Exophthalmos. J. Clin. Endocr. 11:512, 1951.

Beierwaltes, W. H.: The Status of Radioiodine Therapy. In Brucer, M.: Internally Administered Isotopes for Cancer Therapy and New Developments in Teletherapy. Nucleonics 10:46, 1952. Presented in part in Beierwaltes, W. H.: Indications and Contraindications for Treatment of Thyroid Cancer with Radioactive Iodine. Ann. Int. Med. 37:23, 1952.

Beierwaltes, W. H.: X-Ray Treatment for Malignant Exophthalmos: A Report on 28 Patients. J. Clin. Endocr. 13:1090, 1953.

Beierwaltes, W. H., and Johnson, P. C.: Hyperthyroidism Treated with Radioiodine: A Seven-Year Experience. AMA Arch. Int. Med. 97:393, 1956.

Beierwaltes, W. H., and Robbins, J.: Familiar Increase in Thyroxine-Binding Sites in Serum Alpha Globulin. J. Clin. Invest. 38:1683, 1959.

Beling, U., and Einhorn, J.: Incidence of Hypothyroidism and Recurrence Following I[131] Treatment of Hyperthyroidism. Acta Radiol. 56:275, 1961.

Berson, S. A., and Yalow, R. S.: Quantitative Aspects of Iodine Metabolism. The Exchangeable Organic Iodine Pool, and the Rates of Thyroidal Secretion, Peripheral Degradation and Fecal Excretion of Endogenously Synthesized Organically Bound Iodine. J. Clin. Invest. 33:1533, 1954.

Berson, S. A., and Yalow, R. S.: Iodine Metabolism and the Thyroid Gland. New York J. Med. 63:35, 1963.

Berson, S. A., Yalow, R. S., Sorrentino, J., and Roswit, B.: The Determination of Thyroidal and Renal Plasma I[131] Clearance Ratios as a Routine Diagnostic Test of Thyroid Dysfunction. J. Clin. Invest. 31:141, 1952.

Blizzard, R. M., and Chandler, R. W.: The History and Present Concepts of Autoimmunization in Thyroid Disease. J. Pediat. 57:399, 1960.

Blomfield, G. W., Eckert, H., Fisher, M., Miller, H., Munro, D. S., and Wilson, G. M.: Treatment of Thyrotoxicosis with I[131]: A Review of 500 Cases. Brit. Med. J. 1:63, 1959.

Bloom, P. S., and Terpstra, J.: High PBI[131] Concentration in Blood of Patients with Myxedema: Preliminary Report. J. Clin. Endocr. 13:989, 1953.

Bowers, C. Y., Murison, P. J., Gordon, D. L., and Locke, W.: Effect of Thyrotropin on the Serum Protein-Bound Iodine Level in Various Thyroid States (TSH-PBI test). J. Clin. Endocr. 21:465, 1961.

Brown-Grant, K.: Extrathyroidal Iodide Concentrating Mechanisms. Physiol. Rev. 41:189, 1961.

Buchanan, W. W., Alexander, W. D., Crooks, J., Koutras, D. A., Wayne, E. J., Anderson, J. R., and Goudie, R. B.: Association of Thyrotoxicosis and Autoimmune Thyroiditis. Brit. Med. J. 1:843, 1961.

Buchanan, W. W., Koutras, D. A., Alexander, W. D., Crooks, J., Richmond, M. H., MacDonald, E. M., and Wayne, E. J.: Iodine Metabolism in Hashimoto's Thyroiditis. J. Clin. Endocr. 21:806, 1961.

Chapman, E. M., Maloof, F., Moisterrena, J., and Martin, J. M.: Ten Years' Experience with Radioactive Iodine. J. Clin. Endocr. 14:45, 1954.

Chatin, A.: Series of papers. C.R. Acad. Sci. 1850–1876.

Chattaway, F. D.: The Discovery of Iodine. Chem. News 99:193, 1909.

Childs, D. S., Jr., Keating, F. R., Jr., Rall, J. E., Williams, M., and Power, M. H.: The Effect of Varying Quantities of Inorganic Iodide (Carrier) on the Urinary Excretion and Thyroidal Accumulation of Radioiodine in Exophthalmic Goiter. J. Clin. Invest. 29:726,1950.

Clark, D. E., Moe, R. H., and Adams, E. E.: The Rate of Conversion of Administered Inorganic Radioactive Iodine into Protein-Bound Iodine of Plasma as an Aid in the Evaluation of Thyroid Function. Surgery 26:331, 1949.

Clark, D. E., and Rule, J. H.: Radioactive Iodine or Surgery in Treatment of Hyperthyroidism. J.A.M.A. 159:995, 1955.

Clements, F. W., and Wishart, J. W.: A Thyroid-Blocking Agent in the Etiology of Endemic Goiter. Metabolism 5:623, 1956.

Coindet, J. C.: Discouverte d'un Nouveau Remède Contre le Goitre. Bibl. Universelle Sci., Belleslettres, et Arts, Faisant Suites Bibl. Britannique 14:190, 1820.

Crile, G., Jr., and Schneider, R. W.: Diagnosis and Treatment of Thyroiditis with Special Reference to the Use of Cortisone and ACTH. Cleveland Clin. Quart. 19:219, 1952.

Crispell, K. R., Parson, W., Hollifield, G. F., and Alrich, E. M.: The Use of Radioactive Iodine to Prepare Patients with Toxic Nodular Goiter for Surgery. Trans. Amer. Goiter Ass. 1955.

Crooks, J., Aboul-Khair, S. A., Turnbull, A. C., and Hytten, F. E.: The Incidence of Goiter During Pregnancy. Lancet 2:334, 1964.

Curran, R. C., Eckert, H., and Wilson, G. M.: The Thyroid Gland After Treatment of Hyperthyroidism by Partial Thyroidectomy or Iodine-131. J. Path. Bact. 76:541, 1958.

Danowski, T. S.: Thyroiditis. Clin. Endocr. 2:429, 1962.

Degrossi, O., Gotta, H., Olivari, A., Pecorini, V., and Chwojnik, A.: Possibilities of Using Tc-99m in Place of Radioiodine in Thyroid Function Studies. Nuclearmedizin 4:383, 1965.

DeRobertis, E., and Grasso, R.: Peroxidase Activity of the Thyroid Gland Under Normal and Experimental Conditions. Endocrinology 38:137, 1946.

Dobyns, B. M.: The Influence of Thyroidectomy on the Prominence of the Eyes in the Guinea Pig and in Man. Surg. Gynec. Obstet. 80:526, 1945.

Dobyns, B. M., and Lennon, B.: A Study of the Histopathology and Physiologic Function of Thyroid Tumors, Using Radioactive Iodine and Radioautography. J. Clin. Endocr. 8:732, 1948.

Doniach, I.: Experimental Induction of Tumours of the Thyroid by Radiation. Brit. Med. Bull. 14:181, 1958.

Doniach, D., Hudson, R. V., and Roitt, I. M.: Diagnostic Aspects of Lymphadenoid Goiter. Proc. Roy. Soc. Med. 50:946, 1957.

Doniach, D., Hudson, R. V., and Roitt, I. M.: Human Autoimmune Thyroiditis: Clinical Studies. Brit. Med. J. 1:365, 1960.

Doniach, D., and Roitt, I. M.: Auto-Antibodies in Disease. Ann. Rev. Med. 13:213, 1962.

Dowling, J. T., Micoloff, J. T., and Holvey, D. N.: The Use of Iodine[132] in the Rapid Detection of Defective Thyroidal Organic Iodinations. Presented at the American Thyroid Association Meeting, Chicago, 1963.

El Kabir, D. J., Doniach, D., and Turner-Warwick, R.: Serum Content of Thyrothyroiditis: Low TSH Levels with High Radioiodine Uptake in Mild Autoimmune Thyroiditis. J. Clin. Endocr. 23:6, 1963.

Ermans, A. M., Dumont, J. E., and Bastenie, P. A.: Thyroid Function in a Goitrous Endemic. II. Nonhormonal Iodine Escape from the Goitrous Gland. J. Clin. Endocr. 23:550, 1963.

Fitzgerald, P. J., and Foote, F. W.: The Function of Various Types of Thyroid Carcinoma as

Revealed by the Radioautographic Demonstration of Radioactive Iodine (I[131]). *J. Clin. Endocr.* 9:1153, 1949.

Floyd, J. C., Jr., Beierwaltes, W. H., Dodson, V. N., and Carr, E. A., Jr.: Defective Organic Binding of Iodine as a Cause of Nodular Goiter. *J. Clin. Endocr.* 34:133, 1960.

Frantz, V. K.: *In* Clark, D. E., Ed.: Proceedings of the Conference on Radioiodine. Argonne Cancer Research Hospital, USAEC and the Clinics of the University of Chicago, November, 1956.

Fraser, R., Hobson, Q. J. G., Arnott, D. G., and Emry, E. W.: The Urinary Excretion of Radioiodine as a Clinical Test of Thyroid Function. *Quart. J. Med.* 22:99, 1953.

Freedberg, A. S., Blumgart, H. L., Kurland, G. S., and Chamovitz, D. L.: The Treatment of Euthyroid Cardiac Patients with Intractable Angina Pectoris and Congestive Failure with Radioactive Iodine. *J. Clin. Endocr.* 10:1270, 1950.

Fromm, G. A., Lascano, E. F., and Enriori, C.: Estruma Linfoideo (Enfermedad de Hashimoto). *Endocrinología (Buenos Aires)* 1:86, 1950.

Fyfe, A.: Accounts of Some Experiments Made with the View of Ascertaining the Different Substances from Which Iodine Can Be Procured. *Edinburgh Philos. J.* 1:254, 1819.

Goldberg, R. C., and Chaikoff, I. L.: Induction of Thyroid Cancer in the Rat by Radioactive Iodine. *Arch. Path. (Chicago)* 53:22, 1952.

Goldsmith, R. E., Sturgis, S. H., Lerman, J., and Stanbury, J. B.: The Menstrual Pattern in Thyroid Disease. *J. Clin. Endocr.* 12:846, 1952.

Goolden, A. W. G.: A Comparison of Radioiodine Tests With the Diagnosis of Hyperthyroidism. *Brit. J. Radiol.* 31:433, 1958.

Goolden, A. W. G., Mallard, J. R., and Farran, H. E. A.: Radiation Sialadenitis Following Radioiodine Therapy. *Brit. J. Radiol.* 30:210, 1957.

Gordon, E. S., and Goldberg, M.: Carbon-14 Studies of Energy Metabolism in Various Thyroid States. *Metabolism* 13:591, 1964.

Goudie, R. B., Anderson, J. R., and Gray, K. G.: Complement-Fixing Anti-Thyroid Antibodies in Hospital Patients with Asymptomatic Thyroid Lesions. *J. Path. Bact.* 47:389, 1959.

Gould, R. G., LeRoy, G. V., Okita, G. T., Kabara, J. J., Keegan, D., and Bergenstal, D. M.: Use of C[14]-Labeled Acetate to Study Cholesterol Metabolism in Man. *J. Lab. Clin. Med.* 46:372, 1955.

Grayson, R. R.: Factors Which Influence the Radioactive Iodine Thyroidal Uptake Test. *Amer. J. Med.* 28:397, 1960.

Green, M.: Thyrotoxicosis Treated by Surgery or Iodine-131: With Special Reference to Development of Hypothyroidism. *Brit. Med. J.* 1:1005, 1964.

Greer, M. A., and DeGroot, L. J.: The Effect of Stable Iodine on Thyroid Secretion in Man. *Metabolism* 5:682, 1956.

Greer, M. A., and Shull, H. F.: A Quantitative Study of the Effect of Thyrotropin Upon the Thyroidal Secretion Rate in Euthyroid and Thyrotoxic Subjects. *J. Clin. Endocr.* 17:1030, 1957.

Hadjidakis, S. G., Koutras, D. A., and Daikos, G. K.: Endemic Goiter in Greece: Family Studies. *J. Med. Genet.* 1:82, 1964.

Hall, R.: Immunologic Aspects of Thyroid Function. *New Eng. J. Med.* 266:1204, 1962.

Halmi, N. S.: Thyroidal Iodide Transport. *Vitamins Hormones (N.Y.)* 19:133, 1961.

Hamilton, J. G., and Lawrence, J. H.: Recent Clinical Developments in the Therapeutic Application of Radio-Phosphorus and Radio-Iodine. *J. Clin. Invest.* 21:624, 1942.

Hamolsky, M. W., Stein, M., and Freedberg, A. S.: The Thyroid Hormone-Plasma Protein Complex in Man. II. A New In Vitro Method for Study of Uptake of Labeled Hormonal Components by Human Erythrocytes. *J. Clin. Endocr.* 17:33, 1957.

Harington, C. R.: Chemistry of Thyroxine. II. Constitution and Synthesis of Desiodo-thyroxine. *Biochem. J.* 20:300, 1926.

Harland, W. A.: Morphology of the Thyroid Gland in Jamaica. *J. Clin. Endocr.* 24:580, 1964.

Harland, W. A., and Frantz, V. K.: Clinicopathologic Study of 261 Surgical Cases of So-Called "Thyroiditis." *J. Clin. Endocr.* 16:1433, 1956.

Harper, P. V., Beck, R., Charleston, D., and Lathrop, K. A.: Optimization of a Scanning Method Using Tc-99m. *Nucleonics* 22:50, 1964.

Hashimoto, H.: Zur Kenntnis der Lymphomatösen Veränderung der Schilddrüse (Struma Lymphomatosa). *Arch. Klin. Chir.* 97:219, 1912.

Haynie, T. P., Nofal, M. M., and Beierwaltes, W. H.: Treatment of Thyroid Carcinoma with I-131. Results at Fourteen Years. *J.A.M.A.* 183:303, 1963.

Hazard, J. B., and Kaufman, N.: Survey of Thyroid Glands Obtained at Autopsy in So-Called Goiter Area. *Amer. J. Clin. Path.* 22:860, 1952.

Hertz, S., and Roberts, A.: Application of Radioactive Iodine in Therapy of Graves' Disease. *J. Clin. Invest.* 21:624, 1942.

Hertz, S., Roberts, A., and Evans, R. D.: Radioactive Iodine as an Indicator in the Study of Thyroid Physiology. *Proc. Soc. Exp. Biol. Med.* 38:510, 1938.

Hodges, R. E., Evans, T. C., Bradbury, J. T., and Keettel, W. C.: The Accumulation of Radioactive Iodine by Human Fetal Thyroids. *J. Clin. Endocr.* 15:661, 1955.

Hurxthal, L. M., et al.: Ten to Twenty Year Results Following Subtotal Thyroidectomy for Primary Hyperthyroidism Operated on Before 1927. *Surg. Clin. N. Amer.* 25:651, 1945.

Johnson, D. E., Solomon, D. H., and Greer, M. A.: The Effect of Triiodothyronine and Thyroxine Upon the Rate of Release of Thyroid Hormone in Various Thyroid States. *J. Clin. Endocr.* 19:317, 1959.

Johnson, P. C., and Redding, T. R.: Glucose-l-C[14] Oxidation by Blood: A Potential Test for Tissue Effects of Thyrotoxicosis. *J. Nucl. Med.* 4:393, 1963.

Johnson, P. C., Redding, T. R., Wade, L., and Jona, J.: A Metabolic Defect Associated with Exophthalmos and Thyroid Disease. *Clin. Res.* 11:220, 1963.

Kammer, H., and Goodman, M. J.: Sterility After Radioiodine Therapy for Metastatic Thyroid Carcinoma. *J.A.M.A.* 171:1963, 1959.

Keating, F. R., Jr., and Albert, A.: The Metabolism of Iodine in Man as Disclosed with the Use of Radioiodine. *Recent Progr. Hormone Res.* 4:429, 1949.

Keating, F. R., Jr., Patterson, H. A., and Vanderlaan, W. P.: Radioactive Iodine, Surgery or Antithyroid Drugs in Treatment of Graves' Disease. *Postgrad. Med.* 23:78, 1958.

Kelly, F. C., and Snedden, W. W.: Prevalence and Geographical Distribution of Endemic Goiter. *Bull. WHO* 18:5, 1958.

Kelly, F. C., and Snedden, W. W.: Prevalence and Geographical Distribution of Endemic Goiter. *In* Endemic Goiter. WHO, Geneva, 1960.

Kendall, E. C.: The Isolation in Crystalline Form of the Compound Containing Iodine Which Occurs in the Thyroid. *J.A.M.A.* 64:2042, 1915.

Kilpatrick, R., Blomfield, G. W., Neal, F. E., and Wilson, G. M.: Carcinoma of the Thyroid, A Review of 100 Cases. *Quart. J. Med.* 26:209, 1957.

Kilpatrick, R., Milne, J. S., Rushbrooke, M., and Wilson, G. M.: A Survey of Thyroid Enlargement in Two General Practices in Great Britain. *Brit. Med. J.* 1:29, 1963.

Kimball, O. P.: History of the Prevention of Endemic Goiter. *Bull. WHO* 9:241, 1953.

Kinsell, L. W., Michaels, A. D., and Imaichi, K.: Studies with Fat Emulsions. Metabolism of Intravenously Administered ^{14}C-Tripalmitin. *Amer. J. Clin. Nutr.* 16:97, 1965.

Kirland, R. H.: Impaired Organic Binding of Radioiodine by the Thyroid Following Radioiodine Treatment of Hyperthyroidism. *J. Clin. Endocr.* 14:565, 1954.

Koutras, D. A., Alexander, W. D., Buchanan, W. W., Crooks, J., and Wayne, E. J.: Stable Iodine Metabolism in Nontoxic Goiter. *Lancet* 2:784, 1960.

Koutras, D. A., Alexander, W. D., Buchanan, W. W., Crooks, J., and Wayne, E. J.: Studies of Stable Metabolism as a Guide to the Interpretation of Radioiodine Tests. *Acta Endocr.* (*Kbh.*) 37:597, 1961.

Kretchmar, A. L., Gomberg, H. G., Weyant, D. E., and Bethell, F. H.: The Effect of Thyroidectomy on the Mortality and Peripheral Blood Changes of the Rat Subjected to Whole Body X-Irradiation. *Endocrinology* 51:59, 1952.

Kurland, G. S., and Freedberg, A. S.: The Distribution of I[131] in Tissues Obtained at Necropsy or at Surgical Operation in Man. *J. Clin. Endocr.* 11:843, 1951.

Lahey, F. H., and Hurxthal, L. M.: Postoperative End-Results in Three Hundred Thyrocardiacs. *Amer. J. Surg.* 24:225, 1934.

Lindsay, S., Daily, M. E., Friedlander, J., Yee, G., and Soley, M. H.: Chronic Thyroiditis: Clinical and Pathologic Study of 354 Paitents. *J. Clin. Endocr.* 12:1578, 1952.

Lipsky, S. R., Bondy, P. K., Man, E. B., and McGuire, J. S.: Effects of Triiodothyronine on Biosynthesis of Plasma Lipids from Acetate-l-^{14}C in Myxedematous Subjects. *J. Clin. Invest.* 34:950, 1955.

London, W. T., Koutras, D. A., Pressman, A., and Vought, R. L.: Epidemiologic and Metabolic Studies of a Goiter Endemic in Eastern Kentucky. *J. Clin. Endocr.* 25:1091, 1965.

Lowenstein, B. E., Bruger, M., Hinton, J. W., and Lough, W. G.: The Protein-Bound Plasma Iodine in Patients with Thyroid Diseases. II. The Effect of Thiouracil. *J. Clin. Endocr.* 5:181, 1945.

Lowrey, R., and Starr, P.: Chemical Evidence of Incidence of Hypothyroidism. *J.A.M.A.* 171:2045, 1959.

Luxton, R. W., and Cooke, R. T.: Hashimoto's Struma Lymphomatosa; Diagnostic Value and Significance of Serum-Flocculation Reactions. *Lancet* 2:105, 1956.

Macksood, W., Rapport, A. L., and Hodges, F.: The Increasing Incidence of Hashimoto's Disease. *Arch. Surg.* (*Chicago*) 83:384, 1961.

Magalotti, M. F., Hummon, I. F., and Hierschbiel, E.: The Effect of Disease and Drugs on the Twenty-Four Hour I[131] Thyroid Uptake. *Amer. J. Roentgen.* 81:47, 1959.

Maloof, F., and Chapman, E. M.: Responses to Radioactive Iodine Therapy in Hyperthyroidism, with Special Reference to Cardiac Problems. *J. Clin. Endocr.* 11:1296, 1951.

Maloof, F., Dobyns, B. M., and Vickery, A. L.: The Effects of Various Doses of Radioactive Iodine on the Function and Structure of the Thyroid of the Rat. *Endocrinology* 50:612, 1952.

Marine, D.: Endemic Goiter: A Problem in Preventive Medicine. *Ann. Int. Med.* 41:875, 1954.

Marshall, S. F., Meissner, W. A., and Smith, D. C.: Chronic Thyroiditis. *New Eng. J. Med.* 238:758, 1948.

Masi, A. T.: Hashimoto's Disease—An Epidemiological Study Based on a Community-Wide Hospital Survey. *J. Chronic Dis.* 18:35, 1965.

Masi, A. T., Hartmann, W. H., and Shulman, L. E.: Hashimoto's Disease—An Epidemiological Critique. *J. Chronic Dis.* 18:1, 1965.

McConahey, W. M., Keating, F. R., Jr., Beahrs, O. H., and Woolner, L. B.: On the Increasing Occurrence of Hashimoto's Thyroiditis. *J. Clin. Endocr.* 22:542, 1962.

McConahey, W. M., Keating, F. R., Jr., Butt, H. R., and Owen, C. A., Jr.: Comparison of Certain Laboratory Tests in the Diagnosis of Hashimoto's Thyroiditis. *J. Clin. Endocr.* 21:879, 1961.

McConahey, W. M., Owen, C. A., Jr., and Keating, F. R., Jr.: A Clinical Appraisal of Radioiodine Tests of Thyroid Function. *J. Clin. Endocr.* 16:724, 1956.

McCullagh, E. P.: Radioactive Iodine in the Treatment of Hyperthyroidism. *Ann. Int. Med.* 37:739, 1952.

McDermott, W. V., Jr., Morgan, W. S., Hamlin, E., Jr., and Cope, O.: Cancer of the Thyroid. *J. Clin. Endocr.* 14:1336, 1954.

McGirr, E. M.: Sporadic Goitrous Cretinism. *Brit. Med. Bull.* 16:113, 1960.

Means, J. H.: The Thyroid and Its Diseases. J. B. Lippincott Co., Philadelphia, 1948.

Means, J. H., DeGroot, L. J., and Stanbury, J. B.: The Thyroid and Its Diseases. Ed. 3. McGraw-Hill Book Co., New York, 1963.

Means, J. H., and Lerman, J.: The Curves of Thyroxine Decay in Myxedema and of Iodine Response in Thyrotoxicosis: Their Similarity and Its Possible Significance. *Ann. Int. Med.* 12:811, 1938.

Mitchell, M. L., Burrows, B. A., and Ross, J. F.: The Relationship Between Clinical and Laboratory Findings in Hyperthyroidism and the Response to Radio-Iodine Therapy. *Clin. Res. Proc.* 3:121, 1955.

Mitchell, M. L., O'Rourke, M. E., and Harden, A. B.: Resin Uptake of Radiothyroxine from Serum in Thyroid Diseases and in Pregnancy. *J. Clin. Endocr.* 21:1448, 1961.

Modell, W.: Observations on Structures of Blood Vessels Within Thyroid Gland of Dog. *Anat. Rec.* 55:251, 1933.

Morgans, M. E., and Trotter, W. R.: Defective Organic Binding of Iodine by the Thyroid in Hashimoto's Thyroiditis. *Lancet* 1:533, 1957.

Mortensen, J. D., Woolner, L. B., and Bennett, W. A.: Gross and Microscopic Findings in Clinically Normal Thyroid Glands. *J. Clin. Endocr.* 15:1270, 1955.

Mosier, H. D., Armstrong, M. K., and Shultz, M. A.: Measurement of the Early Uptake of Radioactive Iodine by the Thyroid Gland. *Pediatrics* 31:426, 1963.

Murray, I. P., and McGirr, E. M.: Radioactive Iodine Studies in the Diagnosis of Hashimoto's Thyroiditis. *Brit. Med. J.* 1:838, 1960.

Mustacchi, P., and Cutler, S. J.: Some Observations on Incidence of Thyroid Cancer in United States. *New Eng. J. Med.* 255:889, 1956.

Myant, N. B.: Prognostic Value of Early Tests of Thyroid Function After Treatment of Thyrotoxicosis by I[131]. *Brit. J. Radiol.* 26:139, 1953.

Myant, N. B., Corbett, B. D., Honour, A. J., and Pochin, E. E.: Distribution of Radioiodine in Man. *Clin. Sci.* 9:405, 1950.

Myant, N. B., Pochin, E. E., and Goldie, E. A. G.: The Plasma Iodide Clearance Rate of the Human Thyroid. *Clin. Sci.* 8:109, 1949.

Myhill, J., Reeve, T. S., and Figgis, P. M.: Measurement of the Mass of the Thyroid Gland In Vivo. *Amer. J. Roentgen.* 44:828, 1956.

Nadler, N. J., Leblond, C. P., and Bogoroch, R.: The Rate of Iodine Metabolism by the Thyroid Follicle as a Function of Its Size. *Endocrinology* 54:154, 1954.

Nilsson, L. R., and Doniach, D.: Auto-Immune Thyroiditis in Children and Adolescents. I. Clinical Studies. *Acta Pediat.* (*Stockholm*) 53:255, 1964.

Nodine, J. H., Channick, B. J., Sokhos, D., Tassoni, S. D., and Perloff, W. H.: Measurement of the Active Iodine Stores and Daily Hormonal Output of the Intact Human Thyroid. *J. Clin. Endocr.* 17:832, 1957.

Osborn, S. B., and Smith, E. E.: The Genetically Significant Radiation Dose from the Diagnostic Use of X-Rays in England and Wales: A Preliminary Report. *Lancet* 1:949, 1956.

Peltola, P., and Krusius, F. E.: Effect of Cow's Milk from the Goiter Endemia District of Finland on Thyroid Function. *Acta Endocr.* (*Kbh.*) 33:603, 1960.

Pitt-Rivers, R.: Biochemistry and Physiology of the Thyroid Hormones. *New York J. Med.* 63:43, 1963.

Pitt-Rivers, R., and Cavalieri, R. R.: Free Iodotyrosines of the Thyroid. *Biochem. J.* 86:86, 1963.

Pochin, E. E.: The Examination of Thyroid Activity with Radioiodine. *Brit. J. Radiol.* 33:595, 1960.

Pochin, E. E.: Leukemia Following Radioiodine Treatment of Thyrotoxicosis. *Brit. Med. J.* 2: 1545, 1960.

Rall, J. E., et al.: Radiation Pneumonitis and Fibrosis: A Complication of Radioiodine Treatment of Pulmonary Metastases from Cancer of the Thyroid. *J. Clin. Endocr.* 17:1263, 1957.

Rawson, R. W., et al.: The Effect of Total Thyroidectomy on the Function of Metastatic Thyroid Cancer. *J. Clin. Endocr.* 8:826, 1948.

Rawson, R. W., Rall, J. E., and Peacock, W.: Limitations and Indications in the Treatment of Cancer of the Thyroid with Radioactive Iodine. *J. Clin. Endocr.* 11:1128, 1951.

Reinhard, E. H., Moore, C. V., Bierbaum, O. S., and Moore, S.: Radioactive Phosphorus as a Therapeutic Agent: A Review of the Literature and Analysis of the Results of Treatment of 155 Patients with Various Blood Dyscrasias, Lymphomas, and Other Malignant Neoplastic Diseases. *J. Lab. Clin. Med.* 31:107, 1946.

Renda, F., Holmes, R. A., North, W. A., and Wagner, H. N., Jr.: Characteristics of Thyroid Scans in Normal Persons, Hyperthyroidism and Nodular Goiter. *J. Nucl. Med.* 9:156, 1968.

Roitt, I. M., and Doniach, D.: Human Auto-Immune Thyroiditis. Serological Studies. *Lancet* 2:1027, 1958.

Schiff, L., et al.: Gastric (and Salivary) Excretion of Radioiodine in Man. Preliminary Report. *J. Nat. Cancer Inst.* 7:349, 1947.

Schneyer, L. H.: Effect of Administration of Radioactive Iodine on Human Salivary Gland Function. *J. Dent. Res.* 32:146, 1953.

Schultz, A. L., and Jacobson, W. E.: The Effect of Propylthiouracil on the Thyroid Uptake of I^{131} and the Plasma Conversion Ratio in Hyperthyroidism. *J. Clin. Endocr.* 12:1205, 1952.

Schultz, A. L., and Zieve, L.: Early Prediction of Success or Failure of Radioiodine Therapy of Hyperthyroidism. *J. Clin. Endocr.* 15:834, 1955.

Sharp, G.: The History of Iodine, the Iodides and Iodoform. *Pharm. J.* 91:98, 1913.

Skanse, B.: Radioactive Iodine in the Diagnosis of Thyroid Disease. *Acta Med. Scand.* 136:1, 1949.

Skanse, B. N.: Radioactive Iodine, Its Use in Studying the Urinary Excretion of Iodine by Humans in Various States of Thyroid Function. *Acta Med. Scand.* 131:251, 1948.

Skillern, P. G., Crile, G., McCullagh, E. P., Hayard, J. B., Lewis, L. A., and Brown, H.: Struma Lymphomatosa: Primary Thyroid Failure with Compensatory Thyroid Enlargement. *J. Clin. Endocr.* 16:35, 1956.

Skillern, P. G., McCullagh, E. P., and Clamen, M.: Radioiodine in Diagnosis and Therapy of Hyperthyroidism. *Arch. Intern. Med.* 110:6, 1962.

Sloan, L. W.: Of the Origin, Characteristics and Behavior of Thyroid Cancer. *J. Clin. Endocr.* 14:1309, 1954.

Soley, M. H., Miller, E. R., and Foreman, N.: Graves' Disease: Treatment with Radioiodine I^{131}. Symposium on Radioiodine. July, 1948.

Soley, M. H., Miller, E. R., and Foreman, N.: Graves' Disease: Treatment with Radioiodine (I^{131}). *J. Clin. Endocr.* 9:29, 1949.

Sos, J., Szabo, G., and Raksanyi, A.: Endemic Goiter and Its Prevention in Hungary. *Bull. WHO* 15:317, 1956.

Stanbury, J. B., et al.: The Metabolic Fate of I^{131} After Large Therapeutic Doses in Patients with Metastatic Carcinoma of the Thyroid. *J. Clin. Endocr.* 12:1480, 1952.

Stanbury, J. B., Brownell, G. L., Riggs, D. S., Perinetti, H., Itoiz, J., and Del Castillo, E. B.: Endemic Goiter. The Adaptation of Man to Iodine Deficiency. Harvard University Press, Cambridge, Mass., 1954.

Stanbury, J. B., and Chapman, G. M.: Congenital Hypothyroidism with Goitre. Absence of an Iodide Concentrating Mechanism. *Lancet* 1:1162, 1960.

Stanbury, J. B., and DeGroot, L. J.: Problem of Hypothyroidism After I^{131} Therapy of Hyperthyroidism. *New Eng. J. Med.* 271:195, 1964.

Stanbury, J. B., and Hedge, A. N.: A Study of a Family of Goitrous Cretins. *J. Clin. Endocr.* 10:1471, 1950.

Stanbury, J. B., Ohela, K., and Pitt-Rivers, R.: The Metabolism of Iodine in 2 Goitrous Cretins Compared with That in 2 Patients Receiving Methimazole. *J. Clin. Endocr.* 15:54, 1955.

Stanley, M. M.: The Direct Estimation of the Rate of Thyroid Hormone Formation in Man. The Effect of the Iodide Ion in Thyroid Iodine Utilization. *J. Clin. Endocr.* 9:941, 1949.

Sterling, K., and Chodos, R. B.: Radiothyroxine Turnover Studies in Myxedema Thyrotoxicosis and Hypermetabolism without Endocrine Disease. *J. Clin. Invest.* 35:806, 1956.

Sterling, K., and Tabachnick, M.: Resin Uptake of I[131] Triiodothyronine as a Test of Thyroid Function. *J. Clin. Endocr.* 21:456, 1961.

Sturgeon, C. T., et al.: Treatment of Thyroid Cancer Metastases with TSH and I[131] During Thyroid Hormone Medication. *J. Clin. Endocr.* 13:1391, 1953.

Terpstra, J., and Querido, A.: The Endemic Goiter in the Netherlands. *Acta Endocr. (Kbh.)* 31:433, 1959.

Thode, H. G., Jaimet, C. H., and Kirkwood, S.: Studies and Diagnostic Tests of Salivary and Thyroid Gland Function with Radioiodine. Radioisotope Conference 1954. Proceedings of the Second Conference. Oxford, England, 1954.

Triantaphyllidis, E.: Hétérogénéité fonctionelle de le glande thyroïde. *Arch. Sci. Physiol* 12:191, 1958.

Trotter, W. R., Belvayin, G., and Waddams, A.: Precipitating and Complement Fixing Antibodies in Hashimoto's Disease. *Proc. Roy. Soc. Med.* 50:961, 1957.

Trunnell, J. B.: The Treatment of Human Thyroid Disease with Radioactive Iodine. *Trans. N. Y. Acad. Sci.* 2:195, 1949.

Trunnell, J. B., et al.: The Distribution of Radioactive Iodine in Human Tissues: Necropsy Study in Nine Patients. *J. Clin. Endocr.* 10:1007, 1950.

Van Middlesworth, L.: *In* Radioisotopes in Animal Nutrition and Physiology. International Atomic Energy Agency, Vienna, 1965.

Virtanen, A. I.: On the Chemistry of Brassica Factors, Their Effect on the Function of Thyroid Gland, and Their Transfer to Milk. *Experientia* 17:6, 1961.

Visscher, R. P.: T3-I[131] Binding Capacity of Serum Proteins. *Amer. J. Obstet. Gynec.* 86:829, 1963.

Vought, R. L., and London, W. T.: Dietary Sources of Iodine. *Amer. J. Clin. Nutr.* 14:186, 1964.

Vought, R. L., and London, W. T.: Iodine Intake and Excretion in Healthy Nonhospitalized Subjects. *Amer. J. Clin. Nutr.* 15:124, 1964.

Wagner, H. N., Jr.: An Outline of the Use of Iodine in Endemic Goiter. *AMA Arch. Intern. Med.* 103:484, 1959.

Wayne, E., Blackburn, G., and Davis, R. H.: Today's Drugs. Treatment of Thyroid Disorders. *Brit. Med. J.* 5407:493, 1964.

Wayne, E. J.: Clinical and Metabolic Studies in Thyroid Disease. *Brit. Med. J.* 1:1, 1960.

Wayne, E. J., Koutras, D. A., and Alexander, W. D.: Clinical Aspects of Iodine Metabolism. F. A. Davis Co., Philadelphia, 1964.

Werner, S. C.: The Thyroid. Cassell and Co., London, 1955.

Werner, S. C., and Quimby, E. H.: The Use of Tracer Doses of Radioactive Iodine (I[131]) in the Study of Normal and Disordered Thyroid Function in Man. *J. Clin. Endocr.* 9:342, 1949.

Werner, S. C., Quimby, E. H., and Schmidt, C.: Radiactive Iodine, I[131], in the Treatment of Hyperthyroidism. *Amer. J. Med.* 7:731, 1949.

Williams, E. D., and Doniach, I.: The Post-Mortem Incidence of Focal Thyroiditis. *J. Path. Bact.* 83:255, 1962.

Witebsky, E., and Rose, N. R.: Studies on Organ Specificity. IV. Production of Rabbit Thyroid Antibodies in the Rabbit. *J. Immun.* 76:408, 1956.

Wollman, S. H.: Analysis of Radioiodine Therapy of Metastatic Tumors of the Thyroid Gland in Man. *J. Nat. Cancer Inst.* 13:815, 1953.

Wollman, S. H., Scow, R. O., Wagner, B., and Morris, H. P.: Radioactive Uptake by Transplantable Tumors of the Thyroid Gland in C3H Mice. I. Experimental Results. *J. Nat. Cancer Inst.* 13:785, 1953.

Woolner, L. B., McConahey, W. M., and Beahrs, O. H.: Struma Lymphomatosa (Hashimoto's Thyroiditis) and Related Thyroidal Disorders. *J. Clin. Endocr.* 19:53, 1959.

CHAPTER VIII

METABOLIC DISEASES

WALTON W. SHREEVE

E. JAMES POTCHEN

Understanding of dynamic biochemistry and physiology expanded greatly with the use of radioactive and stable isotopes of the common organic elements of the body, i. e., carbon, hydrogen, oxygen, nitrogen, phosphorus, and sulfur. Clinical use of these nuclides has developed more slowly, but undoubtedly they will provide major new diagnostic procedures in the future and, perhaps more important, better understanding of basic mechanisms of disease. Leroy (1955) has commented, "The future description of disease might well be a statement of the abnormality in the size of the (body) compartments, of the rate of exchange between them, and of the concentrations and rates of inter-conversion of substances within the compartments."

Deuterium was the first of this general class of isotopes to be applied to biological investigation (Rittenberg, 1949; Leroy, 1955). With the use of the mass spectrometer, the stable isotopes ^{15}N and ^{13}C were employed to elucidate further the "dynamic state of the body constituents" as it was titled in a famous lecture by a pioneer in this field, Rudolf Schoenheimer (Rittenberg, 1949).

First ^{11}C and then ^{14}C became available for biochemical studies (Buchanan and Hastings, 1946). Carbon-11, with a half-life of 21 min., required a highly organized, rapid sequence of organic synthesis, purification, experimentation, chemical isolation, and radioactivity analysis. Such heroic early efforts became outmoded, since the beta-emitting, long half-lived (5600 years) ^{14}C provided much greater simplicity of investigation. Today, potential applications of whole-body counting and localization by external scanning techniques of ^{11}C-labeled organic compounds may result in a renewed interest in ^{11}C.

Tritium, or ^3H, has largely replaced deuterium for biological and medical usage. It provides greater ease and sensitivity of assay than deuterium, and the low energy of its beta emission permits discrete intracellular localization by autoradiography.

The stable isotope of oxygen, ^{18}O, has not yet been applied in biomedical studies, but it also will probably be used in the future. The very short half-lived radioisotope, ^{15}O, has been used in physiological studies in man. The beta-emitting ^{32}P has been employed in basic biochemical studies in animals, but has been used in man primarily for its therapeutic and diagnostic value, in leukemias, for example, because of its concentration in actively reproducing tissues. The radioisotope of sulfur, ^{35}S, which has a beta emission of approximately the same energy as ^{14}C and a suitable half-life of 87 days, has been used in basic studies in animals, but not often in clinical investigation. The turnover of plasma proteins in Cushing's disease and hypoproteinemia has been studied with ^{35}S-methionine (Kinsell et al., 1949).

In clinical study of metabolic diseases, the most widely used radioisotopes have been ^{14}C and ^3H, and the stable isotope, ^{15}N; these have been used in studies of such conditions as diabetes, gout, hyperlipemia, and obesity. (Metabolic tracer studies in thyroid disease are discussed in Chapter VII.)

CARBOHYDRATE METABOLISM

GLUCOSE

The conversion of ^{14}C-labeled glucose to $^{14}CO_2$ is of interest in diabetes mellitus and related disturbances of carbohydrate metabolism. Baker et al. (1954) first carried out analyses of expired $^{14}CO_2$ and blood glucose-^{14}C at intervals after intravenous injection of a trace amount of glucose-U-^{14}C in normal human subjects. These and later studies (Shreeve et al., 1956; Reichard et al., 1961; Manougian et al., 1964) have indicated that in normal, resting, postabsorptive persons about 20 to 30 per cent of expired CO_2 derives directly from glucose. This indicates that glucose clearly does not provide all, or even most, of metabolic fuel, at least in the resting, postabsorptive state.

The volume of distribution of free glucose was calculated to be about 25 to 30 per cent of body weight. Segal et al. (1961) defined, by kinetic analysis, a first compartment of distribution consisting of about 15 to 20 per cent body weight, and a second compartment almost as large. Frankson et al. (1962) obtained a value for the distribution of glucose similar to that of extracellular water. All these methods use extrapolation of the time curve back to the time of injection and therefore may overestimate the glucose mass and space, because some glucose may be utilized before uniform mixing in the first compartment is completed. Kalant et al. (1963) have used in man a priming continuous infusion of glucose-U-^{14}C which indicates a rapidly mixing (5 minute) glucose pool of about four times the plasma glucose mass, a value similar to that calculated by Segal et al. (1961) for the rapidly mixing volume. According to Kalant et al. (1963), the miscible glucose mass continues to increase slowly with an increase of about 50 per cent above the 5 minute value by the end of 30 minutes. Thus the single-injection and the continuous-infusion methods agree in the estimation of a rapid (5 minute) mixing volume equal to about 15 per

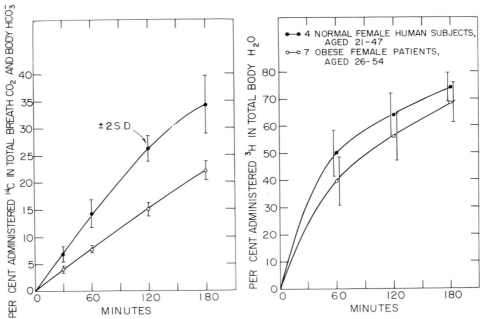

FIGURE 8-1. Simultaneous conversions of glucose-1-^{14}C to $^{14}CO_2$ and glucose-1-^{3}H to ^{3}HOH after combined single intravenous injection in trace amounts. (From Shreeve, W. W.: *Ann. N.Y. Acad. Sci.* 131:464, 1965.)

cent of body weight and an equilibrium value after approximately 30 minutes of about 30 per cent body weight.

Other parameters of interest obtained from measurement of the disappearance of glucose-^{14}C from plasma are the absolute rate of glucose turnover and, together with measurement of the appearance of ^{14}C in CO_2, the percentage of the glucose pool which is oxidized directly to CO_2. In normal persons this averages 50 to 60 per cent (Shreeve et al., 1956; Manougian et al., 1964). Using glucose labeled with both ^{14}C and ^{3}H, Shreeve reported a similar percentage in normal human subjects when he compared the amount of ^{3}H converted to total body water and ^{14}C converted to total expired and body CO_2 (Fig. 8-1; Shreeve, 1965).

The rate of turnover of glucose has been reported to range from 70 to 140 mg./kg./hour in the postabsorptive state (Searle et al., 1959; Reichard et al., 1961; Manougian et al., 1964). By estimating the recycling of glucose from the rate of reappearance of ^{14}C from injected glucose-1-^{14}C into carbons 1, 2, 5, and 6 of blood glucose, Reichard et al. (1963) concluded that the true glucose turnover rate is appreciably higher, since 12 to 20 per cent of glucose was found to be resynthesized from lactate, returned from the peripheral tissues to the liver in the classic "Cori cycle." From data on the rate of lactate formation from glucose in both brain and muscle, Reichard et al. suggested that most of the lactate that enters the blood is resynthesized to glucose. Studies of new glucose formation from injected DL-lactate-2-^{14}C and pyruvate-2-^{14}C indicate that probably less than 25 per cent of the ^{14}C is accountable in glucose or glycogen of normal human subjects (De Meutter and Shreeve, 1963).

Much interest has centered on the question of the relative importance of the oxidative shunt pathway or pentose cycle (PC) pathway for glucose utilization compared to Embden-Meyerhof (EM) glycolytic pathway. Attempts to determine this from the relative rates of appearance of $^{14}CO_2$ from glucose-1-^{14}C and from glucose-6-^{14}C have been somewhat difficult to interpret (Wood et al., 1963). Segal et al. (1961) analyzed the curves of relative specific activity of expired $^{14}CO_2$ after intravenous injection of glucose-1-^{14}C or glucose-6-^{14}C in normal human subjects, and concluded that about 8 per cent of glucose metabolized by the whole body was oxidized via the PC pathway. Gordon and Goldberg (1964a) have reported that the ratio of $^{14}CO_2$ from glucose-1-^{14}C to $^{14}CO_2$ from glucose-6-^{14}C in normal subjects is much higher among premenopausal females than among males of the same age or post-menopausal females (Fig. 8-2). Evidence that estrogen levels affect the activity of the PC pathway is consistent with other data, and is potentially applicable in clinical studies.

The finding of a small percentage of the total glucose ^{14}C in the outer (1, 2, 5, and 6) carbons after metabolic formation of glucose from injected acetate-1-^{14}C (Shreeve, 1958) indicated the occurrence of the PC pathway in the human liver. Similar studies with DL-lactate-2-^{14}C and pyruvate-2-^{14}C indicate that a major route of gluconeogenesis is CO_2 fixation into dicarboxylic acids and suggest other deviations from a simple reversal of the EM glycolytic pathway (Shreeve and De Meutter, 1964).

In a series of studies of brain metabolism using ^{14}C-labeled glucose and various other organic substrates, Sacks (1965) estimated the rate of turnover of the Krebs cycle in normal human brain in vivo and postulated an enlarged Krebs cycle that included a small active component of glutamate as well as gamma-aminobutyrate and succinic semialdehyde.

RIBOSE

This pentose is important in nucleic acid and nucleotide structure and as an intermediate in the PC pathway of glucose oxidation. Segal and Foley (1958)

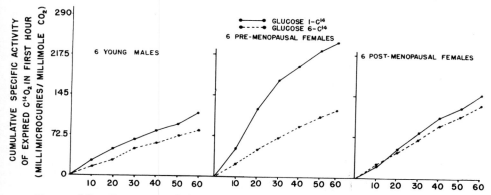

FIGURE 8-2. Comparison of glucose-1-C^{14} and glucose-6-C^{14} oxidation curves. The curves of postmenopausal females for C^{14} glucose oxidation resemble those of males. The center curves from young females illustrate the typical pattern attributed to ovarian production of estrogen. (From Gordon, E. S., and Goldberg, M.: *Metabolism* 13:775, 1964.)

measured the conversion of ribose-1-^{14}C to $^{14}CO_2$ and to glucose in man and concluded that pentose is metabolized promptly and to a large extent via glucose through conversion in the PC pathway.

FUCOSE

Fucose (6-deoxy-L-galactose) is a constituent of mucinous polysaccharides and a free sugar in urine and milk. The formation and utilization of fucose has been measured in lactating females with the aid of ^{14}C-labeled glucose and fucose by Segal and Topper (1958). Fucose was formed from the intact carbon skeleton of glucose and rapidly metabolized to $^{14}CO_2$. Labeled fucose was also found to a considerable extent in urine.

FAT METABOLISM

FREE FATTY ACIDS

Circulating unesterified long-chain fatty acids are a major source of energy. Studies of the disappearance of ^{14}C-labeled fatty acids from the plasma of human subjects (Laurell, 1957; Frederickson and Gordon, 1958) indicated high fractional turnover rates of the order of one half of the entire circulating pool per minute for palmitic and oleic acids. Total turnover rates after fasting could account for the total caloric needs of the person. However, comparison of $^{14}CO_2$ formed with disappearance of plasma free fatty acid-^{14}C suggested that not more than half of the turnover represented direct utilization for energy. Friedberg et al. (1960a) with a single-injection technique and Havel et al. (1963) with a continuous infusion method concluded that in normal human subjects exercise markedly increases the absolute turnover rate of free fatty acids (FFA) as judged by the disappearance of palmitate-1-^{14}C from plasma. By relating these data to respiratory O_2, CO_2, and $^{14}CO_2$, Havel et al. (1963) calculated that during exercise, FFA of plasma accounted for 40 to 50 per cent of energy metabolism, which was double the value when the subjects were at rest. Prior carbohydrate feeding lowered the percentages in both cases to about one fifth of the values found in the fasting state. These studies provide striking evidence that blood glucose is not the only or even the major fuel for working muscle, particularly in the fasting state. Friedberg et al. (1960b) observed extraction of palmitic acid-1-^{14}C by the human arm or leg even when there was a net release of total free fatty acids.

TRIGLYCERIDES

Synthesis of plasma triglycerides in normal man has been evaluated with acetate-^{14}C (Lipsky et al., 1957; Hennes and Redding, 1961), palmitate-^{14}C (Friedberg et al., 1961; Havel, 1961; Farquhar et al., 1965) and glycerol-2-^{3}H (Farquhar et al., 1965) given intravenously and linoleate-1-^{14}C (Ormsby et al., 1963) given orally. These studies indicate that triglyceride fatty acids (TGFA) are labeled rapidly (1 to 4 hour peak of activity) compared to much slower labeling of plasma phospholipids and cholesterol esters. These findings, along with other data from animal studies, suggest that neutral fat rather than phospholipids or cholesterol esters serves to transport fatty acids from the liver to the peripheral tissues. However, the rate of turnover of TGFA in the postabsorptive state, as calculated from the data of Friedberg et al. (1961) and of Farquhar et al. (1965) would not account for more than about 10 to 20 per cent of the energy requirements even if all were directly oxidized to CO_2. The similar rates of disappearance of labeled palmitic, oleic, and stearic acids from plasma TGFA (Lipsky et al., 1957; Friedberg et al., 1961) suggest that triglycerides are utilized intact rather than after undergoing selective exchange of constituent fatty acids. Nestel (1965) noted similar disappearance rates of palmitate-9,10-^{3}H and linoleate-1-^{14}C from TGFA of lipoproteins of very low density in patients with normal plasma triglyceride levels.

Friedberg et al. (1961) and Havel (1961) have made calculations from the amount of FFA label administered, the radioactivity in TGFA, and the flux rates of FFA and TGFA and concluded that most of the plasma TGFA (in the postabsorptive state) is derived from circulating FFA. This may explain correlations in the rise and fall of plasma TG and FFA levels. The studies of Farquhar et al. (1965) have established other interesting relationships among the hepatic triglyceride pool and the plasma pools of triglycerides and free fatty acids. After studies of labeling of the liver and plasma TG by palmitate-1-^{14}C and glycerol-2-^{3}H, they concluded that there is appreciable recycling of the TGFA relative to the TG-glycerol, and that the hepatic TG pool in man has a much higher relative and absolute turnover rate than the plasma TG pool; this has not been the case in animals studied so far (rat, rabbit, and dog). The conclusions of Farquhar et al. linking the hepatic TG pool and the plasma FFA pool suggest a more significant role for the liver in regulating plasma FFA levels.

Fine et al. (1962) studied the incorporation of ^{14}C from glucose-U-^{14}C into human plasma triglycerides. Uptake was considerably greater in subjects on high-carbohydrate diets compared to those on high-fat diets. Hirsch and Goldrick (1965) noted that restriction of calories depresses lipogenesis from ^{14}C-labeled glucose, palmitate, and acetate in human adipose tissue in vitro. More radioactivity from glucose is incorporated into glycerol than into the fatty acid moiety, particularly when the subject is on a low-carbohydrate diet.

The uptake of palmitate-1-^{14}C and synthesis of lipid from acetate-1-^{14}C and glucose-U-^{14}C have been compared in human omental and subcutaneous adipose tissue (Hamosh et al., 1963; Ostman, 1965). Tissue from the omental site was several times more active in taking up long-chain fatty acid, 10 to 20 times more active in synthesizing neutral lipid from acetate-1-^{14}C and two times more active in synthesizing it from glucose-U-^{14}C. Lipomas were found to have 20 times the rate of lipid synthesis from labeled acetate as adjacent normal subcutaneous adipose tissue (Gellhorn and Marks, 1961; Hamosh et al., 1963).

A comparison between glucose-1-^{3}H and DL-lactate-2-^{3}H in conversion to human plasma TG (Ghose et al., 1964) and TGFA (Shreeve, 1965) has indicated a higher specific incorporation (relative to labeling of body water) for the NAD-linked substrate, lactate, than the NADP-linked substrate, glucose. This bears out other findings from animal studies and suggests the need for revision of former concepts concerning the hydrogen sources and coenzymes involved in reduction of fatty acid intermediates.

Various investigators (Balodimos et al., 1962; Bierman and Hamlin, 1963; Kinsell et al., 1965) have studied the characteristics of disappearance of particulate, "artificial chylomicronous" tripalmitin-^{14}C administered intravenously. A rapid removal rate relative to turnover of subsequently formed lipoprotein was found. The peak of $^{14}CO_2$ specific activity occurred at 2 hours, about the same time as the secondary peak of triglyceride activity due to formation of labeled plasma lipoproteins.

CHOLESTEROL AND CHOLESTEROL ESTERS

The synthesis of plasma free and esterified cholesterol from ^{14}C-labeled acetate has been studied by Hellman et al. (1954), Gould et al. (1955) and Hennes et al. (1962). Free cholesterol reached a peak specific activity at 2 to 4 hours after intravenous or oral administration, whereas esterified cholesterol did not reach maximum activity until about 48 hours. Percentages of incorporation of tracer were quite variable for normal subjects, but were generally about 0.1 to 0.4 per cent of dose for plasma cholesterol and 1 per cent or more for total liver-blood cholesterol. Relationships of specific activity curves at various times indicated a direct precursor-product relationship between free and esterified cholesterol. Whereas Lipsky et al. (1957) and Fine et al. (1962) suggested that the fatty acids esterified with cholesterol were related to labeled TGFA in a manner that indicated a precursor-product mechanism, Hennes (unpublished) noted that the pattern of labeling of different fatty acids from acetate-1-^{14}C differs widely between TGFA and cholesterol-FA. Hennes found, as did Lipsky, that palmitate is labeled much more intensively than stearate or oleate in TGFA. However, the C-20 or longer fatty acids, which contain a minor fraction of total ^{14}C in TGFA, constitute 90 per cent of labeled cholesterol-FA.

By using the specific cholesterol precursor, mevalonic acid-2-^{14}C, Gidez and Eder (1961) were able to provide much higher activities of human plasma free and esterified cholesterol and thus could follow the rate of disappearance of radioactivity for 180 days or more. Rates of total daily cholesterol synthesis could be calculated. Similar characteristics of cholesterol metabolism were obtained in man by Kurland et al. (1954) following intravenous infusion of cholesterol-4-^{14}C. Their data, which included some postmortem tissue analyses, led to the hypothesis that the labeled carbon of cholesterol is reutilized in the formation of new cholesterol. By using both ^{14}C and ^{3}H, Kritchevsky et al. (1965) made the important observation in baboons that cholesterol in the alpha or beta lipoproteins of plasma has the same characteristics of transport and turnover whether derived from exogenous sources (labeled cholesterol) or endogeneous sources (labeled mevalonate or acetate).

DIABETES MELLITUS

According to classic concepts, diabetes mellitus is characterized by diminished transfer of glucose into cells. This can be studied in human subjects by measuring the turnover of glucose in the blood and its oxidation to $^{14}CO_2$. However, in diabetes, the amount of the body glucose is increased. Therefore, measurement of the formation of $^{14}CO_2$ without analysis of the ^{14}C concentration in blood glucose would not permit interpretation of a decreased formation of $^{14}CO_2$ as a decreased transfer of ^{14}C from the blood glucose "compartment" to the CO_2 "compartment" of the body. We also need to know the size of the compartment of CO_2.

Shreeve et al. (1956) gave single intravenous injections of glucose-U-^{14}C in trace amounts and analyzed the precursor-product relationship between glucose and CO_2. In mild diabetic patients with moderate hyperglycemia but no ketosis, glucose was oxidized at a normal rate. Ketotic patients with severe hyperglycemia showed a depression of oxidation to about half of normal. Later studies of Reichard et al. (1961) and Manougian et al. (1964) have confirmed these observations.

It is possible that the blood glucose level in diabetic subjects may be high enough to compensate completely and allow a normal rate of glucose metabolism. In any case, the rate of formation of $^{14}CO_2$ from glucose-U-^{14}C in vivo does not appear to be a sensitive criterion for the diagnosis of diabetes mellitus nor is it of value in its management. It is not yet known whether specifically labeled glucose-^{14}C rather than uniformly labeled glucose will yield different results. That this may be the case is suggested by the findings that euglycemic obese persons exhibit a low level of formation of $^{14}CO_2$ when studied with glucose-1-^{14}C or glucose-6-^{14}C (Gordon, 1964; Shreeve, 1965) (Fig. 8-1).

The rate of turnover of glucose-U-^{14}C was not significantly altered in the majority of diabetic patients (Shreeve et al., 1956; Searle et al., 1959; Reichard et al., 1961; Manougian et al., 1964). By using a continuous-infusion rather than a single-injection technique, Kalant et al. (1963) found a slight but insignificant decrease. In juvenile diabetics with ketosis, the turnover rate when measured by the single injection technique was two or more times higher than normal. An increase of hepatic glucose production in diabetes is also suggested by measurements of splanchnic or hepatic arteriovenous differences of glucose concentration.

De Meutter and Shreeve (1963) measured the appearance of ^{14}C in blood glucose after intravenous administration of labeled pyruvate and lactate in normal and diabetic human subjects. There was a progressive increase of ^{14}C content in total glucose with increasing severity of diabetes, up to twice normal in severely diabetic patients. Accelerated hepatic gluconeogenesis or release of glucose into the circulation may contribute significantly to the hyperglycemia of diabetes.

De Meutter and Shreeve (1963) noted a fall (to about 50 per cent of control value) in incorporation of ^{14}C into glucose when insulin or tolbutamide was injected before the labeled lactate or pyruvate. This finding partly supported the results of Jacobs et al. (1958), Searle et al. (1959), and Pollycove (1964), who found "plateauing" of the specific activity of glucose-^{14}C immediately after intravenous insulin or tolbutamide in either diabetic or nondiabetic humans. It was not compatible with the conclusion that complete suppression of glucose output by the liver had been caused by the insulin or tolbutamide. However, in both types of study, alternative explanations are possible (De Meutter and Shreeve, 1963; Pollycove, 1964): in each case equilibria of glucose pools were shifting, which makes interpretation of such in vivo metabolic tracer studies hazardous.

Nondiabetic subjects had approximately a 150 per cent increase in glucose utilization after insulin administration; diabetic subjects showed only a 30 per cent increase (Searle et al., 1959). By analyzing changes in specific activity during continuous infusion of glucose-U-^{14}C, Kalant et al. (1963) observed that diabetic patients showed less increase in utilization after insulin than nondiabetic subjects. Such studies are of significance in elucidation of the extent and nature of insulin insensitivity, a phenomenon of increasing importance in patients with diabetes mellitus, particularly of the type that usually begins after maturity.

In diabetic patients, the total glucose mass as determined by extrapolation of the glucose-^{14}C specific-activity curve to the time of injection, is commensurate with the increase in blood glucose concentration. Apparently there is no abnormality in the size of the "equilibrium" glucose space (about 25 to 30 per cent of body weight). Kalant et al. (1963) found that the rapidly miscible 5 minute glucose pool was only about 60 per cent as large in diabetics as in nondiabetics.

There is no evidence that more extensive recycling of products (e.g., lactate) back into glucose occurs in diabetic patients than in normal persons. However, the increased rate of incorporation of ^{14}C into glucose from labeled lactate or pyruvate (McManus et al., 1961; De Meutter and Shreeve, 1963) provides evidence that at least one phase of the Cori cycle is accelerated. Information on the fate of blood lactate in normal and diabetic subjects can be derived from analysis of the $^{14}CO_2$ formed after injection of the ^{14}C-labeled lactate or pyruvate (McManus et al., 1961; Shreeve et al., 1964). Particularly in ketotic diabetics, one finds a decrease (10 to 20 per cent of the dose), which is of the same order as the increased amount of ^{14}C appearing in glucose. Although well controlled, nonobese diabetics do not show much decrease in the formation of $^{14}CO_2$ from labeled lactate, obese adult diabetic patients do. Determination of a carbohydrate redox ratio by combined analysis of breath $^{14}CO_2$ and blood glucose-^{14}C after injection of labeled pyruvate or lactate may be an indicator of an abnormality in the diabetic liver which tends to divert intermediate carbohydrates away from oxidation and toward reduction to glucose.

LIPID METABOLISM IN DIABETES MELLITUS

FREE FATTY ACIDS

When insulin and glucose are given together to human subjects, a rapid and profound fall in plasma concentration of nonesterified (albumin-bound) free fatty acids (FFA) results (Dole, 1956). Therefore, this lipid fraction of plasma has been of great interest in diabetes. It is possible that the metabolism of FFA is related to the regulation of carbohydrate metabolism by insulin and its antagonists (Randle et al., 1963). Radioactive tracers are particularly useful in answering questions about the turnover, production, and utilization of FFA. When dogs were infused with palmitate-1-^{14}C, the specific activity of the plasma FFA rose sharply after intravenous injection of insulin. There was also a fall in plasma concentration of FFA (Bierman et al., 1957; Armstrong et al., 1961). This may indicate a decrease in formation or decreased release of unlabeled fatty acids into the plasma pool. Increased glucose metabolism may provide glycerol for reesterification of fatty acids in adipose tissue, and prevent or slow their release into the blood stream. The theory of control of FFA release by reesterification is supported by the finding that insulin produces increased A-V differences of FFA in the human forearm Rabinowitz and Zierler, 1962), and in adipose tissue perfused in situ (Scow, 1965). A recent report, however, indicates that after glucose ingestion A-V differences of FFA across the forearm decrease and may become negative (Schless, 1964). To account for the fall in plasma concentration of FFA, there was proposed a rapid turnover theory in which FFA were believed to be metabolized at an accelerated rate rather than being released at a decreased rate.

Turnover rates of FFA using single injection of palmitate-1-^{14}C have been studied in fasting and normal human subjects (Frederickson and Gordon, 1958) and in exercised subjects (Friedberg et al., 1960a; Havel et al., 1963) Frederickson (unpublished) has found that acidotic diabetic patients have a normal fractional turnover rate and presumably an increased absolute turnover rate of FFA, since the plasma concentration of FFA is high. Additional studies are required to characterize further the turnover, formation, release, and utilization of FFA in patients with different types of diabetes, including studies of their response to physiological or therapeutic perturbations. Problems of changing pool sizes, equilibration of labeled and unlabeled materials, and others must be solved, and the sites of changes, such as in muscle, fat, and other tissues, must be delineated. Incubation of biopsy specimens of subcutaneous adipose tissues with labeled substrates (Hirsch and Goldrick, 1965; Ostman, 1965) and studies of omental fat may yield valuable information (Kahlenberg and Kalant, 1964).

Triglycerides

Tissues from diabetic patients have a decreased capacity to synthesize esterified long-chain fatty acids. Hennes and Redding (1961) measured the appearance of ^{14}C in plasma triglyceride fatty acids (TGFA) after injection of ^{14}C-labeled acetate in diabetic and nondiabetic patients. Although the diabetic patients required insulin, they had normal blood glucose concentrations at the time of study. Nevertheless, the uptake of ^{14}C into TGFA was only about one fifth as much in the diabetic patients as in the normal subjects (Fig. 8-3). This was true whether specific activity or total ^{14}C in plasma TGFA was calculated. Various factors might lead to this result, e.g., greater dilution of tracer in expanded precursor pools, defective fatty acid synthesis or esterification of fatty acids, defective transformation of triglycerides into lipoproteins, or their release from the liver into the circulation. Nevertheless, the finding points to some occult defect (presumably in the liver) which may cause abnormal accumulations of lipid and produce some of the degenerative changes found in diabetes.

Prior administration of carbohydrate and insulin produced only slight increases in the conversion of acetate-1-^{14}C to plasma TGFA in diabetic patients

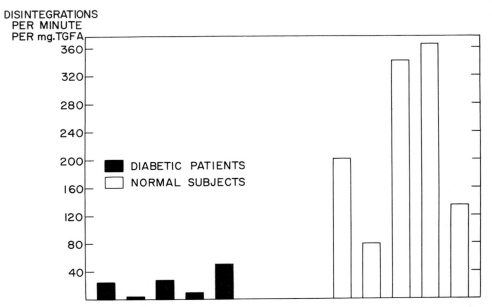

Figure 8-3. Peak specific radioactivity of plasma triglyceride fatty acids (TGFA) after intravenous injection of 100 μc. acetate-1-14C. (From Hennes, A. R., and Redding, T. W.: *Diabetes* 10:85, 1961.)

(Hennes and Redding, 1961; Shreeve, 1965). It had little effect on transfer of glucose-1-3H to circulating triglycerides in a mild diabetic patient but caused an increase in a severely diabetic patient (Shreeve, 1965). Such studies are of interest because of the importance of metabolic systems which use NADPH as a source of reducing hydrogen for fatty acid biosynthesis. The supply of NADPH (via utilization of glucose in the pentose pathway) may be a limiting factor in fatty acid biosynthesis. In subjects with diabetes, this may be a mechanism of decreased formation of fatty acids. Mildly diabetic, obese patients studied both with glucose-1-3H and with DL-lactate-2-3H have not been found to be different from normal in labeling of plasma TGFA (Shreeve, 1965).

Studies of lipogenesis in isolated tissues of diabetic patients have been carried out in adipose tissue (Carlson and Ostman, 1963) and in whole blood cells (Awai et al., 1964; Hennes and Awai, 1965). A lower percentage uptake of palmitic acid-1-14C into an esterified form was found in diabetic subcutaneous adipose tissue compared to normal. The study of incorporation of acetate-1-14C into blood cells (leukocytes and platelets) included separation of individual fatty acids by gas chromatography. Besides having a decrease in total amount of radioactivity in fatty acids per unit quantity of leukocytes, patients with severe diabetic acidosis had a relative decrease in synthesis of fatty acids with 16 or fewer carbon atom chains and an increase in synthesis of 18-carbon fatty acids. This suggested a relatively greater decrease in activity of the cytoplasmic malonyl-CoA pathway of fatty acid synthesis, which has also been found for the liver of the alloxan diabetic rat. Similar changes were found in incubated platelets. In the case of platelets, the abnormalities occurred in nonacidotic diabetic patients and were not fully restored to normal by control of the blood glucose level.

Since metabolism of blood cells may be influenced by certain abnormal constituents of diabetic plasma (Hennes and Awai, 1965), such studies may indicate some basic "diabetic" defects either in the cells or plasma. The suggestion that increased tendency to thrombosis may be related to the abnormalities in lipid metabolism of platelets has stimulated further interest in this possibility.

In view of the elevation of the neutral fat fraction of the blood in diabetics, particularly when in the ketotic state, abnormal utilization of this fraction was suspected. Hennes and Redding (1961) have data that suggest the possibility of a delayed removal of endogenously labeled plasma TGFA. Hennes and Shreeve (1959) observed a more pronounced delay in the fall of specific activity of TGFA in the blood of a patient with lipoatrophic diabetes, a finding that may provide a clue to the nature of the hyperlipemia. However, studies with ^{14}C-labeled tripalmitin administered intravenously in particulate form to diabetic patients (Balodimos et al., 1962; Bierman and Hamlin, 1963) have failed to demonstrate any effects of diabetes or of insulin on the rate of initial disappearance of the particulate triglyceride or on the reappearance of ^{14}C in the beta lipoproteins. These results are different from those obtained in diabetic dogs by Kessler (1962). The possibility remains that abnormal lipemia in diabetes may be in part related to defective removal of certain secondary transport forms of plasma triglyceride.

CHOLESTEROL

Radioisotope methodology has been used relatively little to study the metabolism of cholesterol in diabetic patients. Hennes et al. (1962) found that adult diabetic patients did not differ significantly from normal subjects in the percentage of incorporation of acetate-1-^{14}C into plasma cholesterol. There was a wide range of uptake in both normal and diabetic groups, considerably wider than the range of cholesterol concentration. Treatment of diabetes with chlorpropamide was associated in some cases with decreased incorporation of ^{14}C into plasma free and esterified cholesterol without any significant change in the cholesterol concentration. Studies such as those of Doherty et al. (1962), in which the oral administration of ^{14}C- or ^{3}H-labeled cholesterol to patients with atherosclerosis revealed increased turnover rates and altered percentages of radioisotope in alpha and beta lipoprotein, may prove useful in increasing our understanding of the relationship of diabetes and cardiovascular disease.

KETONE BODIES

Ketogenesis in diabetics with mild and severe ketosis has been studied by analysis of urinary ketone bodies (beta-oxybutyric acids, BOBA) after intravenous injection of acetate-1-^{14}C (Shreeve and Tocci, 1961). Incorporation of ^{14}C did not increase to the same extent as the increase of concentration of BOBA in severe ketosis. This may indicate a larger dilution with endogenous substrate in the case of beta-oxybutyric acids, but could result from decreased utilization. Variations among patients in the rate of decline of specific activity of BOBA seemed to be related to treatment. Measurement of the changes in specific activity of labeled BOBA perhaps could be used to gauge the effect of therapeutic agents on ketogenesis. One might measure urinary BOBA-^{14}C at various intervals. A slowing of the rate of fall of specific activity would indicate a slowing of ketogenesis. Because certain studies in animals have indicated a stimulation of utilization of BOBA by glucose and insulin, Shreeve (1963) tested the effect of intravenous treatment with these agents on the conversion of acetoacetic acid-3-^{14}C to expired $^{14}CO_2$ in a diabetic patient but did not observe any stimulation.

HYPERLIPEMIA

The high incidence of hyperlipemia among patients with cornary artery disease, hypertension, and diabetes has led to a search for abnormalities of fat metabolism in these conditions, as well as in "essential" or "primary" cases of gross hyperlipemia. Recent studies have led to classification of hyperlipemias into carbohydrate-induced and fat-induced categories (Ahrens et al., 1961) or according to their distinctive paper electrophoretic patterns of plasma lipoproteins (Frederickson and Lees, 1965).

Tracer studies may help clarify the nature of the metabolic abnormalities in each category. Fine et al. (1962) measured the incorporation of glucose-U-^{14}C into circulating triglycerides in five hyperglyceridemic patients, who were intolerant of high-fat diets. As a group they did not show significantly abnormal increases in the content of ^{14}C in triglycerides, although there were individual abnormalities. All normal subjects incorporated more ^{14}C into triglycerides when fed a high-carbohydrate diet compared to a high-fat diet; one hyperglyceridemic patient did not. In this patient, D-triiodothyronine decreased the net incorporation of label to about half the control value.

Nestel (1965) measured the turnover rates of injected linoleic acid-1-^{14}C and palmitic acid-9,10-^{3}H before and after their transfer to very low density lipoproteins (VLDLP) in patients with coronary artery disease with varying degrees of hypertriglyceridemia. Whether free or as VLDLP-fatty acid, the linoleate turnover varied inversely with the concentration of triglyceride whereas that of palmitate did not. Halving the triglyceride concentration by reduction of caloric intake in two subjects caused increased turnover of VLDLP triglyceride linoleate but not palmitate. The increase in absolute turnover of palmitate but not linoleate may indicate increased synthesis of lipid from carbohydrate.

The fractional turnover rate of human chylomicra, prepared from thoracic duct lymph after oral ingestion of glyceryl-tripalmitate-1-^{14}C, was determined in two hyperlipemic patients (Nestel et al., 1962). There was an inverse relationship between turnover rate and plasma level of esterified fatty acids, which suggested that triglyceride pool size is an important determinant of fractional turnover rate.

A special type of hyperlipemia is that associated with lipoatrophic diabetes. In a young female patient with a tendency to hyperlipemia, the rate of decrease of specific activity of plasma TGFA after labeling by intravenous injection of acetate-2-^{14}C was much slower than that of other diabetic and nondiabetic subjects (Hennes and Shreeve, 1959). Possibly there was an inability to store circulating triglycerides in adipose tissue. Further studies of this type may improve understanding of the etiology of the gross hyperlipemia commonly associated with diabetic ketoacidosis.

METABOLIC FACTORS IN OBESITY

The growing recognition of metabolic factors in obesity has led to increasing study of possible alterations of metabolism in this condition. Various evidence indicates a wide prevalence of decreased glucose tolerance in obese people. Gordon (1964) found a decrease in the rate of accumulation of $^{14}CO_2$ in the breath of obese patients after injection of glucose-6-^{14}C. Administration of triiodothyronine increased the output of $^{14}CO_2$ from labeled glucose in an obese patient, as it does in hypothyroid subjects (Gordon and Goldberg, 1964). Shreeve (1965), using intravenous injection of glucose-1-^{14}C, has confirmed in adult obese subjects the decreased formation of $^{14}CO_2$ and has estimated the total breath and body $^{14}CO_2$ for normal and obese groups. Concomitant administration of glucose-1-^{3}H showed that appearance of tritium in body water was less depressed in the obese than was the formation of $^{14}CO_2$ (Fig. 8-2). This suggests that an intracellular metabolic abnormality may be more responsible for the depressed formation of $^{14}CO_2$ than a difference in distribution or primary utilization of the labeled glucose. Pollycove (1964) infused one obese subject with glucose-U-^{14}C and found a moderately decreased turnover rate and a decreased oxidation to $^{14}CO_2$ (30 per cent of normal).

Recent studies (Tashjian et al., 1965) of the formation of $^{14}CO_2$ from glucose-1-^{14}C in a standard cortisone-glucose tolerance test indicated that the appearance of $^{14}CO_2$ in the breath provides a criterion for decreased glucose tolerance which compares favorably with the measurement of blood glucose concentration. Further studies of blood glucose content of ^{14}C will aid in establishing the validity of this procedure. The employment of glucose-^{14}C in an oral glucose load followed by analysis of $^{14}CO_2$ in the breath has the important advantage of not requiring venipunctures.

The obese subjects studied by Gordon (1964) and Shreeve (1965) fit into the category of "static" obesity characterized by a fixed impaired glucose tolerance. It has been postulated that a "dynamic" phase characterized by a normal or even enhanced glucose tolerance can occur early in persons with rapidly increasing obesity. An obese 14 year old girl studied with glucose-1-^{14}C may be an example of this condition. Her output of $^{14}CO_2$ was greater than that of two young normal subjects (Cozzetto, 1964).

Gordon (1964) found decreased formation of $^{14}CO_2$ from injected palmitate-1-^{14}C and acetate-1-^{14}C in obese subjects, but other studies (Gordon and Goldberg, 1964b) suggest that the apparent low rate of oxidation to CO_2 is attributable to the expanded fatty acid pool with the elevation of concentration of FFA. This does not explain the decreased conversion of glucose-^{14}C to $^{14}CO_2$, since the blood glucose levels of obese subjects studied under fasting conditions were usually within normal limits. In evaluating studies of subjects with widely differing pool sizes of body constituents, the effect of difference in dilution as well as in rates of circulation and distribution frequently complicates interpretation of the results. Dilution by initial and intermediate substrate pools is an important factor, as is the size of the large, slowly replaced CO_2 pool(s) which determine the pattern of expiration of $^{14}CO_2$. It is advisable to add all breath and body $^{14}CO_2$ (Fig. 8-1) as well as measure the specific activity of expired $^{14}CO_2$. To calculate the data of Figure 8-1 it was assumed that the amount of body CO_2 was 20 mM./liter of body water (the latter measured separately with

^{3}HOH), since studies of several obese and nonobese subjects with NaH^{14}CO$_3$ indicated a closer correlation of the bicarbonate space with body-water space (lean body mass) than with weight (Shreeve, 1965).

Shreeve et al. (1963) noted decreased oxidation to ^{14}CO$_2$ of injected DL-lactate-2-^{14}C in obese subjects (diabetic and nondiabetic). In these patients ^{14}C appeared in greater quantities in the blood glucose. Both findings may signify some abnormality of intermediary metabolism in these obese subjects. Brown (1965) has observed that obese women (4 out of 5) did not respond as did normal subjects to a glucose load by a decrease in oxidation of palmitate-1-^{14}C to ^{14}CO$_2$. This may be attributed to the strong adaptation of obese patients to fat utilization, but the mechanism of this glucose "insensitivity" remains unclear. A similar lack of response was noted in normal subjects following growth hormone administration.

Hirsch and Goldrick (1965) developed a punch biopsy technique to obtain subcutaneous adipose tissue for analysis of in vivo lipid synthesis from ^{14}C-labeled substrates. They have found a dependence of lipogenic activity on the preceding nutritional state of the subject, with a relatively slow response to feeding or intravenous insulin and glucose after fasting.

DISEASES OF THE ADRENALS

Either a deficiency or an excess of adrenal cortical steroids affects the appearance of ^{14}C in plasma lipids and in the carbon dioxide of breath after administration of ^{14}C-labeled acetate to human subjects. Gould et al. (1955) compared patients with collagen diseases on prolonged high doses of cortisone to subjects not receiving cortisone therapy. Intravenous administration of acetate-1-^{14}C resulted in a fourfold to fivefold increase in specific activity of free cholesterol in the plasma of the former group. This effect was not observed with acetate-2-^{14}C after more acute dosage with prednisone (Hennes and Shreeve, 1959); thus it may depend upon secondary metabolic disturbances. Although acute treatment with prednisone increased the specific activity of plasma TGFA, it did not necessarily increase the total amount of labeled TGFA since plasma triglyceride levels were lower in these subjects. Hennes (1962) studied two patients with untreated adrenal insufficiency and made the observation that maximum incorporation of ^{14}C from acetate-1-^{14}C into plasma TGFA was only 12 to 38 per cent of that seen in the same patients when receiving cortisone. A lesser decrease (to 63 per cent) occurred for the conversion of acetate-1-^{14}C to plasma free cholesterol.

Gillman et al. (1962) studied incorporation of ^{14}C from pyruvate-2-^{14}C and acetate-1-^{14}C into serum triglycerides, phospholipids, and cholesterol of infants with kwashiorkor. Increased uptake of acetate-1-^{14}C and decreased uptake of pyruvate-2-^{14}C was observed in patients with kwashiorkor who developed edema and fatty liver. Comparisons with endocrine-manipulated baboons led to suggestions about the state of the adrenal, pituitary, and pancreatic endocrine functions in kwashiorkor.

Administration of prednisone for short periods caused a moderate (15 to 20 per cent) decrease in rate of appearance of ^{14}C from acetate-1 or 2-^{14}C in diabetic patients (Hennes and Shreeve, 1959; Shreeve et al., 1959). In untreated patients with adrenal insufficiency, Hennes (1962) found a moderate *increase* in the rate of output of $^{14}CO_2$ from injected acetate-1-^{14}C. The level of activity of adrenal cortical steroids influenced both the nature and time of appearance of multiple peaks of specific activity of $^{14}CO_2$ in the breath after labeled acetate (Shreeve et al., 1959; Hennes, 1962), presumably owing to different sizes and turnover rates of intermediate pools as well as multiple organ effects. The technique of continuous analysis of expired $^{14}CO_2$ is useful in further characterizing such effects.

Because adrenal glucocorticoids increase gluconeogenesis, measurement of the amount of ^{14}C (or ^{3}H) transferred to blood glucose from an appropriate precursor (e.g., amino acid, lactic acid, or intermediate of the TCA cycle) might be useful as a means of detecting excesses of these hormones. Several animal studies with ^{14}C-labeled compounds both in vitro and in vivo attest to this possibility (Landau et al., 1962; Ashmore et al., 1964; Oji and Shreeve, 1965). Diabetic patients have shown increased conversion of ^{14}C-labeled lactate and pyruvate to blood glucose (DeMeutter and Shreeve, 1963), perhaps a reflection of increased gluconeogenesis.

Precursors of various steroids labeled with ^{14}C or ^{3}H have been incubated with human adrenal cortex, followed by analysis of products in order to characterize the biochemical pathways of adrenal steroid synthesis (Bloch and Benirschke, 1959; Cohn and Mulrow, 1963; Axelrod et al., 1965) and to determine abnormalities associated with clinical syndromes (Axelrod et al., 1965). In the latter study, 5-pregnenolone-4-^{14}C was used to identify a deficiency of 3B-hydroxysteroid dehydrogenase in both adrenal and ovarian tissues of a patient with adrenogenital syndrome. Cohn and Mulrow (1963) combined the use of ^{14}C- and ^{3}H-labeled steroids in studies of adrenal gland slices to provide information about two alternative synthetic pathways.

Other studies with labeled steroids in vivo in man have been designed to measure plasma turnover and renal clearance rates, pool sizes of distribution, or conversion to various metabolites detectable in plasma or urine. For instance, the turnover and metabolism of cortisol-4-^{14}C have been studied by Gold (1962) who noted changes in a patient with Cushing's syndrome. The occurrence of conjugation of aldosterone in kidney as well as in liver and abnormalities of conjugation and renal excretion in patients with cardiac failure have been demonstrated in vivo with aldosterone-1,2-^{3}H (Luetscher et al., 1965).

DISEASES OF THE PITUITARY

Although pituitary growth hormone is "diabetogenic" in the sense of producing hyperglycemia and decreased tolerance to glucose, its particular actions on carbohydrate metabolism are poorly understood. Some effects of growth hormone may be secondary to a direct antagonism to insulin, although in other respects, e.g., nitrogen retention and growth, growth hormone and insulin may act synergistically. Effects on carbohydrate metabolism may be secondary to a direct influence on fat metabolism, e.g., to mobilization of FFA, which according to the concept of the glucose–fatty acid cycle (Randle et al., 1963) could account for the decreased tolerance to glucose. One study of glucose metabolism after injection of glucose-U-^{14}C in hypophysectomized human subjects before and during administration of high doses of human growth hormone for 2 or 3 days (Ikkos and Luft, 1962) indicated a slightly decreased rate of production and utilization of glucose in some patients, but not in others. Since hyperglycemia was produced, an effect that in normal subjects would increase the absolute turnover rate, the authors believe that the results indicate a deficiency in turnover of glucose relative to the elevated plasma glucose concentration. Quite different findings and conclusions were reached by Altszuler et al. (1959) who gave growth hormone to normal, hypophysectomized, and adrenalectomized dogs. According to their study with continuous infusion of glucose-U-^{14}C, the hyperglycemia caused by growth hormone is accompanied by both increased production and increased utilization of glucose. The specific metabolic abnormalities in acromegaly and perhaps other diseases of pituitary growth hormone may be effectively studied with radioisotope methods.

DISEASES OF THE GONADS

The level of endogenous estrogen activity may be characterized by the ratio of formation of $^{14}CO_2$ from glucose-1-^{14}C versus glucose-6-^{14}C in female human subjects in vivo (Gordon and Goldberg, 1964a; Fig. 8–2). This correlation may be of value in defining the menopausal transition and in differentiating pathological disturbances of menstruation.

The conversion of estradiol-1-^{14}C to various urinary metabolites by postmenopausal women with benign and malignant diseases of the breast suggested that those with carcinoma metabolize the administered steroid more rapidly but did not show any useful separation between responders and nonresponders to subsequent estrogen therapy (Crowley et al., 1965). As with other steroid hormones, the plasma production rate has been correlated with urinary production rate of testosterone using the tritiated steroid, making possible estimates of plasma production rate and plasma levels of steroid from the analyses of radioactive testosterone excreted as the glucuronide in urine (Horton et al., 1965).

GOUT

The metabolism of uric acid in patients with gout has been extensively studied with ^{15}N- and ^{14}C-labeled compounds. Benedict et al. (1949) attempted to determine the size and turnover rate of the urate pool by measuring the dilution of injected uric acid-^{15}N and the rate of decline of specific activity. Higher values than normal for the mass of miscible urate in certain gouty patients could be attributed to exchange of soluble urate with large tophaceous deposits. Estimates of synthetic rate in these patients were unreliable because unlabeled urate was mobilized or exchanged from tophi at various rates. This could not be distinguished from uric acid synthesis. On the other hand, since the isotope-dilution technique in some gouty patients gave normal values for size and turnover of the urate pool (Seegmiller et al., 1961), it was reasonable to conclude that such patients did not have an increased rate of synthesis.

Biosynthesis of uric acid in gout has also been studied by measuring the incorporation of labeled precursors into uric acid. Examples are use of glycine-^{15}N (Benedict et al., 1953) and glycine-1-^{14}C (Wyngaarden, 1957); one advantage of ^{14}C was that trace amounts of precursor could be used rather than the larger amounts of nitrogen-labeled glycine. Early results were conflicting. It was uncertain whether all or only some gouty patients showed increased specific activity and urinary excretion of labeled uric acid; later studies (Gutman et al., 1958; Seegmiller et al., 1961) have indicated that only those patients who tend to have abnormally high rates of urinary excretion and serum levels of uric acid incorporate labeled glycine at an abnormal rate. Nevertheless, increased pool sizes may lead to underestimation of synthetic rates by this method.

Seegmiller et al. (1961) simultaneously injected uric acid labeled with a different isotope than precursor glycine. This made possible correction of the values for the amount of isotope from glycine that was excreted as uric acid according to the degree to which extrarenal pathways accounted for disposal of newly formed urate. The fraction removed by an extrarenal route was considerably higher than normal in some gouty patients, particularly those with tophi. These investigators also used another technique that is of general applicability in metabolic studies. After oral administration of sodium benzoate, hippuric acid (benzoyl-glycine) was isolated from the urine; its specific radioactivity was determined and indicated that of the glycine pool in the liver. This provided information on the specific activity of precursor glycine at the time and site of its incorporation into uric acid. Although no consistent abnormality was observed in gouty patients, in one instance an excessive incorporation into uric acid may have been related to a very high specific activity of precursor glycine.

Seegmiller et al. (1961) found a greater difference between gouty and nongouty patients in the rate of incorporation of precursor into uric acid than in the size and turnover rate of the urate pool, the rate of urinary excretion of unlabeled uric acid, and the serum urate levels. Thus radioisotope methods appeared to be more sensitive than chemical methods in detecting differences between diseased and normal persons. The production of uric acid as measured by radioisotope techniques could not be related to the duration of the disease or to the degree of tophaceous involvement.

Another abnormality that can be detected in radioisotope studies of uric acid metabolism in patients with primary gout is early, rapid incorporation with marked decline of specific activity of labeled uric acid after the first day or two. This may be the result of direct synthesis of uric acid from purines without the intermediate formation of nucleic acids. The occurrence of this pathway, even in nongouty patients, has also been suggested in studies with labeled precursors other than glycine (Seegmiller et al., 1963). Patients with gout secondary to increased ribonucleic acid turnover, e.g., myeloid metaplasia or chronic myelocytic leukemia, have a different pattern of incorporation of labeled glycine into uric acid than those with primary gout. In secondary gout, the specific activity of uric acid rises slowly, reaching a maximum about 2 weeks after administration of the precursor, a distinct difference that could be helpful in the differentiation of primary and secondary gout in clinically doubtful cases.

The demonstration of overproduction of uric acid from purine precursors (Seegmiller et al., 1963) has raised the possibility that drugs might be used effectively to regulate this process. The use of ^{14}C-labeled precursors makes these studies quite feasible.

Recent studies of the distribution of ^{15}N in the uric acid molecule synthesized from glycine-^{15}N in gouty patients (Gutman and Yü, 1963) has suggested that an abnormality in glutamine metabolism may be a possible mechanism for secondary overproduction of uric acid.

RADIOASSAY OF HORMONES IN PLASMA

RADIOIMMUNOASSAY

PRINCIPLES OF THE METHOD

The use of ^{131}I-labeled insulin in combination with insulin antiserum led to the highly specific and sensitive measurement of this hormone in human plasma (Berson and Yalow, 1959; Grodsky and Forsham, 1960). The method is based essentially on the principle of isotope dilution. Increasing amounts of unlabeled hormone (in a sample of serum being measured) cause progressively decreasing percentages of binding of insulin-^{131}I by a fixed amount of antibody.

Originally separation of bound and unbound insulin-^{131}I was achieved by chromatoelectrophoresis on filter paper (Berson et al., 1956). Details and subsequent modification of this method by the original authors have been described recently (Yalow and Berson, 1964). Bound insulin-^{131}I moves on the filter paper with antibody gamma globulin but unbound or free insulin-^{131}I remains at the site of origin. Whereas chromatoelectrophoresis provides optimal speed and resolution, hydrodynamic flow chromatography without electrophoresis is almost as satisfactory (Yalow and Berson, 1964). Adequate separation of the two components may be achieved in an hour or less by either of these methods. In the original method, a period of incubation of the reactants at 4° C. for 3 to 4 days is used. Areas under the peaks of radioactivity are calculated after paper-strip counting. A standard curve is prepared, which may be a plot of the ratio of bound insulin-^{131}I (B) to free insulin-^{131}I (F) (Fig. 8-4).

When there is high energy of interaction of hormone and antibody, the curve is steeper and the assay more accurate. Guinea pig antibodies to pork insulin have proved more satisfactory for the assay of human insulin. In the preparation of insulin-^{131}I and in its preincubation with the plasma to be analyzed, the insulin may be altered. Damaged products can be removed and their formation minimized. Purification is almost always necessary to remove products damaged during iodination. Incubation damage is minimized by greater dilution of the unknown plasma. In addition to the use of very active antiserum, high specific activity of tracer insulin-^{131}I increases the sensitivity by sharpening the initial part of the curve (Fig. 8-4). However, the higher the specific activity, the higher may be the preparation damage of insulin-^{131}I.

The original chromatoelectrophoretic method has the advantage (over precipitation methods) of permitting recognition of iodide and damaged ^{131}I-labeled components from free undenatured hormone-^{131}I or antibody-bound hormone-^{131}I. Lack of such recognition may be responsible for apparent inhibition of hormone-antibody reactions (Berson and Yalow, 1964); this can lead to falsely high estimates of hormone concentration in plasma since denatured products are generally not bound by antibody. For this reason, the original method continues to have enduring and unique value (Yalow and Berson, 1964; Berson and Yalow, 1964). However, several investigators have advocated physical separation of the bound from the unbound hormone-131I by making the former insoluble. Grodsky and Forham (1960) used sodium sulfite to salt out the globulins and thus precipitate the insulin-antibody complex. Separation may not be complete by this technique. Meade and Klitgaard (1962) described the attachment of free insulin-131I but not antibody-bound insulin-131I to an anion exchange resin which permitted separation of the two fractions. This method uses low-specific-activity insulin-131I and several ml. of serum for assay. It appears to be relatively simple and rapid. Other investigators (Hales and Randle, 1963; Morgan and Lazarow, 1963; Goetz et al., 1963) have precipitated the insulin-131I-antibody complex with a second antibody (from rabbit serum) directed to the guinea-pig gamma globulin. Morgan et al. (1964) have described a refinement that overcomes the problem of an inhibitor of the precipitin reaction and permits assay of undiluted plasma.

Recent methods include the use of insulinase to solubilize in trichloroacetic acid that fraction of insulin-131I not bound by antibody (Beck et al., 1964) and the use of coated charcoal to absorb free insulin-131I which is separated from antibody bound insulin-131I by centrifugation (Herbert et al., 1965). Rapidity of complete formation of insulin-antibody complex in the various

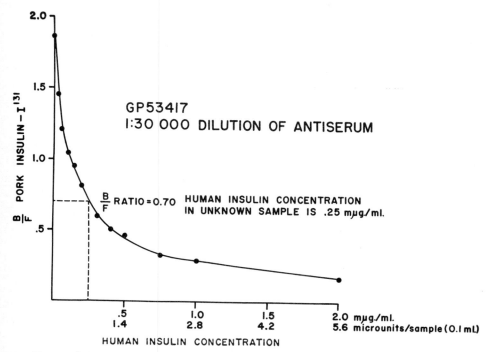

FIGURE 8-4. Varying ratio of antibody-bound (B) to free (F) pork insulin 131I as a function of concentration of human insulin in known standards and unknown plasma sample. (From Yalow, R. S., and Berson, S.A.: Meth. Biochem. Anal. 12:69, 1964.)

modifications is a function of the concentration of the reactants rather than the result of physical separation of free and antibody-bound insulin.

Similar radioassays for other protein hormones in plasma have been developed. Unger et al. (1961) have used both the chromatoelectrophoretic and the two antibody precipitation techniques to assay glucagon using glucagon-[131]I. Grodsky et al. (1961) employed the differential salt precipitation method for assay of glucagon but with less sensitivity. Growth hormone has been analyzed with ^{131}I-iodinated hormone by several investigators. Utiger et al. (1962) and Schalch and Parker (1964) have used antibody precipitation by antibody; Glick et al. (1963) and Hunter and Greenwood (1964a) employed electrophoretic separation. The first method developed for radioassay of adrenocorticotrophic hormone (ACTH) (Felber, 1963) used antibody precipitation and microfiltration for separation and counting of antibody-bound ACTH-^{131}I, but the subsequent analysis of Yalow et al. (1964) with their paper-strip separation technique yields values much lower and closer to those derived from bioassay.

The Berson-Yalow group have also provided a radiochromatoelectrophoretic assay of parathyroid hormone (Berson et al., 1963) which gives good agreement with values from bioassay. Thyroid-stimulating hormone (TSH) has been the subject of radioimmunoassay by Utiger (1965), Odell et al. (1965), and Lemarchand-Beraud et al. (1965). Chromatoelectrophoresis was used in the first two studies, and the two antibody system in the third. Odell et al. found alcohol-saline precipitation preferable for both greater simplicity and greater reproducibility. A starch-gel electrophoretic separation of free and antibody-bound chorionic growth hormone–prolactin (CGP) has recently been used to measure (using CGP-^{131}I) the level of this hormone in the serum and urine of pregnant women (Kaplan and Grumbach, 1965). Greenwood et al. (1964a) studied the growth factor in serum of pregnancy and the placenta by radioimmunoelectrophoresis.

A recent review by Felber et al. (1965) discusses various methods and applications of radioimmunoassay and problems arising in its use.

Applications of radioimmunoassay of hormones

Insulin. The normal level of plasma insulin in fasting subjects averages about 20 μU. (0.7 mμg.)/ml. (Hales and Randle, 1963; Berson and Yalow, 1964) or 60 μU./ml. (Goetz et al., 1963; Elrick et al., 1964). Glucose causes a pronounced increase in plasma insulin levels; sulfonylurea compounds do so to a lesser extent (Yalow and Berson, 1965). Glucose taken orally causes higher levels than the same amount infused intravenously (Elrick et al., 1964). Of considerable interest has been the observation that some mild diabetic patients show delayed but prolonged and excessive secretion of insulin in response to a glucose load (Yalow and Berson, 1965) (Fig. 8-5) and may have increased levels during fasting. Diabetic patients appear to be unable to maintain insulin output during prolonged stimulation (Cerasi and Luft, 1963). Plasma insulin levels of fasting patients with insulinoma are generally high or inappropriate to the blood glucose level (Berson and Yalow, 1964; Yalow and Berson, 1965). Patients with acromegaly may show high fasting levels of plasma insulin and excessive response to glucose loading (Cerasi and Luft, 1964). Obese subjects may also have an exaggerated insulin response to glucose (Karam et al., 1963).

Plasma insulin levels of newborn infants of diabetic mothers have been found to be higher than normal (Stimmler et al., 1964).

Glucagon. This hyperglycemia-producing hormone from the alpha cells of the pancreatic islets is present in the plasma in the normal fasting state at levels detectable by radioimmunoassay. Secretion is increased after the induction of hypoglycemia and following prolonged starvation. It is decreased by administration of glucose, at least in certain amounts. Thus the hormone behaves as if it had a physiological role in maintaining the constancy of the blood glucose concentration. Attempts to identify disorders of glucagon secretion in man have not yet yielded positive results (Unger and Eisentraut, 1964).

Growth Hormone. Radioimmunoassay has revealed that human growth hormone (HGH), like insulin and glucagon, fluctuates with changes in glucose level in the blood. The level of HGH may be markedly increased in response to hypoglycemia, exercise, prolonged fast, and inhibition of glucose utilization by deoxyglucose, and in response to a rapidly falling blood glucose without hypoglycemia (Roth et al., 1963; Hunter and Greenwood, 1964b). Obese subjects may not show a normal elevation during fasting. Hypopituitary dwarfs or hypophysectomized subjects do not respond to hypoglycemia with increases of HGH levels; therefore the method may be useful in assessing pituitary function in various clinical states. Arky and Freinkel (1964) found normal HGH response to induced hypoglycemia in two patients in whom the diagnosis of isolated adrenocorticotrophic defect was confirmed. Greenwood et al. (1964b) found levels of plasma HGH in children and adolescents to be many times those in adult subjects under the same nutritional conditions.

ACTH. Yalow et al. (1964) found that ACTH is normally present in

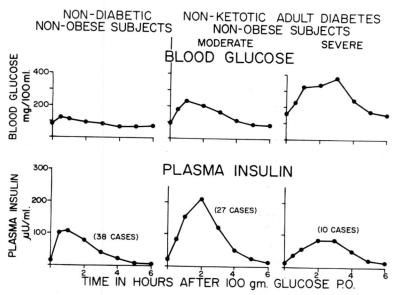

FIGURE 8-5. Mean blood glucose and plasma insulin concentrations in nonobese, nondiabetic or diabetic subjects. Division of diabetics into "moderate" and "severe" classes was based on the criterion of a blood glucose level of 300 mg./100 ml. at two hours. (From Yalow, R. S., and Berson, S. A.: *Diabetes* 14:341, 1965.)

plasma at concentrations averaging 0.6 mU./100 ml. The level was increased in two patients with Cushing's syndrome associated with extrapituitary tumors, in two patients after adrenalectomy, and in three patients with Addison's disease. These findings are consistent with concepts of reciprocal interaction in the adrenal-pituitary axis.

TSH. The plasma level of thyroid-stimulating hormone is inversely related to the functional state of the thyroid gland. Odell et al. (1965) found that the normal level of 3 mμg./ml. was increased to 10 to 150 mμg./ml. in nine patients with primary myxedema and fell to normal levels with replacement therapy. There was no detectable hormone in the plasma of hypophysectomized patients. Similar findings are reported by Utiger (1965).

Parathyroid Hormone. According to the radioimmunoassay of Berman et al. (1963), parathyroid hormone, although detectable in the plasma of hyperparathyroid and some normal subjects, cannot be found in the plasma of parathyroidectomized subjects.

Functional Assay

Insulin-like activity

Martin, Renold, and Dagenais (1958) used the metabolism of a ^{14}C-labeled compound in vitro as an indicator of the extent of insulin-like activity (ILA) in blood or other biological fluids. They used the stimulation of conversion of glucose-1-^{14}C to $^{14}CO_2$ by sections of rat epididymal fat pad as a measure of ILA. Subsequently fat formation from ^{14}C-labeled glucose in this tissue was also used (Leonards, 1959; Samaan et al., 1962). These assays show more ILA in human blood than other methods of measurement. Much of this ILA is not neutralizable by insulin antibodies and it may persist in pancreatectomized animals (Leonards, 1959). Since the latter are acutely diabetic, as are animals given insulin antiserum, the significance for hormonal activity in vivo of this ILA (or that fraction not neutralizable by antibodies) has been questioned (Berson and Yalow, 1964).

Terms such as "atypical insulin" (Samaan et al., 1962), "nonsuppressible ILA" (Froesch et al., 1963), and "bound insulin" (Antoniades et al., 1961) have been applied to fractions of ILA which are not neutralizable by specific antibodies or whose biological activity is released by treatment with alkaline pH or adipose tissue extracts (Antoniades et al., 1961). It is possible that these fractions are an aberrant form of insulin. Immunoreactive insulin does not appear after incubation with adipose tissue extracts (Berson and Yalow, 1964; Meade et al., 1965). It is not known whether, how much, and specifically what fraction of ILA increases in human serum after administration of glucose, which typically causes an increase of immunoreactive insulin. Lyngsoe (1964) has investigated this by separation of serum protein fractions.

Even though the physiological significance and chemical nature of ILA remain in doubt, interesting findings have been made in clinically abnormal states. Steinke et al. (1963) found with the assay of $^{14}CO_2$ from glucose-1 ^{14}C in fat pad that fasting levels of ILA are increased in many youth-onset as well as maturity-onset diabetic patients and also in genetic prediabetic patients. After rapid intravenous infusion of glucose, ILA in the serum of six normal subjects increased sharply at 20 minutes and then fell below normal at 60 min.; a slow increase to a maximum at 60 min. occurred in seven prediabetic subjects. Alp et al. (1964) confirmed the finding of increased fasting levels of ILA in diabetics by the criterion of $^{14}CO_2$ formation and noted average increases in acromegalics and in obese subjects. No significant differences in these groups was obtained for ILA when measured as stimulation of conversion of glucose-6-^{14}C to lipids in vitro. By both criteria adult diabetics had a more exaggerated ILA response to oral glucose load than normal. Obese patients had a greater increment in ILA (by $^{14}CO_2$ analysis) after glucose load. Samaan et al. (1965) have recently reported that atypical ILA (fat pad activity not inhibited by insulin antibody) is excessively increased after oral glucose in obese diabetics as well as obese nondiabetics, although typical ILA is increased only in the nondiabetic. After a 7 day fast glucose load elicits in both groups markedly increased "typical" as well as atypical ILA.

A method for ILA determination in vivo was developed by Rafaelson, who measured the increase in glycogen content of rat diaphragm following intraperitoneal injection of insulin or serum. This method has been modified to include the measurement of incorporation of simultaneously injected glucose-U-^{14}C into glycogen of diaphragm and adipose tissue and lipids of the latter (Cahill et al., 1964; Rafaelson et al., 1965). This development may provide a somewhat more physiological assay of ILA than the in vitro methods, but it is relatively laborious. In addition, the intraperitoneal route of access to metabolizing cells is not truly physiological (Cahill et al., 1964).

The possible future role of the ^{14}C methods of measurement of serum ILA for clinical usage is uncertain, in light of the more specific immunoassay with ^{131}I-labeled insulin. Nevertheless, further investigation of this hormonal-like activity may reveal new possibilities for the management of diabetes.

THYROID HORMONE ACTIVITY

In clinical thyrotoxicosis or following administration of triiodothyronine to euthyroid subjects, the rate of $^{14}CO_2$ production from glucose-1-^{14}C incubated with the patient's blood (Johnson and Redding, 1963) is about half of normal. Administration of TSH to rats for several days has a similar effect. Treatment of thyrotoxic patients with radioactive iodine results in a gradual return of $^{14}CO_2$ production toward normal. This metabolic change may prove useful for the assay of thyroid-like activity or the tissue effectiveness of thyroid hormone, both endogenous and exogenous. The effect cannot be related directly to the level of the thyroid hormone in blood, since addition of triiodothyronine in vitro causes stimulation rather than suppression of $^{14}CO_2$ production from glucose-1-^{14}C by washed human red cells (Necheles and Beutler, 1959). An early effect of thyroxine administration to rabbits is an increase in glucose utilization by red cells followed by depression as treatment continues (Calesnick et al., 1960). Furthermore, with thyrotoxic patients there is an increase rather than a decrease of expiration of $^{14}CO_2$ in the breath after administration of glucose-1-^{14}C (Gordon and Goldberg, 1964b).

TURNOVER OF PROTEIN HORMONES

Besides their use for immunoassay of concentration of protein hormones, hormones labeled with ^{131}I provide a means for the study of their turnover in plasma. Evidence of abnormalities of concentration of hormones has increased interest in the possibility of abnormalities of metabolism of the protein hormones.

Berson et al. (1956) studied the disappearance of insulin-^{131}I from the blood of normal and diabetic subjects. They found that the injected insulin distributed into a space equivalent to about 40 per cent of body weight and disappeared (in normal subjects) at a rate of about 2 per cent per minute. In diabetics treated with insulin for several months, the disappearance of labeled insulin was much slower and was associated with binding of insulin-^{131}I by gamma globulin, probably acquired antibody. Bolinger et al. (1964) studied this phenomenon in treated and untreated diabetics. In the early rapid phase of disappearance from plasma, the half-life of insulin-^{131}I was 15 min. for diabetic patients not treated with insulin, 24 min. for stable, insulin-treated patients, and 59 min. for patients with brittle diabetes. Patients in whom the half-life was longest were found to be best regulated on regular (unmodified) insulin, which in these patients behaved more like the modified, long-acting insulins. This test may serve as a convenient guide to the management of brittle diabetes by helping determine the best proportion of long-acting and regular insulin.

The half-life of human growth hormone in plasma has been estimated by Hunter and Greenwood (1964b) to be about 20 to 30 min. This estimate was based not on disappearance of the ^{131}I-labeled hormone, but on the rate of decline of concentration of HGH either following administration of exogenous hormone or following glucose administration, which presumably halts production of endogenous HGH. Utiger (1965) has observed the rate of fall of TSH in the plasma after acute administration of triiodothyronine and concluded that the half-life of TSH in plasma is about 1 to 2 hours. This estimate agreed well with values from analysis of disappearance of ^{131}I-labeled TSH.

A hormone that is not itself protein in nature (although it is bound to plasma globulin), but which can be labeled with ^{131}I, is thyroxine. The half-time of this labeled hormone in plasma is normally about 5 days and certain abnormalities have been found in thyrotoxicosis, hepatitis, and obesity (Benoit and Durrance, 1965).

Studies of turnover and metabolism of ^{131}I-labeled hormones would be supplemented greatly by the availability through synthetic or biosynthetic processes of hormones labeled with components, (e.g.,[14]C, ^{3}H, or ^{35}S) which would represent more truly (in the case of proteins) the natural hormones and permit further investigation of the details of their metabolism.

THE PARATHYROID GLANDS

E. JAMES POTCHEN

The parathyroid glands, four in number, are usually embedded in the superior and inferior poles of the thyroid. Each is about 6 mm. in length and weighs about 100 mg. in an adult. In 1925, Collip prepared an extract from beef parathyroid glands and found that it produced a marked elevation of the blood calcium concentration. Tetany that developed after surgical removal of the parathyroid glands could be alleviated with parathyroid extract and the blood calcium returned to normal. In man the presence of a tumor or hyperplasia of the parathyroid glands leads to a clinical syndrome characterized by an elevation of the serum calcium concentration, diminished phosphate concentration, and a marked increase in the renal excretion of calcium. This may result in the formation of urinary calculi, together with impairment of renal function. With the excessive loss of calcium in the urine, decalcification of the bones occurs, leading to the formation of bone cysts (osteitis fibrosa cystica). Because of the excessive fragility of the bones, the patient is susceptible to spontaneous and induced fractures. The bone abnormalities are often accompanied by an increase in the serum alkaline phosphatase.

When suspected in a patient with unexplained renal or bone disease, the diagnosis of hyperparathyroidism can usually be confirmed by the biochemical alterations. The problem then becomes one of surgical removal of the hyperplastic gland. If the abnormal gland could be located prior to surgery, its removal would be greatly facilitated.

Two agents have been used in attempts to visualize parathyroid adenomas by radioisotope scanning: ^{57}Co-cyanocobalamine and ^{75}Se-selenomethionine. The latter agent has seemed most promising. Its use is based upon the premise that this amino acid analog will be taken up by a hyperactive parathyroid gland more readily than by neighboring structures (especially the thyroid gland).

METABOLISM OF SELENOMETHIONINE

When injected intravenously, selenomethionine is rapidly removed from the blood and enters into protein synthesis (Awwad et al., 1966). This results in a rapid fall in the plasma activity followed by an increase of activity when the isotope reappears in the form of plasma proteins. Thus the blood concentration is lowest 20 to 30 minutes after injection of the isotope in both man and rat (Potchen et al., 1966).

Selenomethionine is actively taken up by the thyroid gland in man and experimental animals. Administration of thyroxine decreases the uptake of selenomethionine, an effect that can be reversed by thyrotropin. Although the time sequence of thyroid uptake of selenomethionine has not been studied in man, much data has been accumulated in the rat. The specific activity of the thyroid reaches a plateau 4 hours after injection. This plateau value is never as high as the levels in the blood or parathyroid glands.

The selenomethionine concentration in muscle is much lower than in the thyroid, parathyroid, or blood, and reaches an early plateau because of the slow rate of turnover of muscle protein.

The changes in the activity of the human parathyroid gland after selenomethionine injection are not known. An isolated instance of a parathyroid adenoma removed 1 hour after intravenous injection of selenomethionine revealed a parathyroid activity six times greater than blood and seven times greater than the thyroid. Thyroidal uptake had been suppressed by pretreatment with tri-iodothyronine (Potchen et al., 1965).

The time course of the uptake of selenomethionine by the parathyroid of the rat has been analyzed in detail (Potchen and Watts, 1967). The para-thyroid activity reaches a peak 20 minutes after injection and then falls for the next 2 hours. The peak corresponds to the time of lowest blood concentration. The difference between the blood and parathyroid radioactivity is an important factor in selecting the time that scanning should be carried out.

The hyperactive parathyroid gland has a greater than normal number of cells actively synthesizing protein from precursor amino acids. In autoradio-graphic studies, methionine has been found to be taken rapidly into the cells of the hyperactive rat parathyroid (Potchen, 1963). The time of greatest intra-cellular accretion is the best time for scanning, in contrast to the case of highly vascular tumors—such as lymphomas—when it may be best to scan when the blood specific activity is highest.

The *in vitro* uptake of the amino acid, lysine, and the amino acid analog, isobutyric acid, by the parathyroid can be markedly enhanced by decreasing the calcium concentration of the media (Raisz et al., 1965). When rats are placed on a calcium-deficient diet for 21 days, there is a twofold increase in seleno-methionine accretion by the parathyroid. These studies lead to the hypothesis that the hyperactive human parathyroid gland might accumulate the labeled amino acid analog, ^{75}Se-selenomethionine.

PARATHYROID SCANNING

The patient is pretreated for 4 days with triiodothyronine (25 μg. four times a day). A dose of 250 μc. of ^{75}Se-selenomethionine (specific activity 60 to 80 μc. per mg.) is injected intravenously, and scanning is begun 5 minutes later. The field of view extends from the hyoid bone to the end of the sternum. Four serial scans are completed over a period of 2½ hours. Thus the scanning interval extends over the period of lowest blood activity. Each image is evaluated sepa-rately and then all four are superimposed. An area of increased accumulation is indicated by the persistence of a focus of increased activity above the sta-tistical fluctuations of the background. A persistent focus of uptake is best ac-complished by superimposition of the four scans.

The results of parathyroid scanning of 40 patients who have undergone parathyroid surgery for suspected hyperparathyroidism are shown in Table 8-1. In 36 patients parathyroid tissue was identified at surgery, and in 20 instances the site of the abnormally functioning parathyroid was correctly identified on the preoperative scan. In four additional cases, only one or two hyperactive glands were identified on the preoperative scan, and three were found at surgery.

When a focus of increased activity was identified on the scan, a parathyroid adenoma was usually found, but in five instances none was found. In four of these patients, a thyroid adenoma was found at surgery. Therefore, we now carry out a simultaneous ^{125}I-iodide scan of the region to look for a thyroid ade-noma. This should decrease the number of false-positive parathyroid scans (Charkes, unpublished).

TABLE 8-1. THE SURGICAL CORRELATION OF PREOPERATIVE PARATHYROID SCAN LOCALIZATION IN 40 PATIENTS WITH SUSPECTED HYPERPARATHYROIDISM

	TOTAL	ADENOMA	HYPERPLASIA	CARCINOMA	NEGATIVE EXPLORATION
Complete correlation	24	15	3	2	4
Partial correlation	4	2	2	—	—
False positive	5	—	—	—	5
False negative	5	4	1	—	—
Technically unsatisfactory	2	—	—	—	—
	40	21	6	2	9

From the experience in these 40 cases, the following conclusions appear warranted:

1. Preoperative parathyroid scanning, when positive, helps in the management of the patient with hyperparathyroidism.

2. Thyroid suppression with thyroxine, though not essential in some cases of fulminating hyperparathyroidism (Hayne et al., 1964), is helpful.

3. A positive scan is usually found with large parathyroid glands, although a small gland may be so hyperactive that it can be visualized. On the other hand, some large glands are relatively inactive. Therefore, the sicker the patient, the more likely the scan will be positive if he has the disease.

4. There are a significant number of false-negative scans in patients with active hyperparathyroidism.

5. The technique of superimposition of scans carried out at different times after injection had aided in the identification of abnormal foci of radioactivity.

6. Attention to technical detail and rigid diagnostic criteria in interpreting parathyroid scans is essential. Scanning does not help in the diagnosis of hyperparathyroidism but at times is helpful in the preoperative localization of abnormal parathyroid activity.

REFERENCES

Ahrens, E. H., Hirsch, J., Oette, K., Farquhar, J. W., and Stein, Y.: Carbohydrate-Induced and Fat-Induced Lipemia. *Trans. Ass. Amer. Physicians* 74:134, 1961.

Alp, H., Recant, L., Kilo, C., Eggeman, J., and Koch, M. B.: Insulin-like Activity in Serum of Normal and Diabetic Subjects. Results Obtained with Dual Assay Measuring Conversion of C-14 Glucose to CO_2 and to Lipid in Rat Adipose Tissue. *Diabetes* 13:509, 1964.

Altzuler, N., Steele, R., Wall, J. S., Dunn, A., and de Bodo, R. C.: Effect of Growth Hormone on Carbohydrate Metabolism in Normal and Hypophysectomized Dogs; Studies with C14 Glucose. *Amer. J. Physiol.* 196:121, 1959.

Antoniades, H. N., Beigelman, P. M., Tranquada, R. B., and Gunderson, K.: Studies on the State of Insulin in the Blood: "Free" Insulin and Insulin Complexes in Human Sera and Their In Vitro Biological Properties. *Endocrinology* 69:46, 1961.

Arky, R. A., and Freinkel, N.: The Response of Plasma Human Growth Hormone to Insulin and Ethanol-induced Hypoglycemia in Two Patients with "Isolated Adrenocorticotropic Defect." *Metabolism* 13:547, 1964.

Armstrong, D. T., Steele, R., Altszuler, N., Dunn, A., Bishop, J. S., and de Bodo, R. C.: Plasma Free Fatty Acid Turnover During Insulin-Induced Hypoglycemia. *Amer. J. Physiol.* 201:535, 1961.

Ashmore, J., Wagle, S. R., and Uete, T.: Studies on Gluconeogenesis. *Advances Enzym. Regulat.* 2:101, 1964.

Awai, K., Hammarstrand, K., and Hennes, A. R.: Studies of Incorporation of Radioactivity into Lipids by Human Blood. I. Pattern of Incorporation of Radioactivity into Fatty Acids by Blood from Normal Subjects and Patients in Diabetic Acidosis. *Metabolism* 13:328, 1964.

Axelrod, L. R., Goldzieher, J. W., and Ross, S. D.: Concurrent 3β-Hydroxysteroid Dehydrogenase Deficiency in Adrenal and Sclerocystic Ovary. *Acta Endocr. (Kbh.)* 48:392, 1965.

Baker, N., Shreeve, W. W., Shipley, R. A., Incefy, G. E., and Miller, M.: [14]C Studies in Carbohydrate Metabolism. I. The Oxidation of Glucose in Normal Human Subjects. *J. Biol. Chem.* 211:575, 1954.

Balodimos, M. C., Ball, J. J., and Williams, R. H.: Intravenous Triolein-^{131}I and Tripalmitin-[14]C Emulsions in Humans. *Metabolism* 11:365, 1962.

Beck, L. V., Zaharks, D. S., Roberts, N., McNeill, J., King, C., and Blankenbaker, R.: Insulin Assay by Combined Use of ^{131}I-labeled Insulin, Anti-insulin Serum and Insulinase. *Life Sci.* 3:545, 1964.

Benedict, J. D., Forsham, P. H., and Stetten, DeW., Jr.: Metabolism of Uric Acid in Normal and Gouty Humans Studied with Aid of Isotopic Uric Acid. *J. Biol. Chem.* 181:183, 1949.

Benedict, J. D., Yü, T. F., Bien, E. J., Gutman, A. B., and Stetten, DeW., Jr.: A Further Study of the Utilization of Dietary Glycine Nitrogen for Uric Acid Synthesis in Gout. *J. Clin. Invest.* 32:775, 1953.

Benoit, F. L., and Durrance, F. Y.: Radiothyroxine Turnover in Obesity. *Amer. J. Med. Sci.* 249:647, 1965.

Berson, S. A., and Yalow, R. S.: Quantitative Aspects of the Reaction between Insulin and Insulin-binding Antibody. *J. Clin. Invest.* 38:1996, 1959.

Berson, S. A., and Yalow, R. S.: Immunoassay of Protein Hormones. *In:* Pincus, G., Thimann, K. V. and Astwood, E. B., Eds.: The Hormones. Academic Press, Inc., New York, 1964, vol. 4.

Berson, S. A., Yalow, R. S., Aurbach, C. D., and Potts, J. T., Jr.: Immunoassay of Bovine and Human Parathyroid Hormone. *Proc. Nat. Acad. Sci.* 49:613, 1963.

Berson, S. A., Yalow, R. S., Bauman, A., Rothschild, M. A., and Newerly, K.: Insulin-I[131] Metabolism in Human Subjects: Demonstration of Insulin Binding Globulin in the Circulation of Insulin-treated Subjects. *J. Clin. Invest.* 35:170, 1956.

Bierman, E. L., and Hamlin, J. T., III: The Effect of Insulin and Glucagon on the Removal of ^{14}C-Labeled Particulate Triglyceride from Plasma in Man. *Metabolism* 12:666, 1963.

Bierman, E L.., Schwartz, I. L., and Dole, V. P.: Action of Insulin on Release of Fatty Acids from Tissue Stores. *Amer. J. Physiol.* 191:359, 1957.

Bloch, E., and Benirschke, K.: Synthesis *in Vitro* of Steroids by Human Fetal Adrenal Gland Slices. *J. Biol. Chem.* 234:1085, 1959.

Bolinger, R. E., Morris, H., McKnight, F. G., and Diederick, D. A.: Disappearance of ^{131}I-Labeled Insulin from Plasma as a Guide to Management of Diabetes. *New Eng. J. Med.* 270:767, 1964.

Brown, J.: Metabolism of Free Fatty Acids in Obese Humans. *Proc. Soc. Exp. Biol. Med.* 118:901, 1965.

Buchanan, J. M., and Hastings, A. B.: The Use of Isotopically Marked Carbon in the Study of Intermediary Metabolism. *Physiol. Rev.* 26:120, 1946.

Cahill, G. F., Jr., Lauris, V., Soeldner, J. L., Slone, D., and Steinke, J.: Assay of Serum Insulin and Insulin-like Activity on Adipose Tissue and Muscle in Vivo. *Metabolism* 13:769, 1964.

Calesnick, B., Altarelli, V. R., and Spirtes, M. A.: Decrease in Aerobic Glycolysis of Erythrocytes Following the Continuous Administration of L-Triiodothyronine. *Endocrinology* 66:517, 1960.

Cameron, J. S.: The Effect of Insulin on Carbohydrate Metabolism in the Mammalian Liver: A Review. *Guy. Hosp. Rep.* 111:145, 1962.

Carlson, L. A., and Ostman, J.: In Vitro Studies on the Glucose Uptake and Fatty Acid Metabolism of Human Adipose Tissue in Diabetes Mellitus. *Acta Med. Scand.* 174:215, 1963.

Cerasi, E., and Luft, R.: Plasma Insulin Response to Sustained Hyperglycemia Induced by Glucose Infusion in Human Subjects. *Lancet* 2:1359, 1963.

Cerasi, E., and Luft, R.: Insulin Response to Glucose Loading in Acromegaly. *Lancet* 2:769, 1964.

Cohn, G. L., and Mulrow, P. J.: Androgen Release and Synthesis *in Vitro* by Human Adult Adrenal Glands. *J. Clin. Invest.* 42:64, 1963.

Cozzetto, F. J.: Radiocarbon Estimates of Intestinal Absorption. Studies of Breath Excretion of $C^{14}O_2$ after Ingestion of Labeled Fatty Acids, Glucose and Lactose. *Amer. J. Dis. Child.* 107:605, 1964.

Crowley, L. G., Demetriou, J. A., Kotin, P., Donovan, A. J., and Kushinsky, S.: Excretion Patterns of Urinary Metabolism of Estradiol-4-^{14}C in Postmenopausal Women with Benign and Malignant Disease of the Breast. *Cancer Res.* 25:371, 1965.

De Meutter, R. C., and Shreeve, W. W.: Conversion of DL-Lactate-2-C^{14} or -3-C^{14} or Pyruvate-2-C^{14} to Blood Glucose in Humans: Effects of Diabetes, Insulin, Tolbutamide, and Glucose Load. *J. Clin. Invest.* 42:525, 1963.

Doherty, J. E., Perkins, W. H., and Shapira, J.: Radiocarbon and Tritium-Labeled Cholesterol in Alpha and Beta Lipoproteins After Oral Administration to Human Subjects. *J. Lab. Clin. Med.* 59:550, 1962.

Dole, V. P.: A Relation Between Non-Esterified Fatty Acids in Plasma and the Metabolism of Glucose. *J. Clin. Invest.* 35:150, 1956.

Elrick, H., Stimmler, L., Hlad, C. J., Jr., and Arai, Y.: Plasma Insulin Response to Oral and Intravenous Glucose Administration. *J. Clin. Endocr.* 24:1076, 1964.

Farquhar, J. W., Gross, R. C., Wagner, R. M., and Reaven, G. M.: Validation of an Incompletely Coupled Two-Compartment Nonrecycling Catenary Model for Turnover of Liver and Plasma Triglyceride in Man. *J. Lipid Res.* 6:119, 1965.

Felber, J. P.: ACTH Antibodies and Their Use for a Radioimmunoassay for ACTH. *Experientia* 19:227, 1963.

Felber, J. P., Moody, A. J., and Vannotti, A.: Méthodes Immunologiques et Radioimmunologiques de Détermination des Hormones Protidiques. *Schweiz. Med. Wschr.* 95:757, 1965.

Fine, M., Michaels, G., Shah, S., Chai, B., Fukayama, G., and Kinsell, L.: The Incorporation of C^{14} from Uniformly-Labeled Glucose into Plasma Triglycerides in Normals and Hyperglyceridemics. *Metabolism* 11:893, 1962.

Frankson, J. R. M., Ooms, H. A., Bellens, R., Conard, V., and Bastenie, P. A.: Physiologic Significance of the Intravenous Glucose Tolerance Test. *Metabolism* 11:482, 1962.

Frederickson, D. S., and Gordon, R. S., Jr.: The Metabolism of Albumin-Bound ^{14}C-Labeled Unesterified Fatty Acids in Normal Human Subjects. *J. Clin. Invest.* 37:1504, 1958.

Frederickson, D. S., and Lees, R. S.: A System for Phenotyping Hyperlipoproteinemia. *Circulation* 31:321, 1965.

Friedberg, S. J., Harlan, W. R. J., Trout, D. L., and Estes, E. H., Jr.: The Effect of Exercise on the Concentration and Turnover of Plasma Nonesterified Fatty Acids. *J. Clin. Invest.* 39:215, 1960a.

Friedberg, S. J., Klein, R. F., Trout, D. L., Bogdonoff, M. D., and Estes, E. H., Jr.: The Characteristics of the Peripheral Transport of ^{14}C Labeled Palmitic Acid. *J. Clin. Invest.* 39:1511, 1960b.

Friedberg, S. J., Klein, R. F., Trout, D. L., Bogdonoff, M. D., and Estes, E. H., Jr.: The Incorporation of Plasma Free Fatty Acids into Plasma Triglycerides in Man. *J. Clin. Invest.* 40:1846, 1961.

Froesch, E. R., Burgi, H., Ramseier, E. B., Bally, P., and Labhart, A.: Antibody-suppressible and Nonsuppressible Insulin-like Activities in Human Serum and their Physiological Significance. An Insulin Assay with Adipose Tissue of Increased Precision and Specificity. *J. Clin. Invest.* 42:1816, 1963.

Gellhorn, A., and Marks, P. A.: The Composition and Biosynthesis of Lipids in Human Adipose Tissues. *J. Clin. Invest.* 40:925, 1961.

Ghose, A., Shreeve, W. W., Shigeta, Y., and Schwartz, I. L.: Incorporation of Tritium from Glucose-1-^{3}H and DL-Lactate-2-^{3}H into Human Plasma Triglycerides. *Nature* 201:722, 1964.

Gidez, L. I., and Eder, H. A.: Cholesterol Metabolism in Man. *Biochem. Pharmacol.* 8:86, 1961.

Gillman, J., Gilbert, C., and Savage, N.: Endocrine Control of the Fatty Liver and Serum Lipids in Baboons with Special Reference to the Disorder of Lipid Metabolism in Kwashiorkor. *Metabolism* 11:800, 1962.

Glick, S. M., Roth, J., Yalow, R. S., and Berson, S. A.: Immunoassay of Human Growth Hormone in Plasma. *Nature* 199:784, 1963.

Goetz, T. C., Greenberg, B., Ells, J., and Meinert, C.: A Simple Immunoassay for Insulin: Application to Human and Dog Plasma. *J. Clin. Endocr.* 23:1237, 1963.

Gold, N. I.: Kinetic Aspects of Cortisol-1-^{14}C Metabolism in a Patient After Subtotal Adrenalectomy for Cushing's Syndrome Associated with Bilateral Adrenal Hyperplasia. *J. Clin. Invest.* 41:1871, 1962.

Gordon, E. S.: New Concepts of the Biochemistry and Physiology of Obesity. *Med. Clin. N. Amer.* 48:1285, 1964.

Gordon, E. S., and Goldberg, M.: Carbon-14 Studies of Energy Metabolism in Various Thyroid States. *Metabolism* 13:591, 1964a.

Gordon, E. S., and Goldberg, M.: Studies of Energy Metabolism in Human Subjects Using ^{14}C-Labeled Compounds. *Metabolism* 13:775, 1964b.

Gould, R. G., Leroy, G. V., Okita, G. T., Kabara, J. J., Keegan, P., and Bergenstal, D. M.: The Use of C14-Labeled Acetate to Study Cholesterol Metabolism in Man. *J. Lab. Clin. Med.* 46:372, 1955.

Greenwood, F. C., Hunter, W. M., and Klopper, A.: Assay of Human Growth Hormone in Pregnancy at Parturition and in Lactation. *Brit. Med. J.* 1:22, 1964a.

Greenwood, F. C., Hunter, W. M., and Marrian, V. J.: Growth Hormone Levels in Children and Adolescents. *Brit. Med. J.* 1:25, 1964b.

Grodsky, G. M., and Forsham, P. H.: An Immunochemical Assay of Total Extractable Insulin in Man. *J. Clin. Invest.* 39:1070, 1960.

Grodsky, G. M., Hayashide, T., Peng, C. T., and Geschwind, I. I.: Production of Glucagon Antibodies and Their Role in Metabolism and Immunoassay of Glucagon. *Proc. Soc. Exp. Biol. Med.* 107:491, 1961.

Gutman, A. B., and Yü, T. F.: An Abnormality of Glutamine Metabolism in Primary Gout. *Amer. J. Med.* 35:820, 1963.

Gutman, A. B., Yü, T. F., Black, H., Yalow, R. S., and Berson, S. A.: Incorporation of Glycine-1-C^{14}, Glycine-2-C^{14}, and Glycine-N^{15} into Uric Acid in Normal and Gouty Subjects. *Amer. J. Med.* 25:917, 1958.

Hales, C. N., and Randle, P. J.: Immunoassay of Insulin with Insulin-Antibody Precipitate *Biochem. J.* 88:137, 1963.

Hamosh, H., Hamosh, P., Bar-Moor, J. A., and Cohen, H.: Fatty Acid Metabolism by Human Adipose Tissue. *J. Clin. Invest.* 42:1648, 1963.

Havel, R. J.: Conversion of Plasma Free Fatty Acids into Triglycerides of Plasma Lipoprotein Fractions in Man. *Metabolism* 10:1031, 1961.

Havel, R. J., Naimark, A., and Borchgrevink, C. F.: Turnover Rate and Oxidation of Free Fatty Acids of Blood Plasma in Man During Exercise: Studies During Continuous Infusion of Palmitate-1-C^{14}. *J. Clin. Invest.* 42:1054, 1963.

Hellman, L., Rosenfeld, R. S., and Gallagher, T. F.: Cholesterol Synthesis from C^{14}-Acetate in Man. *J. Clin. Invest.* 33:142, 1954.

Hennes, A. R.: Abnormalities of Acetate Metabolism in Adrenal Insufficiency in Man. *Amer. J. Med.* 32:343, 1962.

Hennes, A. R., and Awai, K.: Studies of Incorporation of Radioactivity into Lipids by Human Blood. III. Abnormal Incorporation of Acetate-^{14}C into Fatty Acids by Whole Blood and Platelets from Nonketotic Insulin-Dependent Diabetics. *Metabolism* 14:487, 1965.

Hennes, A. R., Moore, M. Z., and Masters, U. F.: Studies of Cholesterol Metabolism with C^{14}-Acetate in Diabetic Patients and in Patients with Hypercholesterolemia. *Metabolism* 11:925, 1962.

Hennes, A. R., and Redding, T. W.: Defective Synthesis of Triglyceride Fatty Acids from 1-C-14-Acetate in the Well-Controlled Stable Adult Diabetic. *Diabetes* 10:85, 1961.

Hennes, A. R., and Shreeve, W. W.: Hormonal Effects on C-14 Acetate Metabolism in the Human. *Proc. Soc. Exp. Biol. Med.* 100:246, 1959.

Herbert, V., Lau, K. S., Gottbet, C. W., Arky, R. A., and Bleicher, S. J.: Radioimmunoassay of Insulin: A Rapid, Simple Method Using "Instant Dialysis" with Coated Charcoal. *J. Clin. Invest.* 44:1059, 1965.

Hetenyi, G., Jr., Wrenshall, G. A., and Best, C. H.: Rates of Production Utilization, Accumulation and Apparent Distribution Space of Glucose: Effects of Insulin in Dogs Using a Validated Tracer Method. *Diabetes* 10:304, 1961.

Hirsch, J., and Goldrick, B.: Metabolism of Human Adipose Tissue In Vitro. *In* Renold, A. E., and Cahill, G. F., Jr., Eds.: Handbook of Physiology. Sec. 5. Waverly Press, Inc., Baltimore, 1965.

Horton, R., Shinsako, J., and Forsham, P. H.: Testosterone Production and Metabolic Clearance Rates With Volumes of Distribution in Normal Adult Men and Women. *Acta Endocr. (Kbh.)* 48:446, 1965.

Hunter, W. M., and Greenwood, F. C.: A Radio-immunoelectrophoretic Assay for Human Growth Hormone. *Biochem. J.* 91:43, 1964a.

Hunter, W. M., and Greenwood, F. C.: Studies on the Secretion of Human Pituitary Growth Hormone. *Brit. Med. J.* 1:804, 1964b.

Ikkos, D., and Luft, R.: Effects of Short-Term Administration of Large Doses of Human Growth Hormone on Carbohydrate Metabolism in Adult, Non-Diabetic Hypophysectomized Women; Studies with ^{14}C-Labeled Glucose. *Acta Endocr. (Kbh.)* 39:567, 1962.

Jacobs, G., Reichard, G., Goodman, E. H., Jr., Friedman, B., and Weinhouse, S.: Action of Insulin and Tolbutamide on Blood Glucose Entry and Removal Rates. *Diabetes* 7:358, 1958.

Johnson, P. C., and Redding, T. R.: Glucose-1-C^{14} Oxidation by Blood: A Potential Test for Tissue Effects of Thyrotoxicosis. *J. Nucl. Med.* 4:393, 1963.

Kahlenberg, A., and Kalant, N.: The Effect of Insulin on Human Adipose Tissue. *Canad. J. Biochem.* 42:1623, 1964.

Kalant, N., Csorba, T. R., and Heller, N.: Effect of Insulin on Glucose Production and Utilization in Diabetes. *Metabolism* 12:1100, 1963.

Kaplan, S. L., and Grumbach, M. M.: Immunoassay for Human Chorionic Growth Hormone-Prolactin in Serum and Urine. *Science* 147:751, 1965.

Karam, J. H., Grodsky, G. M., and Forsham, P. H.: Excessive Insulin Response to Glucose in Obese Subjects as Measured by Immunochemical Assay. *Diabetes* 12:197, 1963.

Kessler, J. I.: Effect in Insulin on Release of Plasma Lipolytic Activity and Clearing of Emulsified Fat Intravenously Administered to Pancreatectomized and Alloxanized Dogs. *J. Lab. Clin. Med.* 60:747, 1962.

Kinsell, L. W., Margen, S., Tarver, H., Frantz, J. McB., and Flanagan, E. K.: Studies in Protein Metabolism with the Aid of ^{35}S-Labeled Methionine. *J. Clin. Invest.* 28:793, 1949.

Kinsell, L. W., Michaels, A. D., and Imaichi, K.: Studies with Fat Emulsions. Metabolism of Intravenously Administered ^{14}C-Tripalmitin. *Amer. J. Clin Nutr.* 16:97, 1965.

Kritchevsky, D., Werthessen, N. T., and Shapiro, I. L.: Studies on the Biosynthesis of Lipids in the Baboon. Biosynthesis and Transport of Cholesterol. *Clin. Chim. Acta* 11:44, 1965.

Kurland, G. S., Lucas, J. L., and Freedberg, A. S.: The Metabolism of Intravenously Infused C^{14}-Labeled Cholesterol in Man. *J. Clin. Invest.* 33:950, 1954.

Landau, B. R., Mahler, R., Ashmore, J., Elwyn, D., Hastings, A. B., and Zotter, S.: Cortisone and the Regulation of Hepatic Gluconeogenesis. *Endocrinology* 70:47, 1962.

Laurell, S.: Turnover Rates of Unesterified Fatty Acids in Human Plasma. *Acta Physiol. Scand.* 41:158, 1957.

Lemarchand-Béraud, T., Felber, J. P., and Vannotti, A.: Développement d'une Méthode Radio-immunologique pour la Détermination de la Thyréostimuline. *Schweiz. Med. Wschr.* 95:772, 1965.

Leonards, J. R.: Insulin-Like Activity of Blood—What Is It? *Fed. Proc.* 18:272, 1959.

Leroy, G. V., Jr.: Clinical Research Using Compounds Labeled with Radioactive Carbon and Hydrogen as Tracers. *Ann. Intern. Med.* 42:239, 1955.

Lipsky, S. R., Haavik, A., Hopper, C. L., and McDivitt, R. W.: The Biosynthesis of the Fatty Acids of the Plasma of Man. I. The Separation of Certain Chromatographically Separated Higher Fatty Acids of the Major Lipid Complexes from Acetate-1-C^{14}. *J. Clin. Invest.* 36:233, 1957.

Luetscher, J. A., Hancock, E. W., Carnargo, C. A., Dowdy, A. J., and Nokes, G. W.: Conjugation of 1,2-^{3}H-Aldosterone in Human Liver and Kidney and Renal Extraction of Aldosterone and Labeled Conjugates from Blood Plasma. *J. Clin. Endoc.* 25:628, 1965.

Lyngsoe, J.: The Insulin-Like Activity in Serum Determined by the Rat Epididymal Fat Method. V. The Distribution of Insulin-Like Activity in Electrophoretically-Separated Serum Protein Fractions from Normal Fasting Subjects and the Effect of Ingestion of Glucose. *Acta Med. Scand.* 175:401, 1964.

Manougian, E., Pollycove, M., Linfoot, J. A., and Lawrence, J. H.: ^{14}C Glucose Kinetic Studies in Normal, Diabetic and Acromegalic Subjects. *J. Nucl. Med.* 5:763, 1964.

Martin, D. B., Renold, A. E., and Dagenais, Y. M.: An Assay for Insulin-Like Activity Using Rat Adipose Tissue. *Lancet* 2:76, 1958.

McManus, J. R., Sweeney, P., and Olson, R. E.: Metabolism of Pyruvate-2-C^{14} in Normal and Diabetic Humans. *Fed. Proc.* 20:191, 1961.

Meade, R. C., and Klitgaard, H. M.: A Simplified Method for Immuno-assay of Human Serum Insulin. *J. Nucl. Med.* 3:407, 1962.

Meade, R. C., Stiglitz, R. A., and Kleist, T. J.: The State of Pancreatic and Serum Insulin. Results of Immunoassay. *Diabetes* 14:387, 1965.

Morgan, C. R., and Lazarow, A.: Immunoassay of Insulin. Two Antibody System. Plasma Insulin Levels of Normal, Subdiabetic and Diabetic Rats. *Diabetes* 12:115, 1963.

Morgan, C. R., Sorenson, R. L., and Lazarow, A.: Further Studies of an Inhibitor of the Two Antibody Immunoassay System. *Diabetes* 13:579, 1964.

Necheles, T., and Beutler, E.: The Effect of Triiodothyronine on the Oxidative Metabolism of Erythrocytes. I. Cellular Studies. *J. Clin. Invest.* 38:788, 1959.

Nestel, P. J.: Metabolism of Linoleate and Palmitate in Patients with Hypertriglyceridemia and Heart Disease. *Metabolism* 14:1, 1965.

Nestel, P. J., Denborough, M. A., and O'Dea, J.: Disposal of Human Chylomicrons Administered Intravenously in Ischemic Heart Disease and Essential Hyperlipemia. *Circulation Res.* 10:786, 1962.

Odell, W. D., Wilber, J. F., and Paul, W. E.: Radioimmunoassay of Human Thyrotropin in Serum. *Metabolism* 14:465, 1965.

Oji, N., and Shreeve, W. W.: Studies of Gluconeogenesis Using ^{14}C- and ^{3}H-Labeled Compounds in Cortisone-Treated Rats. *Fed. Proc.* 24:537, 1965.

Ormsby, J. W., Schnatz, J. D., and Williams, R. H.: The Incorporation of Linoleic-1-C^{14} Acid in Human Plasma and Adipose Tissue. *Metabolism* 12:812, 1963.

Ostman, J.: A Procedure for In Vitro Studies on Fatty Acid Metabolism by Human Subcutaneous Adipose Tissue. *Acta Med. Scand.* 177:183, 1965.

Pollycove, M.: Glucose Kinetics and Oxidation and the Effects of Insulin, Tolbutamide and Phenethylbiguanide (DBI) in Normal Human Subjects. Symposium on Respiration Pattern Analysis in Intermediary Metabolism Study. Applied Physics Corporation, Berkeley, Calif., 1964.

Rabinowitz, D., and Zierler, K. L.: Role of Free Fatty Acids in Forearm Metabolism in Man, Quantitated by Use of Insulin. J. Clin. Invest. 41:2191, 1962.

Rafaelson, O. J., Lauris, V., and Renold, A. E.: Localized Intraperitoneal Action of Insulin on Rat Diaphragm and Epididymal Adipose Tissue In Vivo. Diabetes 14:19, 1965.

Randle, P. J., Hales, C. N., Garland, P. B., and Newsholme, E. A.: Glucose Fatty-Acid Cycle: Its Role in Insulin Sensitivity and the Metabolic Disturbances of Diabetes Mellitus. Lancet 1:785, 1963.

Reichard, G. A., Jacobs, A. G., Kimbell, P., Hochella, N. J., and Weinhouse, S.: Blood Glucose Replacement Rates in Normal and Diabetic Humans. J. Appl. Physiol. 16:789, 1961.

Reichard, G. A., Moury, N. F., Jr., Hochella, N. J., Patterson, A. L., and Weinhouse, S.: Quantitative Estimation of the Cori Cycle in the Human. J. Biol. Chem. 238:495, 1963.

Rittenberg, D.: Dynamic Aspects of the Metabolism of Amino Acids. The Harvey Lectures. Charles C Thomas, Springfield, Ill. 1949.

Roth, J., Glick, S. M., Yalow, R. S., and Berson, S. A.: Hypoglycemia: A Potent Stimulus to Secretion of Growth Hormone. Science 140:987, 1963.

Sacks, W.: Cerebral Metabolism of Doubly-Labeled Glucose in Humans In Vivo. J. Appl. Physiol. 20:117, 1965.

Samaan, N. A., Dempster, W. J., Fraser, R., Please, N. W., and Stillman, D.: Further Immunological Studies on the Form of Circulating Insulin. J. Endocrinology 24:263, 1962.

Samaan, N. A., Fraser, R., Brown, J., and Trayner, R.: Serum Insulin-Like Activity in Obese Diabetics and Nondiabetics Before and After a Prolonged Fast. Diabetes 14:442, 1965.

Schalch, D. S., and Parker, M. L.: A Sensitive Double Antibody Immunoassay for Human Growth Hormone in Plasma. Nature 203:1141, 1964.

Schless, G. L.: Nonesterified Fatty Acids as a Metabolic Substrate: The Rapid Turnover Theory. Metabolism 13:934, 1964.

Scow, R. O.: Perfusion of Isolated Adipose Tissue: FFA Release and Blood Flow in Rat Parametrial Fat Body. In Renold, A. E., and Cahill, G. F., Jr., Eds.: Handbook of Physiology. Sec. 5. Waverly Press, Inc., Baltimore, 1965.

Searle, G. L., Mortimore, G. E., Buckley, R. E., and Reilly, W. A.: Plasma Glucose Turnover in Humans as Studied with ^{14}C Glucose Influence of Insulin and Tolbutamide. Diabetes 8:167, 1959.

Seegmiller, J. E., Grayzel, A. I., Laster, L., and Liddle, L. W.: Uric Acid Production in Gout. J. Clin. Invest. 40:1304, 1961.

Seegmiller, J. E., Laster, L., and Howell, R. R.: Biochemistry of Uric Acid and Its Relation to Gout. New Eng. J. Med. 268:764, 1963.

Seegmiller, J. E., Laster, L., and Liddle, L. W.: Failure to Detect Consistent Over-Incorporation of Glycine-1-^{14}C into Uric Acid in Primary Gout. Metabolism 7:376, 1958.

Segal, S., Berman, M., and Blair, A.: The Metabolism of Variously ^{14}C-Labeled Glucose in Man and an Estimation of the Extent of Glucose Metabolism by the Hexose Monophosphate Pathway. J. Clin. Invest. 40:1263, 1961.

Segal, S., and Foley, J.: The Metabolism of D-Ribose in Man. J. Clin. Invest. 37:719, 1958.

Segal, S., and Topper, Y. J.: The Biosynthesis and Metabolism of L-Fucose in Man. J. Clin. Invest. 37:930, 1958.

Shreeve, W. W.: Pathways of Carbohydrate Formation in Man. I. Isotope Distribution in Glucose from Nondiabetic Subjects Given 1-C^{14}-Acetate. J. Clin. Invest. 37:999, 1958.

Shreeve, W. W.: Diabetic Ketosis. Ann. N.Y. Acad. Sci. 104:772, 1963.

Shreeve, W. W.: Transfer of ^{14}C and ^{3}H from Labeled Substrates to CO_2, Water, and Lipids in Diabetic and Obese Subjects In Vivo. Ann. N.Y. Acad. Sci. 131:464, 1965.

Shreeve, W. W., Baker, N., Miller, M., Shipley, R. A., Incefy, G. E., and Craig, J. W.: ^{14}C Studies in Carbohydrate Metabolism. II. The Oxidation of Glucose in Diabetic Human Subjects. Metabolism 5:22, 1956.

Shreeve, W. W., and De Meutter, R. C.: Pathways of Carbohydrate Formation in Man. III. Distribution Labeling of Blood Glucose by DL-Lactate-2-^{14}C or Pyruvate-2-^{14}C in Diabetic and Nondiabetic Subjects. J. Biol. Chem. 239:722, 1964.

Shreeve, W. W., De Meutter, R. C., and Shigeta, Y.: Diabetes, Insulin, Tolbutamide, and Glucose Load in the Degradation of C^{14}-labeled Lactate and Pyruvate. Diabetes 13:615, 1964.

Shreeve, W. W., De Meutter, R. C., Shigeta, Y., and Ghose, A.: Formation of C-14-O_2 and H-3-OH from Labeled Lactate, Pyruvate and Glucose in Diabetic and Obese Patients. Diabetes 12:360, 1963.

Shreeve, W. W., Hennes, A. R., and Schwartz, R.: Production of $^{14}CO_2$ from 1- and 2-C^{14}-Acetate by Human Subjects in Various Metabolic States. Metabolism 8:742, 1959.

Shreeve, W. W., and Tocci, P. M.: Conversion of 1-C¹⁴-Acetate to Ketone Bodies in Diabetics. *Metabolism* 10:522, 1961.

Steinke, J., Soeldner, S., Camerini-Davalos, R. A., and Renold, A. E.: Studies on Serum Insulin-Like Activity (ILA) in Prediabetes and Early Overt Diabetes. *Diabetes* 12:502, 1963.

Stimmler, L., Brazie, J. V., and O'Brien, D.: Plasma-Insulin Levels in the Newborn Infants of Normal and Diabetic Mothers. *Lancet* 1:137, 1964.

Tashjian, A. J., Oji, N., and Shreeve, W. W.: Comparison of Intravenous and Oral Cortisone-Glucose Tolerance Tests With Utilization of Glucose-1-¹⁴C and Glucose-1-³H in Obese and Diabetic Patients. *Diabetes* 14:467, 1965.

Unger, R. H., and Eisentraut, A. M.: Studies of the Physiological Role of Glucagon. *Diabetes* 13:563, 1964.

Unger, R. H., Eisentraut, A. M., McCall, M. S., and Madison, I. L.: Glucagon Antibodies and an Immunoassay for Glucagon. *J. Clin. Invest.* 40:1280, 1961.

Utiger, R. D.: Radioimmunoassay of Human Plasma Thyrotropin. *J. Clin. Invest.* 44:1277, 1965.

Utiger, R. D., Parker, M. L., and Daughaday, W. H.: Studies on Human Growth Hormone. I. A Radioimmunoassay for Human Growth Hormone. *J. Clin. Invest.* 41:254, 1962.

Wood, H. G., Katz, J., and Landau, B. R.: Estimation of Pathways of Carbohydrate Metabolism. *Biochem. Z.* 338:809, 1963.

Wyngaarden, J. B.: Over-Production of Uric Acid as the Cause of Hyperuricemia in Primary Gout. *J. Clin. Invest.* 36:1508, 1957.

Yalow, R. S., and Berson, S. A.: Immunoassay for Plasma Insulin. *Meth. Biochem. Anal.* 12:69–96, 1964.

Yalow, R. S., and Berson, S. A.: Dynamics of Insulin Secretion in Hypoglycemia. *Diabetes* 14:341, 1965.

Yalow, R. S., Glick, S. M., Roth, J., and Berson, S. A.: Radioimmunoassay of Human Plasma ACTH. *J. Clin. Endocr.* 24:1219, 1964.

THE PARATHYROID GLANDS

Awwad, H. K., et al.: The Regional Distribution of Se-75 Selenomethionine in the Rat. *Metabolism* 15:370, 1966a.

Awwad, H. K., et al.: Se-75 Selenomethionine Incorporation into Human Plasma Proteins and Erythrocytes. *Metabolism* 15:626, 1966b.

Awwad, H. K., et al.: The Interconversion and Reutilization of Injected Se-75 Selenomethionine in the Rat. *J. Biol. Chem.*

Bartelheimer, H., et al.: Auffindung eines Nebenschilddrusenadenoms erst nach szintigraphischer Darstellung mit ⁷⁵Se-Methionin. *Klin. Wschr.* 16:854, 1965.

Beierwaltes, W. H.: Attempts at Visualization of the Parathyroid and Pancreas by Photoscanning. *Northwest Med.* 63:771, 1964.

Charkes, N. D.: Unpublished Data.

DiGuilio, W., and Morales, J.: An Evaluation of Parathyroid Scanning Using Selenium-75-Methionine. *J. Nucl. Med.* 7:380, 1966.

Gottschalk, A., et al.: Bilateral Intra-arterial Injection in the Thyrocervical Trunk: A Technique to Facilitate Localization of Parathyroid Adenoma with Selenium-75-Methionine. *J. Nucl. Med.* 7:374, 1966.

Haynie, T. P., Otte, W. K., and Wright, J. C.: Visualization of a Hyperfunctioning Parathyroid Adenoma Using Se-75 and the Photoscanner. *J. Nucl. Med.* 5:710, 1964.

Potchen, E. J.: Isotopic Labeling of the Rat Parathyroid as Demonstrated by Autoradiography. *J. Nucl. Med.* 4:480, 1963.

Potchen, E. J., et al.: The Thyroid Uptake of Se-75-Selenomethionine: Effect of L-Thyroxine and Thyroid-Stimulating Hormone. *J. Nucl. Med.* 7:433, 1966.

Potchen, E. J., and Watts, H. G.: The Thyro-Parathyroid Uptake of Selenomethionine in the Rat. *Endocrinology* 80:469, 1966.

Potchen, E. J., Wilson, R. E., and Dealy, J. B., Jr.: External Parathyroid Scanning with Se-75 Selenomethionine. *Ann. Surg.* 162:505, 1965.

Raisz, L. G., et al.: *In* Gaillard, P. J., et al. (eds.): The Parathyroid Glands. University of Chicago Press, Chicago, 1965, p. 37.

Sack, V. H., et al.: Darstellung eines Nebenschilddrusenadenoms mit ⁷⁵Selen-methionin und der Szintillationskamera. *Deutsch. Med. Wschr.* 90:2353, 1965.

IX

THE BLOOD

R. M. KNISELEY

D. R. KORST

W. B. NELP

N. I. BERLIN

THE BONE MARROW

R. M. KNISELEY[1]

INTRODUCTION

Valuable diagnostic information can be obtained from needle aspirations or biopsies of bone marrow, but only small areas can be sampled. By means of radioisotope scanning techniques, we can delineate areas of active bone marrow, showing such features as abnormal expansion of active areas into the extremities, localized or generalized decrease in hematopoiesis, and compensatory marrow activity in sites normally occupied by fat. Although day-to-day problems in hematological practice may often not be solved with marrow scans, the method provides a useful tool in clinical investigation. We can glean valuable information about disorders that destroy bone marrow, visualize responses to stresses, such as infection or blood loss, and evaluate the stage of disease. With suitable instrumentation, relatively small defects in sites of active marrow can be seen.

---

[1] Medical Division, Oak Ridge Institute of Nuclear Studies, under contract with the U.S. Atomic Energy Commission.

Visualization of the distribution of active bone marrow depends on the use of a physiological process that concentrates the radioactive tracer. Two groups of compounds can be used; one group depends for its effect on the function of active marrow as a producer of granulocytes, megakaryocytes (and platelets), and erythrocytes, and the other depends on its function as an important site of reticuloendothelial activity. Iron is incorporated into hemoglobin during eryth-

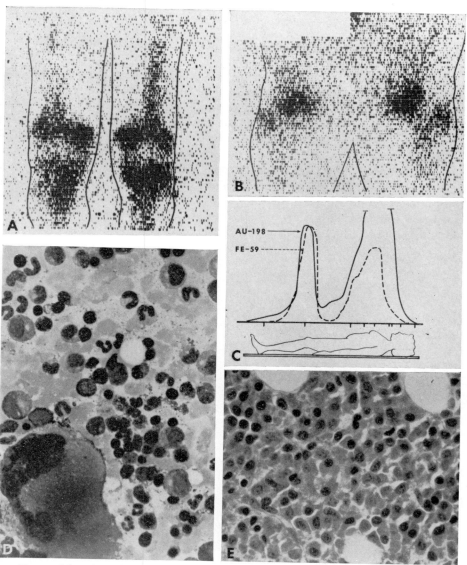

FIGURE 9-1. *A*, Multiple myeloma in a woman, with extensive destruction of the skeleton of the trunk. Area scan of knees shows pronounced activity in lower femora and upper tibias. *B*, Area scan of the pelvis shows greatly diminished marrow in the pelvic bone with increased uptake in proximal femora. *C*, Linear scan showing unusual distribution of the colloidal [198]Au. The high amount of uptake in the knee region corresponds to the active hematopoiesis. This correlates well with the linear scan after a test dose of [59]Fe. *D*, Aspirate from tibia showing cellular marrow with normal hematopoietic elements (Wright stain). *E*, Biopsy of ilium showing the characteristic pattern of multiple myeloma (hematoxylin and eosin stain). (From Edwards, 1964.)

ropoiesis and accumulates in areas of bone marrow that produce red blood cell precursors. However, we must remember that in certain instances disorders of iron metabolism may also influence the sites of localization of radioiron. Phagocytosis of colloidal particles by reticuloendothelial (R.E.) cells of the bone marrow correlates well with hematopoietic activity, and forms the basis for another approach to bone marrow scanning. Fatty marrow usually does not accumulate radioactive colloids.

RADIOPHARMACEUTICALS FOR BONE MARROW SCANNING

Two isotopes of iron have been used. Iron-59, with its long half-life (45 days), is limited to small doses; the number of photons available is too small to permit highly resolved images, but linear or profile scans can be obtained by doses of 10 to 25 μc. (Fig. 9-1C). With a 40 μc. dose it has been possible to obtain an image of poor resolution on a rectilinear scan (Simpson, 1963). Extension of the marrow into the extremities can be detected by this method. Iron-52, a cyclotron-produced positron-emitting isotope with a 6.2 hour half-life, permits administration of higher doses of radioactivity, with a much smaller and quite permissible radiation exposure to the subject. The localization of the ^{52}Fe in the marrow can be clearly shown in positron camera pictures (Anger and Van Dyke, 1964, 1965) (Fig. 9-2). At present, only a few groups have the capabilities

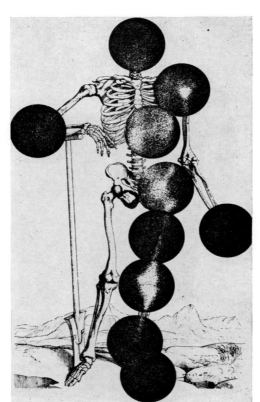

FIGURE 9-2. Positron camera picture of a patient with secondary polycythemia caused by severe cyanotic heart disease. The expansion of the marrow is clearly shown in these multiple views of the skeleton, taken about 16 hours after intravenous administration of 150 μc. of ^{52}Fe, each area requiring a 10 minute exposure. The views are superimposed on a plate of Vesalius's "Fabrica." (Anger and VanDyke, 1964.)

for production of this isotope. Nevertheless, demonstration of the feasibility of this approach is a very important contribution to bone-marrow scanning.

Colloidal gold-198 has been a useful compound for delineating bone marrow. It has the virtues of ready availability and moderate gamma energy (411 kev.). The strong beta emission and the 2.7 day half-life prohibit its wide application in large doses. We have confined its use to doses of 1 to 2 mc. and to patients with serious marrow disorders when the prognosis is limited, or when marrow-depressing irradiation or chemotherapy is required for control of the disease (Edwards et al., 1964; Kniseley et al., 1964, 1966). However, in these doses no hematological alterations have been clinically detectable. With sacrifice of scanning speed or spatial resolution, distributions of the marrow can be ob-

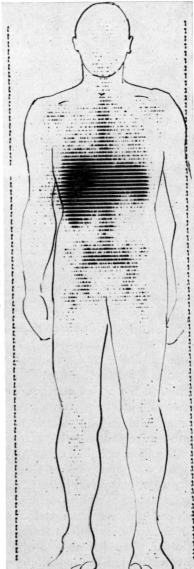

FIGURE 9-3. Whole-body scan after intravenous colloidal [198]Au in a young man without known hematopoietic disorder. A high uptake by the liver and spleen obscures the midtrunk. The active bone marrow is confined mostly to the trunk, the proximal femora, and the humeri.

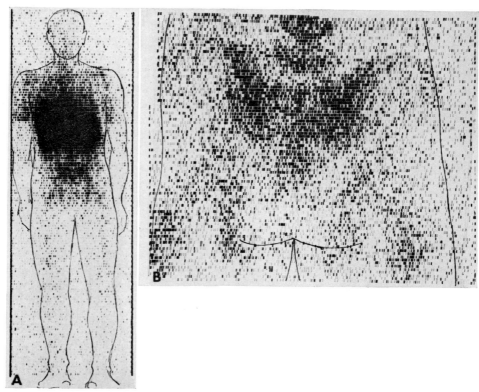

FIGURE 9-4. *A,* Whole-body scan 3.5 hours after intravenous injection of 4 mc of ^{99m}Tc sulfur sol colloid in a patient with chronic granulocytic leukemia. In general, the active marrow has the usual distribution with slight extension into the femora. The bone marrow in the region around the large amount of activity in the liver and spleen is obscured by the right-angle scatter of the low-energy colloid. Scatter is seen also in the upper arms, but was prevented in the lower arms by the placing of a sheet of lead between the forearm and the trunk. *B,* Scan of posterior view of the pelvis in the same patient as in *A,* using the ORNL 37 hole gold-tungsten collimator shield. Scatter observed in the whole-body scan is not obvious with this view. Note that intervertebral disks are visualized.

tained with lower doses (500 μc.) than in our initial studies (Larsson and Jonsson, 1964). After intravenous injection, the blood is cleared of the colloid with a half-time of 3 to 4 minutes; scanning is begun after about 15 minutes. The colloid is fixed in the R.E. cells, mostly in the liver and spleen, with a small fraction in the active marrow. There is no mobilization, transport, or excretion; hence scans can be performed even after a day or two. High concentrations in the liver and spleen obscure the marrow of the midtrunk region and constitute a disadvantage of this radiopharmaceutical for bone-marrow scanning (Fig. 9-3).

The ideal colloidal compound would have a moderately low energy gamma emission, no beta emission, ready availability, a short half-life, a colloidal nature easily reproduced, uniform particle size, and characteristics that would favor localization of a high percentage of the dose in the marrow. Among those compounds that have been tested are colloidal gold-199, iodine-131 heat-treated albumin, technetium-99m sulfur sol colloid, and gadolinium-159 hydroxycitrate. Colloidal ^{199}Au has only a slight theoretical advantage over colloidal ^{198}Au. Heat-treated ^{131}I-labeled albumin has a clearance pattern that resembles that of gold. However, there is early release of the ^{131}I label, leading to radioactivity in the blood, concentration in the thyroid gland (which can be blocked with Lugol's solution), and concentration in the urinary bladder, where it interferes with the view of the pelvis.

Technetium-99m has many characteristics of the ideal nuclide, but its low energy makes quantitative measurements *in vivo* difficult. The low energy gamma emission of technetium also results in directional changes of the photons within tissue with little photon energy loss. This scattering increases the problem of spatial resolution (Fig. 9-4A). Certain of the rare earths at appropriate pH and in the proper chemical form and concentration behave as colloidal preparations and are distributed within the body in a manner that may be useful for marrow localization.

Gadolinium-159 hydroxycitrate has the advantage of a rather short half-life (18 hours), favorable gamma emission (370, 57 kev.), and ready availability by neutron irradiation of enriched [158]Gd. Although the relatively high concentration in the marrow, compared to liver and spleen, has been documented in animals (Kyker and Rafter, 1965), initial clinical trials have not as yet provided better scans than those available with other colloids. Furthermore, shortly after injection some particles concentrate in the lung and some are slowly removed from the blood, indicating that the colloidal particles are not uniform with present methods of preparation.

INSTRUMENTATION

External counting with a stationary radiation detector is a simple and inexpensive way to detect the presence of localized radioactivity at various points in the skeleton after doses of radioiron or radioactive colloids. Radioisotope scanning provides more information, since it gives an image of the distribution of the nuclide. Rectilinear scanners, preferably with 5 in. sodium iodide crystals or larger, and with a selection of collimators optimally designed for the desired resolution and for the gamma-ray energy of the nuclide, are used. One version of a rectilinear scanner for bone marrow scanning provides a view of the entire body. We have developed a scanner at Oak Ridge Institute of Nuclear Studies Medical Division that permits life-size scanning of selected areas or a 5:1 reduction view of the whole body (Morris, 1964).

A positron scintillation camera developed by Anger and Van Dyke (1964) has special advantages for imaging the distribution of positron-emitting [52]Fe. Sixteen hours after administration of 50 to 150 μc. of [52]Fe, a 10 minute exposure produces a view of the marrow over an area 20 cm. in diameter.

Linear or profile scans are made using Pochin's method (Pochin, 1959). A modification of this instrument developed at ORINS consists of two opposed rows of six sodium iodide crystals with a variable slit collimation obtained by movable lead jaws of 3 in. thickness (Morris, 1960). Because of the weight of the lead shields, we move the patient between the rows of crystals rather than moving the detectors. Alfrey et al. (1964) have constructed a version employing two 2 in. sodium iodide crystals between 2 in. lead plate shields, which are moved below the patient. With this equipment, a linear or profile scan can be obtained, and by comparison with suitable phantoms, the whole-body retention of the radionuclide can be estimated. An example of the usefulness of the method is the ease with which we can demonstrate the responses of the bone marrow to treatment.

CLINICAL RESULTS

Although we still do not have the ideal radiopharmaceutical, and the instruments are far from perfect, bone marrow scanning has provided new knowledge in the study of hematological disease. On *a priori* grounds, one would not have expected that ionic iron and colloids would be similarly distributed in patients with hematopoietic diseases involving primarily one cell population. Yet, similar distributions have been found after exposure of the marrow to destructive agents, in the pattern of expansion of marrow into the extremities in a variety of disorders, in the distribution of focal lesions, and in regional hyperplasia.

Hashimoto (1960) has carried out systematic study of the distribution of active marrow in the bones of the normal adult at autopsy and concluded that the marrow of the trunk contains a nonhomogeneous distribution of hematopoietic elements; islands of fatty marrow are found in persons who presumably are normal. Only the proximal portions of the humeri and femora have hematopoietic marrow in the normal adult. The proportion of fatty marrow is believed to increase with age (Custer and Ahlfeldt, 1932, Hartsock et al., 1965). In children there is active hematopoiesis in the marrow of the extremities, but the details of transition from the childhood distribution to the distribution in adults are not well documented. The normal distribution of marrow in adolescents is another unanswered question.

In leukemia, considerable variation exists in the distribution of the active marrow as determined by scanning. Some children and adults with acute leukemia accumulate particles only in the liver and spleen after injections of intravenous colloids, and not in the marrow, which is packed with leukemic cells; yet a majority of the adults with acute leukemia, untreated or treated, have a normal pattern of distribution of marrow (Fig. 9-4) or even distinctly expanded marrow into the extremities. Some patients with chronic myelogenous leukemia show decreased or absent marrow activity after tracer doses of ^{59}Fe, but others have normal uptake. In contrast, the marrow is expanded in some patients with chronic lymphocytic leukemia, there is normal distribution or patchy decrease in distribution of the marrow in some, and occasionally the marrow extends into the long bones, possibly as a compensation for the lymphocytic replacement of the marrow in the trunk.

Simpson and Baker, in 1963, using ^{59}Fe in the study of marrow in 38 patients with active polycythemia vera, observed a normal distribution in 22, expanded marrow in 9, normal distribution accompanied by a slight splenic concentration in 3, and decreased or absent marrow in 4 patients. Larsson and Jonsson (1964), using colloidal ^{198}Au, found most patients with active polycythemia vera to have expansion of the marrow. In secondary polycythemia, the extension of the marrow into the long bones, as observed with ^{52}Fe or ^{59}Fe, is not common, and has been described only in cases of unusually long-standing and severe disease.

Experience with marrow studies in patients with chronic anemias has been small. Expansion of the marrow organ occurs in hemolytic anemia (VanDyke and Anger, 1965) but severe, chronic blood loss or active hemolysis does not always stimulate expansion of marrow into the long bones. At times there is a poor correlation of expansion or contraction of the bone marrow with the findings in the peripheral blood and the clinical syndrome. Profound ineffectual erythropoiesis associated with an expanded marrow organ has been observed in very anemic patients.

Myelofibrosis shows a characteristic pattern of accumulation of activity in an enlarged spleen and liver with absence of activity of the marrow. This pattern is found in both idiopathic myelofibrosis and fibrosis complicating polycythemia vera.

VanDyke and Anger (1965), using ^{52}Fe, have proposed an interesting classification of the distribution of erythropoietic marrow: Type I, normal; Type II, expansion to the proximal portion of the humerus and femur; Type III, extension to the elbow and tibia; Type IV, further extension into extremities with loss of marrow from usual sites; Type V, failure of medullary erythropoiesis with radioiron deposited in the liver and spleen. Although we have occasionally seen

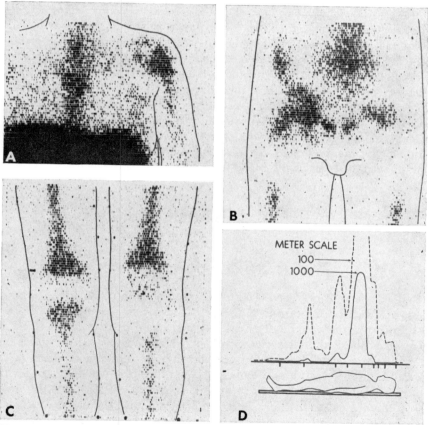

FIGURE 9-5. Hodgkin's disease in a 12 year old boy. The scans followed intravenous injection of colloidal ^{198}Au. Multiple courses of radiation therapy had been given to the chest and pelvis during the previous 2 years. *A*, Chest with normal concentration in the bony thorax. The extension in the humerus may be normal for the patient's age. *B*, Anterior view of the pelvis. Note absence of uptake in the left ilium, which was the site of radiotherapy with 3000 R. of ^{60}Co completed 10 days before scan. *C*, Anterior view of the legs with pronounced extension into the extremities; this is possibly to be expected in a child. Note the defect in the right tibia of a pathological fracture from Hodgkin's disease. *D*, Linear scan showing increased activity in the lower extremity. (From Kniseley et al., 1964.)

peripheral expansion apparently as a consequence of "central atrophy," we have not yet observed enough cases to confirm the hypothesis that atrophy begins centrally and proceeds peripherally.

We have studied a variety of locally destructive lesions of bone marrow. At times, in the course of local radiation therapy to soft tissue tumors, the bone marrow is in the radiation field, and the marrow scan demonstrates the extent and distribution of the loss of functioning hematopoietic tissue (Fig. 9-5). In most instances, marrow hypoplasia in these sites persists for many months or years. Surprisingly, in certain circumstances, the marrow regenerates in these sites. Sites of osseous metastases, both those that have been treated and those that have not, fail to concentrate the tracer. In multiple myeloma, marrow is lost in the trunk and is replaced by proliferating myeloma cells, and some compensatory hematopoiesis develops in the long bones (Fig. 9-1).

In summary, marrow scanning with radioisotopes can provide detailed visualization of the active, functioning bone marrow. Two groups of tracers have been used: radioiron, which is incorporated into red cell precursors and localizes areas of erythropoiesis; and radioactive colloids, which are phagocytosed by the reticuloendothelial (R.E.) cells in the marrow. R.E. function seems to be localized in areas of general hematopoietic activity, and therefore scanning of the distribution of colloids is a useful method for delineating active marrow. Scans in a variety of disorders affecting the hematopoietic system give valuable information about the distribution of the marrow, the responses to a variety of physiological stresses, such as hypoxia, and the extent of disease. In the present state of development, marrow scanning does not have wide application in routine hematological practice, but it contributes new and heretofore unavailable information about the status of the blood-forming organ.

IRON METABOLISM

D. R. Korst

HISTORICAL OUTLINE

Radioactive iron has been used for 25 years (Hahn et al., 1941; Hahn, 1948) to study the distribution of iron in the body and it was among the early methods used to measure the volume of circulating red blood cells (Gibson et al., 1946). As a result of these and later investigations, we now have a better understanding of iron absorption, iron distribution, and the kinetics of iron metabolism (Granick, 1954; Gubler, 1956; Moore and Dubach, 1956). Improved methods of measuring the chemical amounts of iron in serum (Peters et al., 1956 a, b), the invention of the sodium iodide (thallium-activated) crystal, and increased availability of nuclides of iron of high specific activity have made tracer studies more practical and meaningful in a variety of diseases affecting iron metabolism (Finch et al., 1949; Huff et al., 1950, 1951; Wasserman et al., 1952; Elmlinger et al., 1953; Ledlie and Baxter, 1954; Giblett et al., 1956). We have increased our knowledge of polycythemia (Lawrence, 1955), normal mechanisms of iron metabolism (Loeffler et al., 1955), the anemia of infection (Bush et al., 1956), the basic physiology of bone marrow failure (Wetherley-Mein et al., 1956; Bothwell et al., 1956; Berlin et al., 1957; Chodos and Ross, 1958), absorption of oral iron compounds (Garby and Sjolin, 1957), the anemia of a variety of diseases (Freirich et al., 1957), the effect of toxic agents on bone marrow (Bertinchamps et al., 1958), and the metabolism of iron at the cellular level (Noyes et al., 1960).

KINETICS OF IRON METABOLISM

The amount of iron leaving the plasma compartment per unit time is referred to as the *plasma iron turnover,* or PIT. This rate can be measured easily, as can the rate at which iron is being incorporated into the hemoglobin of red blood cells. External measurements at the surface of the body with a scintillation detector directed at specific organs tell us the relative rates of accumulation of iron by organs such as liver, spleen, and bone marrow. Loss of labeled cells into the gastrointestinal tract or other sites of hemorrhage can be measured from the amount of radioactivity in the feces or menstrual blood after radioactive iron has been incorporated into red blood cells.

An outline of the normal pathways and kinetics of iron metabolism is pre-

TABLE 9-1. KINETICS OF IRON METABOLISM IN A NORMAL 70 KG. MAN
WITH 4 TO 5 G. OF TOTAL BODY IRON

% OF TOTAL BODY IRON			METHOD OF MEASUREMENT

Absorption ↓	Daily ingested iron
	
	→
	12–15 mg.
	Fe
		Small intestine
		
		Fe^{++}
		|
		0.6–1.5 µg./day
		↓
			Oral
			^{59}Fe Fe^{++} Citrate
			      Fe^{++} Sulfate
			      Fe^{++} Gluconate
			      Fe^{+++} Chloride
			^{55}Fe Compounds

Transport
 	
0.1%
↓ ↑
	Fe + transferrin
	  Plasma iron 75–125 µg./100 ml.
	  Total iron-binding
	    capacity 300–340 µg./100 ml.
	  Plasma iron pool 3.5 mg.
	  Plasma clearance T/2 = 60–120 min.
	  Daily turnover = 25–50 mg.
			^{59}Fe Citrate
			I.V.
			Plasma samples in
			well counter

Utilization →
65.0%
 	
4.7% →
9.2% →
	Daily turnover = 20–50 mg.
	Hemoglobin 2300 mg.
	  circulating RBC utilization (uptake)
	  70–95% in 7–10 days
	Myoglobin Cytochromes
	Heme enzymes Catalase
			Blood samples in well
			counter
			^{59}Fe heme

↓ ↑ *Storage* 30.0% ↓	RE system 1000 mg. Liver—right flank Spleen—left flank Bone marrow—sacrum		External monitoring scintillation probe
Excretion 0.1% Daily	0.9 mg./day as blood loss and cell exfoliation in bowel plus urine, bile, and sweat loss Menses = 0.5–1.0 mg./day		Whole-body counter

TABLE 9-2.   CHARACTERISTICS OF THE NUCLIDE ^{59}FE

Half-life:	45.1 days
Radiations:	beta: 0.271 mev. 46%
	0.462 mev. 54%
	1.560 mev. 30%
	gamma: 0.191 mev.
	1.098 mev.
	1.289 mev.
Produced by:	^{58}Fe(n,γ)^{59}Fe
Available as:	FeCl$_3$ Chloride
	FeC$_6$H$_5$O$_7$ Citrate
	FeCH$_2$OH(CHOH)$_2 \cdot$ 2H$_2$O
	Gluconate
	FeSO$_4 \cdot$ 2H$_2$O Sulfate

sented in Table 9-1. The rate of absorption depends on whether the iron is in the ferrous or ferric state, and upon the anatomical and physiological status of the small intestine. Iron may also be ingested in the form of organic complexes rather than as a salt. Iron-55 may be used together with ^{59}Fe to measure both absorption and rate of turnover. Detailed discussion of iron metabolism can be found in the text by Bothwell and Finch (1962).

The clearance from plasma of intravenously injected iron is rapid, since it reflects the clearance rate of a small pool of iron (4 mg.), referred to as the *labile* pool (Table 9-3). Iron is bound to an iron-binding beta globulin, called transferrin. In most patients there is enough transferrin in plasma so that there is instantaneous binding of radioactive iron to the circulating transferrin. If the patient's plasma transferrin is already completely saturated, as in hemochromatosis, it is necessary to incubate the radioiron *in vitro* in normal plasma before intravenous administration. The specific activity of most commercially available isotopes of iron is sufficiently high to require only 5 to 10 ml. plasma for complete *in vitro* binding.

Many factors are involved in the clearance of radioactive iron from the blood. Therefore its measurement is not as specific as determining the rate of incorporation of iron into the hemoglobin of red blood cells. For a complete evaluation, we must measure plasma iron clearance, the rate of iron incorporation into red cells, and the rate of accumulation of activity in the liver, spleen, and sacrum over a period of 7 to 10 days.

Incorporation of radioiron into the hemoglobin of erythrocytes is determined from serial measurements of the concentration of radioactivity in the blood, together with the blood volume and the amount of radioactivity administered. Calculation of the daily turnover of hemoglobin iron has not proved to be as useful as the shape of the uptake curve over a 7 to 10 day period.

The rate of appearance of tracer iron in erythrocytes is a function of the activity of the bone marrow at the time the tracer was introduced into the circulation. Cells of the erythrocytic series extending from early precursors to reticulocytes accumulate iron from carrier transferrin. The amount of radioiron in the circulating red blood cells usually reaches a plateau between 7 to 10 days later and remains at this level for as long as the labeled population of cells remains in the circulation. This end point is not sharp because of random destruction of cells and variability in the life span of normal cells. The plateau is

TABLE 9-3. APPROXIMATE COMPOSITION OF THE IRON-CONTAINING COMPOUNDS
IN MAN (70 KG. BODY WEIGHT WITH A BLOOD VOLUME OF 5000 ML.;
PLASMA VOLUME 2000; RBC VOLUME 3000 ML.; AND 15 G. HGB.)

COMPOUNDS	Fe IN G.	% OF TOTAL Fe
Iron porphyrin (heme) compounds:		
Blood hemoglobin (900 g.)		
(3.34 mg. iron/g. hgb.)	3.0	60–70
Muscle hemoglobin (myoglobin 40/gm.)	0.13	3–5
Heme enzymes:		
Cytochrome C (0.8 g.)	0.004	0.1
Catalase (5.0 g.)	0.004	0.1
Noniron porphyrin compounds:		
Transferrin	0.004	0.1
Ferritin (3 g.)	0.4–0.8	15
Total available iron stores	1.2–1.5	15
Total iron	4–5	100

relatively constant for at least a month, and can be determined as a background for a second tracer study. This has been particularly helpful in studying the relative rates of absorption of different iron compounds after oral administration.

Excretion of radioiron is negligible. Only about 0.9 mg. of radioiron is lost per day. Greater amounts appearing in the feces usually indicates an abnormal loss of blood into the gastrointestinal tract.

CALCULATION OF FERROKINETIC DATA

Serum iron concentration is expressed in micrograms per milliliter. Normal values are 0.05 to 1.2 micrograms per milliliter.

Plasma iron clearance is usually expressed as a half-time.

Plasma iron pool (milligrams) is equal to the serum iron concentration $\times$ plasma volume.

Plasma iron turnover (PIT in units of milligrams per day or milligrams per kg. per day) is calculated as the product of the fractional plasma clearance and the plasma iron pool.

The plasma ^{59}Fe disappearance curve yields the fraction (kg.) of the total plasma iron leaving the plasma compartment per unit time (hour).

$$kg. = \frac{0.693 \times 60}{T\frac{1}{2}\ (min.)}$$

Plasma iron turnover (PIT) (milligrams per 24 hours) =

$$\frac{plasma\ iron\ pool \times 997.9}{T\frac{1}{2}\ in\ min.}$$

Daily iron pool turnover =

$$\frac{PIT\ mg./day}{iron\ pool\ mg.}$$

RBC uptake = % uptake at the level at which the iron incorporation curve reaches a plateau.

RBC iron turnover rate = RBC uptake % $\times$ PIT mg./day.

TABLE 9-4.   RADIOIRON TURNOVER STUDIES

NAME John Smith		AGE	24

DIAGNOSIS   Normal person

DATE ^{59}Fe INJECTED	2/12/57	Dose 10 μc. without tagging
		UIBC = 200 TIBC = 250

Serum iron	0.50	μg./ml. (0.05–1.7)	20	% saturation
Plasma vol.	4170	ml.	50	ml./kg. (^{59}Fe method)
				(37–45)
Blood vol.	6423	ml.	77	ml./kg. (calculated)
				(66–77)
Cell vol.	2253	ml.	27	ml./kg. (calculated)
				(28–32)

Hematocrit	49		Av. of	13	determinations
Weight	183	lb.		83	kg.
Hemoglobin	15.0	grams per 100			
Plasma iron clearance (T½)	71	min. (80–120)	1.18	hours	
Plasma iron pool	2.470	mg. (2.4–4.0)			
Plasma iron turnover rate	35	mg./day (32–52)			
	0.42	mg./kg./day (0.46–0.70)			
Daily iron pool turnover	14.2	(9.6–14.0)			
RBC uptake (^{59}Fe)	100	% (70–95) in	7	days (7–10)	
RBC iron turnover rate	3.5	mg./day (30–50)	0.42	mg./kg./day	
				(0.43–0.70)	
Red cell iron (total)	3250	mg. (2500)			
Red cell iron renewal	1.08	% daily			
Mean red cell life span	93	days			
External counting pattern	normal				

Time (days)	¼	1	2	3	4	5	6	7	8	9	10
Sacrum/Liver Ratio	1.7	1.46	1.05	1.08		0.73		0.80			0.77

Red cell iron (total) = Hemoglobin (grams per 100 ml.) × 3.34 × blood volume per milliliter × 10^{-2}.

Red cell iron renewal = percentage red cell iron turnover per day.

Mean red cell life span (days) =

$$\frac{100\%}{\text{red cell iron renewal }\%/\text{day}}$$

Normal values are shown in Table 9-4. This form has been found useful as a record of the routine data.

EXAMPLES OF CLINICAL USEFULNESS

A patient with *pernicious anemia* was studied before and after vitamin B_{12} therapy. Before therapy, a pattern of decreased blood production was found; following vitamin B_{12} administration, there was normal production of hemoglobin by the bone marrow (Fig. 9-6). Before therapy, iron was being removed by marrow and other iron storage sites, but was not being converted to circulating hemoglobin. Serum iron values decreased as iron was utilized by the activated bone marrow.

TABLE 9-5. DISEASE STATES WITH VARIOUS PATTERNS OF RADIOIRON TURNOVER

NORMAL	REFRACTORY	ACCELERATED
Cancer	Marrow failure	Cirrhosis with
Mild lymphoma	Aplastic anemia	hemolytic anemia
Leukemia in remission	Myelophthisic anemia	Acute leukemia
Pernicious anemia in	Fanconi syndrome	Polycythemia vera
remission	Renal disease	Iron deficiency
	Chronic leukemia	Chronic blood loss
	Pernicious anemia in	after acute bleeding
	relapse	
	Thalassemia	
	Hypoplastic anemia	
	Infection	
	Radiation or	
	cytotoxic drug	

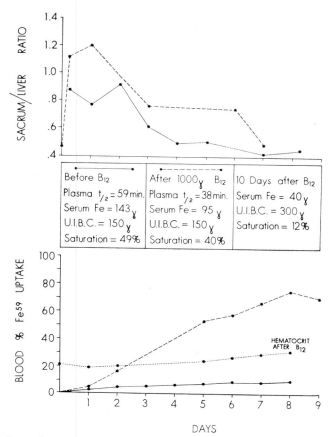

FIGURE 9-6. Radioiron turnover studies in a 70 year old man with pernicious anemia in relapse.

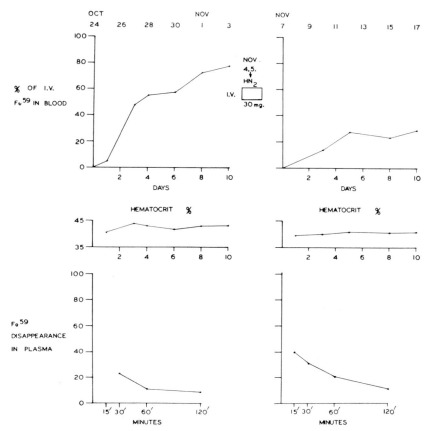

FIGURE 9-7. Intravenous Fe[59] turnover studies before and after intravenous administration of 30 mg. nitrogen mustard in a patient with breast carcinoma.

The use of chemotherapy, such as nitrogen mustard, can cause a transient depression of bone marrow and diminished iron turnover. This is demonstrated in Figure 9-7, which illustrates two studies in the same patient.

A pattern of decreased blood production (refractory) is characterized by a normal or slow plasma iron clearance, a decreased red blood cell ^{59}Fe uptake, a flat sacrum-to-liver ratio curve, and sometimes a high serum iron (Table 9-5).

A pattern of increased blood production (accelerated) is characterized by an accelerated plasma clearance rate, a fast red blood cell uptake that reaches 100 per cent after several days, a low serum iron, and a prompt turnover of ^{59}Fe in the bone marrow.

ORAL IRON ABSORPTION

Studies of iron absorption by various investigators (Dubach et al., 1946; Chodos, 1958; Saylor and Finch, 1953; Badenoch and Callender, 1954; Tati et al., 1956) provided evidence that ferrous iron is better absorbed than ferric iron by patients with iron deficiency. The use of ^{59}Fe and [55]Fe to measure simultaneously intestinal absorption of iron and the incorporation of iron after intravenous injection has indicated that varying the doses of oral iron from 5 to 500 mg. does not change the rate of absorption of oral iron in iron-deficient patients or normal

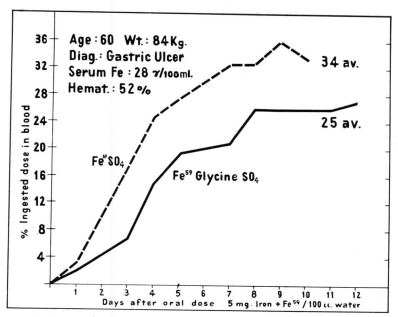

FIGURE 9-8. Comparison of the absorption of two radioisotope-labeled compounds of iron in the same patient at two separate times. The differences shown here are probably not significant.

subjects. However, there is more efficient absorption of iron from doses smaller than 5.0 mg. Under standard conditions, the absorption of iron is reproducible in the same person.

These techniques are useful in comparing the absorption of various iron preparations in the same subject (Fig. 9-8). Serum iron and iron-binding capacities and daily hematocrits were determined in each subject. Blood volume was assumed to be 72 ml. per kilogram. Iron was given in the form of a constant oral dose of 5 mg. of elemental iron in 100 ml. distilled water, together with 40 μc. or less of ^{59}Fe as citrate or sulfate. Two 1 ml. aliquots were retained, diluted to 100 ml., and kept as standards. Feces were collected for 10 to 12 days. Measurements were made with a precision of 0.5 per cent or less.

The total content of iron in the body is maintained at a constant level unless there is blood loss or increased demands for iron during growth or pregnancy. In the normal subject, the daily loss of iron from the body ranges from 0.5 to 1.5 mg., most of which is excreted in the feces. The average diet contains 15 mg. of iron, so that absorption of about 10 per cent of dietary iron will maintain a state of balance. Absorption of tracer iron reflects depletion of iron stores and may be increased in spite of normal hemoglobin values or the acute elevation of serum iron by parenteral iron administration. Bone marrow activity is another controlling factor; the relationship between factors influencing intestinal absorption and bone marrow activity is still uncertain.

ERYTHROPOIETIN ASSAY

During recent years, it has been discovered that a humoral substance produced or activated by the kidney stimulates an increase in erythropoiesis in the

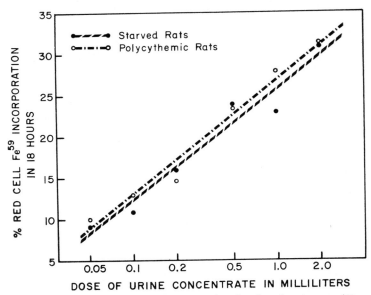

FIGURE 9-9.   Erythropoietin bioassay in starved and polycythemic rats. (From Gallagher, N. I., Hagan, D. Q., McCarthy, J. M., and Lange, R. D.: Response of Starved Rats and Poly-cythemic Rats to Gradual Doses of Erythropoietin. *Proc. Soc. Exp. Biol. Med.* 106:126, 1961.)

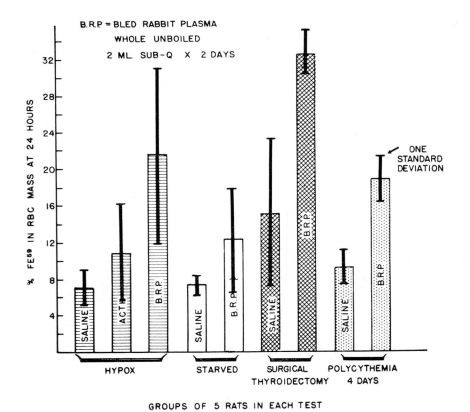

FIGURE 9-10.   Comparison of methods of bioassay of erythropoietin.

bone marrow (Wolstenholme and O'Connor, 1960; Gordon, 1959; Jacobson, 1962; Korst and Bethell, 1957; Linman and Bethell, 1960; Root, 1959; Stohlman, 1959). This substance, called erythropoietin, is found in urine and serum of most patients with anemia except when the anemia is associated with severe kidney disease. Erythropoietin can be measured by bioassay in animals. Measurement of the rate of incorporation of radioiron into circulating hemoglobin provides a fast and accurate method of assay (Plzak et al., 1955). The rat or mouse can be conditioned by starvation, polycythemia, hypophysectomy, or thyroidectomy, procedures that decrease iron turnover so that erythropoietin provides a more striking increase in the uptake of radioiron (Gurney et al., 1957, 1960; Filmanowicz and Gurney, 1961; Gallagher et al., 1960, 1961; Lange and Pavolovic-Kentera, 1964).

The assay using polcythemic rats was compared to that using starved rats in studies summarized in Figure 9-9. A comparison of other bioassay methods is shown in Figure 9-10.

Control plasma is obtained from normal animals; positive or active preparations are obtained from animals that have been bled or treated with phenylhydrazine. More recently, an extract of anemic sheep plasma or extracts from urine from anemic patients have been used as erythropoietin standards. Results in normal and starved rats are shown in Table 9-6. Because of the biologic variation in radioiron turnover, it is necessary to use four or five animals for each erythropoietin assay. At present, only differences greater than 100 per cent can be considered important. Work is in progress to provide better assays of erythropoietin. Recently the British Research Council has proposed the use of an extract of human urine as a standard in which 1.4 mg. of material is equivalent to a unit of erythropoietin activity.

TABLE 9-6. COMPARATIVE RESULTS OBTAINED IN THE NORMAL RAT AND THE STARVED RAT IN WHICH RADIOIRON TURNOVER WAS USED AS AN ASSAY OF ERYTHROPOIETIN[*]

TEST SUBSTANCE	NUMBER OF RATS	MEAN	RANGE	ONE S.D.
Normal Rats				
Physiologic saline	5	26	21–32	4.6
Cobalt (5 μM. CoCl$_2$ · H$_2$O)	3	33	30–37	3.4
Anemic sheep plasma (3% body wt.)	5	22	19–29	2.3
Armour extract of anemic sheep plasma (10 cobalt units)	4	33	30–35	1.8
Starved Rats				
Saline (0.9%)	5	7	5–9	1.7
Normal human plasma	5	5	3–7	2.0
Cobalt	5	12	8–17	3.7
Anemic sheep plasma	5	26	22–30	3.2
Erythropoietin extract	5	33	26–46	8.2
Anemic rabbit plasma	5	18	13–23	4.0

[*] Results expressed as the mean, S.D., and range of per cent uptake

VITAMIN B_{12} METABOLISM

W. B. NELP

OUTLINE OF VITAMIN B_{12} METABOLISM

Vitamin B_{12} was the first active compound to be isolated from a family of related compounds called cobalamins. One important function is an effect on the rate of synthesis of deoxyribonucleic acid (DNA) and cell division. Although many organ systems are affected by deficiency of this important coenzyme, the common clinical manifestations of deficiency are megaloblastic and macrocytic anemia and neurological abnormalities resulting from subacute combined degeneration of the spinal cord.

Vitamin B_{12} has a molecular weight of about 1400 and consists of two basic units, a planar group and a nucleotide chain (Fig. 9-11). The planar group has four pyrrole rings joined to a central atom of cobalt. The union of the cobalt with the remainder of the molecule is quite stable to acid or base, but can be broken down photochemically, catalytically, and chemically. Cobalamin coenzymes are stable only in the dark, and are transformed photolytically to hydroxycobalamin.

Vitamin B_{12} is synthesized by microorganisms growing in soil, in water, and in the intestines or rumens of certain animals. If radioactive cobalt is added to the growth media of appropriate bacteria, such as *Streptomyces griseus,* the radioactive label is incorporated into the vitamin, which can be recovered and purified.

The human liver contains considerable quantities ($\simeq$0.3 to 1.3 μg. per gram) of vitamin B_{12} activity. Human beings require about 1 μg. of vitamin B_{12} per day. Daily parenteral administration of 0.5 to 1.0 μg. to patients with pernicious anemia produces a maximum hematopoietic response; a similar daily amount maintains normal hematopoiesis. The vitamin B_{12} content of diets in the United States varies from 2 to 30 μg. per day, depending primarily on the intake of meat.

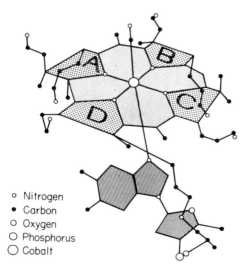

FIGURE 9-11. Vitamin B_{12}.

o Nitrogen
• Carbon
o Oxygen
O Phosphorus
O Cobalt

422

VITAMIN B_{12} METABOLISM

TABLE 9-7. COUNTING CHARACTERISTICS OF COBALT RADIOISOTOPES

ISOTOPE	γ-RAY ENERGIES MEV.	RATIO OF PHOTOELECTRIC TO LINEAR ABSORPTION COEFFICIENTS ρ/μ_a (SODIUM IODIDE)	RATIO OF TRUE ABSORPTION COEFFICIENTS	RATIO OF COUNTING EFFICIENCIES (MEASURED)	COUNTS PER MINUTE PER μC. (MEASURED)
^{57}Co	0.123 (100%)	0.98	1.0	1.0*†	111,640*†
^{60}Co	1.17 (100%)	0.10	0.024	0.818*	91,400*
	1.33 (100%)	0.09			

* Integral count.

† Differential count (50 to 200 kev. window) measured as vitamin B₁₂ in 100 ml. water in glass bottle on top of a scintillation well counter crystal.

DOSAGE CHARACTERISTICS OF COBALT RADIOISOTOPES

ISOTOPE	PHYSICAL HALF-LIFE (DAYS)	EFFECTIVE HALF-LIFE (VITAMIN B₁₂ IN LIVER)	TOTAL LIVER ABSORBED DOSE, RAD/μC. DOSE (EFF. T½)	AVERAGE β-RAY ENERGY $\overline{E}_\beta$, MEV.	γ-RAY DOSE-RATE CONSTANT, Γ, R/MC./HR., 1 CM.	RATIO OF LIVER DOSE OF ISOTOPES
^{57}Co	270	161.2	0.288	0.019‡	0.55	1
^{60}Co	1920	331	8.318	0.093	3.3	28.9

‡ No beta-ray, includes x-rays from electron capture and low-energy (14 kev.) gamma-rays.

Some of the vitamin in food is in a form that may not be biologically active. The metabolically active form of cobalamin is not known precisely.

The metabolism of vitamin B₁₂ is very slow both in normal man and in patients with pernicious anemia. The biological half-life of vitamin B₁₂ is between 400 and 770 days (Bozian et al., 1963). Radioactive vitamin B₁₂ was first produced with cobalt-60 in 1950 (Chaiet et al., 1950).

THE RADIOACTIVE LABELS

Two isotopes of cobalt, ^{60}Co and ^{57}Co, are commonly used labels of vitamin B₁₂. Table 9-7 compares some characteristics of the two nuclides. Cobalt-60 vitamin B₁₂ has a longer physical half-life and decays by beta emission. Therefore, the radiation exposure to the liver is greater than with ^{57}Co. Cobalt-57 can be obtained with a much greater specific activity (microcurie per microgram). Because of its low gamma-photon energy (0.123 mev.), it can be counted more efficiently with sodium iodide detectors. Only with ^{57}Co B₁₂ is it practical to measure the small amounts of radioactivity in plasma following oral doses of the radioactive vitamin.

QUANTITATIVE ASPECTS OF VITAMIN B₁₂ ABSORPTION

When an oral dose contains from 0.1 to 0.5 μg. of vitamin B₁₂, approximately 70 per cent is absorbed. With larger doses, progressively smaller percentages are

TABLE 9-8. QUANTITATIVE RELATIONSHIPS OF B_{12} ABSORPTION*

ORAL DOSE (μg.)	% ABSORBED	AMOUNT ABSORBED (μg.)
0.1	77	0.08
0.5	71	0.35
1.0	56	0.56
5.0	28	1.40
10.0	16	1.60

* Modified from Mollin, 1959.

absorbed, although slightly larger absolute quantities are absorbed (Table 9-8). In diagnostic tests, if one expresses the result as a percentage of the absorbed dose, it is essential to control the microgram quantity of vitamin B_{12} administered. Usually 0.5 μg. of vitamin B_{12}, containing about one μc. of radioactivity, is given.

If 50 to 100 μg. doses of vitamin B_{12} are ingested, a small fraction (approximately 2 per cent) will be absorbed by diffusion through the intestinal wall even in the absence of intrinsic factor. In this case, the time of appearance of the vitamin in the plasma is much earlier (within 1 hour) than following administration of a physiological amount of vitamin.

Absorption of vitamin B_{12} is outlined diagrammatically in Figure 9-12. After ingestion, it combines with gastric intrinsic factor and passes to the terminal ileum, where absorption takes place (Rosenthal and Hampton, 1955; Mollin et al., 1957; Booth and Mollin, 1959). Intrinsic factor (I.F.) is a protein with a molecular weight of about 50,000; it is very stable and relatively resistant to acid, alkali, and the proteolytic enzymes in the gastrointestinal tract. Vitamin B_{12} binds very readily to intrinsic factor. Because the absorption occurs in the ileum (Keuning, 1959; Drapanas et al., 1963), significant amounts of radioactivity do not appear in the plasma until about 4 hours after ingestion. The small amount of vitamin B_{12} not absorbed (20 to 30 per cent) is excreted in the feces. The vitamin B_{12}–intrinsic factor complex is absorbed through the intestinal wall and free vitamin B_{12} is released into the portal venous blood. Once in the blood, vitamin B_{12} forms a firm bond with a specific binding globulin in plasma. Most is transported to the liver; smaller amounts are delivered to other tissues. The firm bond between vitamin B_{12} and the plasma proteins prevents renal excretion of the vitamin.

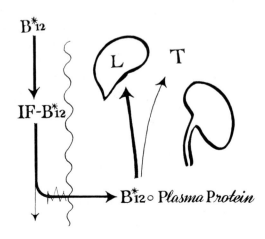

FIGURE 9-12. Absorption of vitamin B_{12}. IF, intrinsic factor; L, liver; T, tissue.

ABNORMALITIES OF VITAMIN B₁₂ ABSORPTION

A *lack of intrinsic factor* is the mechanism of malabsorption of vitamin B_{12} in Addisonian pernicious anemia and following total gastrectomy. Recently antibodies to various human gastric juices have been demonstrated in patients with pernicious anemia, suggesting a possible mechanism for the gastric atrophy characteristic of the disease.

Sometimes measurement of the absorption of radioactive vitamin B_{12} provides the only way of making the diagnosis of pernicious anemia. In the early stages of the disease, when only slight anemia is present, we can demonstrate that vitamin B_{12} absorption is abnormal. Some patients are treated with vitamin B_{12} injections without adequate confirmation of the diagnosis. If the radioactive vitamin B_{12} absorption test is found to be normal, the original diagnosis was in error. Conversely, the finding of a low test value permits proper planning of long-term therapy. Progressive deterioration of the nervous system from subacute combined degeneration can occur without anemia if the patients have received vitamin preparations containing folic acid, which cures the blood abnormalities but does not arrest the neurological damage. In these patients, demonstration of malabsorption of vitamin B_{12} indicates the need for vitamin B_{12} therapy. A specific defect of intrinsic factor can be documented if a low absorption value reverts to normal when intrinsic factor is given in a second absorption test.

Abnormalities within the small intestine can cause malabsorption of vitamin B_{12}. The fish tapeworm (*Diphyllobothrium latum*) can consume so much ingested vitamin B_{12} that the patient develops a deficiency. Small intestinal diverticula, surgical blind loops, and strictures may sequester high concentrations of bacteria which consume or inactivate the vitamin or the intrinsic factor–vitamin B_{12} complex. When such patients are treated with oral broad-spectrum antibiotics for several weeks, vitamin B_{12} absorption will usually become normal.

A third mechanism of vitamin B_{12} deficiency is disease of the intestinal wall at the absorption site in the terminal ileum, as in regional enteritis, sprue, and surgical resection of the terminal ileum. Rapid transit of material through the intestines may aggravate this type of disease.

The vitamin B_{12} absorption test is not a sensitive screening test for intestinal malabsorptive diseases. On the other hand, abnormal test results indicate that the disease involves the terminal ileum. If serial studies are done in patients receiving therapy for intestinal diseases involving the terminal ileum, improvement in vitamin B_{12} absorption usually correlates with clinical and radiographic signs of improvement.

TESTS OF ABSORPTION

One of the earliest diagnostic tests for pernicious anemia was measurement of fecal radioactivity following an oral dose of radioactive vitamin B_{12} (Heinle et al., 1952; Swenseid et al., 1953). Feces were collected for 3 to 5 days and had to be processed for counting. Soon thereafter, a method was proposed in which the rate of accumulation of radioactivity in the liver was measured with an external radiation detector (Glass et al., 1954, 1956). The results were difficult to quantify, and they were abnormally low as the result of disease of the

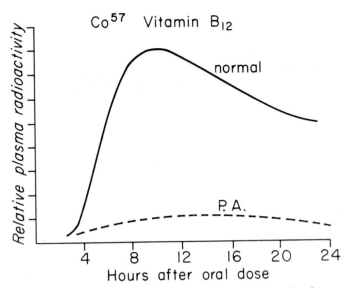

FIGURE 9-13. Time course of plasma radioactivity in a normal subject and a patient with pernicious anemia (P.A.).

liver. Another disadvantage was that 3 to 7 days of observation were needed. Measurement of the urinary excretion of the labeled vitamin following a saturating dose of stable vitamin (the Schilling test) has proved to be a useful and simple method (Schilling, 1953). A recent, but less widely used, method consists of measuring the amount of ^{57}Co B_{12} radioactivity absorbed in the plasma 8 hours following administration of the dose (Booth and Mollin, 1956; Doscher-holmen and Hagen, 1957; Nelp et al., 1963).

THE 8 HOUR PLASMA TEST

Figure 9-13 illustrates the time course of radioactivity in the plasma of a normal person compared to that of a patient with pernicious anemia. Little or no radioactivity can be found in the plasma during the first 4 hours following oral administration, the time required for the material to travel to the ileum and be transported across the intestine. Plasma radioactivity increases thereafter until a peak value is reached between 8 and 14 hours. Then plasma radioactivity decreases slowly. The plasma curve is the net result of absorption of vitamin B_{12} into the plasma and the simultaneous transfer of vitamin B_{12} from the plasma to the tissues.

Figure 9-14 summarizes the result of measuring a single plasma sample 8 hours following a dose of 1 μc. of ^{57}Co vitamin B_{12} containing an average of 0.3 μg. of stable vitamin. Patients represented by the solid dots had pernicious anemia; the open circles represent a group of control patients of all ages with a variety of disease states, including achlorhydria, but without any other known gastrointestinal disease. To standardize the results of variation in body weight, the plasma concentration of radioactivity was expressed in relation to body weight. Patients who had a value lower than 0.18 per cent of the dose per 1 per cent body weight of plasma were considered to have malabsorption of vitamin B_{12}.

Patients with pernicious anemia usually had values less than 0.10 per cent per 1 per cent body weight. The group of hospital "control" patients had an average value of 0.70 per cent dose per 1 per cent body weight. The control and pernicious anemia patients did not show a clear bimodal distribution. Presumably certain patients in the control group had partial defects.

The plasma test is technically easy and does not require the patient to collect urine or feces. The result does not depend on renal function as it does with the urinary test. Some patients with normal results with the plasma test have abnormally low 24 hour urinary excretion values because of impaired renal function. Renal function plays no role in determining the level of plasma radioactivity when small amounts of vitamin are given; the vitamin B_{12} is firmly

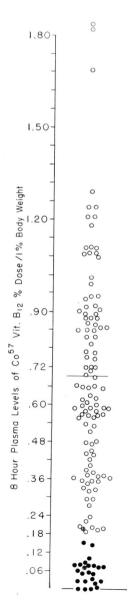

Figure 9-14. Eight hour plasma test results. See text for explanation.

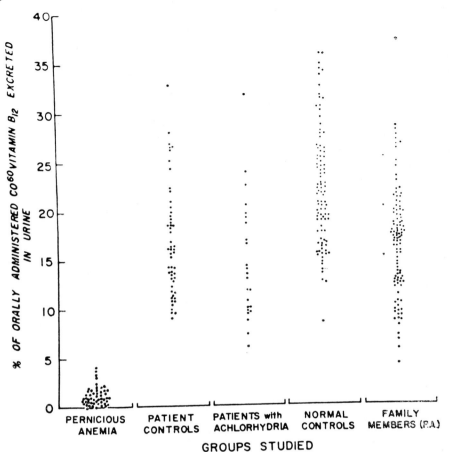

FIGURE 9-15.   Results of the Schilling test in various groups of patients. (From McIntyre et al., 1956.)

bound by plasma protein and is not excreted by the kidneys. A final advantage is that one need not give a therapeutic injection of stable vitamin B_{12}. Diagnostic studies of bone marrow morphology or measurement of the stable vitamin B_{12} concentration in the plasma can be performed after the plasma test if desired. Recent studies by McIntyre and Wagner (1966) indicate that as many as 7 per cent of patients with vitamin B_{12} malabsorption may have 8 hour values that fall within the normal range, a serious limitation to the plasma test.

URINARY EXCRETION MEASUREMENTS

These have been described by many authors (Schilling, 1953, 1955; Callender and Evans, 1955; Best et al., 1956; Bull et al., 1956; Krevans et al., 1956; McIntyre et al., 1956; Rabiner et al., 1956; Reisner et al., 1956; Goldberg et al., 1957; Oxenhorn et al., 1958). In order to promote renal excretion of absorbed vitamin B_{12}, a large dose of stable vitamin, usually 1000 μg., is given intravenously or intramuscularly. Usually the stable vitamin is given 1 to 2 hours after the test dose, and has been called a "flushing dose" or "saturation dose." The stable vitamin B_{12} saturates the tissue and plasma vitamin B_{12} binding sites before the absorption of most of the radioactive vitamin B_{12}. A portion of the radioactive vitamin subsequently absorbed remains unbound and is excreted by the kidney.

Figure 9-15 from McIntyre et al. (1956) is a graph of results of the Schilling test in various groups of patients. Those with pernicious anemia had less than 5 per cent of the dose in the 24 hour specimen. The Schilling test gives a clear distinction between patients with pernicious anemia and normal subjects. Separation of normal subjects from patients with other diseases, from those with achlorhydria, or from family members of subjects with pernicious anemia is not so clear-cut.

With this test, absorption is considered normal if more than 15 per cent of the dose is recovered in the 24 hour urine. Values of less than 7 per cent excretion indicate significant malabsorption of vitamin B_{12}. In patients with renal insufficiency the excretion of the radioactivity may be delayed, giving a falsely low 24 hour urine value. In such patients, urine should be collected for an additional 24 hours.

Because of the delayed absorption of vitamin B_{12}, one can perform a urinary excretion test after withdrawing an 8 hour plasma sample. A dose of 1000 μg. of stable vitamin B_{12} injected even after 8 hours will saturate the binding sites of the plasma so that subsequently absorbed vitamin is excreted in the urine.

BLOOD VOLUME AND RED BLOOD CELL SURVIVAL

D. R. KORST

RADIOACTIVE CHROMIUM (^{51}Cr)

Radioactive chromium (^{51}Cr) became available in high specific activity about 14 years ago (Harbottle and Maddock, 1953). In 1950, Sterling and Gray had reported that radioactive chromium could be used to label plasma and red blood cells. Sodium chromate was used as an erythrocyte label and chromic chloride as a plasma label. Ebaugh, Emerson, and Ross (1953) were the first to measure the rate of survival of red blood cells labeled with radiochromate. A number of excellent articles have confirmed the value of ^{51}Cr in determining red cell volume (Small and Verloop, 1956; Cooper and Owen, 1956), red cell sur-

TABLE 9-9. CHARACTERISTICS OF THE NUCLIDE ^{51}CR

Half-life:	27.8 days
Radiations:	beta: none
	gamma: 0.32 mev. 8%
	other: electron capture
Produced by:	^{50}Cr(n,γ)^{51}Cr
Available as:	^{51}CrCl$_3$ and Na$_2$^{51}CrO$_4$

vival (Donohue et al., 1955; Mollison and Veall, 1955), blood loss via the gastro-intestinal tract, splenic sequestration of red cells, and splenic structure by scanning techniques.

Radioactive chromium-51 decays by K-capture; 8 per cent of the disintegrations are accompanied by gamma-rays. One hundred microcuries of ^{51}Cr administered to a 70 kg. man gives a daily dosage of 0.003 rep (Marinelli et al., 1948). Anionic ^{51}Cr in the form of sodium chromate has a marked affinity for erythrocytes both *in vitro* and *in vivo*. The site of labeling is within the erythrocyte, primarily to the protein fraction of hemoglobin. The affinity of this fraction for chromate varies in the case of abnormal hemoglobins. Chromium-51 in the form of chromic chloride does not penetrate the erythrocyte membrane. The chromate form is readily reduced to chromic form in the circulation and therefore should not be injected directly if one wishes to label the red cells. After entering the erythrocyte, the chromate is presumably reduced to the chromic form. Chromium-51, released from erythrocytes as a result of death of the cells, does not label other erythrocytes. Labeling with chromate is not uniform, since it has been observed that the radioactivity of older cells is about half that of the general population of cells in rabbits and man (Danon et al., 1966). The radioactivity of the younger cell population is about three times higher than the average. Radiochromate also labels leukocytes and platelets, but the difference in size of the populations nullifies most of this artifact in studies of erythrocytes. Consequently, ^{51}Cr is an excellent means of determining the rate of survival of a given population of labeled red blood cells.

The rate of binding of chromate to red blood cells is dependent upon temperature and pH. Reticulocytes have a higher uptake of chromate. Results of simultaneous red blood cell survival studies using ^{51}Cr and Ashby agglutination techniques are not identical. Much of the discrepancy is due to elution of the chromium from the erythrocytes at a rate of about 1 per cent per day. This rate of elution is relatively constant in most disease states in which the chromium method has been compared with the agglutination method (Ebaugh et al., 1955a). Normal values of red cell survival using the chromium method have been obtained in large numbers of subjects. The physical elution is not significant when determining red cell volume or measuring splenic sequestration of red cells several days after injection.

Chromium in the chromic form is readily excreted in the urine; less than 1 per cent of the isotope is excreted in the feces. Organs with high concentrations of reticuloendothelial cells, such as the liver and spleen, temporarily concentrate the radioactive chromium released from effete red blood cells. Subsequently, radioactivity in the form of chromic ion is excreted in the urine over a period of weeks. The spleen may retain radioactivity for several weeks after erythrocyte labeling. In cases of hemolytic anemia, the splenic concentration may be very high.

Chromium-51 (half-life 27.8 days) can be obtained in either the chromic or the chromate form. The amount of chemical chromium in each study does not exceed 1 mg. and is usually less than 0.5 mg. The chromate form should not be kept in acid citrate dextrose (ACD) solution for storage, as it is easily reduced to the chromic form (Cunningham et al., 1957). In erythrocyte labeling, approximately 80 to 90 per cent of the labeled material penetrates the erythrocyte membrane as chromate. The addition of ascorbic acid reduces the extracellular chromate and prevents further labeling of other cells. Total injected doses of radiochromate seldom need to be more than 200 μc.; 100 to 150 μc. is adequate for determination of red blood cell survival by most techniques.

A concentration of radioactive chromium greater than 1000 μc. per milliliter of radioactive material or over 50 μg. of chromium per milliliter of red cells damages the cells. The nuclide has a gamma emission of 0.32 mev. and can easily be counted in standard scintillation counters.

RED CELL VOLUME

Chromium-51 labeling of autologous erythrocytes is an excellent way to measure the absolute volume of erythrocytes in the circulation (Gray and Frank, 1953). The blood volume may then be determined from the hematocrit. Plasma volume may be determined with iodine-labeled albumin (Gurney and Bolt, 1956) or Evans blue dye; the blood volume can be calculated as the sum of the plasma volume and red cell volume.

The red cell volume determination is useful in patients with polycythemia or in patients before and after surgery (Berson, 1955; Berlin et al., 1950b; Davies and Topley, 1959; Lichtman and Rabiner, 1957; McCall and Keller, 1960; Read, 1954; Sterling and Gray, 1950; Reilly et al., 1954). Calculation of total blood volume from the plasma volume determination may be less accurate than when calculated from the red cell volume (Korst et al., 1957; McClenahan et al., 1966).

The reproducibility of the ^{51}Cr method is shown in Figure 9-16. The mean error of 5 per cent is comparable to the accuracy of erythrocyte and leukocyte counting. Labeling of type O blood cells to provide a readily available source of labeled cells has certain drawbacks in that minor incompatibilities may cause a more rapid removal of the cells from the circulation. This could be demonstrated in several patients in whom labeled type O cells were used, as summarized in Figure 9-17. In a random sample of seven tests in five subjects, there

PT.	HEMAT. (%)	RBC VOLUME (ML./KG.)	%ERROR
SB	50 ± 0.2	30 ± 4.3	11
JY	50 ± 0.2	33 ± 3.2	7
AC	51 ± 1.6	25 ± 3.2	9
WL	49 ± 1.2	24 ± 0.5	2
BL	42 ± 0.2	25 ± 0.5	2
HR	42 ± 1.7	17 ± 0.6	2
EA	37 ± 0.2	23 ± 0.2	4
AW	30 ± 0.2	14 ± 1.5	10
FL	71 ± 0.5	53 ± 0.5	2

MEAN PLUS ONE STANDARD DEVIATION   AVE. 5%

FIGURE 9-16. Three consecutive ^{51}Cr RBC volume studies on different days in the same patient.

PT.		TIME	COUNT 1 ML. W.B.
HA	6/12	10'	888
		20'	834
	6/13	10'	547
		20'	496
	6/14	10'	346
		20'	281
HL	5/31	15'	736
		25'	671
RM	7/2	10'	606
		20'	540
DP	5/24	15'	1017
		30'	965
CS	6/27	10'	1179
		20'	1065

FIGURE 9-17.   Red cell volume determinations in normal subjects by ^{51}Cr-labeled O Rh negative cells.

was more than 10 per cent difference between the 10 minute and 20 minute sample in four of the determinations. Maximum counting accuracy is obtained by averaging the results of three samples.

A relatively poor correlation of red cell volume with the peripheral hematocrit is shown in Figure 9-18 and emphasizes the need for direct measurement of red cell volume in some patients. The normal values for red cell volume in our laboratory (Korst) are 28 to 32 ml. per kilogram. In 248 studies of 154 patients (Fig. 9-19) a close correlation between hematocrit and red cell volume was obtained in 38 determinations. The remaining showed a lack of correlation. The numbers within the dotted line represent determinations in which a normal red cell volume was associated with an abnormal hematocrit. Some obese patients (Fig. 9-20) have a high hematocrit; however, the red cell volume per kilogram was normal or low in the majority of these patients. The use of body surface area or ideal weight estimations did not appear to solve the problem.

A correlation of the hematocrit with the red cell volume expressed as a percentage of the normal seemed to indicate that the hematocrit is a useful indicator of the anemia of recent gastrointestinal bleeding (Fig. 9-21). Several patients with polycythemia of primary or secondary type (Fig. 9-22) were studied. A lack of correlation between hematocrit and red cell volume (^{51}Cr) was observed in a patient with secondary polycythemia. Values before and after phlebotomy were more accurately determined by the red cell volume than by the hematocrit.

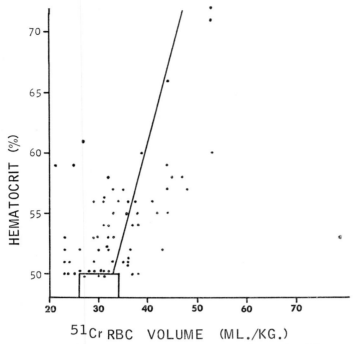

FIGURE 9-18. Correlation of red cell volume with peripheral hematocrit.

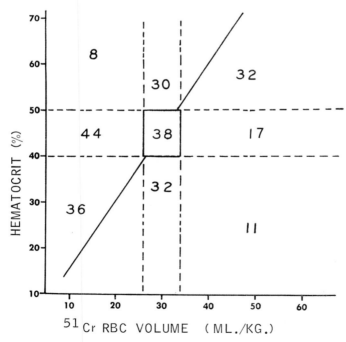

FIGURE 9-19. Correlation between the hematocrit and the ^{51}Cr red cell volume based on 248 studies in 154 patients.

PT.	WT. (KG.)	HEMAT. (%)	WEIGHT ML./KG.	IDEAL WEIGHT ML./KG.	BODY AREA ML./M2
AB	126	59	25	52	1420
RB	91	41	23	30	1054
CC	92	51	23	34	1084
RG	95	46	20	26	948
GH	109	58	32	42	1469
VS	101	49	39	50	1810
WL	91	50	24	27	971
WC	94	61	27	36	1218

FIGURE 9-20.   Studies of ^{51}Cr red cell volume in obesity.

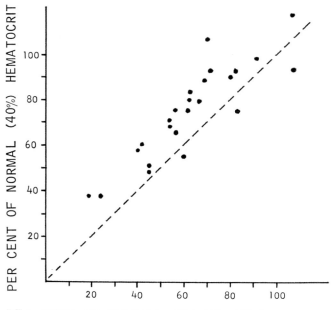

FIGURE 9-21.   Correlation between hematocrit and red cell volume, expressed as a percentage of normal, in anemia due to recent gastrointestinal bleeding.

POLYCYTHEMIA VERA		HEMAT.(%)	RBC(ML./KG.)	(ML./M^2)
F.L.	2/12/57	72	53	1872
	PHLEBOTOMY	1000 ML BLOOD		
	2/19/57	54	37	1278
SECONDARY POLYCYTHEMIA				
J.H.	6/15/56	54	79	3095
	PHLEBOTOMY AND P^{32}			
	8/6/56	55	33	1266
	10/4/56	56	29	1138
	12/6/56	54	31	1216
	2/6/57	55	44	1659
	PHLEBOTOMY	1000 ML BLOOD		
	2/8/57	50	29	1086

Figure 9-22. Correlation between hematocrit and ^{51}Cr red cell volume in patients with primary and secondary polycythemia.

RED CELL SURVIVAL

The determination of the rate of disappearance of labeled red blood cells from the circulation is useful in the diagnosis and management of patients with hemolytic anemia from various causes (Ebaugh et al., 1953; Eadie and Brown, 1955; Strumia et al., 1955; Sutherland et al., 1954; Weinstein et al., 1954; Read et al., 1954; Necheles et al., 1953). Red blood cells disappear from the circulation of normal persons with a mean half-time of approximately 30 days (Fig. 9-23) and a range of between 28 to 32 days (Birkeland, 1958; Remenchik et al., 1958; Aufderheide, 1960). If the data are plotted on semilog paper, it is somewhat easier to estimate the 50 per cent or T½ point (Fig. 9-24). Except in studies of patients with severe hemolytic anemia, one should obtain blood samples for at least 10 days and at least six points, for a sufficiently precise value.

If blood is lost into the gastrointestinal tract after injection of the labeled cells, an error results in the determination of the red cell survival. If blood loss is suspected, several fecal specimens should be obtained and measured for radioactivity. In normal subjects and subjects without gastrointestinal blood loss, the detectable activity in the feces is usually less than 1 per cent of the total administered activity.

A variety of primary or secondary hemolytic anemias as well as a number of hemoglobinopathies have been studied by this method (Ebaugh et al., 1955a; Hughes Jones and Mollison, 1956; Korst et al., 1956; Block and McGaffney, 1957; McClellan et al., 1958; Hollingsworth et al., 1955; Holt et al., 1959). Chromium-51 labeling of red blood cells has also been valuable in improving the survival of bank blood or donor blood. In such studies, gentle handling of the cells is necessary, since washing of the erythrocytes tends to increase their fragility and may

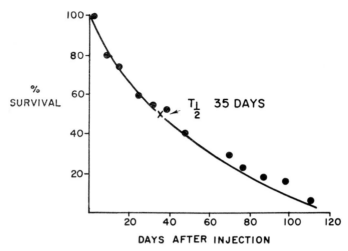

FIGURE 9-23. Normal ⁵¹Cr RBC survival plotted on linear coordinates.

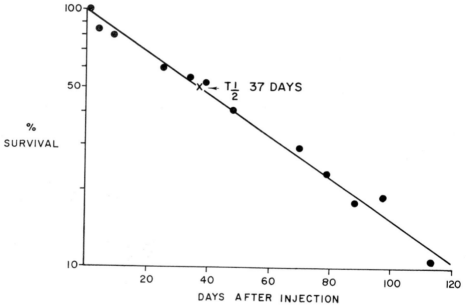

FIGURE 9-24. RBC survival by the ⁵¹Cr method in a normal subject plotted on semilog coordinates.

decrease cell survival. As much as a 5 per cent drop in activity may occur during the first 24 hours.

In brisk hemolytic anemia, red cell disappearance or destruction approaches an exponential function of time. However, the more normal the survival curve, the more curvilinear the graph.

Final results may be corrected for elution, but generally it is satisfactory to compare the results to a normal half-time value of 30 days.

Examples of survival curves are shown in Figure 9-25. Three patients with hemolytic anemia are shown with survival half-times of 9, 16, and 19 days. Half-time cell survivals longer than 32 days are not abnormal, but reflect a variable rate of physical elution from cells. Physical elution of chromium from erythrocytes is estimated at 1 per cent daily but may vary slightly in abnormal erythrocytes.

RED CELL SEQUESTRATION

Measurement of the time course of radioactivity in various organs by external counting presents problems, but liver or splenic activity can be approximated without much difficulty. Accumulation of ^{51}Cr-labeled erythrocytes in the liver and spleen may provide helpful data in the management of certain patients with hemolysis (Jandl et al., 1956; Motulsky et al., 1956, 1958; Schloesser et al., 1957; Hughes Jones and Szur, 1957; McCurdy and Rath, 1958). A wide collimator directed toward the liver, spleen, precordium, and sacrum usually provides the best data. The detector is placed over the second left interspace to obtain a *precordial* count which is used as representative of activity in the blood. The detector is placed over the lateral aspect of the left flank at the costal margin for the splenic activity and over the same area on the right flank for the liver. We calculate the ratio of activity of the spleen to that of the liver and of

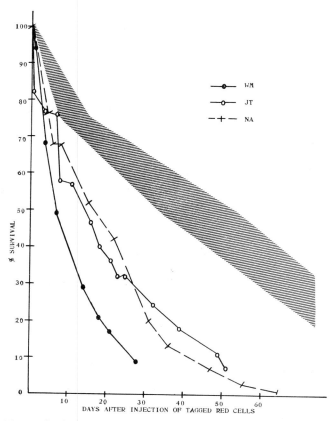

FIGURE 9-25. Radiochromate-tagged red cell survival curves before splenectomy in three patients with acquired hemolytic anemia compared to the normal range (black area).

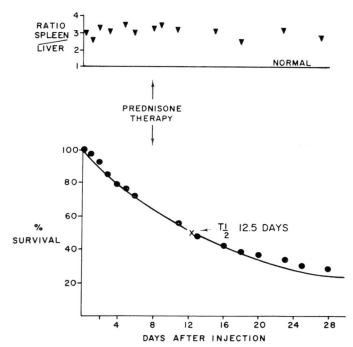

FIGURE 9-26. Studies of ^{51}Cr-labeled RBC survival in acquired hemolytic anemia. A slight change in the slope of the curve is noted after corticosteroid therapy was begun. The splenic activity is abnormally high.

the spleen to the precordium. External counting is done every other day throughout the red cell survival study.

In the normal subject, the spleen-to-liver ratio is approximately 1:1. In patients with active splenic sequestration of cells, this ratio varies from 2:1 to 4:1. An enlarged spleen, as in myelofibrosis or chronic granulocytic leukemia, concentrates the labeled cells with a spleen-liver ratio of about 2:1. Therefore we do not feel that one can diagnose significant selective splenic sequestration of labeled erythrocytes by this method unless the spleen-liver ratio is above 2.5:1, or unless the spleen-to-precordium ratio is greater than 2:1.

It must be remembered that this procedure is qualitative rather than quantitative. External counting in the illustrative case of acquired hemolytic anemia shown in Figure 9-26 revealed that the counts per minute over the spleen were in the range of 4000 to 4500, whereas those over the liver were in a range of 1200 to 1500, and those over the precordium 2000 to 2300. The spleen-liver ratio, therefore, ranged from 2.67:1 to 3.5:1 with a mean ratio of 3.0:1. The spleen-to-precordium counts varied from 1.7:1 to 2.5:1 with a mean ratio of 2:1. Therefore, by either method of calculation there was significant splenic sequestration of cells.

Correct positioning of the scintillation detector over the spleen is extremely important. It is helpful to move the probe slowly over the splenic area to determine the area of greatest activity. A scintillation detector connected to a *howler* that emits a tone with a changing pitch correlated to the amount of activity provides an accurate way of determining the point of highest activity over the spleen.

The highest spleen-to-liver ratios are found in patients who have hereditary spherocytosis. Labeled spherocytes injected into a normal recipient are sequestered with a half-time of 6 to 7 days. Spleen-to-liver ratios may be as high as 5:1. Ratios of 3:1 may be associated with relatively normal red cell survival in patients with splenomegaly associated with myelofibrosis or polycythemia vera (see Fig. 9-28). Acquired hemolytic anemia and hemolytic anemia secondary to lymphoma or leukemia are often characterized by increased splenic sequestration of red blood cells. Patients with paroxysmal nocturnal hemoglobinuria, lead intoxication, lupus erythematosus, and hemolysis associated with cold agglutinins have, in many instances, failed to show selective splenic sequestration in the face of a rapid disappearance of the labeled cells from the circulation. This latter group of patients are not helped by splenectomy.

Chromium-51-labeled hemoglobin injected intravenously into a normal subject does not sequester in the liver or spleen. Unbound ^{51}Cr chloride is rapidly cleared from the circulation and is excreted in the urine with only slight accumulation of activity in the liver and the spleen. Preliminary incubation of chromic chloride with serum before injection results in some increase in the liver uptake.

Patients with sickle cell anemia who have altered splenic function as a

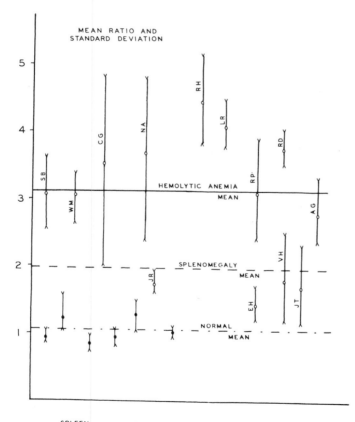

FIGURE 9-27. External spleen and liver radioactivity in patients with hemolytic anemia as compared to normal subjects.

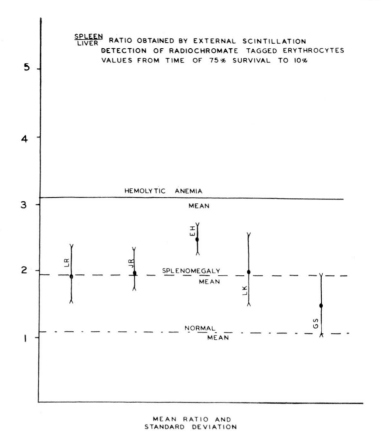

FIGURE 9-28. External spleen and liver radioactivity in patients with splenomegaly without significant hemolytic anemia.

result of infarction have a combination of shortened red cell survival, little activity over the splenic area, and the considerable uptake of activity in the liver. In hemoglobin C disease, splenic sequestration is not increased despite the presence of moderately increased red cell destruction. Patients with liver disease, particularly that associated with chronic alcoholism, may show a significant shortening of cell survival and increased splenic sequestration. This may be a transient process subsiding after the patient's nutrition is improved.

There appears to be a correlation between the degree of red cell damage and the degree of cell sequestration by the spleen and liver, respectively (Wagner et al., 1962b). The degree of hemolysis depends upon the condition of the erythrocyte, the presence of abnormal proteins in the blood, and the condition of the spleen (Palmer et al., 1953; Jandl et al., 1956; Ham et al., 1957; Harris et al., 1957).

There are four patterns of accumulation of labeled red blood cells (Lewis et al., 1960): (1) excessive accumulation in the spleen, as in hereditary spherocytosis; (2) excessive accumulation in the liver, as in sickle cell disease; (3) excessive accumulation in neither liver nor spleen, as in hereditary nonspherocytic hemolytic anemia or paroxysmal nocturnal hemoglobinuria, and (4) excessive severe accumulation in both liver and spleen, as in some patients with severe autoimmune acquired hemolytic anemia. Those patients with the first pattern would be expected to have the greatest benefits from splenectomy.

Splenectomy has about a 50 per cent chance of significantly improving hemolytic anemia (Doan and Wright, 1946; Coller et al., 1950; Dameshek and Welch, 1951; Hayhoe and Whitby, 1955; Wasserman et al., 1955; Chertkow and Dacie, 1956; DeWees and Coller, 1959; Weisman et al., 1953).

Figures 9-27 and 9-28 demonstrate the splenic uptake of radioactivity in subjects with hemolytic anemia, in subjects with splenomegaly but without a shortened cell survival, and in normal subjects. Each point represents studies on one patient. The mean ratio and one standard deviation of 6 to 12 studies in each patient is also shown. The horizontal line represents the average of the mean spleen-to-liver ratios of the entire group. Those patients with hemolytic anemia all had a good response to splenectomy. In a comprehensive study from Western Infirmary in Glasgow, Scotland (Goldberg et al., 1966), 11 of 13 patients with acquired hemolytic anemia had a good response to splenectomy and a positive indication of excessive splenic sequestration of radioactivity. The most clear-cut indication for splenectomy was a spleen-liver ratio of 2.3:1 or more and progressively rising splenic activity.

SPLENIC SCANNING

The spleen can be visualized by radioisotope scanning with a simple procedure (Winkelman et al., 1960; Wagner et al., 1960; Wagner, 1963; Wagner, 1964). Five cubic centimeters of blood is labeled with sodium chromate (^{51}Cr) in the usual manner and heated at 50° C. for 60 minutes in a water bath. Care must be taken not to exceed this temperature. The spleen is scanned 1 to 24 hours after injection of the cells. The normal scan of the spleen is shown in Figure 9-29 and a spleen with multiple filling defects is shown in Figure 9-30.

Splenic scanning is a useful technique in those patients in whom the spleen cannot be felt or when a question arises as to whether or not a palpated mass is

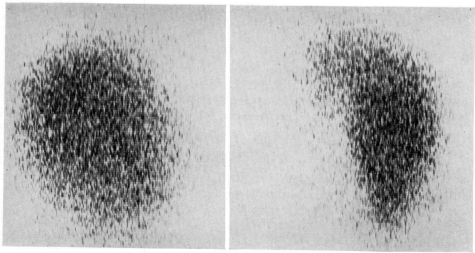

FIGURE 9-29.   *Left,* Lateral and *right,* posterior view of a normal spleen.

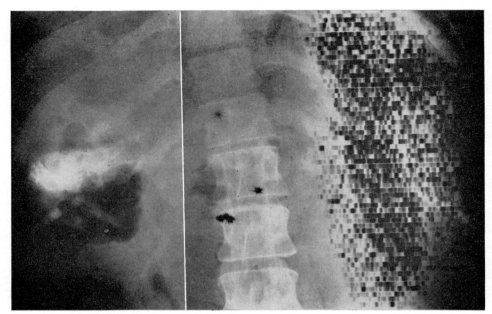

FIGURE 9-30.   Scan of a spleen with multiple filling defects.

actually the spleen. The scanning image of the spleen, correlated with routine radiographs and physical examination, is useful in the differential diagnosis of left upper quadrant masses, in the diagnosis of splenomegaly, and in assessing the absence or abnormal position of the spleen.

Spleen scanning can be performed with the use of mercury-197 mercuri-hydroxypropane-labeled erythrocytes (Wagner et al., 1964). This method does not require heating of the cells and is more reliable and reproducible. Spleen uptake studies with autologous ^{197}HgMHP-labeled red cells may give information similar to the ^{51}Cr method but in a much shorter period of time (Korst et al., 1965).

GASTROINTESTINAL BLOOD LOSS

In the absence of active gastrointestinal bleeding, very little ^{51}Cr is excreted in the feces after injection of labeled red blood cells (Owen et al., 1954; Bannerman, 1957; Roche et al., 1957; Ebaugh et al., 1958, 1959; Jones, 1958; Levin et al., 1959; Izak et al., 1960). When given orally, less than 1 per cent of ^{51}Cr is found in the circulation, whether the ^{51}Cr is given in ionic form in solution or bound to hemoglobin.

Gastrointestinal blood loss may be investigated simultaneously with a red cell survival study or following a red cell volume determination. A minimum of 100 μc. of ^{51}Cr is used, since the study is usually carried out for a week or more. The patient's erythrocytes are labeled and injected intravenously. The patient is provided with containers and instructed to collect all fecal specimens. Urine contamination will result in error. On each day that a fecal specimen is obtained, a 5 cc. sample of venous blood is withdrawn for use as a standard.

This technique makes possible quantitative estimation of fecal blood loss, and is discussed in more detail in Chapter XII.

RESEARCH PROCEDURES

Chromium-51-labeled cell techniques have been widely applied in animal and human studies to determine cell survival (Kraintz and Talmage, 1952; Stohlman and Schneiderman, 1956) and sites of cell destruction, and to study experimental models of splenomegaly and splenic sequestration of cells (Jandl et al., 1956; Painter and Korst, 1959). Chromium-51 has also been used to label ascites tumor cells (Rajam et al., 1958), platelets (Morgan et al., 1955), hemoglobin (Pearson and Vertrees, 1961), and cord blood (Suderman et al., 1957), and to study the absorption of intramuscular, intrapleural, and intraperitoneal erythrocytes (Hollingsworth, 1954; Pritchard and Weisman, 1957). Studies of the spleen after splenectomy in patients with hemolytic anemia has shown that the activity of the isolated spleen closely parallels the activity that was found by external counting.

POLYCYTHEMIA VERA, LEUKEMIA, AND ³²P THERAPY

N. I. BERLIN

HISTORICAL OUTLINE

Radioactive phosphorus, ³²P, was one of the first products of cyclotrons used in biological research. The biochemists of the late 1930's and early 1940's used this new radioisotope to study intermediary metabolism. At the same time, John H. Lawrence and his colleagues studied the tissue and organ distribution of ³²P after administration of the phosphate (Jones et al., 1940a, b; Lawrence et al., 1940). The results indicated that ³²P might be used successfully to treat diseases of the bone marrow and lymph nodes. In 1938, Lawrence, Scott, and Tuttle treated patients with chronic leukemia and shortly thereafter began an extensive series of studies on the therapy of polycythemia vera with ³²P (Lawrence, 1949). Of all the diseases in which ³²P was used as a potential therapeutic agent, in only a few were successful results achieved: polycythemia vera, chronic myelogenous (granulocytic) leukemia, and the rare primary hemorrhagic thrombocythemia. Even in these diseases, the possible leukemogenic role of ³²P in polycythemia vera and the development of chemotherapeutic agents for chronic myelogenous leukemia have resulted in decreased use of ³²P. The therapeutic use of ³²P in carcinoma of the prostate (Maxfield, 1956; Kaplan et al., 1960; Smart, 1964), carcinoma of the breast (Friedell and Storaasli, 1950; Maxfield, 1956), and multiple myeloma (Lawrence and Donald, 1958) has been described, but is not widespread.

Lawrence et al. (1940) studied the metabolic fate of ³²P when given as dihydrogen sodium phosphate to normal and leukemic mice. The uptake of ^{32}P in the lymph glands of the leukemic animals was approximately three times that in normal mice. The bone marrow and bone in the leukemic animals had slightly greater activity but the rate of exchange of phosphorus was about the same as in normal animals. In the leukemic animals, the tissues with increased ^{32}P content were the spleen, bone marrow, lymph node, and liver, or those tissues that were predominantly involved in the leukemic process. Lawrence and his co-workers concluded that the "relatively high concentration of radiophosphorus in leukemic tissues gives us a method of some localization of the irradiation to the infiltrated areas and this should prove valuable in the therapy of this disease."

Subsequently, Erf and Lawrence (1941) found that most tissues infiltrated with malignant cells in patients with a variety of tumors retained as much ^{32}P as other rapidly metabolizing tissues in the same patients. Jones et al. (1940a, b) showed that following intraperitoneal injection of ^{32}P as phosphate into mice, the tissue-specific activity reached a maximum in 5 to 10 hours. Greatest activity occurred in the liver, small intestines, and kidney; the least was found in blood and brain. In mice with transplantable mammary carcinoma, lymphoma, and lymphosarcoma, the neoplastic tissues accumulated radioactive phosphorus to the same degree as the liver, kidney, and small intestine, and appeared to retain it for long periods of time (Jones et al., 1940a, b).

Jones, Wrobel, and Lyons (1944) showed that particles of chromic phosphate 1 micron or less in diameter were cleared from the blood principally (90 per cent) by the liver. The remainder (10 per cent) was found in the spleen and lung. It was postulated that this might make possible selective therapeutic irradiation of the liver and spleen. The radiation dose to these organs was estimated to be at least 100 times greater than that to the lung.

PHYSICAL AND DOSIMETRIC PARAMETERS OF [32]P

Phosphorus-32 is a pure beta-emitter with a maximum beta energy of approximately 1.8 Mev. and an average beta energy of approximately 0.7 Mev. The physical half-life is 14.5 days. The beta-rays of ^{32}P have a maximum range of 8 mm. of soft tissues. Except in small organs of small animals, it can be assumed for purposes of dosimetric calculations that ^{32}P will irradiate only those organs that contain it.

The radiation dose to tissue from a pure beta-emitter can then be calculated from the following formula:

$$d = \frac{\text{dpm/g. tissue} \times \bar{E} \times 1.6 \cdot 10^{-6} \times 1.440 \times 10^3 \text{ rads/day}}{100}$$

where dpm/g. tissue = disintegration per minute per gram tissue, $\bar{E}$ = average energy of beta particle in Mev., 1.6×10^{-6} = a constant for conversion from Mev. to ergs, 1.440×10^3 = minutes/day and 100 ergs/rad. The integrated dose may then be calculated from the following formula

$$d = 1.44 \, d_o \text{ effective } T\frac{1}{2}$$

where d_o = dose rate at t_o, (assumed to be the time when the dose is uniformly distributed and assuming that the time required for distribution is small compared to the biological $T\frac{1}{2}$) and effective $T\frac{1}{2}$ = effective half-life of isotope in the organ; 1.44 = a constant.

POLYCYTHEMIA VERA

Polycythemia vera is a disease characterized by fatigue, headache, ruddy cyanosis, splenomegaly, an elevated red blood cell count, hemoglobin, and hematocrit, leukocytosis with a shift to the left, and thrombocytosis. The bone marrow is hyperplastic and there is an increase in the total circulating red cell volume (Lawrence, 1949; Lawrence et al., 1953; Stroebel et al., 1951; Wiseman et al., 1951; Abbatt et al., 1954; Harman et al., 1955; Erf, 1956; Calabresi and Meyer, 1959; Szur et al., 1959). Polycythemia vera must be distinguished from the other polycythemias, since ordinarily only polycythemia vera can be advantageously treated with ³²P or an equivalent myelosuppressive agent. The symptoms of polycythemia vera are summarized in Table 9-10, which is taken from the report of Calabresi and Meyer (1959) and includes six large series of patients. Weakness, headache, dizziness and vertigo, disturbances of the extremities, psychiatric manifestations, dyspnea, and orthopnea occur in over 35 per cent of the patients. Less common symptoms are a tendency to bleed, visual complaints, paresthesias, and thrombotic manifestations. Intractable pruritus is often associated with polycythemia vera. Symptoms often precede diagnosis by a long time, the average interval ranging from 1 to 2 years. Ruddy cyanosis or plethora of the face, fingertips, nose, ears, lips, and mucous membranes of the mouth and pharynx occurs in 62 to 83 per cent of patients. Distended retinal veins and congestion of the oral and nasal mucosa and conjunctiva are prominent findings.

Approximately two thirds of the patients have splenomegaly; in eight large series of patients, the number ranged between 48 and 93 per cent (Calabresi and Meyer, 1959). Hepatomegaly occurred in 7 to 48 per cent in the same series, with a mean of about 30 per cent. Systolic arterial pressure greater than 150 mm. Hg or diastolic pressure over 90 mm. Hg, or both, was present in 67 per cent of the females and 38 per cent of the males. Peptic ulcer and gout were common complications. An important laboratory finding, in addition to an in-

TABLE 9-10 SYMPTOMS IN POLYCYTHEMIA VERA

	% PATIENTS
Weakness and fatigue	55
Headache	51
Dizziness and vertigo	44
Disturbances of the extremities	43
Psychiatric manifestations	42
Dyspnea and orthopnea	35
Constipation	34
Bleeding tendencies	32
Visual complaints	31
Abdominal pain	31
Thrombotic manifestations	30
Pruritus	26

TABLE 9-11. SPECIFIC FEATURES OF POLYCYTHEMIAS

POLYCYTHEMIA	SPECIFIC FEATURE
Polycythemia vera	
Secondary polycythemia (due to anoxia)	Decreased arterial blood O_2 saturation
"Stress" or relative polycythemia	Normal total red cell volume
Polycythemia with tumors	
Cerebellar hemangioblastoma	Erythropoietin producing
Renal carcinoma	Erythropoietin producing
Renal adenoma	Erythropoietin producing
Uterine myxoma	
Hepatoma	
Ovarian tumors (luteomas)	
Adrenal cortical carcinoma	
Pheochromocytoma	
Polycythemia with renal disease	
Renal cysts	Erythropoietin producing
Hydronephrosis	Erythropoietin producing
Pickwickian syndrome	Massive obesity

crease in red blood cell count, hemoglobin, and hematocrit, is an elevated total red cell volume. Leukocytosis with a shift to the left, thrombocytosis, and hyperplastic bone marrow in which the fat is replaced by cells of the myeloid and erythroid series are also characteristic findings. An important difference between polycythemia vera and secondary polycythemia is that in polycythemia vera the blood oxygen saturation is within normal limits (Wasserman et al., 1949). Other findings that occur occasionally are increases in the vascular markings in the chest radiographs and elevation of the basal metabolic rate.

Polycythemia vera should be differentiated from the other polycythemias tabulated in Table 9-11. The differential diagnosis is most often among polycythemia vera, stress or relative polycythemia, and the polycythemias secondary to decreased arterial oxygen saturation. Stress polycythemia can be differentiated from the other polycythemias *only* by measurement of the total red cell volume. The diagnosis of many conditions that lead to low arterial blood oxygen saturation can often be made on the basis of evidence of congenital heart disease, evidence of acquired pulmonary disease, or residence at high altitude. In some instances an arterial oxygen saturation test should be done. In all cases, a careful neurological examination is necessary to rule out a cerebellar hemangioblastoma and an evaluation of the kidneys to eliminate hypernephroma and other renal diseases that can lead to polycythemia.

TREATMENT OF POLYCYTHEMIA VERA

At present, the method of choice for the treatment of polycythemia vera appears to be bone marrow inhibition by the use of [32]P. The use of venesection and other chemical myelosuppressive agents is frequently discussed. With one very recent exception, Perkins et al. (1964), these remain to be evaluated in terms of long-term results.

Initial therapy may be either ^{32}P plus venesection, or venesection alone. Three millicuries of ^{32}P is the recommended initial dose. In elderly patients when the total red cell volume is markedly elevated (e.g., in the 65 ml. per kilogram range or more) or when the platelet count is markedly elevated, phlebotomy can be performed to reduce the total red cell volume rapidly. This is done to prevent thrombotic complications. The patients are examined at approximately 2 to 3 week intervals, and at 12 weeks after the first administration of ^{32}P they are fully reevaluated in terms of symptomatology, peripheral blood count, and, most important, the total red cell volume. At this time, if the total red cell volume shows a satisfactory reduction, no further therapy need be given. If reduction of total red cell volume is insufficient, the patient should be given a second dose of 3 mc. of ^{32}P. After another interval of approximately 10 to 12 weeks, evaluation of all parameters is made again. Rarely will a patient require more than a third dose of ^{32}P. More than 50 per cent of the patients respond satisfactorily after a single 3 mc. dose. The average dose of radioactive phosphorus necessary to induce a remission is 6.5 to 7 mc. A few patients require a fourth dose. After the disease has been brought under control, examinations should be conducted at approximately 4 to 8 week intervals. If the red count shows a tendency to rise, another blood volume determination is performed and the patient should be re-treated if the total red cell volume increases. In these instances doses less than 3 mc. may be used.

Elective surgical procedures should be postponed until peripheral blood values have been returned to normal by myelosuppressive therapy, either ^{32}P or chemical. In an emergency, phlebotomies can be used to reduce the total red cell volume to the normal level. Both procedures are required to reduce the morbidity and mortality rate associated with surgery in untreated patients (Wasserman and Gilbert, 1964).

To evaluate a therapeutic agent in a chronic disease such as polycythemia vera, one must judge amelioration of symptoms, a return of the physical signs to normal, or at least toward normal, and a correction of the principal laboratory

TABLE 9-12. REPORTED LIFE EXPECTANCIES OF PATIENTS WITH
POLYCYTHEMIA VERA, TREATED BY VARIOUS METHODS

AUTHOR	METHOD	MEDIAN SURVIVAL FROM ONSET
Chievitz and Thiede, 1962	Untreated	1.5 years
Chievitz and Thiede, 1962	Venesection	3.5 years
Videbaek, 1950	Mixed	5.6 years
Chievitz and Thiede, 1962	X-ray and myelosuppression	10.5 years
Chievitz and Thiede, 1962	X-ray	12–13 years
Modan and Lilienfeld, 1965*	No radiation	9.5 years
Modan and Lilienfeld, 1965*	^{32}P	11.5 years
Lawrence, Berlin, and Huff, 1953	^{32}P	13.2 years
Calabresi and Meyer, 1959	^{32}P	11.0 years
Osgood, 1964a	^{32}P	12.6 years
Perkins, Israëls and Wilkinson, 1964	Venesection and myelosuppression	13.6 years

* Selected from patients treated during the year in which diagnosis was made to provide a comparison without bias.

abnormalities. It is equally necessary to determine the long-range effect of the therapeutic regimen, primarily in terms of life expectancy.

Life expectancy can be calculated in two ways: one is to calculate the median survival for the group, and the other is to construct a life table and compare the survival rate of the patient population to that of a control population matched for age and sex. Unfortunately, until recently no large series of patients had been treated with any method of therapy other than ^{32}P. Those who have advocated venesection rather than ^{32}P therapy have not put forth evidence in terms of survival. Recently, Perkins et al. (1964) reported on life expectancy in a large number of patients treated with chemical myelosuppressive agents, plus venesection, rather than radioactive myelosuppressive agents. Life expectancy was almost identical to that previously reported for patients treated with ^{32}P (Table 9-12).

There is no doubt that ionizing radiation is leukemogenic. The question is the relationship between the dose of ^{32}P and the incidence of leukemia. It is particularly difficult to evaluate the problem of acute leukemia in polycythemia vera. The natural history of polycythemia vera includes a phase in which the bone marrow is no longer hyperplastic but becomes fibrotic, the spleen enlarges, and the leukocyte count rises. At this stage the disease resembles chronic myelogenous leukemia, with two important differences: (1) the white cells contain a normal or an increased amount of alkaline phosphatase rather than a subnormal level (Valentine et al., 1952), and (2) the Philadelphia chromosome is absent (Sandberg et al., 1962). However, a small group of patients with chronic myelogenous leukemia do not have the Philadelphia chromosome (Carbone et al., 1963); this group tends to include younger persons and to have a shorter course.

A second problem is that many patients who are finally diagnosed as having acute leukemia pass through a phase characterized only by splenomegaly and an elevated leukocyte count, a confusing diagnostic problem until they finally pass into a "blastic" crisis, a common terminal event in patients with chronic myelogenous leukemia. Whether this chain of events should be classified as acute leukemia, chronic myelogenous leukemia, idiopathic myelofibrosis, myeloid metaplasia, or a phase of polycythemia vera is difficult to decide. Different observers, given the same set of conditions, may categorize the patient in any of the four classes mentioned, depending on the stage at which the patient is examined.

At present, with the exception of the report of Perkins, Israëls, and Wilkinson (1964), there is no evidence to indicate that ^{32}P is not the treatment of choice in polycythemia vera. However, it must be recognized that since 1949 there has been considerable discussion about the potential leukemogenic role of radioactive phosphorus in patients with polycythemia vera. A number of investigators believe it to be a significant factor in the choice of therapy. Others believe that the potential risk is outweighed by the greatly increased life expectancy of patients treated with ^{32}P. The studies of Perkins et al. (1964) indicate that the life span of patients treated with other myelosuppressive agents is not greater, but that acute leukemia appears to be less frequent than in patients treated with ^{32}P. Table 9-12 indicates that either ^{32}P or venesection and chemical myelosuppressive agents are the treatments of choice on the basis of life expectancy.

CHRONIC LEUKEMIA

When ^{32}P was introduced (1938) there were few chemical methods for the treatment of chronic myelogenous and chronic lymphocytic leukemia. Since the initial description by Lawrence and his colleagues (1948, 1949), the use of ^{32}P for the treatment of chronic leukemias has been described and reviewed by Diamond and co-workers (1950, 1951), Lawrence (1954), Chodos and Ross (1958), Reinhard et al. (1959), and Osgood (1964b).

Although chronic myelogenous leukemia and chronic lymphocytic leukemia are separate disease entities, certain aspects can be discussed together. In both diseases the history, the physical findings, and, if ^{32}P is used, the plan of therapy are similar in many respects. The laboratory findings and the course are dissimilar.

Symptoms may range all the way from none to many, particularly those related to anemia and fever. A mass may be noted in the left upper quadrant of the abdomen. The age incidence is approximately the same, with a peak in the forties for chronic myelogenous leukemia and in the fifties for chronic lymphocytic leukemia. Ratios of occurrence by sex (male to female) are 2:1 in chronic lymphocytic leukemia and 1.3 to 1.4:1 in chronic myelogenous leukemia. Physical examination may reveal only lymphadenopathy, hepatomegaly, and splenomegaly.

In chronic myelogenous leukemia, there is an elevated white blood cell count with a shift to the left in the differential count and a decrease in the amount of alkaline phosphatase in leukocytes (Valentine et al., 1952). The specific Philadelphia chromosome is found in the white cells in approximately 90 per cent of patients with chronic myelogenous leukemia (Sandberg et al., 1962). In chronic lymphocytic leukemia, there is a preponderance of lymphocytes, often representing 95 to 98 per cent of the circulating white blood cells. The red blood count is generally slightly reduced in a patient with chronic myelogenous leukemia but may be normal or even slightly greater than normal. Early in the course of the disease, patients with chronic lymphocytic leukemia may have a normal red cell blood count. Initially the platelet count in chronic myelogenous leukemia is usually elevated but in chronic lymphocytic leukemia it is usually normal or decreased. The reticulocyte count may be slightly elevated in patients with chronic myelogenous leukemia, and the bone marrow is hyperplastic with a considerable diminution of the amount of fat. There is a hyperplasia and shift to the left of the cells of myeloid series with a reduction in percentage of cells of the erythroid series. In chronic lymphocytic leukemia the bone marrow is variable. There may be small infiltrates of lymphocytes within a normal marrow architecture, focal collections of lymphocytes that do not disturb the general pattern of hematopoietic tissue and fat. These may progress to larger nodules, which finally coalesce and alter the structure of the marrow. In the extreme cases the entire fat content and virtually all the myeloid, erythroid, and megakaryocytic elements disappear.

The total red cell volume in chronic myelogenous leukemia is usually within the normal range but below average. The plasma volume tends to be high, particularly when the spleen is palpable. In chronic lymphocytic leukemia the blood volume may be in the normal range or markedly reduced. There is no correlation between splenomegaly and an elevated plasma volume in chronic lymphocytic leukemia (Berlin et al., 1950a).

The mechanism of anemia of chronic leukemia was a problem until Huff and co-workers (1950) began to use radioactive iron to measure the rate of formation of red blood cells. In chronic myelogenous leukemia the rate of production of red cells was normal or even greater than normal, and in chronic lymphocytic leukemia the red cell production rate was either normal or increased. Only rarely was the rate of red cell production decreased. This occurred in the late "blastic" phase of chronic myelogenous leukemia.

TREATMENT OF CHRONIC LEUKEMIA

Once the diagnosis of chronic myelogenous leukemia or chronic lymphocytic leukemia is made, treatment with ^{32}P can be started. The principal indications are symptoms and elevation of the white blood count. One millicurie is given weekly until a significant decrease in the white blood count occurs. Patients with chronic myelogenous leukemia may have a complete remission of the abnormalities in the blood with the white blood count in the normal range and very few or no abnormal white blood cells in the peripheral blood. The bone marrow architecture may revert toward normal. Patients with chronic lymphocytic leukemia do not show such striking changes in the peripheral blood or bone marrow but do show a decrease in the white blood count and the percentage of lymphocytes in the peripheral blood with a concomitant increase in the number of polymorphonuclear leukocytes.

The patient should be examined at weekly intervals, and treatment continued until either a remission is obtained or it is judged that further therapy cannot be given. As the white blood cell count falls, judgment is required to decide when therapy should be stopped. In general, the aim is to bring the white blood cell count within the 21,000 or 30,000 range. If no further reduction occurs, additional therapy may be given to bring the white blood cell count to between 10,000 and 20,000. In chronic lymphocytic leukemia the criteria for satisfactory therapy are less well defined. When symptomatic relief and some reduction in the white blood cell count are obtained, therapy should be discontinued. In both diseases, when the patient has had a total of more than 10 to 12 mc. over a 3 month period, it is best to stop therapy.

Some patients may require 2 or even 3 mc. of ^{32}P per week. Easson (1957) determined the dose of ^{32}P by the rate of fall of the white blood cell count. Osgood and Seaman (1952) attempt to maintain the white blood cell count at a particular level.

It is difficult to determine the precise cause of death in patients with chronic myelogenous and chronic lymphocytic leukemia. The "blastic crisis" of chronic myelogenous leukemia occurs frequently, and is characterized by an enlarged spleen and anemia. The white count tends to rise to high levels (100,000 to 200,000) with a marked shift to the left of the myeloid cells both in the bone marrow and the peripheral blood; there is a great increase in the number of myeloblasts in the peripheral blood and bone marrow. These patients are refractory to radiation therapy, but recently after chemotherapy with combined vincristine, methotrexate, 6-mercaptopurine, and prednisone, remissions have been noted (Karon et al., 1965).

In chronic lymphocytic leukemia, on the other hand, a hemolytic phase often intervenes and in about a third of the patients a specific antibody can be demonstrated (Troup et al., 1960). In other instances, alterations in the capacity of the immune mechanisms to respond to bacterial and fungal challenge is markedly decreased and the patients succumb to infection.

The life expectancy in both of these diseases has been analyzed by a number of authors, particularly by Osgood and his co-workers (1952, 1964b). The principal conclusions are that despite therapy in chronic myelogenous leukemia, there has not been a significant increase in life expectancy. There is slight evidence of an increase in the life expectancy in patients with chronic lymphocytic leukemia. Whether this is attributable to specific antileukemia therapy or the availability of agents for supportive therapy, i.e., splenectomy and adrenal cortical steroids for treatment of the hemolytic phase and some of the newer antibiotics for treating the infectious complications, remains conjectural.

PRIMARY HEMORRHAGIC THROMBOCYTHEMIA

This rare disease is characterized by an increase in platelets in the peripheral blood not associated with other hematological abnormalities such as chronic myelogenous leukemia or polycythemia vera. Case reports describing the disease from the time of Di Guglielmo's original description have been summarized by Ozer et al. (1960).

The disease occurs in late middle or old age, with a slightly greater incidence in females. Bleeding in the skin, nose, gums, gastrointestinal tract, and genitourinary tract are common features, with thromboembolic phenomena less frequent. Splenomegaly is characteristic. Hepatomegaly and occasionally lymphadenopathy may be present. Anemia is a common finding and is probably the result of repeated blood loss. There is a moderate leukocytosis and a marked and persistent increase in blood platelets, often associated with marked morphological changes. Fragments of megakaryocytes can be seen in the peripheral blood. The bone marrow is hyperplastic in all elements, with a predominance of megakaryocytes. Urethane and x-radiation have been used to treat this disease, but ³²P appears to be the treatment of choice. These patients should be treated in the same manner as patients with polycythemia vera, that is, given an initial dose of 3 mc. of ³²P with close examination of the effect. Although Ozer and colleagues (1960) tended to use larger doses in their patients, we believe that the effect of smaller doses should be evaluated initially.

COLLOIDAL CHROMIC PHOSPHATE

Radioactive colloidal gold (¹⁹⁸Au), chromic phosphate (³²P), and radioactive yttrium (⁹⁰Y) (Dobson et al., 1949) have been used for the treatment of pleural and peritoneal effusions. The use of ¹⁹⁸Au and ⁹⁰Y colloid has decreased because of the greater physical half-life of ³²P and the relative ease of handling a pure beta-emitter.

Card et al. (1960) collected data from several large series of patients which indicate that in approximately one half of the patients there was a significant therapeutic effect varying from a decrease in rate to complete suppression of the formation of fluid. Intracavitary instillation of chemotherapeutic agents is also useful in the treatment of persistent effusion. Availability and freedom from radiation hazard, together with an approximately equivalent therapeutic efficacy, have resulted in reduction in the use of radioactive agents for this purpose.

AUTORADIOGRAPHY AND OTHER TRACER PROCEDURES

D. R. KORST

TRITIATED THYMIDINE

Radioactive hydrogen, or tritium, has a half-life of 12.4 years and a maximal beta particle energy of 18 kev., with a range of only 0.005 mm. in water. The physical characteristics of this nuclide make it ideal for autoradiography (Fitzgerald et al., 1951). Tritium has been incorporated into a number of organic compounds by direct synthesis or by the method of Wilzbach. The use of tritiated water (Odekwa et al., 1963) has been found useful in measuring total body water. A number of compounds such as leucine, methionine, and glycine are available, but the most commonly used has been labeled thymidine.

Tritiated thymidine is usually introduced into the living animal by parenteral injection or added directly to the tissue *in vitro*. The metabolism is rapid; in a few minutes there is evidence of incorporation into DNA synthesis in the nucleus of the cell. The rapidity of utilization has been referred to as a "flash label." The nonutilized thymidine is converted to water and is reutilized to a very small degree as a nucleic acid precursor. Tissue concentration and localization may

TABLE 9-13. CHARACTERISTICS OF THE NUCLIDE ^{3}H

Half-life:	12.46 years
Radiations:	beta: 0.0179 Mev.
	gamma: none
Produced by:	Li^6 (n, α) ^{3}H
Available as:	Tritiated thymidine

$$\text{(structure of tritiated thymidine)}$$

Specific activity:	2500 mc. per millimole
Concentration:	2.0 mc. per milliliter aqueous solution

be determined by scintillation counting of the tissues (Frenkel et al., 1962) or by scanning paper chromatograms.

In mice (Shorter and Titus, 1962) the highest percentage of labeled nuclei were found in thymocytes, lymphoid tissue, and hematopoietic tissue. In man (Rubini et al., 1960) there is a rapid plasma clearance with half-times of 1 minute or less. As early as 1 minute after injection there is evidence of concentration in the proliferating cells, usually completed by 10 minutes. The label remains in the cell for its lifetime without evidence of radiation damage to the cell; it is concentrated in chromosomes (Lajtha, 1952, 1959). For this reason, the *in vivo* use in man is restricted to studies involving patients with limited life expectancy. About one third of the administered thymidine is catabolized within a few hours to tritiated water.

Labeled thymidine has been particularly useful in studying the localization of DNA synthesis in human tissues (Grass et al., 1951) and in blood cells (Bond et al., 1958) *in vivo* and *in vitro* (Rubini et al., 1961). The label has also been used to trace cells such as lymphocytes (Everett et al., 1960) in the thoracic duct. The effects of irradiation on nucleated cells of marrow, intestinal mucosa cells, and seminal vesicle cells can be closely followed with thymidine labeling and mitotic activity of normal tissue and neoplastic tissue can be compared.

Tritiated thymidine added to fresh marrow or blood *in vitro* or given to patients with lymphocytic leukemia results in labeling of "smudge" cells. Smudge cells are thought to be derived from a pool of primitive proliferating cells in

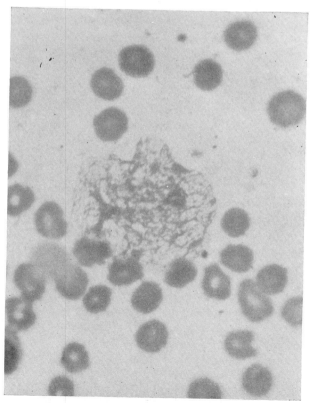

FIGURE 9-31. Basket cells in the blood.

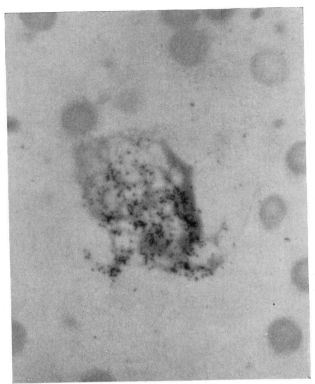

FIGURE 9-32.   Thymidine concentration by basket cells.

marrow or in lymphocytes; the cells in the pool actively synthesize DNA but do not divide and are destroyed *in situ* (Cronkite, 1958). Smudge cells are seen in the blood as *basket* cells (Fig. 9-31) and probably reflect reticuloendothelial activity. They are found in patients or rats with leukemia and concentrate thymidine in a striking fashion (Fig. 9-32).

AUTORADIOGRAPHIC TECHNIQUE

Tissues containing tritiated thymidine are sectioned or smeared on glass slides and covered with photographic emulsion. Following incubation for several weeks, the emulsion is developed and the tissue stained. This results in a preparation of tissue with superimposed black granules of the emulsion formed at loci of tritium concentration. A number of detailed techniques have been published (Boyd, 1955; Joftes, 1963; Kopriwa and Leblond, 1962; Conference on Autoradiography, 1959). Very high resolution may be obtained by combining autoradiography with electron microscopy to yield a maximum resolution of 0.1 micron for tritium and 0.3 micron for ^{32}P (Caro and Schnös, 1965).

Difficulties in interpretation result from background granules lying between cells. Excellent nuclear concentration of granules is shown in Figure 9-33, in which there is very little background. The preparation is a lymphoid cell from the circulation of a patient with leukemia. The cell is thought to be a circulating precursor cell actively synthesizing DNA and occurs in an average of 0.05

per cent of circulating nucleated cells (Rubini et al., 1961). Keeping the tissues and preparation in a frozen or near frozen state helps prevent tritium activity from leaking out of the cell after death (Appleton, 1964; Miller et al., 1965; Darzynkienicz et al., 1966). If one keeps in mind the method of slide preparation, it is easy to see that electrons with a maximum range of 6 microns might appear separate from the cell wall. With tritium, about 90 per cent of the electrons will travel 3 microns or less.

A number of other nuclides are used for autoradiography, including carbon-14, sulfur-35, phosphorus-32, iron-55 (Austoni, 1956), and chromium-51.

The technique used in our laboratory is as follows:

1. Tissue sections or blood films are fixed in absolute methanol for 5 minutes and air dried. They are then stored at 5° C. until the autoradiographs are made.

2. In a darkroom equipped with Kodak Wratten Safelight No. 2, Kodak NTB-3 dipping emulsion is warmed to 45° C. The slides are dipped and drained, and the backs wiped clean of emulsion. The film is allowed to set, and the slides are stored in open boxes in a paper safe containing an open vessel of KNO_2 to provide about 50 per cent humidity. The paper safe is placed in a refrigerator at 5° C.

3. Exposure time is 3 to 6 weeks.

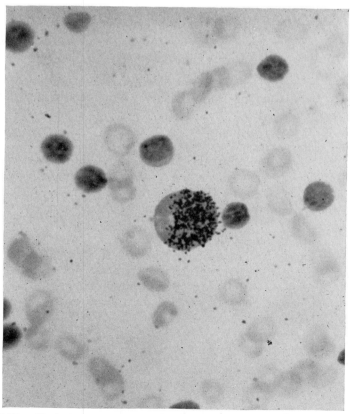

FIGURE 9-33.   Nuclear concentration of granules with very little background; lymphoid cell from the circulation of a patient with leukemia.

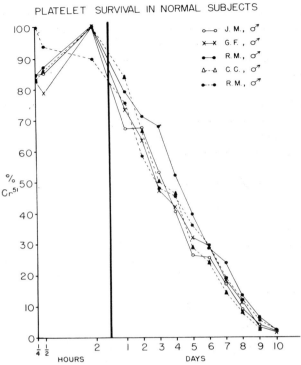

FIGURE 9-34. Normal ^{51}Cr platelet survival with a mean half-time of 4 to 5 days. (Courtesy of R. B. Solomon and D. V. Clatanoff, University of Wisconsin Medical School.)

4. The autoradiographs are developed in Kodak D-19 developer. The schedule is as follows (all solutions are kept at 19° C. to prevent swelling of the gelatin film):

    a. D-19 developer, 2 minutes.
    b. Tap water wash.
    c. Kodak liquid fixer, 1 minute. Then turn on light to time clearing. Allow the slides to remain in the hypo for twice as long as it takes to clear.
    d. Kodak Fixer Clearing Bath, 1 minute.
    e. Wash in running tap water, 10 minutes.
    f. Dry.

5. Slides are then stained with Wright's stain.

A number of good techniques have been described and the one to be used should be chosen according to the aims of the individual project. The above technique is particularly suited to cytologic detail of blood and marrow cells. A significant number of granules per cell must be seen in order to conclude that the cell has concentrated thymidine or other labeled material. We believe that 8 to 10 granules per cell are necessary and that the background must be one granule or less in a 20 micron field.

LEUKOCYTE LABELING

Radioisotopic labeling of the various blood cells can be accomplished by several procedures. Most depend on physical separation of the cells into categories without damaging them. It is necessary to be well versed in the various cellular isolation techniques in addition to the labeling and counting procedures.

A cholinesterase inhibitor, diisofluorophosphate (DFP), labeled with ^{32}P, has been shown to be a useful cell label (Grob et al., 1947). This compound rapidly forms an irreversible bond with a number of enzymes of the cell. When the cell dies, the radioactivity (^{32}P) is rapidly excreted in the urine. DFP has been used for *in vivo* studies of erythrocytes (Cohen and Warringa, 1954), platelets, and leukocytes.

DF[32]P is injected intravenously or intramuscularly and the labeled blood cells are separated to obtain the cell fraction of interest (Leeksma and Cohen, 1956, Athens et al., 1959). Studies in dogs using [32]P (Perry et al., 1957) for labeling leukocytes provided useful information concerning leukokinetics. However, the use of ^{32}P for tracer studies of leukocytes in man requires doses in the therapeutic range.

Leukocyte survival rates and distribution have been reported using [32]P (Craddock et al., 1960), ^{35}S-labeled L-cystine (Weisberger and Levine, 1954), and [51]Cr (McCall et al., 1955; Danon et al., 1966). Radioisotopic labeling has been shown to be a useful tool in the study of leukopoiesis (Bierman, 1964), but the degree of sophistication of laboratory technique prevents the adoption of these tests in the routine clinical radioisotope laboratory.

PLATELET LABELING

Studies of platelet production, life span, and destruction are greatly augmented by the tracer principle. The techniques are quite similar to those for leukocytes, requiring careful separation of the platelets without damaging them and shortening their life span. Labeling with DF[32]P has the advantage of minimizing handling of the cells. However, all the techniques require careful separation of the platelets from the blood before counting since other cells are labeled in various degrees.

Labeling with [51]Cr (Morgan et al., 1955; Aas and Gardiner, 1958; Baldini et al., 1960) requires prior handling of the platelets. Phosphorus-32 (Adelson et al., 1957), DF[32]P (Leeksma and Cohen, 1956; Alfos et al., 1959). [35]S (Lajtha et al., 1953; Odell et al., 1955b), and ^{14}C-labeled serotonin (Heyssel, 1961) have all been used. There is relatively good agreement in estimates of platelet life span among the various methods (Cronkite, 1958). All have limited clinical use and have been applied primarily to investigative purposes.

Radioactive chromate is added to the platelets *in vitro* after separation from other cellular elements of the blood. The mechanism of labeling is similar to that of labeling erythrocytes and the success of the method depends on the skill of handling the fragile platelets before use. The normal life span of the ^{51}Cr-labeled platelet is 4 to 11 days (Fig. 9-34). The technique (Aster and Jandl, 1964) involves preparation of platelet-rich plasma. The anticoagulant of choice is a fresh solution of modified ACD containing 0.085 M trisodium citrate and 2 per cent dextrose sterilized by Seitz filtration. The anticoagulant (95 ml.) plus 500 ml. blood are mixed at pH 6.5. Centrifugation of blood is carried out at 275 G for 14 minutes at room temperature and repeated at 400 G for 5 minutes. The resulting platelet "button" is resuspended in 20 ml. of the remaining serum and incubated for 15 minutes with 250 μc. of radiochromate.

The use of ^{32}P requires *in vivo* doses at therapeutic levels in order to obtain an adequate platelet label; it can be accomplished by separating platelets from the blood of a patient with polycythemia vera just after ^{32}P therapy. This latter procedure has the disadvantage of using homologous rather than autologous platelets.

The DF^{32}P method requires separation of labeled platelets from the labeled leukocytes and erythrocytes. The required doses may be as high as 600 μc. Sulfur-35 is incorporated into megakaryocytes *in vivo* and provides a physiologic label. Again the major drawbacks for clinical use are the large doses required, 7 mc. ^{35}S, and the need for careful platelet separation. The ^{14}C serotonin methods also provide a physiological *in vivo* label but require liquid scintillation counting techniques to detect the small quantities (2 μc. or less) of ^{14}C.

COMBINED STUDIES

Combinations of tracers may be helpful in the investigation of certain hematological disorders. We can measure simultaneously iron absorption and the rate of iron turnover by using ^{55}Fe and ^{59}Fe (Saylor and Finch, 1953; Davis and Koepke, 1964).

A useful combination of value in the diagnosis of obscure anemias is the combined use of ^{51}Cr and ^{59}Fe to measure simultaneously red cell survival and the turnover of iron (Weinstein and Beutler, 1955; Crook and Szur, 1960; Mitchell et al., 1957; Giuliani et al., 1961). The effective half-lives of ^{51}Cr (22 days) and ^{59}Fe (37 days) are similar; however, the differences in the energy spectra allow accurate simultaneous measurement using a single-channel gamma spectrometer. Chromium-51 has a peak at 0.32 Mev. and ^{59}Fe has two peaks at 1.10 and 1.30 Mev. By utilizing a lower window (BLV, baseline voltage) for ^{59}Fe, we eliminate the counts under about 1.00 Mev. A window is then set at the ^{51}Cr peak with the lower window (BLV) just below 0.32 Mev. and the upper limit of the window (ULD, upper limit discriminator) at about 5 volts above the BLV; this cuts off the higher energy peaks of the ^{59}Fe. A factor is established as follows:

$$\text{Mixture } ^{51}\text{Cr} + {}^{59}\text{Fe} = \text{counts/min. at high and low windows}$$
$$\text{Iron } (^{59}\text{Fe}) \text{ standard} = \text{counts/min. at high and low windows}$$
$$\frac{^{59}\text{Fe (low window)}}{^{59}\text{Fe (high window)}} = \text{correction factor}$$

Using this factor, one can subtract the iron activity that is measured when counting ^{51}Cr at the lower window. No activity of ^{51}Cr is detected when ^{59}Fe is being counted at the high window.

SPLENIC FUNCTION MEASURED WITH MERCURI-HYDROXYPROPANE (MHP)

The labeling of 1-mercuri-2-hydroxypropane with ^{197}Hg or ^{203}Hg has provided a useful compound to study the fate of damaged erythrocytes (Wagner et al., 1964). Addition of MHP to erythrocytes in proper concentrations results in damage or alteration in the red cell membrane with binding to protein stroma and globin. Too high a chemical concentration results in gross agglutination or hemolysis of the erythrocytes. When the cells are reinjected, the spleen selectively sequesters the altered cells and in 30 to 60 minutes an excellent scan of

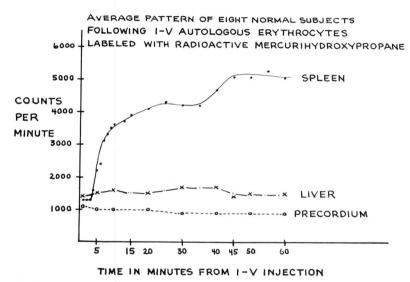

FIGURE 9-35. Spleen and liver uptake of MHP-damaged erythrocytes.

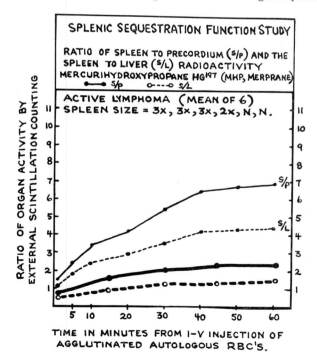

FIGURE 9-36. The external radioactivity over the liver, spleen, and precordium expressed as ratios. The splenic sequestration function in six patients with lymphoma was depressed as shown in the lower two heavy curves.

the spleen can be obtained (Wagner et al., 1964; Croll, 1965; Wang et al., 1965; Herman and Custer, 1966).

By standardizing the amount of damage to the red cells, one can quantify the splenic sequestration function of the spleen with respect to red blood cells (Fig. 9-35) (Korst et al., 1965; Wang et al., 1965).

When the spleen is infiltrated by leukemia or lymphoma, some loss of the red cell sequestration function of the spleen has been found in a small number of preliminary studies (Fig. 9-36) (Korst et al., 1965).

The use of MHP facilitates splenic sequestration studies because the entire test can be carried out within an hour; the test provides information about spleen size as well as spleen function.

Four patterns of uptake of the MHP-labeled cells have been recognized: (1) Patients with infiltration of the spleen with leukemia or lymphoma have a decreased splenic sequestration. (2) Patients with fibrosis of the spleen or who have undergone splenic irradiation have increased hepatic sequestration of cells. (3) Patients with cirrhosis have decreased liver uptake. (4) Patients with hypersplenism have increased splenic sequestration of cells.

The mechanism of action of MHP on the erythrocytes and the fate of labeled cells has been studied. *In vitro* incubation of rat, dog, and human erythrocytes with varying concentrations of MHP indicates that there are slight species differences in agglutination, in hemolysis, and in release of free MHP from the cells.

Rats that had been given injections of methylcellulose to induce splenomegaly and hemolytic anemia and normal rats failed to sequester selectively MHP-damaged red blood cells. Dogs were studied in the normal state and following splenic irradiation. The spleen had fivefold more radioactivity per gram of tissue than liver, kidney, or blood; this difference was reduced by radiation.*

REFERENCES

Aas, K. A., and Gardiner, F. H.: Survival of Blood Platelets Labeled with Chromium-51. *J. Clin. Invest.* 37:1257, 1958.

Abbatt, J. D., Chaplin, H., Jr., Darte, J. M. M., and Pitney, W. R.: Treatment of Polycythemia Vera with Radiophosphorus: Haemological Studies and Preliminary Clinical Assessment. *Quart. J. Med.* 23:91, 1954.

Adelson, E., Rheingold, J. J., and Crosby, W. H.: Studies of Platelet Survival by Tagging In Vivo with P^{32}. *J. Lab. Clin. Med.* 50:570, 1957.

Alfos, L. G., Field, E. O., and Ledlie, E. M.: Clinical Studies with DFP^{32} on the Life Span of Platelets. *Lancet* 2:941, 1959.

Alfrey, C. P.: Personal Communication.

Alfrey, C. P., Jr., Pittman, J., and Fuller, D.: Bone Marrow Distribution in Man. *Clin. Res* 12:345, 1964 (Abstr.).

Anger, H. O., and Van Dyke, D. C.: Human Bone Marrow Distribution Shown In Vivo by Iron-52 and the Positron Scintillation Camera. *Science* 144:1587, 1964.

Appleton, T. C.: Autoradiography of Soluble Labelled Compounds. *J. Roy. Micr. Soc.* 83:277, 1964.

Aster, R. H., and Jandl, J. H.: Platelet Sequestration in Man. I. Methods. *J. Clin. Invest.* 43:834, 1964.

* The author would like to express appreciation for the work and information provided by Mr. Charles Knorpp and Mrs. Mary Rennie of the Veterans Administration Hospital, Ann Arbor, Michigan, and Miss Janet Quirk of Madison General Hospital, Madison, Wisconsin.

Athens, J. W., Mauer, A. M., Ashenbrucker, H., Cartwright, G. E., and Wintrobe, M. M.: Leukokinetic Studies. I. A Method for Labeling Leukocytes with Diisopropyl Fluorophosphate (DFP32). *Blood* 15:303, 1959.

Aufderheide, A. C.: Radiochromium in the Estimation of Survival of Red Blood Cells. Review of the Literature. *Am. J. Clin. Path.* 34:258, 1960.

Badenoch, J., and Callender, S. T.: Iron Metabolism in Steatorrhea; Use of Radioactive Iron in Studies of Absorption and Utilization. *Blood* 9:123, 1954.

Baldini, M., Costea, N., and Dameshek, W.: The Viability of Stored Human Platelets. *Blood* 16:1669, 1960.

Baldini, M., Costea, N., and Small, W.: Platelet Survival and Viability of Stored Platelets. *J. Clin. Invest.* 38:985, 1959.

Bannerman, R. M.: Measurement of Gastrointestinal Bleeding Using Radioactive Chromium. *Brit. Med. J.* 11:1032, 1957.

Berlin, N. I., Lawrence, J. H., and Elmlinger, P. J.: Recent Advances in the Knowledge of Total Red Cell Volume, Production and Destruction. *Blood* 12:147, 1957.

Berlin, N. I., Lawrence, J. H., and Gartland, J.: The Blood Volume in Chronic Leucemia as Determined by P^{32} Labeled Red Blood Cells. *J. Lab. Clin. Med.* 36:435, 1950a.

Berlin, N. I., Lawrence, J. H., and Gartland, J.: Blood Volume in Polycythemia as Determined by P^{32} Labeled Red Blood Cells. *Amer. J. Med.* 9:747, 1950b.

Berlin, R., Berlin, H., Brante, G., and Sjöberg, S. G.: Failures in Long-Term Oral Treatment of Pernicious Anemia with B_{12}-Intrinsic Factor Preparations. *Acta Med. Scand.* 161:2, 1958.

Berson, J. A.: Blood Volume Determination. *Bull. N.Y. Acad. Med.* 30:755, 1955.

Bertinchamps, A., Kenis, Y., and Tognon, J. J.: The Effect of the Administration of HN_2 on the Utilization of Plasma Iron. *Cancer* 2:117, 1958.

Best, W. R., Landmann, W. A., and Limarzi, L. R.: Time Pattern of Vitamin B_{12} Co^{60} Urinary Excretion in Man after Oral Administration and Parenteral "Flushing." *Blood* 11:352, 1956.

Bierman, H. R.: Leukopoiesis in Health and Disease. *Ann. N.Y. Acad. Sci.* 113:511, 1964.

Birkeland, S.: Use of Cr^{51} for Studying Destruction of RBC in Healthy Humans. *Scand. J. Clin. Lab. Invest.* 10:122, 1958.

Block, M., and McGaffney, R.: Red Cell Survival Studies Using Radiochromium. *Rocky Mountain Med. J.* 54:1010, 1957.

Bond, V. P., Cronkite, E. P., Fliedner, T. M., and Schork, P. K.: Deoxyribonucleic Acid Synthesizing Cells in Peripheral Blood of Normal Human Beings. *Science* 128:202, 1958.

Booth, C. C., and Mollin, D. L.: Plasma, Tissue, and Urinary Radioactivity after Oral Administration of ^{56}Co Labelled Vitamin B_{12}. *Brit. J. Haemat.* 2:223, 1956.

Booth, C. C., and Mollin, D. L.: The Site of Absorption of Vitamin B_{12} in Man. *Lancet* 1:18, 1959.

Bothwell, T. H., Callender, S., Mallett, B., and Witts, L. J.: The Study of Erythropoiesis Using Tracer Quantities of Radioactive Iron. *Brit. J. Haemat.* 2:1, 1956.

Bothwell, T. H., and Finch, C. A.: Iron Metabolism. Little, Brown & Co., Boston, 1962.

Boyd, G. A.: Autoradiography in Biology and Medicine. Academic Press, New York, 1955.

Bozian, R. C., Ferguson, J. L., Heyssel, R. M., Meneely, G. R., and Darby, W. J.: Evidence Concerning the Human Requirements for Vitamin B_{12}. *Amer. J. Clin. Nutr.* 12:117, 1963.

Bull, F. E., Campbell, D. C., and Owen, C. A., Jr.: Symposium on Hematologic Disorders: The Diagnosis and Treatment of Pernicious Anemia. *Med. Clin. N. Amer.* 40:1005, 1956.

Bush, J. A., Ashenbrucker, H., Cartwright, G. E., and Wintrobe, M. M.: The Anemia of Infection. XX. The Kinetics of Iron Metabolism in the Anemia Associated with Chronic Infection. *J. Clin. Invest.* 35:89, 1956.

Calabresi, P., and Meyer, O. O.: Polycythemia Vera. *Ann. Intern. Med.* 50:1182, 1202, 1959.

Callender, S. T., and Evans, J. R.: The Urinary Excretion of Labeled Vitamin B_{12}. *Clin. Sci.* 14:2, 1955.

Carbone, P. P., Tjio, J. H., Whang, J., Bloc, J. G., Kremer, W. B., and Frei, E., III: The Effect of Treatment in Patients with Chronic Myelogenous Leukemia—Hematologic and Cytogenetic Studies. *Ann. Int. Med.* 59:622, 1963.

Card, R. Y., Cole, R. H., and Henschke, U. K.: Summary of Ten Years of the Use of Radioactive Colloids in Intracavitary Therapy. *J. Nucl. Med.* 1:195, 1960.

Caro, L. G., and Schnös, M.: Tritium and Phosphorus-32 in High-Resolution Autoradiography. *Science* 149:60, 1965.

Chaiet, L., Rosenblum, C., and Woodbury, D. T.: Biosynthesis of Radioactive Vitamin B_{12} Containing Cobalt-60. *Science* 111:601, 1950.

Challener, W. A., and Korst, D. R.: Pitfalls in the Diagnosis and Treatment of Pernicious Anemia. *Amer. J. Med. Sci.* 240:2, 1960.

Chertkow, G., and Dacie, J. V.: Results of Splenectomy in Auto-Immune Hemolytic Anemia. *Brit. J. Haemat.* 2:236, 1956.

Chievitz, E., and Thiede, T.: Complications and Causes of Death in Polycythemia Vera. *Acta Med. Scand.* 162:513, 1962.

Chodos, R. B.: Clinical Application of Radioiron and Radiochromium in the Diagnosis and Management of Anemias. Proceedings of the International Society of Hematology, Sixth Congress. Grune and Stratton, New York, 1958, p. 277.

Chodos, R. B., and Ross, J. F.: The Use of Radioactive Phosphorus in the Therapy of Leukemia, Polycythemia Vera and Lymphomas: A Report of 10 Years' Experience. *Ann. Int. Med.* 48:956, 1958.

Cohen, J. A., and Warringa, M. G. P. J.: The Fate of P^{32} Labelled Diisopropylfluorophosphonate in the Human Body and Its Use as a Labelling Agent in the Study of the Turnover of Blood Plasma and Red Cells. *J. Clin. Invest.* 33:459, 1954.

Coller, F. A., Blain, A., and Andrews, G.: Indications for and Results of Splenectomy. Charles C Thomas, Springfield, Ill., 1950.

Cooper, M., and Owen, C. A.: Labeling Human Erythrocytes with Radiochromium. *J. Lab. Clin. Med.* 47:65, 1956.

Craddock, C. G., Perry, S., Ventzke, L. E., and Lawrence, J. S.: Evaluation of Marrow Granulocyte Reserve in Normal and Disease States. *Blood* 15:840, 1960.

Croll, M. N.: A New Agent for Splenic Scanning: BMHP. *Radiology* 84:492, 1965.

Cronkite, E. P.: Regulation of Platelet Production in Homeostatic Mechanisms. *Brookhaven Sympos. Biol.* 10:96, 1958.

Crook, A., and Szur, L.: A Simple Method for the *In Vivo* Discrimination of Cr^{51} and Fe^{59}. *Brit. J. Radiol.* 33:447, 1960.

Cunningham, T., McGirr, E. M., and Clement, W. E.: The Effect of Prior Contact Between Acid Citrate Dextrose and Sodium Radiochromate Solutions on the Efficiency with which Cr^{51} Labels Red Cells. *J. Lab. Clin. Med.* 50:778, 1957.

Custer, R. P., and Ahlfeldt, F. E.: Studies on the Structure and Function of Bone Marrow. II. Variations in Cellularity of Various Bones with Advancing Years of Life and their Relative Response to Stimuli. *J. Lab. Clin. Med.* 17:960, 1932.

Dacie, J. V.: The Auto-Immune Haemolytic Anaemias. *Amer. J. Med.* 18:810, 1955.

Dameshek, W., and Welch, C. J.: Hypersplenism and Surgery of the Spleen. Grune and Stratton, New York, 1951.

Danon, D., Marikovski, Y., and Gasko, O.: ^{51}Chromium Uptake as a Function of Red Cell Age. *J. Lab. Clin. Med.* 67:70, 1966.

Darzynkiewicz, Z., Rogers, A. W., and Barnard, E. A.: Autoradiography with Tritiated Methotrexate. *Science* 151:1528, 1966.

Davies, J. W. L., and Topley, E.: A Critical Evaluation of Red Cell and Plasma Volume Techniques in Patients with Civilian Injuries. *J. Clin. Path.* 12:289, 1959.

Davis, B. K., and Koepke, J. A.: A Simple Method for Fe^{55} and Fe^{59} Assay in Mixed Plasma Preparations. *J. Nucl. Med.* 5:209, 1964.

DeWeese, M. S., and Coller, F. A.: Splenectomy for Hematologic Disorders. *Western J. Surg.* 56:129, 1959.

Diamond, H. D., and Craver, L. F.: Radioactive Phosphorus. II. In the Treatment of Myeloid Leukemia. *Cancer* 4:999, 1951.

Diamond, H. D., Craver, L. F., Woodard, H. Q., and Parks, G. H.: Radioactive Phosphorus. I. In the Treatment of Lymphatic Leukemia. *Cancer* 3:770, 1950.

Doan, C. A., and Wright, C. S.: Primary Congenital and Secondary Acquired Splenic Panhematopenia. *Blood* 1:10, 1946.

Dobson, E. L., Gofman, J. W., Jones, H. B., Kelly, L. S., and Walker, L. A.: Studies with Colloids Containing Radioisotopes of Yttrium, Zirconium, Columbium and Lanthanum. *J. Lab. Clin. Med.* 34:305, 1949.

Donohue, D. M., Motulsky, A. G., Giblitt, E. R., Pirzio-Biroli, G., Viranavatti, F., and Finch, C. A.: The Use of Chromium as a Red Cell Tag. *Brit. J. Haemat.* 1:249, 1955.

Doscherholmen, A., and Hagen, P. S.: Radioactive Vitamin B_{12} Absorption Studies Results of Direct Measurement of Radioactivity in the Blood. *Trans. Int. Soc. Hemat.*, 1956, p. 347; *Blood* 12:336, 1957.

Drapanas, T., Williams, J. S., McDonald, J. C., Heyden, W., Bow, T., and Spencer, R. P.: Role of the Ileum in the Absorption of Vitamin B_{12} and Intrinsic Factor (NF). *Clin. Sci.* 184:5, 1963.

Dubach, R., Moore, C. V., and Minnich, V.: Studies of Iron Transport and Metabolism; Utilization of Intravenously Injected Radioactive Iron for Hemoglobin Synthesis, and Evaluation of Radioactive Iron Method for Studying Iron Absorption. *J. Lab. & Clin. Med.* 31:1201, 1946.

Eadie, G. S., and Brown, I. W.: The Potential Life Span and Ultimate Survival of Fresh Red Blood Cells in Normal Healthy Recipients as Studied by Simultaneous Cr^{51} Tagging and Differential Hemolysis. *J. Clin. Invest.* 34:629, 1955.

Easson, E. C.: A Quantitative Study of the Radiosensitivity of Chronic Leukemia. *Brit. J. Radiol.* 30:35, 1957.

Ebaugh, F. G., and Beeken, W. L.: Quantitative Measurement of Gastrointestinal Blood Loss. II. Determination of 24 Hour Fecal Blood Loss by a Chemical Photospectrometric Technique. *J. Lab. Clin. Med.* 53:777, 1959.

Ebaugh, F. G., Clemens, T., Rodnan, G., and Peterson, R. F.: Quantitative Measurement of Gastrointestinal Blood Loss. I. The Use of Radioactive Cr^{51} in Patients with Gastrointestinal Hemorrhage. *Amer. J. Med.* 25:169, 1958.

Ebaugh, F. G., Emerson, C. P., and Rodnan, G. P.: An Evaluation of Na_2 Cr^{51} 04 as an Agent for the Determination of the Erythrocyte Life Span In Vivo in Various Hemolytic States. *J. Clin. Invest.* 34:931, 1955a.

Ebaugh, F. G., Jr., Emerson, C. P., and Ross, J. F.: The Use of Radioactive Chromium 51 as an Erythrocyte Tagging Agent for the Determination of Red Cell Survival In Vivo. *J. Clin. Invest.* 32:1260, 1953.

Ebaugh, F. G., Jr., Peterson, R. E., Rodnan, G. P., and Bunim, J. J.: The Anemia of Rheumatoid Arthritis. *Med. Clin. N. Amer.* 39:489, 1955b.

Edwards, C. L., Andrews, G. A., Sitterson, B. W., and Kniseley, R. M.: Clinical Bone Marrow Scanning with Radioisotopes. *Blood* 23:741, 1964.

Elmlinger, P. J., Huff, R. L., Tobias, C. A., and Lawrence, J. H.: Iron Turnover Abnormalities in Patients Having Anemia: Serial Blood and *in vivo* Tissue Studies with Fe-59. *Acta Haemat.* 9:73, 1953.

Erf, L. A.: Radioactive Phosphorus in the Treatment of Primary Polycythemia (Vera). *Prog. Hemat.* 1:153, 1956.

Erf, L. A., and Lawrence, J. H.: Phosphorus Metabolism in Neoplastic Tissue. *Proc. Soc. Exp. Biol. Med.* 46:694, 1941.

Everett, N. B., Reinhardt, W. O., and Yoffee, J. M.: The Appearance of Labeled Cells in the Thoracic Duct Lymph of the Guinea Pig After Administration of Tritiated Thymidine. *Blood* 15:82, 1960.

Filmanowicz, E., and Gurney, C. W.: Studies on Erythropoiesis. XVI. Response to a Single Dose of Erythropoietin in a Polycythemic Mouse. *J. Lab. Clin. Med.* 47:65, 1961.

Finch, C. A., Gibson, J. G., Peacock, W. C., and Flaharty, R. G.: Iron Metabolism Utilization of Intravenous Radioactive Iron. *Blood* 4:905, 1949.

Fitzgerald, P. J., Eidinoff, M. L., Knoll, H. E., and Simmel, E. B.: Tritium in Radioautography. *Science* 115:595, 1951.

Freireich, E. J., Ross, J. F., Bayles, T. B., Emerson, C. P., Finch, S. C., and MacDonald, C.: Radioactive Iron Metabolism and Erythrocyte Survival Studies of the Mechanism of the Anemia Associated with Rheumatoid Arthritis. *J. Clin. Invest.* 36:1043, 1957.

Frenkel, E. P., Whalley, B. E., Knorpp, C. T., and Korst, D. R.: On the Counting of Tritiated Thymidine in Tissues. *J. Lab. Clin. Med.* 59:174, 1962.

Friedell, H. L., and Storaasli, J. P.: The Use of Radioactive Phosphorus in the Treatment of Carcinoma of the Breast with Widespread Metastases to Bone. *Amer. J. Roentgen.* 64:559, 1950.

Gallagher, N. I., McCarthy, J. M., and Lange, R. D.: Erythropoietin Production in Uremic Rabbits. *J. Lab. Clin. Med.* 57:281, 1961.

Gallagher, N. I., McCarthy, J. M., and Lange, R. C.: Observations on Erythropoietic-Stimulating Factor (ESF) in the Plasma of Uremic and Nonuremic Anemic Patients. *Ann. Intern. Med.* 52:1201, 1960.

Garby, L., and Sjolin, S.: Some Observations on the Distribution Kinetics of Radioactive Colloidal Iron (Imferon and Ferric Hydroxide). *Acta Med. Scand.* 157:319, 1957.

Giblett, E. R., Coleman, D. H., Pirzio-Biroli, G., Donohue, D. M., Motulsky, A. G., and Finch, C. A.: Erythrokinetics: Quantitative Measurements of Red Cell Production and Destruction in Normal Subjects and Patients with Anemia. *Blood* 11:291, 1956.

Gibson, J. G., II, Peacock, W. C., Seligman, A. M., and Sack, T.: Circulating Red Cell Volume Measured Simultaneously by the Radioactive Dye and Iron Method. *J. Clin. Invest.* 25:838, 1946.

Giuliani, E. R., Hagedorn, A. B., Owen, C. A., and Scudamore, H. H.: Anemia of Nontropical Sprue Studied with Radioiron and Radiochromium. *J. Nucl. Med.* 2:297, 1961.

Goldberg, A., Hutchison, H. E., and MacDonald, E.: Radiochromium in the Selection of Patients with Haemolytic Anemia for Splenectomy. *Lancet* 1:109, 1966.

Goldberg, S. R., Trivedi, B. K., and Oliner, L.: Radioactive Vitamin B_{12} Studies. *J. Lab. Clin. Med.* 49:4, 1957.

Gordon, A. S.: Hematopoietin. *Physiol. Rev.* 39:1, 1959.

Granick, S.: Iron Metabolism. *Bull. N.Y. Acad. Med.* 30:81, 1954.

Grass, J., Bogoroch, R., Nadler, N. J., and Teblond, C. P.: The Theory and Methods of Radiographic Localization of Radioelements in Tissues. *Amer. J. Roentgen.* 54:420, 1951.

Gray, S. J., and Frank, H.: The Simultaneous Determination of Red Cell Mass and Plasma Volume in Man with Radioactive Sodium Chromate and Chromic Chloride. *J. Clin. Invest.* 32:1000, 1953.

Grob, D., Lilienthal, J. L., Jr., Harvey, A. M., and Jones, B. F.: The Administration of Diisopropyl fluorophosphate (DFP) to Man. *Bull. Johns Hopkins Hosp.* 81:217, 1947.

Gubler, C. J.: Absorption and Metabolism of Iron. *Science* 123:87, 1956.

Gurney, C. W., and Bolt, R. J.: The Simultaneous Use of Chromium Labeled Erythrocytes and I^{131} Tagged Human Serum Albumin in Blood Volume Determinations. *Univ. Mich. Med. Bull.* 22:319, 1956.

Gurney, C. W., Goldwasser, E., and Pan, C.: Studies on Erythropoiesis. VI. Erythropoietin in Human Plasma. *J. Lab. Clin. Med.* 50:534, 1957.

Gurney, C. W., and Pan, C.: Studies on Erythropoiesis in Experimental Polycythemia. *Proc. Soc. Biol. Med.* 98:789, 1959.

Gurney, C. W., and Pan, C. Studies on Erythropoiesis. XIII. A Comparison of Methods of Bioassay of Erythropoietin in Human Plasma. *J. Lab. Clin. Med.* 55:67, 1960.

Hahn, P. F.: The Use of Radioactive Isotopes in the Study of Iron and Hemoglobin Metabolism and the Physiology of the Erythrocyte. *Advances Biol. Med. Phys.* 1:288, 1948.

Hahn, P. F., Balfour, W., Ross, J. F., and Bale, W. M.: Red Cell Volume, Total and Circulating, as Determined by Radioiron. *Science* 93:87, 1941.

Hahn, P. F., Carothers, E. L., Hilliard, G. W., Bernard, L., and Jackson, M.: Treatment of Chronic Leukemias by Intravenously Administered Radioactive Colloids. *In* Hahn, P. F., Ed.: Therapeutic Use of Artificial Radioisotopes. John Wiley and Sons, Inc., New York, 1956, p. 128.

Hahn, P. F., Laureau, D. G., Feaster, B. L., Carothers, E. L., Gollan, F., Meneely, G. R., and Sherman, D.: Intravenous Radioactive Gold in the Treatment of Chronic Leukemia. *Acta Radiol.* 50:565, 1958.

Ham, T. H., Weisman, R., and Hinz, C. F.: Mechanisms of Destruction of Red Cells in Certain Hemolytic Conditions. *AMA Arch. Intern. Med.* 98:574, 1957.

Harbottle, G., and Maddock, A. G.: The Preparation of Chromium^{51} of High Specific Activity. *J. Chem. Phys.* 21:1686, 1953.

Harman, J. B., Hart, P. L. de V., and Ledlie, E. M.: Treatment of Polycythaemia with Radioactive Phosphorus. *Brit. Med. J.* 1:930, 1955.

Harris, I. M., McAlister, J. M., and Prankerd, T. A. J.: The Relationship of Abnormal Red Cells to the Normal Spleen. *Clin. Sci.* 16:223, 1957.

Hartsock, R. J., Smith, E. B., and Petty, C. S.: Normal variations with aging of the amount of hematopoietic tissue in bone marrow from the anterior iliac crest. *Am. J. Clin. Path.* 43:326, 1965.

Hashimoto, M.: The distribution of active marrow in the bones of normal adult. *Kyushu J. Med. Sci.* 11:103, 1960.

Hayhoe, F. G. F., and Whitby, L.: Splenic Function. A Study of the Rationale and Results of Splenectomy in Blood Disorders. *Quart. J. Med.* 24:354, 1955.

Heinle, R. W., Welch, A. D., Scharf, V., Meashan, G. C., and Prusoff, W. H.: Studies of Excretion (and absorption) of Co^{60}-Labeled Vitamin B$_{12}$ in Pernicious Anemia. *Trans. Ass. Amer. Physicians* 65:214, 1952.

Hempelmann, L. A., Jr., Reinhard, E. H., Moore, C. V., Bierbaum, O. S., and Moore, S.: Hematologic Complications of Therapy with Radioactive Phosphorus. *J. Lab. and Clin. Med.* 29:1020, 1944.

Hermann, G., and Custer, R. P.: Splenic Scintiscans with Merisoprol Hg 197 *J.A.M.A.* 195:1015, 1966.

Heyssel, R. M.: Determination of Human Platelet Survival Utilizing C^{14}-Labelled Serotonin. *J. Clin. Invest.* 40:2134, 1961.

Hollingsworth, J. W.: Disappearance of Radioactive Chromium Tagged Erythrocytes from Tissues and Body Cavities of Rabbits. *Proc. Soc. Exp. Biol. Med.* 87:493, 1954.

Hollingsworth, J. W., and Hollingsworth, D. R.: Study of Total Red Cell Volume and Erythrocyte Survival Using Radioactive Chromium in Patients with Advanced Pulmonary Tuberculosis. *Ann. Int. Med.* 42:810, 1955.

Holt, F. J., and Korst, D. R.: Transient Hemolytic Anemia Associated with Liver Disease. *Univ. Mich. Med. Bull.* 25:79, 1959.

Huff, R. L., Elmlinger, P. J., Garcia, J. F., Oda, J. M., Chocrell, M. C., and Lawrence, J. H.: Ferrokinetics in Normal Persons and in Patients Having Various Erythropoietic Disorders. *J. Clin. Invest.* 30:1512, 1951.

Huff, R. L., Hennessy, T. G., Austin, R. E., Garcia, J. F., Roberts, B. M., and Lawrence, J. H.: Plasma and Red Cell Iron Turnover in Normal Subjects and in Patients Having Various Hematopoietic Disorders. *J. Clin. Invest.* 29:1041, 1950.

Hughes Jones, N. C., and Mollison, P. L.: The Interpretation of Measurements with Cr^{51} Labeled Red Cells. *Clin. Sci.* 15:207, 1956.

Hughes Jones, N. C., and Szur, L.: Determination of the Sites of Red Cell Destruction Using Cr^{51}-labeled Cells. *Brit. J. Haemat.* 3:320, 1957.

Izak, G., Stein, Y., and Karshai, A.: A Quantitative Determination of Gastrointestinal Bleeding Using Cr^{51}-Labeled RB Cells. *Amer. J. Dig. Dis.* 5:24, 1960.

Jacobson, L. O., Ed.: Erythropoietin. Second Conference on Cellular Kinetics. Grune & Stratton, New York, 1962.

Jacobson, L. O., Gurney, C. W., and Goldwasser, E.: The Control of Erythropoiesis. *Advances Intern. Med.* 10:297, 1960.

Jandl, J. H., Greenberg, M. S., Yonemoto, R. H., and Castle, W. B.: Clinical Determination of the Sites of Red Cell Sequestration in Hemolytic Anemias. *J. Clin. Invest.* 35:842, 1956.

Jandl, J. H., Richardson Jones, A., and Castle, W. B.: The Destruction of Red Cells by Antibodies in Man. *J. Clin. Invest.* 36:1428, 1957.

Jerzy Glass, G. B.: Differentiation of Macrocytic Anemias and Detection of Pernicious Anemia and Sprue in Remission by Accelerated Measurement of Hepatic Uptake of Radioactive Co^{60} B_{12}. *Trans. Int. Soc. Hemat.*, 1956, p. 334.

Jerzy Glass, G. B., Boyd, L. J., and Stephanson, L.: Intestinal Absorption of Vitamin B_{12} in Humans as Studied by Isotope Technique. *Proc. Soc. Exp. Biol. Med.* 86:522, 1954.

Jerzy Glass, G. B., Goldbloom, A. A., Boyd, L. J., Laughton, R., Rosen, S., and Rich, M.: Intestinal Absorption and Hepatic Uptake of Radioactive Vitamin B_{12} in Various Age Groups and the Effect of Intrinsic Factor Preparations. *Amer. J. Clin. Nutr.* 4:2, 1956.

Joftes, D. L.: Radioautography, Principles and Procedures. *J. Nucl. Med.* 4:143, 1963.

Johnson, P. M., Wood, E. H., and Mooring, S. L.: Splenic Scintillation Scanning. *Amer. J. Roentgen.* 86:757, 1961.

Jones, H. B., Chaikoff, I. L., and Lawrence, J. H.: Phosphorus Metabolism of the Soft Tissues of the Normal Mouse as Indicated by Radioactive Phosphorus. *Amer. J. Cancer* 40:235, 1940a.

Jones, H. B., Chaikoff, I. L., and Lawrence, J. H.: Phosphorus Metabolism of Neoplastic Tissues (Mammary Carcinoma, Lymphoma, Lymphosarcoma) as Indicated by Radioactive Phosphorus. *Amer. J. Cancer* 40:243, 1940b.

Jones, H. B., Wrobel, C. J., and Lyons, W. R.: A Method of Distributing Beta-Radiation to the Reticulo-Endothelial System and Adjacent Tissues. *J. Clin. Invest.* 23:783, 1944.

Jones, H. C. H.: Measurement of Red Cell Loss from the Gastrointestinal Tract Using Radioactive Chromium. *Brit. Med. J.* 1:493, 1958.

Kaplan, E., Fels, I. G., Kotlowski, B. R., Greco, J., and Walsh, W. S.: Therapy of Carcinoma of the Prostate Metastatic to Bone with P^{32} Labeled Condensed Phosphate. *J. Nucl. Med.* 1:1, 1960.

Karon, M., Freireich, E., and Carbone, P.: Effective Combination Therapy of Adult Acute Leukemia. *Proc. Amer. Ass. Cancer Res.* 6:34, 1965.

Keuning, F. J., Arends, A., Mandema, E., and Nieweg, H. O.: Observations on the Site of Production of Castle's Intrinsic Factor in the Rat. *J. Lab. Clin. Med.* 53:127, 1959.

Kniseley, R. M., Andrews, G. A., Edwards, C. L., and Tanida, R.: Scanning of Bone Marrow in Hematopoietic Disorders. *In* Medical Radioisotope Scanning, Proceedings of a Symposium on Medical Radioisotope Scanning, Athens, 1964. Vienna, International Atomic Energy Agency, 2:207, 1964.

Kniseley, R. M., Andrews, G. A., Tanida, R., Edwards, C. L., and Kyker, G. C.: Delineation of Active Marrow by Whole-Body Scanning with Radioactive Colloids. *J. Nucl. Med.*, in press.

Kopriwa, B. M., and Leblond, C. P.: Improvements in the Coating Technique of Radioautography. *J. Histochem. Cytochem.* 10:269, 1962.

Korst, D. R., and Bethell, F. H.: Assay of Erythropoietic Factor(s) Using Radioiron Uptake in the Nitrogen Mustard Treated Rat. Erythrocyte Radioiron Uptake in the Rat and the Effects of Cobalt. *J. Lab. Clin. Med.* 52:356, 364, 374, 1957.

Korst, D. R., Clatanoff, D. V., and Schilling, R. F.: On Myelofibrosis. *Arch. Intern. Med.* 96:169, 1956.

Korst, D. R., Knorpp, C. T., and Bolt, R. J.: Circulating Red Cell Mass Determination Using Radiochromate. *Int. J. Appl. Radiat.* 2:156, 1957.

Korst, D. R., Nixon, J. C., Boblitt, D. E., and Quirk, J.: Studies of Selection Splenic Sequestration of Erythrocytes Labeled with Radioactive Mercurihydroxypropane (MHP). *J. Lab. Clin. Med.* 66:788, 1965.

Kraintz, L., and Talmage, R. N.: Distribution of Radioactivity Following Intravenous Administration of Trivalent Chromium 51 in the Rat and Rabbit. *Proc. Soc. Exp. Biol. Med.* 81:490, 1952.

Krevans, J. R., Conley, C. L., and Sachs, M. V.: Radioactive Tracer Tests for Recognition and Identification of Vitamin B_{12} Deficiency States. *J. Chronic Dis.* 3:234, 1956.

Kriss, J. P., Bierman, H. R., Thomas, S. F., and Newell, R. R.: Treatment of Multiple Myeloma with Radioactive Iodine and Radioactive Iodinated Serum Albumin. *Radiology* 65:241, 1955.

Kyker, G. C., and Rafter, J. J.: Scanning of Bone Marrow in Animals. *J. Nucl. Med.* 6:361, 1965 (Abstr.).

Lajtha, L. G. Isotope Uptake of Individual Cells. *Exp. Cell Res.* 3:696, 1952.

Lajtha, L. G.: The Culture of Bone Marrow Cells In Vitro. *Brit. Med. Bull.* 15:47, 1959.

Lajtha, L. G., Ellis, F., and Oliver, R.: Isotope Uptake in Individual Cells: Uptake of S35 Sulfate by Human Bone Marrow Cells In Vitro. *Brit. J. Cancer* 7:401, 1953.

Lange, R. D., and Pavolovic-Kentera, V.: Erythropoietin. *In* Moore, C. V., and Brown, E. B., Eds.: Progress in Hematology. Vol. 4. Grune and Stratton, New York, 1964.

Larsson, L.-G., and Jonsson, L.: Bone-Marrow Scanning after Intravenous Injection of Colloidal 198Au. *In* Medical Radioisotope Scanning, Proceedings of a Symposium on Medical Radio-isotope Scanning, Athens, 1964. Vienna, International Atomic Energy Agency, 2:193, 1964.

Lawrence, J. H.: The Control of Polycythemia by Marrow Inhibition. A Ten Year Study of 172 Patients. *J.A.M.A.* 141:13, 1949.

Lawrence, J. H.: The Treatment of Chronic Leukemia. *Med. Clin. N. Amer.* 38:525, 1954.

Lawrence, J. H.: Polycythemia: Physiology, Diagnosis and Treatment Based on 303 Cases. Modern Medical Monographs. Grune and Stratton, New York, 1955.

Lawrence, J. H., Berlin, N. I., and Huff, R. L.: The Nature and Treatment of Polycythemia. *Medicine* 32:323, 1953.

Lawrence, J. H., Dobson, R. L., Low-Beer, B. V. A., and Brown, B. R.: Chronic Myelogenous Leukemia. A Study of 129 Cases in Which Treatment Was with Radioactive Phosphorus. *J.A.M.A.* 136:672, 1948.

Lawrence, J. H., and Donald, W. G., Jr.: Giant Follicular Lymphoblastoma: Its Treatment with Radioisotopes. *Ann. Intern. Med.* 49:1, 1958.

Lawrence, J. H., Low-Beer, B. V. A., and Carpender, J. W. J.: Chronic Lymphatic Leukemia: A Study of 100 Patients Treated with Radioactive Phosphorus. *J.A.M.A.* 140:585, 1949.

Lawrence, J. H., Scott, K. G., and Tuttle, L. W.: Studies on Leukemia with the Aid of Radio-active Phosphorus. *New Int. Clinics* 3:33, 1939.

Lawrence, J. H., Tuttle, L. W., Scott, K. G., and Connor, C. L.: Studies on Neoplasma with the Aid of Radioactive Phosphorus. I. The Total Phosphorus Metabolism of Normal and Leu-kemic Mice. *J. Clin. Invest.* 19:267, 1940.

Lawrence, J. H., and Wasserman, L. R.: Multiple Myeloma: A Study of 24 Patients Treated with Radioactive Isotopes (P^{32} and Sr^{89}). *Ann. Intern. Med.* 33:41, 1950.

Ledlie, E. M., and Baxter, C. F.: Some Clinical Applications of Techniques with Tracer Doses of Fe-59. *Harwell Radioisotope Conference* 1:97, 1954.

Leeksma, C. H. W., and Cohen, J. A.: Determination of the Life Span of Human Blood Platelets Using Labeled Diisopropylfluorophosphonate. *J. Clin. Invest.* 35:964, 1956.

Levin, N. W., Hart, D., and Bothwell, T. H.: The Measurement of G.I. Bleeding Using Radio-active Chromium. *S. Afr. J. Lab. Clin. Med.* 5:93, 1959.

Lewis, S. M., Szur, L., and Dacie, J. V.: The Pattern of Erythrocyte Destruction in Hemolytic Anemia as Studied with Radioactive Chromium. *Brit. J. Haemat.* 6:122, 1960.

Lichtman, H. C., and Rabiner, S. F.: The Circulating Red Blood Cell Volume. *AMA Arch. Intern. Med.* 99:8, 1957.

Linman, J. W., and Bethell, F. W.: Factors Controlling Erythropoiesis. Charles C Thomas, Springfield, Ill., 1960.

Loeffler, R. K., Rappoport, D. A., and Collins, V. P.: Radioiron Citrate as Tracer to Determine Disappearance Rate of Plasma Iron in Normal Subjects. *Proc. Soc. Exp. Biol. Med.* 88:441, 1955.

Low-Beer, B. V. A.: Radioisotope Therapy. *In* Low-Beer, B. V. A.: The Clinical Use of Radio-active Isotopes. Charles C Thomas, Springfield, Ill., 1950.

Low-Beer, B. V. A., and Bell, H. G.: Surgical and Radiation Treatment of Carcinoma of the Breast. A New Concept. *Amer. J. Roentgen.* 75:1162, 1956.

Low-Beer, B. V. A., Blais, R. S., and Scofield, N. E.: Estimation of Dosage for Intravenously Ad-ministered P^{32}: Calculation Based on Two Compartment Distribution of the Isotope. *Amer. J. Roentgen.* 67:28, 1952.

Marinelli, L. D., Quimby, E. H., and Hine, G. J.: Dosage Determination with Radioactive Iso-topes. II. Practical Considerations in Therapy and Protection. *Amer. J. Roentgen.* 59:269, 1948.

Maxfield, J. R., Jr.: The Use of Radioactive Phosphorus and Testosterone in the Treatment of Metastatic Lesions in Bone from Breast and Prostate. *Int. J. Appl. Radiat.* 1:133, 1956.

McCall, M. S., and Keller, S.: An Abbreviated Method for Blood Volume Measurement Employing Cr[51]. *J. Lab. Clin. Med.* 55:149, 1960.

McCall, M. S., Sutherland, D. A., Eisentraut, A. M., and Lanz, H.: The Tagging of Leukemic Leukocytes with Radioactive Chromium and Measurement of the In Vivo Cell Survival. *J. Lab. Clin. Med.* 45:717, 1955.

McClellan, J. E., Donegan, C., Thorup, O. A., and Leavell, B. S.: Survival Time of the Erythrocyte in Myxedema and Hyperthyroiditis. *J. Lab. Clin. Med.* 51:91, 1958.

McClenahan, J. B., Yamauchi, H., and Roe, B. B.: Blood-Volume Studies in Cardiac-Surgery Patients. *J.A.M.A.* 195:356, 1966.

McCurdy, P. R., and Rath, C. E.: Splenectomy in Hemolytic Anemia: Results Predicted by Body Scanning After Injection of Cr[51]-Tagged Red Cells. *New Eng. J. Med.* 259:459, 1958.

McIntyre, P. A., Sachs, M. V., Krevans, J. R., and Conley, O. L.: Pathogenesis and Treatment of Macrocytic Anemia. *AMA Arch. Intern. Med.* 96:541, 1956.

Miller, A., Corbus, H. F., and Sullivan, J. F.: The Plasma Disappearance, Excretion, and Tissue Distribution of Cobalt-60 Labeled Vitamin B_{12} in Normal Subjects and Patients with Chronic Myelogenous Leukemia. *J. Clin. Invest.* 1:18, 1957.

Miller, O. L., Stone, G. E., and Prescott, D. M.: Autoradiography of Soluble Materials. *J. Cell Biol* 23:654, 1965.

Mitchell, T. G., Spencer, B. P., and King, E. R.: The Use of Radioisotopes in Diagnostic Hematologic Procedures. III. Simultaneous Cr[51] and Fe[59] Studies. *Amer. J. Clin. Path.* 28:461, 1957.

Modan, B., and Lilienfeld, A. M.: Polycythemia Vera and Leukemia—The Role of Radiation Treatment. *Medicine* 44:305, 1965.

Mollin, D. L.: Radioactive Vitamin B_{12} in the Study of Blood Diseases. *Brit. Med. Bull.* 15:8, 1959.

Mollin, D. L., Booth, C. C., and Baker, S. J.: The Absorption of Vitamin B_{12} in Control Subjects in Addisonian Pernicious Anemia and in the Malabsorption Syndrome. *Brit. J. Haemat.* 3:412, 1957.

Mollison, P. L., and Veall, N.: The Use of the Isotope Cr[51] as a Label for Red Cells. *Brit. J. Haemat.* 1:62, 1955.

Moore, C. V., and Dubach, R.: Metabolism and Requirements of Iron in the Human. *J.A.M.A.* 162:197, 1956.

Morgan, M. C., Keating, R. P., and Reisner, E. H., Jr.: Survival of Radiochromate Labeled Platelets in Rabbits. *J. Lab. Clin. Med.* 46:521, 1955.

Morris, A. C., Jr.: A Linear Scanner for Human Radioisotope Research. USAEC Report ORINS-33, 1960.

Morris, A. C., Jr.: The Whole-Body Scanner. *In* USAEC Report ORINS-49, 1964, p. 124.

Motulsky, A. G., Casserd, F., and Giblett, E.: In Vivo Measurement of Splenic Circulation: A Rapid Method for the Demonstration of Splenic Red Cell Sequestration. *J. Clin. Invest.* 35:625, 1956.

Motulsky, A. G., Casserd, F., Giblett, E. R., Braun, G. O., and Finch, C. A.: Anemia and the Spleen. *New Eng. J. Med.* 259:1164, 1958.

Neal, F. E.: Some Experiences with Radioactive Phosphorus in the Treatment of Mycosis Fungoides. *Proc. Roy. Soc. Med.* 47:859, 1954.

Necheles, T. F., Weinstein, I. M., and LeRoy, G. V.: Radioactive Sodium Chromate for the Study of Survival of Red Blood Cells. I. The Effect of Radioactive Sodium Chromate on Red Cells. II. The Rate of Hemolysis in Certain Hematologic Disorders. *J. Lab. Clin. Med.* 43:358, 368, 1953.

Nelp, W. B., McAfee, J. G., and Wagner, H. N.: Single Measurement of Plasma Radioactive Vitamin B_{12} as a Test for Pernicious Anemia. *J. Lab. Clin. Med.* 61:158, 1963.

Noyes, W. D., Bothwell, T. H., and Finch, C. A.: The Role of the Reticulo-Endothelial Cell in Iron Metabolism. *Brit. J. Haemat.* 4:43, 1960.

Odekwa, F. A. O., Kozoll, D. D., and Meyer, K. A.: Determination of Total Body Water with Tritium Oxide. *J. Nucl. Med.* 4:60, 1963.

Odell, T. T., Jr., Tausche, F. G., and Furth, J.: Platelet Life Span as Measured by Transfusion of Isotopically Labeled Platelets into Rats. *Acta Hemat.* 13:45, 1955a.

Odell, T. T., Jr., Tausche, F. G., and Gude, W. D.: Uptake of Radioactive Sulfate by Elements of the Blood and Bone Marrow of Rats. *Amer. J. Physiol.* 180:491, 1955b.

Osgood, E. E.: Contrasting Incidence of Acute Monocytic and Granulocytic Leukemias in P[32]-treated Patients with Polycythemia Vera and Chronic Lymphocytic Leukemia. *J. Lab. Clin. Med.* 64:560, 1964a.

Osgood, E. E.: Treatment of Chronic Leukemias. *J. Nucl. Med.* 5:139, 1964b.

Osgood, E. E., and Seaman, A. J.: Treatment of Chronic Leukemias—Results of Therapy by Titrated, Regularly Spaced Total Body Radioactive Phosphorus, or Roentgen Irradiation. *J.A.M.A.* 150:1362, 1952.

Osgood, E. E., Seaman, A. J., and Tivey, H.: Comparative Survival Times of X-ray Treated versus P[32] Treated Patients with Chronic Leukemias under the Program of Titrated, Regularly Spaced Total-Body Irradiation. *Radiology* 64:363, 1955.

Owen, C. A., Jr., Bollman, J. L., and Grindlay, J. H.: Radiochromium-Labelled Erythrocytes for the Detection of Gastrointestinal Hemorrhage. *J. Lab. Clin. Med.* 44:238, 1954.

Oxenhorn, S., Estren, S., Wasserman, L. R., and Adlersberg, D.: Malabsorption Syndrome: Intestinal Absorption of Vitamin B[12]. *Ann. Intern. Med.* 48:1, 1958.

Ozer, F. L., Truax, W. E., Miesch, D. C., and Levin, W. C.: Primary Hemorrhagic Thrombocythemia. *Amer. J. Med.* 28:807, 1960.

Painter, T. S., and Korst, D. R.: Studies on Acquired Hypogammaglobulinemia. *New Eng. J. Med.* 260:15, 1959.

Palmer, J. G., Eichwald, E. G., Cartwright, G. E., and Wintrobe, M.: The Experimental Production of Splenomegaly, Anemia, and Leukopenia in Albino Rats. *Blood* 8:72, 1953.

Pearson, H. A., and Vertrees, K. M.: Site of Binding of Cr[51] to Hemoglobin. *Nature* 189:1019, 1961.

Perkins, J., Israëls, M. C. G., and Wilkinson, J. F.: Polycythemia Vera: Clinical Studies on a Series of 127 Patients Managed without Radioactive Therapy. *Quart. J. Med.* 33:499, 1964.

Perry, S., Weinstein, I. M., Craddock, C. G., and Lawrence, J. S.: The Combine Use of Typhoid Vaccine and P[32] Labeling to Assess Myelopoiesis. *Blood* 12:549, 1957.

Peters, T., Giovanniello, T. J., Apt, L., and Ross, J. F.: A New Method for the Determination of Serum Iron-Binding Capacity. *J. Lab. Clin. Med.* 48:278, 1956a.

Peters, T., Giovanniello, T. J., Apt, L., and Ross, J. F.: A Simple Improved Method for the Determination of Serum Iron. *J. Lab. Clin. Med.* 48:280, 1956b.

Plzak, L. F.: Plasma Proteins with Radioactive Chromium. *J. Clin. Invest.* 29:1604, 1950.

Plzak, L. F., Fried, W., Jacobson, L. O., and Bethard, W. F.: Studies on Erythropoiesis: Demonstration of Stimulation of Erythropoiesis by Plasma Iron Anemic Rats Using Fe-59. *J. Lab. Clin. Med.* 46:671, 1955.

Pochin, E. E.: Profile Counting. *In* Medical Radioisotope Scanning, Proceedings of a Seminar, Vienna, 1959. Vienna, International Atomic Energy Agency, 1959, p. 143.

Pritchard, J. A., and Weisman, R.: The Absorption of Labeled Erythrocytes from the Peritoneal Cavity of Humans. *J. Lab. Clin. Med.* 49:756, 1957.

Rabiner, S. F., Lichtman, H. C., Messite, J., Watson, J., Ginsberg, V., Ellenbogen, L., and Williams, W. L.: The Urinary Excretion Test in the Diagnosis of Addisonian Pernicious Anemia. *Ann. Intern. Med.* 44:3, 1956.

Rajam, P. C., Jackson, A., and Black, S. H.: The Intracellular Labeling of Ehrlich Mouse Ascites Tumor Cells with Radiochromate. *J. Lab. Clin. Med.* 51:767, 1958.

Rath, C. E., McCurdy, P. R., Duffy, B. J., and Howley, J. R.: Value and Limitations of Cobalt[60] B[12] Test. *Amer. J. Med.* 20:954, 1956.

Rath, C. E., McCurdy, P. R., Schreiner, G. E., and Duffy, B. J.: The Effect of Renal Disease on the Urinary Excretion of Cobalt 60 Vitamin B[12]. *Trans. Int. Soc. Hemat.,* 1956, p. 329.

Read, R. C.: Studies of Red-Cell Volume and Turnover Using Radiochromium. *New Eng. J. Med.* 250:1021, 1954.

Read, R. C., Wilson, G. M., and Gardner, F. H.: The Use of Radioactive Sodium Chromate to Evaluate the Life Span of the Red Blood Cell in Health and Certain Hematologic Disorders. *Amer. J. Med. Sci.* 228:40, 1954.

Reilly, W. A., French, R. M., Lau, F. Y. K., Scott, K. G., and White, W. E.: Whole Blood Volume Determined by Radiochromium-Tagged Red Cells. Comparative Studies on Normal and Congestive Heart Failure Patients. *Circulation* 9:571, 1954.

Reinhard, E. H., Moore, C. V., Bierbaum, O. S., and Moore, S.: Radioactive Phosphorus as a Therapeutic Agent. *J. Lab. Clin. Med.* 31:107, 1946.

Reinhard, E. H., Neely, C. L., and Samples, D. M.: Radioactive Phosphorus in the Treatment of Chronic Leukemias: Long-Term Results over a Period of 15 Years. *Ann. Intern. Med.* 50:942, 1959.

Reisner, E. H., Jr., Gilbert, J. P., Rosenblum, C., and Morgan, M.: Applications of the Urinary Tracer Test (of Schilling) as an Index of Vitamin B[12] Absorption. *Amer. J. Clin. Nutr.* 4:134, 1956.

Remenchik, A. P., Schuckmell, N., Dyniewicz, J. M., and Best, W. R.: The Survival of Cr[51] Labeled Autogenous Erythrocytes in Children. *J. Lab. Clin. Med.* 51:753, 1958.

Roche, M., Perez-Gimenez, M. E., Layrisse, M., and Deprisio, E.: Study of Urinary and Fecal Excretion of Radioactive Chromium Cr[51] in Man. Its Use in the Measurement of Intestinal Blood Loss Associated with Hookworm Infection. *J. Clin. Invest.* 36:1183, 1957.

Root, W. S., Ed.: Hematopoietic Mechanisms. *Ann. N.Y. Acad. Sci.* 77:407, 1959.

Rosenberg, S. A., Diamond, H. D., and Craver, L. F.: Lymphosarcoma: The Effects of Therapy and Survival in 1269 Patients in a Review of 30 Years' Experience. *Ann. Intern. Med.* 53:877, 1960.

Rosenthal, H. L., and Hampton, J. K., Jr.: The Absorption of Cyanocobalamin (Vitamin B$_{12}$) from the Gastrointestinal Tract of Dogs. *J. Nutr.* 56:67, 1955.

Rubini, J. R., Bond, V. P., Keller, S., Fliedner, T. M., and Cronkite, E. P.: DNA Synthesis in Circulating Blood Leukocytes Labeled In Vitro with H3-Thymidine. *J. Lab. Clin. Med.* 58:751, 1961.

Rubini, J. R., Cronkite, E. P., Bond, V. P., and Fliedner, T. M.: The Metabolism and Fate of Tritiated Thymidine in Man. *J. Clin. Invest.* 39:909, 1960.

Sandberg, A. A., Ishihara, T., Crosswhite, L. H., and Hauschka, T. S.: Comparison of Chromosome Constitution in Chronic Myelocytic Leukemia and Other Myeloproliferative Disorders. *Blood* 20:393, 1962.

Saylor, L., and Finch, C. A.: Determination of Iron Absorption Using Two Isotopes of Iron. *Amer. J. Physiol.* 172:372, 1953.

Schilling, R. F.: The Effect of Gastric Juice on the Urinary Excretion of Radioactivity after the Oral Administration of Radioactive Vitamin B$_{12}$. *J. Lab. Clin. Med.* 84:860, 1953.

Schilling, R. F.: The Absorption and Utilization of Vitamin B$_{12}$. *Amer. J. Clin. Nutr.* 3:1, 1955.

Schilling, R. F., Clatanoff, D. V., and Korst, D. R.: Further Observations Utilizing the Urinary Radioactivity Test in Subjects with Achlorhydria, Pernicious Anemia, or a Total Gastrectomy. *J. Lab. Clin. Med.* 45:926, 1955.

Schilling, R. F., Muckerheide, M. M., Jacob, E., and Abels, J.: Multiple Autoantibodies to Gastric Juice. Presented at American College of Physicians, 24 March 1965; *Ann. Intern. Med.* 62:1085, 1965 (Abstr.).

Schloesser, L. L., Deshpande, P., and Schilling, R. F.: Biologic Turnover Rate of Cyanocobalamin (Vitamin B$_{12}$) in Human Liver. *AMA Arch. Intern. Med.* 101:306, 1958.

Schloesser, L. L., Korst, D. R., Clatanoff, D. V., and Schilling, R. F.: Radioactivity Over the Spleen and Liver Following the Transfusion of Chromium[51] Labeled Erythrocytes in Hemolytic Anemia. *J. Clin. Invest.* 36:1470, 1957.

Schwartz, M., Lous, P., and Meulengracht, E.: Absorption of Vitamin B$_{12}$ in Pernicious Anemia. *Lancet* 2:1200, 1958.

Shorter, R. G., and Titus, J. L.: The Distribution of Tritiated Thymidine in Adult Mice. *Proc. Staff Meet. Mayo Clin.* 37:669, 1962.

Simpson, W. J., and Baker, R. G.: Total-Body Scanning. *In* Kniseley, R. M., Andrews, G. A., and Harris, C. C., Eds.: Progress in Medical Radioisotope Scanning, Proceedings of a Symposium, Oak Ridge, Tennessee, 1962. USAEC Report TID-7673: 1963, p. 205.

Small, W. J., and Verloop, M. C.: Determination of the Blood Volume Using Radioactive Cr^{51}. *J. Lab. Clin. Med.* 46:255, 1956.

Smart, J. G.: Radioactive Phosphorus Treatment of Bone-Metastatic Carcinoma of the Prostate. *Lancet* 2:882, 1964.

Steinkamp, R. C., Lawrence, J. H., and Born, J. L.: Long-Term Experiences with the Use of P^{32} in the Treatment of Chronic Lymphocytic Leukemia. *J. Nucl. Med.* 4:92, 1963.

Sterling, K., and Gray, S. J.: Determination of the Circulating Red Cell Volume or Mass by Radioactive Chromium. *J. Clin. Invest.* 29:1614, 1950.

Stohlman, F., Jr., Ed.: The Kinetics of Cellular Proliferation. Grune and Stratton, New York, 1959.

Stohlman, F., and Schneiderman, M. A.: Application of the Cr^{51} Technique to the Study of Experimental Hemolysis in the Dog. *J. Lab. Clin. Med.* 47:72, 1956.

Stroebel, C. F., Hall, B. E., and Pease, G. L.: Evaluation of Radiophosphorus Therapy in Primary Polycythemia. *J.A.M.A.* 146:1301, 1951.

Strumia, M. M., Taylor, L., Sample, A. B., Colwell, L. S., and Dugan, A.: Uses and Limitations of Survival Studies of Erythrocytes Tagged with Cr^{51}. *Blood* 10:429, 1955.

Sturgis, C. C.: Hypersplenism, A Clinical Evaluation. Charles C Thomas, Springfield, Ill., 1953.

Suderman, H. J., White, F. D., and Israels, L. G.: Elution of Chromium^{51} from Labeled Hemoglobins of Human Adult and Cord Blood. *Science* 126:650, 1957.

Sutherland, D. A., McCall, M. S., Groves, M. T., and Muirhead, E. E.: The Survival of Human Erythrocytes Estimated by Means of Cells Tagged with Radioactive Chromium. *J. Lab. Clin. Med.* 43:717, 1954.

Swenseid, M. E., Halsted, J. A., and Libby, R. L.: Excretion of Cobalt^{60} Labeled Vitamin B$_{12}$ after Total Gastrectomy. *Proc. Soc. Exp. Biol. Med.* 83:226, 1953.

Szur, L., Lewis, S. M., and Goolden, A. W. G.: Polycythemia Vera and Its Treatment with Radioactive Phosphorus. A Review of 90 Cases. *Quart. J. Med.* 28:397, 1959.

Tati, M. N., Straebel, C. F., and Owen, C. A., Jr.: Some Clinical Uses of Radioactive Iron. *M. Clin. N. Amer.* 40:993, 1956.

Taylor, K. B., and Oxon, M. A.: Inhibition of Intrinsic Factor by Pernicious Anemia Sera. *Lancet* 2:106, 1959.

Toporek, M., Bishop, R. C., Nelson, N. A., and Bethell, F. H.: Urinary Excretion of Co^{60}-Vitamin B_{12} as a Test for Effectiveness of Intrinsic Factor Preparations. *J. Lab. Clin. Med.* 46:665, 1955.

Troup, S. B., Swisher, S. N., and Young, L. E.: The Anemia of Leukemia. *Amer. J. Med.* 28:751, 1960.

Valentine, W. N., Follette, J. H., Mills, H., and Lawrence, J. S.: Biochemical Studies in Chronic Myelocytic Leukemia, Polycythemia Vera and Other Idiopathic Myeloproliferative Disorders. *Blood* 7:959, 1952.

Van Dyke, D., and Anger, H. O.: Patterns of Marrow Hypertrophy and Atrophy in Man. *J. Nucl. Med.* 6:109, 1965.

Videbaek, A.: Polycythemia Vera—Course and Prognosis. *Acta Med. Scand.* 138:179, 1950.

Visek, W. J., Whitney, I. B., Kuhn, U. S. G., III, and Comar, C. L.: Metabolism of Cr^{51} by Animals as Influenced by Chemical State. *Proc. Soc. Exp. Biol. Med.* 84:610, 1953.

Wagner, H. N., Jr.: Radioisotope Scanning of the Spleen. *In* Kniseley, R. M., Andrews, G. A., and Harris, C. C., Eds.: Progress in Medical Radioisotope Scanning, Proceedings of a Symposium, Oak Ridge, Tennessee, 1962. USAEC Report TD-7673: 1963.

Wagner, H. N., Jr.: Splenic Scanning. *Northwest Med.* 63:767, 1964.

Wagner, H. N., Jr., McAfee, J. G., and Mozley, J. M.: Medical Radioisotope Scanning. *J.A.M.A.* 174:162, 1960.

Wagner, H. N., Jr., McAfee, J. G., and Winkelman, J. W.: Splenic Disease Diagnosis by Radioisotope Scanning. *Arch. Intern. Med.* 109:673, 1962a.

Wagner, H. N., Jr., Weiner, I. M., McAfee, J. G., and Martinez, J.: 1-Mercuri-2-Hydroxypropane (MHP). *AMA Arch. Intern. Med.* 113:696, 1964.

Wagner, H. N., Jr., Razzak, M. A., Gaertner, R. A., Caine, W. P., Jr., and Feagin, O. T.: Removal of Erythrocytes from the Circulation. *Arch. Intern. Med.* 110:90, 1962b.

Wang, Y., Westerman, M. P., and Heinke, E. W.: Spleen-Function Study with 1-Mercuri-2-Hydroxypropane Labeled with Mercury 197. *J.A.M.A.* 194:1254, 1965.

Wasserman, L. R., and Bassen, F.: Polycythemia. *J. Mount Sinai Hosp.* 26:1, 1959.

Wasserman, L. R., Dobson, R. L., and Lawrence, J. H.: Blood Oxygen Studies in Patients with Polycythemia and in Normal Subjects. *J. Clin. Invest.* 28:60, 1949.

Wasserman, L. R., and Gilbert, H. S.: Surgical Bleeding in Polycythemia Vera. *Ann. N.Y. Acad. Sci.* 115:122, 1964.

Wasserman, L. R., Rashkoff, I. A., Leavitt, D., Mayer, J., and Port, S.: The Rate of Removal of Radioactive Iron from the Plasma. An Index of Erythropoiesis. *J. Clin. Invest.* 31:32, 1952.

Wasserman, L. R., Stats, D., Schwartz, L., and Fudenberg, H.: Symptomatic and Hemopathic Hemolytic Anemia. *Amer. J. Med.* 18:961, 1955.

Weinstein, I. B., and Watkin, D. M.: Co^{58} B_{12} Absorption, Plasma Transport and Excretion in Patients with Myeloproliferative Disorders, Solid Tumors and Non-Neoplastic Diseases. *J. Clin. Invest.* 39:1667, 1960.

Weinstein, I. M., and Beautler, E.: The Use of Cr^{51} and Fe^{59} in a Combined Procedure to Study Erythrocyte Production and Destruction in Normal Human Subjects and in Patients with Hemolytic or Aplastic Anemia. *J. Lab. Clin. Med.* 45:616, 1955.

Weinstein, I. M., Spurling, C. L., Klein, H., and Necheles, T. F.: Radioactive Sodium Chromate for the Study of Survival of Red Blood Cells. III. The Abnormal Hemoglobin Syndromes. *Blood* 9:1155, 1954.

Weisberger, A. S., and Levine, B.: Incorporation of Radioactive L-cystine by Normal and Leukemic Leukocytes In Vivo. *Blood* 10:1082, 1954.

Weisman, R., Jr., Hurley, T. H., Harris, J. W., and Ham, T. H.: Studies of the Function of the Spleen in the Hemolysis of Red Cells in Hereditary Spherocytosis and Sickle Cell Disorders. *J. Lab. Clin. Med.* 42:965, 1953.

Wetherley-Mein, G., Hutt, S. R., Langmead, W. A., and Hill, M. J.: Radioactive Iron Studies in Routine Hematological Practice. *Brit. Med. J.* 1:1459, 1956.

Winkelman, J. W., Wagner, H. N., Jr., McAfee, J. G., and Mozley, J. M.: Visualization of the Spleen in Man by Radioisotope Scanning. *Radiology* 75:465, 1960.

Wiseman, B. K., Rohn, R. J., Bouroncle, B. A., and Myers, W. G.: The Treatment of Polycythemia Vera with Radioactive Phosphorus. *Ann. Int. Med.* 34:311, 1951.

Wolstenholme, G. E. W., and O'Connor, M., Eds.: Haemopoiesis, Cell Production and Its Regulation. Ciba Foundation Symposium. Little, Brown & Co., Boston, 1960.

GENERAL REFERENCES

Briggs, R.: Hematology. *In* Dyke, S. C.: Recent Advances in Clinical Pathology. Series III. Little, Brown & Co., Boston, 1960.

Dacie, J. V.: The Haemolytic Anaemias. Part I. Ed. 2. Grune and Stratton, New York, 1960, pp. 59. 65, and 135.

X

THE LUNG

HENRY N. WAGNER, Jr.

RICHARD A. HOLMES

VINCENT LOPEZ-MAJANO

DONALD E. TOW

INTRODUCTION

It is extremely probable that the blood takes in air in its course through the lungs and owes its bright colour to the admixture of air. Moreover, after the air has left the blood again within the body, it is equally consistent with reason that the venous blood, which has lost its air, should forthwith appear darker and blacker. Without such intercourse, anyone would be able to live in as good health in the stench of a prison as among the most pleasant vegetation. In a word, wherever a fire can burn well, there we can equally breathe well. (Lower, 1669.)

In 1875, Cohnheim and Litten suggested that, because of the low pressure in the pulmonary circulation, the slightest variation of resistance in the lungs would affect local pulmonary blood flow; thus they anticipated the current concept of the delicate balance between alveolar ventilation and capillary perfusion.

The crucial respiratory function of the lung—exchange of oxygen for carbon dioxide—takes place far down the respiratory tree. Each alveolar duct terminates in a rotunda-like space, the alveolar sac, which bears several terminal alveoli. Each of these is surrounded by the body's richest capillary network. The epithelial lining of alveoli is exceedingly thin; in places it is no thicker than 0.2 micron (Krahl, 1963). During gaseous exchange, the tissues traversed by the respiratory gases comprise: the alveolar epithelium; its basement membrane;

a narrow connective tissue space; the basement membrane of the capillary endothelium; and the capillary endothelium itself.

As a result of both anabolic and catabolic chemical reactions, the body produces large quantities of carbon dioxide that must be exchanged for oxygen. Part of the required oxygen is stored in the form of oxyhemoglobin and is available during short bursts of activity, but for more prolonged activities, oxygen must be taken into the body simultaneously with the performance of work. And, of course, when such work is increased, the exchange of carbon dioxide and oxygen is increased by more active pulmonary ventilation. For this gaseous exchange to be efficient, changes in regional blood flow must match the changes in ventilation. In certain diseases, there may be an imbalance between ventilation and the perfusion of various alveoli, despite compensatory mechanisms that act to restore the balance.

A major contribution of radioactive tracers is that they make possible the measurement of *regional* pulmonary function, supplementing the tests of *total* function. Although bronchospirometry is still used in measuring the ventilation and oxygen uptake of each lung, that method is often too complex for routine clinical or research use, particularly with severely ill patients. Knipping and his colleagues (1955) first suggested the use of radioactive gases, an important technical advance that has been greatly extended since that time. In addition to radioactive gases, radioactive particles have also been used to study the regional circulation in a variety of diseases and physiological conditions. At times, external radiation detectors permit the diagnosis of disease of certain regions before impairment of total function can be detected. Or, we can locate areas of greatest involvement in generalized disease of the lungs. This information is not only of diagnostic value; it can also help the surgeon decide which parts of a lung may need to be removed.

Also, the effectiveness of some of the nonrespiratory functions of the lungs— such as coughing, mucociliary activity, and alveolar phagocytosis—can be measured with radioactive tracers. In general, radioactive tracers are an aid in the study of the lungs in four ways: (1) in the measurement of physiological abnormalities in precise quantitative terms; (2) in locating areas of malfunction; (3) in the planning of the optimum management of a patient's illness; and (4) in the objective evaluation of the results of treatment.

RADIOACTIVE GASES

The function of various regions of the lungs can be determined without the use of radioactive tracers. Sampling of the gases from individual lobes of the lung can be carried out by means of radiopaque polyvinyl catheters placed into selected lobar bronchi (Martin et al., 1953). Or, we can use a triple-lumen catheter to study gaseous exchange in the upper and lower lobes (Mattson and Carlens, 1955). But both these methods are difficult for the patient, and have not been used widely.

The first use of radioactive gases to study pulmonary disease was by Knipping et al. (1957); they were concerned primarily with the early diagnosis of bronchial carcinoma, and they developed a procedure called "radio-xenon thorakography." By placing radiation detectors over various regions of the lung and observing the change in radioactivity as the patient breathed radioactive xenon through a closed system, they could detect impairment in regional ventilation caused by local bronchial stenosis or pleural thickening. In intrapulmonary diseases not resulting in bronchial narrowing there was only slight impairment of regional ventilation. These earlier methods, although novel and ingenious, were qualitative rather than quantitative; they have been greatly improved by subsequent modifications.

The three principal respiratory gases—oxygen, carbon dioxide, and nitrogen—can be made radioactive by deuteron bombardment of nitrogen, boron, or carbon in a cyclotron. The use of oxygen-15, carbon-11, and nitrogen-13 for lung function studies was introduced by West et al. (1962), Dollery (1960), and Dyson et al. (1960). Unfortunately, these nuclides cannot be produced in appreciable quantities in a nuclear reactor and they decay within minutes; for these reasons their clinical usefulness is limited.

Radioactive carbon dioxide was prepared by passing ^{15}O through copper tubing as the radioactive gas evolved from a cyclotron. Despite the 2.5 minute physical half-life of ^{15}O, it was possible to measure the initial concentration and rate of disappearance of inhaled radioactive carbon dioxide by means of two pairs of crystal scintillation detectors arranged in front of and behind the chest. By moving the detectors from one position to another, it was possible to record the rate of clearance of the radioactive gas from different parts of the lungs, and to determine the relative distribution of ventilation and perfusion in different regions.

Since ^{15}O and its derivatives $C^{15}O_2$ and $C^{15}O$ were available only in medical units located near cyclotrons, the application of the xenon-133 method was modified and extended by Ball et al. (1962). This radioactive gas is readily available and inexpensive, and it can be injected in aqueous solution intravenously. The patient holds his breath during the injection, and when the xenon reaches the pulmonary capillary bed it diffuses into the air within the alveoli. If the patient holds his breath for 5 to 10 seconds after the injection, intrapulmonary distribution of radioactivity is determined primarily by regional pulmonary blood flow, which can be measured with external radiation detectors.

After the initial distribution has been measured, a second determination is made after a period of rebreathing, during which time the gas is distributed evenly throughout the alveoli and thus provides an indication of the lung volume being viewed by the collimated detector.

An example of physiological information obtained with radioactive gases is the finding that perfusion of the lungs in normal persons is usually greater in the lower regions of the lung compared to the upper regions when the person is in an upright position, but that this difference disappears when he is supine.

To measure the ventilation of different regions of the lungs, instead of injection of the xenon solution (as in the perfusion studies), the patient can be instructed to take a single breath of the radioactive gas and hold his breath for 10 to 15 seconds. Scintillation detectors located in front of or behind the chest record the time course of radioactivity in various regions of the lungs in a manner similar to the regional perfusion studies. During inspiration the radioactive gas enters various regions of the lung at a rate directly related to ventilation. A modification of the single-breath technique consists of measuring the time required for the radioactivity to reach equilibrium when the patient breathes from a closed system (Bentivoglio et al., 1963a, b). In contrast to the single-breath method, which measures primarily dead-space ventilation, the equilibration time method gives a better indication of alveolar ventilation.

In the measurement of both ventilation and perfusion, an important advantage of the xenon method is that it lets the air within the lungs become uniformly labeled with the radioactive gas. This provides an indication of the volume of lung within the field of the detector, and makes it possible to determine the ventilation and perfusion per unit volume of lung.

RADIOACTIVE PARTICLES

Instead of using radioactive gases, regional pulmonary arterial blood flow can be measured by the *particle distribution method*. The technique is easy, relatively inexpensive, and free of significant danger or discomfort to the patient. The method is based on a principle somewhat similar to that used in measurement of regional blood flow by determination of the fractional distribution of injected potassium-42, or iodine-131 antipyrine (Sapirstein, 1958). However, the use of particulate rather than soluble indicators obviates the problem of recirculation, and the detection instruments are simpler. With the particle distribution method, the particles are injected under the particular physiological condition to be studied, and measurements can be made at a later time. The fractional distribution within the lungs of particles that were injected intravenously is determined by the regional pulmonary arterial blood flow at the time of injection, and this can be quantified by radioisotope scanning. Macroaggregates of human serum albumin (MAA) labeled with ^{131}I have been the most widely used radioactive particles (Taplin et al., 1964; Wagner et al., 1964).

An important advantage of the use of metabolizable macroaggregates of albumin, rather than the ceramic microspheres that were used formerly (Ariel, 1963), is that the albumin particles can be safely administered to man. The use of this material for the measurement of regional pulmonary blood flow developed from the use of similar but smaller particles in study of the reticuloendothelial system. In 1956, Halpern and his associates began to use human protein aggregates rather than insoluble particles—such as carbon, thorium dioxide, saccharated iron oxide, chromic phosphate, and colloidal gold—that remain in phagocytic cells almost indefinitely.

An essential preliminary to the application of lung scanning was the demonstration of its safety. Macroaggregates of albumin might be toxic in any of three ways: (1) the material might be antigenic because of the alteration in the structure of the albumin molecule; (2) obstruction of pulmonary capillaries and arterioles might have harmful cardiovascular effects; and (3) there might be a radiation hazard. Therefore, extensive testing for potential toxicity was carried out before the substance was used in man, and subsequent experience with thousands of patients has confirmed the safety of the method.

The absence of hemodynamic effects of the macroaggregates of this size range (10 to 50 microns) is due to the small amount injected and to the structural characteristics of the lung. Weibel (1963) established that the human lung contains about 280 billion capillary segments that arise from arterioles at about the twenty-eighth consecutive branching of the pulmonary artery. In carrying out a lung scan, fewer than one million particles are injected.

Gold and McCormack (1966) measured pulmonary function of 11 patients before and after lung scans; they found that scans produced no effect on lung volumes, pulmonary diffusing capacity, wasted ventilation, arterial oxygen and carbon dioxide pressures and pH, or the cardiopulmonary response to exercise. Lung scanning was a safe procedure even in the presence of preexisting pulmonary vascular disease.

VALIDITY OF THE PARTICLE DISTRIBUTION METHOD

The particle distribution method is based on the assumptions that: (1) the particles are uniformly mixed in the blood in the course of their passage from the point of injection to the pulmonary artery; (2) hemodynamic and gravitational forces affect the distribution of the particles in a manner similar to that of red blood cells; (3) the particles are nearly completely extracted from the pulmonary circulation in a single passage through the lung; (4) the particles, in the small quantities administered, do not themselves alter the distribution of blood flow; (5) the particles are not metabolized so rapidly that the initial distribution is significantly altered before their detection by the external radiation detectors; and (6) proper calibration can be made to correct for the effects of variations in chest wall thickness, lung volume, and other geometric factors affecting the quantification of radioactivity by the scanning method.

Indirect evidence of adequate mixing was obtained by measurement of the variability in amount of radioactivity per unit weight of lung in multiple specimens of tissue obtained from different regions of the lungs of experimental animals. In several hundred observations of the lungs of 12 dogs and 14 rats, the relative standard deviation of the radioactivity per unit weight of lung specimen in the same animal was about 20 per cent. This suggested that mixing with the blood was probably complete before the arrival of the particles in the capillary bed of the lungs. Preliminary studies in which MAA labeled with iodine-125 and red cells labeled with chromium-51 were injected simultaneously, and the animals then killed within 10 seconds of the intravenous injection, indicate a close correlation between the distribution of MAA and red blood cells (Tow et al., 1964). Evidence of nearly complete extraction is the finding of 80 to 100 per cent of the injected dose within the lungs of experimental animals.

Differential spirometry is an accepted method for evaluating the distribution of pulmonary blood flow between the right and left lungs. With this technique an index of the vascular perfusion through each lung is obtained by measurement of the percentage of the total oxygen consumption by each lung. In the estimation of the percentage of the total blood flow to the right and left lungs, the correlation between spirometry and scanning was excellent (r = 0.96; P < 0.001) (Lopez-Majano et al., 1964). This provides evidence that the particle distribution method is as reliable as the differential oxygen uptake for estimating the relative distribution of pulmonary artery blood flow to each lung.

Additional studies were carried out by Chernick et al. (1965). The two methods for estimating the percentage of total pulmonary vascular perfusion to each lung were compared in 27 patients during rest and exercise. At rest, the correlation between oxygen uptake of each lung and the percentage of pulmonary blood flow obtained from the lung scan was excellent ($r = 0.98$; $P < 0.001$), and there was also excellent agreement between the two methods during exercise ($r = 0.95$; $P < 0.001$). We therefore concluded that pulmonary scanning is as reliable and accurate as differential spirometry in measuring the percentage of pulmonary blood flow to each lung during rest and exercise. Also, spirometry is unpleasant and potentially hazardous, whereas scanning is safer and simpler.

USE OF INDIUM-113m LABELED PARTICLES

Recently particles of iron hydroxide labeled with radioactive indium have been used (Stern et al., 1966). Among the advantages of ^{113m}In are that it decays with a half-life of 1.7 hours and emits 390 kev. gamma-rays without emission of beta particles—thus resulting in a lower radiation dose than ^{131}I. Carrier-free quantities of ^{113m}In can be obtained from tin-113, which has a half-life of 118 days (Fig. 10-1).

Iron hydroxide particles labeled with ^{113m}In are made as follows. Ferric chloride in acidified solution is added to an aliquot from the ^{113}Sn column, so that the final ferric ion concentration is ~ 10 μg. per ml. The solution is titrated to pH 10.5 to 11.5 with sodium hydroxide. Gelatin (20 per cent solution) is added so that the final concentration of gelatin is 20 mg. per ml. The pH is adjusted to 7.5 with dilute hydrochloric acid. The final product is sterilized by autoclaving for 20 minutes. The majority of the particles range from 20 to 40 microns in diameter, with no particles in excess of 60 microns.

In addition to providing excellent lung scans, ^{113m}In-labeled iron hydroxide has the following advantages:

1. The absorbed radiation dose to the lungs from 1 mc. of ^{113m}In is about 0.75 rads, instead of 2 to 4 rads from a 300 μc. dose of ^{131}I MAA.

2. The radionuclide is available from a long-lived parent.

3. The particles are easy to prepare.

4. The final product can be sterilized by autoclaving.

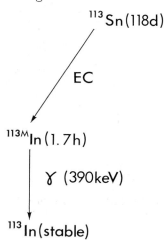

FIGURE 10-1.   Decay scheme of tin-113.

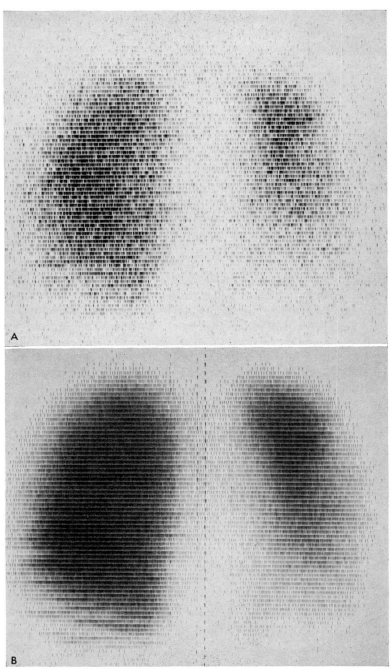

FIGURE 10-2.   Pulmonary embolus to the left lower lung. A, Posterior lung scan after injection of 300 μc. of ^{131}I macroaggregated albumin. B, Lung scan in same patient using 2.4 mc. of ^{113m}In (FeOH$_3$) complex. It can be seen that with the increased photon yield of indium the statistical fluctuations are less.

5. The larger dose that can be administered provides increased numbers of emitted photons and decreases image distortion resulting from statistical fluctuations (Fig. 10-2).

EXTERNAL DETECTION

The regional distribution of radioactivity in the human lungs after the injection of labeled particles can be measured by multiple stationary detectors, by a camera device, or by a single detector that scans the thorax in a rectilinear pattern. We usually have the patient lie supine during the scanning procedure, with the detector mounted beneath the subject and capable of moving at a relatively high speed. Patients can be scanned with an over-the-table detector, but occasionally they have difficulty in lying prone for the posterior view.

Quantification of the regional distribution of radioactivity can be accomplished in several ways. One method is to count the number of dots printed automatically on paper at a rate proportional to the counting rate. The method is tedious, and thus is not often used. A second method is to use the density of the film on which the scanning image is obtained for quantification; this can be done if the system is calibrated to correct for the nonlinear response of the film. Another method is recording of the counting rates by two scalers, each recording the activity from one lung. The radioactivity in particular segments of lung is usually expressed as a percentage of the total radioactivity in the lungs (Fig. 10-3).

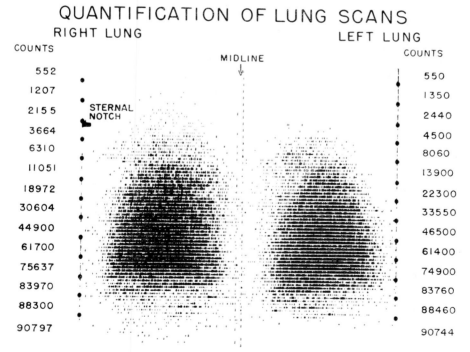

FIGURE 10-3. Quantification of activity in various segments of lung determined by summing the counts over 2 cm. intervals for each lung.

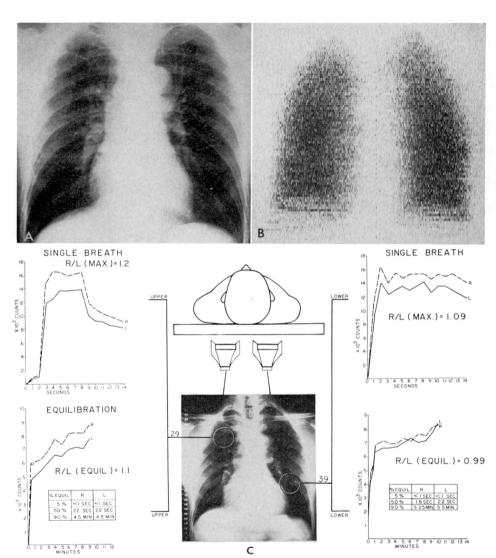

FIGURE 10-4. *A,* Chest radiograph in a normal patient. *B,* Posterior lung scan showing normal particle distribution. *C,* Xenon-133 study of ventilation in a normal person. Upper left tracing: The activity over the right and left apices after a single breath of xenon gas followed by 8 seconds of breath holding. The ratio of the maximum activity of the right and left lung was 1.2. Lower left tracing: The course of activity over the right and left apices during tidal breath of a xenon-oxygen mixture. The time required to reach half of the 10 minute values was 22 seconds on each side. The results indicated symmetrical ventilation of both apices. Upper right tracing: Single breath of ¹³³Xe followed by 12 seconds of breath holding. During this study the detector was over the lower lungs. Lower right tracing: Equilibration study during tidal breathing of xenon with the detectors over the lower lungs. The half-time of equilibration was 18 seconds on the right and 22 seconds on the left. These results indicated symmetrical ventilation.

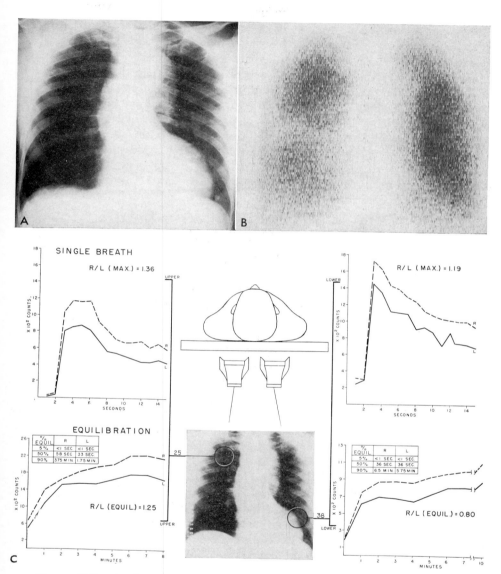

FIGURE 10-5. *A,* Chest radiograph in a patient with dyspnea, chest pain, and hemoptysis. The clinical diagnosis was pulmonary embolus. *B,* Multiple areas of diminished perfusion in both lungs, more marked on the right. *C,* Position of detectors for the xenon-133 study. In cases of suspected pulmonary embolism, when the lung scan indicates large areas of decreased perfusion, it is helpful to determine whether ventilation is normal in the involved areas. In this patient, whose lung scan showed greatly diminished blood flow to the right lower lung field, the ratio of the plateaus of activity after a single breath of xenon-133 (1.19) and the time required to reach 50 per cent of the equilibration value (36 seconds) during normal breathing of xenon-133 showed that ventilation was symmetrically distributed in the lower lung fields. In view of the perfusion defect at the right, this finding made pulmonary embolism the most likely diagnosis.

A rectilinear scanner can be used to measure the distribution of radioactive particles within the lung, but it cannot be used to measure the rapid changes in radioactivity that occur with the use of radioactive gases. With the gases, three types of instrument systems have been used. The first is a battery of two to six detectors arranged over the front or back of the chest. The output of the detectors can be stored in an intermediate system, such as magnetic or paper punched tape, and then played back one channel at a time through a single or dual recording system. A second method is to use a single pair of counters that rapidly scan the chest in two vertical lines from the bottom to the top of the lungs in a period of about 7 seconds. The time response of the detection and recording system must be fast (about a third of a second) because changes in activity occur in a matter of seconds. The third method of measuring the distribution of rapidly changing concentrations of radioactivity in the lungs is to use one of the newer stationary imaging devices or cameras. A suitable instrument should cover the entire lung field, have a spatial resolution of about 1 cm., and a fast time response.

Up to the present time, radioactive xenon has been used primarily to study the ventilatory physiology of the lungs in normal persons and patients with obstructive lung disease. It is predictable that with simplification of the techniques, the radioactive gases will be used more and more to solve clinical problems. Justification for simpler methods arise from basic investigations which have revealed that the degree of spatial resolution obtained with six or more detectors is usually not necessary for the solution of most clinical problems, particularly since identification of the detailed size and shape of the blood flow defects can be determined by scanning after the injection of radioactive particles. To solve a diagnostic problem, it is necessary to determine whether ventilation to a particular area is normal or reduced. This can be accomplished with equipment that is readily available in most departments of nuclear medicine. The most readily adaptable equipment is the dual-detector system widely used for the detection of unilateral renal disease (see Chapter XIII). If the temporal response is fast enough (measurements must be made at 1 second intervals), regional ventilation can readily be determined.

The technique is as follows: the patient lies quietly in a supine position with the two detectors positioned first over the upper halves of the lungs and then, in a repeated study, over the lower halves of the lungs. A 10 liter spirometer is filled with oxygen or room air and several millicuries of ^{133}Xe. The ^{133}Xe can be introduced into the spirometer from a shielded tank containing oxygen (or compressed air) and xenon. The patient's nostrils are occluded with a padded clamp and he breathes through a two-way valve connected to the spirometer. After several practice breaths, the patient takes a single deep breath of the xenon and oxygen mixture and holds his breath for 10 seconds. The time course of radioactivity in the two regions of the lungs is recorded at 1 second intervals. The counting rates are graphed on linear graph paper. In the second phase of the study, the patient breathes at a normal tidal volume. After a period of time, the valve connecting the mouthpiece to the spirometer is turned so that the patient breathes from the closed system containing the xenon. The system contains a carbon dioxide absorber and rebreathing continues until equilibrium has been reached or for at least 10 minutes. The counting rates are recorded from each of the detector sites at 1 second intervals, and are graphed as a function of time on linear graph paper.

The lung volume in the field of view of the detector can be estimated from the counting rate at the end of the equilibration period. The plateau values after the single breath are related to both ventilation and the lung volume viewed by the detector. If the lung volumes are the same, differences in the single breath plateau values can be used to determine the relative ventilation of the two regions. The rate with which equilibration is reached is also used as an index of regional ventilation. The time required to reach 5, 50, and 90 per cent of the final equilibration activity is also measured.

In practice, the regional perfusion of the lung is first assessed by scanning and then ventilation is measured. The finding of decreased perfusion with relatively normal ventilation may help in distinguishing pulmonary embolism from chronic obstructive pulmonary disease. Figures 10-4 and 10-5 are examples of the use of radioactive xenon together with the particle distribution technique.

PULMONARY ARTERIAL BLOOD FLOW IN NORMAL PERSONS

When a person is upright, pulmonary arterial blood flow per unit volume of lung is less in the top of the lungs than in the bottom (West, 1962); but when a person lies down, the apical and basilar flows become virtually the same. With exercise, the apical flow increases more than basilar flow, and thus the distribution may become uniform, even in the upright position. Different phases of the respiratory cycle also influence the distribution of pulmonary arterial blood flow. In clinical studies, therefore, in order to achieve a more even distribution of blood flow per unit volume of lung, we inject the radioactive particles with the patient lying quietly in a supine position. We also inject the particles slowly over a period of several seconds, to average the effect of the different phases of the respiratory cycle. We do not ask the patient to breathe deeply or hold his breath, to avoid his becoming conscious of his breathing. The distribution of particles within the lung is determined by scanning shortly after the injection, although the relative concentrations of the particles change little over a period of up to at least a few hours.

The typical appearance of the lung scan made with the detector in front of the chest is illustrated in Figure 10-6A. Usually, the outline of the heart can be seen in the anterior view as an area without radioactivity. Respiratory motion may give a serrated appearance to the lower borders, but the remainder of the lung fields usually have smooth convex borders. We look carefully at the borders for concavities, which are often seen in pulmonary embolism (see Fig. 10-25). The lower lateral borders of the scan often have a rounded contour, even in normal persons.

In the posterior view (Fig. 10-6B) the cardiac image is less prominent, and the two lungs appear more symmetrical. The apices may have slightly less radioactivity than the bases, although this is usually not pronounced if the injection was made with the patient in a supine position. In the posterior view, the medial borders of the lungs appear straight, except in such conditions as cardiomegaly, distention of the pulmonary arteries, and hilar adenopathy.

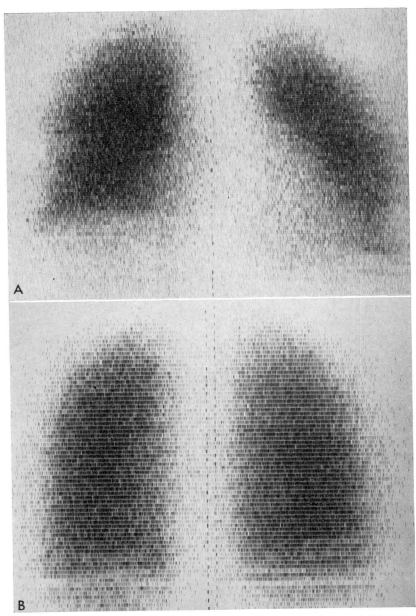

FIGURE 10-6. A, Anterior lung scan performed with indium-113m labeled particles.
B, Posterior lung scan performed with indium-113m labeled particles.

The lateral views (Fig. 10-7) are very helpful and should be performed
routinely; at the very least, they should be performed whenever an abnormality
is noted in the anterior or posterior view. In the left lateral view, the heart
may produce a concave indentation of the anterior borders of the lung, particularly if the heart is enlarged. On both lateral views, the inferior margin of
the lung is usually concave because of the diaphragm; respiratory movements
may produce serrations of this concave border. To avoid an image that is diffi-

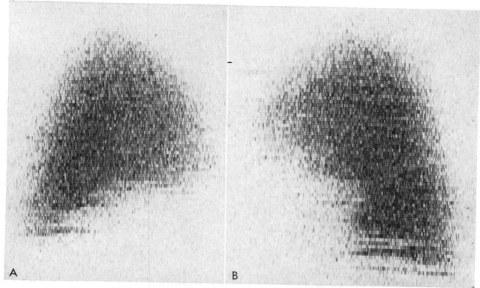

FIGURE 10-7. A, Right lateral lung scan. B, Left lateral lung scan.

cult to interpret, the lateral views require the utmost care to ensure that the patient's position is truly lateral rather than oblique.

ARTIFACTS AND FREQUENT NORMAL VARIANTS

If the particles are not shaken immediately before injection, or if blood is allowed to clot within the syringe, the result may be a bizarre scan showing large masses of radioactivity. Movement of the patient during the scanning procedure will distort the scan, but this can usually be recognized by corresponding changes at the lateral and medial borders of each lung. If the patient is breathing rapidly, respiratory artifacts at the bases become more prominent and may even be seen along the vertical borders of the lungs as well.

A common error is the use of excessive contrast enhancement in the performance of the lung scan. Unlike brain scanning, in which high contrast is essential, lung scanning usually requires little data processing because of the high counting rates and the great differences in the amount of radioactivity in the lesions compared to the normal lung. Therefore we prefer that the optical density of the scan be as linearly related to the counting rate as possible. If excessive contrast is used, areas of decreased activity may appear completely clear, as if they contained *no* activity. Excessive contrast can also make the lungs appear abnormally small. In high-contrast scans, lesions may be erroneously interpreted as having *no* pulmonary arterial blood flow, when they actually have only *reduced* blood flow (Fig. 10-8). Contrast can be evaluated by looking for evidence of the background radiation surrounding the chest. If no background activity is visible in the scanning image, the contrast was probably excessive, and the scan should be repeated with less contrast.

Multiple views of the lungs are needed because of the limited depth of focus of most focusing collimators. An example of a lesion that might have been

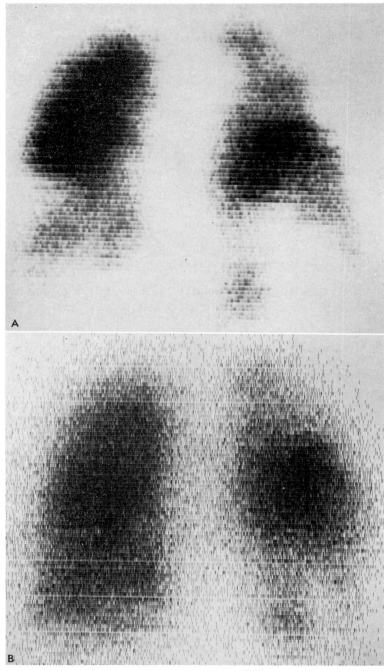

FIGURE 10-8. *A*, High-contrast scan suggesting multiple areas of *no* perfusion in a patient with pulmonary emboli. *B*, Scan with less contrast in same patient. Blood flow is reduced, not completely absent, in areas such as the right base.

misinterpreted if reliance had been placed on a single view is illustrated in Figure 10-9. Despite the small infiltrate in the left midlung field on the radiograph, the posterior scan suggested that the abnormality included the entire midlung field. The left lateral view, however, showed the lesion to have the concave appearance often seen in embolism.

The particle distribution technique has confirmed the results of the radioactive gas studies: that regional shifts in pulmonary blood flow occur as the result of minor changes, such as shifting the body position (Fig. 10-10).

Awareness of the sensitivity of the method in detecting changes in regional pulmonary blood flow is helpful in interpreting lung scans. Unilateral pleural effusion may result in a marked reduction in blood flow, particularly if the fluid is free and impinges upon the pulmonary vessels when the patient is lying down (Fig. 10-11).

Another variant is the decrease in regional blood flow resulting from an enlarged heart. The area of decreased activity does not usually extend to the periphery of the lung (Fig. 10-12) except in cases of extreme enlargement. The effects of cardiomegaly should not be interpreted as pulmonary lesions. The left lateral view is particularly helpful in determining whether there is a pul-

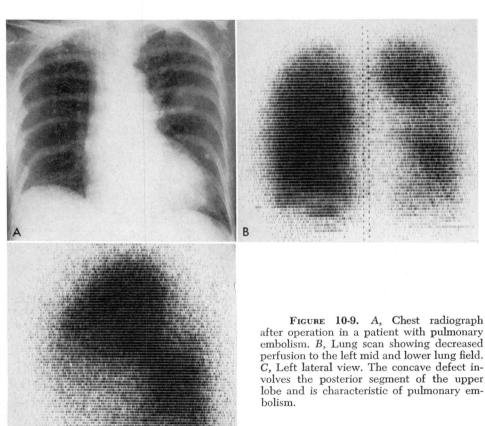

FIGURE 10-9. A, Chest radiograph after operation in a patient with pulmonary embolism. B, Lung scan showing decreased perfusion to the left mid and lower lung field. C, Left lateral view. The concave defect involves the posterior segment of the upper lobe and is characteristic of pulmonary embolism.

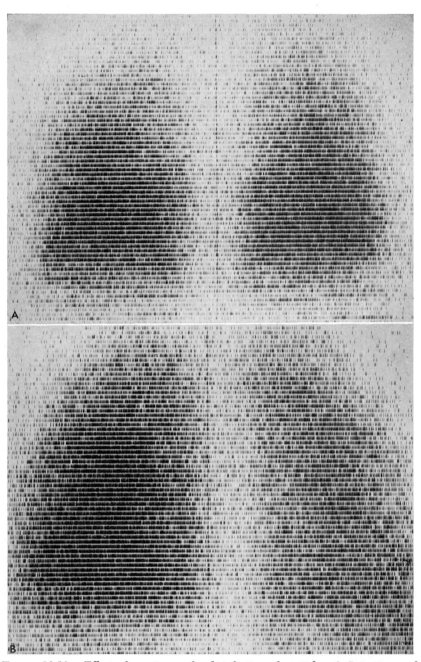

FIGURE 10-10.   Effect of gravity on the distribution of particles. A, Injection made with the patient seated. B, Injection made with the patient lying on his right side. The apices are better perfused when the patient is lying down. In A (sitting position) the distribution of injected particles between the right and left lung was 50.1 and 49.9 per cent. In B (right lateral decubitus position) 59.1 per cent of the particles went to the dependent lung.

monary lesion in the left lower field in patients with cardiomegaly. Lesions of the left lower lung will often be missed if only an anterior view is obtained.

Developmental (or acquired) abnormalities of the chest wall, thoracic spine, or sternum—such as hemithorax, kyphoscoliosis, pectus excavatum, and pectus carinatum—may alter the appearance of the lung scan. These conditions emphasize one of the first principles of lung scanning: one should *never* interpret a scan without examining the patient and the chest radiograph.

CONGENITAL DISEASES

Some congenital disorders (Table 10-1) alter the pulmonary circulation in ways that provide diagnostic information. Proper interpretation of lung scans

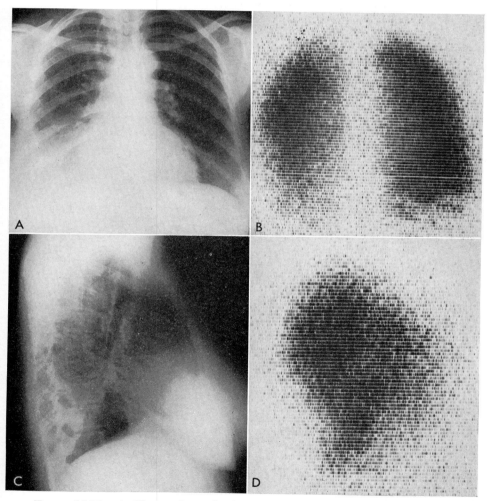

FIGURE 10-11. *A*, Chest radiograph of a patient with pleural effusion on the right. *B*, Posterior lung scan showing decreased perfusion, particularly at the right base; 42 per cent of the blood flow went to the right lung, as determined by the quantitative data. *C*, Right lateral lung radiograph with density in lower posterior lung field. *D*, Right lateral scan in the same patient.

TABLE 10-1. CONGENITAL INTRATHORACIC ANOMALIES

A. *Bronchoalveolar anomalies*
  1. Primary tracheomalacia
  2. Aplasia (agenesis) and hypoplasia of the lung
  3. Azygous lobe (tracheal lobe and accessory lobe)
  4. Pulmonary sequestration
    a. Intralobar
    b. Extralobar
  5. Congenital atelectasis
  6. Miscellaneous
    a. Situs inversus and bronchiectasis (Kartagener's syndrome)
    b. Fibrocystic disease of the pancreas, with lung involvement
    c. Esophageal atresia and tracheo-esophageal fistula
B. *Vascular anomalies*
  1. Aplasia and hypoplasia of the pulmonary artery
  2. Unilateral transradiancy of the lung (Macleod's or Swyer-James syndrome)
  3. Hemangiomas (hamartomas)
  4. Arteriovenous fistula of the lung
  5. Vascular encirclement of major airways
    a. Aortic ring
    b. Aberrant subclavian and innominate arteries ("dysphagia lusoria")
    c. Congenital cardiac lesions
  6. Cardiopulmonary defects
    a. Without shunt
      (1) Fixed obstruction of the pulmonary artery: valvular, supravalvular, or sub-
          valvular (infundibular) pulmonary stenosis
      (2) Primary pulmonary hypertension
      (3) Idiopathic dilatation of the pulmonary artery
      (4) Absence of the pulmonary valve
      (5) Ebstein's anomaly of the tricuspid valve
      (6) Tricuspid stenosis; isolated, or associated with pulmonary stenosis
    b. With shunt
      (1) Acyanotic
        (a) Atrial septal defect (ostium secundum; ostium primum)
        (b) Atrial septal defect in combination with: pulmonary stenosis, partial anom-
            alous venous connection, or mitral stenosis (Lutembacher's syndrome)
      (2) Cyanotic
        (a) Tricuspid atresia with pulmonary or infundibular stenosis
        (b) Pulmonary stenosis with patent foramen ovale or with atrial septal defect
            (trilogy of Fallot)
        (c) Tetralogy of Fallot
        (d) Taussig-Bing complex
        (e) Total anomalous pulmonary venous connection
        (f) Transposition of the great vessels
        (g) Persistent truncus arteriosus
C. *Chest wall anomalies*
  1. Sternum: bifid sternum, pectus carinatum, pectus excavatum
  2. Spine: kyphoscoliosis, hemivertebrae
  3. Rib cage: rib aplasia or hypoplasia, supernumerary ribs, synostosis of ribs
D. *Diaphragm anomalies*
  1. Diaphragmatic hernia (foramen of Bochdalek; foramina of Morgagni)
  2. Eventration of the diaphragm
E. *Congenital mediastinal cysts*
  1. Bronchogenic cysts (paratracheal, carinal, hilar, or paraesophageal)
  2. Esophageal cysts
  3. Gastric cysts

in patients with congenital cardiac defects requires an understanding of the relationship between the pulmonary and bronchial circulation. Except when there is an abnormal communication between the right and left side of the heart, such as a ventricular septal defect, the bronchial circulation does not contain radioactive particles after intravenous injection; the distribution of the particles within the lungs is a function only of the pulmonary arterial blood flow. However, if right-to-left shunting is present, and especially if the bronchial circulation is increased, particles can reach the lungs by way of both the pulmonary and the bronchial circulations. For example, in patients with total pulmonary atresia, all the particles are shunted into the systemic circulation and reach the lungs only via the bronchial circulation.

If a single pulmonary artery is missing, the scanning image will be similar to that seen in unilateral aplasia of the lung (Atwood et al., 1966), that is, no perfusion of the involved side. In unilateral lung hypoplasia some activity is usually observed on the affected side though a major portion of the blood flow to the lung may be from the bronchial arteries. In the young, reduced or absent unilateral pulmonary blood flow can result from acquired disease, as represented

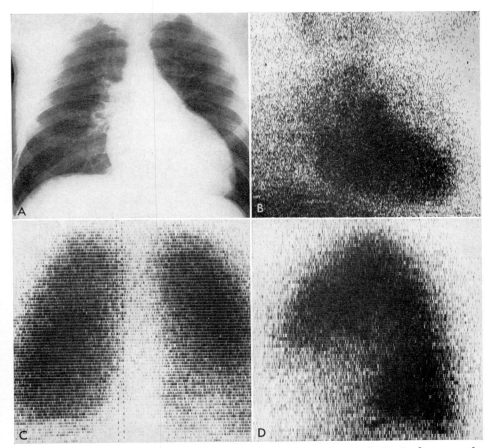

FIGURE 10-12.   A, Chest radiograph in a patient with cardiomegaly. B, Cardiac scan after 4.0 mc. of 99mTc-labeled albumin. C, Lung scan showing diminished perfusion of the left lower lung. D, Left lateral view showing the effect of cardiomegaly on pulmonary arterial blood flow.

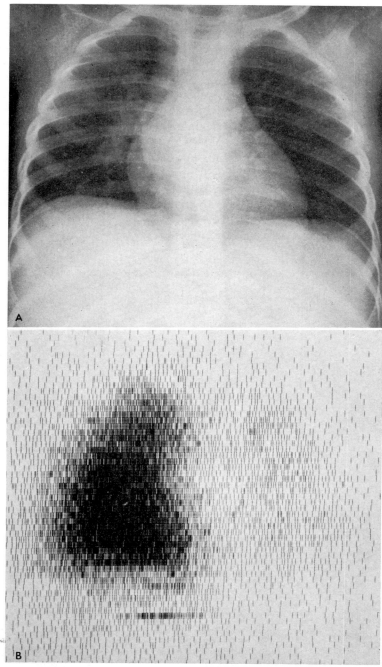

FIGURE 10-13. *A,* Chest radiograph of a child with a positive tuberculin skin test, cough, and negative bronchoscopy, showing decreased vascular markings in the left lung. *B,* Scan showing absent perfusion to the left lung that revascularized after several months of therapy for tuberculosis.

by the child in Figure 10-13. The absent perfusion of the left lung in this case resulted from large hilar tuberculous nodes compressing the left main pulmonary artery.

The lung scan is also helpful in adult patients with "hyperlucency" of one lung. Ueda and his associates (1965) reported the scan of a patient with unilateral hyperlucency of the lung as described by Macleod (1954) and Swyer and James (1953). Figure 10-14 is the scan that we obtained in an asymptomatic 20 year old male who showed hyperlucency of the left lung on the radiograph and diminished perfusion of the left lung in the arteriogram. Whether this condition results from agenesis of the pulmonary artery or from bronchial aplasia has been discussed by Rakower and Moran (1962).

When right-to-left shunting is pronounced, radioactivity often appears in organs with high systemic blood flow, such as the liver and kidneys. An example is the scan in Figure 10-15, obtained from a child with tetralogy of Fallot. In our experiments with dogs, and in the studies of Kennady et al. (1965) in monkeys, doses of particles far greater than the doses reaching the cerebral circulation in cases of pulmonary artery atresia (even when complete) were not associated with any detectable side effects. Consequently, we do not believe that right-to-left shunting is a contraindication to lung scanning.

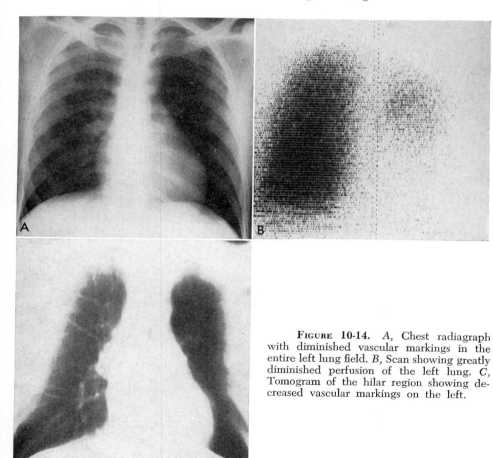

FIGURE 10-14. A, Chest radiagraph with diminished vascular markings in the entire left lung field. B, Scan showing greatly diminished perfusion of the left lung. C, Tomogram of the hilar region showing decreased vascular markings on the left.

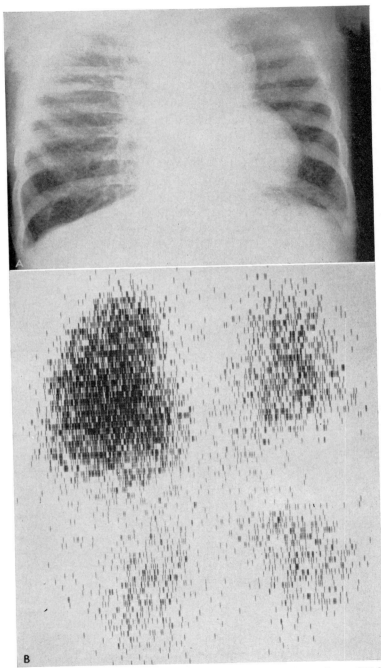

FIGURE 10-15.   A, Chest radiograph of a 2 year old girl with tetralogy of Fallot. B, Posterior lung scan indicating decreased activity on the left. The activity in the kidneys is the result of marked right-to-left shunting.

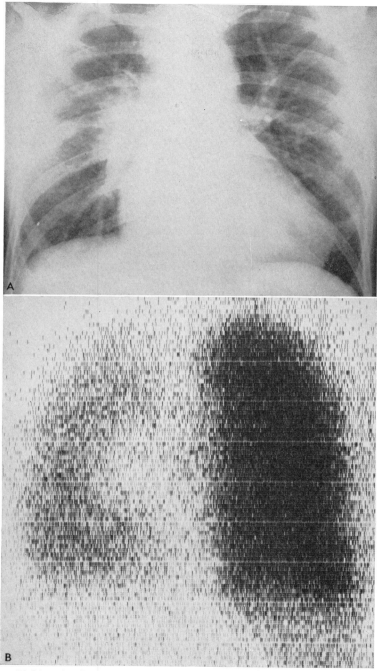

FIGURE 10-16.   A, Chest radiograph and B, lung scan of a patient with tetralogy of Fallot after right subclavian–pulmonary artery anastomosis. The decrease in activity in the right lung field is the result of perfusion of the right lung with systemic blood that does not contain particles. The study provides evidence of the patency of the Blalock-Taussig anastomosis.

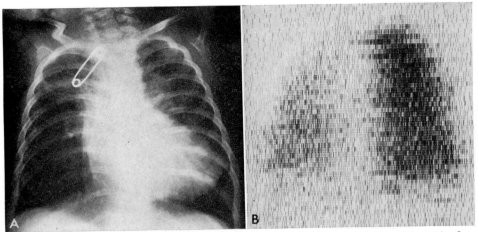

FIGURE 10-17.   *A,* Chest radiograph of an infant with a truncus arteriosus (Type I) whose right pulmonary artery was banded. *B,* Scan showing slight perfusion to the right lung.

An example of the use of the particle distribution technique in congenital heart disease is the evaluation of patients with tetralogy of Fallot who have undergone subclavian–pulmonary artery anastomoses. If pulmonary atresia is present, all of the intravenously injected particles reach the lungs by way of the anastomosis, and the distribution of particles in the lungs is no different after operation than before. On the other hand, if pulmonary atresia is not complete, most of the particles reach the lungs by way of the pulmonary artery. In such cases, no significant change occurs postoperatively if the anastomosis functions poorly or not at all. In patients in whom the anastomosis functions well, the lung of the same side as the anastomosis receives a *decreased* number of intravenously injected particles. Thus it is an indication of an unsatisfactory result if the number of particles reaching the lung on the side of the anastomosis is not decreased postoperatively. In some patients, this decrease may not occur until several months after operation. The improvement in the circulation to the side of the anastomosis can be readily demonstrated by injection of the radioactive particles into the aortic root (Friedman and Braunwald, unpublished). The shunt changes the distribution of blood entering the main pulmonary artery from the right ventricle, diverting most of the unsaturated systemic venous return to the lung on the side *opposite* the anastomosis.

Friedman and Braunwald (unpublished) have proposed that serial lung scans after intravenous injection of particles can be a simple means of evaluating the natural history of a palliative subclavian anastomosis. If the distribution of particles becomes more symmetrical after intravenous injection of particles, this is evidence that the anastomosis has become smaller or has closed completely.

Serial scans also permit estimation of the patency of superior vena cava–pulmonary anastomoses. If the shunt is working properly, particles injected into a vein of the upper arm will produce a scan of the lung on the same side as the anastomosis; the opposite lung will be visualized after injection into a lower extremity.

Another example of the use of lung scanning as a means of evaluating the pulmonary circulation in congenital heart disease is shown in Figure 10-17. This patient had a truncus arteriosus treated by banding of the right pulmonary artery, which resulted in markedly diminished perfusion of the right lung. Spleen and liver scanning may also be helpful in the preoperative evaluation of patients with congenital heart disease (Shah et al., 1964). As pointed out by Ivemark (1955), congenital abnormalities associated with splenic agenesis are usually of a severe truncus type that are not amenable to surgery. Splenic scanning is helpful in the diagnosis of these conditions.

OBSTRUCTIVE PULMONARY DISEASE

Although imbalance between ventilation and perfusion may occur and result in inefficient perfusion and deficient oxygenation of blood, the body is usually quite efficient in balancing changes in regional ventilation by adjustments in the regional pulmonary blood flow. Thus, regional decreases in blood flow will usually be found in bronchial and alveolar diseases as well as in primary disorders of the pulmonary circulation. Bronchial obstruction often produces demonstrable perfusion abnormalities that are detectable by the particle distribution method. In such cases, the defect can be further characterized by the study of regional ventilation with radioactive xenon.

The consequences of bronchial obstruction depend upon (1) the *type* of obstruction—whether it is intrabronchial, extrabronchial, or a combination of the two; (2) the *extent* of the obstruction—whether it affects one or more bronchi; (3) the *degree* of obstruction—whether it is partial or complete, or whether there is a ball-valve type of lesion; (4) the *frequency* of obstruction—whether it is temporary, repetitive, or permanent; and (5) any *complications* of the obstruction. Table 10-2 outlines some types of bronchial obstruction. Tenacious se-

TABLE 10-2. TYPES OF BRONCHIAL OBSTRUCTION*

A. *Intrabronchial obstruction*
  1. Endogenous: bronchitis, tracheobronchitis, bronchiolitis, postoperative atelectasis
  2. Exogenous: foreign bodies
B. *Endobronchial obstruction*
  1. Congenital anomalies (maldevelopments, duplications, constrictions, and evaginations)
  2. Nonspecific inflammations: bronchostenosis in asthmatics, cicatrices following the healing of ulcers or chemical burns, bronchiectasis
  3. Specific inflammation: tuberculosis, mycoses, sarcoidosis
  4. Bronchogenic neoplasms: benign and malignant
  5. Distortion of bronchial lumen: as a result of pulmonary, vertebral, or intrathoracic dislocations of viscera; in association with pneumothorax, thoracoplasty, and other thoracic surgical procedures
C. *Obstruction of extrabronchial origin*
  1. Enlarged lymph nodes of inflammatory or neoplastic origin
  2. Mediastinal suppuration, emphysema, neoplasm, or cysts
  3. Neoplasms of the lungs or esophagus; intrathoracic goiters
  4. Cardiovascular diseases: dilatation of an atrium, aneurysms of the aorta or pulmonary artery, anomalous vascular constriction
  5. Foreign bodies in the esophagus
D. *Combined forms*
  1. Tuberculous and neoplastic lymph nodes
  2. Broncholithiasis

* Modified from Rubin and Rubin, 1961.

cretions, foreign bodies, and bronchial carcinoma are common causes of intrabronchial obstruction. Extrabronchial disease may produce obstruction from extrinsic pressure or invasion of a bronchus.

Chronic Bronchitis and Bronchial Asthma

Chronic bronchitis has been defined as a disease of the lungs characterized by recurrent productive cough of indeterminate cause, occurring without impairment of ventilation or recurrent chest disease (Rubin and Rubin, 1961). If the patient has recognizable elements of an allergic disease accompanying bronchitis, the term "asthmatic bronchitis" is often used, particularly if the patient has symptom-free periods. Asthmatic bronchitis is believed to occur in susceptible persons as the result of sequential sensitization of the tracheobronchial mucosa to one or more specific antigens. Subsequent exposure to the antigen is believed to result in the release of pharmacologically active substances, such as histamine, which affect the mucous glands and smooth muscles of the bronchi and pulmonary blood vessels (Middleton, 1965). In many patients, a clear-cut connection with exposure to specific antigen is not found, and then the term "intrinsic" asthma is often used. Bronchial narrowing, accumulation of secretions, and swelling of the respiratory mucosa result in the characteristic clinical picture of severe expiratory wheezing with cough.

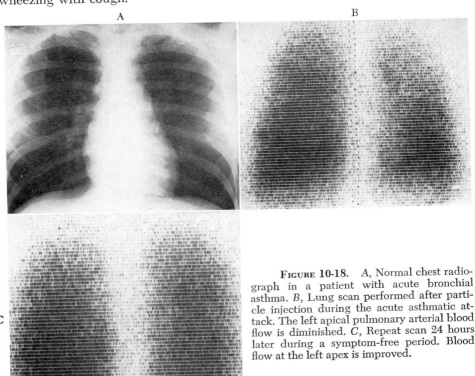

FIGURE 10-18. A, Normal chest radiograph in a patient with acute bronchial asthma. B, Lung scan performed after particle injection during the acute asthmatic attack. The left apical pulmonary arterial blood flow is diminished. C, Repeat scan 24 hours later during a symptom-free period. Blood flow at the left apex is improved.

Bentivoglio and his associates (1963a) used the xenon-133 method to study patients with acute asthma, and found regional defects in *ventilation* even when the patients were free of symptoms between acute asthmatic attacks. The 6 patients (out of 12) in whom the regional defects were noted had a significantly greater degree of impairment of forced expiratory volume (FEV_1), maximum midexpiratory flow rate (MMFR), and helium mixing efficiency than did the 6 who did not show the regional ventilatory abnormalities. The investigators did not find regional *perfusion* defects in these patients between acute attacks.

In most of their patients studied during acute attacks of asthma, Mishkin and Wagner (1967) found regional defects in pulmonary arterial blood flow. An example is shown in Figure 10-18. The study of asthmatic patients during acute attacks illustrates an important advantage of pulmonary scans. The particles are simply injected during an acute episode. Immediately thereafter, the patient can be treated; and after his symptoms have been relieved, the distribution of the previously injected particles can be determined. Between asthmatic attacks, the patients' scans usually appeared normal. Focal defects were found during acute attacks, but often they were found in different regions during different attacks. This suggested that the changes found were the result of temporary structural alterations, such as mucous plugs, or of physiological redistribution of blood flow.

EMPHYSEMA

Chronic obstructive pulmonary emphysema is a pathological condition characterized by abnormal enlargement of the respiratory air spaces and by destructive changes in the alveolar walls. It can occur alone or in association with other diseases. The lungs appear large, pale, and less vascular, and they often have superficial blebs. When the function of the lungs is examined, the findings include increased resistance to air flow, imbalance between ventilation and perfusion, and reduced diffusing capacity.

The disease is most commonly found in males between the ages of 50 and 70 years, usually in heavy smokers. It is the most rapidly increasing cause of death in the United States. In 1963, death records indicate that it was the underlying cause of death in about 20,000 persons and contributed to the death of 40,000 others. According to estimates by the U.S. Public Health Service, not less than 10 per cent of middle-aged and elderly Americans suffer from this disease. The physician should suspect emphysema in any patient in this age category who is found to have had several respiratory infections over a period of a few years, accompanied by a persistent heavy cough. If treated early, many cases could probably be arrested by proper preventive and therapeutic means, but most escape detection until it is too late. The most commonly used screening procedures are questionnaires, chest x-rays, and measurement of the maximum breathing capacity, which is often less than 50 per cent of normal values.

The characteristic x-ray findings in emphysema are enlargement of the lungs and increased radiolucency. The ribs are often found to be more nearly horizontal, and more widely separated, than normal. The diaphragm is often low and flattened, which gives the heart shadow a somewhat long and narrow appearance. In the advanced stages of the disease, the heart begins to enlarge (particularly

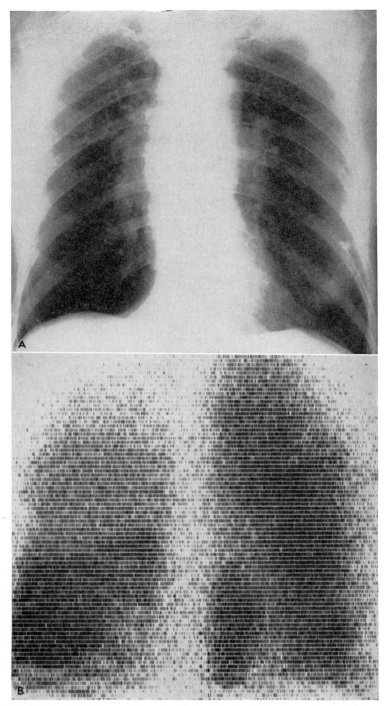

FIGURE 10-19.   A, Chest radiograph of a patient with pulmonary emphysema. B, Lung scan showing long lungs with focal areas of diminished perfusion, most marked in the right upper lung.

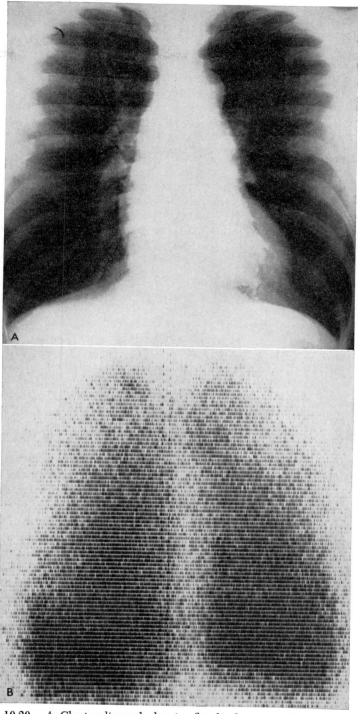

FIGURE 10-20. A, Chest radiograph showing flat diaphragms and horizontal ribs suggesting the diagnosis of emphysema. B, Lung scan showing decreased perfusion at both apices.

the right ventricle) and the pulmonary arteries become more prominent. Fluoro-scopic examination of the lungs can be helpful in making the diagnosis, since in emphysema the lungs may not deflate normally during expiration, and the diaphragm is relatively immobile or may even move upward paradoxically during inspiration. After rapid expiration, areas of focal radiolucency may be observed as a result of trapping of air in those regions.

Some physicians believe that a diagnosis of emphysema can never be made with certainty in a living person unless there are vascular alterations, such as attenuation or disappearance of the normal pulmonary vasculature. Tomography, particularly hilar tomography, may be helpful (Dulfano and DiRienzo, 1962). Bentivoglio and his co-workers (1963b, 1965) found a good correlation between tomography and the regional distribution of pulmonary arterial blood flow as measured with ^{133}Xe. However, the value of tomography is limited by the fact that the smaller blood vessels cannot be seen, and the disease most often affects the arterioles and capillaries. Ball and his associates (1962), using ^{133}Xe, found focal abnormalities of both ventilation and perfusion in patients with emphysema. Delineation of these areas may be of practical value in indicating those patients in whom total lung function might be improved by surgery. Lopez-Majano et al. (1966) used lung scans to study 62 patients with severe pulmonary emphysema, and they confirmed the high incidence of perfusion abnormalities.

The lung scan is particularly useful because its simplicity makes it readily applicable to large numbers of patients. Figures 10-19 and 10-20 show two patients with moderate and far-advanced emphysema, respectively. In the first patient the disease was predominantly in one lung; in the second, a patchy in-volvement of both lungs was apparent.

BRONCHIECTASIS

Bronchiectasis is frequently focal, and areas of decreased perfusion can be seen in the lung scan. For unknown reasons, bronchiectasis affects the left lung more often than the right; this may in some way be related to the encroachment upon the left lower lobe by an enlarging heart. Since hemoptysis from an unknown site is often the presenting complaint in patients with focal bronchiectasis, it is pos-sible that abnormalities may be found in the lung scan even before they are seen on the radiograph. The most specific examination for bronchiectasis is, of course, bronchography with radiopaque contrast media.

PULMONARY INFECTIONS

In the early diagnosis of pulmonary infections, such as pneumonia or tuberculosis, the sensitivity of lung scanning as compared to chest radiography has not yet been determined. It is clear, however, that pulmonary infections associated with radiographic opacifications lead to decreases in concentration of intravenously injected particles. In most cases, the area of decreased radio-

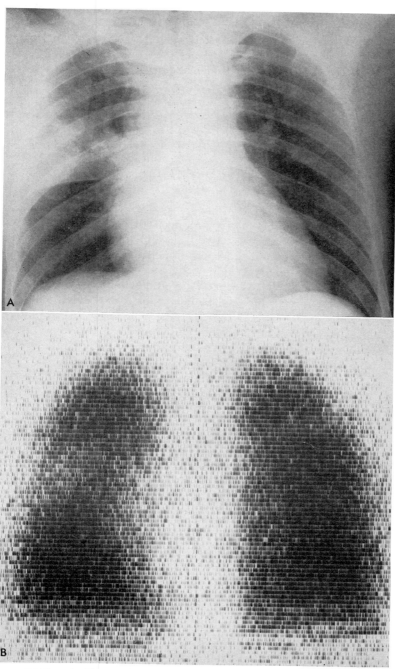

FIGURE 10-21.   A, Chest radiograph of patient with pneumonia in right midlung field.
B, Lung scan showing decreased perfusion of the involved area.

activity is larger than would be suspected from the lesion of the chest radiograph (Lopez-Majano et al., 1965). Figure 10-21 is the scan and chest radiograph of a patient with pneumococcal pneumonia. The diminished radioactivity corresponds to the infiltrate in the radiograph. This does not necessarily indicate a decrease in total perfusion of this region, since it is likely that the bronchial circulation is adequate or even increased. In the absence of a right-to-left shunt, none of the particles reach the lungs via the bronchial circulation after an intravenous injection. The regional decrease in pulmonary arterial blood flow in pulmonary infections is perhaps the result of interstitial or alveolar exudation, or of compression of the pulmonary capillary or arteriolar bed. Tissue necrosis and scarring can also be a cause of decreased regional blood flow.

Pulmonary Tuberculosis

Chronic pulmonary tuberculosis produces an obliterative endarteritis, not only in the immediate vicinity of active disease, but also in areas of scar tissue, interstitial fibrosis, and bronchial and peribronchial fibrosis (Estrada et al., 1956). Although early lesions, miliary tuberculosis, and exudative lesions do not affect the larger pulmonary vessels, arteriographic studies indicate that the pulmonary circulation is nearly always reduced in the presence of cavitation.

In lung scans of 67 patients with chronic pulmonary tuberculosis (Lopez-Majano et al., 1965), the most significant finding was a decrease in the pulmonary arterial blood flow to the diseased areas, which were usually larger than had been expected from the size of the lesion in the chest radiograph. Thus, the scans were of value in delineating the extent or severity of disease. Figure 10-22 compares the lung scan and chest radiograph of a patient with apical pulmonary tuberculosis.

Cancer of the Lung

Cancer of the lung is the most common form of malignancy in the American male and is increasing in frequency more rapidly than any other malignancy. The ratio of involvement of males to females is about five to one, perhaps reflecting the fact that females have only recently begun to smoke as heavily as males. The tumors are squamous cell carcinomas in about 50 per cent of the cases; adenocarcinoma in 15 to 20 per cent; anaplastic or undifferentiated tumors in about 20 per cent; and mixed patterns in about 10 per cent.

Only 5 patients of every 100 with lung cancer live 5 years after diagnosis, and most deaths occur within the first 2 years. A major challenge of modern medicine is to improve these results by earlier diagnosis. High incidence rates are to be expected among the following: older men, very heavy smokers, persons with respiratory symptoms, and those with x-ray abnormalities (whether or not the abnormalities seem suggestive of neoplasm).

Screening of such patients should include: (1) a thorough general history; (2) a careful history regarding respiratory disease, with special attention to

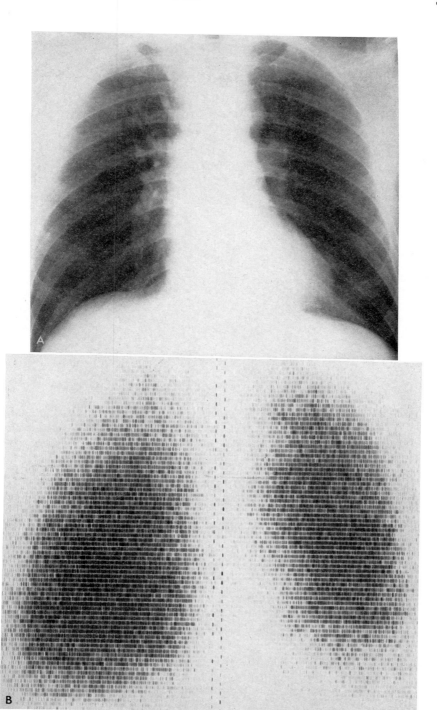

FIGURE 10-22. *A*, Chest radiograph in a patient with active tuberculosis. *B*, Lung scan with diminished perfusion of the right apex. Scanning is helpful in the early diagnosis of pulmonary tuberculosis.

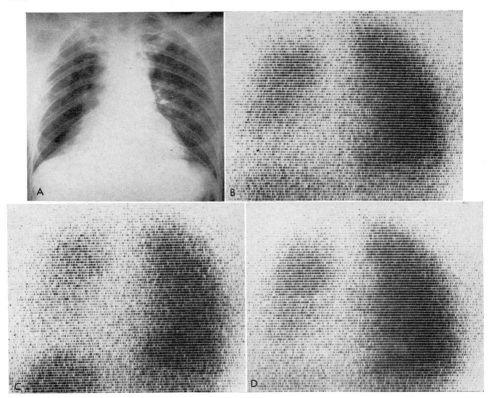

FIGURE 10-23. *A,* Chest radiograph of a patient with hemoptysis initially thought to have pulmonary embolism. *B, C,* and *D,* The lack of improvement, as shown by serial scans, led to questioning of the original diagnosis. Bronchoscopy and biopsy revealed bronchogenic carcinoma. Changing pattern of avascularity is characteristic of pulmonary embolism.

signs and symptoms of dyspnea, blood-streaked sputum, cough, unilateral wheeze, chest discomfort, smoking, and the chronology of symptoms and roentgenographic abnormalities; (3) a thorough general physical examination; and (4) radiographic screening.

According to Boucot et al. (1964) most older men who develop lung cancer have symptoms even before the first x-ray evidence of lung tumor. They found *dyspnea* to be the most frequent symptom. *Chronic cough* was also common and was related to the type, amount, and duration of smoking.

Lung cancer seldom arises spontaneously in healthy lungs. In 45 patients in whom new lung cancers developed, there were only three in whom the first x-ray evidence of malignancy was not preceded by either scarred lungs or respiratory symptoms.

The use of lung scanning in the early diagnosis of bronchogenic carcinoma was first reported by Wagner et al. (1965b), who found that avascular areas in the lung scan were far larger than the radiograph abnormalities. In a few patients the scans were markedly abnormal in patients with unexplained hemoptysis and positive cytology at a time when the radiograph was entirely within normal limits. Characteristically, the vascular defects in carcinoma of the lung did not change significantly for periods up to a month or more. This helps in distinguishing these abnormalities from the changing defects characteristic of pulmonary embolism. The persistence of the defect in the scanning image of the patient with a bronchogenic carcinoma (Fig. 10-23) suggested the possibility that the defect might be a tumor, rather than an embolus as had been suspected clinically.

PULMONARY EMBOLISM

Massive pulmonary embolism was the first disease in which the value of lung scanning was demonstrated (Wagner et al., 1964). The diagnosis of this disease is often difficult and uncertain, primarily because the symptoms and signs may mimic those of other diseases, such as myocardial infarction or pneumonia. Ancillary examinations, including x-ray study of the chest and electrocardiography, are rarely definitive. The diagnosis can be suspected when sudden dyspnea, tachycardia, pleural pain, hemoptysis, syncope, or a bloody pleural effusion occur in patients who are predisposed to pulmonary embolism— that is, those who are suffering from congestive heart failure or polycythemia, or who are bedridden during the postoperative or postpartum state.

Pulmonary embolism is the most common of the serious disorders affecting the pulmonary circulation. When therapeutic measures were relatively non-specific, absolute accuracy in diagnosis was not necessary. Today, however, the need for improved diagnostic ability has increased because new means of treating pulmonary thromboembolism are available. These include: *anticoagulant drugs* to prevent further thrombosis; *proteolytic agents* to dissolve thrombi that have already formed; and specific *surgical therapy,* including ligation or plication of the inferior vena cava (to prevent passage of peripheral thrombi into the lungs) and pulmonary embolectomy (to remove obstructing clots from the pulmonary arteries themselves).

Despite our knowledge of certain predisposing factors, such as prolonged bed rest and mechanical obstruction of the venous return from the legs, the incidence of pulmonary embolism remains about the same—possibly because of an increasing life span, increasing numbers of surgical procedures, and increasing numbers of chronically ill people. Evidence of pulmonary embolism was found in postmortem study of more than half of adult patients who died from all causes (Freiman et al., 1965). In many patients the diagnosis of fatal pulmonary embolism was made for the first time at necropsy. The difficulty in establishing a firm clinical diagnosis is explained by the fact that the signs and symptoms of pulmonary embolism often resemble those of other serious cardiorespiratory diseases.

Pathophysiology of Pulmonary Embolism

Patients with pulmonary embolism can be classified into two groups: those with pulmonary hypertension after repeated embolic episodes, and those with acute massive pulmonary embolism, the result of large emboli occluding one or both of the major pulmonary arteries.

An early sign in experimental massive pulmonary embolism is elevation of pulmonary arterial pressure. Sixty to eighty per cent of the pulmonary vascular bed must be occluded before the circulation is seriously impaired (Dexter and Smith, 1964). Thus, either the right or left main pulmonary artery can be ligated without serious hemodynamic consequences. However, this is usually done under general anesthesia, in which some of the reflex changes of a conscious patient might not occur.

It is not certain whether the elevation of pulmonary arterial pressure is entirely from mechanical obstruction or partly from reflex changes. There is evidence that afferent fibers from the pulmonary vessels produce constriction of the pulmonary arterioles when there is sudden occlusion of a vessel. Injection of particles into one lobe of the lung in dogs usually leads to elevation of pulmonary arterial pressure (Haynes et al., 1947). Some of these experiments have been criticized on the grounds that even though the particles were injected into one lobe of the lung, some particles refluxed into other areas of the lung (Daley et al., 1951). But, even when this is specifically prevented, there is evidence that reflex changes produce pulmonary vasoconstriction (Aramendia et al., 1963).

Systemic hypotension with pulmonary embolism results from two mechanisms: reflexes between the pulmonary and the systemic circulation; and, in the case of severe pulmonary embolism, decreased cardiac output with a secondary fall in systemic arterial pressure.

In both experimental animals and human patients, there is right heart failure only in extensive obstruction. Such failure is caused by the increased work required of the right ventricle in pumping blood against the high pulmonary arterial pressure, by decreased myocardial oxygenation, and by impairment of the general circulation (Sasahara et al., 1965). There is good experimental and clinical evidence that tachypnea is a sensitive sign of embolism, particularly of miliary embolism. The tachypnea is almost certainly of reflex origin, and it is helpful in distinguishing conditions such as acute myocardial infarction from pulmonary embolism. Severe hyperpnea and dyspnea occur only if the pulmonary embolism is massive, leading to right ventricular failure. Tachycardia is frequently present. Bronchoconstriction can occur in pulmonary arterial obstruction, and though serotonin has been implicated, the exact mechanism remains uncertain (Boyer and Curry, 1944; Gurewich et al., 1963, 1965; Webster et al., 1966). Pathological studies point out the importance of mechanical factors in massive pulmonary embolism. In a postmortem study of 100 consecutive patients with massive pulmonary embolism, Gorham (1961) found that 85 had occlusion of one pulmonary artery and, in addition, involvement of the opposite lung. Only 15 patients had emboli restricted solely to one lung, and 12 of the 15 had severe underlying cardiac and respiratory disease.

Thus, pathophysiological studies suggest that most of the clinical manifestations of massive pulmonary embolism result from occlusion of the larger pulmonary arteries (Hyman et al., 1964). Although there is evidence that arteriolar obstruction may lead to reflex vasoconstriction (Hyland et al., 1963) and pulmonary hypertension, when acute right heart failure and systemic hypotension occur, the lung scan will usually indicate obstruction of the large pulmonary arteries.

CLINICAL AND LABORATORY SIGNS OF PULMONARY EMBOLISM

In 1933, White and Brenner described the consequences of pulmonary embolism—tachycardia, accentuation of the second pulmonic sound, dilatation of the cervical veins, and an enlarged and pulsating liver. The triad of sudden chest pain, dyspnea, and hemoptysis is rare in massive embolism and is more often seen with pulmonary infarction. Chest pain results from involvement of the parietal pleura; the pulmonary vessels do not contain pain receptors. Obstruction of the larger pulmonary arteries rarely leads to infarction, presumably because collateral vessels permit adequate oxygenation of the lung tissue. However, emboli that are more peripheral, particularly when they are associated with an impaired systemic circulation, often lead to infarction of the affected regions. Infarction is particularly likely to occur in patients with congestive heart failure or shock.

In massive embolism, the chest radiograph may show, on the side of the pulmonary artery obstruction, diminished vascular markings, a sign first described in 1938 by Westermark and later by Torrance (1959). Despite its usefulness, this sign is not reliable enough to serve as definitive evidence of embolism. Interest has recently focused upon the change in size of the pulmonary artery radiographically in pulmonary embolism, and Chang and Davis (1965) have found abnormal dilatation in all patients with pulmonary infarction and in patients with fatal pulmonary embolism.

The electrocardiogram in pulmonary embolism is neither a sensitive nor a specific means of diagnosis (Littmann, 1965). Alterations may include disturbances of rhythm (atrial fibrillation, ectopic beats, heart block), enlargement of the P wave, ST segment depression, or T wave inversion (especially in leads III, aVF, V_1, V_4, and V_5). The most common abnormality is ST segment depression, a result of accompanying myocardial ischemia (Wolff, 1959). Although frequently helpful, the electrocardiogram cannot be relied upon for a certain diagnosis of pulmonary embolism.

Changes in serum enzymes may be helpful in the diagnosis of pulmonary embolism. A triad consisting of an elevated serum lactic dehydrogenase (LDH) activity, an increased serum bilirubin concentration, and a normal serum glutamic oxaloacetic transaminase (SGOT) activity has been described (Wacker et al., 1961). However, in a recent series of patients with pulmonary embolic disease (Figure 10-24), only 18 per cent showed this triad. The more commonly en-

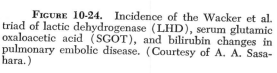

FIGURE 10-24.   Incidence of the Wacker et al. triad of lactic dehydrogenase (LHD), serum glutamic oxaloacetic acid (SGOT), and bilirubin changes in pulmonary embolic disease. (Courtesy of A. A. Sasahara.)

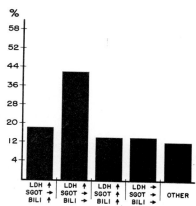

countered triad pattern (42 per cent) consisted of elevated LDH and normal SGOT and bilirubin. Approximately 25 per cent of patients can be expected to show no change in the LDH and SGOT activities (Sasahara et al., 1967). It was further shown that bilirubin elevation in patients with pulmonary embolism correlated best with the presence of right heart failure. Although the enzyme changes may be helpful, Sasahara (1964) has emphasized that in patients with massive embolism and acute cardiovascular changes, clinical urgency may require faster methods of diagnosis.

Pulmonary embolism alters the delicate balance between ventilation and perfusion of the lungs. Occlusion of a major pulmonary arterial branch decreases gaseous exchange in the corresponding segment of the lung, although alveolar ventilation continues (Robin et al., 1959, 1960). In a ventilated but underperfused segment of lung, the composition of the alveolar air tends to approach that of inspired air and has a low partial pressure of carbon dioxide. During expiration, this air is mixed with that from the normal areas of the lung, but the mean alveolar carbon dioxide tension is reduced to a degree that can be detected in the expired air. Arterial carbon dioxide tension remains at a nearly normal level because there are enough normal areas of lung. Measurement of the difference between the arterial and alveolar carbon dioxide tensions has therefore been proposed as an aid in the diagnosis of pulmonary embolism. Robin has emphasized, however, that a compensatory decrease of ventilation in the underperfused areas can occur, which tends to restore the balance of the ventilation-perfusion ratio. Therefore complete reliance cannot be placed in this method.

Table 10-3 lists some of the commonly encountered signs of massive embolism, and Table 10-4 lists some of the important laboratory tests. The major problems of pulmonary arteriography are its technical complexity and the complications that may occur in a critically ill patient. However, this test is specific because it permits visualization of the obstructed arteries themselves. For optimum structural detail, right heart catheterization is preferred to injection of contrast media in a peripheral vein. A characteristic finding in massive embolism is that the appearance of the vessels changes within a few days, because of clot retraction, thrombolysis, or other factors (Fred et al., 1965).

TABLE 10-3. INCIDENCE OF SIGNS OF PULMONARY EMBOLIC DISEASE[*]

Loud pulmonic second sound	95%
Tachypnea	90
Tachycardia	88
Fever	75
Intercostal tenderness	55
Râles	55
Pleural friction rub	45
Pleural effusion (bloody)	30
Gallop rhythm	15
Cyanosis	15
Bronchospasm	?

* Adapted from Dexter et al., 1960, and Gorham, 1961.

TABLE 10-4. LABORATORY FINDINGS IN PULMONARY EMBOLIC DISEASE

A. Leukocytosis (10,000–15,000)
B. Normoblasts in peripheral blood smear
C. Increased serum lactic dehydrogenase (LDH)
D. Increased serum bilirubin
E. Normal serum glutamic oxaloacetic acid transaminase (SGOT)
F. Electrocardiogram abnormalities
    1. Arrhythmias
    2. S wave in lead I; Q wave in lead III; T wave in lead III
    3. T wave inversion $V_1 - V_3$
    4. Clockwise rotation
    5. ST depression
    6. Transient right bundle branch block
    7. Large P waves
G. Roentgenography
    1. Chest x-ray
        a. Elevation of diaphragm on affected side
        b. Pleural effusion
        c. Hemispherical consolidation along pleural surface (Hampton's hump)
        d. Engorgement of pulmonary vessels ⎫
        e. Dilatation of RA and RV   ⎬cor pulmonale
        f. "Oligemic lung" (Westermark-Torrance sign) ⎭
    2. Pulmonary angiography
H. Lung scanning
    1. Avascular areas without corresponding infiltrates on radiograph
    2. Concave lesions at periphery of lung
    3. Changing patterns of decreased blood flow

LUNG SCANS IN PULMONARY EMBOLISM

Lung scanning is a simple and effective procedure for the diagnosis of pulmonary embolism. Although it is not sufficiently specific by itself, when the proper question is asked it provides the right answer. Lung scanning indicates the regional distribution of pulmonary arterial blood flow. It clearly delineates areas where pulmonary arterial blood flow is impaired—a universal finding in massive pulmonary embolism. However, if pulmonary arterial blood flow is reduced generally, as in multiple small embolism or in acute pulmonary edema, pulmonary blood flow will retain an essentially normal distribution. An advantage of the scanning procedure is that, because of its safety and simplicity, it can be performed readily and repeatedly. It can also provide information that cannot be obtained by other means, such as the determination of the rate of return of blood flow to affected areas—either with or without therapy.

It is true that many other diseases besides pulmonary embolism result in regional decreases in pulmonary arterial blood flow. A lung scan does not have the specificity of arteriography, which often shows encroachment of an embolus upon a pulmonary artery, but the scan does provide information concerning the perfusion of the pulmonary capillary bed. Thus, lung scanning and pulmonary arteriography should always be considered as complementary rather than competitive procedures.

At times, the lung scan can be relatively specific for pulmonary embolism, if the findings meet certain criteria. First, we look for large areas of greatly dimin-

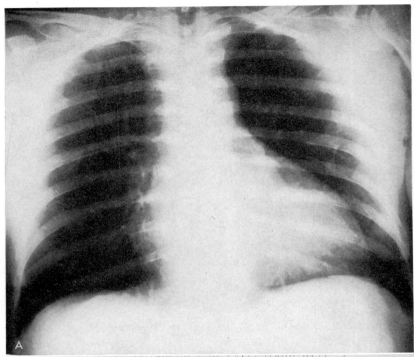

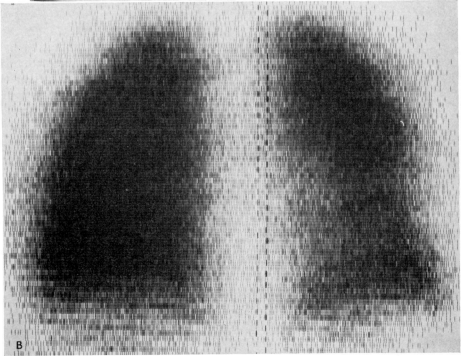

FIGURE 10-25.   A, Normal chest radiograph in a patient with classic clinical signs of pulmonary embolism. B, Characteristic concave (crescent) deformity along the left lateral border.

ished pulmonary arterial blood flow in regions that do not appear affected in the chest radiograph. This is particularly helpful because pneumonia and other infiltrative lesions that have been found to be associated with a decrease in pulmonary arterial blood flow can usually be seen in the radiograph. If the scan shows the characteristic pattern of avascularity, one can usually be certain of the diagnosis. However, if the avascular areas correspond to opacities on the chest x-ray, one cannot distinguish between primary vascular disease and secondary involvement of the pulmonary vasculature. Particularly troublesome lesions are lung cysts and bullae, which may appear as areas of increased radiolucency in a manner similar to pulmonary emboli.

We also look for concave defects at the lateral borders of the scan. These characteristic defects correspond to the hemispherical lesions found at the lung periphery on postmortem examination (Hampton and Castleman, 1940); presumably they represent areas in which the collateral circulation is inadequate (Fig. 10-25). Since large areas of the lung must be compromised before pulmonary hypertension and right ventricular failure result, we look for large defects on the scan before we attribute severe systemic hypotension to massive embolism. The scan is often helpful in ruling out massive embolism in a pa-

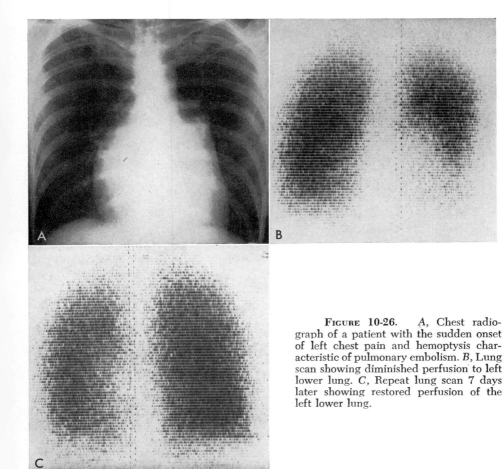

FIGURE 10-26. *A*, Chest radiograph of a patient with the sudden onset of left chest pain and hemoptysis characteristic of pulmonary embolism. *B*, Lung scan showing diminished perfusion to left lower lung. *C*, Repeat lung scan 7 days later showing restored perfusion of the left lower lung.

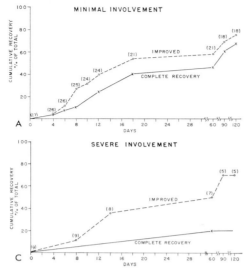

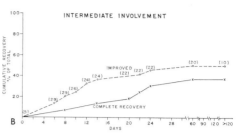

FIGURE 10-27. Rate of recovery of patients with acute pulmonary embolism. *A, Minimal Involvement* (less than 15 per cent of lung involved). Nearly 50 per cent of patients had marked improvement within 18 days. About 40 per cent had complete recovery as indicated by a return to a completely normal lung scan. The numbers in parentheses refer to the number of patients. *B, Intermediate Involvement* (greater than 15 per cent and less than 30 per cent lung involvement). *C, Severe Involvement* (greater than 30 per cent lung involvement).

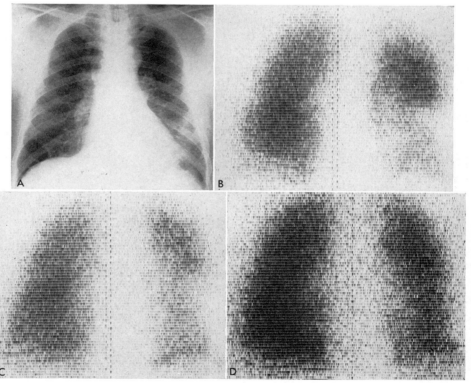

FIGURE 10-28. *A,* Chest radiograph of a patient with pulmonary embolism. Infiltrate in left lower lung field. *B,* Initial lung scan with decreased perfusion, most marked in left lower lung. *C,* Scan after 17 hours of parenteral heparin administration. *D,* Lung scan immediately following 6 hour urokinase infusion. Considerable improvement can be seen.

tient who develops hypotension following surgery or delivery. If the scan is normal, we look elsewhere for the cause of the hypotension.

Figure 10-26 shows serial lung scans in a patient with pulmonary embolism. The changing pattern of defects is characteristic of pulmonary embolism and is a helpful sign in distinguishing embolism from emphysema, carcinoma of the lung, and other lung diseases.

Tow and Wagner have used lung scanning to determine the rate of return of blood flow in embolism. The results are shown in Figure 10-27. One of the major contributions of lung scanning has been in documenting the fact that blood flow often returns spontaneously to affected areas in patients with massive embolism. This finding makes necessary carefully controlled evaluation of therapeutic agents. Figure 10-28 illustrates serial scans from a patient with multiple pulmonary emboli who received a 6 hour infusion of urokinase (a fibrinolytic agent) in an effort to restore blood flow to the involved areas (Tow et al., 1964). In contrast to the results in untreated patients, a scan repeated 24 hours later indicated that considerable restoration of local blood flow had occurred. Similar results have been observed in other patients.

PULMONARY HYPERTENSION

Although pulmonary artery pressure is usually below 30/15 mm. Hg, the clinical picture of pulmonary hypertension often does not develop until the pressure exceeds 50/25 (Wood, 1959). Pressures above 50/25 can occur if cardiac output increases to more than 15 liters per minute, or if there is a reduction of the size of the pulmonary vascular bed, or through a loss of elasticity of the

TABLE 10-5. CLASSIFICATION OF PULMONARY HYPERTENSION*

A. *Increased blood flow in the pulmonary artery*
  1. Heart disease with left-to-right shunt (with or without transmission of the systemic blood pressure)
  2. Postpneumonectomy states
  3. Congenital absence of one of the main branches of the pulmonary artery
B. *Increased pulmonary vascular resistance (organic, functional, or both)*
  1. Postcapillary area
     a. Left atrium
     b. Pulmonary veins
  2. Capillary and precapillary area
     Parenchymatous and interstitial diseases of the lung (emphysema, fibrosis, and granulomatosis)
  3. Arterial and precapillary area
     Vascular diseases of the lung (thromboembolism, arteritis, and primary pulmonary hypertension)
  4. Arterial area
     Stenosis or compression of the pulmonary artery
  5. Combined
     Extrinsic diseases of the lung (pulmonary compression; restriction of the thoracic movements)

* Adapted from Galland, 1961.

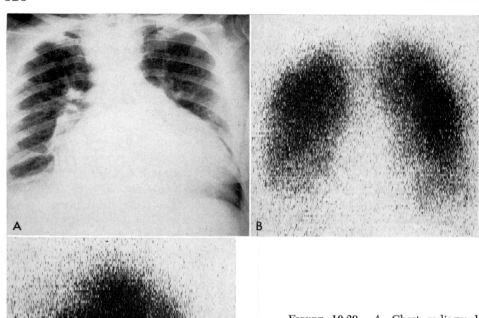

FIGURE 10-29. *A*, Chest radiograph of a patient with rheumatic heart disease and mitral stenosis and insufficiency. *B*, Lung scan showing reversal of flow (greater in the upper than lower lung field) characteristic of pulmonary venous hypertension. *C*, Left lateral lung scan showing large cardiac indentation and reversal of flow.

vessels. On this same pathophysiological basis, Galland (1961) classified pulmonary hypertension in further detail (Table 10-5).

In pathological conditions, such as severe mitral stenosis and left ventricular failure, when the pulmonary venous pressure is raised, there is a reversal of the normal distribution of flow when the patient is erect. In normal persons in the erect position, the blood flow per gram of lung is less in the apex than in the base (West, 1965). In severe pulmonary hypertension, this is reversed and a distinct pattern of distribution of flow is found associated with advanced mitral valve disease. This was confirmed by Dollery and West (1960) using radioactive oxygen, carbon dioxide, and carbon monoxide and later by Dawson et al. (1965) with the ^{133}Xe method.

Friedman and Braunwald (1966) studied the alterations in regional pulmonary blood flow in mitral valve disease with the particle distribution technique. When left-to-right shunting was present in patients with pulmonary hypertension, the ratio of radioactivity in the upper zones of the lung to that in the lower zones was significantly higher than when pulmonary arterial pressure was normal. This was also true in patients with primary pulmonary hypertension.

Pulmonary *venous* hypertension not only increased the blood flow to the apices of the lung, but also caused a decrease in perfusion to the lung bases. This produced a clear-cut pattern in the scanning image (Fig. 10-29) in which the radioactivity in the apices was clearly greater than that in the bases, even when the patients were injected while in an upright position. The upper:lower zone ratios correlated best with mean left atrial pressure when compared to other hemodynamic parameters.

In patients with mitral valve disease the results were different from those in patients with elevated pulmonary arterial pressure but normal left atrial pressures. Above a mean pulmonary arterial pressure of 30 mm. Hg, the upper:lower ratios were significantly higher in patients with elevated pulmonary *venous* pressure than in those with pulmonary *arterial* hypertension alone. The upper: lower ratio never exceeded one in the absence of pulmonary venous hypertension, regardless of the pulmonary arterial pressure. The lung scan alone was able to show whether pulmonary venous pressure was elevated in patients with known severe pulmonary arterial hypertension.

Friedman and Braunwald have summarized the role of scanning in the management of patients with heart disease as follows: In patients with mitral valve disease, the close correlation with the upper:lower ratio and the mean left atrial pressure indicates that it is possible to predict the latter within rea-

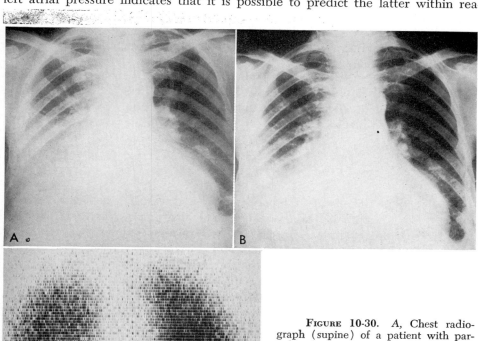

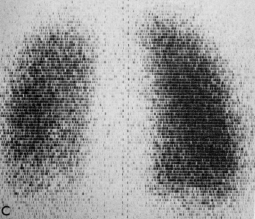

FIGURE 10-30. *A,* Chest radiograph (supine) of a patient with partial right lung opacification secondary to the pleural effusion. *B,* Upright chest radiograph showing shift of effusion in the right lower lung field. *C,* Lung scan showing decreased perfusion of the entire right lung.

sonable limits. The method is particularly useful in the screening of patients with the clinical findings of mitral valve disease whose symptoms are not severe enough to warrant cardiac catheterization. Lung scanning is also useful in the preoperative study of patients so ill that left heart catheterization would be unusually hazardous. The method can show whether pulmonary venous pressure is elevated in patients with known severe pulmonary arterial hypertension. In these patients, it is often difficult to measure pulmonary arterial wedge pressure reliably and the more extensive manipulations necessary for left heart catheterization may be poorly tolerated. Assessment of the distribution of pulmonary arterial blood flow by scanning affords a means of determining the existence of pulmonary venous hypertension, which may lead to the diagnosis of potentially correctable lesions such as mitral stenosis or cor triatriatum.

DISEASES OF THE PLEURA

Nonpurulent effusions are classified as transudates or exudates, according to their protein content (less or greater than 3 g. per 100 ml). In many instances, lesions of the pleura originate from diseases of underlying structures. The effect of pleural effusion on the distribution of pulmonary arterial blood flow as seen in the lung scan has recently been studied by Tow and others (unpublished), who observed a diminished blood flow to the involved lung in cases of large pleural effusions. They concluded from their studies that the diminished perfusion was probably the result of hilar pulmonary artery compression by the accumulated free fluid in the paravertebral gutter. Figure 10-30 shows the chest radiographs and lung scans in the supine and upright positions of a patient with a large pleural effusion.

OTHER DISEASES

Included in this group are pneumothorax; disease entities with "alveolar capillary block"; diffusion abnormalities, including sarcoidosis and interstitial pulmonary fibrosis (Hamman-Rich syndrome); pneumoconioses such as silicosis, asbestosis, and berylliosis; connective tissue diseases (dyscollagenoses); and diseases of the mediastinum and diaphragm, including injuries of the heart and great vessels. In all these conditions lung scanning has been used infrequently, and its exact role has not yet been defined.

TABLE 10-6. RESEARCH APPLICATIONS OF PULMONARY SCANNING

A. Effect of parenchymal diseases on pulmonary circulation
B. Effect of posture, exercise, hypoxia, etc., on pulmonary circulation
C. Effect of abnormal gravitational forces on the pulmonary circulation
D. Effect of drugs on the pulmonary circulation
E. Natural history of pulmonary embolism in man and experimental animals
F. Evaluation of therapy of pulmonary embolism, e.g., fibrinolytic agents and anticoagulant drugs

PATHOPHYSIOLOGICAL STUDIES

Table 10-6 lists some of the research applications of lung scanning.

PULMONARY ARTERIAL BLOOD FLOW IN PARENCHYMAL DISEASE OF THE LUNG

In studies of thousands of patients with a variety of pulmonary disorders—including tuberculosis, carcinoma, pneumonia, lung abscess, sarcoidosis, bullous emphysema, and atelectasis—a consistent finding was absent or decreased pulmonary arterial blood flow to the diseased area. The exact mechanism of the decreased blood flow in these diseases remains conjectural. In certain cases there is mechanical obstruction of the blood vessels, and in others, obliteration of the lung tissue itself. At times the decreased vascularity may result from physiological shifts in the distribution of blood flow. Redistribution of pulmonary arterial blood flow has been shown to result from regional hypoxia or changes in posture (Wagner et al., 1966).

EFFECT OF REGIONAL ALVEOLAR HYPOXIA ON PULMONARY BLOOD FLOW

The idea that respiratory gases themselves affect pulmonary vascular resistance and local blood flow has been one of the most fruitful hypotheses concerning the control of the pulmonary circulation (Riley and Cournand, 1949). Von Euler and Liljestrand (1946) first proposed that the partial pressure of respiratory gases in the alveoli and in capillary blood regulates the regional vascular resistance in such a way that an optimum relationship is maintained between ventilation and perfusion. Himmelstein et al. (1958) administered 5 per cent oxygen to one lung in five normal persons and found a reduction in the fraction of the blood perfusing the hypoxic lung in three. In the fourth, the results were inconclusive, and in the fifth, pulmonary hypertension developed with no change in the partition of flow. Using the scanning technique, we have been able to demonstrate that reproducible decreases in regional blood flow follow local hypoxia. The experimental design is illustrated in Figure 10-31. The administration of 100 per cent nitrogen for 7 minutes to one lung resulted in an average decrease of 42 per cent in the blood flow to the hypoxic lung; when given for 2 minutes, the average decrease was 16 per cent. Local hypercapnia had a smaller, but similar, effect.

EFFECT OF POSTURE AND GRAVITY ON PULMONARY ARTERIAL BLOOD FLOW

In a series of normal persons, the distribution of labeled particles was determined by scanning after the injection had been made with the patient seated. These were compared with scans made after injection with the patient supine. Striking differences were observed. The distribution of the particles was more uniform when the patients were supine. In the sitting position, a greater fraction of the particles was found in the lower third of the lungs. When injection

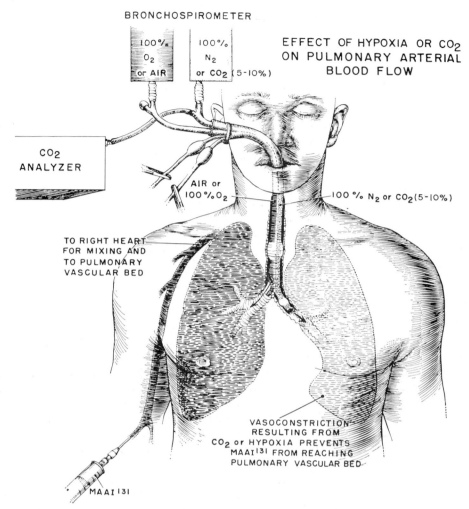

BRONCHOSPIROMETER

100% O₂ or AIR

100% N₂ or CO₂ (5-10%)

EFFECT OF HYPOXIA OR CO_2 ON PULMONARY ARTERIAL BLOOD FLOW

CO_2 ANALYZER

AIR or 100% O_2

100% N_2 or CO_2 (5-10%)

TO RIGHT HEART FOR MIXING AND TO PULMONARY VASCULAR BED

VASOCONSTRICTION RESULTING FROM CO_2 or HYPOXIA PREVENTS MAAI¹³¹ FROM REACHING PULMONARY VASCULAR BED

MAAI¹³¹

FIGURE 10-31. Use of lung scanning to study effects of regional hypoxia or increased alveolar pCO_2 on the distribution of pulmonary arterial blood flow.

was made with the patient in the right and the left lateral decubitus position, the increased blood flow to the downside lung was apparent (Fig. 10-32).

In collaboration with Warren and Stone of the U.S. Air Force, we carried out studies during weightlessness, produced by parabolic flight in a high-speed airplane (Wagner et al., 1966). Labeled particles were injected into six persons after 20 seconds of weightlessness, which then continued for another 40 seconds. The distribution of radioactivity was determined by scanning within 1 hour of injection. Control studies were performed in the same persons, in the sitting position, on the ground and when flying at +1G (straight and level flight) under the same circumstances as during the study of weightlessness. These studies illustrate an important advantage of the particle distribution technique, since the studies would not be possible with other methods.

Bryan and his associates (1965) used the same technique in a study of the effect of up to +4G of gravitational force on the lungs of persons in a human

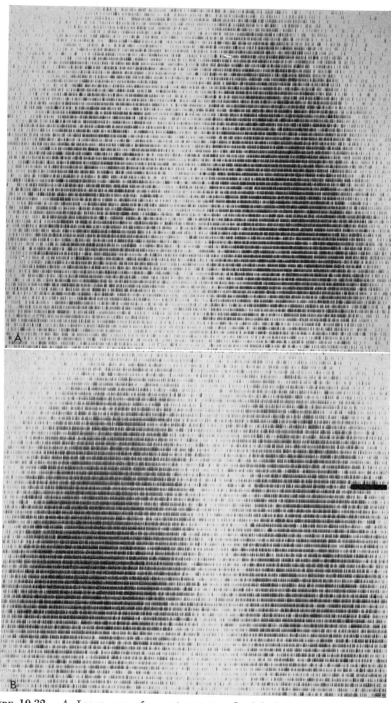

FIGURE 10-32. A, Lung scan of a patient injected while lying on his left side. Greater activity in the dependent left lung, 59 per cent of the total lung activity. B, Same patient injected while lying on his right side; 59 per cent of the total activity in the right lung.

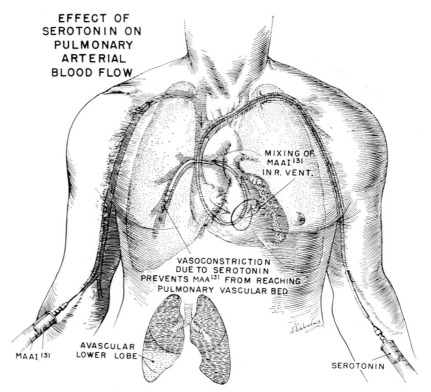

FIGURE 10-33. Use of lung scanning to study the effects of drugs on the pulmonary circulation.

centrifuge. The results indicated that a progressive reduction in upper zone perfusion occurred with increasing acceleration up to $+2G$; but thereafter the perfusion became fixed, suggesting that the vessels were then maximally dilated.

REGIONAL VASOMOTOR ACTIVITY STUDIED BY THE PARTICLE DISTRIBUTION TECHNIQUE

In the past, study of pulmonary vasomotor activity required measurement of changes in the pressure gradient across the pulmonary vasculature. This entailed measurement of left atrial as well as pulmonary arterial pressure, both of which were relatively low and therefore subject to errors in measurement. When substances are instilled into one pulmonary artery, the effect on regional pulmonary blood flow can be measured by scanning after the injection of labeled particles. Doses of the vasoactive material can be adjusted to avoid systemic effects. The experimental design is shown in Figure 10-33.

This method demonstrated that in dogs serotonin in doses of approximately 0.1 mg. cause marked focal vasoconstriction, whereas acetylcholine causes vasodilatation. The method was particularly useful because problems of measurement of pressure gradients were avoided. The pressures across both lungs were identical at any particular time. Therefore changes in vascular resistance could be determined by quantification of regional changes in flow.

NONRESPIRATORY FUNCTIONS

The respiratory functions of the lung can be classified into three major categories: *ventilation, diffusion,* and *perfusion.* In addition, certain nonrespiratory functions are of importance, including mechanisms for protecting the lungs from various atmospheric impurities and microorganisms, and for maintaining the cleanliness of the respiratory tree. Abnormalities of one or more of these subsidiary mechanisms can seriously alter the efficiency of the primary function of the lung, i.e., gaseous exchange.

The respiratory tree is lined with epithelial cells, many of which are columnar in shape and some of which are ciliated. Each ciliated columnar cell bears approximately 270 cilia, which beat with a rapid forward stroke, followed by a slower recovery stroke, 1000 times or more per minute (Krahl, 1963). The effect of the coordinated activities of countless millions of beating cilia is to produce a propulsive wave that carries a film of mucus upward toward the larynx. Scattered among the ciliated cells are tall, vacuolated *goblet* cells, which produce the sheet of mucus that rests upon and is propelled by the beating cilia. Particles that are propelled up to the oropharynx are then expectorated or swallowed.

A secondary mechanism by which foreign particles are eliminated from the lung is coughing.

The importance of the physiological mechanisms for clearing dust and other particulate matter from the lungs and tracheobronchial tree is illustrated by the fact that, although a coal miner may in his lifetime inhale 6000 g. of coal dust particles that are less than 4 microns in size, only about 100 g. of particles will be found in his lungs at postmortem examination (Schiller, 1961). In a typical English industrial town, a person inhales about 100 g. of carbon in a lifetime, but only 0.5 to 1.0 g. is found in his lungs and bronchial glands at autopsy (Blacklock et al., 1954). From experimental investigations of the behavior of particulate matter in the respiratory tract, it is known that larger particles (10 microns or more in size) are trapped in the nose, but smaller particles penetrate farther into the lungs and settle on the mucous blanket that lines the tracheobronchial tree (Pattle, 1961). About 90 per cent of particles less than 1 micron in size reach the lungs.

In the past, quantitative investigation of these mechanisms of removal of particles from the respiratory tract to determine their relative importance and degree of derangement under various physiological and pathological conditions has been difficult, particularly in man. External radiation detectors, combined with the ability to label a variety of particles with gamma-emitting radioactive isotopes, have made possible a new approach to these problems.

Solutions or particles containing radionuclides can be injected at various positions along the tracheobronchial tree in man by means of a fine radiopaque catheter inserted through a needle in the cricothyroid membrane (Wagner et al., 1965a). With this method, the rate and pattern of movement is measured in two ways: by serial radioisotope scanning of the chest or by the use of two stationary crystal scintillation detectors with slit collimators (3.0 × 0.3 cm.). Investigations in the study just cited were carried out in afebrile male patients with chronic pulmonary tuberculosis in various stages of activity. The scanning image of the distribution of the particles was obtained at various times after

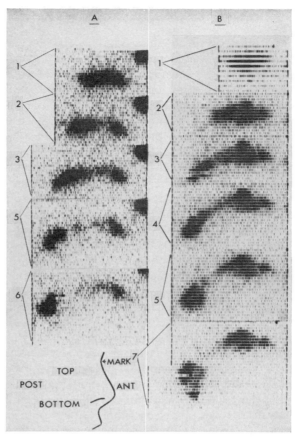

FIGURE 10-34. Serial nasal scans. A, A 52 year old woman. Time in minutes after instillation of 0.06 ml. of a solution containing 20 μc. of ^{131}I macroaggregated albumin: (1) 0.94–3.49 (2) 3.72–6.24 (3) 6.9–9.73 (5) 13.73–17.93 (6) 19.75–24.88. B, A 51 year old normal man. Time in minutes after instillation of 0.02 ml. of solution containing 20 μc. of ^{131}I macroaggregated albumin: (1) 1.22–2.51 (2) 3.42–5.75 (3) 6.33–9.7 (4) 9.56–13.25 (5) 14.60–16.0 (7) 29.48–34.72. (From Proctor, D. F., and Wagner, H. N., Jr.: Clearance of Particles from the Human Nose. *Arch Environ. Health* 11:366, 1965.)

placement of the particles. In many of the tubercular patients, foci of accumulation of the particles were observed to form as the particles moved. Most often these were at the carina, but they were also in other regions along the tracheobronchial tree. The effect of ciliary activity and cough could be readily quantified, and both were effective in clearing the lungs of this type of particle.

The frequent finding of areas of decreased ciliary activity where the particles seem to gather is of interest, since these may indicate areas where cilia or ciliated cells have been destroyed or where changes of the type described by Hilding (1960) may be found—areas of squamous epithelial cells scattered throughout the lower respiratory tract, particularly at the carina. It has been known for many years that islands of metaplasia of ciliated columnar epithelium result from chronic inflammation. In these areas, squamous epithelium replaces the ciliated mucous-covered epithelium, and the regions of diminished motility may correspond to such areas.

In addition to placing test particles along the tracheobronchial tree, it is also possible to administer radioactive aerosols to investigate their distribution and clearance under more physiological conditions. In 1948, Wilson and LaMer estimated the relative deposition of inhaled glycerol particles tagged with sodium-24 by measuring the gamma radiation from the chest. They showed that the deposition of particles in the bronchial tree depends on the size and uniformity of particles, the constancy of flow of air, and the functional status of the lung. Findeisen (1935) also studied the regional distribution of inhaled particles.

Landahl and Herrmann (1950) and later Altshuler et al. (1957, 1959) studied the deposition effect of particle size. Particles measuring 0.5 microns in diameter had a total deposition of 20 per cent, of which 95 per cent was in the alveolar region. In the range from 0.5 to 4.0 micron diameter of particles both total and alveolar deposition increased with particle size, achieving a maximum total deposition of 70 per cent, of which 80 per cent was alveolar. Beeckmans (1965a, b) estimated the size of particle for maximum alveolar deposition to be approximately 2.5 microns in diameter, in agreement with the work of Landahl.

Clearance of radioactive particles from the lung was first measured by Albert and Arnett (1955) with radioactive iron oxide particles of small (1.4 to 2.3 microns) and larger (3.5 to 4.3 microns) size. They found that a greater number of the larger particles were eliminated from the lung in the first 2 hours. Morrow et al., using $^{54}MnO_2$ (in press) and $^{239}PuO_2$ (1961) aerosols, found both an early clearance (lasting 2 to 3 hours) and a late (or slow) clearance that lasted 93 to 120 days. Using ferric oxide labeled with chromium-51 in dogs, they found a biological clearance half-time similar to that obtained with iron oxide labeled with iron-59 (Gibb and Morrow, 1962).

Proctor and Wagner (1965), using aggregates of human serum albumin labeled with iodine-131 varying in particle size from 5 to 100 microns, measured the mucociliary migration and later extraction in the nasopharynx (Fig. 10-34). They found the transport to vary widely from patient to patient, apparently independent of the size of the aggregates. Additional aerosol studies employing macroaggregates of albumin, labeled with iodine-131 and technetium-99m, have been made to evaluate the luminal patency of the tracheobronchial tree by scanning (Taplin et al., 1966; Quinn and Head, 1966).

CONCLUSIONS

Present scientific knowledge of the pulmonary circulation and the mucociliary activity of the tracheobronchial tree is based to a large extent on observations made on anesthetized animals, isolated lung preparations, and patients with cardiopulmonary diseases. Although such studies have produced fundamental contributions to our understanding, the circumstances of study have usually involved altered, impaired, or absent function. Even studies in normal and conscious humans frequently necessitate abnormal conditions—such as bronchospirometry, cardiac catheterization, and arterial cannulation. The most significant advantage of tracer methods is the minimal disturbance of the patient's normal physiology by the technique itself. Also, quantification of findings can be made readily, although some spatial geometric problems are encountered. The techniques are comparatively easy and relatively inexpensive, and they can be repeated in the same person.

The studies of weightlessness and of patients with acute asthma illustrate a unique advantage of the particle distribution method: its applicability under difficult experimental conditions. The primary requirement is that the injection of the particles be made under the conditions of the experiment. If it can be established that the internal mixing is completed during the experiment, one can derive the distribution of regional pulmonary blood flow that was present at the time of the injection, despite the fact that the fractional distribution is determined after a period of time (up to 1.5 hours or more).

Further, using the scanning technique with injected particles, we have confirmed the data obtained from studies with radioactive gases—the changes in the distribution of pulmonary blood flow that occur when a person stands up or lies down. We have found in thousands of patients that various diseases of the lungs result in a shift of pulmonary arterial blood away from the diseased area. The mechanism is not fully known, but mechanical obstruction, obliteration of the vascular bed, and functional changes such as alveolar hypoxia are probable factors.

Vasoactive substances such as serotonin and acetylcholine have been demonstrated in dogs to have a vasomotor effect when perfused through various parts of the pulmonary vascular bed. The particle distribution technique has made it quite easy to demonstrate vasomotor changes, because the problem of monitoring the pressure gradient across the pulmonary vascular bed can be avoided. The effect on regional flow is measured, not changes in pressure. The technique is a simple and effective way to study the circulation and the other physiological activities in various regions of the lungs of healthy persons and of patients with disease.

REFERENCES

Albert, R. B., and Arnett, L. C.: Clearance of Radioactive Dust from the Human Lung. *AMA Arch. Indust. Health* 12:99, 1955.

Altshuler, B., Palmes, E. D., Yarmus, L., and Nelson, N.: Intrapulmonary Mixing of Gases Studied with Aerosols. *J. Appl. Physiol.* 14:321, 1959.

Altshuler, B., Yarmus, L., Palmes, E. D., and Nelson, N.: Aerosol Deposition in the Human Respiratory Tract. I. Experimental Procedures and Total Deposition. *AMA Arch. Indust. Health* 15:293, 1957.

Aramendia, P., Taquini, C. M., Fourcade, A., and Taquini, A. C.: Reflex Vasomotor Activity During Unilateral Occlusion of the Pulmonary Artery. *Amer. Heart J.* 66:53, 1963.

Ariel, I. M. Quoted in Highlights of the Society of Nuclear Medicine Meeting. *J.A.M.A.* 183:32, 1963.

Atwood, R. M., Burchell, H. B., and Tauxe, W. N.: Pulmonary Scan Achieved with Macroaggregated Radioiodinated Albumin: Use in Diagnosis of Pulmonary Artery Agenesis. *Amer. J. Med. Sci.* 252:122, 1966.

Ball, W. C., Stewart, P. B., Newsham, L. G. S., and Bates, D. V.: Regional Pulmonary Function Studied with Xenon-133. *J. Clin. Invest.* 41:519, 1962.

Beeckmans, J. M.: The Deposition of Aerosols in the Respiratory Tract. I. Mathematical Analysis and Comparison with Experimental Data. *Canad. J. Physiol. & Pharmacol.* 43:157, 1965a.

Beeckmans, J. M.: Correction Factor for Size-Selective Sampling Results, Based on a New Computed Alveolar Deposition Curve. *Ann. Occup. Hyg.* 8:221, 1965b.

Bentivoglio, L. G.: Studies of Regional Ventilation and Perfusion Using Radioactive Xenon in Emphysema. *Dis. Chest* 48:502, 1965.

Bentivoglio, L. G., Beerel, F., Bryan, A. C., Stewart, P. B., Rose, B., and Bates, D. V.: Regional Pulmonary Function Studied with Xenon-133 in Patients with Bronchial Asthma. *J. Clin. Invest.* 42:1193, 1963a.

Bentivoglio, L. G., Beerel, F., Stewart, P. B., Bryan, A. C., Ball, W. C., and Bates, D. V.: Studies of Regional Ventilation and Perfusion in Pulmonary Emphysema Using Xenon-133. *Amer. Rev. Resp. Dis.* 88:315, 1963b.

Blacklock, J. W. S., Kennaway, E. L., Lewis, G. M., and Urquhart, M. E.: Carbon Content of Human Lungs and Bronchial Glands. *Brit. J. Cancer* 8:40, 1954.

Boucot, K. R., Cooper, D. A., Weiss, W., and Carnahan, W. J.: Appearance of First Roentgenographic Abnormalities Due to Lung Cancer. *J.A.M.A.* 190:1103, 1964.

Boyer, N. H., and Curry, J. J.: Bronchospasm Associated with Pulmonary Embolism. *Arch. Intern. Med.* 73:403, 1944.

Bryan, A. C., Macnamara, W. D., Simpson, J., and Wagner, H. N., Jr.: Effect of Acceleration on the Distribution of Pulmonary Blood Flow. *J. Appl. Physiol.* 20:1129, 1965.

Chang, C. H., and Davis, W. C.: A Roentgen Sign of Pulmonary Infarction. *Clin. Radiol.* 16:141, 1965.

Chernick, V., Lopez-Majano, V., Wagner, H. N., Jr., and Dutton, R. E.: Estimation of Differential Pulmonary Blood Flow by Bronchospirometry and Radioisotope Scanning During Rest and Exercise. *Amer. Rev. Resp. Dis.* 92:958, 1965.

Cohnheim, J., and Litten, M.: Ueber die Folgen der Embolie der Lungenarterien. *Virchow Arch. Path. Anat.* 65:99, 1875.

Daley, R., Wade, J. O., Maraist, F., and Bing, R. J.: Pulmonary Hypertension in Dogs Induced by Injection of Lycopodium Spores into the Pulmonary Artery, with Special Reference to the Absence of Vasomotor Reflex. *Amer. J. Physiol.* 164:380, 1951.

Dawson, A., Kaneko, K., and McGregor, M.: Regional Lung Function in Patients with Mitral Stenosis Studied with Xenon-133 During Air and Oxygen Breathing. *J. Clin. Invest.* 44:999, 1965.

Dexter, L., Dock, D. S., McGuire, L. B., Hyland, J. W., and Haynes, F. W.: Pulmonary Embolism. *Med. Clin. N. Amer.* 44:1251, 1960.

Dexter, L., and Smith, G. T.: Quantitative Studies of Pulmonary Embolism. *Amer. J. Med. Sci.* 247:641, 1964.

Dollery, C. T., and West, J. B.: Regional Uptake of Radioactive Oxygen, Carbon Monoxide and Carbon Dioxide in the Lungs of Patients with Mitral Stenosis. *Circ. Res.* 8:765, 1960.

Dulfano, M. J., and DiRenzo, A.: Laminographic Observations of the Lung Vasculature in Chronic Pulmonary Emphysema. *Amer. J. Roentgen.* 88:1043, 1962.

Dyson, N. A., Hugh-Jones, P., Newbery, G. R., Sinclair, J. D., and West, J. B.: Studies of Regional Lung Function Using Radioactive Oxygen. *Brit. Med. J.* 1:231, 1960.

Estrada, A. S., et al.: La angiografía en las neumopatías. *An. Inst. Nac. Neum.* 2:199, 1956.

Euler, U. S. von, and Liljestrand, G.: Observations on the Pulmonary Arterial Blood Pressure in the Cat. *Acta Physiol. Scand.* 12:301, 1946.

Findeisen, W.: Über das Absetzen kleiner in der Luft suspendierter Teilchen in der menschlichen Lunge bei der Atmung. *Pflüger Arch. Ges. Physiol.* 236:367, 1935.

Fred, H. L., Axelrad, M. A., Lewis, J. M., and Alexander, J. K.: Rapid Lysis of Pulmonary Thromboemboli in Man: Angiographic Study. *Clin. Res.* 13:25, 1965.

Freiman, D. G., Suyemoto, J., and Wessler, S.: Frequency of Pulmonary Thromboembolism in Man. *New Eng. J. Med.* 272:1278, 1965.

Friedman, W. F., and Braunwald, E.: Alterations in Regional Pulmonary Blood Flow in Mitral Valve Disease Studied by Radioisotope Scanning. *Circulation* 34:363, 1966.

Galland, F.: Classification of Pulmonary Hypertension. (Editorial.) *Amer. J. Cardiol.* 7:471, 1961.

Gibb, F. R., and Morrow, P. E.: Alveolar Clearance in Dogs after Inhalation of an Iron-59 Oxide Aerosol. *J. Appl. Physiol.* 17:429, 1962.

Gold, W. M., and McCormack, K. R.: Pulmonary-Function Response to Radioisotope Scanning of the Lungs. *J.A.M.A.* 197:146, 1966.

Gorham, L. W.: Study of Pulmonary Embolism. I. Clinicopathological Investigation of 100 Cases of Massive Embolism of the Pulmonary Artery; Diagnosis by Physical Signs and Differentiation from Acute Myocardial Infarction. II. Mechanism of Death. III. Mechanism of Pain. *Arch. Intern. Med.* 108:8, 189, 418, 1961.

Gurewich, V., Sasahara, A. A., and Stein, M.: Pulmonary Embolism, Bronchoconstriction and Response to Heparin. *In* Sasahara, A. A., and Stein, M. (eds.): Pulmonary Embolic Disease. Grune and Stratton, New York, 1965, p. 162.

Gurewich, V., Thomas, D., Stein, M., and Wessler, S.: Bronchoconstriction in the Presence of Pulmonary Embolism. *Circulation* 27:339, 1963.

Halpern, B. N., Biozzi, G., Benacerraf, B., Stiffel, C., and Hillemand, B.: Cinétique de la phagocytose d'une sérum albumine humaine spécialement traitée et radiomarquée et son application à l'étude de la circulation hépatique chez l'homme. *C. R. Soc. Biol.* (*Paris*) 150:1307, 1956.

Hamman, L., and Rich, A. R.: Acute Diffuse Interstitial Fibrosis of the Lungs. *Bull. Johns Hopkins Hosp.* 74:177, 1944.

Hampton, A. O., and Castleman, B.: Correlation of Postmortem Chest Teleroentgenograms with Autopsy Findings. *J. Roentgen. and Radium Ther.* 43:305, 1940.

Haynes, F. W., Kinney, T. D., Hellems, H. K., and Dexter, L.: Circulatory Changes in Experimental Pulmonary Embolism. *Fed. Proc.* 6:125, 1947.

Hilding, A. C.: Air-Flow as an Etiologic Factor in Metaplasia in the Tracheobronchial Tree. *Arch. Path.* 70:550, 1960.

Himmelstein, A., Harris, P., Fritts, H. W., Jr., and Cournand, A.: Effect of Severe Unilateral Hypoxia on the Partition of Pulmonary Blood Flow in Man. *J. Thorac. Surg.* 36:369, 1958.

Hyland, J. W., Smith, T. G., McGuire, L. B., Harrison, D. C., Haynes, F. W., and Dexter, L.: Effect of Selective Embolization of Various Sized Pulmonary Arteries in Dogs. *Amer. J. Physiol.* 204:619, 1963.

Hyman, A. L., Myers, W. D., and Meyer, A.: The Effect of Acute Pulmonary Embolus upon Cardiopulmonary Hemodynamics. *Amer. Heart J.* 67:313, 1964.

Ivemark, B. I.: Implications of Agenesis of the Spleen on the Pathogenesis of Cono-Truncus Anomalies in Childhood, an Analysis of the Heart Malformations in the Splenic Agenesis Syndrome, with Fourteen New Cases. *Acta Paediat.* Suppl. 104, 44:1, 1955.

Kartagener, M.: Zur Pathogenese der Bronchiektasien: Bronchiektasien bei Situs viscerum inversus. *Beitr. Klin. Tuberk.* 83:489, 1933.

Kennady, J. C., and Taplin, G. V.: Albumin Macroaggregates for Brain Scanning (Experimental Basis and Safety in Primates). *J. Nucl. Med.* 6:566, 1965.

Knipping, H. W., Bolt, W., Valentin, H., Venrath, H., and Endler, P.: Regionale Funktionsanalyse in der Kreislauf- und Lungenklinik mit Hilfe der Isotopenthorakographie und der selektiven Angiographie der Lungengefäbe. *München. Med. Wschr.* 99:1, 1957.

Knipping, H. W., Bolt, W., Venrath, H., Valentin, H., Ludes, H., and Endler, P.: Eine neue Methode zur Prüfung der Herz- und Lungenfunktion; die regionale Funktionsanalyse in der Lungen- und Herzklinik mit Hilfe des radioaktiven Edelgases Xenon-133. *Deutsch. Med. Wschr.* 80:1146, 1955.

Krahl, V. E.: Microstructure of the Lung. *Arch. Environ. Health* 6:37, 1963.

Landahl, H. D., and Herrmann, R. G.: Retention of Vapors and Gases in Human Nose and Lung. *Arch. Indust. Hyg.* 1:36, 1950.

Littmann, D.: Observations on the Electrocardiographic Changes in Pulmonary Embolism. *In* Sasahara, A. A., and Stein, M. (eds.): Pulmonary Embolic Disease. Grune and Stratton, New York, 1965, p. 136.

Lopez-Majano, V., Chernick, V., Wagner, H. N., Jr., and Dutton, R. E.: Comparison of Radioisotope Scanning and Differential Oxygen Uptake of the Lungs. *Radiology* 83:697, 1964.

Lopez-Majano, V., Tow, D. E., and Wagner, H. N., Jr.: Regional Distribution of Pulmonary Arterial Blood Flow in Emphysema. *J.A.M.A.* 197:81, 1966.

Lopez-Majano, V., Wagner, H. N., Jr., Tow, D. E., and Chernick, V.: Radioisotope Scanning of the Lungs in Pulmonary Tuberculosis. *J.A.M.A.* 194:1053, 1965.

Lower, R.: Tractus de corde. Allestry, London, 1669.

Macleod, W. M.: Abnormal Transradiancy of One Lung. *Thorax* 9:147, 1954.

Martin, C. J., Cline, F., Jr., and Marshall, H.: Lobar Alveolar Gas Concentrations; Effects of Body Position. *J. Clin. Invest.* 32:617, 1953.

Mattson, S. B., and Carlens, E.: Lobar Ventilation and Oxygen Uptake in Man; Influence of Body Position. *J. Thorac. Surg.* 30:676, 1955.

Middleton, E.: The Anatomical and Biochemical Basis of Bronchial Obstruction in Asthma. *Ann. Intern. Med.* 63:695, 1965.

Mishkin, F. S., and Wagner, H. N., Jr.: Regional Abnormalities in Pulmonary Arterial Blood Flow During Acute Asthmatic Attacks. *Radiology* 88:142, 1967.

Morrow, P. E., and Casarett, L. J.: An Experimental Study of the Deposition and Retention of a Plutonium-239 Dioxide Aerosol. *In* Davies, C. N. (ed.): Inhaled Particles and Vapours. Vol. 1. Pergamon Press, New York, 1961, p. 167.

Morrow, P. E., and Gibbs, M. S.: The Clearance of Dust from the Lower Respiratory Tract of Man. *In* Davies, C. N. (ed.): Inhaled Particles and Vapours. Vol. 2. Pergamon Press, New York, in press.

Pattle, R. E.: The Lining Complex of the Lung Alveoli. *In* Davies, C. N. (ed.): Inhaled Particles and Vapours. Vol. 1. Pergamon Press, New York, 1961, p. 70.

Proctor, D. F.: Airborne Disease and the Upper Respiratory Tract. *Bact. Rev.* 30:498, 1966.

Proctor, D. F., and Wagner, H. N., Jr.: Clearance of Particles from the Human Nose. *Arch. Environ. Health* 11:366, 1965.

Quinn, J. L., III, and Head, L. R.: Radioisotope Photoscanning in Pulmonary Disease. *J. Nucl. Med.* 7:1, 1966.

Rakower, J., and Moran, E.: Unilateral Hyperlucent Lung (Swyer-James Syndrome). *Amer. J. Med.* 33:864, 1962.

Riley, R. L., and Cournand, A.: "Ideal" Alveolar Air and the Analysis of Ventilation-Perfusion Relationships in the Lungs. *J. Appl. Physiol.* 1:825, 1949.

Robin, E. D., Forkner, C. E., Jr., Bromberg, P. A., Croteau, J. R., and Travis, D. M.: Alveolar Gas Exchange in Clinical Pulmonary Embolism. *New Eng. J. Med.* 262:283, 1960.

Robin, E. D., Julian, D. G., Travis, D. M., and Crump, C. H.: A Physiologic Approach to the Diagnosis of Acute Pulmonary Embolism. *New Eng. J. Med.* 260:586, 1959.

Rubin, E. H., and Rubin, M.: Thoracic Diseases. W. B. Saunders Co., Philadelphia, 1961.

Sapirstein, L. A.: Regional Blood Flow by Fractional Distribution of Indicators. *Amer. J. Physiol.* 193:161, 1958.

Sasahara, A. A., Cannilla, J. E., Morse, R. L., Sidd, J. J., and Tremblay, G. M.: Clinical and Physiologic Studies in Pulmonary Thromboembolism. *Amer. J. Cardiol.* In press.

Sasahara, A. A., Stein, M., Simon, M., and Littmann, D.: Pulmonary Angiography in the Diagnosis of Thromboembolic Disease. *New Eng. J. Med.* 270:1075, 1964.

Sasahara, A. A., Tremblay, G. M., and Leland, O. S., Jr.: Cardiopulmonary Alterations in Acute Pulmonary Thromboembolism. *Circulation Suppl.* 32:II-187, 1965.

Schiller, E.: Inhalation, Retention and Elimination of Dust from Dogs' and Rats' Lungs with Special Reference to the Alveolar Phagocytes and Bronchial Epithelium. *In* Davies, C. N. (ed.): Inhaled Particles and Vapours. Vol. 1. Pergamon Press, New York, 1961, p. 342.

Shah, K. D., Neill, C. A., Wagner, H. N., Jr., and Taussig, H. B.: Radioisotope Scanning of the Liver and Spleen in Dextrocardia and in Situs Inversus with Levocardia. *Circulation* 29:231, 1964.

Stern, H. S., Goodwin, D. A., Wagner, H. N., Jr., and Kramer, H. H.: In-113m—a Short-Lived Isotope for Lung Scanning. *Nucleonics* 24:57, 1966.

Swyer, P. R., and James, G. C. W.: A Case of Unilateral Pulmonary Emphysema. *Thorax* 8:133, 1953.

Taplin, G. V., Dore, E. K., Poe, N. D., Swanson, L. A., Johnson, D. E., and Greenberg, A.: Lung Perfusion and Bronchial Patency Evaluation by Radioisotope Scanning. *Picker Scintillator* March 14, 1966.

Taplin, G. V., Johnson, D. E., Dore, E. K., and Kaplan, H. S.: Lung Photoscans with Macroaggregates of Human Serum Radioalbumin. Experimental Basis and Initial Clinical Trials. *Health Phys.* 10:1219, 1964.

Torrance, D. J., Jr.: Roentgenographic Signs of Pulmonary Artery Occlusion. *Amer. J. Med. Sci.* 237:651, 1959.

Tow, D. E., Mishkin, F. S., Wagner, H. N., Jr., Baker, R. B., and Jensen, A. D.: Effect of Free Pleural Fluid on the Pulmonary Circulation. Unpublished data.

Tow, D. E., and Wagner, H. N., Jr.: Recovery of Pulmonary Arterial Blood Flow in Patients with Pulmonary Embolism. *New Eng. J. Med.* 276:1053, 1967.

Tow, D. E., Wagner, H. N., Jr., Lopez-Majano, V., Smith, E. M., and Migita, T.: Validity of Measuring Regional Pulmonary Arterial Blood with Macroaggregates of Human Serum Albumin. *Amer. J. Roentgen.* 96:664, 1966.

Tow, D. E., Wagner, H. N., Jr., Sabiston, D. C., Jr., and Meyer, J. K.: Lysis of Experimental Pulmonary Thrombi in Dogs by Urokinase. *Clin. Res.* 12:467, 1964.

Ueda, H., Kaihara, S., Iio, M., and Togashi, M.: Abnormal Transradiancy of One Lung Studied by Pulmonary Scintiscanning. *Jap. Heart J.* 6:268, 1965.

Wacker, W. E. C., Rosenthal, M., Snodgrass, P. J., and Amador, E.: A Triad for the Diagnosis of Pulmonary Embolism and Infarction. *J.A.M.A.* 178:8, 1961.

Wacker, W. E. C., and Snodgrass, P. J.: Serum LDH Activity in Pulmonary Embolism Diagnosis. *J.A.M.A.* 174:2142, 1960.

Wagner, H. N., Jr., Lopez-Majano, V., and Langan, J. K.: Clearance of Particulate Matter from the Tracheobronchial Tree in Patients with Tuberculosis. *Nature* 205:252, 1965a.

Wagner, H. N., Jr., Lopez-Majano, V., Tow, D. E., and Langan, J. K.: Radioisotope Scanning of Lungs in Early Diagnosis of Bronchogenic Carcinoma. *Lancet* 1:344, 1965b.

Wagner, H. N., Jr., Sabiston, D. C., Jr., Iio, M., McAfee, J. G., Meyer, J. K., and Langan, J. K.: Regional Pulmonary Blood Flow in Man by Radioisotope Scanning. *J.A.M.A.* 187:601, 1964.

Wagner, H. N., Jr., Sabiston, D. C., Jr., McAfee, J. G., Tow, D. E., and Stern, H. S.: Diagnosis of Massive Pulmonary Embolism in Man by Radioisotope Scanning. *New Eng. J. Med.* 271:377, 1964.

Wagner, H. N., Jr., Tow, D. E., Lopez-Majano, V., Chernick, V., and Twining, R.: Factors Influencing Regional Pulmonary Blood in Man. *Scand. J. Resp. Dis.* Suppl. 62, 1966.

Webster, J. R., Jr., Saadeh, G. B., Eggum, P. R., and Suker, J. R.: Wheezing Due to Pulmonary Embolism: Treatment with Heparin. *New Eng. J. Med.* 274:931, 1966.

Weibel, E. R.: Morphometry of the Human Lung. Academic Press, New York, 1963.

West, J. B.: Regional Differences in Gas Exchange in the Lung of Erect Man. *J. Appl. Physiol.* 17:893, 1962.

West, J. B.: Ventilation/Blood Flow and Gas Exchange. F. A. Davis Co., Philadelphia, 1965.

West, J. B., and Dollery, C. T.: Distribution of Blood Flow and Ventilation-Perfusion Ratio in the Lung, Measured with Radioactive CO_2. *J. Appl. Physiol.* 15:405, 1960.

West, J. B., Holland, R. A. B., Dollery, C. T., and Matthews, C. M. E.: Interpretation of radioactive Gas Clearance Rates in the Lung. *J. Appl. Physiol.* 17:14, 1962.

Westermark, W.: On the Roentgen Diagnosis of Lung Embolism. *Acta Radiol.* 19:357, 1938.

White, P. D., and Brenner, O.: Pathological and Clinical Aspects of Pulmonary Circulation. *New Eng. J. Med.* 209:1261, 1933.

Wilson, I. B., and LaMer, V. K.: Retention of Aerosol Particles in Human Respiratory Tract as Function of Particle Radius. *J. Indust. Hyg. Toxicol.* 30:265, 1948.

Wolff, L.: The Electrocardiogram in Pulmonary Embolism. *Heart Bull.* 8:111, 1959.

Wood, P.: Pulmonary Hypertension. *Mod. Conc. Cardiov. Dis.* 28:513, 1959.

XI

THE CIRCULATION

LUIGI DONATO*

RICHARD A. HOLMES

HENRY N. WAGNER, JR.

PRINCIPLES

Luigi Donato

INTRODUCTION

The use of indicator techniques in studies of the circulation began long before the discovery of nuclear energy and the availability of radioactive tracers. Most of the principles of indicator use had already been established by the pioneer work of Fick, Stewart, Henriques, Hamilton, and Kety. However, radio-isotopes have greatly enhanced the practical value of tracer techniques in studies of the circulation, so that presently they are the methods of choice for measuring blood flow and circulating blood volumes in intact animals and men.

BASIC HEMODYNAMIC PARAMETERS

When describing the status of a patient's circulatory system, the physician often thinks in terms of pressures or pressure gradients. This is quite under-standable since the concept of pressure gradients lends itself to simple hydraulic analogies. These would be perfectly adequate if blood were propelled by the heart through rigid tubes, in which pressure and flow would be related to each

* This study was supported by Euratom Association Contract 026–63–4 BIAC.

other simply by the diameter of the tubes and the characteristics of the flowing blood. In such a system, the measurement of the rate of blood flow would give the cardiac output; and the pressure measurements, for a given flow rate, would provide an adequate description of the hemodynamic characteristics of the vessels. These are implicit assumptions in methods of studying the circulation that estimate resistance by dividing pressure into flow; resistance changes are estimated by relating pressure changes to flow changes.

This approach, although undoubtedly useful in practice, becomes inadequate when one attempts to interpret changes in calculated resistance as changes in vessel diameter. Since the circulatory system consists of distensible tubes, with a consequent nonlinearity of the pressure-flow relationship, local adjustment and variation of cross section can occur. Moreover, estimates based on calculated resistance are necessarily confined to the resistive vessels. Ideally, one would like to be able to measure directly the cross section of the vessels, but this is obviously impossible in the living subject. However, we can measure the volume of blood in a given part of the circulatory system, and this will be related to the average cross section of that portion. Similarly, if one assumes that adaptation of the entire circulatory system, or part of the system, to a stimulus will result in changes of the average radius of vessels, with only minor changes in length, measurement of volume changes will permit the detection of changes in vessel radius; and the latter will be magnified in the volume change.

Thus, we can characterize a hemodynamic system if we know the blood pressure, the flow rate, and the circulating blood volume. Indicator techniques enable us to measure the latter two parameters.

GENERAL ASPECTS OF CIRCULATION STUDIES WITH INDICATOR TECHNIQUES

To illustrate the principles of indicator methods for circulatory studies, let us consider a system that has one input and one output through which blood flows at a rate, F, and which contains a blood volume, V_B. Further, this vascular system perfuses a mass of tissue, V_T, which tissue can be reached by indicators diffusing through the capillaries.

The most general equation describing the kinetics of an indicator substance flowing into the system is the following:

$$Q'(t) = FC_i - FC_o \tag{1}$$

which simply states that the change in the indicator content of the system $Q'(t)$ equals the difference between the amounts of inflowing and outflowing indicator, which is indicated by the product of flow, F, times the input and output concentrations, C_i and C_o, respectively, with flow F assumed to be constant.

No assumptions are made as to the distribution of indicator within the system: this will depend primarily on the type of indicator employed, including its ability to diffuse ultimately across the capillaries of the system. Since equation 1 is a general one for the kinetics of the system, various indicator methods can be examined on the basis of this equation, and the assumptions underlying each method can be examined. The following discussion is largely based on the concepts first developed by Meier and Zierler (1954).

A unit amount of indicator entering the system at time 0, and becoming thoroughly mixed with the flowing blood, will appear at the outflow of the system after a certain time, and, depending on the flow pattern within the system, the outflow of the indicator will have a variable spread in time. This concept can be visualized by considering the circulatory system as composed of a series of vascular circuits connected in parallel with each other—each characterized by the fraction of the total flow going through it, and by a typical transit time. If we indicate by $\phi(t)$ the flow through the channel with transit time t, then the equa-

$$h(t) = \frac{\phi(t)}{F} \tag{2}$$

tion indicates the probability that a particle of indicator entering the system at time 0 will leave it at time t.

Integration of the frequency function of transit times h(t), from 0 to infinity, yields:

$$\int_0^\infty h(t)dt = 1 \tag{3}$$

which simply states that ultimately the entire amount of indicator that entered the system at time 0 will leave the system.

The product of the flow $\phi(t)$ through each channel *times* the transit time t of the channel gives the volume of blood in the channel having transit time t.

When all the channel volumes are added, the volume of the system, V, is obtained. Therefore, multiplying both terms of equation 2 by t and integrating from 0 to infinity:

$$\int_0^\infty th(t)dt = \frac{1}{F}\int_0^\infty t\phi(t)dt = \frac{V}{F} \tag{4}$$

The integral in equation 4 is therefore the volume-flow ratio of the system. It has the dimension of time and is, in fact, the *mean circulation time*, $T = V/F$, of the system, or the mean time of the distribution of transit times, h(t). This is evident if one writes equation 4 as:

$$\int_0^\infty th(t)dt = \int_0^\infty t\left(\frac{\phi(t)}{F}\right)dt = T \tag{5}$$

In the integral, every value of time is weighed by the fraction of total flow going through the ideal channel with transit time t.[1]

The value of T, as well as its significance, depends on the type of indicator used. If there are no stagnant pools in the system, the volume indicated in equation 4 corresponds to the blood volume of the system, V_B, in the case of a non-diffusible indicator; it corresponds to the entire mass of the organ (including the blood volume) for a diffusible indicator.[2]

---

[1]It will be useful to consider the following developments of equation 5. Integrating by parts:

$$\int th(t)dt = t\int h(t)dt - \int\int h(t)dt \tag{5.1}$$

Since the first integral at the second member tends to 1, one may write

$$\lim_{t\to\infty} \int th(t)dt = t - \int\int h(t)dt \tag{5.2}$$

$$\lim_{t\to\infty} \int th(t)dt = \int^\infty[1 - \int h(t)dt]dt \tag{5.3}$$

---

[2] This statement is strictly correct only if the indicator has the same solubility per unit volume of blood or tissue of the organ. Otherwise, the volume in equation 4 equals $[V_B + V_T\lambda]$, where λ is the partition coefficient of the indicator between tissue and blood.

It is important to point out that the mean transit time for any vascular system can be defined as the difference between the mean transit time between the entrance and the exit of the system. Thus, if $h_A(t)$ and $h_B(t)$ are the frequency functions of transit times at points A and B, point B being downstream to A, and the injection point being upstream to both:

$$\int_0^\infty th_B(t)dt - \int_0^\infty th_A(t)dt = T_B - T_A = T_{B-A} \tag{6}$$

where T_B and T_A indicate the mean circulation times between the injection point and points B and A, respectively. Their difference is the mean time of the frequency function of transit times for a unit impulse of indicator entering at point A and leaving the system at point B.[3]

Studies of the circulation with indicator techniques can be performed in several different ways. Two groups of techniques will be considered: methods based on the observation of the first transit of the indicator through the circulatory system being investigated; and methods based on observation of the distribution of the indicator within the system at equilibrium.

From the viewpoint of radioisotope techniques, this grouping seems more adequate than the traditional one based on the distinction between the dilution of nondiffusible indicators and the distribution of diffusible indicators.

In traditional applications of indicator techniques, blood sampling is essential, and the site of sampling is critical; but radioisotope techniques of external counting have overcome this limitation, thus enlarging tremendously the effectiveness of these techniques.

METHODS BASED ON THE FIRST TRANSIT OF THE INDICATOR

These methods are based on the measurement of the amount of indicator entering the system during the first transit and measurement of the mean concentration attained by the indicator in the blood flowing into (or out of) the system during the transit. The ratio of the two gives the volume of blood in which the indicator is mixed. The ratio of the volume of flowing blood with which the indicator has mixed during its transit *to* the duration of the transit is a measure of rate of blood flow of the system. It is important to the test that none of the indicator enter the system twice; i.e., recirculation must not occur. Basic requirements of these methods, therefore, are: (a) measurement of the amount of indicator entering the system during the entire first transit; and (b) measurement of the concentration curve of the indicator during the first transit, at a site which can be considered as representative of the whole system.

The present principle is often applied to measurement of blood flow by directly injecting the indicator in such manner that the whole injectate will go through the system under study. In other instances the indicator mixes first with the entire

---

[3]It will be useful to consider the following developments of equation 6. If the proper substitutions from equation 5.3 are made for the two integrals at the first member of equation 6, one obtains:

$$T_{B-A} = \int_0^\infty [1 - \int h_B(t)dt]dt - \int_0^\infty [1 - \int h_A(t)dt]dt \tag{6.1}$$

$$T_{B-A} = \int\int_0^\infty [h_A - h_B]dt \tag{6.2}$$

cardiac output; then it is transferred, already mixed, to the part of the circulatory system that one wishes to measure.

DIRECT INJECTION OF INDICATOR INTO THE SYSTEM

These techniques can be applied to the study of the central or the peripheral circulation, to measure either the total or the regional blood flow. In the first case, the indicator can be injected anywhere in the venous circulation, since mixing with the total blood flow will take place in the central circulation; but when peripheral flow is to be measured, the indicator must be injected directly into the inflow of the system under study. The indicator can be given either by instantaneous injection or by constant infusion, for such purposes as the following.

Instantaneous Injection. BLOOD FLOW. After a single injection, without subsequent input of indicator into the system, equation 1 becomes simplified to:

$$Q'(t) = - FC_o(t) \tag{7}$$

The term $FC_o(t)$ indicates the amount of indicator leaving the system at time t, following injection of an amount $Q(o)$ at 0 time. On the other hand, since $h(t)$ represents the fraction of a unit amount of indicator that entered the system at time 0 and is leaving the system at time t (see equation 2), we may write

$$FC_o(t) = Q(o)h(t) \tag{8}$$

whence

$$C_o(t) = \frac{Q(o)}{F} h(t) \tag{9}$$

Equation 9 establishes an important relationship between the concentration of the indicator at the outflow of the system and the frequency function of transit times.

Assuming absence of recirculation of the indicator, and integrating equation 9 to include the entire first transit of the indicator, one obtains:

$$\int_0^\infty C_o(t)dt = \frac{Q(o)}{F} \tag{10}$$

whence

$$F = \frac{Q(o)}{\int_0^\infty C_o(t)dt} \tag{11}$$

The flow F is obtained by dividing the amount of indicator injected *by* the integral of the first concentration curve at the outflow of the system, carried to completion of the curve. The method requires extrapolation of the recorded outflow curve if recirculation occurs.

It will be noted from equation 10 that the same principles apply no matter in which outflow branch the integral of the concentration curve is measured, provided the amount of indicator q(o) and flow (f) through that branch are in the same proportion as the entire injected indicator and total flow:

$$f/q(o) = F/Q(o) \tag{12}$$

MEAN CIRCULATION TIME. From equations 9 and 10, the frequency function of transit times may be defined as:

$$\frac{C_o(t)}{\int_0^\infty C_o(t)dt} = h(t) \tag{13}$$

As a consequence, according to its definition in equation 5, the mean circulation time of the system, from injection to sampling point, may be obtained as:

$$T = \int_0^\infty th(t)dt = \frac{\int_0^\infty tC_o(t)dt}{\int_0^\infty C_o(t)dt} \tag{14}$$

whence the equivalent volume of blood with which the indicator has mixed between injection and sampling point is obtained as:

$$V = F \cdot T \tag{15}$$

It can also be shown from equation 14 that the mean circulation time measured by using the curve recorded at site B downstream to site A, equals the mean circulation time from injection point to A plus the mean circulation time from A to B. Intermediate volumes may be obtained by a single injection, and sampling at two such points, immediately upstream and downstream from the region of interest; or by double injection immediately above and below the region of interest, with sampling farther downstream.

The mean circulation time of the intermediate region is given (see equations 6.1 and 6.2) simply as:

$$T_{B-A} = \frac{\int_0^\infty tC_B(t)dt}{\int_0^\infty C_B(t)dt} - \frac{\int_0^\infty tC_A(t)dt}{\int_0^\infty C_A(t)dt} = \frac{\int\int_0^\infty (C_A - C_B)dt}{\int_0^\infty C(t)dt} \tag{16}$$

where the integral in the denominator can be measured at any level, with the same restrictions as in equation 12.

MEASURING RESIDUAL RADIOACTIVITY IN THE REGION OF INTEREST. Instead of measuring the concentration in the blood flowing out of the region, measurements can be made of the residual radioactivity, $Q(t)$, in the region of interest.

Equation 7, which describes the change in the indicator content of the system, can also be written:

$$Q'(t) = -Q(o)h(t) \tag{17}$$

By two successive integrations:

$$\int_0^{t'} Q(t)dt = Q(o) \int_0^{t'} \left[1 - \int_0^t h(\tau)d\tau\right]dt \tag{18}$$

Since at $t = \infty$ the term between brackets equals the turnover time of the system (see equation 5.3):

$$\int_0^\infty Q(t)dt = Q(o)T = Q(o)(V/F) \tag{19}$$

which may be written:

$$\frac{1}{V} \int_0^\infty Q(t)dt = \frac{Q(o)}{F} \tag{20}$$

It is of interest to compare equation 20 with equation 10: since $Q(t)$ is the total amount of indicator in the volume V at any one time, it may be written as:

$$Q(t) = \int_v c_v(t)dv \qquad (21)$$

or, indicating with $\bar{c}_v$ the mean concentration in the system:

$$Q(t) = \bar{c}_v(t)V \qquad (22)$$

Substituting from equation 22 into 20, and equating equation 20 with equation 10, it is seen that:

$$\int_0^\infty \bar{c}_v(t)dt = \int_0^\infty C_o(t)dt = Q(o)/F \qquad (23)$$

which states the important fact that the integral of the mean concentration within the entire volume of the system equals the integral of the outflowing concentration.

Equations 19 and 20 show how measurements of indicator content of the system may be used to evaluate its hemodynamic parameters. From equation 19 it is seen that:

$$T = \frac{V}{F} = \frac{\int_0^\infty Q(t)dt}{Q(o)} \qquad (24)$$

which permits the measurement of the turnover time of the indicator in the organ. When the volume of distribution of the indicator V corresponds to the organ mass, results can be expressed in terms of mass by equating V to the organ mass M. The flow per unit organ mass is then:

$$F/M = \frac{Q(o)}{\int_0^\infty Q(t)dt} \qquad (25)$$

If V is measurable, the absolute flow F can be obtained from equation 20 as:

$$F = \frac{Q(o)V}{\int_0^\infty Q(t)dt} \qquad (26)$$

This approach can be used to evaluate the hemodynamic characteristics of a region by recording the time course of the radioactivity in the region by means of γ-emitting indicators and external radiation detectors (Zierler, 1965).

Radiocardiography and most of the modern techniques for measuring peripheral blood flow depend on these principles. However, application of equations 24, 25, and 26 to external counting depends on the counting efficiency of the external detector and on its sensitive volume with respect to the distribution of the radioactive indicator in the region of interest. This problem will be considered in detail later.

Constant Infusion. If the indicator is administered as a constant infusion, the change of the content of indicator in the region will be described by:

$$Q'(t) = I - FC_o(t) \qquad (27)$$

where I is the rate of infusion of the indicator per unit time, and (as in the case of the instantaneous injection) recirculation is neglected.

This type of input can be dealt with as a series of instantaneous injections at infinitely small time intervals. The outflow of indicator $FC_o(t)$ can be obtained from equation 8, which indicates the outflow after an instantaneous injection at time 0. In the case of a constant infusion, at any time t a fraction $h(\theta)$ of the amount I that entered the system θ time units earlier—that is, at time $(t - \theta)$—will leave the region. The total outflow of indicator at any particular time can be obtained by adding, from time 0 to time t, the amounts injected per unit time multiplied by the proper h value. Thus the amount I that entered at time 0 will contribute to the output by an amount Ih_t; and the amount I that entered at time 1, by an amount Ih_{t-1}; whereas that entering at time t will contribute by an amount Ih_o, as follows:

$$FC_{o_t} = I\ (h_o + h_1 + \ldots + h_{t-1} + h_t)$$

or, more appropriately:

$$FC_o(t) = I \int_0^t h(\tau)d\tau \tag{28}$$

whence:

$$C_o(t) = \frac{I}{F} \int_0^t h(\tau)d\tau \tag{29}$$

Inspection of equation 29 indicates that $C_o(t)$ increases progressively from time 0, to attain a maximum value $C_o(max.)$ after the first transit has been completed. At that moment:

$$C_o(max.) = \frac{I}{F} \tag{30}$$

whence:

$$F = \frac{I}{C_o(max.)} \tag{31}$$

Flow can be obtained by dividing the infusion rate into the concentration attained at the outflow. It should be noted that, provided I mixed with F at the inflow, the ratio (I/F) also indicates the inflowing concentration C_i.

Solving equation 29 for the integral of the frequency function of transit times, the mean transit time through the system, according to its expression from equation 5.3, can be obtained as:

$$T = \int_0^\infty \left[1 - \int_0^t h(\tau)d\tau\right]dt = \int_0^\infty \left[1 - \frac{C_o(t)}{I/F}\right]dt \tag{32}$$

or, from equation 30:

$$T = \frac{V}{F} = \frac{\int_0^\infty [C_o(max.) - C_o(t)]dt}{C_o(max.)} \tag{33}$$

Methods based on the first transit of a constant infusion do not differ in their assumptions, their value, or their limitations from the instantaneous-injection method. Therefore, the single-injection method is usually preferred to the more cumbersome infusion technique.

INDIRECT INJECTION OF INDICATOR INTO THE SYSTEM

In this case the indicator is injected in such a way that it mixes with the entire blood flow through the central circulation. From the standpoint of the circulation in the peripheral region of interest, the situation differs from the case of the direct injection; the indicator entering the peripheral region is already mixed with the inflowing blood, and the inflowing concentration curve into the region corresponds to the outflowing concentration curve from the central circulation.

Indicating with c_i and c_o the inflowing and outflowing concentrations, the equation describing the amount of indicator in the peripheral region under study is obtained by integration of equation 1, with $c_i = C_o$, where C_o is the output concentration of the central system in which the indicator is diluted in the total flow F, f being the flow of the peripheral region to be measured:

$$q(t) = f \int C_o(t)dt - f \int c_o(t)dt \tag{34}$$

The possibility of measuring the flow f through the system depends on the possibility of knowing the amount of indicator entering the system with the first indicator transit curve. This possibility can be achieved in some special instances.

Total Extraction of the Inflowing Indicator by the Region. If the blood flowing through the region is completely cleared of its indicator content during its passage through the system, the change in the indicator content of the system, and the content of indicator in the system, are given by:

$$q'(t) = fC_o(t) \tag{35}$$

$$q(t) = f \int C_o(t)dt \tag{36}$$

It should be noted that, since every particle of indicator entering the system is cleared from the circulation, the first indicator transit actually lasts until no indicator is left in the entire circulation; this statement agrees with the previously stated requirement for the definition of first indicator transit through a system, since it is obvious that all indicator particles may enter the system only once. The total amount of indicator is then:

$$q(\infty) = f \int_0^\infty C_o(t)dt \tag{37}$$

If the total flow to the organs that clear the indicator from the circulation is small in comparison to the total blood flow, the indicator will attain an essentially uniform concentration in the entire systemic circulation as soon as the indicator has been subject to the mixing effect of total blood flow. This is the case, for instance, of indicators used to measure renal plasma flow, such as PAH or Hippuran (Smith et al., 1945), or to measure liver blood flow, such as BSP (Bradley et al., 1945) or particulate material (Dobson et al., 1953).

It is obvious from equations 35, 36, and 37 that flow f can be obtained if both the amount of indicator taken up by the organ and the concentration in the systemic circulation can be measured. In this procedure, an example of which is the measurement of renal clearance, venous blood usually provides a sufficiently accurate estimate of C_o, since mixing is rapidly attained in the blood volume.

Since:

$$C_o(t) = \frac{Q(o)}{F} h(t) \tag{9}$$

and

$$Q'(t) = - Q(o)h(t) \tag{17}$$

where $Q(o)$ and $Q(t)$ indicate the amount of indicator injected and that remaining in the circulation, respectively, and F now indicates the total clearance rate of the indicator from the circulation, equations 35 through 37 may be written as:

$$q'(t) = -(f/F)Q'(t) \tag{38}$$

$$q(t) = (f/F)[Q(o) - Q(t)] \tag{39}$$

$$q(\infty) = (f/F)Q(o) \tag{40}$$

These equations relate the amount of indicator accumulated in the region under study to the amount of indicator left in the circulation. From equations 39 and 40 we derive:

$$q(\infty) - q(t) = \frac{f}{F} Q(t) \tag{41}$$

In the special case in which the region under study is the only one clearing the indicator from the circulation ($f = F$), the flow through the system can be obtained from the blood curve or from the organ uptake only. In fact, since $q(\infty)$ will equal $Q(o)$, equation 37 reduces to:

$$f = \frac{Q(o)}{\int_0^\infty C_o(t)dt} \tag{42}$$

Flow can then be obtained by dividing the amount of indicator injected *into* the integral of the blood concentration curve. On the other hand, equation 41 becomes:

$$q(\infty) - q(t) = Q(t) \tag{43}$$

From equation 19 it is then seen that:

$$\frac{q(\infty)}{\int_0^\infty [q(\infty) - q(t)]dt} = \frac{f}{V_i} \tag{44}$$

where V_i is the volume of distribution of the indicator; if this volume can be approximated or independently measured, the absolute flow can be obtained solely from measurements of the activity taken up by the organ. In the case of the liver uptake of colloidal ^{198}Au, the ratio of liver blood flow to total blood volume can then be obtained if the liver uptake can be measured.

Partial or No Extraction of Indicator by the Region. If the organ does not completely extract the indicator from the blood flow, the problem of assessing the amount of indicator reaching the organ during the first passage becomes very complex. In this case, the first transit is limited to the first circulation of the indicator through the organ, and the integral of the indicator concentration curve equals the integral of the first outflow curve from the central circulation. The problem of measuring the corresponding amount of inflowing indicator can be solved only in special cases. The following are examples.

MEAN CIRCULATION TIME OF A BLOOD POOL HAVING A TRANSIT TIME SHORTER THAN ANY OTHER. Under these conditions the amount of a nondiffusible indicator leaving the region will appear in the venous side of the central circulation before the arrival of indicator from any other circuit. Assuming for the moment that no indicator except the portion that has gone through the region under study returns to the mixed venous blood, this indicator will be diluted in the total venous blood flow F to a concentration $\bar{c}_m$, as follows:

$$\bar{c}_m(t) = \frac{fc_o(t)}{F} \tag{45}$$

Since, on the other hand:

$$f\int_0^\infty c_o(t)dt = q(o) \tag{46}$$

where $q(o)$ is the amount of indicator corresponding to the first transit, integrating equation 45 and making the substitutions from equation 46, the following is obtained:

$$q(o) = F\int_0^\infty \bar{c}_m(t)dt \tag{47}$$

On the other hand, since the ratio of indicator to flow during the first transit is the same for the main flow and all secondary branches, it is also true that:

$$q(o) = f\int_0^\infty C_o(t)dt \tag{48}$$

Equating equations 47 and 48 and solving for f:

$$f = F\frac{\int_0^\infty \bar{c}_m(t)dt}{\int_0^\infty C_o(t)dt} \tag{49}$$

which indicates that the flow can be measured if the mixed venous concentration curve resulting from indicator returning from the region of interest can be separated from the rest of the recirculation (Henly et al., 1956).

Attempts to use this approach to measure coronary flow have been unsuccessful because of the practical impossibility of accurately separating the coronary return of indicator from that of the rest of the body (Marchioro et al., 1961). However, the method can be successfully used to measure left-to-right shunts (Donato et al., 1966a).

ORGAN UPTAKE PROPORTIONAL TO BLOOD FLOW. Radioactive potassium and rubidium have an unusual pattern of distribution in the body after they are injected intravenously. Although their final distribution is determined by the size of the various potassium compartments in the body, the initial distribution (as observed shortly after injection) is proportional to the distribution of blood flow to the various organs and tissues (Sapirstein, 1956). However, the brain is an important exception to this rule.

For any organ other than the brain, it has been observed that, after injection of the tracer, the indicator content of the organ rises rapidly to a level that remains essentially constant for an appreciable time, after which the equilibrium is disrupted and distribution proceeds toward attainment of uniform specific activity in the body. Indicating with $q(\tau)$ the indicator content of the organ during the initial equilibrium, it is observed that:

$$\frac{q(\tau)}{f} = \frac{Q(o)}{F} \tag{50}$$

Then, recalling the earlier statement:

$$\frac{Q(o)}{F} = \int_0^\infty C_o(t)dt \tag{10}$$

equation 50 would seem to indicate 100 per cent extraction of the indicator by the organ during the first transit. If $q(\tau)$ could be measured, the flow f could be obtained as:

$$f = \frac{q(\tau)}{\int_0^\infty C_o(t)dt} \tag{51}$$

The validity of equation 51 does not result, however, from the complete extraction of the indicator during the first transit, since this has been shown not to occur. The validity of equation 51 derives from the fact that during the initial circulations of the indicator through most organs, these organs extract the *same* fraction of the inflowing indicator. As a result, the integrals of the concentrations of the outflowing indicator from various organs are quite similar to each other and to the integral of indicator concentration in mixed venous blood.

Since there is no appreciable loss of indicator in the pulmonary circulation, every indicator transit through an organ after the first transit will bring back to the organ an amount of indicator similar to the amount that left the organ during the preceding transit. Because the potassium pool in the organs is extremely large in comparison to the plasma potassium, diffusion of indicator back from organ to blood occurs at a negligible rate during this phase, and extraction continues. If one assumes an infinitely large potassium pool in the perfused organs, *at the end of a few successive transits, each organ would contain an amount of indicator proportional to its blood flow, whereas no indicator would be left in the blood.* In other words, the system would behave as if the entire amount of indicator that entered with the first transit had been extracted (Sapirstein, 1958).

Actually, however, such a situation is not strictly true to life, because not all organs behave similarly (the brain, which has a low potassium content, diffuses the indicator back to the blood very quickly) and the potassium pool in organs is finite, and therefore the indicator slowly diffuses back into the blood. However, the fraction of total flow going to organs that deviate from the ideal activity (such as the brain) is sufficiently small, and the rate at which indicator is returned from the other organs to the blood is sufficiently slow, that the method can be used effectively if measurements are made within the proper periods of time.

This method has been used successfully to measure regional blood flow in animals and man. Its particular value for testing certain regions, such as the myocardium, derives from the fact that both terms of equation 51 can be assessed by external counting (Donato et al., 1964a).

Special Forms of the Frequency Functions of Transit Times. In the preceding paragraphs, no assumptions have been made concerning the analytical form of the frequency function of transit times of the systems studied. In some instances, however, the transfer function has a definite analytical form; this is an important advantage in hemodynamic studies, not only because the information about the system is increased but also because other approaches become available for estimating the hemodynamic parameters.

The most important type of frequency function is the exponential function, in which:

$$h(t) = ke^{-kt} \tag{52}$$

where k is a constant equal to the flow-volume ratio of the system, or the reciprocal of the turnover time. This is easily demonstrated by introducing ke^{-kt} into equation (4), thus:

$$\int_0^\infty t[ke^{-kt}]dt = \frac{1}{k} \tag{53}$$

Since this integral equals the volume-flow ratio of the system, we can write:

$$k = F/V \tag{54}$$

When the exponential transfer function is introduced into equation 17, one obtains:

$$Q'(t) = -(F/V) Q(o) e^{-(F/V)t} \tag{55}$$

whence, integrating:

$$Q(t) = Q(o) e^{-(F/V)t} \tag{56}$$

Taking the natural logarithm of equation 56 and solving for F/V, we get:

$$-\ln\left(\frac{Q(t)}{Q(o)}\right)/t = F/V \tag{57}$$

i.e., the logarithm of the indicator content in the system decays linearly, and the slope per unit time equals the flow-volume ratio.[4]

It is important to consider some significant implications of exponential frequency functions. By combining equations 55 and 56 we get:

$$Q'(t) = -(F/V)Q(t) \tag{58}$$

i.e., the amount of indicator leaving the system at any time is a constant fraction of the amount in the system.

Further, since:

$$Q'(t) = -FC_o(t) \tag{7}$$

equating equation 7 with 58 and solving for $C_o(t)$, the result is:

$$C_o(t) = \frac{Q(t)}{V} \tag{59}$$

i.e., the outflowing concentration is constantly equilibrated with the concentration in the system. Dividing both terms of equation 56 by the volume of the system, then substituting from equation 59 and solving for F/V, we get:

$$-\ln\left(\frac{C_o(t)}{C_o(o)}\right)/t = F/V \tag{60}$$

---

[4] When $Q(t)/Q(o) = 0.5$ equation 57 takes the well known form: $0.693/t_{1/2} = F/V$, where $t_{1/2}$ is the half-time of the indicator content of the system.

which is similar to equation 57, showing that F/V can be calculated from the rate of decrease of the outflowing concentration, as well as from the rate of decrease of the indicator content of the system.

The advantages of this type of approach stem from the fact that one need not obtain the entire concentration or residual-amount curve, from 0 to infinity, but only for a time interval long enough to permit the measurement of the slope with the required precision. The validity of this approach depends on the assumption that the outflowing concentration equals the mean concentration of the indicator in the system.

Exponential Washout from Well Mixed Chambers. The washout of a nondiffusible indicator from a system in which adequate mixing insures uniform distribution of the indicator within the system can be described by a single exponential equation representing the first transit of the indicator.

The washout of an indicator injected into one of the ventricles of the heart is a good approximation of the situation. The concentration curve at the outflow of the ventricle can be assumed to be representative of the concentration curve within the ventricle, with a constant fraction of the residual indicator in the chamber being ejected at each cycle. The slope k of the resulting exponential curve yields the flow-volume ratio in the ventricle. The discontinuity of ventricular emptying does not affect the validity of this procedure.[5]

Exponential Clearance from a Homogeneously Perfused Tissue. The clearance of a diffusible indicator from a homogeneously perfused tissue, in which instantaneous diffusion equilibrium can be assumed to occur between blood and tissue, takes place according to a single exponential frequency function.

The clearance of an indicator injected subcutaneously is an example. Indicating with ϕ_i/v_i the flow-volume ratio in a volume v_i of the system, and assuming the diffusion equilibrium between blood and tissue to be instantaneous, in every volume v_i the indicator content will decrease according to equation:

$$q_i(t) = q_i(o)e^{-(\phi_i/v_i)t} \tag{65}$$

The total amount of indicator in the system will be:

$$Q(t) = \sum_{o}^{n} q_i(o)e^{-(\phi_i/v_i)t} \tag{66}$$

If the tissue is homogeneously perfused, ϕ_i/v_i is the same throughout the system, and:

---

[5]In fact, the residual amount of the indicator in the ventricle after the nth ejection is:

$$Q_n = Q(o)(1 - r)^n \tag{61}$$

where r is the rate of emptying of the ventricle, or the ratio of stroke volume to end-diastolic volume. Logarithmic transformation of equation 61 yields:

$$\ln[Q_n/Q(o)] = n[\ln(1 - r)] \tag{62}$$

which shows that the ln of residual indicator decreases linearly, as a function of n with a slope equal to ln (1−r). The washout curve can be interpolated by a continuous function:

$$Q(t) = Q(o)e^{-kt} \tag{63}$$

where

$$k = \ln(1 - r)\frac{n}{t} \tag{64}$$

$$\phi_i/v_i = F/V \tag{67}$$

Since:

$$\sum_{o}^{n} q_i(o) = Q(o) \tag{68}$$

it is readily seen that equation 66 reduces to equation 56, and F/V can be obtained from the log plot of the indicator content or the concentration at the outflow tract (Kety, 1949).

It is important to point out that, if perfusion is truly uniform, the entire first transit of the indicator should decay with a single exponential slope. The use of this kind of analysis when only a part of the first transit has been measured is open to criticism. One should always be alert to the possibility that the single exponential clearance may not be real but only apparent, or it may not appear in the observed part of the curve.

Indicator Transit from Tissues Perfused Nonhomogeneously. The exponential analysis of the curves for first transit of indicator may also yield useful information in the case of nonhomogeneously perfused tissue if every component behaves as in equation 65; i.e., venous blood from any volume v_i contains indicator at a concentration $q_i(t)/v_i$. In this case the indicator content of the system and the concentration in the outflow tract will decrease at a progressively slowing rate, as a result of the increasing contribution of the lower values of ϕ_i/v_i as time elapses.

ZERO TIME TANGENT. The change in the indicator content of the system is obtained by taking the first derivative of equation 66; thus:

$$Q'(t) = -\sum q_i(o) \frac{\phi_i}{v_i} e^{-(\phi_1/v_1)t} \tag{69}$$

If the concentration in the tissue at time 0 is the same for all the tissue components, every $q_i(o)$ can be written as: $q_i(o) = C(o)v_i$. Then equation 69 at time 0 becomes:

$$Q'(o) = -C(o) \sum v_i \left(\frac{\phi_i}{v_i}\right) \tag{70}$$

whence, since $C(o) = Q(o)/V$, we may write:

$$Q'(o) = -(F/V)Q(o) \tag{71}$$

and

$$\frac{Q'(o)}{Q(o)} = -F/V \tag{72}$$

which is similar to equation 58. The difference is that, whereas in equation 58 F/V represents the slope at which the indicator is cleared from the system at any time t, in the present case F/V is only the initial slope of the indicator transit, and can be obtained by drawing a tangent to the indicator curve at time 0 (Lassen and Ingvar, 1961).

The flow-volume ratio of the system can be obtained from the mean concentration of the indicator in the system, as can be shown upon dividing both terms of equation 72 by V. This approach, although sound in principle, may be uncertain in application because of the frequent occurrence of differences in the interval between time 0 and the time of maximal downslope in the experimental curves; also, it may be difficult to obtain a uniform initial concentration in non-homogeneously perfused tissues. This uniformity can be approximated (for example, in the brain) by infusing a diffusible gas, such as ^{133}Xe, into an afferent artery for a period sufficiently long to approach equilibration of the gas with the various tissues, followed by sudden cessation of the infusion. The negligible degree of recirculation of the gas, as a result of its rapid clearance from the lung, simplifies measurement of the slope (Lassen and Ingvar, 1961).

It is important to point out that under these conditions the outflow concentration curve does not give the same information as the residual indicator curve, although the initial concentration at the outflow tract is the same as C(o), because of the uniform initial concentration throughout the entire system. The outflowing concentration is obtained from equation 69, keeping in mind the fact that $Q'(t) = - FC_o(t)$. Therefore:

$$C_o(t) = \frac{C_o}{F} \sum \phi_i e^{-(\phi_i/v_i)t} \tag{73}$$

The initial slope will then be:

$$\frac{C'_o(o)}{C(o)} = - \sum \frac{\phi_i}{F} \left(\frac{\phi_i}{v_i} \right) \tag{74}$$

It is evident that equation 74 approximates equation 72 only if ϕ_i/v_i is constant and therefore equal to F/V, as in the case of a homogeneously perfused tissue.[6]

MULTIEXPONENTIAL ANALYSIS. Indicator transit in nonhomogeneously perfused tissues can frequently be described analytically as the sum of several exponential terms. This requires the entire curve or, as is frequently the case, the assumption that the last observed rate of disappearance of the indicator from the region, or the concentration in the outflow tract, adequately describes the subsequent unknown parts of the transit. "Peeling off" exponentials from such a curve is a simple and variably accurate procedure, its accuracy depending on the scatter of the experimental points. Description of the curve as a sum of exponentials may simplify the calculation of flow and flow-volume ratios by means of the methods reported in the previous sections. Thus, if the curves for outflow concentration are described as:

$$C_o(t) = \sum a_i e^{-b_i t} \tag{75}$$

where a_i and b_i are the intercepts and slopes of the individual exponential terms, we have:

$$\int_0^\infty C_o(t)dt = - \sum \frac{a_i}{b_i} \tag{76}$$

---

[6] It is of interest to point out the difference between the initial slope of the mean concentration curve and that of the outflowing concentration curve. For the mean concentration, from equation 70 one may write:

$$\frac{c_m(o)}{C(o)} = \sum \frac{v_i}{V} \left(\frac{\phi_i}{v_i} \right) \tag{70.1}$$

which indicates that in this case the individual flows (ϕ_i/v_i) are weighted by the corresponding relative volume, whereas in the case of equation 74 they are weighted by the corresponding relative flow.

and

$$\int_0^\infty tC_o(t)dt = \sum \frac{a_i}{b_i^2} \tag{77}$$

The solution may simplify the calculation of the integral expressions of equations 11, 14, 16, 24, and so forth. *It should be understood, however, that this approach simply represents a computational simplification and is not a representation of the physical parameters involved.* One must therefore avoid the temptation of trying to relate the individual exponential components, into which the curves have been resolved, to various physical components of the region.

If the indicator is injected into the inflowing artery, and if $c_i(o)$ is the mixed inflowing concentration, $\phi_i c_i(o)$ would represent the amount of indicator reaching the tissue component having flow ϕ_i and volume v_i at time 0.

With the assumption that each exponential term corresponds to a definite component of the system, the intercept and slope of every exponential term can be indicated as:

$$\left. \begin{aligned} a_i &= \phi_i c_i(o) \\ b_i &= \phi_i/v_i \end{aligned} \right\} \tag{78}$$

From equations 78 it follows that:

$$\frac{a_i}{b_i} = v_i c_i(o) \tag{79}$$

whence

$$\frac{v_n}{V} = \frac{a_n/b_n}{\sum a_i/b_i} \tag{80}$$

yields the relative volume of the nth component and

$$\frac{\phi_n}{F} = \frac{a_n}{\sum a_i} \tag{81}$$

gives the relative flow of the nth component.

It cannot be overemphasized that this sort of analysis rests entirely on the assumption that the system can be resolved into a limited number of physical components (with a homogeneous flow) that are distinct from the other components. The fact that the indicator curve can be resolved into a sum of exponential functions gives no basis for conclusions about the number of components, however, or about their relative flow and volume. In using this approach, one should make every effort to obtain as much independent information as possible regarding the physical parameters of the system under study.

METHODS BASED ON DISTRIBUTION OF THE INDICATOR AT EQUILIBRIUM

We have considered the problems involved in using techniques for the study of peripheral circulation based on the first transit of an indicator because of the difficulty of determining the amount of indicator that entered the system in the first transit. With the exception of the cases in which the uptake of ^{42}K or ^{86}Rb by the organ can be measured during the early transit equilibrium, or when the organ extracts the indicator from blood completely, direct injection of the indicator into the regional circulation to be studied is required. This is not always feasible, and it frequently presents a technical limitation.

The advantage of methods based on the first transit of the indicator is the reduction of the number of variables from three to two—i.e., the amount of indicator entering the system (or some function of that amount) and the outflowing or inflowing concentration curve. If the simplifications on which the first transit methods are based are not applicable, it becomes necessary to measure both the inflowing and outflowing concentration, as well as the indicator content of the system.

In principle, there are various ways of handling the problem: one way is to measure flow independently. In practice, however, the instances in which this can be done are few. On technical grounds, since the concentration of the outflow tract must be measured, all methods necessitate catheterization of an outflow vessel of the system under study.

Equation 1 can be directly solved for flow thus:

$$F = \frac{dq/dt}{C_i(t) - C_o(t)} \tag{82}$$

But this equation is not applicable in practice, except in the special case in which all the terms involved (dq/dt, C_i, and C_o) are constant for a given flow rate. This is the case in the direct Fick method, in which dq/dt represents the oxygen consumption per unit time, and the difference at the denominator is the arteriovenous oxygen difference. Under steady-state conditions, all terms involved are constant and can therefore be accurately measured.

For any other indicator, even if dq/dt were measurable, equation 82 would be difficult to apply because the concentration of indicator is changing in both the inflowing and outflowing blood, and even small errors in the time of measurement of the three terms could result in large errors in flow.

Equation 1 can be integrated and solved for flow, to give:

$$F = \frac{q(t)}{\int c_i(t)dt - \int c_o(t)dt} \tag{83}$$

If the indicator content and the curves for outflowing and inflowing concentration are measurable, equation 83 provides a suitable method for measurement of flow.[7]

Methods based on the attainment of equilibrium of indicator distribution in the system to be studied overcome in part the limitation that results from the impossibility of measuring $q(t)$. The methods are based on the observation of the kinetics of the indicator in the system during the entire period of time required to reach an equilibrium state in which inflowing and outflowing blood

---

[7] It is of interest to point out that, as in the first-transit methods, the ratio of the total amount of indicator that entered the system *to* the integral of the inflowing concentration yields the rate of blood flow to the system. In fact, equation 83 can be written as:

$$F = \frac{q(t) + F\int_0^t c_o(t)dt}{\int_0^t c_i(t)dt} \tag{83.1}$$

The numerator represents the amount of indicator that entered the system during the entire period, and the denominator represents the integral of the inflowing concentration.

(as well as perfused tissue) contain indicator at the same concentration.[8] It makes no difference if the process is measured in reverse—i.e., in equilibrium-to-zero concentration, rather than from zero concentration to equilibrium.

To be certain that one has attained a state of equilibrium, one can infuse at a constant rate a diffusible indicator that will be cleared from the circulation at a rate proportional to its concentration in blood. Inert gases cleared by the lungs, or indicators excreted by the kidney or the liver, can be used for this purpose—the only assumption being that they are not metabolized, so that one can safely assume that the total amount of infused indicator will ultimately leave the system. In such a case, the entire circulation can be considered as one system through which the indicator is being perfused at a constant rate, I. Equilibrium will be attained after completion of the *first transit* of the indicator through the entire circulation. Also, as in any other case of the first transit of a constantly infused indicator, the final concentration that is attained will be maximal, and will be equal to the ratio of the rate at which indicator is added to the system *to* the sum of the clearance rates of the indicator from the system. During this time, corresponding to the first transit for the entire circulation, several recirculations of the indicator will occur through peripheral vascular beds.

On the other hand, if we indicate with c_{eq} the equilibrium concentration that will be attained in blood and tissue, and with V the volume of tissue and blood in which the indicator contained in the system at equilibrium is distributed, we can write:

$$q(eq) = c(eq)V \qquad (84)$$

where $q(eq)$ represents the amount of indicator in the organ at equilibrum. Once equilibrium is attained, the concentrations in the inflowing and outflowing blood are the same as in tissue; therefore, $c(eq)$ can be estimated from the outflowing concentration, and the flow-volume ratio in the system can be obtained by rewriting equation 83 thus:

$$\frac{F}{V} = \frac{c_{eq}}{\int_0^\infty \left[c_i - c_o \right] dt} \qquad (85)$$

or, for the mean transit time:

$$T = \frac{V}{F} = \frac{\int_0^\infty \left[c_i - c_o \right] dt}{c_{eq}} \qquad (86)$$

Equations 85 and 86 both permit us to obtain hemodynamic information concerning a peripheral vascular system, without needing to measure the amount of indicator in the system itself. The so-called indirect Fick method, using inert gases or other nonmetabolized indicators, is based on equation 86. The inflowing concentration $c_i(t)$ is measured by sampling arterial blood; the outflowing concentration is measured in the venous blood from the organ, collected by catheterization (Kety and Schmidt, 1945).

The *technical requirements* for the applications of this method are, therefore: the need to sample blood from the venous outflow of the system under

---

[8]The equality of concentration in blood and tissue is subject to the restrictions resulting from differences in solubility of the indicator in the two media.

study, as well as from an artery; and the need to carry out the observation of the indicator kinetics until full equilibrium has been attained in the system.

The *main limitations* of this approach are: It does not measure absolute flow, but only the mean transit time of the system; therefore, it is usually preferable to express the results as flow per 100 g. of tissue, by equating the volume V of equation 85 to the organ mass and multiplying F/V by 100. A long period is needed for equilibration, during which it is assumed that steady-state conditions are maintained; this assumption seriously limits the possibility of repeated studies.

The *main sources of error* result from the foregoing limitations and can be summarized as the failure to attain equilibration of venous outflow concentration with the concentration in the tissue. If distribution of flow is not proportional to the distribution of mass in the organ—that is, if there are parts of the organ that receive more than their "share" of blood flow—equilibration will not be attained at the same time in all areas. This will be evidenced by the continuing rise of the venous concentrations; but the situation may not be apparent, with resultant errors. The greater the discrepancy between the fraction of blood flow and the fraction of mass, the more important will be the errors from unattained equilibration. Two extreme cases are represented by the presence of arteriovenous shunts within the circulation (zero mass per unit flow) and unperfused tissue (zero flow per unit mass). This problem has been examined in detail by Sapirstein and Ogden (1956).

It is important to realize that *any deviation from the required equilibrium state will result in overestimates of the mean flow per unit mass, from equation 85.*[9] And in the two limiting cases cited, arteriovenous shunts and unperfused tissue, the actual flow-mass value will be overestimated even after equilibrium has been effectively attained.

---

[9] This statement can be verified by introducing in equation 85 the term $C_o(t)$ in place of $c(eq)$, and by taking the first derivative of the ratio

$$c_o(t)/\int(c_i - c_o)dt \tag{87}$$

having assumed nonuniformity of the F/V ratio within the system. The first derivative is negative from time 0 to equilibrium time, when it becomes zero; consequently, calculation using the values of the ratio at any time before equilibration will yield values larger than the actual flow-volume ratio in the organ, whereas the correct value of F/V is progressively approached as equilibration time nears.

Thus, assuming constant input concentration c_i, and indicating with ϕ_i/v_i the flow-volume ratios in different parts of the organ, equilibrium state will be reached earlier in the sections with larger values of ϕ_i/v_i; in fact, $c_o(t)$ will rise as:

$$c_o(t) = c_i \int \frac{\phi_i}{F} [1 - e^{-(\phi_i/v_i)t}]dt \tag{88}$$

and the mean concentration will rise as:

$$c_m(t) = c_i \int \frac{v_i}{V} [1 - e^{-(\phi_i/v_i)t}] \tag{89}$$

Thus, c_o will equal c_m at any time only if every $v_i/V = \phi_i/F$, or if $\phi_i/v_i = F/V$. If this is not the case, $c_o(t)$ will equal $c_m(t)$ only at infinite time, when both will equal the input concentration.

At a time t, at which equilibrium is attained everywhere except in the nth section, equations 88 and 89 can be written as:

$$c_o(t) = c_i[1 - (\phi_n/F)e^{-(\phi_n/v_n)t}] \tag{88.1}$$

$$c_m(t) = c_i[1 - (v_n/V)e^{-(\phi_n/v_n)t}] \tag{89.1}$$

APPLICATIONS

Luigi Donato

Radioactive tracers are particularly useful for studies of the circulation by means of external radiation detectors. This obviates the need to obtain blood samples by means of a catheter or indwelling needle. It also permits measurement of the content of a radioactive indicator within a specific organ or vascular segment.

At the same time, the use of external detectors in studies of the circulation introduces new problems. The first problem stems from the fact that a detector directed at an organ from outside of the body can never attain true selectivity of detection. In all instances, despite collimation, the detector will measure radiations arising from areas other than the organ or tissue under investigation. The second problem is to relate the counts recorded by the external detector to the true content of the tracer in the organ under study.

Collimation and *calibration* are the two chief problems that must always be considered in the use of external counting in studies of the circulation. Although these problems apply to all external measurements, they are particularly troublesome in the case of studies of the circulation, owing to the rapid changes of distribution of the radioactivity in the body.

In this section, the technical problems of external counting of radioactive tracers in the study of the circulation will be discussed. Methods based solely on blood sampling techniques will not be considered, since they do not differ from the methods using nonradioactive indicators.

COLLIMATION

Ideal spatial selectivity can never be achieved in external counting. However, there are several ways in which we can minimize the contribution to the counting rate from organs or structures other than those of interest.

The counting rate R recorded by a collimated counter directed toward an activity containing body is

a condition in which

$$c_o(t) > c_m(t) \tag{90}$$

since

$$\phi_n/v_n < F/V \tag{91}$$

whence

$$\phi_n/F < v_n/V \tag{92}$$

The sign of the first derivative of the ratio in equation 87 is determined in this condition by the ratio:

$$\sum_{o}^{n-1} \left[\frac{\phi_n/v_n}{\phi_i/v_i} - 1 \right] \tag{93}$$

which is obviously negative, since ϕ_n/v_n is by definition smaller than any other ϕ_i/v_i.

$$R = K \int_V c(v)\, g(v)\, T(v)\, dv \qquad (94)$$

where: K = a coefficient depending on the characteristics of the radioisotope
and detector used;

V = the volume of tissues which contributes to the counting rate;

$c(v)$ = the concentration of radioactivity at any point in V;

$g(v)$ = the geometrical efficiency, i.e., the fraction of the primary radiations
emitted from any point in V in the direction of the crystal;

$T(v)$ = the overall transmission coefficient for radiations emitted from any
point in V, and includes scattering towards the crystal of radiations
primarily directed elsewhere, and absorption of radiations primarily
directed toward the crystal.

Given a certain body of volume V' contained in a greater volume, the problem of reducing to a minimum the contribution to the counting rate of radiations coming from outside V' can be approached by modifying certain factors in the equation (94).

In principle, one could: (1) limit the volume contributing to the counting rate to V' (or less); (2) reduce the geometrical efficiency for the points outside V' (which is practically the same as point 1) or increase the relative count rate for points within V'; or (3) reduce the transmission from the points outside V'.

These three effects depend on collimator size and shape, on the selection of which radiations will be detected, and on analysis of pulses prior to counting.

The reduction of V can be achieved by reducing the diameter of the collimating channel, or by increasing its length, which results in a reduction of g. This may give rise to the problem of excessive reduction of the counting rate.

Scattered radiations reaching the crystal have lower energy than primary radiations. A lead filter in front of the detector reduces the scattered radiations more than the primary radiations. Pulse-height analysis has the same effect, since only pulses corresponding to the energy of the primary radiations are selected for counting.

In principle, coincidence counting of positron-emitting nuclides is the best approach to spatial selectivity (Bing et al., 1964). Unfortunately, its applications have been rather limited. Other types of collimation have also been used. Provided the γ energy of the isotope is high enough, a counting system consisting of two scintillation detectors, aligned on the same axis, with the crystals facing each other, can provide high selectivity if the two crystals are recessed to produce a cylindrical field of view. The output of the two detectors is added. This system is referred to as a twin counter system (TCS) (Donato et al., 1964a).

Thus we can see that the choice of the tracer influences the way in which one can achieve spatial localization.

None of the methods described reduce the contribution to the counting rate from tracer that is present within the field of view of the detector, but not in the volume of interest, V'.

In general, collimation is always a compromise between ideal spatial selectivity and counting efficiency; the relative importance of one or the other depends upon the particular type of measurement, and is largely a function of the relative amounts of activity in the organ of interest and in the surrounding areas at the time of the study. The route of administration of the tracer often affects the relative amounts of indicator in the organ of interest and the surrounding area.

CALIBRATION

In examining the calibration problem, i.e., the relation between $R(t)$ values obtained by the external counter and the concentration $c(t)$ or the content $Q(t)$ of the indicator in the organ of interest, we shall assume: (1) that perfect spatial selectivity has been attained, i.e., that all the radiations detected externally come from the organ of interest; and (2) that the indicator concentration in the organ is uniform. Equation (94) can be rewritten as:

$$R = K\bar{c} \int_v g(v) \, T(v) dv \tag{95}$$

Let us now indicate with $\eta(v) = Kg(v) \, T(v)$, the overall counting efficiency for radioactivity at point v, defined as the fraction of the radiations emitted from a source in v which are effectively detected as pulses.

For activity uniformly distributed in V, the average counting efficiency $\bar{\eta}$ can be defined, so that

$$R = \bar{c}(\bar{\eta}V) = \bar{c} \, W \tag{96}$$

where $W = \eta V$ is the *effective volume of counting;* it represents a virtual volume, which would be equal to V if all radiations emitted from V were detected as pulses ($\eta = 1$) (Donato et al., 1962a).

If, instead of concentration, we consider the total amount Q of indicator in V, since $Q = \bar{c}V$ we may write:

$$R = Q\eta \tag{97}$$

These last two equations define the relationship between the external counting rate due to activity in a volume V and the average concentration and total content of activity in V, respectively. Thus,

$$\frac{R}{Q} = \frac{W}{V} \tag{98}$$

i.e., the external counting rate and radioactive content of the organ are in the same proportion as the effective volume and true volume of the organ.

If it can be assumed that radioactivity outside V does not contribute to R, and if an average counting efficiency η can be considered as representative of the efficiency with which radioactivity in the organ under study is detected, equations 96 and 97 can be used to calibrate external counts in terms of radioactive concentration or content of the organ, provided η or W or both can be measured and they are representative of the system to be studied.

Whenever estimates of η or W are available, and stay constant during the entire period of the measurement (i.e., the internal distribution of activity in V does not change appreciably), external measurements can easily be converted to tracer concentrations or tracer content within the organ. Thus the principles outlined in the first section of this chapter become immediately applicable.

On the other hand, if η and W remain constant during the measurement, even if they are not known, we can take advantage of the fact that external counting data are proportional at any time to the concentration and content values, and the rate of change of R, c, and Q is the same.

In some cases, internal calibration of the system is not possible. In such cases, we often use suitable phantoms to supply the information required for calibration.

METHODS BASED ON THE FIRST TRANSIT PRINCIPLE

DIRECT INJECTION INTO THE SYSTEM UNDER STUDY

Measurement of Flow. In the case of a γ-emitting tracer, if the injection is made in such a way that the whole injectate, $Q(o)$, mixes with the entire flow to be measured, F, external counting will permit the determination of F provided that: (1) it is possible, from the external measurements, to obtain a tracing of the first passage of the indicator through the region under study (this can be any vascular network—consisting of parallel or sequential channels, or combinations of both—in which each vessel receives tracer in proportion to its blood flow); and (2) an effective counting volume W can be defined as representative of the entire curve and its value can be determined.

To understand the first condition, we should remember that the integral from zero to infinity of the concentration of an indicator in a system equals the same integral for any output vessel from the system and both equal the in-jectate-to-flow ratio, $Q(o)/F$.

If the external curve is due to activity in the entire region, it will be:

$$\int_0^\infty R(t)dt = W \int_0^\infty \bar{c}_v(t)dt \tag{99}$$

and in the case of the network:

$$\int_0^\infty R(t)dt = \sum w_i \int_0^\infty c_i(t)dt \tag{100}$$

In both cases, we may write:

$$F = \frac{Q(o)W}{\int_0^\infty R(t)dt} \tag{101}$$

where W is the effective volume of the region in the first case, and the sum of the effective volumes of each vessel in the region in the second.

In order to measure W and thus meet the second condition, we need to measure the mean concentration in the counting volume and the external counts simultaneously. Since the counting volume is more often a composite, and the concentration may be different in the various components at the same instant of time during recording of the curve, to measure the $R/\bar{c} = W$ ratio, we wait until a constant concentration is attained throughout the system. This approach is used in measuring cardiac output (radiocardiograms).

RADIOCARDIOGRAPHIC MEASUREMENT OF CARDIAC OUTPUT. The radiocardio-gram (RCG) is the curve recorded by a collimated counter, positioned over the precordium, during the passage through the heart chambers of a γ-emitting tracer injected into the venous side of the circulation (Prinzmetal et al., 1948; Waser and Hunzinger, 1948). In general, it is a double-peaked curve, the two peaks representing the passage of the tracer through the right- and left-sided chambers.[10] Veall et al., in 1954, first proposed the use of RCG for the determination of cardiac output.

Adequate mixing of the indicator occurs by the time it reaches the right ventricle. As a consequence, the precordial counting rate is:

$$\int R(t)dt = W_{RA}\int C_{RA}(t)dt + W_{RV}\int C_{RV}(t)dt + W_{LA}\int C_{LA}(t)dt + W_{LV}\int C_{LV}(t)dt \quad (102)$$

where the subscripts of the terms indicate the four heart chambers.

Addition of a fifth term, indicating the contribution of activity in the pulmonary circulation, does not affect the validity of using the area of RCG (first members of the equation) for measurement of cardiac output. When carried to infinity, all integrals of the second member are equal to $Q(o)/F$, whence

$$F = \frac{Q(o)W_T}{A_{RCG}} \quad (103)$$

where W_T is the *total effective volume*, i.e., the sum of the effective volumes of the individual chambers contributing to the curve (Donato et al., 1962a).

A_{RCG} is calculated by adding the individual R values to the time at which recirculation of indicator (i.e., its reappearance in the right-sided chambers) interrupts the downslope of the left curve of the RCG. The area is completed by semilog extrapolation beyond the point of recirculation.

The total effective volume W_T is determined by taking a precordial count and a blood sample 5 to 10 minutes after the injection. At that time, if the indicator is a nondiffusible one, such as ^{131}I HSA, its concentration is uniform throughout the circulation and the final precordial counting rate R_f is related to the blood concentration of the indicator c_f according to:

$$R_f = W_f c_f \quad (104)$$

W_f is greater than W_T, the effective volume during the RCG curve, because it includes vascular regions (e.g., vessels of the chest wall) that did not contribute to the primary curve. A simple way of approximating W_T is to take a counting rate over the thigh immediately after R_f has been taken, and use the difference of the two to determine W_T (Donato et al., 1962b). It has been repeatedly shown that W_T averages 83 per cent of W_f. The results obtained for cardiac output have been shown to compare well with both Fick and arterial dilution methods (Lewis et al., 1962; Mariani et al., 1966).

Measurement of Circulation Times, Specific Flow and Circulating Blood Volume. Under special circumstances, mean circulation times and hence their reciprocal F/V ratios (flow per unit volume) can be determined from the external record without the need of calibrating the curves (i.e., without determining W). This can be done whenever the externally recorded curves are proportional (through a W or η factor) to the concentration or residual activity curves.

This method demands first of all a high degree of spatial selectivity, so that "pure" curves are obtained, in which the contribution of the indicator from regions other than those of interest is fully excluded or accounted for. The second requirement is that the proportionality factor η or W be constant for the entire curve, i.e., that redistribution of the tracer within the region from which one is counting does not affect the external counting rate.

---

[10] The resolution of the two peaks of the RCG depends on: (1) collimation—the smaller the contribution from the lung, the better the resolution; and (2) the injection site and volume— the smaller the dilution of the injectate before it reaches the lungs, the better the resolution. The latter can be accomplished by injecting a small volume of tracer into the right ventricle.

This approach can be applied in two ways.

1. *By injecting the indicator directly into the system to be investigated and recording externally a curve proportional to the residual activity in the system, under conditions in which reappearance of the indicator into the counting field is excluded or is late enough to permit adequate description of the "pure" curve of the system.*

Under such circumstances, $R(t)$ is proportional to $Q(t)$ at all times, the initial counting level $R(o)$ is proportional to the amount of tracer injected, and the F/V ratio of the system can be obtained, according to equation 25, as:

$$\frac{F}{V} = \frac{1}{T} = \frac{R(o)}{\int_0^\infty R(t)dt} \tag{105}$$

In case of frequency functions that are exponential, it is also possible to replace R for Q in equation 57 and derive F/V from the slopes of the semilogarithmic record of the external curves.

Obviously, if only one part of the system is seen by the counter, the specific flow thus obtained refers to that volume only, and any generalization regarding the entire system makes the assumption that the flow per unit volume (F/V) is the same throughout the entire system.

2. *By injecting the indicator upstream from the system of interest, and recording externally two curves, proportional to the indicator flow into and out of the system, under conditions in which the contribution from the system itself is excluded.*

Under such circumstances, the mean transit time of the intermediate section (hence its reciprocal F/V) can be obtained as the difference of the mean circulation times of the two curves, replacing the values of the externally recorded output and input curves (R_o and R_i) for $C_B(t)$ and $C_A(t)$, respectively, in equation 16:

$$T_{B-A} = \frac{\int t R_o(t)dt}{\int R_o(t)dt} - \frac{\int t R_i(t)dt}{\int R_i(t)dt} \tag{106}$$

The first approach is the basis of techniques for measuring specific organ or tissue blood flow by direct injection of the indicator into the afferent artery or directly into a tissue mass, as well as those for measuring the volume of cardiac chambers, recording the RCG after direction injection. The second approach is the basis of methods for measuring mean pulmonary circulation time from the radiocardiogram.

Intra-arterial Injection of Radioactive Inert Gases (^{133}Xe). Radioactive xenon or krypton (^{133}Xe, ^{79}Kr, or ^{85}Kr) can be used to estimate specific flow (flow per unit mass) in various organs, by injecting the gas dissolved in solution into one of the afferent arteries to the organ and recording the passage of the indicator through the organ by means of an external counter (Zierler, 1965).

Recirculation of indicator through the organ is assumed to be negligible, since, because of its low blood-air partition coefficient, it is rapidly cleared from the circulation during its first passage through the pulmonary capillaries. Departure from this ideal condition, resulting in incomplete clearance of the indicator from the lungs, will affect the measurement by increasing the area of the curve being recorded by the detector directed at the organ. This decreases the value of specific flow calculated from equation 105 or by means of the semilogarithmic slope methods. The smaller the fraction of cardiac output that the organ receives, the smaller will be the error resulting from this recirculation of the tracer.

The assumption that the external curve is proportional to the activity within the organ is a crucial assumption, particularly when specific flow is calculated from equation 105. The collimation must be such that movement of the radioactivity tracer within the organ does not change the counting rate. For instance, if the counter includes in its field of view the afferent artery into which the injection is made, and only part of the organ under study, the initial rise of the curve to $R(o)$ would be affected, and specific flow determined from equation 105 would yield falsely high values. Despite these limitations, the method has yielded satisfactory results in the estimation of blood flow to the brain (Hoedt-Rasmussen et al., 1966), myocardium (Ross et al., 1964), kidneys (Kemp et al., 1963), and other organs.

VENTRICULAR VOLUMES. Radiocardiogram curves make possible measurement of the rate of turnover of blood (F/V) of the ventricles. We derive this from the slope k of the exponential ventricular washout curve. The method requires direct injection of the indicator into the ventricle and a high degree of collimation, so that the vascular sections immediately downstream from the ventricle are out of the field of view of the detector. Injection of small volumes of tracer into the right atrium is preferable to a ventricular injection (except for very large fibrillating hearts) because transfer of tracer from atrium to ventricle is rapid, mixing is facilitated, and the occurrence of premature beats is less likely. Measurements are usually made together with an electrocardiographic tracing, to facilitate the evaluation of the fractional drop of the counting rate with successive heart cycles. As indicated in equations 61 to 64, this fraction r (fractional rate of emptying of the ventricle) is related to the slope k of the exponential washout curve. The fraction r is the fraction of the ventricular end-diastolic volume (VDV) ejected with each beat of the heart; we can use this value to estimate both VDV and VRV (the ventricular postsystolic residual volume) if the stroke volume (SV) is also known:

$$VDV = SV/r$$
$$VRV = VDV - SV \tag{107}$$

Measurements can be made for both the right and left ventricle (Donato et al., 1962a; Folse and Braunwald, 1962).

PULMONARY BLOOD VOLUME. With the same collimation and injection technique used for determining right ventricular volumes, we can estimate mean pulmonary circulation time, T_{PC}, from RCG curves. We can calculate the pulmonary blood volume ($PVB = F \cdot T_{PC}$), if cardiac output F is measured at the same time. If the right and left curves of the radiocardiogram were truly representative of the input and output curves of the blood flow through the lungs, T_{PC} could be obtained by replacing right and left external curve values for $R_o(t)$ and $R_i(t)$, respectively, in equation 106. This assumption is not warranted, however, because the left RCG curve is proportional to the activity in the left heart, and not truly proportional to the output of tracer from the lungs. Therefore the mean circulation time of the left curve includes the mean transit time of the indicator through the left side of the heart.[11] Therefore, in order to use the two

---

[11] If only the atrium or the ventricle were seen by the detector directed toward the left heart, the mean circulation time of the left RCG curve would include the left atrium or the left atrial plus the left ventricular mean transit times, respectively. If both are seen, the mean circulation time of the curve varies between the two extremes.

RCG curves to derive information concerning the pulmonary circulation, we have to make some assumptions about the distribution of pulmonary transit time or about the size of the left heart blood volumes, or about both (Donato et al., 1964).

We use as time 0 the R wave of the first heart cycle when activity is ejected from the right ventricle (initial drop in the right RCG curve). The "mid time" method assumes that the pulmonary circulation time (T_{PC}) must be longer than the time of appearance of activity in the left heart (foot of the left curve) and shorter than its peak time; it therefore takes the average of these two values as the most probable pulmonary circulation time (Donato et al., 1962a). The "left peak" method neglects the difference between the volume of the right ventricle and the combined left heart volume (Giuntini et al., 1963). With this assumption, if there were no pulmonary circulation, the left peak time would correspond to the turnover time of the right ventricle, T_{RV}, which is the reciprocal of the down-slope of the right curve. This method assumes that the difference between actual left peak time and T_{RV} equals T_{PC}. To investigate the effect of possible deviations from the assumptions, comparisons have been made of this method and methods in which input and output concentration curves are directly obtained. These studies have all shown the method to be sufficiently reliable to be of practical clinical value (Lewis and Giuntini).

INDIRECT INJECTION OF THE INDICATOR INTO THE SYSTEM

These techniques are based on the selective extraction of the radioactive indicator by the organ under study or on the proportionality between organ blood flow and the rate of uptake of an indicator. They are particularly suited to the use of external detectors to estimate the content of radioactivity within the organ or its rate of change.

Total Extraction. The problem of spatial localization of activity during external detection is relatively easy to solve when the external detector is placed directly over the specific site of accumulation of the indicator. After the injection of the radioactive indicator, the activity tends to become progressively more concentrated in the organ of interest, whereas in the rest of the body the level of activity decreases progressively as more and more indicator is extracted by the organ. If organs other than the one of interest contribute significantly to the effective volume from which activity is being measured, the external record needs to be corrected by subtracting values obtained from a curve simultaneously recorded from a nonextracting area. This necessitates normalization of the initial values of both curves.

If the indicator is given as a single injection, a "pure" uptake curve will progressively and asymptotically rise to a maximum. A linear increase of activity is recorded if the indicator is given by continuous infusion so that a constant blood concentration is maintained after equilibration.

If after a single injection the uptake curve is followed until extraction is complete and if the effective counting volume stays constant during the entire measurement, $R(t)$ values can be introduced instead of $q(t)$ values in equation 44 and the ratio of the organ blood flow to the volume of distribution of the indicator can be obtained directly. If the volume of distribution can be estimated, organ blood flow in milliliters per minute can be obtained:

$$f = \frac{R(\infty)V_i}{\int_0^\infty [R(\infty) - R(t)]dt} \tag{108}$$

A semilog plot of $[R(\infty) - R(t)]$ results in a curve suitable for exponential analysis according to equation 57.

It is important to realize that changing the placement of the detector over differently perfused areas of the organ does not influence the flow value obtained from equation 108, provided no part of the organ becomes saturated with the indicator; in fact, the rate of uptake everywhere in the extracting organ is determined by the ratio of the total organ blood flow to the volume of the distribution of the indicator. The value for the regional perfusion is a multiple of the uptake curve, affecting its amplitude but not its time course. Thus uptake curves recorded at different sites and normalized for their asymptotic values are superposable.

The use of this approach to estimate differences in perfusion in different parts of the extracting organ is not possible unless we know the counting efficiency at the various counting sites. On the other hand, if R values can be calibrated or the counting efficiency is uniform, $R(t)$ and $R'(t)$ values may replace $q(t)$ and $q'(t)$ values in equations 38 to 40; under such conditions, by comparing $R(t)$ or $R'(t)$ values in two different extracting areas, the relative perfusion of the two areas can be obtained.

Estimates of liver blood flow, total and regional renal blood flow, and the distribution of blood flow per unit lung volume are all based on these principles.

LIVER BLOOD FLOW. Several radiocolloids are nearly completely extracted by the Kupffer cells during their passage through the liver. Gold-198 colloids (Vetter et al., 1954), iodine-131 heat-denatured albumin (Halpern et al., 1958), and other particles with suitable characteristics can be used to obtain an uptake curve by means of an external detector placed over the liver. Liver blood flow can be obtained from such a curve using equation 105 or by the slope method. In the latter, $f = (0.693/T_{1/2})V$, where V can be taken as the total blood volume and $T_{1/}$ is the time at which the uptake curve attains one half of the maximum. If extraction by the organ of interest is not complete, the flow values equal true flow multiplied by the extraction index.

RENAL BLOOD FLOW. Hippuran-131 is nearly completely extracted by the kidneys and its renal clearance can be used to measure renal blood flow. Classic clearance methods, based on equation 35, relate the amount of indicator excreted during a certain time to the mean blood concentration during that time; they can be simplified by measuring the increment of the counting rate over the bladder rather than collecting the urine by means of a catheter (Bianchi and Toni, 1963). Blood activity contributes very little to the measurement of the external counting rate if the increment in bladder activity is measured some time after injection. Subtraction of the counting rate at the beginning of the clearance period is used to correct for activity present in the bladder at the start and for the contribution from surrounding tissues. Calibration of the counting rate in the bladder is required in order to relate excreted activity to blood concentration, as indicated in equation 35. This is obtained by having the patient urinate and measuring the eliminated activity $\Delta X(t)$ and the corresponding drop of counting rate over the bladder $\Delta R(t)$. The relation

$$\Delta R(t) = \bar{\eta}\Delta X(t) \tag{109}$$

permits us to obtain $\bar{\eta}$, which may then be used to obtain q from R and calculate flow from equation 35. With special wide-angle collimators, external counting rate is linearly related to the content of radioactivity within the bladder up to volumes of 200 to 300 ml.

The same method can be used to obtain blood flow of one kidney if the measurement of bladder activity is performed while the urine flow into the bladder from the other kidney is obstructed by means of a compressing wedge. Alternate compression and release on both sides in successive clearance periods permits the estimate of the blood flow of each kidney (Bianchi et al., 1967).

DISTRIBUTION OF REGIONAL LUNG PERFUSION.[12]   Both ^{133}Xe dissolved in saline and radioactive particles, such as heat-denatured macroaggregates of human serum albumin, labeled with ^{131}I (MAA ^{131}I) when injected intravenously mix with the cardiac output and are distributed to different lung regions in proportion to their blood flow. The two agents differ in that most of the radioactive gas passes in the alveolar space of the lungs during the first circulation through the pulmonary capillaries whereas the radioactive particles are retained in the pulmonary microcirculation for an appreciable length of time. External counting over different lung zones (during breath-holding immediately after injection of the gas, and before metabolism of the particles) yields counting rates proportional to regional perfusion and effective volume being viewed by the detector. The following equation describes the principles of the method:

$$R_{(inj)i} = \frac{f_i}{v_i} \left(\frac{Q(o)}{F} \right) w_i \tag{110}$$

where f_i v_i is the perfusion per unit lung volume in the ith zone, and w_i is the $(Q(o)/F)$ is corresponding effective volume; the ratio injectate to cardiac output is a normalization factor that is constant throughout the lung.

In the case of ^{133}Xe (Ball et al., 1962; West, 1962), the readings over the various zones after injection can be calibrated by measuring the counting rates over the same areas after rebreathing ^{133}Xe from a spirometer until equilibration is attained throughout the lung. The counting rate will be:

$$R_{(eq)i} = c_s w_i \tag{111}$$

where c_s is the final concentration in the spirometer.

The ratio ρ_i of R_{inj} and R_{eq} in corresponding areas is therefore:

$$\rho_i = \frac{R_{inj}}{R_{eq}} = \frac{f_i}{v_i} H \tag{112}$$

where H is a normalization factor that is constant throughout the lung and which can be determined if $Q(o)$, F, and c_s are measured. In any case, the distribution of ρ values over different lung areas can be used as an index of perfusion per unit lung volume. Radioactivity in the chest wall is a source of error with the xenon method.

In the case of MAA ^{131}I (Taplin et al., 1964; Wagner et al., 1964), integration of area or profile scans over symmetrical regions of the two lungs gives data that may be used for comparing relative perfusions, under the assumption that differences in counting efficiency can be neglected. Both methods have proved valuable in physiological and clinical studies.

---

[12]Despite the fact that the injectate mixes with the entire pulmonary blood flow, these methods are classified with those based on indirect injection of the indicator since the aim is measurement of regional and not total lung flow. Other similarities with the methods outlined in this section should be noted.

Organ Uptake Proportional to Blood Flow. The use of external counting to estimate the fraction of the cardiac output perfusing an organ from the fraction of the injectate taken up by the organ during the initial distribution of rubidium-86, potassium-42, or other types of indicator poses important problems from the point of view of both collimation and calibration of the measurement.

From equation 50 it is seen that for external counting to be used successfully to measure blood flow, it is necessary that:

$$\frac{R(\tau)}{R(o)} = \frac{q(\tau)}{Q(o)} = \frac{f}{F} \tag{113}$$

i.e., uptake of indicator $q(\tau)$ and injectate dose $Q(o)$ should be measured with the same counting efficiency $\bar{\eta}$. This implies that: (1) no activity except that taken up by the organ contributes to $R(\tau)$; (2) all the activity in the organ contributes externally detectable counts with the same counting efficiency; and (3) the external counts corresponding to Q_o are measured with the same counting efficiency with which the uptake is measured.

These problems require attention to collimation to achieve selective spatial localization, which is particularly important since we often wish to obtain the flow of the entire organ and not just part of it, and attention to calibration, since measuring the injectate and uptake with the same counting efficiency makes it necessary to determine $\bar{\eta}$. A further complication, from the point of view of spatial selectivity, is the possibility that a significant amount of tracer may remain in the circulating blood at the time when uptake is measured.

CORONARY BLOOD FLOW BY SINGLE INJECTION OF RUBIDIUM OR POTASSIUM. The use of external counting for the measurement of coronary blood flow in man by the single injection of radioactive rubidium requires a counting system that affords counting of the activity of the entire mass of the heart with the same efficiency. It also requires a method of subtracting the external counts and the contribution of radioactivity within the heart chambers at the time of the measurement.

The first requirement is met by using coincidence counting of the positron-emitter [84]Rb; the same arrangement of detectors can also be used for ^{86}Rb or [42]K. Two identical opposing detectors are sometimes referred to as a twin counter system (TCS). In order to encompass all the heart, the placement of the TCS with respect to the patient's chest should be determined by fluoroscopy or x-ray. Activity in the chest wall and lungs contributes little to the external counts, because of their low flow per unit volume, which results in little uptake of tracer per unit mass. On the other hand, activity in the heart chambers is not negligible; it can be corrected for by injecting simultaneously a nondiffusible tracer such as ^{131}I human serum albumin and measuring both external and arterial blood counts of the two isotopes at the same time, with a two-channel spectrometer. The contribution of the chambers themselves can then be subtracted. The effective volume of circulating blood W can be determined from the external and blood counts of the nondiffusible tracer. From this value and the arterial concentration of ^{86}Rb, the contribution of intravascular tracer that is to be subtracted from the external counts can be obtained, provided the difference in counting efficiency for the two radionuclides in both the well detector and the external detection system are considered.

An estimate of the relative efficiency for the two tracers can be made with a plastic phantom, the thickness of which can be varied to match the chest diameter. The same phantom is used to obtain R(o), by counting the injectate under the same conditions as the uptake measurement (Donato et al., 1964a, 1966; Chwojnik et al., 1966).

INHALATION OF RADIOACTIVE GASES

The main limitation of this group of techniques is the lack of methods for measuring the indicator content of the organ under study. Thus we can obtain only the blood flow per unit volume, and even this measurement requires that an equilibrium distribution of the tracer be achieved so that the tissue concentration may be assumed to be equal to both arterial and venous concentrations.

External counting of gamma-emitting nuclides makes it possible to overcome these limitations, since we can estimate the radioactive content of the organ under study or its rate of change during or after inhalation of radioactive inert gases, such as ^{79}Kr or ^{133}Xe.

Compared to the methods in which the same tracers are given in the form of a direct injection into the organ or into its afferent artery, gas inhalation methods present some special problems of collimation. The indicator is no longer selectively distributed in the organ of interest, but is also in other perfused structures within the counting field. This often affects the estimate of the radioactive content of the organ or its rate of change.

Calibration of the external measurement is required if we wish to calculate flow from equations 82 or 83; it can be determined with the aid of a phantom.

In practice, this approach has been used only for estimates of cerebral blood flow using ^{79}Kr.

CEREBRAL BLOOD FLOW BY DIRECT FICK USING ^{79}Kr

Equation 82 has been used for the measurement of cerebral blood flow with inhalation of ^{79}Kr, continuous measurement of arterial and venous concentrations by repeated sampling, and external counting to estimate the amount of indicator in the brain (Lewis et al., 1960). A cylindrical counter is designed to exclude as much as possible of the contribution from tissues other than the brain. Calibration is performed by counting a known quantity of the radioactive tracer in a plastic phantom of the skull placed in front of the counter. One of the potentially most valuable uses of this approach, which justifies its complexity, is to monitor continuously circulatory changes in the brain. We must assume, however, that changes in external counting rate reflect only changes in the radioactive content of the organ and not changes in the internal distribution of the tracer. The latter could cause variations in the efficiency with which the same amount of indicator is detected by the external counter.

BRAIN CLEARANCE OF INHALED ^{133}Xe

A simple method of assessing the regional cerebral blood flow by external counting is the inhalation of ^{133}Xe for a period sufficiently long to attain an essentially steady level of counting over the brain. The xenon administration is then stopped abruptly and the radioactive gas is rapidly exhaled. Arterial concentration falls very rapidly. The method assumes that no recirculation of ^{133}Xe occurs, and that the external record reflects only the rate of washout of activity from the brain (Mallett and Veall, 1965).

Under the assumption that uniform distribution of the indicator has been attained in the various tissue components, the tangent at the time 0 of the curve of equation 72 can be used for determining the blood flow.

The flow value represents blood flow to the mass of brain viewed by the detector and measurements may be made simultaneously over different areas for purposes of comparison.

The method is valuable because of its simplicity and because errors due to interference from activity in other tissues are not a problem.

DELINEATION OF BLOOD POOLS

RICHARD A. HOLMES
HENRY N. WAGNER, JR.

THE HEART

The density of blood is similar to that of most soft tissues, so that x-rays are often ineffective in delineating the size and shape of blood pools. Injection of radiopaque contrast media helps to outline the intracardiac blood pool (Robb and Steinberg, 1939a, b). Rejali, MacIntyre, and Friedell (1958) first suggested the use of radioisotope scanning in the diagnosis of pericardial effusion. By comparing the scanning image of the distribution of ^{131}I-labeled human serum albumin with the radiographic image of the heart, they were able to detect the presence of pericardial fluid. Although the effusion had the same radiographic density as the heart muscle and intracardiac blood, it appeared as a zone of decreased concentration of radioactivity in the scanning image. Using a special radiographic procedure that minimized magnification of the radiographic image of the heart, Wagner et al. (1961) found the method useful in the diagnosis of 40 patients with suspected pericardial disease. The criteria used to diagnose pericardial effusion were: (1) a discrepancy between the transverse diameter of the radiographic image of the heart and the image of the distribution of radioactive albumin (or other radioactive agents that are retained in the cardiac blood pool during the study); (2) a reduction in the absolute diameter of the scanning image of the cardiac blood pool (in contrast to that observed with hypertrophy or dilatation); and (3) a greater than normal zone of decreased activity between the heart and the liver, corresponding to the decreased radioactivity in the pericardial fluid. The test was quite specific, but a few other diseases produced the image characteristic of an effusion. These included amyloidosis of the heart and fibrous constrictive pericarditis. On the other hand, the test was insensitive since only large effusions could be detected. Bonte and his associates (1962) studied phantoms made of balloons immersed in water and were unable to detect effusions of less than 200 ml. Charkes and Sklaroff (1963) reported similar limitations in the sensitivity of the method. In studies of patients who were operated upon shortly after the scanning procedure, they were consistently able to detect effusions only when they were greater than 200 ml.

The use of Cholografin labeled with ^{131}I, which was slowly extracted by the liver, decreased the radiation dose below that received from ^{131}I albumin, but did

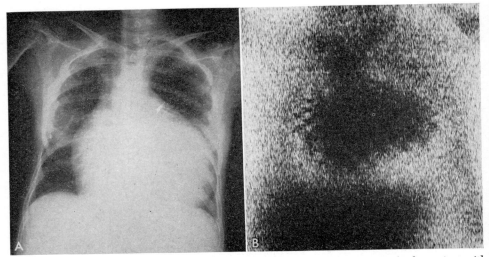

FIGURES 11-1 and 11-2.   Chest radiograph and heart scan (indium-113m) of a patient with tetralogy of Fallot and pericardial effusion.

not improve the quality of the images. The number of emitted photons remained quite low (MacIntyre et al., 1963; Sklaroff et al., 1964).

The radionuclide technetium-99m was introduced into clinical use by Harper et al. (1964). Shortly thereafter, McAfee et al. (1964) labeled human serum albumin with this nuclide to increase the photon yield in cardiac and other blood-pool scanning. Bonte and Curry (1965, 1966) used ^{99m}Tc albumin to determine whether mediastinal masses were vascular, as well as to diagnose pericardial effusion. Holmes et al. (1966) found that this radiopharmaceutical not only improved the sensitivity of the method in the diagnosis of pericardial effusion, but also often gave greatly improved images of the structure of the heart. The method could be applied to the diagnosis of pericardial effusion and used in other cardiac diseases. For example, left ventricular hypertrophy, enlargement of the left atrial appendage, and giant left atrium could easily be recognized in patients with rheumatic disease of the mitral valve.

More recently, scintillation cameras have been used to obtain images of blood pools. Technetium-99m pertechnetate has been used (Rosenthal, 1966), and Stern et al. (1967) have recently used carrier-free indium-113m, which can be injected in a form that is bound to a plasma transferrin, which remains in the vascular space for sufficiently long periods to permit detailed studies of the size and shape of vascular pools. Figures 11-1 and 11-2 show a cardiac scan performed with [113m]In transferrin.

CLINICAL USES

CARDIAC DILATATION

One of the early signs of heart failure is dilatation of the heart, which may result from structural lesions within the heart or disease of the cardiac muscle. Intracardiac volume during diastole is closely related to the degree of heart failure and impairment of cardiac output. It produces the characteristic blood-pool image illustrated in Figure 11-3. Delineation of individual cardiac chambers is often difficult with single-plane scanning of the distribution of radioactivity, which gives a two-dimensional representation of a three-dimensional distribution of activity.

CARDIAC HYPERTROPHY

As the result of an increased work load, the muscles of the heart hypertrophy from enlargement of individual muscle fibers. Premortem diagnosis of hypertrophy is difficult, because the radiographic images of dilatation and hypertrophy are usually indistinguishable. Hypertrophy can be established at autopsy from measurements of the thickness of the walls of the cardiac chambers, from histological evaluation of the size of the individual muscle fibers, and from the gross weight of the heart. A hypertrophied heart in an adult is defined as one weighing more than 400 g. in a male or more than 375 g. in a female (Friedberg, 1966).

The detection of hypertrophy of specific chambers of the heart is helpful

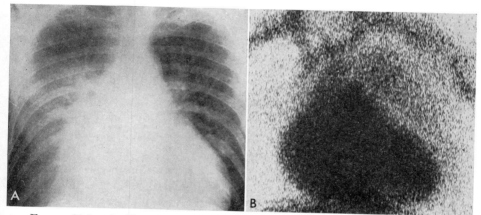

FIGURE 11-3. *A,* Chest radiograph showing cardiac enlargement and an infiltrate in the middle of the right lung. *B,* Heart scan (technetium-99m albumin) of the same patient. The scan reveals a decrease in the radioactivity at the right hilus as well as cardiac dilatation.

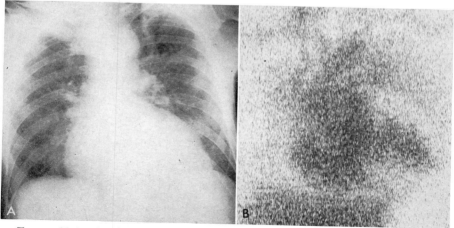

FIGURE 11-4. *A,* Chest radiograph and *B,* heart scan in a patient with hypertension and left ventricular hypertrophy. The cardiac muscle is relatively avascular compared to the intracavitary blood pool.

in diagnosis, since specific diseases often result in characteristic patterns of hypertrophy. The hypertrophied heart may be able to maintain cardiac output at adequate levels so that functional impairment is slight. Thus, the diagnosis of compensatory hypertrophy may be of value in the early diagnosis of heart disease, before it has reached the more advanced, functionally decompensated stage.

The scanning image of the hypertrophied heart is characterized by a slightly lower concentration of activity in the muscle than within the cardiac chambers (Rejali et al., 1958; Holmes et al., 1966). An example is illustrated in Figure 11-4. This distinction between the intracardiac blood pool and cardiac muscle is possible only with the improved photon yields obtainable from millicurie doses of short-lived radiopharmaceuticals. One distinguishing feature of hypertrophy as compared to dilatation is that the strong contractions of the hypertrophied heart can at times be distinguished from the weak contractions of the dilated heart. The strong contractions of the hypertrophied heart can occasionally be seen as multiple serrations in the scanning image.

PERICARDIAL EFFUSION

The pericardium is thought to aid in distributing evenly the pressures associated with cardiac contraction. Its inner surface produces a serous secretion. Inflammation of either the parietal or visceral pericardium may result from infection or other diseases listed in Table 11-1. Effusion may or may not accompany inflammation of the pericardium. At times, pericarditis may result in symptoms and signs that escape detection during life. The condition is often unexpectedly found at autopsy (4 to 10 per cent of all autopsies).

If a large effusion develops, compression of the heart may decrease cardiac output and lead to symptoms of heart failure. If an effusion reaches a critical amount, a condition known as cardiac tamponade results. This is characterized by systemic hypotension, reduced pulse pressures, and elevated venous pressure.

The electrocardiogram is a sensitive and relatively specific test for acute

TABLE 11-1. CAUSES OF PERICARDIAL DISEASE

  1. Idiopathic (acute benign) pericarditis
  2. Infectious pericarditis
     a. Suppurative bacterial pericarditis (staphylococcus, streptococcus, pneumococcus)
     b. Viral pericarditis (varicella, Coxsackie virus)
     c. Tuberculous percarditis
     d. Fungal pericarditis (actinomycosis, histoplasmosis, aspergillosis)
     e. Other infections (parasitic disease—echinococcus and cysticercus, syphilitic gummatous pericarditis, toxoplasmosis)
  3. Rheumatic pericarditis
  4. Uremic pericarditis
  5. Pericarditis with myocardial infarction; postmyocardial infarction syndrome
  6. Collagen disease pericarditis
     a. Pericarditis in rheumatoid arthritis
     b. Pericarditis in polyarteritis nodosa
     c. Pericarditis in Libman-Sacks disease (systemic lupus erythematosus)
  7. Postpericardiatomy syndrome
  8. Traumatic and post-traumatic pericarditis
  9. Radiation pericarditis
 10. Neoplastic pericarditis

pericarditis, and may indicate the diagnosis in patients with a normal chest radiograph and heart scan.

One of the characteristics of pericardial effusion in serial chest radiographs is progressive enlargement of the cardiac image without evidence of congestion of the lungs. If the enlargement is the result of sudden cardiac dilatation, the associated heart failure often results in detectable pulmonary congestion. The most conclusive evidence of pericardial effusion is aspiration of fluid with a needle, together with a radiograph of the chest after injection of air equal in volume to about one half the amount of air removed. This will usually produce a characteristic fluid level and the pericardial membrane itself can be seen above the level of the fluid (Fig. 11-5). The aspiration procedure is not completely innocuous, however, particularly in the presence of myocardial disease that may have precipitated the cardiac dilatation. If the fluid is loculated, the needle may miss it. Failure to obtain fluid is not absolute evidence of the absence of a pericardial effusion.

The diagnosis of a pericardial effusion is even more difficult if pleural effusion is also present. Thus, the diagnosis of pericardial effusion is often suspected from the chest radiograph but the image is not sufficiently characteristic to permit the diagnosis with a sufficient degree of certainty. Therefore, ancillary procedures must be used to confirm or refute the diagnosis. These include cinefluoroscopy, fluoroscopy, angiocardiography, radiography after intravenous injection of carbon dioxide (Stauffer et al., 1960), and, more recently, ultrasound cardiography (Feigenbaum et al., 1965).

Radioisotope scanning is helpful, and has the important advantage that the procedure is harmless and easy to perform. The main problem is that small effusions cannot be detected with present techniques. On the other hand, if the ratio of the scanning image of the cardiac blood pool is less than 80 per cent of the image of the heart in the chest radiograph (taken with care to minimize magnification of the cardiac image), and if there is a zone of decreased radioactivity separating the cardiac blood pool from the liver and lung fields, the diagnosis can be made (Fig. 11-6). Other characteristics of a large pericardial effusion are elevation of the hilar vessels of the lung and a typical halo of decreased activity surrounding the blood pool.

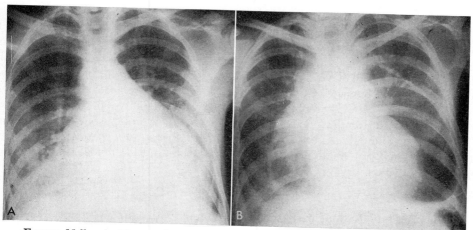

FIGURE 11-5. *A,* Chest radiograph before and *B,* after pericardiocentesis in a patient with uremia and pericardial effusion. Air was injected into the pericardial sac.

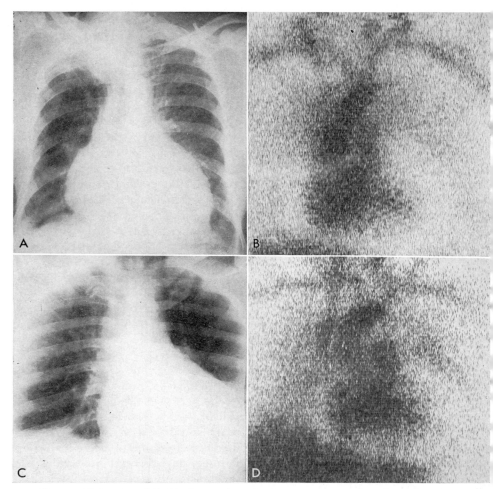

FIGURE 11-6.   A and B, The large relatively clear area surrounding the cardiac blood pool is diagnostic of a pericardial effusion. C and D, A myxedematous patient with clinical signs of pericardial disease. The "halo" of diminished activity surrounding the heart is the result of a pericardial effusion.

Loculated pericardial effusions (Fig. 11-7), intracardiac tumors (Fig. 11-8) (Bonte and Curry, 1967), and pericardial cysts also appear on the scan as localized areas of decreased activity within or next to the cardiac blood pool. Usually these do not have the same configuration as an effusion, but rather displace the intravascular pool to one side.

The heart scan usually appears normal in constrictive pericarditis unless there is great thickening of the pericardium or epicardium. An example is the patient with tuberculous pericarditis who eventually required pericardial surgery (Fig. 11-9), in whom angiocardiography with carbon dioxide revealed a thickened fibrous epicarditis.

MYOCARDIAL DISEASE

Figure 11-10 is the heart scan of a patient with chronic congestive heart failure and cardiomegaly due to idiopathic cardiomyopathy. The left oblique view demonstrates the thickened interventricular septum, which separates the right and left ventricular cavities. This can be demonstrated by angiography only if the contrast medium is injected simultaneously into both ventricular cavities.

ACQUIRED VALVULAR DISEASE

In advanced mitral insufficiency, the cardiac scan often has a characteristic pattern as a result of the giant left atrium and large auricular appendage (Fig. 11-11). Left ventricular enlargement also can be seen.

Aortic valvular disease leads to enlargement of the left ventricular blood pool and thickening of the muscle. In some cases of muscular subaortic stenosis, the ventricular blood pool is comparatively small, reflecting the rapid emptying.

A nonspecific cardiac scan pattern is seen in tricuspid valvular disease because of the superimposition of the involved heart chambers on the frontal plane view; however, in tricuspid insufficiency there is a suggestion of right atrial enlargement, but the pattern is much less characteristic that that of left atrial enlargement.

Pulmonic valvular disease, whether it be stenosis or insufficiency, often leads to dilatation of the main pulmonary artery and is easily seen on the heart scan (Fig. 11-12). Poststenotic dilatation is usually the result of congenital, rather than acquired, heart disease.

CONGENITAL HEART DISEASE

Congenital heart diseases are divided into cyanotic and acyanotic types (Table 11-2). The cyanotic diseases are usually detectable during infancy and childhood, but the acyanotic diseases may have such nonspecific manifestations that they often go undiagnosed until adulthood. Heart scanning has been used infrequently in the diagnosis of congenital diseases, but with new radionuclides,

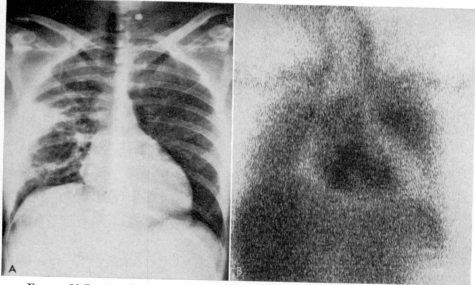

FIGURE 11-7. *A*, Chest radiograph showing right middle lung infiltrate and *B*, heart scan showing large clear area along left lateral border of cardiac blood pool. Repeated aspirations showed this to be a loculated pericardial effusion.

such as ^{99m}Tc and ^{113m}In, the resolution of the heart scan is improving to the degree that some congenital heart lesions can be suspected from the scan patterns. Figure 11-13 shows a child with tetralogy of Fallot; the image of the heart, unlike that on the usual radiograph, which often has a "boot-shaped" configuration, is similar to the configuration of acquired mitral insufficiency but with a much less prominent left atrium and left ventricle.

The scanning patterns in patients with septal defects and intracardiac shunts are variable and depend on which chambers are involved. Congenital valvular stenosis gives patterns indistinguishable from acquired lesions.

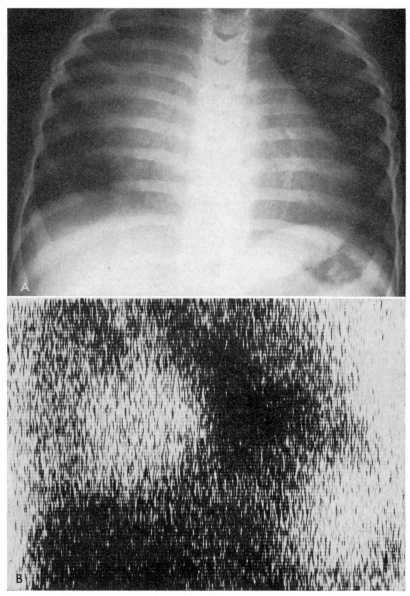

FIGURE 11-8.   A, Chest radiograph and B, heart scan of a patient with a teratoma involving the right heart. The tumor appears as a clear area on the scan.

In the diagnosis of congenital heart disease, it is helpful to know the distribution of the pulmonary arterial circulation. This has been discussed in Chapter X. Lung scanning with either ^{131}I macroaggregates of albumin or ^{113m}In iron hydroxide particles has been used: (1) to provide evidence of right-to-left shunting of the blood by measuring the fraction of the dose of injected particles in organs such as the brain or kidneys that are supplied by the systemic circulation; (2) to provide evidence of pulmonary venous hypertension, which reverses the normal blood flow gradient of the lung and results in higher concentrations of particles in the lung apices; (3) to provide evidence of pulmonary arterial hypertension, which decreases the normal gradient of blood flow from the top to the bottom of the lung when the injection is made with the patient erect; (4) to evaluate the patency of subclavian-pulmonary artery anastomoses, which usually decrease perfusion to the lung on the side of the anastomosis because of its greater systemic perfusion; and (5) to provide evidence of alterations in pulmonary arterial blood flow after cardiac surgery.

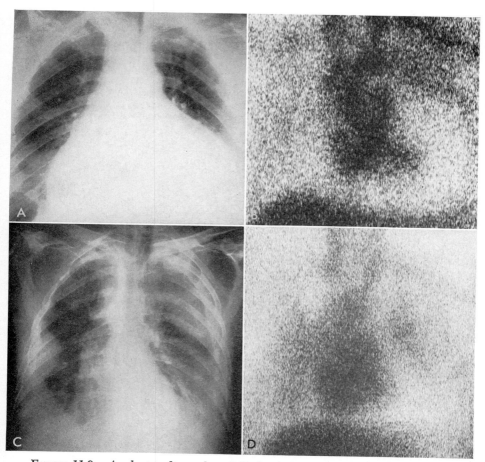

FIGURE 11-9. *A,* chest radiograph and *B,* heart scan of a patient with a tuberculous pericardial effusion. *C,* Chest radiograph and *D,* heart scan one year later of the same patient with continued evidence of pericardial effusion. Carbon dioxide angiocardiography showed this to be thickened epicarditis.

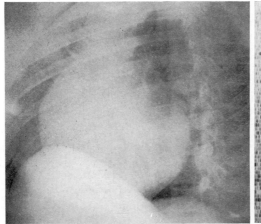
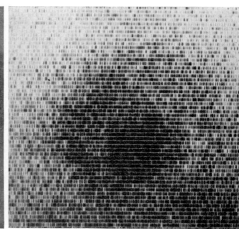

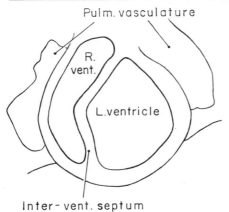

Pulm. vasculature

R. vent.

L.ventricle

Inter-vent. septum

FIGURE 11-10. The left anterior oblique chest radiograph and heart scan of a patient with idiopathic cardiomyopathy. The scan reveals the thickened intraventricular septum separating the two ventricular blood pools.

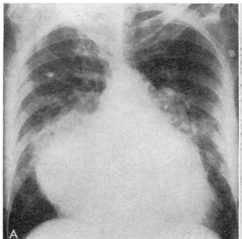
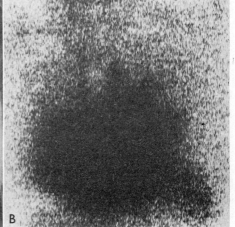

FIGURE 11-11. A and B, Typical giant left atrium and prominent left atrial appendage in a patient with rheumatic mitral insufficiency.

CORONARY ARTERY DISEASE

Rubidium-86 was first used for myocardial scanning by Carr et al. (1962b), although it had previously been used to measure coronary blood flow (Nolting et al., 1958; Love and Burch, 1959; Levy and DeOliveira, 1961). Carr and his associates also used mercury-203 chlormerodrin (1962a), which showed a positive defect on the heart scan in the areas of myocardial necrosis. In 1964, Carr et al. injected ionic cesium-131 into patients to differentiate the normally perfused from the unperfused areas of myocardium. Like rubidium, cesium is distributed in the same manner as potassium and can be used as an index of blood flow. The nonperfused areas resulting from coronary artery occlusion appear on the scan as a zone of absent activity, as seen in Figure 11-14, which was obtained from a dog heart whose anterior branch of the left coronary artery was ligated

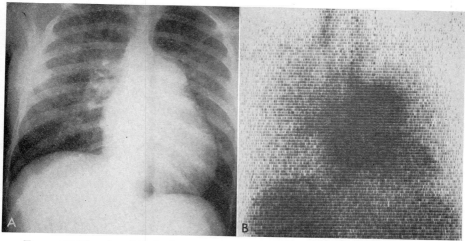

FIGURE 11-12.   *A* and *B,* Radiograph and scan showing dilatation of the main pulmonary artery caused by rheumatic heart disease with mitral stenosis and pulmonic valvular insufficiency.

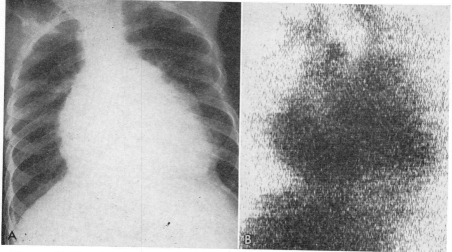

FIGURE 11-13.   *A* and *B,* Tetralogy of Fallot in a 9 year old child. There is poststenotic dilatation of the pulmonary artery and a small left ventricular blood pool.

TABLE 11-2. CONGENITAL HEART DISEASE

A. CYANOTIC
  1. Tetralogy of Fallot
  2. Pulmonic stenosis with interatrial communication and intact ventricular septum
  3. Eisenmenger complex (bidirectional shunt through ventricular septal defect)
  4. Tricuspid atresia with nonfunctioning right ventricle
  5. Complete transposition of the great vessels
  6. Taussig-Bing syndrome (partial transposition of great vessels)
  7. Truncus arteriosus
  8. Ebstein's anomaly (downward displacement of tricuspid valve)
  9. Total anomalous pulmonary venous return
  10. Hypoplastic left heart syndrome
      a. Mitral atresia
      b. Aortic atresia
  11. Miscellaneous types:
      a. Pulmonary atresia with intact ventricular septum
      b. Hypoplasia of the right ventricle
      c. Systemic venous return to the left atrium
      d. Trilocular and bilocular hearts
      e. Levocardia with situs inversus
      f. Atresia or stenosis of the pulmonary veins
      g. Double-outlet right ventricle
      h. Asplenia
B. NONCYANOTIC
  1. Patent ductus arteriosus
  2. Atrial septal defect (ostium primum, ostium secundum, foramen ovale, sinus venosus defect)
  3. Atrioventricularis communis
  4. Ventricular septal defect
  5. Corrected transposition of the great vessels
  6. Coarctation of the aorta
  7. Pulmonic stenosis without shunt
  8. Congenital aortic stenosis
  9. Sinus of Valsalva fistula
  10. Coronary arteriovenous fistula
  11. Congenital mitral stenosis
  12. Congenital mitral insufficiency
  13. Endocardial fibroelastosis
  14. Miscellaneous types:
      a. Aortic septal defect
      b. Congenital absence of the pulmonary valve
      c. Congenital defect of the pericardium
      d. Anomalous left pulmonary artery
      e. Dextrocardia (five types)
      f. Cor triatriatum
      g. Anomalous coronary artery arising from the pulmonary artery
      h. Congenital diverticulum of the left ventricle
      i. Aortic left ventricular tunnel
      i. Parachute mitral valve

before the ^{131}Cs injection. Relatively good resolution was achieved by scanning when the heart had been removed from the chest, but the beating heart in the living dog results in much poorer resolution than that seen in these studies. Clinical application will require the use of scintillation cameras that can be activated during restricted portions of the cardiac cycle, e.g., triggered by the electrocardiogram.

Other nuclides, such as [84]Rb (Cohen et al., 1965) and radioiodinated fatty acids (Evans et al., 1965; Gunton et al., 1965) have also been used as myocardial scanning agents, but none of the procedures can be considered ready for clinical use.

THE GREAT VESSELS

With blood-pool scanning, one can delineate the aorta and in some instances detect aneurysmal dilatation of the aorta when the lumen is patent and saccular. The smaller muscular arteries cannot be seen because of their size. The great veins are usually seen in a heart scan but are at times poorly resolved because of their angulation and variable depth within the body. The superior vena cava is usually seen as it enters the cardiac blood pool. Figure 11-15 is the chest radiograph, venous angiogram, and blood-pool scan of a patient with a Pancoast tumor and superior vena caval obstruction. The superior mediastinal mass caused narrowing of the superior vena cava and was seen on both the venous angiogram and the scan.

Attempts at radioisotope venography have been reported by Rosenthal (1966), who used ^{99m}Tc pertechnetate and the scintillation camera. By serial scintiphotographs he was able to detect obstructing lesions of the inferior vena

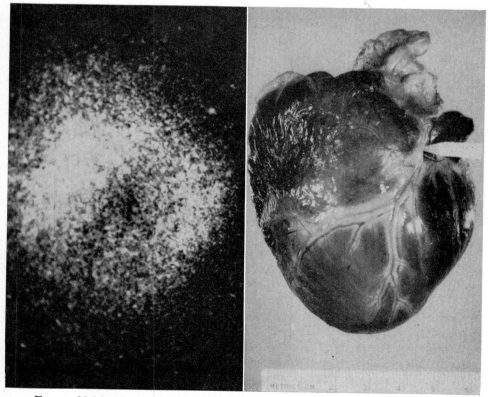

FIGURE 11-14. Cesium-131 camera image of a dog heart showing a central area of diminished activity, the result of absent perfusion produced from ligation of the anterior branch of the left coronary artery.

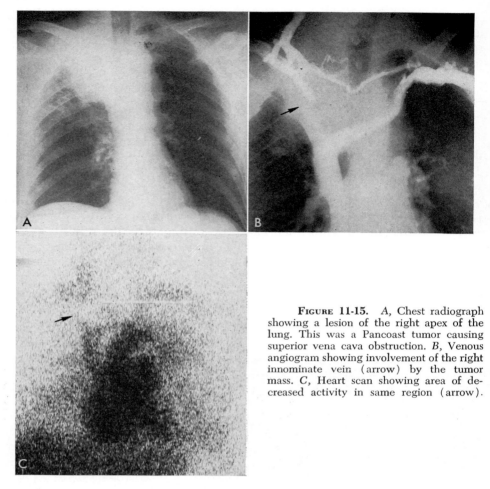

FIGURE 11-15. *A,* Chest radiograph showing a lesion of the right apex of the lung. This was a Pancoast tumor causing superior vena cava obstruction. *B,* Venous angiogram showing involvement of the right innominate vein (arrow) by the tumor mass. *C,* Heart scan showing area of decreased activity in same region (arrow).

cava and the common iliac veins and advocated use of the procedure as a screening test in suspected venous obstructive lesions.

THE PLACENTA

Accurate placental localization is important in differentiating placenta previa from other causes of bleeding in the third trimester of pregnancy. Several established techniques are available, such as sterile vaginal examination and thermography (Johnson et al., 1966; Birnbaum and Kliot, 1964, 1965). Another method is radiographic placentography, which provides only indirect evidence of placental implantation. Radioisotope placentography has gained wide acceptance since its accuracy is greater than 90 per cent (Hibbard, 1961; Swartz et al., 1963; Thaidigsman and Schulman, 1964). A variety of radiopharmaceuticals have been used, including iodine-131- and iodine-132-labeled human serum albumin (HSA) (Weinberg et al., 1957; Hibbard, 1961); sodium-24 chloride (Browne and Veall, 1950); chromium-51-labeled red cells (Paul et al., 1963);

chromium-51-labeled HSA (Johnson et al., 1964); technetium-99m-labeled human serum albumin (McAfee et al., 1964); and indium-113m transferrin (Stern et al., 1967). Because of their physical characteristics, technetium-99m and indium-113m are the nuclides of choice.

The placenta can be localized in two ways. The first and most widely used is multiple point counting over from 9 to 21 selected sites of the abdomen with a collimated scintillation detector (Cavanagh et al., 1961; Durfee and Hovieson, 1962). A recent comparison of this method with scanning in the same patient revealed the inferiority of the point-counting method (Cooper et al., 1966). The improved spatial resolution of placental scanning is exemplified in the scan in Figure 11-16 performed with ^{99m}Tc human serum albumin. The normal upper uterine implantation of the vascular placenta is easily seen but bladder excretion of the technetium gives an additional area of increased activity that could be confusing. A scan made after the injection of [113]In transferrin in a patient with placenta previa is shown in Figure 11-17. The important advantage of [113m]In transferrin over ^{99m}Tc albumin is that bladder activity is absent. Both maternal and fetal radiation exposure is low with both [113m]In and [99m]Tc. Placental scanning is also helpful in locating the placenta before amniocentesis.

PERIPHERAL BLOOD FLOW

Forssmann (1929, 1931) first delineated vascular blood pools with radiopaque media and thus introduced the technique of angiography, which is widely employed today. The method consists of the direct injection of the material into an artery. By means of rapid sequential x-rays or cinefluoroscopy, the vessel is outlined as the material proceeds along the artery into its distal branches. Dilu-

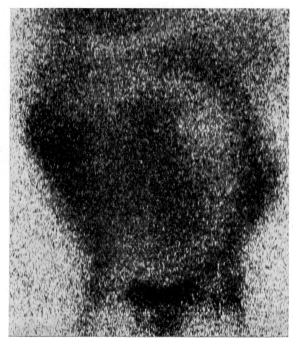

FIGURE 11-16. Placental scan (^{99m}Tc-albumin, 1.0 mc.) showing a normal intra-uterine implantation and bladder activity from free pertechnetate.

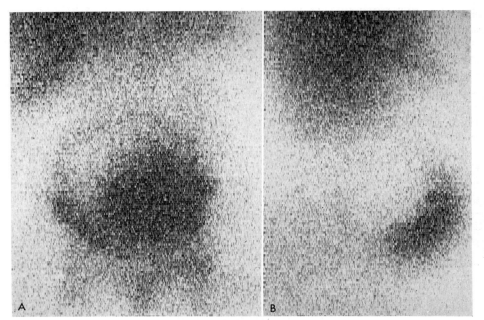

FIGURE 11-17.   A, Placental scan [113m]In transferrin, 1.0 μc.) showing low implanation of the placenta. B, Lateral scan of the same patient showing the implantation to be anterior.

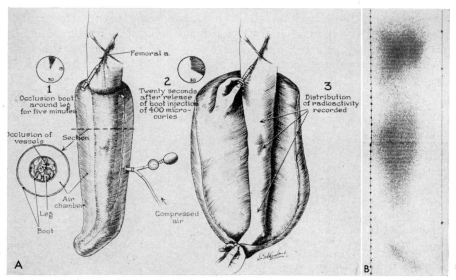

FIGURE 11-18.   A, Leg cast method for producing reactive hyperemia. B, Scan of the leg after a 300 μc. injection of ^{131}I MAA into the femoral artery of a normal person during reactive hyperemia.

tion makes the visualization transient. A venous phase is frequently observed but is usually much less distinct.

Peripheral blood flow in man has been measured by several tracer and other methods (Kramer et al., 1963; Whitney, 1953; Andres et al., 1954). Lassen and his associates (1964) used ^{133}Xe and [85]Kr to measure blood flow in peripheral muscle by determining the rate of clearance of the gases. Lindbjerg (1965) measured the muscle blood flow with ^{133}Xe after histamine injection as a diagnostic method in peripheral arterial disease.

The particle distribution method developed for clinical lung scanning by Wagner et al. (1964) has also been used to measure regional blood flow in the extremities (Wagner et al., 1965; Jones et al., 1965). Quantification of the distribution of intra-arterially injected particles can be accomplished by point counting or by quantitative scanning. Bardfeld and Wagner (1967) have used this method to study the circulation of the lower extremities in patients with peripheral arteriosclerosis. Using reactive hyperemia produced by a long-leg arm-compression boot, which applied circumferential pressure to all areas of the extremity beneath it, to simulate exercise, they found a markedly diminished leg activity in the arteriosclerotic patient compared to the much greater activity seen in the leg of a healthy person (Fig. 11-18). The difference is thought to be the result of increased peripheral shunting as suggested by the work of Liebow (1963). Bardfeld et al. (1967) have also applied their method in studying clubbing of the fingers and Raynaud's disease of the upper extremity. After brachial artery injection of iodinated macroaggregated albumin, no significant difference was found in the deposition in diseased and normal persons (Fig. 11-19).

The rapid intravenous injection of a radiopharmaceutical such as ^{99m}Tc pertechnetate has been used in rapid-sequence studies with either a stationary detector or a scintillation camera to detect unilateral carotid artery insufficiency. Renal blood flow can also be measured by this method.

The venous circulation of the lower extremity was first studied by Wright et al. in 1948 using ^{24}Na chloride. Fabrikant and his associates (1962),

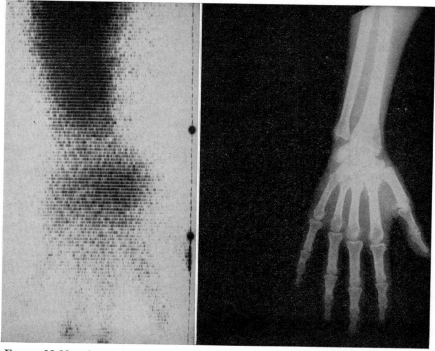

FIGURE 11-19. Arm scan of a normal patient after brachial artery injection of iodine-131-labeled macroaggregated albumin.

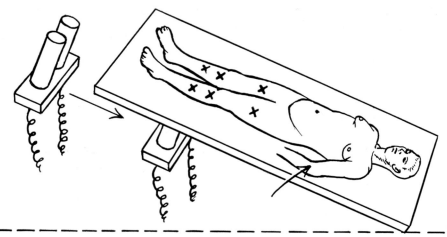

FIGURE 11-20. Method of elevation of the legs after the intravenous injection of technetium-99m-labeled albumin with quantification of the change in count rate at selected points (**x**) of each leg to determine deep venous obstruction.

using [131]I Diodrast, made the method clinically applicable in determining the extent of deep vein involvement, in distinguishing the superficial collaterals of primary varicose veins and incompetent postphlebitic veins, and in evaluating venous surgery. Tow et al. (1967) have studied venous insufficiency in patients with lower extremity thrombophlebitis using ^{99m}Tc-labeled albumin. While counting over the calf of the affected leg, they elevated the leg 15 and 30 degrees and established new vascular volumes reflected by the change in count rate. Comparing these results with those of the unaffected leg, studied in the same way, they could quantify obstruction or retardation of flow. The level of obstruction could be determined by counting at various levels. The degree of leg elevation was optimum at 15 degrees, with little change noted up to 30 degrees, at which point the run-off caused collapse of the veins (Fig. 11-20).

REFERENCES

Andres, R., Zierler, L., Anderson, H. M., Stainsby, W. N., Cader, G., Ghrayyeb, A. S., and Lilienthal, J. L.: Measurement of Blood Flow and Volume in the Forearm of Man with Notes on the Theory of Indicator Dilution and on Production of Turbulence, Hemolyses and Vasodilatation by Intravascular Injection. *J. Clin. Invest.* 33:482, 1954.

Ball, W. C., Stewart, P. B., Newsham, L. G. S., and Bates, D. V.: Regional Pulmonary Function studied with Xenon[133]. *J. Clin. Invest.* 41:519, 1962.

Bardfeld, P. A., Lopez-Majano, V., and Wagner, H. N., Jr.: Measurement of the Regional Distribution of Arterial Blood Flow in the Human Forearm and Hand. *J. Nucl. Med.* 8:542, 1967.

Bardfeld, P. A., and Wagner, H. N., Jr.: The Regional Circulation of the Extremities in Normal Man and Patients with Peripheral Arteriosclerosis. (Abstr.) *J. Nucl. Med.* 8:279, 1967.

Bianchi, C., Coli, A., Giannotti, P., and Lenaers, A.: A New Approach to the Measurement of Divided Renal Plasma Flow by [113]I-Hippuran and External Counting in Humans. Radio-acktive Isotope in Klinik und Forschung. *Strahlentherapie,* 65:136, 1967.

Bianchi, C., and Toni, P.: L'usage des indicateurs radioactifs et de la gammagraphie dans la mesure du débit plasmatique rénal et du taux de filtration glomérulaire. Radioaktive Isotope in Klinik und Forschung. *Strahlentherapie* 53:301, 1963.

Bing, R. J., Bennish, A., Bluemchen, G., Cohen, A., Gallagher, J. P., and Zaleski, E. J.: The Determination of Coronary Flow Equivalent with Coincidence Counting Technique. *Circulation* 24:833, 1964.

Birnbaum, S. J., and Kliot, D. A.: Thermography—Obstetrical Applications. *Ann. N. Y. Acad. Sci.* 121:209, 1964.

REFERENCES

Birnbaum, S. J., and Kliot, D. A.: Thermoplacentography: Placental Localization by Infrared Sensing Techniques. *Obstet. Gynec.* 25:515, 1965.

Bonte, F. J., Andrews, G. J., Elmendorf, F. A., Presley, N. L., and Krohmer, J. S.: Radioisotope Scanning in the Detection of Pericardial Effusions. *Southern Med. J.* 55:577, 1962.

Bonte, F. J., and Curry, T. S., III: Blood Pool Scanning with Tc-99m Human Serum Albumin. *Radiology* 85:1120, 1965.

Bonte, F. J., and Curry, T. S., III: The Radioisotope Blood Pool Scan. *Amer. J. Roentgen.* 96:690, 1966.

Bonte, F. J., and Curry, T. S., III: Technetium-99m HSA Blood Pool Scan in Diagnosis of an Intracardiac Myxoma. *J. Nucl. Med.* 8:35, 1967.

Bradley, S. E., Ingelfinger, F. J., Bradley, G. P., and Curry, J. J.: The Estimation of Hepatic Blood Flow in Man. *J. Clin. Invest.* 24:890, 1945.

Browne, J. C. M., and Veall, N.: A Method of Locating the Placenta in the Intact Human Uterus by Means of Radioactive Sodium. *J. Obstet Gynaec. Brit. Emp.* 57:566, 1950.

Carr, E. A., Jr., Beierwaltes, W. H., and Bartlett, J. D., Jr.: Detection of Myocardial Infarcts by Scans. (Abstr.) Given at the 9th Annual Meeting of the Society of Nuclear Medicine, June 27, 1962a.

Carr, E. A., Jr., Beierwaltes, W. H., Wegst, A. V., and Bartlett, J. D., Jr.: Myocardial Scanning with Rubidium-86. *J. Nucl. Med.* 3:76, 1962b.

Carr, E. A., Jr., Gleason, G., Shaw, J., and Krontz, B.: The Direct Diagnosis of Myocardial Infarction by Photoscanning after Administration of Cesium-131. *Amer. Heart J.* 68:627, 1964.

Cavanagh, D., Powe, C. E., and Gibson, A. J.: Placenta Previa: Modern Methods of Diagnosis with Special Reference to Isotopic Placentography. *Obstet. Gynec.* 18:403, 1961.

Charkes, N. D., and Sklaroff, D. M.: Radioisotope Photoscanning as a Diagnostic Aid in Cardiovascular Disease. *J.A.M.A.* 186:920, 1963.

Chwojnik, A., Torreggiani, G., Bartolomei, G., and Donato, L.: Improvement of the [86]Rb Single Injection Method for the Measurement of Coronary Blood Flow in Man Using a Double Tracer Technique. *J. Nucl. Biol. Med.* 10:89, 1966.

Cohen, A., Zaleski, E. J., Luebs, E. D., and Bing, R. J.: Use of Positron Emitter in Determination of Coronary Blood Flow in Man. *J. Nucl. Med.* 6:651, 1965.

Cooper, R. D., Jr., Izenstark, J. L., Branyon, D. L., Bowen, E. G., and Weens, H. S.: Isotopic Placentography or Placental Scanning. *Radiology* 87:291, 1966.

Dobson, E. L., Warner, G. F., Finney, C. R., and Johnston, M. E.: The Measurement of Liver Circulation by Means of the Colloid Disappearance Rate. I. Liver Blood Flow in Normal Young Men. *Circulation* 7:690, 1953.

Donato, L., Bartolomei, G., and Giordani, R.: Evaluation of Myocardial Blood Perfusion in Man with Radioactive Potassium and Rubidium and Precordial Counting. *Circulation* 29:195, 1964.

Donato, L., Giuntini, C., Lewis, M. L., Durand, H., Rochester, D. F., Harvey, R. M., and Cournand, A.: Quantitative Radiocardiography. I. Theoretical Considerations. *Circulation* 26:174, 1962a.

Donato, L., Giuntini, C., Mariani, M., Maseri, A., and Micheli, G.: Un metodo per la determinazione della portata cirolatoria di shunts sinistro-destri. *Atti del XXVII Congresso della Società Italiana di Cardiologia.* 1966, Vol. 2, p. 20.

Donato, L., Rochester, D. F., Lewis, M. L., Durand, J., Parker, J. O., and Harvey, R. M.: Quantitative Radiocardiography. II. Technique and Analysis of Curves. *Circulation* 26:183, 1962b.

Durfee, R. B., and Howieson, J. L.: Localization of the Placenta with Radioactive Iodinated Serum Albumin. *Amer. J. Obstet. Gynec.* 84:577, 1962.

Evans, J. R., Gunton, R. W., Baker, R. G., Beanlands, D. S., and Spears, J. C.: Use of Radioiodinated Fatty Acid for Photoscans of the Heart. *Circulation Res.* 16:1, 1965.

Fabrikant, J. I., Anlyan, W. G., Baylin, G. J., and Isley, J. K.: Isotope Studies for the Evaluation of Venous Disease of the Lower Extremity. *J. Nucl. Med.* 2:136, 1962.

Feigenbaum, H., Waldhausen, J. A., and Hyde, L. P.: Ultrasound Diagnosis of Pericardial Effusion. *J.A.M.A.* 191:711, 1965.

Folse, R., and Braunwald, E.: Determination of Fraction of Left Ventricular Volume Ejected per Beat and of Ventricular End-Diastolic and Residual Volumes. Experimental Clinical Observations with a Precordial Dilution Technique. *Circulation* 25:674, 1962.

Forssmann, W.: Die Sondierung des rechten Herzens. *Klin. Wschr.* 8:2085, 1929.

Forssmann, W.: Über Kontrastdarstellung der Höhlen des lebenden rechten Herzens und der Lungenschlagader. *München Med. Wschr.* 78:489, 1931.

Friedberg, C. K.: Diseases of the Heart. Ed. 3. W. B. Saunders Co., Philadelphia, 1966.

Giuntini, C., Lewis, M. L., Sales Luis, A., and Harvey, R. M.: A Study of the Pulmonary Blood Volume in Man by Quantitative Radiocardiography. *J. Clin. Invest.* 42:1589, 1963.

Gunton, R. W., Evans, J. R., Baker, R. G., Spears, J. C., and Beanlands, D. S.: Demonstration of Myocardial Infarction by Photoscans of Heart in Man. *Amer. J. Cardiol.* 16:482, 1965.

Halpern, B. N., Biozzi, G., Pequignot, G., Stiffel, C., Delaloye, B., and Mouton, D.: La cinétique de L'épuration sanguine des suspensions colloidale comme mésure de la circulation hépatique. *Rev. Franç. Etud. Clin. Biol.* 3:549, 1958.

Harper, P. B., Beck, R., Charleston, D., and Lathrop, K. A.: Optimization of a Scanning Method Using Tc-99m. *Nucleonics* 22:50, 1964.

Henly, W. S., Creech, O., Couves, C. M., Morgan, M. D., Chapman, D. W., and Allen, H. C.: Determination of Myocardial Blood Flow Utilising Iodinated (I^{131}) Human Serum Albumin. *Surg. Forum* 7:306, 1956.

Hibbard, B. M.: Placental Localization Using Radioiodinated Serum Albumin (RISA). *J. Obstet. Gynaec. Brit. Comm.* 68:481, 1961.

Høedt-Rasmussen, K., Sveinsdottir, E., and Lassen, N. A.: The Inert Gas Intra-arterial Injection Method for Determining Regional Cerebral Blood Flow in Man Through the Intact Skull. *Circ. Res.* 18:237, 1966.

Holmes, R. A., Silbiger, M. L., Karmen, A., Wagner, H. N., Jr., and Stern, H. S.: Cardiac Scanning with Technetium-99m-Labeled Albumin. *J.A.M.A.* 198:67, 1966.

Johnson, P. M., Bragg, D. G., and Sciarra, J. J.: Placental Localization: A Comparison of Radiopharmaceutic and Thermographic Methods. *Amer. J. Roentgen.* 96:681, 1966.

Johnson, P. M., Sciarra, J. J., and Stickley, E. E.: New Radiopharmaceutical for Placentography. *Radiology* 83:346, 1964.

Jones, E. L., Wagner, H. N., Jr., and Zuidema, G. D.: New Method for Studying Peripheral Circulation in Man. *Arch. Surg.* 91:725, 1965.

Kemp, E., Høedt-Rasmussen, K., Bjerrum, J. K., Fahrenkrug, A., and Ladefoged, J.: A New Method for Determination of Divided Renal Blood Flow in Man. *Lancet* 1:1402, 1963.

Kety, S. S.: Measurement of Regional Circulation by the Local Clearance of Radioactive Sodium. *Amer. Heart J.* 38:321, 1949.

Kety, S. S., and Schmidt, C. F.: The Determination of Cerebral Blood Flow in Man by the Use of Nitrous Oxide in Low Concentrations. *Amer. J. Physiol.* 143:53, 1945.

Kramer, K., Lochner, W., and Wetterer, E.: Methods of Measuring Blood Flow, *In* Handbook of Physiology. Sec. 2, Circulation. Vol. II. Hamilton, W. F., and Dow, P. (eds.). American Physiological Society, Washington, 1963, pp. 1281–1293.

Lassen, N. A., and Ingvar, D. H.: The Blood Flow of the Cerebral Cortex Determined by Radioactive Krypton-85. *Experientia* 17:42, 1961.

Lassen, N. A., Lindbjerg, J., and Munck, O.: Measurement of Blood-Flow through Skeletal Muscle by Intramuscular Injection of Xenon-133. *Lancet* 1:686, 1964.

Levy, M. N., and DeOliveira, J. M.: Regional Distribution of Myocardial Blood Flow in the Dog as Determined by Rb^{86}. *Circulation Res.* 9:96, 1961.

Lewis, M. L., and Giuntini, C.: Unpublished data.

Lewis, M. L., Giuntini, C., Donato, L., Harvey, R. M., and Cournand, A.: Quantitative Radiocardiography. III. Results and Validation of Theory and Method. *Circulation* 26:189, 1962.

Liebow, A. A.: Situations Which Lead to Changes in Vascular Patterns: Methods of Measuring Blood Flow. *In* Handbook of Physiology. Sec. 2, Circulation. Vol. II. Hamilton, W. F., and Dow, P. (eds.). American Physiological Society, Washington, 1963, pp. 1254–1256.

Lindbjerg, I. F.: Measurement of Muscle Blood Flow with ^{133}Xe after Histamine Injection as Diagnostic Method in Peripheral Arterial Disease. *Scand. J. Clin. Lab. Invest.* 17:371, 1965.

Love, W. D., and Burch, G. E.: Influence on the Rate of Coronary Plasma Flow on the Extraction of Rb^{86} from Coronary Blood Flow. *Circulation Res.* 7:24, 1959.

MacIntyre, W. J., Crespo, G. G., and Christie, J. H.: The Use of Radioiodinated (I^{131}) Iodipamide for Cardiovascular Scanning. *Amer. J. Roentgen.* 89:315, 1963.

Marchioro, T., Feldman, A., Owens, J. C., and Swan, H.: Measurement of Myocardial Blood Flow. Indicator Dilution Techniques. *Circ. Res.* 9:541, 1961.

Mariani, M., Maseri, A., and Giuntini, C.: Precordial Counting Versus Arterial Sampling for Measuring the Cardiac Output in Man. *J. Nucl. Biol. Med.* 10:66, 1966.

McAfee, J. G., Stern, H. S., Fueger, G. F., Baggish, M. S., Holzman, G. B., and Zolle, I.: ^{99m}Tc Labeled Serum Albumin for Scintillation Scanning of the Placenta. *J. Nucl. Med.* 5:936, 1964.

Meier, P., and Zierler, K. L.: On the Theory of the Indicator Dilution Method for Measurement of Blood Flow and Volume. *J. Appl. Physiol.* 6:731, 1954.

Nolting, D., Mack, R., Luthy, E., Kirsch, M., and Hogancamp, C.: Measurement of Coronary Blood Flow and Myocardial Rubidium Uptake with Rb^{86}. *J. Clin. Invest.* 37:921, 1958.

Paul, J. D., Jr., Gahres, E. E., Albert, S. N., Terrell, W. D., Jr., and Dodek, S. M.: Placenta Localization Using Cr-51 Tagged Erythrocytes. *Obstet. Gynec.* 21:33, 1963.

Prinzmetal, M., Corday, E., Bergman, H. C., Schwartz, L., and Sprizler, R. J.: Radiocardiography: A New Method for Studying the Blood Flow Through the Chambers of the Heart in Human Beings. *Science* 108:340, 1948.

Rejali, A. M., MacIntyre, W. J., and Friedell, H. L.: A Radioisotope Method of Visualization of Blood Pools. *Amer. J. Roentgen.* 79:129, 1958.

Robb, G. P., and Steinberg, I.: Visualization of the Chambers of the Heart. *Amer. J. Roentgen.* 41:1, 1939a.

Robb, G. P., and Steinberg, I.: Visualization of the Chambers of the Heart, the Pulmonary Circulation and the Great Blood Vessels in Heart Disease; Preliminary Observations. *Amer. J. Roentgen.* 42:14, 1939b.

Rosenthal, L.: Radionuclide Venography Using Technetium-99m Pertechnetate and the Gamma-Ray Scintillation Camera. *Amer. J. Roentgen.* 97:874, 1966.

Ross, R. W., Ueda, K., Lichtlen, P. R., and Rees, J. R.: Measurement of Myocardial Blood Flow in Animals and Man by Selective Injection of Radioactive Inert Gas into the Coronary Arteries. *Circ. Res.* 15:28, 1964.

Sapirstein, L. A.: Fractionation of the Cardiac Output of Rats with Isotopic Potassium. *Circ. Res.* 4:689, 1956.

Sapirstein, L. A.: Regional Blood Flow by Fractional Distribution of Indicators. *Amer. J. Physiol.* 193:161, 1958.

Sapirstein, L. A., and Ogden, E.: Theoretic Limitations of the Nitrous Oxide Method for the Determination of Regional Blood Flow. *Circ. Res.* 4:245, 1956.

Sklaroff, D. M., Charkes, N. D., and Morse, D.: Measurement of Pericardial Fluid Correlated with I^{131} Cholografin and IHSA Heart Scan. *J. Nucl. Med.* 5:101, 1964.

Smith, H. W., Finkelstein, N., Aliminosa, L., Crawford, B., and Graber, M.: The Renal Clearance of Substituted Hippuric Acid Derivatives and Other Aromatic Acids in Dog and Man. *J. Clin. Invest.* 24:388, 1945.

Stauffer, H. M., Soloff, L. A., Zatuckni, J., and Carter, B. L.: Gas and Opaque Contrast in Roentgenographic Diagnosis of Pericardial Disease. *J.A.M.A.* 172:1122, 1960.

Stern, H. S., Goodwin, D. A., Scheffel, U., Wagner, H. N., Jr., and Kramer, H. H.: In ^{113m} for Blood Pool and Brain Scanning. *Nucleonics* 25:62, 1967.

Swartz, D. P., Platt, M. A., and Heagy, F. C.: Radioisotope (I^{131}) Studies of Placental Localization and Circulation. *Amer. J. Obstet. Gynec.* 85:338, 1963.

Taplin, G. V., Johnson, D. E., Dow, E. K., and Keplon, H. S.: Suspensions of Radioalbumin Aggregates for Photoscanning the Liver, Spleen, Lung, and Other Organs. *J. Nucl. Med.* 5:259, 1964.

Thaidigsman, J. H., and Schulman, H.: Placenta Localization using Radioactive I^{131} Tagged Human Serum Albumin. *Obstet. Gynec.* 23:757, 1964.

Tow, D. E., Wagner, H. N., Jr., and North, W. A.: Detection of Venous Obstruction in the Legs with ^{99m}Tc-Albumin. (Abstr.) *J. Nucl. Med.* 8:277, 1967.

Veall, N., Pearson, J. D., Henley, T., and Lowe, A. E.: A Method for the Determination of Cardiac Output (Preliminary Report). *In* Radioisotopes Conference, Oxford—Medical and Physiological Applications. Butterworth & Co., London, 1954, Vol. 1, p. 183.

Vetter, H., Falkner, R., and Neumayr, A.: The Disappearance Rate of Colloidal Radiogold from the Circulation and its Application to the Estimation of Liver Blood Flow in Normal and Cirrhotic Subjects. *J. Clin. Invest.* 33:1594, 1954.

Wagner, H. N., Jr., Jones, E. L., Tow, D. E., and Langan, J. K.: Preliminary Report: A Method for Study of Peripheral Circulation in Man. *J. Nucl. Med.* 6:150, 1965.

Wagner, H. N., Jr., McAfee, J. G., and Mozley, J. M.: Diagnosis of Pericardial Effusion by Radioisotope Scanning. *Arch. Intern. Med.* 108:679, 1961.

Wagner, H. N., Jr., Sabiston, D. C., Jr., Iio, M., McAfee, J. G., Meyer, J. K., and Langan, J. K.: Regional Pulmonary Blood Flow in Man by Radioisotope Scanning. *J.A.M.A.* 187:601, 1964.

Wagner, H. N., Jr., Sabiston, D. C., Jr., McAfee, J. G., Tow, D. E., and Stern, H. S.: Diagnosis of Massive Pulmonary Embolism in Man by Radioisotope Scanning. *New Eng. J. Med.* 271:377, 1964.

Waser, P., and Hunzinger, W.: Bestimmung von Kreislaufgrösser mit $Na^{24}Cl$. *Helv. Physiol. Acta* 7:62, 1948.

Weinberg, A., Rizzi, J., McManus, R., and Rivera, J.: Localization of the Placental Site by Radioactive Isotopes. *Obstet. Gynec.* 9:692, 1957.

West, J. B.: Regional Differences in Gas Exchange in the Lung of Erect Man. *J. Appl. Physiol.* 17:893, 1962.

Whitney, R. J.: The Measurement of Volume Changes in Human Limbs. *J. Physiol.* 121:1, 1953.

Wright, H. B., Osborn, S. B., and Edmonds, D. G.: Rate of Flow of Venous Blood in the Leg Measured with Radioactive Sodium. *Lancet* 2:767, 1948.

Zierler, K. L.: Equations for Measuring Flow by External Monitoring of Radiosotopes. *Circ. Res.* 16:309, 1965.

XII

THE GASTROINTESTINAL TRACT, LIVER, AND PANCREAS

HENRY N. WAGNER, Jr.

FRED MISHKIN

SHIGEKOTO KAIHARA

THOMAS WALDMANN

THE GASTROINTESTINAL TRACT

INTRODUCTION

As the result of studies begun in the nineteenth century, it has been possible to isolate the most important chemical constituents of food and relate them to health. For example, protein starvation can result in various diseases, such as kwashiorkor, first recognized in the 1940's. This disease develops in babies soon after they are weaned, when they shift from mother's milk to the thin starchy gruel that is standard fare in many underdeveloped areas.

Although protein deficiency is the most widespread and serious nutritional disease in the world, other deficiencies are also important. In addition to proteins, carbohydrates, and fats, man needs at least 40 other nutrients, including minerals and vitamins. A deficiency of any one of them can cause illness. Loss of dietary constituents from infestation with worms or other parasites can also cause disease even if the diet itself is adequate.

Laster and Ingelfinger (1961) have summarized the physiological processes believed to be involved in the movement of a dietary constituent from the bowel lumen to the blood or lymph as follows:

1. Intraluminal digestion.
2. Binding of the substance to the surface of the intestinal columnar cell.
3. Transport across the luminal surface of the columnar cell membrane.
4. Intracellular metabolism and transcellular transport.
5. Release from the cell.
6. Migration across the basement membrane of the mucosal epithelium and through the lamina propria.
7. Penetration to blood or lymph capillaries.

Radioisotope techniques help define specific abnormalities—resulting from both faulty absorption and abnormal losses. They enable us to pinpoint the *type* and *site* of biochemical abnormalities. For example, we can determine when proteins are being lost from the body through focal lesions of the intestinal tract, when vitamin B_{12} is lacking because of a specific defect of the stomach, and when triglycerides are not being adequately absorbed from the jejunum.

Tracer techniques have also been useful in defining more precisely over-nutrition, a new type of nutritional disorder becoming increasingly common in certain western countries. It has been estimated that one out of five men and one out of four women in the United States are overweight; and obesity has been strongly linked with a shorter life expectancy and increased susceptibility to atherosclerosis, hypertension, diabetes, and other diseases. The metabolic consequences of chronic overfeeding are being studied from the viewpoint of altered digestion, absorption, and metabolism.

In the process of absorption from the gastrointestinal tract, a dietary component or its breakdown product leaves the intestinal lumen, traverses the epithelium and connective tissue stroma of the intestinal wall, and enters either the lymphatic or the vascular system. Before radioactive tracer techniques were available, measurement of intestinal absorption required administration of large quantities of the substance under study. At times, this procedure was useful in detecting abnormalities—as in the glucose tolerance test—but, at other times, the unphysiological quantities used for testing did not permit clear-cut interpretation of the results.

Classic techniques, such as the measurement of the fat and nitrogen content of the feces, are accurate ways of assaying absorption, but the methods are time-consuming, laborious, and expensive. Radioactive tracers have helped solve some of these problems.

PHYSIOLOGICAL PRINCIPLES OF INTESTINAL ABSORPTION

The transfer of the products of digestion from the intestinal lumen into the mucosal blood and lymph vessels takes place by the process of membrane transport, a phenomenon readily studied with radioactive tracers. Laster and Ingelfinger (1961) have classified the underlying processes of intestinal absorption as passive diffusion, facilitated transport, and active transport.

Passive or *simple diffusion* describes the passage of a molecule across a membrane from a region of higher chemical concentration to one of lower concentration, or passage of a charged particle from a region relatively high in electric charge to a region of lesser similar charge or of opposite charge to that of the particle. The diffusion process is modified by the physical properties of the membrane, but it requires no expenditure of energy by the membrane, since the movement is in the direction of the electrochemical gradient. In general, substances with high lipid solubility (such as many drugs) are rapidly absorbed from the intestine, whereas lipid-insoluble substances are poorly absorbed. The nonionized form of a given drug is more rapidly absorbed than the ionized form, because the former is more soluble in lipid.

Since the intestine can effectively absorb many dietary constituents that are water-soluble and lipid-insoluble, it is clear that mechanisms exist for circumventing the lipoid barrier of the intestinal mucosa. One hypothesis is that biological membranes, such as the intestinal mucosa, contain pores through which water and some water-soluble solutes can pass. Increased water flow accelerates the diffusion of dissolved substances and sweeps solutes along by a process called "solvent drag." This process, a form of facilitated transport, can explain the enhanced absorption of sugars during periods of rapid water absorption. Other factors—such as electrical charge, molecular size and water solubility of the solutes, the presence of electrical charges on the walls of the pores themselves, and the size of the pores—are also believed to be important factors in absorption.

In contrast to passive diffusion across a hypothetical lipoid membrane, or through hypothetical pores, *active transport* requires the expenditure of energy by the membrane itself. This is necessary in order to achieve net movement against the direction of the chemical concentration gradients or against electrical gradients. This type of transport often has a high degree of "stereospecificity"— that is, it requires that the transported molecule have a specific configuration. Minor alterations in molecular structure, such as a change in the direction in which a hydroxyl group projects, can prevent active transport of the molecule. This stereospecificity is not only of fundamental importance in our concept of the nature of the processes, but it is also of practical importance when we label molecules with radioactive tracers. The burden is on the investigator to prove that the radioactive label has not altered the molecule with respect to the biological property under investigation.

Pinocytosis, the local invagination of the cell membrane to form a vesicle that contains the substance being absorbed, and phagocytosis, the ingestion of a particle rather than a droplet, have been considered as possible mechanisms of active transport, but their role in the process of absorption remains uncertain.

TESTS OF INTESTINAL ABSORPTION

Sugars

Certain monosaccharides, such as glucose and galactose, are rapidly absorbed by the process of active transport. Other sugars, such as mannose, sorbose, and the pentoses, are slowly absorbed, probably by passive diffusion. Carbon-14 glucose can be used to measure the absorption of glucose in place of the classic glucose tolerance test; but one must be aware that the test reflects many metabolic processes, only one of which is intestinal absorption. The particular advantage of ^{14}C-labeled molecules is that the basic structure of the molecule has not been altered by the presence of the tracer.

Lipids

Dietary lipids include triglycerides such as tripalmitate, phospholipids such as lecithin, sterols such as cholesterol, terpene derivatives such as carotene, cerebrosides, and a variety of alcohol and aldehyde derivatives of fatty acids. Malabsorption of lipids can result from impaired digestive function, from deranged intestinal motility, from excessive secretion (exudative enteropathy), or from an inadequate absorptive surface as the result of inflammation or surgical ablation. Absorption may be impaired by alterations in the fine structure of the intestine, or from failure of biochemical reactions essential for normal function. The latter is the basis of the so-called primary malabsorption states, such as celiac disease, idiopathic steatorrhea (nontropical sprue), and tropical sprue. Evidence of structural lesions of the intestinal mucosa can be obtained by peroral biopsy techniques. Yet the appearance of the biopsy specimen often does not correlate with the degree of functional impairment in a given patient. The morphological abnormalities in a single biopsy specimen—such as flattened, coalesced villi—can be extremely marked and yet steatorrhea may be slight. Laster and Ingelfinger (1961) pointed out that both the degree and extent of involvement of specific regions of the small intestine determine the severity of the functional derangements. For example, glucose is absorbed primarily in the jejunum, whereas vitamin B_{12} is absorbed in the ileum.

A time-honored test for malabsorption of fat is the gross and microscopic examination of a fecal specimen. Although this method is of value in overt steatorrhea, it is often misleading since even a large amount of fat may not be readily visible. Measurement of vitamin A and carotene levels in plasma are useful as screening procedures, but the levels are dependent on the diet. Chemical analysis of the lipids in plasma, measurement of plasma turbidity, and chylomicron counts have also been used, but fecal fat determination remains the most widely accepted method.

Radioactive tracers were first used to study intestinal absorption in human beings by Stanley and Thannhauser (1949), who labeled olive oil with iodine-131 and measured the radioactivity in blood, urine, and the thyroid after oral administration of the oil. In 10 normal subjects, the concentration of total ^{131}I in the serum was greatest 3 to 6 hours after ingestion. In patients with hyperlipemia, the peak values were two to five times higher than normal, and there was an abnormally slow fall in the blood radioactivity during the next 24 hours. They did not use this method for the diagnosis of malabsorption.

In 1955, Baylin et al. proposed that ^{131}I-labeled fat be used for diagnosis of disturbances of fat absorption. They measured the percentage of administered radioactivity in the blood at intervals up to 6 hours after oral ingestion of ^{131}I-triolein. Patients with pancreatic disease, including pancreatitis or carcinoma, and patients with postgastrectomy steatorrhea, had decreased activity in the blood compared to normal subjects.

After these studies, ^{131}I-labeled triolein and oleic acid became available commercially; subsequent studies were performed by many authors, including McKenna et al. (1957), Reemtsma (1957), Fierst et al. (1958), Berkowitz (1957), Malm et al. (1956), and George (1961). Their results are summarized in Table 12-1.

Malm et al. (1956) proposed a way to distinguish whether an abnormality was due primarily to lack of proper digestive enzymes or to an intrinsic disorder

TABLE 12-1. FAT ABSORPTION

LABELED FAT	PEAK TIME IN BLOOD	% OF INGESTED DOSE IN BLOOD AT PEAK TIME	EFFICIENCY OF ABSORPTION	REPORTED BY
[131]I olive oil	3 hr.	10%		Stanley and Thannhauser, 1949
[131]I triolein	3–6 hr. (usually 3–4)	14–16%	96–99%	Baylin et al., 1955; Shingleton et al., 1955, 1957; McKenna 1957; Malm et al., 1956; etc.
[131]I oleic acid	3–4 hr.	15%	89–99%	Malm et al., 1956.

in the absorption process. If there was a lack of digestive enzymes, a triglyceride (such as triolein) that could not be digested would not be absorbed, but a fatty acid (such as oleic acid) would be absorbed without difficulty. Since their original description, these tests have been changed very little despite certain problems that have arisen. Grossman and Jordan (1958) found that 10 of 14 patients with steatorrhea had blood radioactivity levels in the normal range, and they concluded that the finding of a normal blood level of radioactivity after oral administration of a commercial radioiodinated triolein preparation does not exclude the presence of steatorrhea. Shingleton et al. (1957b) reported that in a series of patients with gastric resection and abnormally elevated fecal fat, only 20 out of 38 had depressed levels of radioactivity in the blood.

Lakshminarayana et al. (1960) analyzed commercial samples of ^{131}I triolein and ^{131}I oleic acid chromatographically and found methyl esters, monoglycerides, and diglycerides as impurities. Tuna et al. (1963) studied five commercially available preparations of radioiodinated triolein chromatographically and found that 30 to 60 per cent of the radioactivity was due to diglyceride impurities. Although Tuna et al. reported a method of purification of ^{131}I triolein that gave more reliable results, recent studies have used ^{14}C-labeled fat as a substitute for radioiodinated fat.

Rothfeld and Rabinowitz (1964) compared [131]I- and ^{14}C-labeled fats in the study of the malabsorption syndrome produced by the antibiotic neomycin in man. They measured the ^{131}I and ^{14}C radioactivity in feces after the administration of ^{131}I-labeled glyceryl trioleate and ^{14}C-labeled tripalmitate and compared the results with chemical measurements of fat. In all subjects, ^{14}C radioactivity showed good correlation with fecal fat, whereas only two of seven patients with steatorrhea showed abnormal fecal or blood levels of ^{131}I-labeled fat.

The use of ^{14}C-labeled compounds in the study of metabolic diseases in man has been greatly simplified by a method of analyzing [14]CO_2 in expiratory air. Von Schuching and Abt (1965) measured ^{14}C specific activity by absorption of CO_2 in 1 ml. of Hyamine hydroxide using phenolphthalein as an indicator (Fig. 12-1). This method is easily applied using ^{14}C-labeled tripalmitate or trioleate. After oral ingestion of 5 $\mu c.$ of ^{14}C-labeled fats, expiratory CO_2 is collected periodically for 24 hours and its specific activity is determined. This reflects the blood level of tripalmitate and makes possible the diagnosis of malabsorption of fat. Problems associated with radiochemical purity are avoided when ^{14}C compounds are used.

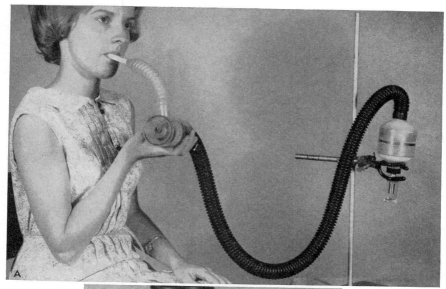

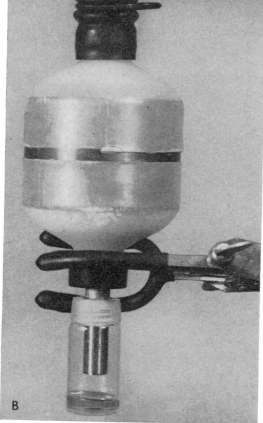

FIGURE 12-1. A, Equipment for sampling of $^{14}CO_2$ in expired air. Liquid scintillation counting vial is attached to a bottle containing calcium chloride to remove water. Carbon dioxide is absorbed by Hyamine in the vial. B, Detail of attachment of liquid scintillation vial containing Hyamine.

XYLOSE

Another example of the use of ^{14}C-labeled compounds is the D-xylose absorption test, which has also been of value in the differential diagnosis of malabsorption syndromes (Benson et al., 1957; Fowler and Cooke, 1960). The use of D-xylose labeled with ^{14}C solves the difficult problem of measuring D-xylose chemically.

CALCIUM

The amount of calcium absorbed from the intestinal tract is related to the amount of calcium in the diet. When the calcium intake is increased, a new metabolic equilibrium is reached after a few days. A decreased intake results in an increase in the percentage of calcium absorbed by the intestine. Absorption is also increased when greater amounts of calcium are required for purposes of repair or growth.

Calcium absorption can be measured after an oral dose of calcium gluconate containing a small amount of ^{45}Ca or ^{47}Ca. In some tests, the oral administration of one nuclide is combined with the intravenous injection of the other (Rich and Ivanovich, 1964).

Avioli et al. (1965) reported a simple 4 hour test for calcium absorption in man. A significant correlation was found between the 1 hour plasma radioactivity and the percentage of ^{47}Ca absorbed when measurements of fecal radioactivity were made over a period of 6 days. Normal subjects rapidly absorbed ^{47}Ca and showed maximum plasma values at 1 hour followed by a gradual decline over the next 3 hours. Patients with malabsorptive disorders had lower levels of radioactivity in the plasma at 1 hour. The abnormal patterns of absorption in these patients returned toward normal when vitamin D was given. Patients could also be characterized by patterns of increased calcium absorption. Serial 4 hour oral tests with ^{47}Ca in these patients showed suppression of the increased calcium absorption during sodium phytate therapy. The technique was as follows: at the end of a 12 to 15 hour overnight fast, 1 hour before breakfast, 5 to 10 μc. of ^{47}CaCl$_2$ (specific activity greater than 150 mc. per gram of Ca) was administered orally in 5 ml. of distilled water containing 20 mg. of calcium as CaCl$_2$.

Bhandarker et al. (1961) found that the maximum plasma radioactivity after an oral dose of 250 mg. of calcium as CaCl$_2$ labeled with ^{47}Ca was reached after about 2 hours, and the activity ranged from 0.3 to 3 per cent of the dose per liter of plasma. There was a good correlation between the plasma activity at 2 hours and the net calcium absorption as determined by calcium balance in 19 subjects. The great majority of patients with osteoporosis or steatorrhea were found to absorb calcium normally.

VITAMIN B$_{12}$

The absorption of vitamin B$_{12}$ can be measured as a test for intestinal absorption; its principal use is in studies of patients with anemia, described in Chapter IX.

EXUDATIVE ENTEROPATHY

Thomas Waldmann

Abnormal loss of serum proteins into the gastrointestinal tract is a common disorder that plays a major role in the pathogenesis of the hypoproteinemia associated with gastrointestinal diseases (Jeffries et al., 1962; Waldmann, 1966). When serum proteins pass into the gastrointestinal tract, they are catabolized rapidly into their constituent amino acids, which are reabsorbed. Hypoproteinemia occurs when the rate of catabolism of a protein exceeds the body's capacity to synthesize that protein.

Study of gastrointestinal protein loss has provided a better understanding of the pathogenesis of the hypoproteinemia of gastrointestinal diseases. The use of the techniques for demonstrating gastrointestinal protein loss may be the only way of pinpointing the intestinal tract as diseased since many patients have hypoproteinemia and edema as their only symptoms. The techniques for quantification of gastrointestinal protein loss have also been of value in determining the site of disease in the intestinal tract, in determining the activity of the gastrointestinal disease, and in studying the efficacy of therapy of the intestinal disorder. A number of new clinical syndromes involving protein loss into the gastrointestinal tract have been discovered in the past few years, a development of special importance.

Gastrointestinal protein loss should be considered in any patient with an unexplained reduction in the serum concentrations of albumin and gamma globulin. Abnormal losses are suggested since these proteins are synthesized at different sites. Other chemical abnormalities in patients with intestinal protein loss are low serum levels of transferrin, beta$_{2A}$ globulin, gamma macroglobulin, and cholesterol. The concentrations of fibrinogen and total alpha globulins are usually normal.

A number of techniques have been proposed for the detection, quantification, and localization of gastrointestinal protein loss. The most valuable involve the use of radioactive macromolecules including serum proteins labeled with ^{131}I or ^{125}I, polyvinylpyrrolidone labeled with ^{131}I, albumin labeled with chromium-51, and ceruloplasmin labeled with copper-67.

An ideal label for the detection of gastrointestinal protein loss should fulfill the following requirements: First, one should be able to attach the label to serum proteins without altering the metabolic behavior of the protein in terms of either survival or distribution. Second, there should be no absorption of the radioactive label from the gastrointestinal tract after catabolism of the protein since this would result in an underestimation of the extent of the gastrointestinal protein loss. Third, there should be no excretion of the label into the gastrointestinal tract except when bound to protein. Such secretion in the salivary, gastric, or biliary fluids would result in overestimation of the magnitude of the gastrointestinal protein loss. Although none completely fulfills all requirements, the materials used at present do provide a great deal of useful information.

The first widely used radioactive macromolecules, the radioiodinated serum proteins, fulfill the first requirement. One can iodinate proteins without altering their metabolism or distribution in the body. To perform a study of the rate of turnover of iodinated protein, the labeled protein is administered intravenously

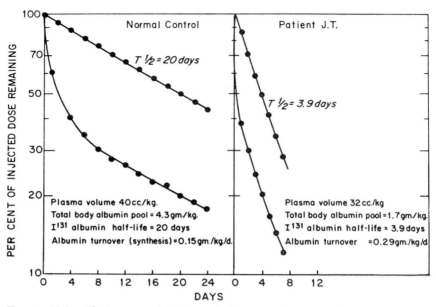

FIGURE 12-2. The turnover of I^{131} albumin in a normal person and in a patient, J.T., with gastrointestinal protein loss secondary to intestinal lymphangiectasia. The upper curves represent the decline in total body radioactivity with time. The lower curves represent the decline in plasma radioactivity. The total body albumin pool was markedly reduced in patient J.T. The survival half-life of iodinated albumin was markedly shortened and the albumin synthetic rate was slightly greater than normal.

to a patient who has been given an iodide solution orally to block thyroidal uptake of the radioisotope. After the iodinated protein is catabolized, the radio-iodine label is released and excreted in the urine. Complete urine collections and intermittent blood samples are obtained for 2 to 3 weeks following administration of the radioisotope. Graphs of radioactivity retained in the plasma and the cumulative radioactivity excreted in the urine are used for the analysis (Fig. 12-2). One can calculate the total body pool of a protein and, in the steady state, the synthetic rate of the protein. In general, patients with gastrointestinal protein loss have a reduced body pool of albumin, 7S gamma globulin (IgG), gamma macroglobulin (IgM), beta$_{2A}$ globulin (IgA) and ceruloplasmin (Schwartz and Jarnum, 1959; Barth et al., 1964). The half-time of survival of each of these proteins in the blood is markedly reduced, indicating an increase in the fraction of the intravascular pool of protein catabolized per day. Normal subjects catabolize from 6 to 10 per cent of their intravascular pool of albumin or gamma globulin per day. In contrast, patients with excessive gastrointestinal protein loss may lose 60 per cent of their plasma pool of these proteins each day into the gastrointestinal tract. In patients with gastrointestinal protein loss, all proteins studied are lost into the intestinal tract at the same rate, irrespective of molecular size. This is in contrast to the protein metabolism in patients with nephrosis; in these people small proteins are lost from the plasma into the urine at more rapid rates than large proteins.

The rate of synthesis of albumin in patients with gastrointestinal protein loss is normal or increased to a maximum of twice normal (Waldmann et al., 1961). A similar limited capacity to accelerate albumin synthesis occurs in patients with nephrosis (Gitlin et al., 1956) and in normal subjects following plasmaphoresis. The rate of synthesis of the three immunoglobulins (IgG, IgA, and IgM) is usually normal in patients with gastrointestinal protein loss. Thus, although there can be a marked acceleration of immunoglobulin synthesis following antigenic stimulation, a low plasma concentration does not appear to be an effective stimulus to immunoglobulin production.

Although iodinated proteins have been very valuable in the study of protein metabolism, they have certain limitations. There is rapid absorption of the radioiodide label following catabolism of the protein in the intestinal lumen, as well as active secretion of radioiodine in salivary and gastric secretions. In an effort to overcome the problem of absorption of the radioiodide label, Citrin et al. (1957) used intubation to collect the gastric secretions from a patient with giant gastric rugae who had previously received iodinated albumin intravenously. They were able to show that sufficient protein-bound radioiodine appeared in the gastric secretions to explain the hypercatabolism of albumin in this patient. This technique has not had wide use since one cannot collect all gastrointestinal secretions, especially when there are lesions in the small and large intestines. Furthermore, the intubation procedure itself may traumatize the bowel and lead to transient protein loss. Jeejeebhoy and Coghill (1961) gave an ion exchange resin (Amberlite IRA-400) orally in conjunction with intravenous ^{131}I albumin in an attempt to bind the free radioiodine released during catabolism of protein within the gastrointestinal lumen. In this way, reabsorption of the radioiodine is prevented and the radioactivity is excreted with the resin in the feces. Unfortunately, one of the requirements for a suitable test substance has not been met, namely, that there be no secretion of the radioiodine into the intestinal tract. If sodium radioiodide is injected intravenously, up to 50 per cent of the radioactivity will be bound to the resin and excreted in the feces (Waldmann and Wochner, 1964; Freeman and Gordon, 1964). Because of this secretion of iodide into the gastrointestinal lumen in the salivary and gastric secretions, catabolism of proteins at other body sites cannot be differentiated from gastrointestinal loss. Thus, this technique does not provide any information not obtainable using ^{131}I albumin turnover data alone and cannot be used to quantify gastrointestinal protein loss.

A number of other labeled macromolecules have been proposed to circumvent the problems in using ^{131}I-labeled proteins. Gordon (1959) introduced iodinated polyvinylpyrrolidone (PVP), a large polymer that is not metabolized by mammalian or bacterial enzymes and is poorly absorbed following oral administration. In testing for gastrointestinal protein loss, iodinated PVP is administered intravenously and the percentage of the administered dose appearing in the feces in the subsequent 4 days is determined. Normal subjects excrete from none to 1.5 per cent of the dose in the feces during this period; patients with gastrointestinal protein loss excrete 2 to 30 per cent of the injected dose. Although ^{131}I PVP has proved very useful in the detection of gastrointestinal protein loss, it is subject to several criticisms. PVP is not a natural serum protein but rather a polymer with a wide spectrum of molecular weights. Its survival in the blood is much shorter than that of most serum proteins and it is rapidly cleared by the reticuloendothelial system or excreted in the urine. The iodine-PVP bond is unstable, and variable amounts (10 to 64 per cent) of the radioactive label that enter the gastrointestinal tract are absorbed.

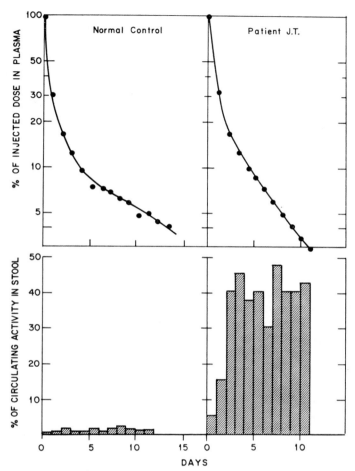

FIGURE 12-3. The fecal clearance of ⁵¹Cr following intravenous ⁵¹Cr albumin in a normal subject and a patient, J.T., with gastrointestinal protein loss. The normal person cleared 0.8 per cent of the plasma pool of labeled albumin into the gastrointestinal tract each day; patient J.T. cleared over 30 per cent of the plasma pool into the gastrointestinal tract each day, indicating severe gastrointestinal protein loss.

Human serum albumin labeled with ⁵¹Cr appears to be more satisfactory for studies of intestinal protein loss (Waldmann, 1961). The ⁵¹Cr label is neither significantly absorbed from nor secreted into the gastrointestinal tract. From 93 to 98 per cent of the radioactivity of an oral dose of ⁵¹Cr albumin appears in the subsequent fecal collections. Initially the test was performed in a manner similar to the PVP procedure, i.e., the dose was administered intravenously and the subsequent fecal radioactivity determined over the next 4 days. Normal subjects excreted less than 0.7 per cent of the administered radioactivity during this period. Patients with intestinal protein loss excreted a greater amount, from 2 to 40 per cent. There was a close correlation between the fecal ⁵¹Cr excretion and the fractional catabolic rate of ¹³¹I albumin in these patients (Waldmann and Wochner, 1964). Quantification of enteric protein loss may be obtained if the daily fecal excretion of ⁵¹Cr is related to the serum radioactivity curve (Fig. 12-3). This is comparable in principle to the use of ⁵¹Cr red blood cells in measuring loss of blood. The data may be expressed as the fraction of the plasma protein pool lost or as milliliters of plasma lost into the intestine per day. The volume of plasma cleared into the intestine per day may be determined from the ratio of the ^{51}Cr counts in the stool of that day and the counts per milliliter of plasma of the same day. The mean of the clearance values for days 2 through 12 after administration of the isotope is used. A normal person clears the albumin from 5 to 25 ml. of plasma into the intestinal tract each day; patients with protein-losing enteropathy may lose from 800 to 1800 ml. of plasma each day. Chromium-51 albumin cannot be used to determine the albumin turnover because the chromium label is gradually eluted from the albumin and the apparent survival of the protein is shortened.

Recently ^{67}Cu-labeled ceruloplasmin has been used to study gastrointestinal protein loss. It fulfills the major requirements for an adequate indicator for this purpose (Waldmann et al., 1967). Following oral administration of ^{67}Cu-labeled ceruloplasmin to dogs and man, 80 to 100 per cent of the administered radioactivity appeared in the feces, indicating that gastrointestinal absorption of the radioactivity was slight. The metabolism of intravenously administered ^{67}Cu-labeled ceruloplasmin was similar to that of ^{131}I-labeled ceruloplasmin, indicating that the labeling of ceruloplasmin with ^{67}Cu did not alter its metabolism.

To measure enteric protein loss, ^{67}Cu ceruloplasmin is administered intravenously and the radioactivity remaining in the serum and excreted daily in the feces is determined over the subsequent 12 days. The fecal clearance of ^{67}Cu ceruloplasmin is determined in the same way as clearance of ^{51}Cr albumin. Normal persons lose less than 2 per cent of the circulating pool of ^{67}Cu ceruloplasmin into the intestinal tract each day. This intestinal loss represents about 10 per cent of the total catabolism of this protein in these subjects. Patients with excessive intestinal protein loss may lose up to 60 per cent of their plasma pool of ceruloplasmin per day into the gastrointestinal tract. Copper-67 ceruloplasmin is difficult to produce and too expensive for routine clinical studies. We therefore use ^{51}Cr albumin for the routine diagnosis of intestinal protein loss. A more exact analysis may be achieved by the simultaneous use of ^{51}Cr labeled albumin and ^{125}I labeled albumin.

Through the use of these techniques, gastrointestinal protein loss has been shown to occur in over 30 common gastrointestinal diseases, including giant gastric rugae (Citrin et al., 1957), gastric carcinoma, (Jarnum and Schwartz, 1959), sprue (Parkins, 1960), Whipple's disease, regional enteritis, and ulcerative colitis (Steinfeld et al., 1960). In many of the patients studied, hypoproteinemia and edema were the only manifestations of the gastrointestinal disease process.

Gastrointestinal protein loss may be a prominent feature of a number of diseases not usually thought of as involving the gastrointestinal tract. A most important one is constrictive pericarditis (Davidson et al., 1961). We have studied nine patients with this disease who had severe gastrointestinal protein loss. All had serum albumin levels of 1.0 to 2.0 g. per 100 ml., increased albumin clearance, and abnormal leakage of ^{51}Cr albumin and ^{131}I PVP. All disorders of protein metabolism were cured by pericardiectomy.

Patients with agammaglobulinemia may develop chronic gastrointestinal infections, ileocolitis, or a spruelike syndrome. Intestinal protein loss may be superimposed on their basic disorders of immunoglobulin production (Vesin et al., 1960; Waldmann and Laster, 1964). When detected and treated, the gastrointestinal protein loss can be successfully reversed. Some patients with nephrosis, amyloidosis, and scleroderma have been found to have enteric protein loss.

A number of new syndromes have been detected by the study of intestinal protein loss. The most common of these is intestinal lymphangiectasia (Schwartz and Jarnum, 1959; Holman et al., 1959; Waldmann et al., 1961). Of 44 patients seen at the National Institutes of Health with idiopathic hypoproteinemia, 20 have had intestinal lymphangiectasia, a disorder of early onset with first symptoms appearing from birth to 28 years. Edema was usually marked and often asymmetrical. The patients had marked hypoalbuminemia and hypogammaglobulinemia with markedly accelerated protein clearance and abnormal ^{131}I PVP and ^{51}Cr albumin tests. The patients were not anemic and did not have eosinophilia but almost all had lymphocytopenia and skin anergy. The gastrointestinal symptoms were relatively mild. A striking feature of the disease was the presence of markedly dilated lymphatic channels in the small bowel. Biopsy of the small intestine revealed dilated telangiectatic lymphatic channels in the submucosa. These frequently contained macrophages filled with fat, some of which completely occluded the lymphatic channels. There were no PAS-positive cells in the submucosa comparable to those seen in Whipple's disease.

The disorder of lymphatic channels is not limited to the gastrointestinal tract. Eight of the 20 patients had chylous effusion. Lymphangiograms revealed significant hypoplasia of peripheral lymphatics and, in some patients, aplasia of the thoracic duct or absence of all abdominal lymph nodes. Intestinal lymphangiectasia is a generalized disorder of the lymphatic system with associated loss of lymph together with its proteins and lymphocytes into the intestinal tract. The following case illustrates the typical clinical features.

J. T. was a 35 year old male admitted for study of generalized edema of 20 years' duration and marked blurring of vision of 3 months' duration. There was no history of cardiac, renal, or hepatic disease. Occasional mild diarrhea was the only gastrointestinal symptom. Physical examination revealed marked edema of the ankles and legs, moderate edema of the hands, and significant macular edema. The visual acuity was 20/200.

Laboratory analysis revealed a hemoglobin of 16.1 g. per 100 ml.; white blood cells 6000 per cu. mm.; lymphocytes 500 per cu. mm. The serum cholesterol was 124 mg. per 100 ml. The total protein was 3.4 g. per 100 ml. with the albumin 1.9 g. per 100 ml., alpha$_1$-globulin 0.28 g. per 100 ml., alpha$_2$-globulin 0.64 g. per 100 ml., beta globulin 0.64 g. per 100 ml., and gamma globulin 0.52 g. per 100 ml. Renal and hepatic function studies were normal.

The metabolism of albumin was studied using ^{131}I-labeled albumin (Fig. 12–2). The plasma volume and total body albumin pool were determined by isotope dilution methods. The plasma volume was 32 cc. per kg., slightly below normal. The total exchangeable albumin was 1.7 g. per kg., markedly below the normal range of 3.6 to 4.4 g. per kg. The half-time of albumin in blood determined from the slope of the whole-body radioactivity curve and from the slope of the serum radioactivity curve was 3.9 days compared to a normal range of 14 to 20 days (Fig. 12–2). The fraction of the total body albumin catabolized per day determined from the ratio 0.693/albumin half-time was 17 per cent per day, markedly greater than the normal of 4 per cent per day. The albumin turn-over (synthetic rate) determined from the product of the total exchangeable albumin and the fraction of the body albumin catabolized per day was 0.29, slightly greater than the normal rate of 0.15 to 0.20 g. per kg. per day. The turnover of 7S gamma globulin (IgG), gamma macroglobulin (IgM), and beta$_{2A}$ globulin (IgA) showed a comparable reduction in total body protein pools with markedly reduced protein survival half-times. Five per cent of an intravenous dose of ^{131}I PVP was excreted in the feces in the subsequent 4 days; the upper limit of normal is 1.5 per cent. Fifteen per cent of an intravenous dose of ^{51}Cr albumin was found in the subsequent 4 day stool collection; the upper limit of normal is 0.7 per cent. The ^{51}Cr clearance showed that the patient lost 40 per cent of the circulating albumin pool per day into the gastrointestinal tract (Fig. 12–3).

The metabolism of ceruloplasmin studied with [67]Cu-labeled ceruloplasmin showed a comparable gastrointestinal clearance of 35 per cent of the circulating pool per day, compared to a mean of 2 per cent in normal subjects. All of the protein turnover studies indicated that the hypoproteinemia was secondary to gastrointestinal protein loss with a normal or slightly accelerated rate of protein synthesis. Roentgenograms of the gastrointestinal tract showed only edema of the small intestinal mucosa. At laparotomy the jejunum and ileum were edematous with dark brown pigmentation over the serosal surface of the ileum. The involved ileal segment was resected. Histological examination revealed marked dilatation of the lymphatic channels in the submucosa. A lymphangiogram revealed hypoplastic lymphatics of the leg with dermal backflow similar to that seen in lymphedema. There was no filling of the thoracic duct. The patient's gastrointestinal protein loss was not affected by the surgical procedure, by a gluten-free or a low-fat diet, or by corticosteroid administration. Following administration of chlorothiazide and spironolactone, the patient lost 18 kg. and the macular edema disappeared, and visual acuity returned to 20/40.

Another syndrome that we have seen in six children is allergic gastroenteropathy. Patients with this syndrome had marked hypoalbuminemia, hypogammaglobulinemia, anemia, extreme eosinophilia, and growth retardation. They had few gastrointestinal symptoms and did not have malabsorption. The peroral small intestinal biopsies were normal except for an increased number of eosinophils in the submucosa. Many patients had asthma or eczema and a familial history of allergies. The symptoms of most patients were aggravated by the ingestion of milk. In three of the patients studied there was a complete return to normal protein metabolism following steroid administration. In three other patients there was a marked amelioration of the hypoproteinemia and eosinophilia when the patient was placed on a hypoallergenic diet. The withdrawal of milk from the diet appeared to be the major factor. Thus allergy, or at least an abnormal response to milk, appeared to initiate the anemia, eosinophilia, and gastrointestinal protein loss.

In summary, gastrointestinal protein loss is a common clinical entity comparable to proteinuria in both its nonspecificity and its importance. It can be diagnosed by simple tests using either ^{51}Cr-labeled albumin or iodinated PVP. The study of gastrointestinal protein loss has led to the discovery of new clinical syndromes including intestinal lymphangiectasia and allergic gastroenteropathy. It is important to try to make a specific diagnosis after gastrointestinal protein loss has been demonstrated since at least half of the patients can be cured by appropriate dietary, drug, or surgical therapy.

DETECTION OF GASTROINTESTINAL BLEEDING

HENRY N. WAGNER, JR.

FRED MISHKIN

Quantitative evaluation of gastrointestinal bleeding by chemical methods is difficult, if not impossible. A sensitive method, such as the use of benzidine, may give positive results in the absence of bleeding. A less sensitive method, such as the use of guaiac, may fail to reveal small amounts of bleeding. In 1954, Owen et al. first proposed the use of ^{51}Cr for the quantitative measurement of gastrointestinal bleeding. They labeled erythrocytes from two normal dogs with about 100 μc. of ^{51}Cr and reinjected them intravenously. They found less than 0.1 per cent of the injected radioactivity in the feces per day, which was equivalent to less than 1 ml. of blood. Chromium-51-labeled erythrocytes were placed in the stomach of another dog; most of the dose appeared in the feces in 48 hours (88 per cent in 48 hours; 92 per cent in 96 hours). During the same period only 2 per cent appeared in the urine, and the observed radioactivity in the blood was low. It was concluded that the amount of blood entering the intestine in pathological conditions could be evaluated with a sensitivity equal to a volume of 5 ml.

In a subsequent report (1954b), Owen and his colleagues showed the validity of this method in clinical cases of portal cirrhosis with esophageal varices. In 1957, Roche et al., Hughes-Jones, and also Bannerman confirmed the results in patients with anemia from chronic gastrointestinal bleeding. Roche reported that the fecal recovery of ^{51}Cr was 96.7 per cent in man. In Hughes-Jones' series, six anemic patients were studied with this method and the estimated blood loss from the intestine correlated well with the rate of loss of ^{51}Cr from the blood.

A simple method for the measurement of fecal radioactivity is described in Chapter XXI, Technical Details of Common Procedures. Because of the unpleasantness of preparing and transferring fecal homogenates, and the inefficiency of counting small aliquots in a well scintillation counter, Buchanan and Sampson (1962) described an easily constructed, gas-fired, laboratory incinerator that is capable of reducing stool specimens and other large organic samples to ashes of small volume. Complete combustion is achieved by surrounding the sample and its container by gas flames and then venting any distilled gases through an incandescent wire screen. The ashes are transferred to test tubes for measurement in a well scintillation counter. The method is considerably more sensitive than the counting of aliquots of homogenized feces, and most of the unpleasantness of former methods is eliminated. Its chief use has been the quantification of gastrointestinal hemorrhage with the use of ^{51}Cr-labeled erythrocytes, but it has also been used successfully with labeled vitamin B$_{12}$.

Determination of the site of upper gastrointestinal bleeding is sometimes difficult, but it is important for diagnosis as well as for surgical treatment. Bleeding sites can sometimes be localized using the technique of Ebaugh et al. (1958) who intubated patients with a Miller-Abbott tube and collected samples at various intestinal sites. In eight of nine cases, the technique was of value in diagnosis. Ariel (1962) used a double-lumen tube with holes inferior and superior to a balloon. Its use in 15 patients revealed gastric or duodenal bleeding in six and esophageal bleeding in five. The test was not satisfactory in four patients, because active bleeding had ceased.

Healey et al. (1960) used three small Geiger counters, which were inserted directly into the three different parts of the gastrointestinal tract. After injection of ^{32}P-labeled red cells, they determined successfully the site of hemorrhage in seven dogs. But because of limitations of the Geiger-Müller counter, the technique was not applied clinically. Brown et al. (1962) studied the possibility of using ^{131}I Hippuran and external counting with scintillation detectors during explorative laparotomy. He reported that the method was useful in localizing bleeding sites in the small intestine.

THE LIVER

Henry N. Wagner, Jr.
Fred Mishkin

The polygonal cells of the liver serve as a storage center for glycogen, proteins, neutral fats, vitamins, and certain minerals. Breakdown and inter-conversion of the storage products also occur in the liver. Breakdown of carbohydrates through the tricarboxylic acid cycle and hexose monophosphate shunt provides energy for the body. The resulting acetyl coenzyme A molecules can be used as energy sources or as building blocks for fats. The ribosyl groups from the hexose monophosphate shunt provide a substrate for nucleic acid production. The liver is the chief site of urea production. Transamination links protein and carbohydrate synthesis. Through a balance of these processes, the liver furnishes the body needed carbohydrates, proteins, enzymes, and coagulation factors. The polygonal cells detoxify and metabolically inactivate substances by conjugation with cysteine, glycine, or sulfate, or by acetylation. The polygonal cells produce and secrete bile acids to aid in fat digestion and absorption.

The Kupffer cells, the principal site of the reticuloendothelial system (RES), are chiefly concerned with phagocytosis. Here blood pigment is broken down to form bilirubin and here the first stages of antibody formation are believed to take place. Because the function of both polygonal cells and reticuloendothelial cells depends upon an adequate blood supply, functional impairment by disease tends to affect both types of cells.

The blood flow to an organ such as the liver can be looked at in several ways: as the fraction of the cardiac output that it receives, as the absolute blood flow in milliliters per unit time, and in terms of the regional distribution of blood flow throughout various parts of the organ. Measurement of one or more of these indices with radioactive tracers is based on one of the following principles: (1) the Fick principle; (2) the clearance of particles by the RES or by capillary blockade; (3) the clearance of a substance accumulated by polygonal cells; or (4) the clearance of an appropriate tracer injected into an afferent blood vessel. The Fick principle is the basis of the measurement of liver blood flow with the use of Bromsulphalein (BSP) and will not be considered in detail. In essence, the method requires hepatic vein catheterization and cannot be performed effectively in jaundiced patients because of the chemical interference with the colorimetric determination. The simplification of the BSP method—in which a single blood sample is obtained after intravenous injection of 5 mg. per kg. of BSP—has the advantage of great sensitivity and ease of performance but is not useful in jaundiced patients.

Certain mononuclear cells that line the sinusoids of the liver and spleen, and to a lesser degree the blood vessels of certain other regions of the body, have a special ability to remove particulate matter from the circulation by the process of phagocytosis. These cells constitute the reticuloendothelial system (RES).

After intravenous injection, particles of all types—gold, silver, chromic phosphate, carbon, thorium dioxide, and so on—are phagocytized with great efficiency. Most inorganic particles remain in phagocytic cells almost indefinitely because they cannot be metabolized; organic particles, such as bacteria, effete blood cells, and aggregates of proteins, are metabolized after ingestion. The nearly complete extraction of particles by these cells and their predominant location in the liver and spleen provide the basis for the colloidal clearance method of estimating liver blood flow.

If we measure the rate of removal from the blood of radioactive particles that are completely removed during a single passage through the liver and spleen, but are not significantly removed from the circulation by any other organ, we have an index of the blood flow to the liver and spleen. The degree to which the radioactive particles are not completely extracted during a single circulation and the degree to which there is uptake of particles in RES cells in areas other than the liver and spleen are factors that result in errors in the estimation of liver blood flow. Errors are also introduced if some of the particles are sufficiently large to become trapped in the pulmonary capillary bed. A partial solution to the problem of extrahepatic uptake of particles is the direct measurement of the rate of accumulation of radioactivity over the liver by means of an external radiation detector.

In 1952, Dobson and Jones first measured the rate of clearance of ^{32}P-labeled chromic phosphate particles from the blood to estimate liver blood flow. The main problem was difficulty in preparing particles of proper size. Furthermore, since ^{32}P is a beta-emitter, it could not be measured satisfactorily by external radiation detectors. To obviate these difficulties, Vetter and his associates (1954) used colloidal gold particles, labeled with a gamma-emitting radioisotope (^{198}Au). However, the gold particles also varied in size, resulting in variable clearance rates and, at times, accumulation of particles in sites such as the lungs. Trying to obtain a particle more suitable than colloidal gold, Halpern and others (1956) used colloidal aggregates of albumin.

Colloidal clearance techniques can be used to provide a rough estimate of hepatic blood flow even though we still do not have the ideal particle for this purpose (Razzak and Wagner, 1961). Such a particle should be less than 1 micron in diameter, of uniform size, and labeled with a gamma-emitting radionuclide to permit easy detection. The radionuclide should have a short physical half-life, since the radiation dose to the liver is limited to permissible levels either by rapid radioactive decay or by excretion after metabolism of the particles. Of the particles used to date, only aggregated albumin and iron colloids are metabolized readily by the body.

A major limitation of the colloidal clearance method of estimating liver blood flow is that patients with liver disease may have a reduced efficiency of the reticuloendothelial cells of the liver and a significantly increased efficiency of the RES in other parts of the body (Fig. 12-4). Since the basic postulates of the method are no longer fulfilled, the estimation of liver blood flow in the presence of liver disease is unreliable. In the dog, after hepatectomy in which 70 per cent of the liver was removed (Baker et al., 1967), the clearance of colloidal particles returned to normal control values within a few days, before the regenerating liver had achieved its original mass.

After Halpern and his colleagues (1956) proposed the use of heat-denatured human serum albumin particles labeled with radioiodine, preliminary results in animals and man suggested that extrahepatic removal was minimal and hepatic extraction was over 90 per cent (Shaldon et al., 1961). In normal subjects, measurements of the rates of clearance of these particles proved suitable for estimating liver blood flow and the results correlated well with those from the indocyanine green method, previously shown to be adequate.

In Sherlock's method (Shaldon et al., 1961), approximately 0.1 mg. per kg. body weight of aggregated albumin (AA) labeled with 20 to 50 μc. of ^{131}I is injected intravenously after the thyroid has been blocked by the administration of Lugol's solution. Arterial samples are obtained at 3, 4, 5, 6, 8, 10, 15, 20, and 30 minutes after injection; venous samples are also suitable. The radioactivity of the samples is determined in a well-type scintillation counter, and the proteins

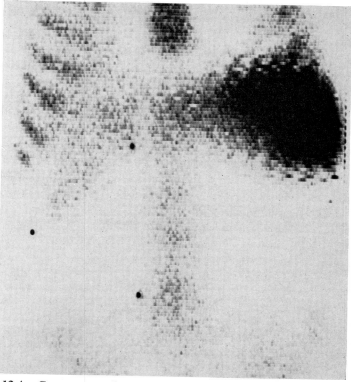

FIGURE 12-4. Compensatory hyperactivity of the reticuloendothelial system. Liver scan performed with ^{99m}Tc-S colloid in a cirrhotic patient. There is poor uptake of the colloid by the severely damaged reticuloendothelial cells of the liver, with increased uptake in the spleen and bone marrow. The half-time of clearance of the particles from the blood was 5 minutes, which is prolonged; the normal range is 2.5 to 3.5 minutes.

are then precipitated. The protein-free supernatant is measured to correct for the presence of free iodine. Coprecipitation of some free iodide occurs, and more precise determinations can be carried out if a Sephadex or ion-exchange column is used. Protein-bound activity after 25 minutes is considered to be due to un-aggregated albumin molecules, and this value is subtracted from each value for the earlier samples. The total activity is plotted on semilog paper as a function of time, and the half-time of clearance ($T\frac{1}{2}$) is calculated. Plasma volume is calculated by dividing the activity at time zero into the total amount of radioactivity injected. Hepatic blood flow is equal to k $\times$ blood volume, where $k = \dfrac{0.693}{T\frac{1}{2}}$.

Since the extraction of the colloid by the liver is not 100 per cent, the value of k underestimates the fraction of the blood volume perfusing the liver. On the other hand, extrahepatic removal of the particles increases the value of k and overestimates the hepatic blood flow. The latter problem is partially solved by the use of external counting techniques, in which an external scintillation counter is directed toward the liver and the time course of radioactivity is measured after intravenous injection. Usually a collimated detector is directed toward the right lateral chest wall perpendicular to the anterolateral surface of the liver. The count rate is recorded by means of a rate meter or recording scaler. Almost immediately after the injection, the count rate increases rapidly, but after 10 minutes it approaches a limiting value. The log of the difference between this value and the values measured at 30 second intervals is plotted as a function of time, and a single exponential uptake is determined. Torrance and Gowenlock (1962) found that the half-time in 24 anesthetized subjects was 2.88 minutes (S.E. 0.14); and in 21 conscious subjects, 1.61 minutes (S.E. 0.17). This compares with the findings of Biozzi and others (1958) of a mean half-time of 2.05 minutes in six unanesthetized control subjects. Although the external detection method solves partially the problem of extrahepatic removal of the colloidal particles, it introduces the problem of variations in the sensitivity of the detector and the structure of the liver and its surroundings.

In 1909, Abel and Rowntree observed that phenoltetrachlorphthalein is excreted almost entirely through the biliary system, and they developed a clinical liver function test based on measurement of the fecal excretion of the dye. In 1922, Rosenthal measured colorimetrically the blood clearance of dyes, and the method of measuring fecal elimination of dye was discarded. Rosenthal and White (1925) prepared a wide spectrum of related halogenated phenolphthalein dyes, studied their relative affinity for the liver and discovered that sulfobromophthalein sodium (Bromsulphalein, BSP) does not leave the blood in significant amounts after the hepatic blood supply has been ligated. The dye rose bengal was studied at the same time, and, although Rosenthal and White believed it to be inferior to BSP, many other investigators found it equally effective in estimating hepatic damage.

Beginning in 1945, Bradley and his associates applied Fick's principle to the indirect estimation of hepatic blood flow in man, and the method became widely used to obtain fundamental information about liver blood flow; it was useful in a simplified form in the solution of the difficult problem of detecting early and marginal hepatic dysfunction. It was clear that rose bengal concentrated only in the polygonal cells and not in the reticuloendothelial cells (Mendeloff, 1949). However, the colorimetric measurements of rose bengal never achieved the popularity of BSP, for reasons that are not clear. The lack of clinical interest in rose bengal continued until 1954, when Taplin and his associates labeled rose bengal with [131]I. The test with radioactive rose bengal could be readily applied to large numbers of patients, and numerous reports of its use appeared in the literature.

Lushbaugh and his associates (1964) pointed out that rose bengal is an ideal dye for the assessment of hepatic function. They also described the numerous modifications of technique that have been used to measure hepatic function with this radiopharmaceutical. One of the important uses of ^{131}I rose bengal has been in neonatal pediatrics. By means of a stationary detector with minimum spatial resolution or by means of serial scans with a higher degree of spatial resolution, together with collection of feces and urine, we can track the movement of radioactivity from the liver into the intestine within a period of 6 hours. In complete biliary atresia, the hepatic image of the radioactivity remains essentially unchanged, and less than 5 per cent of the dose is found in the feces over a 72 hour period. In contrast, in other forms of obstruction, such as congenital hepatitis, the obstruction is less complete and more than 5 per cent of the activity reaches the feces (Brent and Geppert, 1959). Whereas less than 4 per cent of the radioactivity is found in the urine of the normal infant, increasing amounts (up to 35 or 40 per cent of the dose) are found in the urine when varying degrees of intrahepatic or extrahepatic obstruction are present. Successive rose bengal scans of a normal person are illustrated in Figure 12-5. The progressive movement into the biliary tract can be seen.

Measurements of the rates of blood disappearance and liver accumulation of rose bengal can be used as rough indices of function of the hepatic polygonal cells. It is possible to measure the function of the entire liver or of particular regions by serial quantitative scanning techniques. Measurements of the rate of blood clearance or hepatic accumulation of rose bengal are better indices of function if a loading dose of BSP is given simultaneously with the tracer dose of rose bengal (Mena et al., 1959). In patients without jaundice, the BSP test is

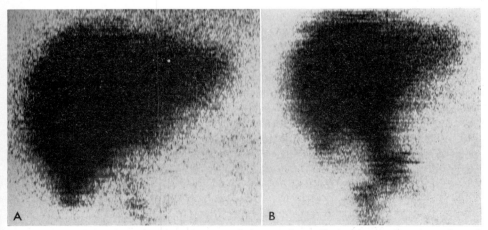

FIGURE 12-5. *A,* Liver scan of a normal person after administration of ^{131}I rose bengal. Normal contour is outlined 20 minutes following injection of the radionuclide with a trace of activity in the area of the extrahepatic biliary system. *B,* Repeat scan in the same person 1 hour later. The dense accumulation of the radionuclide in the extrahepatic biliary system and small bowel is a result of excretion of rose bengal through the biliary system.

preferable because of its high sensitivity and simplicity. In patients with jaundice, the rose bengal test provides information about the patency of the biliary system and the flow of bile, which are difficult to evaluate by other methods. An abdominal detector, used together with serial scanning, can record the changing levels of radioactivity in the intestinal tract. Normally, rose bengal begins to enter the intestine within 10 to 20 minutes after injection and its half-time of excretion from the liver is about 90 minutes. In certain patients, particularly those with complete biliary obstruction, it is easy to demonstrate retention of labeled rose bengal in the liver for prolonged periods of time.

HISTORICAL OUTLINE OF LIVER SCANNING

Rose bengal is the prototype of successful liver scanning agents that localize in the polygonal cells of the liver. In addition to using this radiopharmaceutical for the study of liver function, Taplin et al. (1955) suggested that it might be used to locate tumors, cysts, or abscesses. Earlier, studies of the localization of intravenously injected radioactive colloids (Sheppard et al., 1951; Dobson and Jones, 1952; Root et al., 1954) had revealed that neoplasms seemed to result in a failure of the involved regions of the liver to concentrate the colloidal particles, in striking contrast with the high activity in the remaining normal tissue. Cassen et al. (1951) introduced a collimated scintillation detector automated to scan in a rectilinear manner. Stirret and his co-workers (1954) performed the first scans to demonstrate metastases and abscesses. Originally Stirrett et al. (1953a) employed iodinated ^{131}I human serum albumin patterned after the method of Moore (1953) for detecting cerebral neoplasms. The method consisted of measuring the radioactivity over various points of the abdomen with a collimated scintillation detector 24 hours after the injection of the iodinated albumin. This attempt to survey the liver, point by point, and to demonstrate a lesion depended upon increased uptake of the tracer by the neoplasm. This technique was soon replaced with an automatic scanning method employing [198]Au colloid as the scanning agent (Stirrett et al., 1954). Using a background suppression technique to enhance contrast, Friedell and co-workers (1957) demonstrated the efficacy of both ^{131}I rose bengal and [198]Au colloidal gold in visualizing the structure of the liver. The development of heat-denatured human serum albumin labeled with ^{131}I as an agent for investigating liver phagocytosis and blood flow by Benacerraf et al. (1957) and by Biozzi et al. (1958) quickly led to its use as a scanning agent (Delaloye et al., 1959). Harper and his co-workers (1965) recently introduced a colloidal form of technetium-99m-labeled sulfur. Technetium-99m is an excellent nuclide for scanning because of emission of a monoenergetic gamma ray, lack of particulate emission, short half-life, convenient availability, and cheapness. Recently indium-113m has been introduced as a liver scanning agent in a colloidal form that offers many advantages (Goodwin et al., 1966). Other agents that have had clinical trials include ^{131}I iodipamide (Charkes and Shansky, 1964), ^{64}Cu in both the ionic and complexed form (Aronow et al., 1959), zinc-64 (Aronow et al., 1959), ^{125}I-iodinated rose bengal (Endlich et al., 1962), and molybdenum-99 (Sorensen and Archambault, 1963).

ANATOMY OF THE LIVER

Sixty per cent of the mass of the liver is made up of the polygonal cells; the remaining tissue consists of reticuloendothelial cells. The parenchymal cells are arranged in double-layered plates interlaced with sinusoids so that a spongelike structure results. The right side of the liver is dome-shaped and its lateral border is indented by the rib cage (Fig. 12-6). The inferior border is

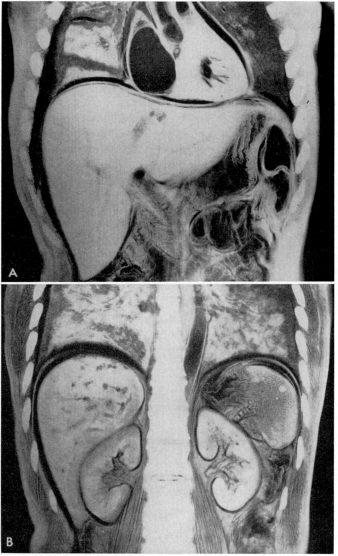

FIGURE 12-6. *A*, Midcoronal section of a cadaver. The rib cage indents the right margin of the liver. The heart rests in a depression in the top of the left lobe of the liver. The major branches of the portal vein at the porta hepatis are outlined with air. There is air in the hepatic veins which coalesce at the foot of the medial slope of the diaphragm. *B*, A coronal section posterior to that in *A*. The left lobe is not seen since it lies anterior to the spine. The kidney indents the midportion of the under surface of the liver.

indented where the ligamentum teres, the rounded free margin of the falciform ligament, enters the hepatic parenchyma, forming the umbilical notch, and continues dorsally to form the longitudinal fissure. The portal vein, hepatic artery, and bile duct come together at the porta hepatis. The gallbladder lies in an indentation along the right anterior-inferior margin parallelling the longitudinal fissure and lined up with the inferior vena cava posteriorly. These structures seem to form an H, lying under the liver, the right side formed by the gallbladder and vena cava, the left side by the longitudinal fissure, and the crossbar by the porta hepatis. The inferior surface of the liver slants sharply upward from front to back; the bottom edge is quite thin, and increases in thickness as it proceeds in a cephalad direction. The liver is also thin in anterior-posterior dimension where it crosses the spine, since the anterior-posterior dimension of the body cavity is narrowest here. The hepatic veins coalesce at the medial foot of the slope of the hepatic dome to enter the inferior vena cava. The heart fits into an impression along the superior margin of the liver. Viewed from the right lateral position, the liver has a convex anterior margin. The inferior margin of the liver slopes sharply upward in an anterior to posterior direction forming a blunted point at the anterior-inferior margin. The right kidney and adrenal are adjacent to the inferior surface of the liver.

Healy et al. (1953) have indicated the value of dividing the liver according to its segmental arterial supply and biliary drainage. This is useful in the case of partial hepatectomy since there are no intrahepatic anastomoses between the intraparenchymal branches of the hepatic arteries. Thus, the right lobe is demarcated by an oblique major fissure extending down from the fossa of the inferior vena cava to that of the gallbladder. The right lobe may be divided into an anterior and posterior portion, each of which may be subdivided into superior and inferior areas. The left lobe is divided into a medial and lateral segment by the falciform ligament and its intrahepatic extension. These segments are divided into superior and inferior areas. The caudate lobe, bounded on the right by the inferior vena cava, on the left by the transverse fissure, and anteriorly by the porta hepatis, may be divided into a right and left portion and a separate caudate process.

SCANNING AGENTS

Radiopharmaceuticals used in liver scanning fall into two major categories: those taken up by the polygonal cells and those phagocytized by the Kupffer cells of the reticuloendothelial system. Agents taken up by the polygonal cells, rose bengal and iodipamide, are excreted into the biliary tree. The concentration of these agents in the liver changes during the time the liver is being scanned, leading occasionally to confusing images, especially if scanning time is prolonged. Excretion into the intestine via the biliary tract may result in confusing abdominal activity. On the other hand, these agents provide a means of demonstrating biliary obstruction. The rate of disappearance of the agent from the liver may be documented by scans at intervals of 1, 6, and 24 hours. Failure of hepatic activity to appear in the intestine in one hour suggests biliary obstruction. In complete obstruction, a scan of the liver performed at 24 hours may not be significantly different from the scan performed shortly after injection,

(Fig. 12-7). However, intrahepatic and extrahepatic obstruction cannot be accurately differentiated in this way.

Except for albumin aggregates and certain iron colloids, which are metabolized, phagocytized particles remain in the Kupffer cells of the liver almost indefinitely. Consequently, short-lived radionuclides must be used to reduce radiation dose. In addition to the liver, other organs containing phagocytic cells, notably the spleen, will accumulate particles and may be visualized by scanning. At times, this may lead to confusion, for example, in deciding whether a concentration of radioactivity is in the left lobe of the liver or the spleen.

Molybdenum (Sorensen and Archambault, 1963) is of interest since it is the only agent used in liver scanning that localizes in the parenchymal cells and is not excreted in the biliary tract but remains in the cells.

Discrepancy in the images of the structure of the liver may occasionally result when different agents are used. For example, in severe cirrhosis, large functional defects apparent on the colloid scan may not be seen on the rose bengal scan (Fig 12-8A and B). In cases of hepatitis, cirrhosis, or obstructive jaundice with severe impairment of parenchymal cell function, clearance of radioactive rose bengal from the blood is often prolonged whereas reticuloendothelial function remains relatively undisturbed, as evidenced by a normal blood clearance of the colloid. Certain properties of the more commonly used hepatic scanning agents are summarized in Table 12-2.

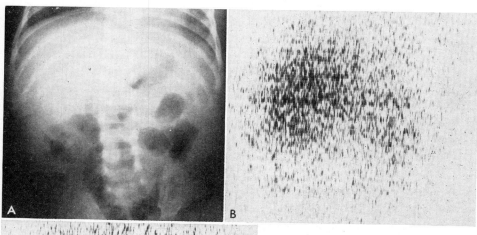

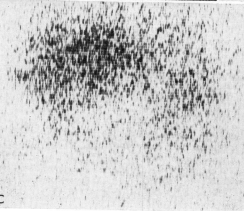

FIGURE 12-7. Neonatal hepatitis with obstruction. A, Plain abdominal film. B, Iodine-131 rose bengal scan 6 hours after injection, showing no appreciable accumulation of activity in the intestine. C, Scan 24 hours after injection, showing little change from the 6 hour scan, indicating obstruction of the biliary tree, but not the site of obstruction. The patient was a 26 day old boy with jaundice, hypoglycemic episodes, and a normal-sized liver. Laboratory studies indicated obstructive jaundice and hepatocellular damage. At surgery, the extrahepatic biliary system was normal.

TABLE 12-2. PROPERTIES OF COMMONLY USED LIVER SCANNING AGENTS

RADIOPHARMACEUTICAL	SYSTEM VISUALIZED	ADMINISTERED DOSAGE	PHYSICAL HALF-LIFE	PHOTON ENERGY (KEV.)	LIVER HALF-TIME (EFFECTIVE)	TIME OF MAXIMAL LIVER CONCENTRATION	BLOOD DISAPPEARANCE HALF-TIME	LIVER DOSE, RADS	WHOLE-BODY DOSE RADS
99mTc-S colloid	Kupffer cells	2 mc.	6 hr.	140	6 hr.	5–10 min.	2.5–3.5 min.	0.66–0.72*	0.03
198Au colloid	Kupffer cells	150 μc.	2.7 days	411	2.7 days	5 min.	4.5 min.	5.7†	0.35†
131I aggregated albumin	Kupffer cells	500 μc.	8.1 days	364	40–60 min. initially, then 10 hr.	10–15 min.	3 min.	0.30*	0.06*
131I rose bengal	Polygonal cells	150 μc.	8.1 days	364	2 hr.‡	20–30 min.	7.5 min.	0.25–0.50	0.05–0.15
113mIn colloid	Kupffer cells	2 mc.	1.7 hr.	390	1.7 hr.	5–10 min.	3 min.	1.10	

* Doses after Smith, 1965. The larger dose assumes that 90 per cent of the particles are trapped by the liver; the smaller dose assumes that the liver traps 70 per cent of the particles, as would happen in liver disease.

† After Quimby, 1960.

‡ The half-time in the liver will be prolonged and hence the radiation will be increased if there is biliary obstruction.

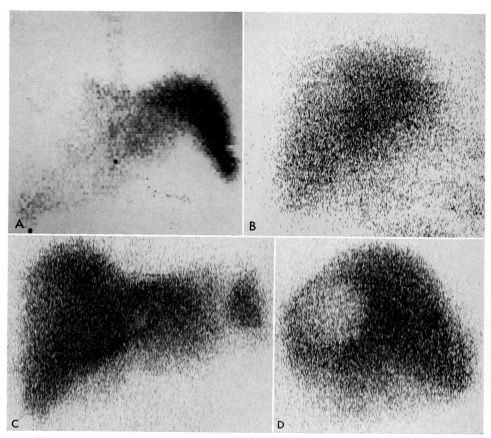

FIGURE 12-8. *A,* Laennec's cirrhosis in a 59 year old alcoholic woman with ascites. The scan with 99mTc-S colloid shows a large defect in the right lobe of the liver and increased uptake of colloid in the spleen and bone marrow (cf. Fig. 12-4). *B,* Repeat scan 72 hours later. In this scan performed with I131 rose bengal, there is a nonuniform distribution of activity, but no evidence of a mass. Rose bengal blood clearance half-time was normal. *C,* Frontal view in a 48 year old woman with unexplained fever. The liver appears normal. *D,* Lateral view reveals a large focal defect in the posterosuperior aspect of the right lobe of the liver.

TECHNIQUE OF LIVER SCANNING

Usually, we inject intravenously 2 mc. of ^{99m}Tc sulfur colloid or 2 mc. of ^{113m}In particles. The patient is placed prone on the scanning table approximately 15 minutes following injection. The detector is beneath the table. With a gamma spectrometer limiting the recorded energies to the appropriate gamma-photon range (135 to 170 kev. in the case of technetium), the maximum count rate is determined by moving the detector over the hepatic area. Scanning speed is chosen according to count rate. The line spacing is chosen so that consecutive lines overlap by half. After the anterior scan, a right lateral view is obtained. With the right side down, there is a tendency for the left side to roll forward, projecting the left lobe of the liver anteriorly. This is avoided by the use of parallel supports. Figure 12-8C and D shows the importance of obtaining a lateral view as a routine procedure; it may reveal lesions that are not seen on the frontal view.

Immediately after the scans are obtained, roentgenograms of the abdomen are made for comparison with the scan. These should be made without moving the patient from the scanning position. Three points marked on the scanning image are identified with lead markers on the patient to provide accurate means of correlation of the scans and roentgenograms.

THE NORMAL LIVER SCAN

The typical appearance of the anterior, posterior and right lateral scan in a normal person is illustrated in Figure 12-9. The rippled or checkerboard appearance in the region of the dome of the liver is a result of respiratory motion. Certain areas of normally decreased radioactivity can be seen. There is an area of decreased activity at the medial foot of the slope of the dome of the liver which represents the site of emergence of hepatic veins from the liver parenchyma to join the inferior cava. The left lobe of the liver contains less functioning tissue than the right and for this reason is often less dense on the photoscan than the right lobe. The left lobe may be quite thin as it crosses the midline area of the spine. This may result in a broad vertical zone of decreased activity, the nature of which becomes readily apparent when the scan is compared with the roentgenogram (see Fig. 12-12). The thin inferior margin of the liver is seen on the scan as a uniform gradient of progressively decreasing density. An area of decreased density is often seen at the porta hepatis, which may appear as a notch. The decrease in activity results from displacement of hepatic parenchyma by the large vascular and biliary conduits entering and emerging from the liver. Lateral to the porta hepatis the inferior margin of the right lobe may display a small concavity representing the bed of the gallbladder (Fig. 12-10). In approximately 4 per cent of normal persons the most inferior margin of the right lobe of the liver extends downward in a tonguelike process to form a Riedel's lobe. The right side of the liver may be indented by the rib cage. The spleen is often visualized when colloidal particles are given. On the lateral view, the anterior border of the liver is convex. The posterior border tends to be straight,

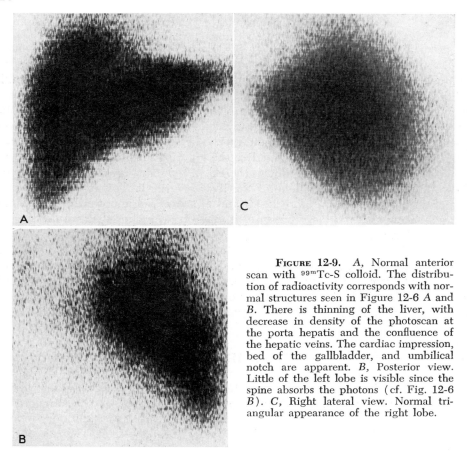

FIGURE 12-9. *A*, Normal anterior scan with ^{99m}Tc-S colloid. The distribution of radioactivity corresponds with normal structures seen in Figure 12-6 *A* and *B*. There is thinning of the liver, with decrease in density of the photoscan at the porta hepatis and the confluence of the hepatic veins. The cardiac impression, bed of the gallbladder, and umbilical notch are apparent. *B*, Posterior view. Little of the left lobe is visible since the spine absorbs the photons (cf. Fig. 12-6 *B*). *C*, Right lateral view. Normal triangular appearance of the right lobe.

slanting forward from back to front. The kidney may cause a concavity in the middle of the posterior margin. The anterior and posterior borders of the liver come together to form a blunted inferior border.

Variations in the configuration of the frontal plane projection of the normal liver are frequent (Fig. 12-11). The liver is readily subject to impressions of its surface by adjacent structures. A flattened diaphragm, such as in massive pleural effusion, carcinoma of the lung, or emphysema, may cause flattening of the hepatic dome, as seen in Figure 12-12. A high diaphragm resulting from splinting of the right chest may exaggerate the dome of the liver; localized diaphragmatic weakness also results in a localized upward bulging of the liver, often beneath the anteromedial portion of the diaphragm. This may occur following surgery of the neck with possible injury to the phrenic nerve (Felson, 1960). The left lobe, usually thin and triangular, may display varying degrees of development. A well developed left lobe may give the liver a quadrilateral shape in the frontal projection. If the circulation through the left main branch of the portal vein is impaired, there may result a very small left lobe with a thickened capsule and signs of atrophy, which give the liver a globular configuration in the frontal view. A kidney that is placed high in the abdomen or

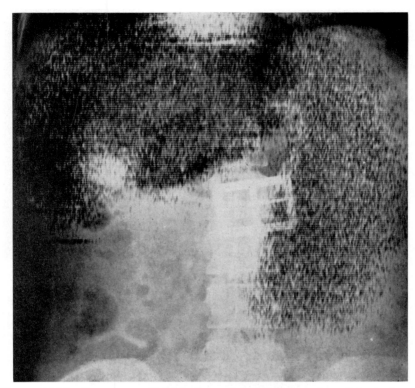

FIGURE 12-10.   Prominent gallbladder fossa. Scan superimposed on abdominal roentgenogram. Gallstones are radiopaque and fit into hepatic defect. The spleen is huge. Patient was a 29 year old woman with thalassemia minor of the alpha chain and hemoglobin H disease.

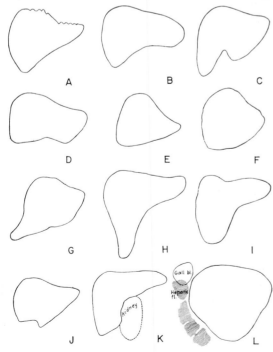

FIGURE 12-11.   Normal variations of hepatic configuration. A, B, and C, Triangular configuration seen in two thirds of normal persons. A, Respiratory scalloping. B, Concave inferior border. C, Prominent umbilical notch. D, Good development of the left lobe. E, Prominent dome associated with a high diaphragm. F, Globular configuration associated with poor development of the left lobe. G, Impression of right margin by the rib cage. H, Liver with Riedel's lobe. I, Localized upward bulging of the liver secondary to a localized diaphragmatic weakness. J, Notching or absence of the inferior tip. K, High kidney indenting the inferior margin of the liver. L, Interposition of the colon between the lateral abdominal wall and the liver. (From McAfee et al., 1965.)

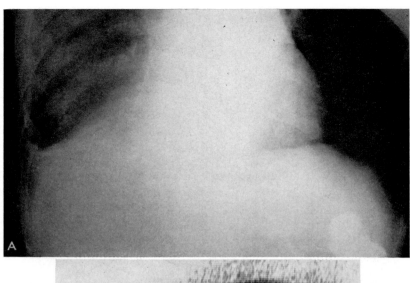

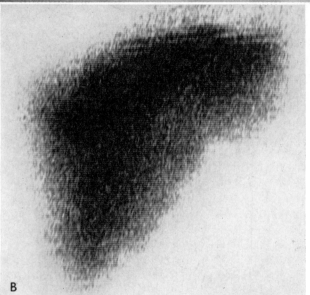

FIGURE 12-12.   *A*, Portion of chest roentgenogram showing calcified pleura from old oleothorax. *B*, Flattening of hepatic dome by calcified pleura. Similar changes may be seen with pleural fluid or emphysema.

enlarged may indent the midportion of the inferior hepatic margin. Colonic interposition displaces and alters the right lateral margin of the liver.

Size may be estimated with a reasonable degree of accuracy from the hepatic scan if care is taken to avoid excessive data processing, such as background suppression (McAfee et al., 1965; Yagan et al., 1962). Liver weight can be calculated by considering the liver to be made up of trapezoids, which are differentiated by using progressively higher cut-off levels. Each separate trapezoid is integrated by planimetry. The technique is laborious, but liver areas may be obtained. No significant correlation between body habitus and liver configuration has been documented.

ABNORMAL LIVER SCANS

MALPOSITION

The size, shape, and position of the liver within the abdomen can furnish significant clues to the nature of congenital heart disease associated with hepatic anomalies (Shah et al., 1964). The liver scan can also reveal the position of the liver in the presence of abnormalities in the height of the two hemidiaphragms. Although precise delineation and classification of cardiac malformation depends upon localizing the dextral or venous atrium by angiographic methods (Rosenbaum et al., 1962), much useful information can be obtained from a knowledge of the position of the abdominal organs together with a chest film (Elliott et al., 1966). If the descending aorta and the stomach are on the left with the major lobe of the liver and gallbladder on the right, situs solitus exists, regardless of the position of the cardiac apex. If the descending aorta and the stomach are on the right side of the body cavity, and the major lobe of the liver and gallbladder located on the left, situs inversus exists, regardless of the position of the cardiac apex. Although any of the four possible combinations of situs solitus and situs inversus and right and left sided cardiac apex can occur with a physiologically normal heart, certain statistical predictions can be made. With situs solitus and a right-sided cardiac apex, there is an extraordinarily high incidence

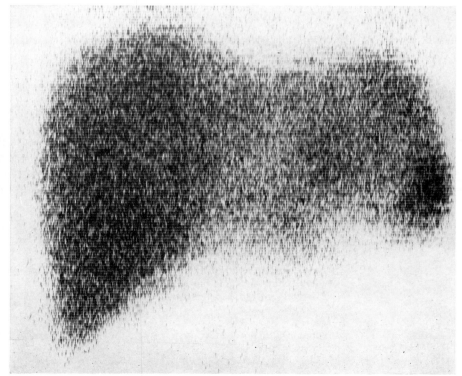

FIGURE 12-13. Chronic active hepatitis. Liver is enlarged, with nonhomogeneous uptake of colloid due to parenchymal damage. The broad vertical zone of decreased activity in the midportion of the hepatic outline is caused by the spine. Patient was a 24 year old woman with recurring jaundice and intrahepatic cholestasis related to hepatocellular damage from hepatitis.

of congenital heart disease, usually corrected transposition and associated anomalies in 80 to 95 per cent of autopsied series. Situs inversus is associated with a 4 to 5 per cent incidence of congenital heart disease. When the descending aorta and stomach lie on opposite sides of the body, this classification breaks down, although the systemic atrium generally lies on the same side as the aorta. This occurs in the syndrome of asplenia or polysplenia, as described by Ivemark (1955), which is associated with severe congenital cardiac malformations and interruption of the inferior systemic venous drainage. In this condition, the hepatic scan characteristically shows a trilobed liver in a median position. Thus, the scanning data provide important prognostic information: most patients with this syndrome die before 9 months of age and their complex anomalies are usually not amenable to surgical intervention.

Displacement of the right side of the liver from the abdominal wall on the right occurs most commonly with ascites, but may also indicate interposition of the colon. A subphrenic abscess is the most common cause of downward and medial displacement of the liver (McAfee et al., 1965). Displacement of the liver into the thorax can occur from a congenital hernia through the retrosternal space of Morgagni or Larrey, through the posterolateral defect of Bochdalek, or through a traumatic rupture with eventration of the diaphragm.

Enlargement of the liver is the most common abnormality revealed by the scan (McAfee et al., 1965). When the left lobe of the liver appears larger than the right and when its density equals or surpasses that of the right lobe, the diagnosis of hepatomegaly can be made. A maximum horizontal diameter of 18.3 cm. and a vertical diameter of 16.7 cm. is given by McAfee et al. The most common causes of hepatomegaly are malignancies, Laennec's cirrhosis, fatty infiltration, chronic passive congestion, and acute and subacute hepatitis (Fig. 12-13).

FOCAL AREAS OF DYSFUNCTION

Localized loss of function of hepatic cells has many causes (Table 12-3). It is impossible to distinguish benign from malignant lesions by means of the scan (Figs. 12-14 and 12-15). Occasionally a diffuse disease of the liver such as cirrhosis may be nonuniform and mimic focal disease (Johnson and Sweeney, 1966). Scanning after administration of both rose bengal and colloidal particles may clarify the diagnosis since parenchymal cell damage may not parallel Kupffer

TABLE 12-3.   CAUSES OF FOCAL DEFECTS OF HEPATIC FUNCTION

1. Metastatic neoplasms
2. Cysts—simple, echinococcus, polycystic
3. Hamartomas (multiple bile duct adenomas)
4. Abscesses—pyogenic, amebic, actinomycosis
5. Large granulomas
6. Infarcts
7. Hodgkin's disease
8. Hemangiomas
9. Primary hepatic carcinoma
10. Trauma—subcapsular hematoma, laceration
11. Postsurgical defects
12. Cirrhosis

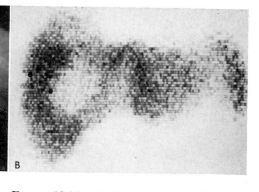

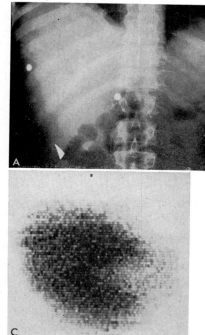

FIGURE 12-14. *A,* Hepatic pyogenic abscess. The plain abdominal film shows a gas shadow projected over the hepatic area. *B,* Focal loss of parenchymal function on the scan, which coincides with the gas shadow. The combination of a parenchymal defect and a corresponding gas shadow suggests the diagnosis of an intrahepatic pyogenic abscess. The patient had a partial right hepatectomy 6 months previously for a traumatic hepatic laceration. There has been complete hepatic regeneration since surgery. *C,* Right lateral view. The abscess lies in the anterior surface of the liver.

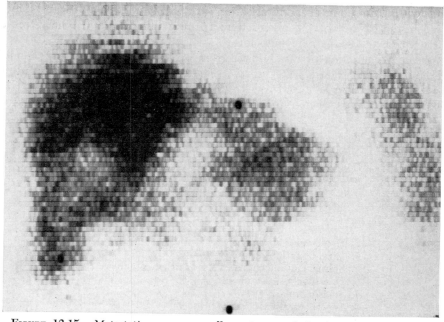

FIGURE 12-15. Metastatic squamous cell carcinoma of the cervix. There are multiple areas of focal loss of function in the liver, which is large.

cell damage in cirrhosis (Fig. 12-8). Cirrhotic livers may be the site of hepatomas (Fig. 12-16) as well as metastases from intra-abdominal neoplasms. One third of autopsied patients with abdominal neoplasms have hepatic metastases. This is true in the cirrhotic as well as the normal liver (Norkin et al., 1962).

Extrahepatic masses may impinge upon the liver (O'Donnell, 1963). These may alter the border of the liver and produce a thinning and compression of normal liver cells or may suggest the appearance of a rim of activity concentrically surrounding the defect (Fig. 12-17). By correctly localizing a hepatic lesion, the scan may improve the accuracy of needly biopsy in focal hepatic disease.

DIFFUSE PARENCHYMAL DISEASE

A nonuniform distribution of radioactivity within the liver may accompany diffuse parenchymal disease from many causes (Table 12-4; Figs. 12-8, 12-13, and 12-18). Cirrhosis is a most common abnormality and is usually accompanied by hepatomegaly. Uptake of activity by the damaged liver may be so poor that large statistical variations in counting rate may occur (Christie and MacIntyre, 1962). When the reticuloendothelial function of the liver is severely impaired, there is compensatory hyperactivity of the rest of the RES, mainly in the spleen and bone marrow. The spleen concentrates colloidal particles to a higher degree than the liver in severe hepatic damage. This finding, together with the mottled appearance of the liver and appearance of radioactivity in the bone marrow, provides a method of assessing liver damage that correlates well with the arterial ammonia concentration (Castell and Johnson, 1966). As a rule, alterations of the scan occur late in the course of a diffuse hepatic dysfunction.

Serial scans are useful in the differential diagnosis of jaundice (Eyler et al., 1965). In the absence of obstruction, rose bengal is detected in the upper small bowel within an hour of administration (Fig. 12-5). Delayed scans may be helpful in the case of partial obstruction. If the gallbladder and biliary tree can be visualized, the scans may help localize the site of obstruction. If this is not the case, differentiation of intrahepatic from extrahepatic obstruction cannot be made with certainty (Fig. 12-7). In the diagnosis of infantile jaundice, one may

TABLE 12-4. CAUSES OF NONUNIFORM DISTRIBUTION OF ACTIVITY IN THE LIVER

1. Cirrhosis
2. Metabolic disease
   a. Fatty infiltration
   b. Amyloidosis
   c. von Gierke's disease
   d. Galactosemia
   e. Niemann-Pick disease
   f. Wilson's disease
3. Hemochromatosis
4. Viral hepatitis—acute, subacute, chronic
5. Spirochetal infections—Weil's disease, syphilis
6. Granuloma—histoplasmosis, sarcoidosis, brucellosis
7. Schistosomiasis
8. Whipple's disease
9. Diffusely invading metastases

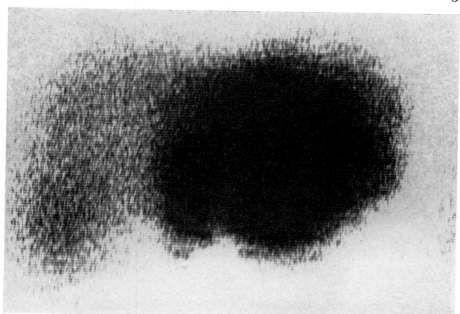

FIGURE 12-16.   Hepatoma, replacing most of the right lobe, in a 61 year old man with a heavy alcoholic intake, postnecrotic cirrhosis, and hemosiderosis. Liver function studies indicated severe hepatocellular damage.

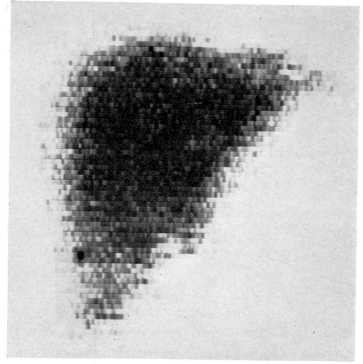

FIGURE 12-17.   Pancreatic pseudocyst in a 52 year old man with persistent abdominal pain, vomiting, cachexia, and jaundice. Note thinned liver surrounding pseudocyst. A narrow concentric rim of increased activity seems to surround this area in the inferior portion of the left lobe.

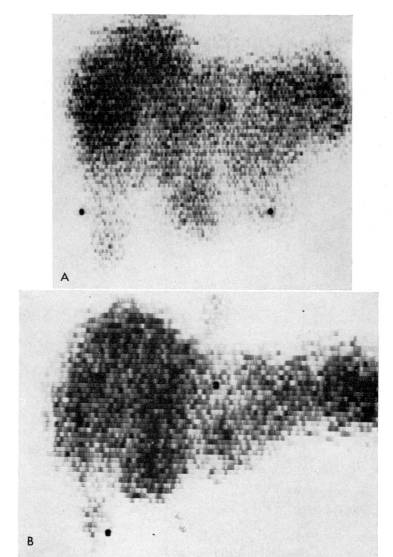

FIGURE 12-18.   *A*, Acute alcoholic hepatitis and septicemia. There is nonuniform distribution of radioactivity and the left lobe is markedly enlarged. *B*, Two weeks later, the left lobe is reduced in size, but the distribution of activity is still nonuniform. Liver function tests returned toward normal.

also collect a fecal sample over a 72 hour period. Less than 4 per cent of the administered dose is excreted in biliary atresia (Brent and Geppert, 1959).

ACCURACY OF THE SCAN IN METASTATIC NEOPLASMS

In metastatic disease approximately 80 to 90 per cent of proved metastases are detectable by scanning (McAfee et al., 1965; Nagler et al., 1963; Czerniak, 1964; Baum et al., 1966). This is considerably higher than the accuracy of enzyme studies, other liver function tests (Baum et al., 1966), and blind hepatic punch biopsy, which yields an accurate diagnosis in 65 to 75 per cent of cases of metastasis (Parets, 1959). Liver punch biopsies guided by the data of scans should prove to be more accurate. Spencer (1966) has pointed out that the scan is most useful in the case of a single discrete lesion and least useful when the pathological process is uniformly distributed, in which case the punch biopsy has its highest yield. Of 33 cases, the biopsy and scan agreed in 27. In 4 cases of diffuse, uniform disease, the scan was normal but the biopsy was abnormal. In 2 cases of localized disease, the scan was abnormal but the biopsy was normal. The incidence of scans falsely indicating localized disease ranges from 10 to 22 per cent (McAfee et al., 1965; Nagler et al., 1963; Czerniak, 1964; Baum et al., 1966). Such false-positive studies usually occur in patients with severe, non-uniform parenchymal disease such as cirrhosis (Johnson and Sweeney, 1966). The wide variation of error may be attributed to differences of technique. Higher doses of the new shorter-lived radiopharmaceuticals should result in better counting statistics with less chance of mistaking artifacts due to statistical variation as lesions.

SOURCES OF ERROR

Poor counting statistics from low concentrations of radioactivity is the most common source of error. Wagner and his associates (1961) have demonstrated

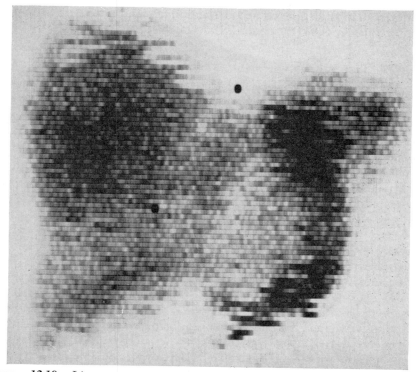

FIGURE 12-19. Liver scan, anterior view (agent ^{99m}Tc colloid), showing generalized enlargement with nonuniform distribution and an irregular strip of increased activity along the left lateral border. Histological examination indicated congestive hepatomegaly. Left border activity was the result of pertechnetate in the stomach from an injection of pertechnetate (15 mc.) for brain scanning the previous day.

that lesions smaller than 2.5 cm. at a depth of 10 cm. within the liver and 1.7 cm. on the surface of the liver are beyond the limits of resolution of present equipment. Development of equipment with better resolution, rotational scanning, and section scanning (Kuhl and Edwards, 1964) may improve spatial resolution. Digital presentation of data (Corey and Benua, 1966) or a color printout (Baum et al., 1966) may help avoid subjective errors. One must be aware of normal areas of lessened activity in order not to interpret them as lesions. Lesions occurring in these areas may easily be overlooked.

If pertechnetate is administered for another purpose, such as for a brain scan, before a liver scan with ^{99m}Tc sulfur colloid, an increased activity may be noted along the lateral border of the left lobe conforming to the stomach (Fig. 12-19). In the patient with chronic decompensated arteriosclerotic heart disease shown in Figure 12-19, the liver was markedly enlarged and the isotope was nonuniformly distributed.

In summary, liver scanning is a simple technique without danger or discomfort to the patient. It has proved useful in the differential diagnosis of right upper quadrant pain and abdominal masses, in the detection of malposition and displacement of the liver, in the detection of metastatic disease, in the differentiation of obstructive from parenchymal causes of jaundice, in distinguishing focal from diffuse parenchymal disease, and as a means of following hepatic parenchymal abnormalities during the course of treatment. It is not a means of making a histological diagnosis of liver disease. Future improvement in instrumentation and scanning agents should increase the already high accuracy of the procedure in detecting abnormalities of the liver.

THE PANCREAS

Because of its location in the retroperitoneal space deep in the epigastrium, the pancreas is not available for clinical examination. It is surrounded by organs and tissues of equal density, and cannot be visualized radiographically except in the unusual circumstances in which marked calcification occurs. The diagnosis of acute pancreatitis is often difficult and occasionally pancreatitis is confused with other intra-abdominal disease. The diagnosis of carcinoma of the pancreas is usually possible only in the advanced stages of the disease or when obstruction of the biliary tract occurs, at a time when surgical therapy is not possible. For these reasons, the search for a pancreatic scanning agent has been one of the important areas of research in nuclear medicine.

The pancreas is one of the most active sites of protein synthesis in the body, and it produces great quantities of digestive enzymes. Consequently, Blau and Manske (1961) postulated that administration of a precursor amino acid labeled with a suitable gamma-emitting radionuclide might result in sufficiently high concentrations of radioactivity in the pancreas to permit its visualization by scanning. Since no suitable radionuclide of sulfur was available, Blau synthesized the selenium analog of methionine by means of a biosynthetic procedure.

Selenomethionine was extracted from the protein products of yeast grown on a sulfur-poor medium enriched with selenium-75 of high specific activity. When injected intravenously, about 7 per cent of the compound was accumulated in the pancreas at a concentration eight to nine times that in the liver. In 1962,

Blau and Bender described a procedure for scanning the pancreas in man that was found successful in two thirds of the cases. The patients were fed a high-protein breakfast—2 glasses of skim milk—followed 3 hours later by intravenous administration of Cecekin, which is a mixture of secretin, pancreozymin, and cholecystokinin. The purpose was to empty the pancreas of digestive enzymes before administration of the radiopharmaceutical. One hour later ^{75}Se seleno-methionine was given intravenously.

Sodee (1964) used a high-protein, low-fat, low-carbohydrate meal followed by injection of ^{75}Se selenomethionine together with 900 mg. of glutamic acid to stimulate secretion of the small intestine. He also proposed the use of a lead shield to prevent confusing hepatic activity with that of the pancreas. Rodriguez-Antunez (1964a) gave morphine to constrict the sphincter of Oddi and prolong retention of the labeled selenomethionine in the pancreas but now finds it is not helpful (Rodriguez-Antunez et al., 1966). Tabern et al. (1965) found Pro-Banthine more suitable than morphine and used it together with an infusion of amino acids. Burdine and Haynie (1965) reported that they did not require dietary preparation or pharmacological stimulation. Kaplan et al. (1966) have used a dual isotope scan subtraction technique to distinguish hepatic from pancreatic activity.

ANATOMY AND PHYSIOLOGY OF THE PANCREAS

The pancreas extends across the abdomen at the level of the first and second lumbar vertebral bodies. Its globular head fits into the duodenal C loop and extends downward to form the uncinate process or lingula, which passes around the superior mesenteric vessels from the right. The body is prism-shaped and slopes upward from right to left, tapering progressively to form a short tail, which ends at the splenic hilum.

Scanning images of the pancreas often show variations, such as a high elliptical transverse shape, a horseshoe shape, or a sigmoid shape (King et al., 1966). The pancreatic ducts, acini, and islet cells are supplied by parasympathetic nerves via the vagus. Sympathetic nerves from the fifth and through the ninth dorsal ganglia are distributed to the pancreatic blood vessels.

The vagus nerve stimulates enzymatic activity of the acinar cells. Administration of the hormone secretin (from the duodenum) increases the volume of the pancreatic juice and, to a lesser degree, its electrolyte content. The enzymatic activity of the pancreatic secretions—amylase, lipase, carboxypeptidase, trypsinogen, and chymotrypsinogen—is increased by pancreozymin, another intestinal hormone. Production and secretion of these digestive enzymes are necessary for proper digestion of food. The production of insulin and glucagon by the islet cells is not related to the technique used at present for pancreatic scanning.

Selenium-75 has a half-life of 128 days and a principal photon energy of 270 kev. After intravenous injection, the concentration of ^{75}Se selenomethionine in the pancreas reaches a peak $\frac{1}{2}$ hour after administration and remains at this level for about 4 hours. The biological half-time in man of ^{75}Se is estimated to be about 144 days. With a scanning dose of 250 μc., Sodee (1964) has estimated the total body dose to be 2.2 rads, gonadal dose 2.5 rads, kidney dose 14 rads, pancreas dose 0.6 rad, and liver dose 0.5 rad.

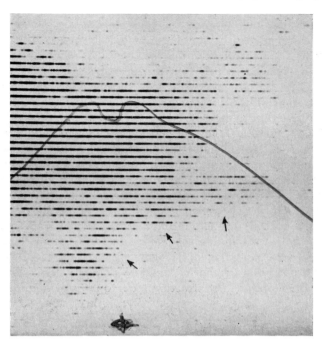

FIGURE 12-20. Photoscan 30 minutes after injection of ^{75}Se-selenomethionine demonstrating normal visualization of the pancreas (arrow). A retroperitoneal neoplasm was found at exploration but the pancreas was not involved. (Courtesy of Dr. T. Haynie, Anderson Hospital, Houston, Texas.)

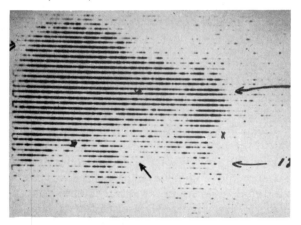

FIGURE 12-21. Pancreas scan revealing concentration of radioactivity in the liver and pancreas 30 minutes after injection of ^{75}Se-selenomethionine. The continuity of the pancreas is interrupted by a rounded "cold" area at the junction of the head and body of the pancreas (arrow). Exploratory celiotomy revealed a 2 to 3 cm. tumor in the pancreas in this location. (Courtesy of Dr. T. Haynie, Anderson Hospital, Houston, Texas.)

Various techniques have been used (Blau and Bender, 1962; Burdine and Haynie, 1965; Sodee, 1964; Tabern et al., 1965). Starvation enhances hepatic uptake of selenomethionine; therefore a high protein meal before scanning increases the relative pancreas-liver concentration ratio, presumably by increasing the availability of selenomethionine for synthesis of pancreatic enzymes. Stimulating the pancreas to secrete its nonlabeled enzymes may be helpful. Morphine administration can result in contraction of the sphincter of Oddi, producing a stable concentration of labeled pancreatic enzymes in the pancreas. Serial scans are sometimes performed between ½ and 4 hours following the intravenous administration of selenomethionine, which is given in a dosage of 3 μc. per kg.

Many laboratories obtain a liver scan as an aid in interpretation of the pancreatic scan.

The pancreas can be visualized in approximately 65 to 90 per cent of people, according to different series. Areas damaged by pancreatitis do not seem to concentrate the radiopharmaceutical, nor do neoplasms (Figs. 12-20 and 12-21).

Sodee (1965) reported the results of 566 scans of 185 patients. Ten scans were unsatisfactory; in 109 of 114 patients without clinical pancreatic disease the scan was normal; the scan was abnormal in 11 of 12 patients with carcinoma of the pancreas and in 13 of 14 patients with pancreatitis. The pancreatic scan is often difficult to interpret, and a normal scan does not exclude pancreatic disease.

REFERENCES

Abel, J. J., and Rowntree, R. G.: On the Pharmacological Action of Some Phthaleins and Their Derivatives with Special Reference to Their Behavior as Purgatives. *J. Pharmacol. Exp. Ther.* 1:233, 1909.

Ariel, I. M.: The Site of Upper Gastrointestinal Bleeding. Detection by Radioactive Tagged Red Blood Cells. *J.A.M.A.* 180:212, 1962.

Aronow, S., Thors, R., and Brownell, G. L.: Positron Scanning of the Liver and Pancreas. *In* Medical Radioisotope Scanning. International Atomic Energy Agency, Vienna, 1959, pp. 105–112.

Avioli, L. V., McDonald, J. E., Singer, R. A., and Henneman, P. H.: A New Oral Isotopic Test of Calcium Absorption. *J. Clin. Invest.* 44:128, 1965.

Baker, R. R., Migita, T., and Wagner, H. N., Jr.: To be published.

Bannerman, R. M.: Measurement of Gastro-intestinal Bleeding Using Radioactive Chromium. *Brit. Med. J.* 2:1032, 1957.

Barth, W. F., Wochner, R. D., Waldmann, T. A., and Fahey, J. L.: Metabolism of Human Gamma Macroglobulins. *J. Clin. Invest.* 43:1036, 1964.

Baum, S., Silver, L., and Vouchides, D.: The Recognition of Hepatic Metastases Through Radioisotope Color Scanning. *J.A.M.A.* 197:675, 1966.

Baylin, G. J., Saunders, A. P., Isley, J. K., Shingleton, W. W., Hymans, J. C., Johnston, P. H., and Ruffin, J. M.: I-131 Blood Levels Correlated with Gastric Emptying Determined Radiographically. *Proc. Soc. Exp. Biol. Med.* 89:51, 1955.

Benacerraf, B., Biozzi, G., Halpern, B. N., Stiffel, C., and Mouton, D.: Phagocytosis of Heat-Denatured Human Serum Albumin Labeled with I-131 and its Use as a Means of Investigating Liver Blood Flow. *Brit. J. Exp. Path.* 38:35, 1957.

Bender, M. A., and Blau, M.: Pancreas Scanning with Se[75] L-Selenomethionine. *In* Quinn, J. L., III (ed.): Scintillation Scanning in Clinical Medicine. W. B. Saunders Co., Philadelphia, 1964, pp. 87–92.

Benson, J. A., Jr., Culver, P. J., Ragland, S., Jones, G. M., Drummey, G. D., and Bougas, E.: D-Xylose Absorption Test in Malabsorption Syndromes. *New Eng. J. Med.* 256:335, 1957.

Berkowitz, D.: The Use of Radioactive Fat in the Study of Absorption in Various Disease States. *Arch. Intern. Med.* 100:951, 1957.

Bhandarker, S. D., Bluhm, M. M., MacGregor, J., and Nordin, B. E. C.: An Isotope Test of Calcium Absorption. *Brit. J. Med.* 2:1539, 1961.

Biozzi, G., Benacerraf, B., Halpern, B. N., Stiffel, C., and Hillemand, B.: Exploration of the Phagocytic Function of the Reticuloendothelial System with Heat Denatured Human Serum Albumin Labeled with I-131 and Applications to the Measurement of Liver Blood Flow in Normal Man and in Some Pathologic Conditions. *J. Lab. Clin. Med.* 51:230, 1958.

Blau, M.: Pancreas Scanning with Se[75] Selenomethionine. *In* Medical Radioisotope Scanning. Vol. 2. International Atomic Energy Agency, Vienna, 1964, pp. 275–287.

Blau, M., and Bender, M. A.: Se[75] Selenomethionine for Visualization of the Pancreas by Isotope Scanning. *Radiology* 78:974, 1962.

Blau, M., and Manske, R. F.: The Pancreas Specificity of Se[75] Selenomethionine. *J. Nucl. Med.* 2:102, 1961.

Bradley, S. E., Ingelfinger, F. J., Bradley, G. P., and Curry, J. J.: The Estimation of Hepatic Blood Flow in Man. *J. Clin. Invest.* 24:890, 1945.

Brent, R. L., and Geppert, L. J.: The Use of Radioactive Rose Bengal in the Evaluation of Infantile Jaundice. *AMA J. Dis. Child.* 98:720, 1959.

Brown, H., Cameron, J., Fumimo, T., Schmidt, E. R., and Brown, J.: Localization of Gastrointestinal Hemorrhage with Radioiodine. Amer. J. Surg. 103:370, 1962.

Buchanan, D. L., and Sampson, L. T.: Incineration of Fecal Specimens for Radioactivity Measurement. J. Lab. Clin. Med. 59:169, 1962.

Burdine, J. A., and Haynie, T. P.: Diagnosis of Pancreatic Carcinoma by Photoscanning. J.A.M.A. 194:979, 1965.

Cassen, B., Curtis, L., Reed, C., and Libby, R.: Instrumentation for I-131 Medical Studies. Nucleonics 9:46, 1951.

Castell, D. O., and Johnson, R. B.: The Au-198 Liver Scan, an Index of Portal-Systemic Collateral Circulation in Chronic Liver Disease. New Eng. J. Med. 275:188, 1966.

Charkes, N. D., and Shansky, F.: Liver Scanning with Radioactive Isotopes. J. Einstein Med. Cent. 12:126, 1964.

Christie, J. H., and MacIntyre, W. J.: Liver Scanning. In Kniseley, R. M., et al. (eds.): Progress in Medical Radioisotope Scanning. U. S. Atomic Energy Commission (TID-7673), 1962, pp. 405–432.

Citrin, Y., Sterling, K., and Halsted, J. A.: The Mechanism of Hypoproteinemia Associated with Giant Hypertrophy of the Gastric Mucosa. New Eng. J. Med. 257:906, 1957.

Corey, K. R., and Benua, R.: Progress in Radioactive Isotope Scanning. Med. Clin. N. Amer. 50:3, 689, 1966.

Czerniak, P.: Scanning Study of 700 Livers: Evaluation of Existing Diagnostic Procedures. In Medical Radioisotope Scanning. International Atomic Energy Agency, Vienna, 1964, pp. 401–424.

Davidson, J. D., Waldmann, T. A., Goodman, D. S., and Gordon, R. S., Jr.: Protein-Losing Gastroenteropathy in Congestive Heart Failure. Lancet 1:899, 1961.

Delaloye, B., Magnenat, P., and Cruehaud, S.: L'hépatoscintillogramme après injection d'albumine humaine denaturée marquée à l'I-131. Schweiz. Med. Wsch. 89:1305, 1959.

Dobson, E. L., and Jones, H. B.: The Behavior of Intravenously Injected Particulate Material: Its Rate of Disappearance from the Blood Stream as a Measure of Liver Blood Flow. Acta Med. Scand. 144 (Suppl. 273):1, 1952.

Durand, P.: Disorders Due to Intestinal Defective Carbohydrate Digestion and Absorption. Il Pensiero Scientifico, Rome, 1964.

Ebaugh, F. G., Jr., Clemens, T., Rodnan, G., and Peterson, R. E.: Quantitative Measurement of Gastrointestinal Blood Loss. I. Use of Radioactive Cr-51 in Patients with Gastrointestinal Hemorrhage. Amer. J. Med. 25:169, 1958.

Elliott, L. P., Sue, K. L., and Amplatz, K.: A Roentgen Classification of Cardiac Malpositions. Invest. Radiol. 1:17, 1966.

Endlich, H., Harper, P. V., Beck, R., Siemens, L. O., and Lathrop, K.: The Use of I-125 to Increase Isotope Scanning Resolution. Amer. J. Roentgen. 87:148, 1962.

Eyler, W. R., Schuman, B. A., DuSault, L. A., and Hinson, R. E.: The Radioiodinated Rose Bengal Liver Scan as an Aid in the Differential Diagnosis of Jaundice. J.A.M.A. 194:990, 1965.

Felson, B.: Fundamentals of Chest Roentgenology. W. B. Saunders Co., Philadelphia, 1960.

Fierst, S. M., et al.: An Evaluation of the Isotopic Iodotriolein Method: Its Correlation with Vitamin A Absorption. Gastroenterology 35:381, 1958.

Fowler, D., and Cooke, V. T.: Diagnostic Significance of D-Xylose Excretion Test. Gut 1:67, 1960.

Freeman, T., and Gordon, A. H.: Human and Rat Intestine as a Site of Catabolism of Albumin. In Peeters, H. (ed.): Protides of the Biological Fluids. Proceedings of the Eleventh Colloquium, Bruges. Elsevier, Amsterdam, 1964, p. 226.

Friedell, H. L., MacIntyre, W. J., and Rejali, A. M.: A Method for the Visualization of the Configuration and Structure of the Liver. Amer. J. Roentgen. 77:455, 1957.

George, E. P.: Radiotriolein Test in Steatorrhea. Brit. Med. J. 2:1650, 1961.

Gitlin, D., Janeway, C. A., and Farr, L. E.: Studies on the Metabolism of Plasma Proteins in The Nephrotic Syndrome. I. Globulin and Iron-Binding Globulin. J. Clin. Invest. 35:44, 1956.

Goodwin, D. A., Stern, H. S., Wagner, H. N., Jr. and Kramer, H. H.: Indium-133m: A New Radiopharmaceutical for Liver Scanning. Nucleonics 24:65, 1966.

Gordon, R. S., Jr.: Exudative Enteropathy: Abnormal Permeability of the Gastrointestinal Tract Demonstrable with Labelled Polyvinylpyrrolidone. Lancet 1:325, 1959.

Grenier, J. H.: Résultats comparés des tests de l'absorption intestinale utilisant la trioléine ou l'acid oléique marqués à l'I-131 et au C-14. Radioaktive Isotope Klin. Forschung 6:337, 1965.

Grossman, M., and Jordan, P. H.: The Radioiodinated Triolein Test for Steatorrhea. Gastroenterology 34:892, 1958.

Halpern, B. N., Biozzi, G., Benacerraf, B., Stiffel, C., and Hillemand, B.: Cinétique de la phagocytose d'une sérum albumine humaine spécialement traitée et radiomarquée et son application à l'étude de la circulation hépatique chez l'homme. *C.R. Soc. Biol.* (*Paris*) 150:1307, 1956.

Harper, P. V., Lathrop, K. A., Jiminez, F., Fink, R., and Gottschalk, A.: Technetium-99m as a Scanning Agent. *Radiology* 85:101, 1965.

Healey, W. V., Riggins, R. C., White, R., Habif, D. V., and Stewart, W. B.: Experimental Method of Localizing Gastrointestinal Hemorrhage. *Surg. Forum* 11:323, 1960.

Healy, J. E., Jr., Schroy, P. C., and Sorenson, R. J.: The Intrahepatic Distribution of the Hepatic Artery in Man. *J. Int. Coll. Surg.* 20:133, 1953.

Holman, H., Nickel, W. F., Jr., and Sleisenger, M. H.: Hypoproteinemia Antedating Intestinal Lesions and Possibly Due to Excessive Serum Protein Loss into Intestine. *Amer. J. Med.* 27:963, 1959.

Hughes Jones, N. C.: Measurement of Red Cell Loss from Gastrointestinal Tract Using Radioactive Chromium. *Brit. Med. J.* 1:493, 1958.

Ivemark, B. I.: Implications of Agenesis of the Spleen on the Pathogenesis of Cono-Truncus Anomalies in Childhood, an Analysis of the Heart Malformations in the Splenic Agenesis Syndrome with Fourteen New Cases. *Acta Paediat.* 44 (Suppl. 104):1, 1955.

Jarnum, S., and Schwartz, M.: Hypoalbuminemia in Gastric Carcinoma. *Gastroenterology* 38:769, 1960.

Jeejeebhoy, K. N., and Coghill, N. F.: The Measurement of Gastrointestinal Protein Loss by a New Method. *Gut* 2:123, 1961.

Jeffries, G. H., Holman, H. R., and Sleisenger, M. H.: Plasma Proteins and the Gastrointestinal Tract. *New Eng. J Med.* 266:652, 1962.

Johnson, P. M., and Sweeney, W. A.: The False Positive Liver Scan. Presented at the 13th Annual Meeting of the Society of Nuclear Medicine, Philadelphia, June 25, 1966.

Kaplan, E., Ben-Porath, M., Fink, S., Clayton, G. D., and Jacobson, B.: Elimination of Liver Interference from the Selenomethionine Pancreas Scan. *J. Nucl. Med.* 7:387, 1966.

Kennedy, J. A., and Kinloch, J. D.: The Impurity of Radioiodinated Triolein. *J. Clin. Path.* 17:160, 1964.

King, E. R., et al.: A Study of the Morphology of the Normal Pancreas Using Se[75] Methionine Photoscanning. *Amer. J. Roentgen.* 96:657, 1966.

Kuhl, D. E., and Edwards, R. Q.: Cylindrical and Section Radioisotope Scanning of the Liver and Brain. *Radiology* 83:926, 1964.

Lakshminarayana, G., Kruger, F. A., Campbell, D. G., and Brown, J. B.: Chromatographic Studies on the Composition of Commercial Samples of Triolein-I-131 and Oleic Acid-I-131 and the Distribution of the Label in Human Serum Lipids Following Oral Administration of These Lipids. *Arch. Biochem.* 88:318, 1960.

Laster, L., and Ingelfinger, F. J.: Intestinal Absorption—Aspects of Structure, Function and Disease of the Small Intestine Mucosa. *New Eng. J. Med.* 264:1138, 1192, 1246, 1961.

Lushbaugh, C. C., Kretchmar, A., and Gibbs, W.: Liver Function Measured by the Blood Clearance of Rose Bengal-I-131: A Review and a Model Based on Compartmental Analysis of Changes in Arm, Blood and Liver Radioactivity. *In* Kniseley, R. M., and Tauxe, W. N. (eds.): Dynamic Clinical Studies with Radioisotopes. U.S. Atomic Energy Commission (TID-7678), pp. 319–354, 1964.

Mallard, J. R., and Peachey, C. J.: A Quantitative Automatic Body Scanner for Localization of Radioisotopes In Vivo. *Brit. J. Radiol.* 32:652, 1959.

Malm, J. R., Reemtsma, K., and Barker, H. G.: Comparative Fat and Fatty Acid Intestinal Absorption Test Utilizing Radioiodine Labeling—Results in Normal Subjects. *Proc. Soc. Exp. Biol.* 92:471, 1956.

McAfee, J. G., Ause, R. G., and Wagner, H. N., Jr.: Diagnostic Value of Scintillation Scanning of the Liver. *Arch. Intern. Med.* 116:95, 1965.

McKenna, R. D., et al.: The Use of I-131 Labeled Fat in the Study of Fat Digestion and Absorption in Normal Individuals and in Patients with Diseases of Fat Absorption. *Gastroenterology* 32:17, 1957.

Mena, I., Kivel, R., Mahoney, P., Mellinkoff, S. M., and Bennett, L. R.: A Method for Increasing the Sensitivity of the Rose Bengal I-131 Liver Function Test with the Use of Bromsulfalein. *J. Lab. Clin. Med.* 54:167, 1959.

Mendeloff, A. I.: Fluorescence of Intravenously Administered Rose Bengal Appears Only in Hepatic Polygonal Cells. *Proc. Soc. Exp. Biol. Med.* 70:556, 1949.

Moore, G.: Diagnosis and Localization of Brain Tumors. A Clinical and Experimental Study Employing Fluorescent and Radioactive Tracer Methods. Charles C Thomas, Springfield, Ill., 1953.

Nagler, W., Bender, M. A., and Blau, M.: Radioisotope Photoscanning of the Liver. *Gastroenterology* 44:36, 1963.

Norkin, S. A., Heimann, R., and Fahimi, H. D.: Neoplasms, Cirrhosis and Hepatic Metastases. *Cancer* 15:1004, 1962.

O'Donnell, T. A.: Liver Scanning for Extrahepatic Tumors. *Amer. J. Roentgen.* 90:1063, 1963.

Owen, C. A., Jr., Bollman, J. L., and Grindlay, J. H.: Radiochromium-labeled Erythrocytes for Detection of Gastrointestinal Hemorrhage. *J. Lab. Clin. Med.* 44:238, 1954a.

Owen, C. A., Jr., Cooper, M., Grindlay, J. H., and Bollman, J. L.: Quantitative Measurement of Bleeding from Alimentary Tract by Use of Radiochromium Labeled Erythrocytes. *Surg. Forum* 5:663, 1954b.

Parets, A. D.: Detection of Intrahepatic Metastases by the Blind Needle Liver Biopsy. *Amer. J. Med. Sci.* 237:335, 1959.

Parkins, R. A.: Protein-Losing Enteropathy in the Sprue Syndrome. *Lancet* 2:1366, 1960.

Quimby, E. H.: Some Problems Regarding Permissible Doses with Radioisotopes. *J. Nucl. Med.* 1:14, 1960.

Razzak, M. A., and Wagner, H. N., Jr.: Measurement of Hepatic Blood Flow by Colloidal Gold Clearance. *J. Appl. Physiol.* 16:1133, 1961.

Reemtsma, K.: Comparative Absorption of Labeled Fat and Fatty Acid in the Study of Pancreatic Disease. *Surgery* 42:22, 1957.

Rich, C., and Ivanovich, P.: Radioisotope Tests of Calcium Absorption. *Northwest Med.* 63:792, 1964.

Roche, M., Perz-Gimenez, M. E., Layrisse, M., and Di Prisco, E.: Study of Urinary and Fecal Excretion of Radioactive Chromium Cr-51 in Man: Its Use in the Measurement of Intestinal Blood Loss Associated with Hookworm Infection. *J. Clin. Invest.* 36:1183, 1957.

Rodriguez-Antunez, A.: Pancreatic Scanning with Selenium-75 Methionine, Utilizing Morphine to Enhance Contrast. A Preliminary Report. *Cleveland Clin. Quart.* 31:213, 1964a.

Rodriguez-Antunez, A.: Use of Morphine in Pancreatic Scanning with Se^{75} Methionine. *J. Nucl. Med.* 5:729, 1964b.

Rodriguez-Antunez, A., Filson, E. J., Sullivan, B. H., Jr., and Brown, C. H.: Photoscanning in Diagnosis of Carcinoma of the Pancreas. *Ann. of Intern. Med.* 65:730, 1966.

Root, S. W., Andrews, G. A., Knisely, R. M., and Tyor, M. D.: Distribution and Radiation Effects of Intravenously Administered Colloidal Au-198 in Man. *Cancer* 7:856, 1954.

Rosenbaum, H. D., Pellingrino, E. D., and Treciokas, L. L.: Acyanotic Levocardia. *Circulation* 26:60, 1962.

Rosenthal, S. M.: An Improved Method for Using Phenoltetrachlorphthalein as a Liver Function Test. *J. Pharmacol. Exp. Ther.* 19:385, 1922.

Rosenthal, S. M., and White, E. C.: Studies in Hepatic Function. VI. The Pharmacological Behavior of certain Phthalein Dyes. The Value of Selected Phthalein Compounds in the Estimation of Hepatic Function. *J. Pharmacol. Exp. Ther.* 24:265, 1925.

Rothfeld, B., and Rabinowitz, J. L.: Comparison of Measurement of Fat Absorption Using I-131 and C-14 Labeled Fats. *Amer. J. Dig. Dis.* 9:263, 1964.

Schwartz, M., and Jarnum, S.: Gastrointestinal Protein Loss in Idiopathic (Hypercatabolic) Hypoproteinemia. *Lancet* 1:327, 1959.

Shah, K. D., Neill, C. A., Wagner, H. N., Jr., and Taussig, H. B.: Radioisotope Scanning of the Liver and Spleen in Dextrocardia and in Situs Inversus with Levocardia. *Circulation* 29:231, 1964.

Shaldon, S., Chiandussi, L., Guevara, L., Caesar, J., and Sherlock, S.: The Estimation of Hepatic Blood Flow and Intrahepatic Shunted Blood Flow by Colloidal Heat-Denatured Human Serum Albumin Labeled with I-131. *J. Clin. Invest.* 40:1346, 1961.

Sheppard, C. W., Jordan, G., and Hahn, P. P.: Disappearance of Isotopically Labeled Gold Colloid from the Circulation of the Dog. *Amer. J. Physiol.* 164:345, 1951.

Shingleton, W. W., Baylin, G. J., Isley, J. K., Saunders, A. P., and Ruffin, J. M.: Evaluation of Pancreatic Function by Use of I-131 Labeled Fat. *Gastroenterology* 32:28, 1957a.

Shingleton, W. W., Isley, J. K., Floyd, R. D., Saunders, A. P., and Baylin, G. J.: Studies on Postgastrectomy Steatorrhea Using Radioactive Triolein and Oleic Acid. *Surgery* 42:12, 1957b.

Shingleton, W. W., Wells, M. H., Baylin, G. J., Ruffin, J. M., and Saunders, A. P.: The Use of Radioactive Labeled Protein and Fat in the Evaluation of Pancreatic Disorders. *Surgery* 38:134, 1955.

Smith, E. M.: Internal Dose Calculation for ^{99m}Tc. *J. Nucl. Med.* 6:231, 1965.

Sodee, D. B.: Radioisotope Scanning of the Pancreas with Selenomethionine (Se-75). *Radiology* 83:910, 1964.

Sodee, D. B.: Scientific exhibit at the 12th Annual Meeting of the Society of Nuclear Medicine, Bal Harbour, Florida, June, 1965.

Sorensen, L. B., and Archambault, M.: Visualization of the Liver by Scanning with Mo-99 Molybdate as Tracer. *J. Lab. Clin. Med.* 62:330, 1963.

Spencer, R. H.: Personal Communication. 1966.

Stanley, M. M., and Thannhauser, S. B.: The Absorption and Disposition of Orally Administered I-131 Labeled Natural Fat in Man. *J. Lab. Clin. Med.* 34:1634, 1949.

Steinfeld, J. L., Davidson, J. D., Gordon, R. S., Jr., and Greene, F. E.: The Mechanism of

Hypoproteinemia in Patients with Regional Enteritis and Ulcerative Colitis. *Amer. J. Med.* 29:405, 1960.

Stirrett, L. A., and Yuhl, E. T.: Clinical Evaluation of Hepatic Radioactivity Survey. *Ann. Surg.* 138:857, 1953.

Stirrett, L. A., Yuhl, E. T., and Cassen, B.: Clinical Applications of Hepatic Radioactive Surveys. *Amer. J. Gastroent.* 21:310, 1954.

Stirrett, L. A., Yuhl, E. T., and Libbey, R. L.: New Technique for Diagnosis of Carcinoma Metastatic to the Liver. *Surg., Gynec. and Obstet.* 96:210, 1953a.

Stirrett, L. A., Yuhl, E. T., and Libbey, R. L.: The Hepatic Radioactive Survey. *Radiology* 61: 930, 1953b.

Tabern, D. L., et al.: The Use of Intravenous Amino Acids in the Visualization of the Pancreas with Seleno-75-Methionine. *J. Nucl. Med.* 6:762, 1965.

Taplin, G. V., Hayashi, J., Johnson, D., and Dore, E.: Liver Blood Flow and Cellular Function in Hepatobiliary Disease. Tracer Studies with Radiogold and Rose Bengal. *J. Nucl. Med.* 2:204, 1961.

Taplin, G. V., Meredith, O. M., and Kade, H.: The Radioactive (I-131 Tagged) Rose Bengal Uptake Excretion Test for Liver Function Using External Gamma Ray Scintillation Counting Techniques. U.S. Atomic Energy Commission Report UCLA-319, University of California at Los Angeles, 1954.

Taplin, G. V., Meredith, O. M., and Kade, H.: The Radioactive I-131 Tagged Rose Bengal Uptake Excretion Test for Liver Function Using Gamma Ray Scintillation Counting Techniques. *J. Lab. Clin. Med.* 45:665, 1955.

Torrance, H. B., and Gowenlock, A. H.: Radioactive Colloidal Clearance Techniques to Measure Liver Blood Flow in Man. *Clin. Sci.* 22:413, 1962.

Tuna, N., Mangold, H. K., and Mosser, D. G.: Re-evaluation of the I-131-Triolein Absorption Test. Analysis and Purification of Commercial Radioiodinated Triolein and Clinical Studies with Pure Preparation. *J. Lab. Clin. Med.* 61:620, 1963.

Vetter, H., Falkner, R., and Neumayr, A.: The Disappearance Rate of Colloidal Radiogold from the Circulation and Its Application to the Estimation of Liver Blood Flow in Normal and Cirrhotic Subjects. *J. Clin. Invest.* 33:1594, 1954.

Vesin, P., Troupel, S., Acar, J., Renault, H., Desbuquois, G., and Cattan, R.: Entéropathie avec perte de protéines et stéatorhée: Étude par le PVP-I[131] et la trioléine I[131]. Action du régime sans gluten. *Bull. Soc. Med. Hop. Paris* 76:261, 1960.

Von Schuching, S. L., and Abt, A. F.: Carbon-14 Fat Oxidation Test: A New Method for Measuring Fat Utilization in the Human. *In* Rothchild, S. (ed.): Advances in Tracer Methodology. Vol. 2. Plenum Press, New York, 1965.

Wagner, H. N., Jr., McAfee, J. G., and Mozley, J. M.: Diagnosis of Liver Disease by Radioisotope Scanning. *Arch. Intern. Med.* 107:324, 1961.

Waldmann, T. A.: Gastrointestinal Protein Loss Demonstrated by ^{51}Cr-Labelled Albumin. *Lancet* 2:121, 1961.

Waldmann, T. A.: Protein-Losing Enteropathy. *Gastroenterology* 50:422, 1966.

Waldmann, T. A., and Laster, L.: Abnormalities of Albumin Metabolism in Patients with Hypogammaglobulinemia. *J. Clin. Invest.* 43:1025, 1964.

Waldmann, T. A., Morell, A. G., Wochner, R. D., Strober, W., and Sternlieb, I.: Quantitation of Gastrointestinal Protein Loss with [67]Copper-Labeled Ceruloplasmin. *J. Clin. Invest.* 46:10, 1967.

Waldmann, T. A., Steinfeld, J. L., Dutcher, T. F., Davidson, J. D., and Gordon, R. S., Jr.: Role of Gastrointestinal System in "Idiopathic Hypoproteinemia." *Gastroenterology* 41:197, 1961.

Waldmann, T. A., and Wochner, R. D.: The Use of ^{51}Cr-Labeled Albumin in the Study of Protein-Losing Enteropathy. *In* Peeters, H. (ed.): Protides of the Biological Fluids. Proceedings of the Eleventh Colloquium, Bruges. Elsevier, Amsterdam, 1964, p. 224.

Walker, W. F.: Clinical Assessment of Intestinal Fat Absorption Using Radioactive Fat. *Brit. Med. J.* 1:1403, 1960.

Wheeler, J. E., Lukens, E. D. W., and Gyorgy, D.: Studies on the Localization of Tagged Methionine within the Pancreas. *Proc. Soc. Exp. Biol. Med.* 70:187, 1949.

Yagan, R., McIntyre, W. J., and Christie, J. H.: Estimation of Liver Size by Multiple Cut-off Scintillation Scanning Technique. *Amer. J. Roentgen.* 88:289, 1962.

CHAPTER XIII

THE KIDNEY

HENRY N. WAGNER, Jr.

RICHARD C. REBA

DAVID A. GOODWIN

INTRODUCTION

The value of radioisotope techniques in the diagnosis of renal disease depends upon: (1) the ability to detect and quantify gamma radiation by means of external detectors directed at each kidney, and (2) the ability to measure radioactivity in biological specimens with extreme precision and sensitivity. External detection makes possible localization of disease of an individual kidney or part of a kidney; measurement of radioactivity makes chemical determinations much simpler and more precise.

The most frequent use of radioisotopes in renal disease has been in screening hypertensive patients to find those who may have surgically correctable abnormalities. The magnitude of the problem is shown by the fact that cardiovascular-renal disease accounted for well over half of the 934,000 deaths in the United States during 1960 (Lerner and Anderson, 1963). In persons over the age of 45 years who died of heart disease, more than 10 per cent had hypertension. Thus the detection of hypertensive patients is a large health problem, as is the screening of these patients to detect surgically correctable unilateral renal disease.

To detect unilateral renal disease, external radiation detectors are positioned at the surface of the body and directed toward each kidney. A gamma-emitting radiopharmaceutical is administered intravenously, and the rate of accumulation and disappearance of the radioactivity over the two kidneys is recorded. The technique does not involve any patient discomfort and can be performed with ease. The tests are used primarily as screening procedures; they cannot be used to indicate that hypertension in a given patient has resulted from unilateral renal disease. An abnormal result indicates only that there are functional or structural differences between the two kidneys.

OUTLINE OF THE DEVELOPMENT OF TECHNIQUES FOR LOCALIZATION OF RENAL DISEASE

One year after the discovery of x-rays by Röntgen in 1895, radiography was used to detect kidney stones. Ten years later the first retrograde pyelogram was performed. In 1923, physicians at the Mayo Clinic administered contrast media intravenously to visualize the urinary tract. The first application of radio-isotope methods to diagnose renal disease was in 1952, when Oeser and Billion measured the rate of excretion of ^{131}I-labeled sodium iodomethramate from each kidney. At about the same time, Smith, Rush, and Evans (1951) reported their results with translumbar aortography, first carried out by Dos Santos and his associates in 1929. Howard and his colleagues (1954) reawakened interest in the diagnosis of renovascular hypertension by demonstrating the effective use of bilateral ureteral catheterization. They proposed that the cure rates reported by Smith in 1948 (47 of 242; 19 per cent) and again in 1956 (149 of 575; 26 per cent) might be improved with better criteria for selection of patients. Maxwell and Prozan (1962) also emphasized that, at most, 14 of 149 cured patients in Smith's second series had lesions of the renal arterial system. The disease in two thirds of the patients was pyelonephritis, atrophic kidney, or hydronephrosis.

The radioisotope renogram was designed in 1956 by Taplin and his co-workers to avoid the necessity of using bilateral ureteral catheterization or arteriography. It was the first use of external radiation detectors in the evaluation of individual kidney function. The test was performed originally by recording the activity over each kidney after the intravenous injection of ^{131}I-labeled Diodrast (iodopyracet) and Urokon. In the following years several other ^{131}I-labeled compounds were used.

Diodrast ^{131}I was found to be better for assessing renal function than Urokon ^{131}I because the latter was too slowly excreted in man (Dennenberg et al., 1960; Porporis et al., 1954). Winter (1956), Winter and Taplin (1958), and Kinter and Pappenheimer (1956) evaluated the Diodrast renogram and outlined the advantages of Diodrast ^{131}I over Hypaque ^{131}I, Urokon ^{131}I, and Miokon [131]I. However, Hypaque ^{131}I was preferred by others because it concentrated to a lesser degree in the liver (Winter et al., 1959; Montandon et al., 1962; Stokes et al., 1962). Several methods were developed to solve the problem of hepatic accumulation of radioactivity. One attempt at solving the problem was to inject a large dose of stable Diodrast before injection of [131]I Diodrast. The nonradio-active material competed with hepatic uptake of the active material but did not prevent plasma protein binding (Block and Burrows, 1959).

Clinical studies of the Diodrast ^{131}I renogram indicated that it might be a more sensitive test for unilateral disease than the intravenous pyelogram (Serrato et al., 1959; Block et al., 1960), but the procedure was not fully accepted. Spencer et al. (1961) repeated the test five times in each of four normal subjects and found that the renogram was not reproducible; Dollery (1960) concluded that it was not a suitable screening test for unilateral renal disease.

Early in 1960, Tubis synthesized ^{131}I-labeled o-iodohippurate. This substance is extracted from the blood with great efficiency, in a manner similar to para-aminohippurate (PAH), and accentuates the difference between the two kidneys in unilateral disease (Nordyke et al., 1960; Whitely et al., 1961).

In 1960, McAfee and Wagner used [203]Hg-labeled chlormerodrin to delineate the kidneys by scanning as a means of detecting focal lesions such as cysts, infarcts, and ischemic segments, as well as generalized renal atrophy. Subsequently, Reba, Wagner, and McAfee (1962, 1963) used the same radiopharmaceutical to measure the function of each kidney by monitoring the rate of accumulation of the labeled chlormerodrin with a pair of external radiation detectors.

RADIOISOTOPE RENOGRAPHY

Renography is the measurement of the time course of radioactivity over each kidney, using paired scintillation detectors after radioiodinated ortho-iodo-hippurate (OIH) has been injected intravenously. A typical pair of tracings are illustrated in Figure 13-1. The radioactivity over the kidneys reaches a maximum in 5 minutes, followed by an approximately exponential decline during the next 10 to 15 minutes. Three segments of the tracing were originally de-

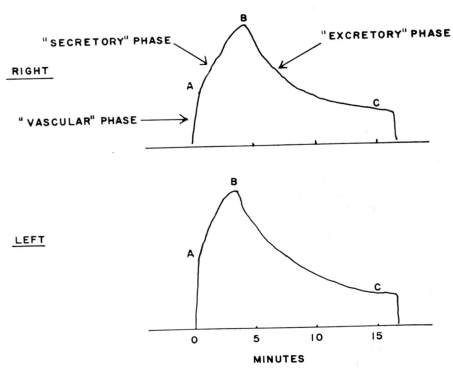

FIGURE 13-1. O-Iodohippurate (Hippuran) renogram in a normal person, illustrating what was originally believed to be the three separate phases of the tracing.

scribed: segment A was believed to result from activity in the vascular bed; segment B, which coincided with a rapid fall in blood OIH levels, was thought to indicate accumulation by the kidneys; and segment C, the phase of rapid decrease, was believed to indicate excretion. Although it is true that the initial rise is determined largely by renal blood flow, and the fall in count rate is primarily affected by urine flow, it is clear that multiple factors influence the entire tracing, and that no single physiological parameter can be separated entirely from the others.

The state of hydration of the patient is an important determinant of the shape of the tracing, but there is disagreement about the optimum state of hydration. Some investigators hydrate their patients, whereas others dehydrate them. Dehydration usually increases the differences between normal and abnormal kidneys; however, it may result in abnormal tracings in some normal persons.

Meade and Shy (1961) evaluated the renogram in normal subjects and found a slightly higher amplitude on the right side, which they attributed to the blood pool in the liver, since radioiodinated human serum albumin also gave a higher value on the right side.

Many criteria have been proposed to evaluate the renogram. Hirakawa et al. (1961) used the same parameters as Winter (1961a, b) and interpreted the results primarily on the basis of the amplitude of the peaks and the 15 minute level of activity. Stewart and Haynie (1962) used the interval between the time of maximum amplitude (T_{max}) and the time of one half of maximum amplitude. Tauxe et al. (1962) studied various diseases under standardized conditions, and Pircher et al. (1963a, b) analyzed 28 different parameters of the Hippuran renogram. The maximum amplitude (B) minus the amplitude at 15 minutes (C) was believed the most reliable criterion for the diagnosis of unilateral renal vascular disease.

Other methods of quantification have included: the percentage of maximum activity remaining 10 minutes after injection, and the slope of the "second segment" of the renogram. Taplin and his associates reported experimental evidence that the rise of the second segment is the most satisfactory index of renal blood flow (Dore et al., 1963). These authors stated that the renogram in unilateral renal artery stenosis is characteristic when renal blood flow to one kidney is less than 40 per cent of total renal blood flow; i.e., it shows prolonged renal transit time (the time between injection and maximum count rate), and delayed urinary excretion, manifest by a slower than normal decrease in count rate.

The position of the patient during performance of the renogram has varied in different laboratories: some keep the patient supine, others use the prone or the sitting position. The first two positions are the most widely used, because of greater ease of localization of the kidneys and less movement of the patient.

It is essential to have the detectors correctly positioned over the kidneys; failure to achieve this is the largest single cause of error. The location of the kidneys can be determined by a preliminary radiograph or by scanning the kidneys immediately before performing the renogram. When one is certain of renal position, scintillation detectors are placed over each kidney. It is essential to balance the two detection systems before the test. Flat-field collimation is usually used to achieve a uniform response across the field of view. The detectors should be at least 7 inches from the face of the collimator, to minimize the effect of differences in distance of the kidneys from the body surface. The detectors are usually connected to dual rate meters and rectilinear chart recorders. A dose of 100 μc. of Hippuran is given intravenously, and a 15 to 20 minute tracing is made at a paper speed of 12 inches per minute.

Certain of the causes of variability of the renogram tracings can be controlled:

    (a) dose and volume injected;
    (b) rate of injection;
    (c) position of patient and crystal;
    (d) sensitivity and collimation of the detector.

Uncontrollable variables include:

    (a) exact distance from patient's kidney to detector;
    (b) size and proximity of liver;
    (c) blood volume;
    (d) mixing time in the circulation.

Apprehension on the part of the patient can cause a decrease in excretion of Hippuran. A change in body position can also affect the tracing (Meade and Shy, 1961). *Each laboratory should determine the range of normality with its own equipment on a series of normal patients,* rather than relying only upon some "ideal normal" curve. A statistical analysis of the renogram in normal subjects is shown in Figure 13-2.

It must be stressed that abnormal tracings in a renogram are not diagnostic of any specific disease. In some cases, however, a characteristic pattern may occur. For example, a normal uptake with a continually rising third phase is

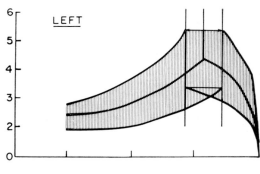

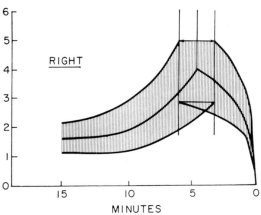

FIGURE 13-2. Hippuran renogram: mean values $\pm$ 1 standard deviation in 19 normal persons.

MINUTES

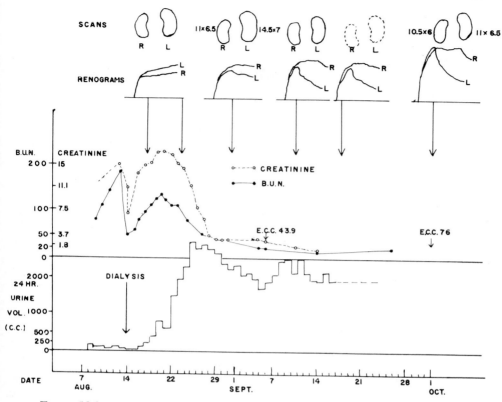

FIGURE 13-3. Acute tubular necrosis in a 28 year old woman following a blood transfusion reaction. Serial scans and renograms are correlated with renal function, showing recovery (more complete in the left kidney) during a period of 2 months.

suggestive of ureteral obstruction (O'Conor, 1961; Beall et al., 1963); but this may also occur in acute tubular necrosis (Fig. 13-3).

Several renogram patterns have been reported in renal hypertension. The most common is an increase in "transit time" (Taplin et al., 1963) and a decrease in the rate of excretion of Hippuran, resulting in a prolongation of the third phase (Block et al., 1960; Tauxe, 1961; Yasky and Volpe, 1963; Burbank and Tauxe, 1963; Taplin et al., 1963). An overall decrease in amplitude on the affected side has also been reported in dogs with a Goldblatt clamp on the renal artery. The value of the test as a screening method has been the subject of widely varying reports; some find no useful application (Moses et al., 1961) and others claim 90 per cent accuracy (Morgan et al., 1962). The radioisotope renogram alone is not an ideal screening procedure, chiefly because of false-negative results. For example, Maxwell and Prozan (1962) reported 16 per cent false-negative results (5 of 40), a rather high figure for a screening procedure.

CHLORMERODRIN ACCUMULATION TEST

This test consists of measuring the rate of accumulation of mercury [197]Hg-labeled chlormerodrin, using the same type of external detectors as in Hippuran renography. The main difference between the two procedures is the radio-pharmaceutical used.

The theoretical advantage of the chlormerodrin accumulation test (CAT) over the ortho-iodohippurate renogram is that the time-concentration tracings are not influenced by so many variables. With iodohippurate, the external detector records a summation of the effects of physical mixing of the radiopharmaceutical in the circulation, renal blood flow, renal tubular extraction efficiency, and the rate of urine flow. Because the rate of accumulation of chlormerodrin is much slower, it can be observed for a period of up to 1 hour rather than for only minutes. Thus, variations in the rate of physical mixing of the radiopharmaceutical in the circulation do not influence the tracings after 3 to 5 minutes. Chlormerodrin is bound temporarily in the renal tubules, rather than being excreted immediately into the urine. The chlormerodrin tracing reflects primarily two parameters of renal function: renal blood flow and renal tubular efficiency. An additional advantage is that measurement of the rate of accumulation of chlormerodrin can be followed by scanning, which supplements the functional data with structural information.

Many organic mercurial compounds form mercaptides with sulfhydryl-containing enzymes of the renal tubular cells. The renal clearance of ^{203}Hg chlormerodrin is about one half of the glomerular filtration rate, or about 40 cc. per min. (Burch et al., 1950); this value is decreased in congestive heart failure and renal disease (Threefoot et al., 1949). In 1951, Weston et al. described renal protein binding of a fraction of intravenously injected mercurial diuretics, with later release of this fraction. In view of the fact that 5 to 10 per cent of the injected mercurial could be retained up to 47 days, Grossman et al. (1951) suggested that repeated injections could lead to accumulation in the body. Borghgraef and his associates (1956) showed that the kidneys of dogs bind 100 to 150 μg. of ^{203}Hg chlormerodrin per gram of tissue, whereas the liver and the spleen bind the material to a lesser degree. Greif and his colleagues (1956) found the concentration of ^{203}Hg chlormerodrin to be highest in the outer renal cortex, less in the medulla, and lowest in the renal papillary tissue. Stop-flow experiments have shown that ^{203}Hg chlormerodrin is excreted by the proximal tubule (Fig. 13-4), and cellular studies have shown this substance to be concentrated in the cells of the proximal tubule (Cafruny et al., 1961).

These considerations of the renal handling of chlormerodrin are very important in the calculation of the radiation dose to the kidney from renal uptake tests or scanning procedures. A lack of knowledge of the biological half-life of ^{203}Hg chlormerodrin led originally to erroneously low estimates of renal radiation dosage. Five to ten per cent of the injected dose is retained in the kidneys after the first 24 hours, with a relatively long effective half-life of about 28 days. Therefore, an intravenous dose of 100 to 150 μc. of ^{203}Hg-labeled chlormerodrin delivers approximately 23 rads to the kidneys, whereas the remainder of the body gets only about 0.13 rad.

Chlormerodrin labeled with the nuclide ^{197}Hg instead of ^{203}Hg is now commercially available. The radioisotope ^{197}Hg has many characteristics that are ideal for external scintillation counting and scanning. It emits a gamma photon of 77 kev., and a characteristic x-ray of 69 kev. Because of its short physical half-life of 2.7 days, and lack of beta emission, the radiation to the kidneys from 150 μc. of ^{197}Hg is only about 1.5 rads, and the total body dose only

0.012 rad. For these reasons, [197]Hg should supplant [203]Hg for clinical uptake tests and scanning.

In performing the chlormerodrin accumulation test, no preliminary preparation of the patient is necessary. Neither food nor fluid need be restricted. The rate of accumulation of [197]Hg chlormerodrin is recorded by means of paired scintillation detectors, scintillation spectrometers, count-rate meters, and chart recorders. The scintillation detectors are sodium iodide crystals (Tl-activated) surrounded by lead shields. The spectrometer is centered on the photopeak energy of [197]Hg, or slightly above the photopeak, according to the recommendations of Harris et al. (1965). The preferred position of the patient is supine, with the detector mounted under the table.

As in radioisotope renography performed with ^{131}I-labeled ortho-iodohippurate, the greatest sources of error are improper positioning of the detector and changes in position of the patient during the study. If serial studies are performed on the same patient, varying the body position as little as 5 cm. can result in abnormal tracings even if renal function is normal.

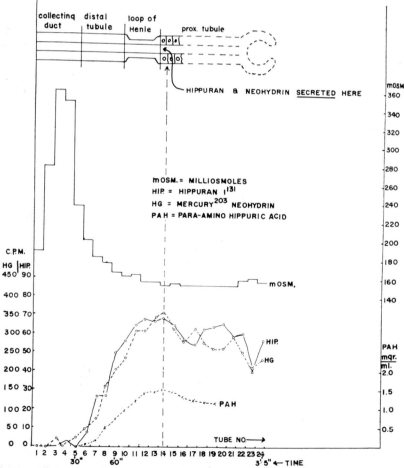

FIGURE 13-4. Stop-flow experiment in a dog: showing that the site of excretion of PAH, ortho-iodohippurate and [203]Hg chlormerodrin (Neohydrin) is the distal part of the proximal tubule.

A preliminary radiograph is obtained while the patient is lying supine on the renogram table. External landmarks are insufficient for locating the kidneys precisely. The position of the kidneys is determined by means of a radiopaque centimeter scale on the table and a scout radiograph. After performance of the scan, a check is made of the position of the detectors relative to the scanning image of the kidneys. If the detectors were misplaced, the accumulation test is considered invalid and is repeated. The patient is instructed to lie motionless during the study; restless patients and young children are sedated to minimize motion.

Contamination of the organic mercurial with free mercuric ions will result in abnormally slow rates of accumulation of radioactivity. Commercial preparations rarely contain significant amounts of free mercury, and solutions may be kept for several months if the pH is 8 or greater; in acidic solutions, free mercury is liberated. The accumulation rate is not influenced by the dose of mercurial within the limits of 0.004 mg. and 0.1 mg. of mercury per kilogram of body weight. Most commercial preparations fall within this limit for doses of radioactivity up to 150 μc.

The accumulation test should be carried out before ureteral catheterization, if this is to be performed, because a transient decrease in uptake may follow this manipulation. Renal arteriography can also depress renal blood flow, so that studies shortly after arteriography should be avoided.

Within 10 to 30 seconds after the intravenous injection of ^{197}Hg chlormerodrin, the count rate frequently rises and falls abruptly as the bolus of radioactivity enters the abdominal arteries and viscera. The rise is usually higher on the right than the left and is similar to that observed with ^{131}I Hippuran. Thereafter, there is a slow progressive increase in count rate for the remainder of the 1 hour study. This gradual rise continues for 2 to 4 hours, because the concentration of the radioactive mercury in the renal tubular cells increases more rapidly than the excretion in the urine. Within the first hour, only 5 to 10 per cent of the administered radioactivity is recovered in the urine. This temporary retention of chlormerodrin in the kidneys contrasts with the rapid decrease in count rate following the injection of ^{131}I Hippuran. The absolute count rates are usually slightly higher on the right than on the left because of the presence of hepatic radioactivity in the field of the right detector. For chlormerodrin, the ratio of kidney to liver concentration per gram of tissue is about 35:1.

The absolute count rate over each kidney depends on the size of the dose, the rate of accumulation of the radioactive material by the kidney, and the geometry and efficiency of the detection system. During the first 3 to 5 minutes, the count rate is also influenced by variations in the rate of mixing of chlormerodrin in the vascular system.

To minimize some of the variability resulting from the use of absolute counting rates, relative count rates are used; i.e., the count rate at various times, t, is compared to the count rate 5 minutes after the intravenous injection.

To compare the rates of accumulation of ^{197}Hg chlormerodrin by the two kidneys, the C_t/C_5 ratios of the right kidney are divided by the corresponding ratios of the left. In our experience both the mean values and the upper and lower limits of these ratios were nearly identical for the normotensive and essential hypertensive patients (Table 13-1, and Fig. 13-5). In both groups the right to left ratios varied little between 20 and 60 minutes after injection; the

TABLE 13-1. RATIO OF C_t/C_5 OF THE RIGHT KIDNEY TO THAT OF THE LEFT KIDNEY

TIME (MINUTES)	10	20	30	40	50	60
			Normal			
$\bar{x} \pm 1$ S.D.	.98 ± .04	.95 ± .03	.94 ± .04	.94 ± .04	.94 ± .04	.95 ± .06
95% conf. limits	.89–1.06	.89–1.01	.87–1.02	.86–1.02	.85–1.02	.83–1.06
(N)	(19)	(19)	(19)	(19)	(17)	(13)
			Essential Hypertension			
$\bar{x} \pm 1$ S.D.	.98 ± .05	.95 ± .04	.94 ± .05	.95 ± .05	.93 ± .05	.93 ± .06
95% conf. limits	.90–1.06	.88–1.03	.85–1.04	.84–1.04	.83–1.04	.82–1.05
(N)	(63)	(63)	(63)	(61)	(55)	(40)

95 percentile range of both groups extended from 0.85 to 1.05; the mean was 0.95.

The ratio of the count rates over the two kidneys (C_t right/C_t left) averaged 1.14 in the normotensive group (95 percentile, 0.78 to 1.5) between 30 and 60 minutes. The slight differences in mean values between the group of normo-

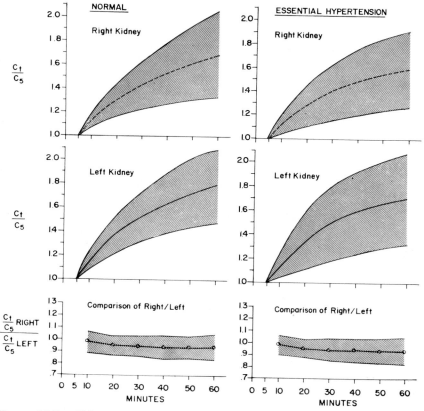

FIGURE 13-5. Chlormerodrin accumulation test: normal values ± 2 standard deviations in normal persons. The tracings are normalized by dividing count rates at various times by 5 minute rate (C_t/C_5). Note relatively narrow 95 percentile range (shaded areas) in both normotensive patients and those with essential hypertension.

tensive patients and those with essential hypertension were not statistically significant.

Sufficiently high concentrations of labeled chlormerodrin are maintained from 1 to 3 hours to permit delineation of the kidneys by scanning after the chlormerodrin accumulation test. The scanning procedure may be repeated without another dose for as long as 24 hours after the study, although the counting rates are significantly lower. Commercially available scanners are useful for renal scanning, although the energy characteristics of [197]Hg make this nuclide satisfactory for nuclear image amplifiers as well.

RENAL SCANNING

Renal scanning has been attempted using Hippuran ^{131}I, but this agent is very rapidly excreted in the urine and does not satisfactorily outline the renal parenchyma. Haynie et al. (1960) were able to lessen this difficulty by using a constant infusion of Hippuran intravenously during the time of scanning. Camera devices have also been used because of their rapid response time. [131]I Hippuran scans of dogs before and after branch renal-artery ligation outlined the area of infarction demonstrated at autopsy. Westphal et al. (1962) used Diodrast ^{131}I as well as Hippuran ^{131}I for renal scanning. Large doses were necessary, however, and good visualization was not obtained.

McAfee and Wagner (1960) introduced [203]Hg-labeled chlormerodrin for visualization of the renal parenchyma by renal scanning. Only a single injection is required because passage of radioactivity through the kidney is slow enough to outline the organ for several hours. Chlormerodrin [203]Hg is very sensitive in the detection of viable renal tissue, since this compound is concentrated in the renal tubular cells. Maximum concentration occurs in the kidney in 1 to 6 hours following injection, and visualization of the kidney is possible even in moderately uremic patients. With depressed renal function, increased hepatic uptake is noted. Other investigators have confirmed the advantages of chlormerodrin [203]Hg for renal scanning (Haynie et al., 1961; Carr, 1961a, b).

Renal scanning is clinically useful for detecting abnormalities in the size, shape, and position of the kidneys; problems caused by overlying gaseous shadows, overlapping organs, and confusion with other structures are thereby avoided. The accumulation of chlormerodrin is highly specific for functioning renal parenchymal tissue, a specificity that is frequently helpful.

Figure 13-6 is an example of a renal scan in a normal person. The position of the kidney varies considerably in different persons. The center of the right kidney in an adult is usually opposite the transverse process of the second lumbar vertebra. The longitudinal axis usually diverges laterally about 15 to 20 degrees, although in some normal persons the divergence may be as little as 9 degrees or as much as 24 degrees. The top of the right kidney is usually at the level of the twelfth rib, whereas the left is at the level of the eleventh. The upper poles of the kidneys are immediately beneath the diaphragm, which causes them to move during respiration. The anterior surface of the upper pole of the right kidney lies immediately below the liver, and may produce an invagination of the liver's inferior surface, which in some people is visible in liver scans. The lateral border of the top of the right kidney is sometimes flattened as the result of the adjacent liver. In such cases, the lower pole usually has a thick, rounded appearance. A similar appearance may be noted on the left.

Immediately adjacent to the upper pole of the left kidney is the spleen. The anterior surface of the left kidney lies immediately behind the body of the pancreas and the lower border of the stomach. Changing from a supine to erect position frequently results in movement of the kidneys, at times as much as 5 cm. (or approximately the size of 1.5 vertebral bodies in a normal adult male).

Except for the region of hilus, the contour of the kidney is usually smooth, but it may be distorted by fetal lobulation. Lobulation usually regresses after age 4, but may persist and result in an irregular shape that causes concern when detected on radiographs. The shape of the kidneys may vary from long and narrow to short and thick, with considerable variability even between the kidneys of the same person.

To obtain criteria for diagnosing abnormalities of renal size, Simon (1964) studied a series of kidneys from 100 persons whose kidneys were without evidence of renal disease at autopsy. As measured on roentgenograms, the length of the kidneys ranged between 9.4 and 13.7 cm., with a mean of 11.7 cm. The ratio of renal length to the height of the radiographic image of the second lumbar vertebral body was 3.7 ± 0.37 (S.D.).

In his studies of 165 normal persons between 20 and 55 years of age, Moell (1956) correlated the roentgenographic dimensions of the kidneys during life with measurements at autopsy. When examined under standard conditions, the average measurements of kidneys of men were: right, 12.7 by 6.3 cm.; left, 13.2 by 6.4 cm. The corresponding figures for women were: right, 12.4 by 5.9 cm.; left, 12.8 by 6.1 cm. In men the total area of the kidneys (determined by assuming the kidney was elliptical) measured 70.1 ± 5.4 sq. cm. per sq. meter of body surface; in women, the area was 72.2 ± 6.6 sq. cm. per sq. meter of body surface. Similar values were obtained when the areas were measured by planimetry.

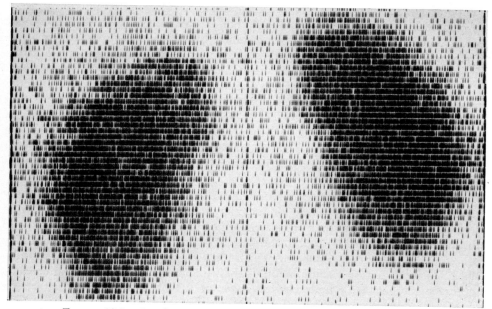

FIGURE 13-6. Renal scan using [197]Hg chlormerodrin in a normal person.

Moell found a linear relationship between the renal area and logarithm of the body weight.

In our own series of chlormerodrin scans of 190 patients with essential hypertension, 28 patients had greater than 1 cm. difference in the length of the two kidneys: 23 had more than 1.5 cm. difference; 5 had greater than 2 cm.; and one had greater than 3 cm. The finding of a difference in length greater than 2 cm. should be considered abnormal.

CONGENITAL DISEASES

Anomalies of the kidney vary from slight hypoplasia to complete agenesis. Hypoplasia is a local or general structural underdevelopment, with retention of normal function. Aplasia denotes a severely underdeveloped or maldeveloped kidney with little or no remaining function. These defects are frequently not visible on abdominal radiographs but may be first observed by retrograde pyelography, renal scanning, or angiography. At times these abnormalities are the focus of infection in patients with pyuria of obscure origin. In its most severe form, aplasia may be associated with cyst formation, a rare condition known as "congenital unilateral polycystic disease" (Nagle and Allen, 1965). The relationship between this disease and bilateral polycystic disease is uncertain. Although pyelonephritis is the most common cause of an abnormally small kidney, congenital hypoplasia must also be considered in the differential diagnosis.

The term ectopic means displacement or malrotation. In extreme cases, the kidney may be found in the thorax or deep in the pelvis; but the most common abnormality is a moderate downward displacement. Malrotation can occur, with the renal pelvis assuming a more anterior or posterior position as the kidney rotates on its longitudinal axis; it is frequently associated with other anomalies. Rotation of the kidney may result in impairment of the arterial blood supply, a factor of clinical importance in certain patients with hypertension.

Sometimes the kidneys are fused; the most common type is a horseshoe kidney, in which the lower poles are joined but the upper poles are separate This may produce vascular anomalies or hydronephrosis from ureteral obstruction. There may be a double kidney on one side, each with its own pelvis.

With conventional radiographic techniques, some of these abnormalities may appear to be tumors. Renal scanning can be used to demonstrate that the tissue is renal, not neoplastic, often obviating the necessity of more difficult procedures. In a large series of renal tumors, none has been found to accumulate chlormerodrin. Visualization of the kidney in an unusual location may prevent confusion of ectopia with aplasia, the latter being suspected when no kidney is seen in the normal location.

In patients with chronic obstruction to urine flow, the demonstration by renal scanning of a horseshoe kidney may indicate ureteral obstruction from structural defects rather than from some other condition, such as a calculus, and this information may be useful in the patient's management. Renal scanning may occasionally be helpful in defining which regions of a defective kidney are functional, as indicated by accumulation of the radioactivity. It can also be of value to screen patients with undescended testes or with hypospadias, to detect the frequently associated congenital defects of the upper urinary tract (Felton, 1959).

Congenital arteriovenous fistulae are rare; but they may be associated with hypertension, high-output congestive heart failure, unusual murmurs, and hematuria (Gold et al., 1965). Such fistulae can be differentiated from those that occur from trauma or renal biopsy. Scanning may be useful as an initial procedure before definitive diagnosis by arteriography.

ABNORMALITIES OF RENAL SIZE

Table 13-2 lists diseases that may cause bilateral abnormalities of renal size. In addition to congenital causes of abnormal positions of the kidney, one must consider displacement by intrarenal tumors or cysts, as well as nonrenal conditions such as enlargement of the liver or spleen, retroperitoneal or intraperitoneal tumors, and perinephric and other abscesses.

The degree of distortion of size of the kidneys in renal scanning is dependent on the technique that is used. As in other scanning procedures in which high counting rates are obtained, it is unwise to use excessive distortion in data processing. If this is done, the edges of the normal kidney may disappear and a spuriously small image will result.

As mentioned, a difference in length of 2 cm. or more must be present before interpreting the difference as abnormal. Don (1961) studied 100 normotensive persons by intravenous pyelography and compared them to a series of patients with unilateral renal-artery disease. He concluded that asymmetry in length

TABLE 13-2. DISEASES THAT MAY CAUSE BILATERAL ABNORMALITIES
OF RENAL SIZE

I. DISEASES CAUSING BILATERAL RENAL ENLARGEMENT
   A. *Congenital Diseases*
      1. Polycystic renal disease
      2. Bilateral hydronephrosis (urinary stasis)
   B. *Diseases Due to Infection*
      1. Acute and subacute glomerulonephritis
      2. Acute bilateral pyelonephritis
      3. Tuberculosis
      4. Sarcoidosis
   C. *Diseases Due to Trauma or Physicochemical Agents*
      1. Acute tubular necrosis: Burns, nephritis, hepatorenal syndrome, traumatic anuria, "lower nephron nephrosis"
   D. *Diseases Due to Circulatory Disturbances*
      1. Bilateral renal vein thrombosis
      2. Bilateral cortical necrosis
   E. *New Growths*
      1. Leukemia, myeloma
   F. *Diseases Due to Unknown or Uncertain Cause*
      1. Amyloidosis
      2. Toxemia of pregnancy

II. DISEASES CAUSING BILATERAL SMALL KIDNEYS
   A. *Hypoplasia and Aplasia*
   B. *Chronic Pyelonephritis*
   C. *Chronic Glomerulonephritis*
   D. *Chronic Nephrosclerosis*

alone, even when 1 cm. or more, is a frequent finding in normotensive persons and is not in itself significant. Study of six cases of main renal-artery disease suggested that asymmetry of length of 1 cm. is significant if accompanied by parenchymatous thinning of the shorter kidney.

RENAL TRAUMA

Hematuria following trauma to the abdomen or back may be a sign of damage of the urinary tract and must be investigated. The renal vein may be transected, and yet the intravenous pyelogram may be normal if the renal artery is intact (McCort, 1964). Complete avulsion of the renal vasculature can occur, and yet the retrograde pyelogram may be normal if the calyces and renal pelvis are undamaged. Renal scans are helpful in the management of these patients.

A blow to the renal area may result in thrombosis of the main renal artery or one of its branches, or less frequently to a hematoma or arteriovenous fistula. Partial obstruction of a calyx from trauma may result in a cyst or hematoma formation. Trauma may cause herniation of the kidney into the thorax. In one patient with hematuria following an automobile accident, the kidneys could not be visualized by renal scanning for 6 weeks after the accident. In three other patients, injury to the kidney from ureteral catheterization markedly impaired renal function for 2 to 3 weeks, as revealed by scanning.

When renal trauma is slight, retrograde and intravenous pyelography are frequently normal, even though the patient may have considerable pain and gross or microscopic hematuria. Major fractures of the parenchyma or damage to the vascular pedicle may produce severe pain, abdominal rigidity, prolonged gross hematuria, shock, anuria, and, if untreated, death. In these cases, pyelography is helpful, because it usually reveals extravasation of urine. The most severe injury, the "shattered kidney," leads to massive perirenal hemorrhage and destruction of the entire kidney.

Renal scans are helpful not only to evaluate the suspected kidney, but also to ascertain whether the contralateral kidney is normal. This is imperative if surgery is contemplated. Demonstration of segmental defects in an injured kidney may prevent unnecessary removal of normal tissue. Recovery of renal function may be indicated earliest by return of ability to concentrate chlormerodrin.

Radioisotope renography, the chlormerodrin accumulation test, and renal scanning plus intravenous pyelography can be performed with ease without unnecessary manipulation of the patient or, in the case of the radioisotope studies, without having to dehydrate the patient.

Late complications of renal trauma include perirenal collections of urine, blood, or pus; hydronephrosis; cyst formation; intrarenal and extrarenal calcification; partial or complete occlusion of the renal arteries; subcapsular hematomas; arteriovenous fistulae; and atrophy and fibrosis of part or all of the kidney. Following renal trauma, some patients develop hypertension.

The urinary tract may be damaged in the course of abdominal or pelvic surgery. Radioisotope techniques can eliminate the need for cystoscopy or the dehydration necessary for pyelography.

Radiation damage to the kidneys may occur as a result of abdominal radiation therapy. Quinn et al. (1962) used radioisotope renography to follow patients undergoing radiation therapy, to detect evidence of urinary obstruction.

RENAL TUMORS

Scanning is a useful procedure in revealing abnormal morphology of the renal parenchyma, although lesions smaller than 2 cm. in diameter usually cannot be detected with present instruments. Figure 13-7 is an example of a hypernephroma. Both renal cysts and tumors fail to concentrate chlormerodrin, and consequently they cannot be differentiated. Renal scans are helpful in distinguishing between fetal lobulations and peripheral tumors. Fetal lobulations

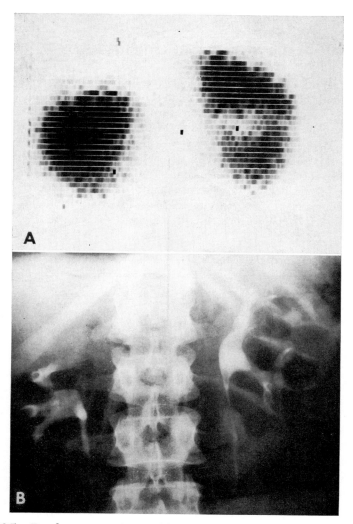

FIGURE 13-7.   Renal scan in a 38 year old Negro female with accompanying intravenous pyelogram. A filling defect is shown in the left kidney, which proved to be a hypernephroma measuring 4.5 cm. at nephrectomy. The chlormerodrin accumulation test and the Hippuran renogram were normal.

accumulate chlormerodrin, whereas tumors do not. Renal scans may also demonstrate peripheral tumors that do not distort the calyceal system. In patients allergic to iodine-containing contrast media, renal scanning may be the only available method to supplement plain films of the abdomen.

A frequent clinical problem is the management of a patient suspected of having a renal tumor, on the basis of urinalysis or suspicious lesion on intravenous pyelogram. If calyceal distortion is absent, a retrograde pyelogram may not be helpful; but renal scanning is frequently positive in these patients. In some cases, the size of a renal tumor as estimated from a scan differs from that obtained by the pyelogram. The scan gives a more accurate picture of the extent of destruction of normal renal tissue; this information is helpful to the surgeon at the time of operation. However, lesions at the extreme periphery of the kidney are difficult to diagnose by scanning.

RENOVASCULAR HYPERTENSION

The cause of essential hypertension remains uncertain, although it has been established with certainty that both bilateral and unilateral renal disease in man may result in elevation of arterial pressure. Table 13-3 lists the bilateral renal diseases that may produce hypertension; Table 13-4, the unilateral renal lesions.

The physician's attention should be directed to the possibility of treatable unilateral renal disease in any patient with hypertension. The probability of renal etiology is increased if the hypertension is of sudden onset, if there is acceleration of preexisting "benign" hypertension into malignant hypertension, or if the patient has one of the predisposing diseases listed in Table 13-4.

Table 13-5 lists the various tests that have been used to diagnose unilateral

TABLE 13-3. BILATERAL RENAL DISEASES ASSOCIATED WITH HYPERTENSION

A. CONGENITAL DISEASES
1. Hydronephrosis (obstructive uropathy)
2. Polycystic disease

B. INFECTIOUS DISEASES
1. Pyelonephritis
2. Glomerulonephritis

C. CIRCULATORY DISEASES
1. Arterial and arteriolar nephrosclerosis
2. Vasculitis (systemic lupus, periarteritis, scleroderma, and others)

D. DISEASES OF UNKNOWN OR UNCERTAIN CAUSE
1. Amyloidosis
2. Toxemia of pregnancy

E. METABOLIC DISEASES
1. Intercapillary glomerulosclerosis
2. Gout
3. Nephrosclerosis
4. Toxic nephritis

F. DISEASES CAUSED BY PHYSICAL AGENTS
1. Radiation nephritis

TABLE 13-4. TYPES OF UNILATERAL RENAL LESIONS ASSOCIATED WITH SYSTEMIC HYPERTENSION (MODIFIED FROM STRAUSS AND WELT)

A. DISEASES OF PRENATAL INFLUENCE
   1. Parenchymal
      a. Congenital hypoplastic kidney
      b. Renal ptosis
   2. Vascular
      a. Hypoplastic renal artery or branch
      b. Aberrant renal artery
      c. Fibromuscular hyperplasia
      d. Renal artery aneurysm
      e. Congenital arteriovenous fistula
B. DISEASES DUE TO INFECTION
   1. Parenchymal
      a. Unilateral chronic pyelonephritis
      b. Unilateral tuberculosis
      c. Perirenal abscess
      d. Perinephritis
      e. Hydatid cyst
   2. Vascular
      a Syphilitic occlusion
      b. Septic emboli
      c. Renal-vein thrombosis secondary to infection
C. DISEASES DUE TO TRAUMA OR PHYSICAL AGENTS
   1. Parenchymal
      a Radiation injury
      b. Compression of kidney by traumatic cyst
   2. Vascular
      a. Thrombosis of renal artery
      b. Arteriovenous fistula
      c. Hematoma
      d. Foreign body in renal artery
D. DISEASES DUE TO CIRCULATORY DISTURBANCES
   1. Atherosclerotic plaque with renal arterial thrombosis
   2. Ischemia of kidney from renal arterial thrombosis
      a. Thromboangiitis obliterans of the renal arteries
      b. Thrombosis of the renal artery; undetermined cause
      c. Thrombosis of the renal veins
   3. Ischemia of the kidney from renal arterial embolism
      a. Aseptic emboli
      b. Mural emboli
      c. Cholesterol emboli
   4. Arteriovenous fistula
   5. Ischemia of the kidney due to renal artery occlusion secondary to dissection of aorta
   6. Ischemia of the kidney secondary to obliterative arteritis
      a. Takayashu's disease of the aorta causing occlusion of renal artery ostia
      b. Polyarteritis
   7. Dissecting aneurysm of renal artery
E. DISEASES INVOLVING STATIC MECHANICAL ABNORMALITY
   1. Parenchymal
      a. Hydronephrotic contracted kidney
      b. Perirenal cyst
   2. Vascular
      a. Torsion of pedicle of kidney
      b. Ganglioneuroma of renal pedicle
      c. Lymphosarcoma of renal pedicle
   3. Fibrous or muscular bands

Table 13-4. (*Continued*)

F. NEOPLASM
1. Carcinoma (hypernephroma)
2. Sarcoma
3. Wilms' tumor
4. Metastatic

renal disease in patients with hypertension. The tests can be divided into screening tests and definitive or predictive tests—that is, those designed to indicate which patients will benefit from surgery. Obviously, ureteral catheterization and aortography are too complicated to apply to all the patients with hypertension. The purpose of radioisotope methodology has been to fill the need for a procedure that will adequately screen all patients with hypertension and select those requiring more extensive study. The renal scan may, for example, reveal an area of infarction, as shown in Figure 13-8.

In our experience with 190 patients with essential hypertension, compared to 51 with unilateral renal disease and hypertension, measurement of the rate of accumulation of chlormerodrin by each kidney followed by scintillation scanning was a reliable screening procedure for hypertension; it proved to be better than Hippuran renography (carried out by us) in the same patients. Figure 13-9 shows a small kidney with decreased chlormerodrin uptake in a hypertensive patient.

TABLE 13-5. TESTS FOR DIAGNOSING UNILATERAL KIDNEY DISEASE

A. DIFFERENTIAL RENAL FUNCTION BY URETERAL CATHETERIZATION
Howard—decreased urine volume and decreased sodium concentration
Birchell—decreased urine volume and decreased tubular rejectate
Schlegel—decreased urine volume and increased urine osmolality
Rapoport—ratio of fractional tubular rejectate

B. UROGRAPHY
Intravenous pyelography (excretory urogram)
Rapid sequence intravenous pyelography
Pyelogram—urea washout test

C. ANGIOTENSIN INFUSION TEST (Kaplan)

D. AORTOGRAPHY
Aortography with measurement of pressure gradient at surgery
Selective renal angiography

E. CIRCULATING PRESSOR SUBSTANCES
Angiotensin II
Plasma renin
Other pressor substances

F. RENAL BIOPSY
Hyperplasia of the juxtaglomerular apparatus

G. RADIOISOTOPE METHODS
Renography
Chlormerodrin uptake test and scanning
Rubidium-86 and other tests

According to our studies, the final diagnosis of a unilateral renal lesion is based on a combination of procedures, including clinical evaluation, intravenous pyelography, renal arteriography and differential ureteral catheterization data, and (in many patients) renal surgery. The most reliable criterion for comparing the function of one kidney with the other is the ratio of the rate of chlormerodrin

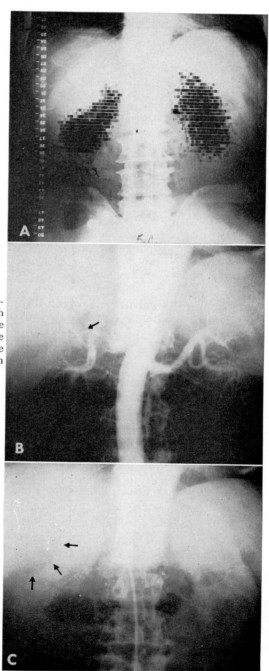

FIGURE 13–8. Renal scan and arteriogram in 56 year old Negro male with renal hypertension. The scan shows the area of infarcted kidney, illustrated on the arteriogram, in the right upper pole. The intravenous pyelogram and chlormerodrin accumulation test were normal.

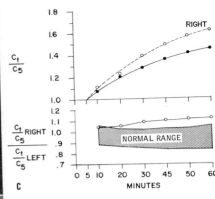

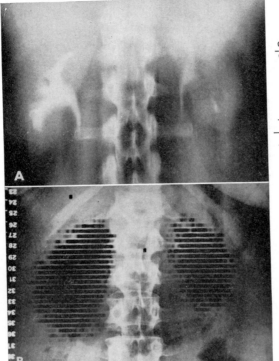

FIGURE 13-9. Labile hypertension and left renal ischemia. Atrophy of the left kidney not revealed by intravenous pyelogram, but demonstrated by nephrotomography and renal scan. Impaired accumulation rate of chlormerodrin in the left kidney. Urine flow reduced by 50 per cent on left. Nephrectomy revealed focal narrowing of intrarenal arteries and cortical scarring.

accumulation of the right kidney and the left. Scintillation scanning alone does not constitute a suitable screening procedure for unilateral renal disease.

Of the 51 patients with unilateral renal disease, 5 false-negative chlormerodrin accumulation tests were obtained (90 per cent accuracy); 2 of the 5 patients were studied for only 30 minutes after the chlormerodrin injection, rather than the usual 60 minute tracings. Although 5 patients had false-negative scans, fortunately in only one patient were both the scan and the chlormerodrin accumulation test falsely negative. Of the 190 patients finally diagnosed as having essential hypertension, 9 had falsely positive chlormerodrin accumulation tests and 8 had false-positive scans. Of the 8 false-positive scans, 5 were the result of interpreting a difference in size of over 2 cm. as abnormal. Only 3 patients with essential hypertension had focal areas of decreased concentration. Over 95 per cent of these patients were hospitalized for study; all were followed for a minimum of 1 year.

The [197]Hg-labeled chlormerodrin accumulation test and scan are not designed for the same purpose as renal arteriography or differential excretion studies. The latter tests attempt to predict the possible effect of corrective surgery. Both arteriography and differential excretion studies are definitive tests in that they occasionally reveal the etiology of the hypertension, but neither method alone detects all instances of correctable unilateral renal disease. On the other hand, radioisotopic techniques are screening procedures and have no value in indicating the etiology of hypertension or the possible effectiveness of renal surgery. For example, in unilateral pyelonephritis, abnormalities demonstrated by both the renogram and the [197]Hg-labeled chlormerodrin accumulation tests are identical to those of unilateral ischemia from renal arterial stenosis.

Bilateral renal damage of moderate severity produces impairment in the rate of accumulation of labeled chlormerodrin by both kidneys, although the right to left ratio is usually within normal limits.

In the presence of moderate renal failure, the size and location of the kidneys may be delineated by scanning when intravenous urography fails to visualize them. In marked renal insufficiency, however, the mercurial fails to concentrate in the kidneys and an abnormally large fraction concentrates in the liver. Blood levels remain high for a longer period of time; this usually occurs when the serum urea nitrogen is over 80 mg. per 100 ml.

Two modified techniques sometimes succeed in visualizing the kidneys when the usual method fails. In the first, cysteine is dissolved in 0.01N NaOH solution and added to the labeled chlormerodrin in a proportion of 20:1. The solution is sterilized by filtration before injection. The formation of chlormerodrin-cysteine complexes decreases the accumulation of uptake of chlormerodrin by nonrenal sulfhydryl binding sites, and increases the eventual renal concentration. In the second modification, renal scans are obtained 1 to 3 days after injection of the radioactive material. These delayed scans give better resolution than those obtained within a few hours of injection.

RENAL CLEARANCE WITH RADIOPHARMACEUTICALS

RENAL BLOOD FLOW

Homer Smith (1945) showed that the clearance of Hippuran and other substituted hippuric acid derivatives, including para-aminohippuric acid (PAH), were essentially the same. The reason he chose PAH to measure "effective renal plasma flow" (E.R.P.F.) was the ease of determination of this compound in the plasma; very small amounts of plasma PAH can be measured by colorimetry. The clearance method of measuring effective renal plasma flow required collection of timed urine samples during continuous infusion of PAH. The calculation was based on the Fick principle, which states that the blood flow is directly proportional to the rate of excretion and inversely proportional to the arterio-venous difference.

$$\text{Flow} = \frac{\text{Rate of excretion}}{\text{A-V difference}}$$

In practice, a continuous infusion of a substance such as PAH is administered until equilibrium occurs between arterial and peripheral venous blood. In normal persons, the arteriovenous difference in renal-artery and renal-vein blood is between 85 to 95 per cent, since the material is nearly completely extracted (Smith, 1945). One measures the amount of PAH in the urine ($U \times V$, where U = urine concentration of PAH, and V = urine flow) and divides by the concentration in venous blood obtained simultaneously. The renal plasma flow is calculated from the relation: $\text{R.P.F.} = \frac{U \times V}{P}$.

The simultaneous clearances of ortho-iodohippurate and para-aminohippurate are similar. Several studies have shown the former to be 81 to 92 per cent of the latter (Meschan et al., 1963; Schlegel et al., 1962; Schwartz and Madeloff, 1961; and Burbank et al., 1961), the average clearance being about 85 per cent of PAH clearance. Protein binding of Hippuran (Schlegel et al., 1962), uptake of

Hippuran by red blood cells, and contaminating free ^{131}I have all been suggested to explain the difference. Protein binding and RBC uptake seem unlikely causes, according to studies by Blaufox et al. (1963) and Magnusson (1962). That contaminating free ^{131}I is the most critical factor was shown by Meschan et al. (1963) and Burbank et al. (1961), who demonstrated that the Hippuran clearance fell with increasing amounts of free [131]I. This is because free ^{131}I clearance is much lower (30 cc. per minute) than Hippuran clearance. For this reason, solutions of Hippuran ^{131}I containing 2 per cent or more of the free iodide should not be used to estimate renal plasma flow (and solutions with greater than 10 to 15 per cent should not be used to perform the routine renogram test). Separation of ^{131}I from the Hippuran molecule occurs with time and exposure to sunlight, but fortunately it does not occur in vivo (Magnusson, 1962).

Further evidence for the similarity in renal handling of PAH and [131]I Hippuran is supplied by stop-flow experiments in dogs. Hippuran and PAH (as well as [203]Hg Neohydrin) are actively secreted in the distal part of the proximal tubule, as shown in Figure 13-4.

When urine cannot be obtained for technical reasons (as in some children) or for pathological reasons (as in shock or severe renal disease), the clearance techniques cannot be applied effectively. Renal blood flow can be approximated in these cases by measuring the rate of accumulation of Hippuran ^{131}I in the kidney by means of external radiation detectors. The tracings may simulate obstructive renal disease (ureteral obstruction) in acute tubular necrosis (Fig. 13-3).

GLOMERULAR FILTRATION RATE

Determination of the glomerular filtration rate (G.F.R.) is important for several reasons; it is the first step in urine formation, and its determination is important in the evaluation of renal tubular reabsorption and secretion. In the steady state, the rate of excretion of a substance that is neither reabsorbed, secreted, nor metabolized by the kidney must be equal to the rate at which it is filtered. If such a substance can be accurately measured in plasma and urine its clearance will be a valid estimate of glomerular filtration rate. It is now accepted that inulin, an oligosaccharide (molecular weight, 5500), is a substance that can be used effectively to estimate the rate of glomerular filtration in all vertebrates including man. Thus, G.F.R. $\times$ (P_{in}) = excretion rate ($U_{in} \times V$) where G.F.R. is the glomerular filtration rate in ml. per minute; (P_{in}) and (U_{in}) are the plasma and urine concentration of inulin per ml.; and V is the urine flow rate (ml. per minute). This expression can be stated: $C_{in} = \dfrac{U_{in} \times V}{P_{in}}$. To compare individual persons, the values are normalized for a total body surface area of 1.73 sq. meters.

Because of technical difficulties in the chemical determination of inulin in plasma and urine, attempts have been made to simplify the analytic procedure. Mannitol and creatinine have been used to approximate the glomerular filtration rate, although these are not completely satisfactory substitutes for inulin.

Renal clearance can be determined in either of three ways. The first is the classical method, UV/P. The second is based on the fact that in the steady state the rate of excretion must equal the rate of infusion of the injected substance therefore, one need determine only the plasma level of the substance being cleared. In the third method, the rate of clearance from the blood is used as a measure of renal clearance if the substance is cleared from the blood exclusively by the kidneys.

Measurement of glomerular filtration rate can be used to determine the presence of bilateral renal disease, in following the course of the disease, and in evaluating therapy. Several radiopharmaceuticals have been used to provide a means of measuring renal clearances that is as accurate as the classical techniques and technically simpler. These include: ^{14}C inulin, ^{57}Co vitamin B_{12}, ^{131}I diatrizoate, and ^{125}I allyl inulin.

Cotlove (1955) first demonstrated that the clearance of ^{14}C inulin is similar to that of the natural substance. The analytical technique is considerably easier and much more precise than the chemical method.

Nelp, Wagner, and Reba (1964) established that free vitamin B_{12} in plasma is neither secreted nor reabsorbed by the renal tubule, and that it is excreted solely by glomerular filtration. Correlation with simultaneous inulin clearance measurements was excellent throughout a wide range of G.F.R. in patients with renal disease.

There is contradictory evidence concerning the validity of using sodium diatrizoate to measure glomerular filtration rate. Stokes et al. (1962) and Woodruff and Malvin (1960) found that significant tubular reabsorption, protein binding, and variation with urine flow and osmotic load complicated the use of this substance. Tauxe and associates (1964) reported a significant amount of free iodide in addition to other unidentified labeled contaminants in this material. Despite these problems, this group has reported a good correlation with inulin clearances in both man and dog.

Recently, Concannon and co-workers (1964) modified the original technique of Brooks et al. (1960) and used an iodine-labeled allyl ether analogue of inulin. Although freshly prepared solutions did not give accurate clearance values, it was found that storage for several days, followed by passage through an anion resin exchange column just before infusion, effectively removed free and loosely bound iodide and resulted in an excellent correlation between this compound and inulin.

REFERENCES

Beall, A. C., Jr., et al.: The Use of the Renogram in Differential Diagnosis of Renal Insufficiency Following Vascular Surgery. *J. Nucl. Med.* 4:106, 1963.

Birchall, R., Batson, H. M., and Brannan, W.: Contribution of Differential Renal Studies to the Diagnosis of Renal Arterial Hypertension with Emphasis on the Value of U Sodium/U Creatinine. *Amer. J. Med.* 32:164, 1962.

Blaufox, M. D., Orvis, A. L., and Owen, C. A., Jr.: Compartment Analysis of the Radiorenogram and Distribution of Hippuran I-131 in Dogs. *Amer. J. Physiol.* 204:1059, 1963.

Block, J. B., and Burrows, B. A.: Diagnostic Use of ^{131}I Diodrast in Hypertension Due to Unilateral Kidney Disease. *Circulation* 18:696, 1958.

Block, J. B., and Burrows, B. A.: Hepatic Transport of ^{131}I Diodrast. *Clin. Res.* 7:34, 1959.

Block, J. B., Hine, G. J., and Burrows, B. A.: ^{131}I Diodrast Studies in Unilateral Renal Disease. *Circulation* 22:913, 1960.

Borghgraef, R. R. M., Kessler, R. H., and Pitts, R. F.: Plasma Regression, Distribution and Excretion of Radiomercury in Relation to Diuresis Following Intravenous Administration of Hg^{203} Labelled Chlormerodrin to Dog. *Clin. Invest.* 35:1055, 1956.

Brooks, S. A., Davies, J. W. L., Graves, I. J., and Rickets, C. R.: Labelling Inulin with [131]I. *Nature* 188:675, 1960.

Burbank, M. K., et al.: Evaluation of Radioiodinated Hippuran for the Estimation of Renal Plasma Flow. *Proc. Mayo Clin.* 36:372, 1961.

Burbank, M. K., and Tauxe, W. N.: The Renogram in Renal Artery Disease in Hypertensive Patients. *Circulation* 27:328, 1963.

Burch, G., Thorpe, R., Threefoot, S., Kelly, F., and Svedberg, A.: The Urinary Excretion and Biological Decay Periods of Radiomercury Labeling Mercurial Diuretic in Normal and Diseased Man. *J. Clin. Invest.* 29:1131, 1950.

Cafruny, E. J., Kormorn, R. M., and Hendrix, R. C.: Pharmacology at the Cellular Level: A Study of Renal Distribution of Mercury Compounds. *Univ. Mich. Bull.* 27:263, 1961.

Carr, E. A., Jr., Haynie, T. P., Stewart, B., Beierwaltes, W. H., and Nofal, M.: The Diagnostic Value of Scintillation Scanning of the Human Kidney (abstract). *Clin. Res.* 9:199, 1961a.

Carr, E. A., Jr., et al.: The Diagnostic Value of Scintillation Scanning of the Human Kidney. *Univ. Mich. Med. Bull.* 27:244, 1961b.

Concannon, J. P., Summers, R. E., Brewer, R., Cole, C., Weil, C., and Foster, W. D.: [125]I Allyl Inulin for Glomerular Filtration Rate. *Amer. J. Roentgen.* 92:302, 1964.

Cotlove, E.: C^{14} Carboxyl Labelled Inulin. *Fed. Proc.* 14:32, 1955.

Dennenberg, T., et al.: On the Distribution and Excretion of Some I^{131} Labelled Renal Contrast Media. *Acta Med. Scand.* 166:351, 1960.

Dollery, C. T.: Detection of Unilateral Renal Disease in Hypertension with Diodrast I^{131}. *Proc. Roy. Soc. Med.* 53:969, 1960.

Don, C.: Unilateral Manifestations of Bilateral Renal Artery Disease. *Canad. Med. Ass. J.* 85:188, 1961.

Dore, E. K., Taplin, G. U., and Johnson, D. E.: Current Interpretation of the Hippuran Renogram. *J.A.M.A.* 185:925, 1963.

Dos Santos, R., Lamas, C., and Caldas, P.: Recent Progress in the Technique of the Arteriography of the Abdominal Aorta. *Presse Med.* 39:574, 1931.

Felton, L. M.: Should Intravenous Pyelography Be a Routine Procedure for Children with Cryptorchidism or Hypospadias? *J. Urol.* 81:335, 1959.

Gold, D., Latts, E. M., and Wexler, H. M.: Congenital A-V Fistulae of Kidney: A Case Report and Review of the Literature. *Arch. Intern. Med.* 115:208, 1965.

Goodrich, J. K., Stone, H. L., and Harris, C. C.: Clinical Applications of Low Energy, High Transmission Collimator. *J. Nucl. Med.* 6:409, 1965.

Goodwin, D. A.: Renal Function Using Hippuran ^{131}I and Neohydrin [203]Hg. Unpublished data (M.S. thesis), 1963.

Greif, R. L., Sullivan, W. J., Jacobs, G. S., and Pitts, R. F.: Distribution of Radiomercury Administration as Labelled Chlormerodrin (Neohydrin) in the Kidneys of Rats and Dogs. *J. Clin. Invest.* 35:38, 1956.

Grossman, J., et al.: Urinary and Fecal Excretion of Mercury in Man Following Administration of Mercurial Diuretics. *J. Clin. Invest.* 30:1208, 1951.

Haynie, T. P., Nofal, M., Carr, E. A., Jr., and Beierwaltes, W. H.: Scintillation Scanning of the Kidney with Radioiodine-131 Contrast Media. *Clin. Res.* 8:288, 1960.

Haynie, T. P., Stewart, B. H., Nofal, M. M., Carr, E. A., Jr., and Beierwaltes, W. H.: Renal Scintiscans in the Diagnosis of Renal Vascular Disease. *J. Nucl. Med.* 2:272, 1961.

Hirakawa, A., et al.: Radioisotope Renogram as a Sensitive Test of Renal Function. *J. Lab. Clin. Med.* 58:825, 1961.

Howard, J. E., Berthrong, M., Gould, D. M., and Yendt, E. R.: Hypertension Resulting from Unilateral Vascular Disease and Its Relief by Nephrectomy. *Bull. Johns Hopkins Hosp.* 94: 51, 1954.

Kinter, W. B., and Pappenheimer, J. R.: Renal Extraction of PAH and Diodrast ^{131}I as a Function of Arterial Red Cell Concentration. *Amer. J. Physiol.* 185:391, 1956.

Lerner, M., and Anderson, O. W.: Health Progress in the United States 1900–1961. University of Chicago Press, Chicago, 1963.

Magnusson, G.: Kidney Function Studies with [131]I Tagged Sodium Ortho-Iodohippurate. *Acta Med. Scand.* 171 (Suppl. 378):1, 1962.

Maxwell, M. H., and Prozan, G. B.: Renovascular Hypertension. *Progr. Cardiov. Dis.* 5:81, 1962.

McAfee, J. G., and Wagner, H. N., Jr.: Visualization of Renal Parenchyma by Scintiscanning with Hg^{203} Neohydrin. *Radiology* 75:820, 1960.

McCort, J. J.: Radiologic Examination in Blunt Abdominal Trauma. *Radiol. Clin. N. Amer.* 2:121, 1964.

Meade, R. C., and Shy, C. M.: The Evaluation of Individual Kidney Function Using Radiohippurate Sodium. *J. Urol.* 86:163, 1961.

Meschan, I., Hosick, T., Schmid, H., and Watts, F. C.: Variability in Renal Clearance Rate Studies Using Fresh OI^{131} H.A., Purified Product and Stored Product. *J. Nucl. Med.* 4:70, 1963.

Moell, H.: Size of Normal Kidneys. *Acta Radiol.* 46:640, 1956.

Montandon, A., Wenger, P., and Roth, H. W.: Le nephrogramme isotopique à l'Hypaque marqué, avantages de l'Hypaque, importance de l'analyse semi-quantitative, valeur clinique. *Schweiz. Med. Wschr.* 92:35, 1962.

Morgan, J. M., et al.: Diagnosis of Renal Hypertension: Use of Renogram and Role of Kidney Biopsy. *Amer. J. Cardiol.* 9:760, 1962.

Moses, J. J., et al.: Evaluation of the Renogram in Hypertension. *J. Urol.* 85:679, 1961.

Nagle, W. C., and Allen, W. H.: Unilateral Multicystic Kidney Disease. *New York J. Med.* 65:681, 1965.

Nelp, W. B., Wagner, H. N., Jr., and Reba, R. C.: Renal Excretion of Vitamin B-12 and Its Use in Measurement of Glomerular Filtration Rate in Man. *J. Lab. Clin. Med.* 63:480, 1964.

Nordyke, R. A., Tubis, M., and Blahd, W. H.: Use of Radioactive Hippuran for Individual Kidney Function Tests. *J. Lab. Clin. Med.* 56:438, 1960.

O'Conor, V. J., Jr.: Role of the Ureter in Renal Transplantation. *J. Urol.* 86:51, 1961.

Oeser, H., and Billion, H.: Funktionelle Strahlendiagnostik durch etikettierte Röntgenkontrast-mittel. *Fortschr. Roentgenstr.* 76:431, 1952.

Pircher, F. J., Carr, E. A., and Patno, M. D.: Evaluation of Quantitative Aspects of the Radioisotope Renogram. *J. Nucl. Med.* 4:117, 1963a.

Pircher, F. J., Wegst, A. V., and Dodson, V. N.: In Vitro Analysis of the Radioisotope Renogram Test. *J. Nucl. Med.* 4:45, 1963b.

Porporis, A. A., et al.: The Mechanism of Urokon Excretion. *Amer. J. Roentgen.* 72:995, 1954.

Quinn, J. L., III, Meschan, I., Blake, D. D., and Witcofski, R. L.: The Usefulness of the Radioisotope Renogram in Radiation Therapy. *Radiology* 78:266, 1962.

Rapoport, A.: Modification of "Howard Test" for Detection of Renal-Artery Obstruction. *New England J. Med.* 263:1159, 1960.

Reba, R. C., McAfee, J. G., and Wagner, H. N., Jr.: Radiomercury-Labeled Chlormerodrin for In Vivo Uptake Studies and Scintillation Scanning of Unilateral Renal Lesions Associated with Hypertension. *Medicine* 42:269, 1963.

Reba, R. C., Wagner, H. N., Jr., and McAfee, J. G.: Measurement of ^{203}Hg Chlormerodrin Accumulation by the Kidneys for Detection of Unilateral Renal Disease. *Radiology* 79:134, 1962.

Schlegel, J. U., Savlov, E., and Gabor, F.: Studies in Renal Hypertension. *J. Urol.* 81:581, 1959.

Schlegel, J. U., Smith, B. G., and O'Dell, R. M.: Estimation of Effective Renal Plasma Flow Using ^{131}I-Labelled Hippuran. *J. Appl. Physiol.* 17:80, 1962.

Schwartz, F. D., and Madeloff, M. S.: Simultaneous Renal Clearances of Radio-Hippuran and PAH in Man. *Clin. Res.* 9:208, 1961.

Serrato, M., Grayback, T. V., and Earle, D. P.: Clinical Evaluation of Diodrast Renogram. *Arch. Intern. Med.* 103:851, 1959.

Simon, A.: Normal Renal Size: an Absolute Criterion. *Am. J. Roentgen.* 92:270, 1964.

Smith, H. W.: Hypertension and urologic disease. *Amer. J. Med.* 4:724, 1948.

Smith, H. W.: Unilateral Nephrectomy in Hypertensive Disease. *J. Urol.* 75:685, 1956.

Smith, H. W. et al.: Renal Clearances of Substituted Hippuric Acid Derivatives and Other Aromatic Acids in Dog and Man. *J. Clin. Invest.* 24:388, 1945.

Smith, P. G., Rush, T. W., and Evans, A. T.: An Evaluation of Translumbar Arteriography. *J. Urol.* 65:911, 1951.

Spencer, C. C., Callendine, G. W., and Vincent, D. J.: Reproducibility of Radioisotope Renogram. *J. Lab. Clin. Med.* 57:350, 1961.

Stamey, T. A.: Diagnosis of Curable Unilateral Renal Hypertension by Ureteral Catheterization. *Postgrad. Med.* 29:496, 1961.

Stewart, B. H., and Haynie, T. P.: Critical Appraisal of the Renogram in Renal Vascular Disease. *J.A.M.A.* 180:454, 1962.

Stokes, J. M., Conklin, J. W., and Huntley, H. C.: Measurement of Glomerular Filtration Rate by Contrast Media Containing I^{131} Isotopes. *J. Urol.* 87:630, 1962.

Strauss, M. B., and Welt, L. G. (eds.): Diseases of the Kidney. Little, Brown & Co., Boston, 1963.

Taplin, G. V., Dore, E. K., and Johnson, D. E.: The Quantitative Radiorenogram for Total and Differential Renal Blood Flow Measurements. *J. Nucl. Med.* 4:404, 1963.

Taplin, G. V., et al.: Radioisotope Renogram: External Test for Individual Function and Upper Urinary Tract Patency. *J. Lab. & Clin. Med.* 48:886, 1956.

Tauxe, W. N.: Renogram in Renal Artery Disease. *Proc. Mayo Clin.* 36:684, 1961.

Tauxe, W. N., Burbank, M. K., Maher, F. T., and Hunt, J. C.: Renal Clearances of ^{131}I-Hippuran and ^{131}I-Diatrizoate. *Proc. Mayo Clin.* 39:761, 1964.

Tauxe, W. N., Hunt, J. C., and Burbank, M. K.: The Radioisotope Renogram (Ortho-Iodohippurate ^{131}I). Standardization of Technique and Expression of Data. *Amer. J. Clin. Path.* 37:567, 1962.

Threefoot, S. A., et al.: Concentration Time Course (Plasma) of Man of ^{203}Hg-Neohydrin. *J. Clin. Invest.* 28:661, 1949.

Tubis, M., Posnick, E., and Nordyke, R. A.: Preparation and Use of [131]I Labelled Hippuran in Kidney Function Tests. *Proc. Soc. Exp. Biol. Med.* 103:497, 1960.

Weston, R. E., et al.: Renal Excretion of Mercury in Man Following Intravenously Administered Mercurial Diuretics. *J. Clin. Invest.* 30:1221, 1951.

Westphal, R. D., et al.: Delineation of Human Kidneys by Scintillation Scanning. *Amer. J. Roentgen.* 87:161, 1962.

Whitely, J. E., Witcofski, R. L., and Meschan, I.: Experimental Comparison of Hippuran and Diodrast in Renal Function Evaluation. *Radiology* 76:464, 1961.

Winter, C. C.: A Clinical Study of a New Renal Function Test. *J. Urol.* 76:182, 1956.

Winter, C. C.: Diagnosis of "Renal" Hypertension and Prediction of Surgical Outcome. Application of Supplementary Renal Tests to Confirm a Positive Screening Survey. *J.A.M.A.*, 178: 1108, 1961a.

Winter, C. C.: Advances in the Radioisotope Renogram Test. *J. Urol.* 85:631, 1961b.

Winter, C. C.: and Taplin, G. V.: A Clinical Comparison and Analysis of Radioactive Diodrast, Hypaque, Miokon and Urokon Renograms as Tests of Kidney Function. *J. Urol.* 70:573, 1958.

Winter, C. C., et al.: Results of Radioisotope Renogram and Comparison with Other Kidney Function Tests in Hypertension. *J. Urol.* 82:674, 1959.

Woodruff, M. W., and Malvin, R. L.: Localization of Renal Contrast Media Excretion by Stop-Flow. *J. Urol.* 84:677, 1960.

Yasky, J., and Volpe, R.: An Assessment of the "Radioactive Renogram" Using O-Iodohippurate Sodium (Hippuran) Labelled with Radioactive Iodine. *Canad. Med. Ass. J.* 88:1055, 1963.

CHAPTER XIV

THE NERVOUS SYSTEM

HENRY N. WAGNER, Jr.

RICHARD A. HOLMES

Detection and proper interpretation of signs and symptoms of altered function provide the basic approach to localizing and characterizing disorders of the nervous system. Often, however, the diagnosis cannot be established with certainty by clinical means alone, and ancillary techniques are required. It is not enough just to detect intracranial mass lesions; we would like to be able to characterize the size, shape, location, and, if possible, the nature of the abnormality. It is easy to recognize certain symptoms of intracranial tumor, such as headache, vomiting, and failing vision—produced by increasing intracranial pressure—but, if possible, a diagnosis should be established before these advanced symptoms develop. Whenever there is an alteration of nervous system function, a focal mass lesion such as a tumor should be suspected and further studies carried out to confirm or exclude the diagnosis. The earlier the diagnosis, the better the chances of successful treatment.

As in other areas of medicine, increasing emphasis on diagnostic skill has followed demonstrated success in treatment. Contrary to the widespread belief in the hopeless prognosis associated with brain tumors, analysis of the results of two large series comprising 1603 and 1814 cases indicated that following operation approximately one third of the patients were able to carry out prolonged and useful activity (Grant, 1953; Horrax, 1954). Presumably even better results would have been obtained had earlier diagnosis been made, since in many patients there was a delay of more than a year in establishing the definitive diagnosis (Redlich et al., 1948). Often the patients were thought to have psychosomatic disorders or functional psychoses.

McLaurin and Helmer (1962) analyzed some of the frequent causes of errors in the diagnosis of intracranial tumors. A major problem was confusion of tumors with vascular disease in the older age group, attributable to the unusual manifestations of intracranial tumors in the elderly. Many doctors assume that a cerebrovascular accident can usually be differentiated from intracranial tumors by the abrupt onset of symptoms followed by a stationary or gradually improving neurological picture. Yet symptoms may appear with great suddenness in tumors. Moersch et al. (1941) analyzed the symptoms of tumors in a review of 100 patients over 60 years of age and noted the relative infrequency of headache and papilledema. Mental symptoms (dullness, confusion, stupor) constituted the most common presenting features. Glioblastomas were the most difficult to diagnose because their more rapid course simulated vascular disease. In 11 of 35 patients with proved glioblastomas, a diagnosis of vascular disease was seriously considered.

When any person, regardless of age, develops a sudden hemiparesis or a deteriorating neurological state, a clinical diagnosis of stroke should be made only with some reservation. If seizures have occurred, the diagnosis of vascular accident becomes more tenuous, since approximately 12 per cent of the patients with cerebrovascular accidents have seizures, whereas the incidence approaches 50 per cent in patients with tumors. Hoefer et al. (1946) state that approximately 41 per cent of patients with meningiomas, 31 per cent with glioblastomas, and 55 per cent with astrocytomas manifest seizures.

The importance and difficulty of detecting and localizing intracranial tumors by clinical means alone have led to the application of numerous ancillary procedures. Pneumoencephalography, ventriculography, and arteriography are often of great value, but because of their complexity cannot fill the important need for a screening procedure. Electroencephalography, although important in the study of epilepsy, has been somewhat disappointing in the detection of brain tumors, its localizing value being limited almost entirely to supratentorial lesions. The introduction of techniques using radionuclides has been of great help, particularly since they can be used in outpatients without the need for hospitalization and without discomfort or danger to the patient.

DiChiro (1961) has emphasized that the neuroradiological evidence of an intracranial mass lesion (bone erosion and displacement of the ventricular system or blood vessels) is mainly indirect. The only direct evidence is the occasional occurrence of abnormal calcifications or increased vascularity of tumors or vascular malformations. Of course, it is useful for the surgeon to know how contiguous structures, especially vessels, are displaced. Consequently the information of pneumography and cerebral angiography is of great value. But both procedures have a low but definite incidence of morbidity and mortality. Brain scanning has provided a simple, safe, and accurate method that often makes possible *direct* demonstration of the intracranial lesion.

Radioisotope techniques have not been used often enough in cerebrovascular disease or in cerebral trauma to permit a clear-cut understanding of their eventual role in these disorders. But because of their safety and simplicity, they may be useful when arteriography is too risky. Radioisotope techniques have also been used in the detection and localization of cerebrospinal fluid fistulae and in the evaluation of the patency of shunts used to treat hydrocephalus. Table 14-1 summarizes the proved and potential uses of radioisotope techniques in the management of patients with diseases of the central nervous system.

TABLE 14-1. PROVED AND POTENTIAL USEFULNESS OF RADIOISOTOPE TECHNIQUES
IN DISEASES OF THE CENTRAL NERVOUS SYSTEM

1. Screening and characterization of primary brain tumors.
2. Detection of cerebral metastases.
3. Evaluation of therapy, i.e., surgery, radiation, and chemotherapy.
4. Evaluation of cerebrovascular disease, i.e., extent and location of encephalomalacia; cerebral blood flow.
5. Differentiation of diffuse and focal inflammatory diseases, i.e., distinguishing between meningoencephalitis and brain abscess or subdural empyema.
6. Evaluation of cranial trauma, i.e., differentiating epidural, subdural, or intracerebral hemorrhage and contusion from simple concussion; detection of subdural hematoma; diagnosis of cerebrospinal fluid fistulae.
7. Evaluation of shunts in the treatment of hydrocephalus.

HISTORICAL OUTLINE

Neurosurgery developed rapidly following Dandy's discovery that mass lesions within the cranium can be localized by outlining the ventricles with air. The next great advance was arteriography. Yet even with both techniques, it was not possible to solve all diagnostic problems, and simple detection of lesions was often not enough, since it was important to know the position and size of the tumor. Because of the uncertainty and dangers in blindly probing with a needle in the region where a tumor was suspected, Moore and his colleagues (1947) injected the dye fluorescein, which concentrated in the tumor and made possible its visualization at operation. Later the radioactive analog, iodine-131 diiodofluorescein, was used.

Neither fluorescein nor other dyes were completely satisfactory. Iodine-containing fluorescein derivatives were introduced with the hope that their opacity to x-rays would make them readily detectable. This approach failed because it was impossible to achieve sufficiently high chemical concentrations in the tumors. Radioisotope techniques do not have this inherent problem of contrast radiography. An important difference between contrast radiography and radioisotope techniques is that the latter do not depend on achieving a high *absolute* concentration of the labeled substance. Because of the extreme sensitivity of the instruments used to measure radioactivity, the concentration of the radioactivity in the tumor *relative* to its surroundings, rather than the absolute concentration, is the important criterion.

Sodium diiodofluorescein (DIF) labeled with ^{131}I provided the initial breakthrough in the localization of brain tumors by radioisotope methods. Between 1947 and 1951, Moore studied a series of 500 patients, initially with Geiger-Müller detectors and subsequently with scintillation detectors. Moore's studies, supplemented by those of Ashkenazy and others (1951), indicated the feasibility and potential value of the methods, although technical problems remained. Progress over the subsequent years has been the result of improved radiopharmaceuticals and better detection instruments.

In 1949, Selverstone and his associates used a Geiger-Müller detector and later a proportional counter to probe the depths of the brain to locate increased concentrations of radioactive phosphorus (^{32}P) in brain tumors. The principal disadvantage of ^{32}P was that localization was not possible except at the time of operation, because the beta radiation could not be detected through the skull. Another problem was that the tiny needle-shaped detector was insensitive and necessitated large doses of ^{32}P, much of which concentrated in the bone marrow, testes, and other tissues.

Radioactive potassium (^{42}K) was also used by Selverstone, and had the important advantage of being measurable with an extracranial detector. However, because of its short half-life (12 hours), it was not readily available at that time, and its high-energy gamma rays (1.5 and 0.64 Mev.) were difficult to localize with accuracy.

Radioiodinated human serum albumin was first used for brain scanning in 1953 by Moore and his colleagues, who concluded that it was then the best available material. Other substances have been used subsequently. For example, Mundinger (1961) recommended bismuth-206, administered either as the nitrate or the lecithin-camphor-carbonate, and Blau and Bender (1959) introduced mercury-203-labeled chlormerodrin. In 1964, Harper and his associates introduced technetium-99m pertechnetate. Other radionuclides such as chelates of indium-113m are currently under development.

Improvements have also been made in the detection instruments. Geiger-Müller detectors were gradually replaced by crystal scintillation counters introduced by Cassen and his co-workers in 1950. Early workers had used heavily shielded detectors that were manually moved from point to point over the skull, but these were eventually replaced by motor-driven detectors. Sweet et al. (1959) used paired radiation detectors and positron-emitting radionuclides. Positron scanning is but one example of a detection system for brain scanning. The development of improved collimators, such as the multihole focusing collimator, was another important advance, improving the sensitivity of the instruments without undue loss of resolution. Collimators gave directional sense to the detectors by enclosing the crystals in shielding materials with multichannel openings directed toward the area immediately beneath the detector. Improvements were also made in the methods of recording data and of presenting an image of the distribution of radioactivity. Various means, such as the use of photographic film, were devised to display the distribution of the radioactivity in easily interpreted patterns. Another recent development is the scintillation camera, which obviates the need to move the detector mechanically from point to point, and yet retains the ability to produce an image of the distribution of radioactivity in the body.

THE DIAGNOSTIC PROBLEM

In the case of mass lesions, the diagnostic problem consists of three parts: *detection* of the presence of the lesion, *characterization* of its size, shape, and position, and finally, *identification* of its nature. At times, a lesion can be detected and localized by specific alterations in the function of the nervous system. For example, the diagnosis of an acoustic neurinoma is based largely on a characteristic progression of symptoms resulting from a lesion at the cerebellopontine angle. There is progressive involvement of the eighth, fifth, seventh, ninth, and tenth nerves, together with symptoms of involvement of the cerebellum on the same side. We would like to make the diagnosis when only the eighth nerve is involved, producing unilateral tinnitus, deafness, and vertigo. But usually the diagnosis is not established until trigeminal paresthesias, facial spasm, suboccipital discomfort, unsteadiness of gait, or other symptoms point to an expanding lesion.

Localization on the basis of altered function of the nervous system is often impossible for two reasons. First, we still have an imperfect understanding of the localization of function, particularly in the cerebral hemispheres. Second, localizing signs may be produced by involvement of structures remote from the original lesion. For example, a frequently encountered sign that may lead to false localization is a sixth nerve palsy. An expanding hemispheral lesion can compress the third nerve and cerebral peduncles against the edge of the ten-

TABLE 14-2. RADIOGRAPHIC EVIDENCE OF INTRACRANIAL MASS LESIONS*

I. *Routine skull x-rays* (AP, PA, lateral views or stereo laterals)
  1. Increased intracranial pressure
    a. Increase in the size of the skull and widening of the sutures in those under 16 years of age.
    b. Increase in convolutional markings (not diagnostic as an isolated finding). This is a normal finding in some children and has a tendency to disappear after 12 years.
    c. Atrophy or erosion of the cranial bones
        Localized—bones of the base, particularly the sella turcica; earliest change in the posterior clinoids
        Diffuse—involving the vault most commonly in children

        Atrophy of the sella turcica, particularly the posterior clinoid, is the most important evidence of increased intracranial pressure after the age of 12 years
  2. Displacement of normal intracranial calcifications, particularly the pineal, falx cerebri or choroid plexus
  3. Presence of abnormal intracranial calcifications, particularly meningioma, oligodendroglioma, astrocytoma, or craniopharyngioma
  4. Presence of abnormal vascular channels, particularly in meningioma and angiomatous malformations
  5. Local changes in bone
    a. Erosion—meningioma, astrocytoma, subdural hematoma, chordoma, osteochondroma, acoustic neurinoma, and pituitary adenoma
    b. Hyperostosis—meningioma
II. *Special views of specific areas*
  1. Base—changes in bone density, particularly nasopharyngeal carcinoma, meningioma, and fractures
  2. Internal auditory meatus—acoustic neurinoma
  3. Optic foramen—gliomas of optic nerve
  4. Sella—tumors of the sella and parasellar regions
  5. Odontoid process and atlanto-occipital junction—platybasia, congenital anomalies
  6. Sinuses
  7. Mastoid and temporal bone

    Tomograms of these areas and other regions are employed for more detailed examination and are particularly helpful in demonstrating obscure fractures of the odontoid process and the temporal bone as well as discrete erosions produced by tumor and inflammatory disease.
III. *Contrast studies*
  1. Air encephalography—pneumoencephalography, ventriculography
  2. Opaque media—angiography, ventriculography

*From Teasdale, R.: Personal communication.

TABLE 14-3. INTRACRANIAL TUMORS*

TYPE	ORIGIN	INCI-DENCE	LOCATION	COMMENT
I. Glioma	Glia	45%		Prognosis is poor for all types
Astrocytoma			Cerebrum Cerebellum	Slowly growing tumor of adults and children
Glioblastoma			Cerebrum	Rapidly growing; adults
Medulloblastoma			Cerebellum	Rapidly growing; children
Oligodendroglioma			Cerebrum	Rare; slowly growing; adults; prone to calcify
Ependymoma			Intraventricular	Very rare; slowly growing
II. Meningioma	Arachnoid villi	20%	Meningeal Parasagittal Suprasellar Olfactory	Good prognosis; slowly growing; prone to calcify; hyperostosis of overlying skull; rare under age 20
III. Pituitary adenoma	Adenohypophysis	10%	Intra-, para-, suprasellar	Slowly growing; rare before the age of 20
IV. Metastatic	Lung, breast and kidney	10%	Cerebrum and cerebellum	Poor prognosis; often multiple tumors; late adult life
V. Others Angiomas	Blood vessels	15%	Cerebrum, cerebellum, and meninges	Prone to calcify
Pinealomas	Glia		Pineal	Rare; slowly growing; 3:1 males; precocious puberty
Cranial nerve tumors; acoustic neurinoma	Schwann		VIII nerve	Defects of hearing and equilibrium
Papilloma of choroid plexus	Choroid		Intraventricular	Slowly growing; only in childhood
Chordoma	Notochord		Clivus	Compression adjacent brain tissue; erosion of base of skull

* Modified from Teasdale, R.: Personal communication; Zülch, 1965.

torium. Internal hydrocephalus may disturb frontal lobe function, yielding extensor plantar responses and bilateral grasp reflexes. The hypothalamus and pituitary may be compressed by distention of the third ventricle to produce symptoms of hypopituitarism. Cerebellar ataxia may be found in patients with frontal lobe tumors and signs of midbrain damage may result from a cerebellar tumor.

After the initial clinical evaluation, it is customary to obtain skull x-rays, electroencephalography, and brain scans, since these procedures are innocuous. Table 14-2 summarizes the radiographic evidence of intracranial mass lesions. Certain features warrant emphasis. Displacement of the pineal gland is detectable in about 10 per cent of patients with mass lesions. Calcification occurs in approximately 10 per cent of patients with glioma; about 50 per cent of the patients with meningioma have alterations of the skull that are visible on routine radiographs. In general, carotid angiography should be employed in patients suspected of having supratentorial lesions, whereas ventriculography is indicated in patients suspected of lesions in the posterior fossa. Frequently both examinations are necessary.

A particularly troublesome diagnostic problem is presented by the patient with benign intracranial hypertension, also known as *pseudotumor cerebri,* a condition almost entirely limited to obese, middle-aged females. Papilledema, headache, and drowsiness are prominent features of this condition, the cause of which is unknown. Usually no localizing neurological signs are observed, although occasionally third and sixth nerve palsies may occur.

At times, focal disturbances of the brain, such as seizures, motor and sensory disturbances, and visual field defects may be found in patients who have cerebral arteriosclerosis. In these patients, it is important to rule out an intracranial mass lesion, such as a tumor, abscess, or hematoma. Both focal and generalized convulsions can occur with mass lesions, particularly meningiomas. Table 14-3 outlines some of the major points that are useful in predicting the nature of intracranial tumors. The table also lists the approximate incidence of these

TABLE 14-4. NON-NEOPLASTIC MASS LESIONS

I. Inflammatory
   Abscess
      Direct extension
         Mastoid
         Nasal sinuses
         Osteomyelitis
         Fracture of skull
      Metastatic infection
         Lung—bronchiectasis
            abscess
         Heart—bacterial endocarditis
            congenital heart disease
   Granuloma
      Tuberculosis
      Syphilis
      Fungi (torula)
      Sarcoidosis
      Parasitic (cysticercosis)
II. Hematoma
   Spontaneous
      Intrinsic—cerebral hemorrhage
      Extrinsic—berry aneurysm
         angioma
   Traumatic
      Epidural
      Subdural
      Intracerebral
      Contusion

lesions in the general population. Table 14-4 lists non-neoplastic mass lesions that must be considered in the differential diagnosis.

RADIOPHARMACEUTICALS

The two fundamental properties of radioactive tracers used for brain scanning are: (1) their ability to be precisely measured when present in exceedingly small concentrations, and (2) their emission of gamma rays that can penetrate the skull and make possible the accurate spatial localization of the radioactivity by means of external radiation detectors. The first step in brain scanning is to inject a radioactive tracer that is distributed in a manner that results in a difference in concentration of radioactivity in the lesion (the target area) and its surroundings (the nontarget area). Radiopharmaceuticals used for brain scanning today are characterized by the fact that *normal* brain tissue is either relatively or completely impermeable to their passage from the blood. In contrast, brain tumors and most other mass lesions of the brain are much more permeable than normal brain, the degree of permeability varying with the type of lesion and the radiopharmaceutical. The difference in permeability of the tumor and normal brain tissue results in a significantly higher concentration of radioactivity in the tumor relative to normal brain. In general, meningiomas, metastatic tumors, and rapidly growing glioblastomas are the most permeable. Of the substances that have been tested in experimental tumors, [206]Bi nitrate achieves the highest tumor-to-brain ratios but its high-energy gamma photons cannot be precisely localized by scanning devices. The next highest ratio is achieved by iodinated albumin; both [203]Hg chlormerodrin and ^{99m}Tc pertechnetate achieve lesser tumor-to-brain ratios than albumin or albumin-bound substances (Long et al., 1963; Matthews and Mallard, 1965; Tator et al., 1965).

It is important to select the optimum time after administration of the radiopharmaceutical to achieve the greatest precision in measuring the activity in the tumor relative to the normal brain. This varies from one radiopharmaceutical to another. One determines this optimum time in the case of a particular agent on the basis of studies in animals with experimental tumors, determinations of radioisotope concentrations in specimens of tumor removed from patients at operation, and evaluation of clinical results. Unfortunately, we do not yet have a radiopharmaceutical that concentrates in brain tumors to a high degree, in a manner analogous to the accumulation of radioiodine by the thyroid gland.

It has been known for decades that the electronegative colloidal dye Evans blue does not enter normal brain tissue but diffuses quite readily into experimental tumors. The dye fluorescein behaves in a similar fashion. Unfortunately, most dyes are actively retained in the phagocytic cells of the reticuloendothelial system. To retain the property of tumor permeability without the complication of persistent staining of the skin by the dyes, Moore substituted albumin labeled with radioactive iodine (1953).

[131]I ALBUMIN

When properly labeled, radioactive albumin retains the biological behavior of normal serum albumin. Following intravenous injection, it diffuses slowly into brain tumors, but not into normal brain. The blood level remains high since labeled albumin is not excreted and is catabolized at a relatively slow rate. The persistence of a high blood level of radioactivity enhances the diffusion of albumin into the tumor.

Radioiodinated (^{131}I) human serum albumin was at one time the most widely used substance for brain scanning despite its many undesirable features. Iodine-131 emits two high-energy gamma rays (640 kev., 9 per cent; 720 kev., 3 per cent) in addition to its principal energy of 360 kev. (87 per cent). As it passes through tissues, gamma-ray energy is reduced; some of the high-energy radiations from nontarget areas impinge on the crystal with a reduced energy that may fall in the primary energy range (i.e., 320 to 390 kev.) being measured. This decreases contrast and impairs spatial resolution.

Another disadvantage of iodinated albumin is that it remains in the body for several weeks, thereby continuing to irradiate the patient even after the scan is completed. The high initial concentration of labeled albumin in the vasculature of the skull and brain makes it desirable to delay the scanning procedure for as long as 24 hours to allow the blood level to fall as the albumin diffuses into the extracellular fluid.

^{203}Hg CHLORMERODRIN AND ^{99m}Tc PERTECHNETATE

Because of these problems, other substances, such as ^{203}Hg chlormerodrin and ^{99m}Tc pertechnetate, have been used. With these agents, the blood level falls rapidly as they are excreted by the kidneys. This decreases the concentration in the nontarget areas of the skull, but also decreases the diffusion of radioactivity into the tumor. Radioactive mercury (^{203}Hg) has more desirable physical characteristics than radioiodine (^{131}I) since the former emits only a single gamma ray with a relatively low energy (280 kev.). Unfortunately, prolonged retention of a part of the dose of radioactive mercury in the kidneys is an important undesirable feature; thus, many persons using chlormerodrin for brain scanning prefer the ^{197}Hg label, because it has a half-life of 65 hours and no beta radiation (Sodee, 1963).

CLASSIFICATION OF BRAIN SCANNING AGENTS

Substances such as ^{131}I albumin, ^{203}Hg chlormerodrin, and copper-64 comprise a group that may be referred to as *protein-bound substances*. A second group, referred to as *intracellular substances,* includes potassium-42, phosphate-32, rubidium-84, bismuth-206, arsenic-74, and manganese-52; these are characterized by a more rapid rate of diffusion into brain tumor than into normal brain (Matthews and Molinaro, 1963). A third group consists of the *ionic extracellular substances,* technetium-99m pertechnetate, gallium-68, bromine-82, zirconium-95, antimony-112, iodide-131, and niobium-95. These substances equilibrate with the extracellular fluid space of the tumor. With the latter two groups of substances (except for ^{206}Bi), maximum tumor-to-brain ratios are usually of the order of 10 to 20:1.

The classification into *protein-bound, intracellular,* and *ionic extracellular* radiopharmaceuticals for brain scanning is based on the biological properties of the materials; a second classification depends on the physical properties of the radioactive nucleus, i.e., upon whether the radionuclide emits positrons or gamma

TABLE 14-5. CALCULATED RADIATION DOSE FOR VARIOUS BRAIN SCANNING AGENTS

AGENT	INTRAVENOUS DOSE	RADIATION DOSE	
		Total Body	Critical Organ
[131]I albumin	375 μc.	0.04 rad	2 rads (blood)
[203]Hg chlormerodrin	750 μc.	0.18 rad	165 rads (kidney)
[197]Hg chlormerodrin	750 μc.	0.08 rad	13 rads (kidney)
[99m]Tc pertechnetate	15 mc.	0.18 rad	1–3 rads (large bowel)

radiation. This distinction is important since the means of localization of the two types of radiations differ. Spatial resolution of gamma radiation is achieved by means of heavy shielding materials, such as lead, with specially designed collimators and gamma spectrometers. The latter limit the response of the detector to a narrow band of gamma-ray energies and help eliminate the problem of scattered radiations from nontarget areas. Radiopharmaceuticals that emit positrons simplify the problem of precise spatial localization. Positron emissions interact with electrons and are transformed into paired gamma rays, which emerge at precisely 180° to each other with identical 0.51 Mev. energies. Paired scintillation counters can be faced toward each other on each side of the head and made to respond only when both are activated *simultaneously*, or in *coincidence*. Since gamma rays that impinge on a single crystal are not counted, only the area exactly between the two opposing crystal faces can yield coincident gamma rays; therefore spatial resolution can be obtained without heavy lead shielding or gamma spectrometry.

At the present time, many hospitals in the United States routinely use ^{99m}Tc pertechnetate for brain scanning; others use [203]Hg or [197]Hg chlormerodrin. It is widely accepted that ^{99m}Tc pertechnetate is superior to ^{131}I albumin because of the increased number of photons emanating from the area under study. Albumin and pertechnetate are similar in that the blood level of radioactivity is relatively high at the time the scanning procedure is performed. Consequently, the vascular structures of the face, scalp, and superior longitudinal sinus, the temporal muscles, the lateral dural sinuses, and the superficial cerebral veins close to the vertex appear as areas of relatively high concentrations of radioactivity. With ^{99m}Tc pertechnetate, however, contrast and resolution of these structures is sufficiently good that these areas are not likely to cause confusion in interpretation.

A nuclide such as ^{99m}Tc, which decays by isomeric transition without emitting a beta particle, can be safely given in millicurie doses. An additional advantage of ^{99m}Tc, and to a lesser degree of [197]Hg chlormerodrin, is the short physical half-life (6 hours for ^{99m}Tc, 3 days for [197]Hg). Table 14-5 lists the calculated radiation dosage for commonly used brain scanning agents.

INSTRUMENTATION

When the relative concentration in the target and nontarget areas is optimum, the next problem is to detect, characterize, and, if possible, identify the nature of any area in which the concentration of radioactivity is abnormally

TABLE 14-6. TYPES OF INSTRUMENTS USED FOR BRAIN SCANNING

1. Single- or dual-crystal, moving detector scanners
2. Dual-crystal, moving detector positron scanners
3. Multiple stationary detectors ("gamma encephalography")
4. Stationary scintillation camera (Anger-Nuclear Chicago)
5. Stationary positron scintillation camera (Anger-Nuclear Chicago)
6. Image intensification camera (Ter-Pogossian, Picker)
7. Multiple-crystal stationary "rank-and-file" array (Bender-Blau, Baird-Atomic)

high. The data must be accurately recorded and displayed in a manner that is readily interpretable. The procedure must not be so time-consuming or expensive that it cannot be applied to the examination of large numbers of patients.

If the radiopharmaceutical were concentrated only in the brain tumor and not in the surrounding normal brain, skull, scalp, and face, we could utilize a detector that would view the entire head and determine whether the concentration of radioactivity was higher than normal. Unfortunately, the concentration of radioactivity in normal brain, although less than in tumors, is not negligible. Therefore with radiopharmaceuticals currently available, the increase in *total* radioactivity in the head as a result of the lesion is not sufficiently great to be detectable. Therefore we must use a highly collimated, i.e., directional, detector that will indicate the increased concentration of radioactivity when it is directed toward the tumor. The increased concentration in the tumor must be differentiated from the surrounding normal brain in order to be detected. Collimation is accomplished by means of shielding that absorbs radiation from all directions except those coming directly from beneath the detector. Since one usually does not know in advance where the lesion may be, the detector has to be moved systematically over the entire skull. When the detector is moved in a single line across the skull, a "profile" of the concentration of the radioactivity across the line is obtained. A series of such parallel lines is obtained until the whole skull is covered and an image of the distribution of radioactivity is obtained.

The instrument most commonly used is a radioisotope scanner, made up of the following components: a *radiation detector* consisting of a highly directional scintillation crystal varying in size from 3 to 8 inches; a *data processing system,* consisting of an amplifier, a pulse-height selector and a counting device, often with the capability of transforming the data in a preselected fashion; and a *data display system,* consisting of a mechanical solenoid tapper that forms a dot pattern on paper, a light source that activates photographic film, or a cathode-ray tube, or a television screen, or a digital recorder.

Newer devices (scintillation cameras) do not scan, but consist of a large single stationary detector or a battery of multiple small detectors. These are described in Chapter V. Table 14-6 lists the instruments that have been most often used for brain scanning.

THE NORMAL BRAIN SCAN

The appearance of the brain scan from normal persons depends on the radiopharmaceutical used and the spatial resolution obtained by the detection

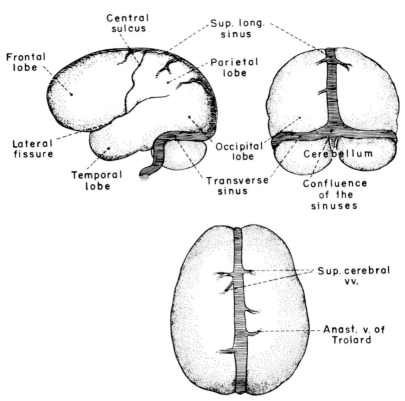

FIGURE 14-1. Normal anatomy of structures seen on the brain scan.

instrument. We shall describe the normal appearance of the various views usually obtained in brain scanning when ^{99m}Tc pertechnetate is used.

Figure 14-1 illustrates the frequently observed anatomical landmarks of the calvaria and its contents. The most prominent features are the large venous sinuses, which contain three fourths of the total blood volume of the brain.

Anterior View (Fig. 14-2). High concentrations of activity are seen in the mouth, the pharynx, and the mucous membranes of the nasal turbinates. The cerebral hemispheres appear as areas of decreased radioactivity. Just above the nasion in the midline, we often see an area of increased activity that represents the cavernous sinus. The frontal sinus may occasionally be seen as an area of increased activity above the nasion. The anterior scan must extend downward below the level of the superior orbital ridges to include the inferior portion of the temporal fossa. At the top of the anterior view is an area of increased activity, which is the superior longitudinal sinus viewed tangentially. The superficial cerebral veins may produce a slight asymmetry on either side of the superior longitudinal sinus.

Lateral View (Fig. 14-3). A band of radioactivity becoming progressively wider as it extends posteriorly can be seen surrounding the cerebral hemispheres. This activity is due to the scalp vasculature, the underlying calvaria, and the superior longitudinal sinus, which becomes progressively larger toward the back of the skull. Just below the vertex a small area of activity is frequently seen at the entrance of the large cerebral veins, called the anastomotic veins of

Trolard, into the superior longitudinal sinus. An area of increased activity is also seen below the line joining the nasion and the external auditory meatus. This is due to the vascularity of the muscles of mastication, the orbit, the face, the lacrimal glands, and the mucous membranes of the nasal cavities and sinuses. Near the middle of the nasiomeatal line an area of lesser activity is frequently observed in the region of the pituitary sulcus. The parotid glands contain high concentrations of pertechnetate. The lateral dural sinus is seen as a band of activity connecting the external auditory meatus with the inion. It usually bows upward and is occasionally asymmetrical from one side to the other. Below the lateral sinus is an area of decreased activity representing the posterior fossa. The small area of activity in the middle of the cerebral hemisphere is the choroid plexus, which will be discussed in the section on Normal Variants.

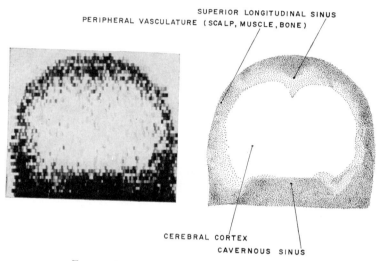

FIGURE 14-2.   Normal brain scan, anterior view.

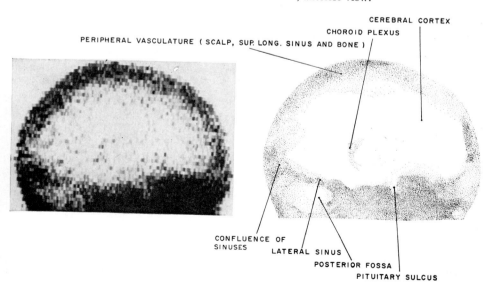

FIGURE 14-3.   Normal brain scan, lateral view.

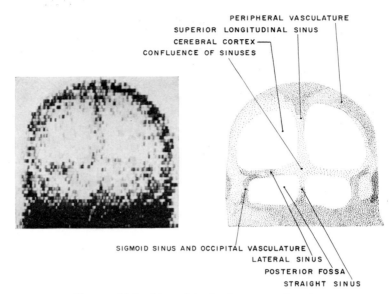

PERIPHERAL VASCULATURE
SUPERIOR LONGITUDINAL SINUS
CEREBRAL CORTEX
CONFLUENCE OF SINUSES

SIGMOID SINUS AND OCCIPITAL VASCULATURE
LATERAL SINUS
POSTERIOR FOSSA
STRAIGHT SINUS

FIGURE 14-4. Normal brain scan, posterior view.

Posterior View (Fig. 14-4). The superior longitudinal sinus is seen as a vertical band of activity that extends from the vertex to below the inion. The lateral dural sinuses are seen as horizontal bands of increased activity that extend from the base of the superior longitudinal sinus to the sides of the skull.

Below the confluence of the superior longitudinal sinus and the lateral sinuses, the straight sinus can sometimes be seen. It occupies the junction of the falx cerebri and the tentorium cerebelli. As it branches at the internal occipital protuberance, the right branch joins the superior longitudinal sinus; the left branch continues as the left lateral sinus. The lateral sinuses run along the posterior border of the tentorium until they reach the petrous pyramids and then curve downward to pass out through the jugular foramen as the internal jugular veins.

Vertex View (Fig. 14-5). In this view, the longitudinal sinus is seen as a band of activity extending down the center of the skull with a somewhat irregular contour caused by insertion of the superior cerebral veins. As it extends backward it progressively enlarges until finally it becomes a large venous lake, the confluence of sinuses (torcula). The longitudinal sinus frequently joins the right branch of the lateral sinus with a smaller channel draining into the left transverse sinus.

Occasionally an indistinct X shaped pattern of activity is seen extending out from the middle of the vertex view into the areas of the sphenoid wings and the petrous ridges. Located at the base of the brain in this area are the cavernous and petrosal sinuses. The cavernous sinus is a broad venous cavity surrounding the sella turcica and draining via the inferior and superior petrosal sinus into the lateral sinuses. Anatomically the choroid plexuses of the lateral ventricles are located in these areas but are rarely seen on the scan.

When the patient is scanned after the administration of pertechnetate, usually two large areas of activity can be seen in the temporal regions, corresponding to the parotid glands. In the frontal area as well, there are areas of

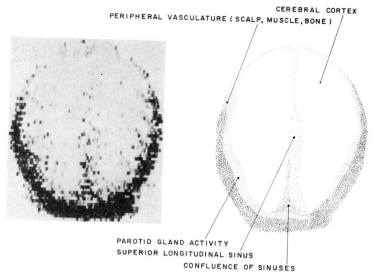

FIGURE 14-5. Normal brain scan, vertex view.

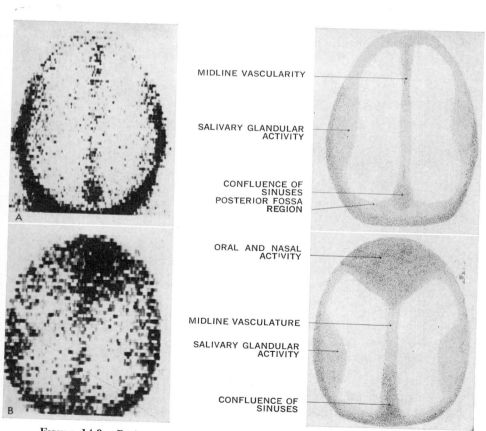

FIGURE 14-6. Brain scan, vertex view. *A,* With atropine. *B,* Without atropine.

increased activity as the result of salivary gland and nasal and oral mucosal secretions. Since these areas interfere with the detection of lesions, 1 mg. of atropine per 70 kg. is administered prior to scanning in order to minimize these areas. The appearance of the vertex view with and without prior administration of atropine is shown in Figure 14-6.

NORMAL VARIANTS

Use of ^{99m}Tc pertechnetate makes possible improved resolution of vascular structures, which must be recognized in order to be distinguished from lesions. Certain areas are particularly troublesome. One example is an area just in front of the pituitary sulcus, where occasionally a narrow vertical lip of increased activity can be seen (Fig. 14-7). This is the region of the middle meningeal veins which drain the pachymeninges. It should not be mistaken for a suprasellar lesion. The anterior view helps the interpretation of this area. This error in interpretation is likely to be made when this region of activity is seen on only one of the two lateral views, which occasionally occurs.

Another difficult area is the region of the coronal suture where the superior frontal cerebral veins drain into the superior longitudinal sinus. Increased activity occasionally is noted along the suture line on the lateral projection and can be mistaken for a focal lesion. Occasionally these veins may be seen alongside the longitudinal sinus at the top of the anterior view.

The superior longitudinal sinus begins anteriorly at the crista galli and extends caudad along the superior sagittal fissure ending in the confluence of sinuses. It frequently drains into the right transverse sinus (DiChiro, 1962),

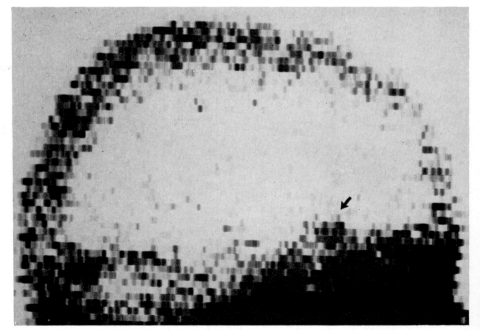

FIGURE 14-7.   Normal variant: area of activity in front of the sella, presumably middle meningeal vessels.

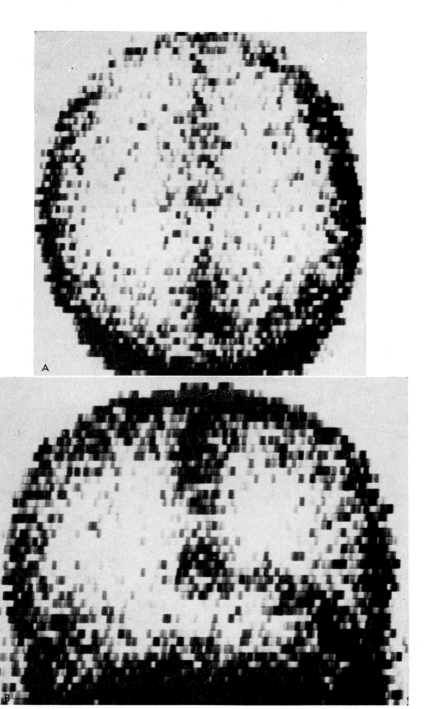

Figure 14-8. Normal variant: *A*, Vertex view. Increased activity in the right posterior fossa area due to the lateral sinus. *B*, Posterior view. Prominent right lateral sinus.

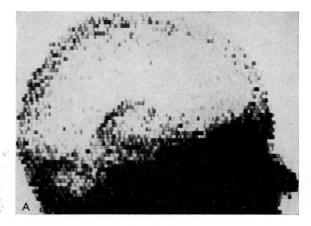

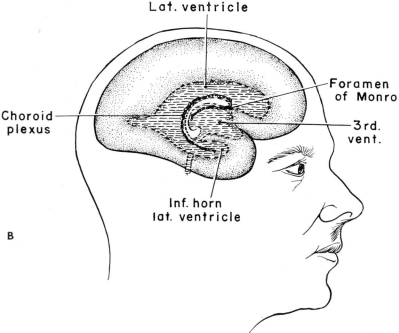

FIGURE 14-9.   Lateral scan with C-shaped posterior temporal activity (choroidal activity) and an illustration of the choroid plexus in the lateral and third ventricles of the brain.

which often gives an asymmetrical focus of increased activity in the posterior fossa region (Fig. 14-8). This is evident on the vertex and posterior views, and must be distinguished from a lesion. In the patient in Figure 14-8, a late-phase cerebral arteriogram proved that this was a large right lateral sinus.

Another common variant observed when pertechnetate is used as a brain scanning agent results from the fact that pertechnetate is concentrated by the choroid plexus (Wolff, 1964). In more than two thirds of the patients, an area of increased activity can be seen in the posterior temporal region on the lateral view. In about 5 per cent of patients, for no apparent reason, choroidal concentration is markedly increased and can be seen to follow the contour of the lateral and third ventricles (Fig. 14-9). When the resolution of the choroid plexus is poor, this activity may fuse into a larger area of increased activity occupying most of the temporal area on the lateral view. This may represent the area referred to as "temporal muscle" (Webber, 1965).

The area of activity in the choroid plexus often causes confusion in interpretation and should be eliminated by the prior oral administration of 200 mg. of potassium perchlorate. An example of a brain scan without and with the administration of perchlorate is shown in Figure 14-10. It can be seen that the suspicious area is not seen on the scan obtained after perchlorate.

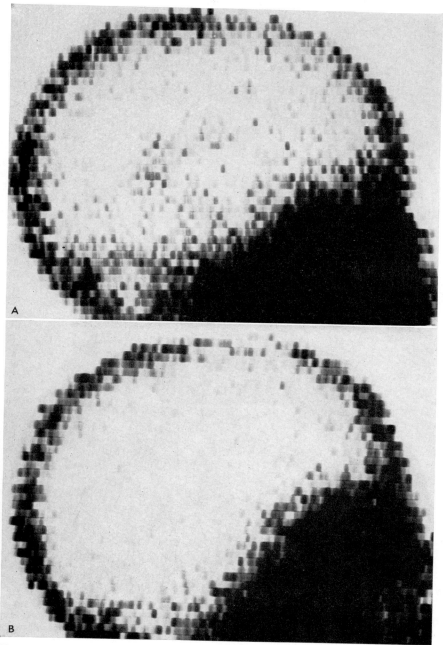

FIGURE 14-10.   Brain scan, lateral view. A, Without perchlorate. B, With perchlorate.

TABLE 14-7. INTRACRANIAL VASCULAR TUMORS AND MALFORMATIONS

Parenchymal
   Telangiectasia (Rendu-Osler-Weber disease)
   Cavernous angioma (venous and arterial)
   Parenchymal varix (single or multiple)
   Retinocerebellar angiomatosis (Lindau-von Hippel disease)
   Ataxia-telangiectasia (Louis-Bar syndrome)
   Arteriovenous malformation (angioma)
Meningeal
   Angioblastic meningioma
   Angiomatous meningioma
   Meningeal varix
   Trigeminofacial hemangiomatosis (Sturge-Weber-Dimitri syndrome)
Miscellaneous
   Sinus pericranii
   Angioglioma

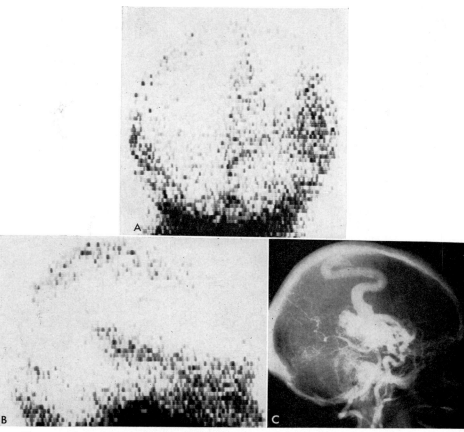

FIGURE 14-11.   Brain scan in congenital vascular lesion. *A*, Vertex view. In reased activit
in the right temporoparietal area. *B*, Right lateral view. Increased activity in the temporal region
C, Angiogram. Calcified racemose lesion in the temporal region with a large draining serpentine
vein.

CONGENITAL ABNORMALITIES

Most congenital lesions of the brain are easily diagnosed on the basis of clinical examination alone. Nevertheless, in specific instances, scanning may be helpful.

In hydrocephalus, brain scanning can be helpful in diagnosing and localizing the cause and in characterizing complications of therapy. Direct intraventricular instillation of gamma-emitting radiopharmaceuticals can be used to determine the degree of dilatation of the ventricles and the patency of natural and surgical shunts (DiChiro et al., 1964; and Schlesinger et al., 1963).

In most congenital vascular lesions (Table 14-7), brain scanning has not been widely used because of the high specificity of cerebral arteriography, but it may be useful as a screening procedure. Planiol and Akerman (1965) concluded that supratentorial arteriovenous aneurysms could be detected by external radiation detection. The early appearance of focal activity, the persistence or slight decrease in maximal activity at the focus, and hypoactivity adjacent to the lesion were indications that the lesions were vascular. Gilson (1966) emphasized the need for early and serial scanning in arteriovenous malformations. A typical vascular lesion is shown in Figure 14-11. The patient had left-sided weakness. On the scan a diffuse area of activity was noted in the midtemporoparietal region on the right extending diagonally toward the vertex. The cerebral arteriogram defined a partially calcified racemose lesion in this area and a large serpentine vessel that extended superiorly toward the longitudinal sinus.

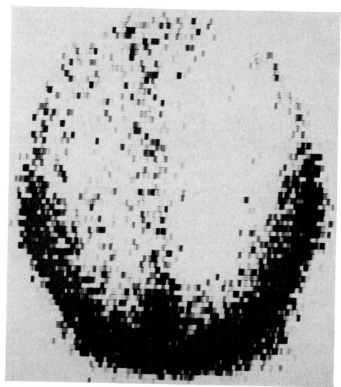

Figure 14-12. Brain scan, vertex view. Porencephalic cyst of the right hemisphere.

TABLE 14-8. INTRACRANIAL CYSTIC LESIONS

Arachnoidal cysts (postmeningitis serosa circumscripta)
Porencephalic cysts (developmental or acquired)
Colloid cyst of third ventricle
Cyst of septum pellucidum
Cystic craniopharyngioma
Infectious cysts (e.g., toxoplasmosis)
Neoplastic cysts (e.g., cystic glioma)
Parasitic cysts (hydatid and *Cysticercus cellulosae*)
Traumatic cysts (e.g., cystic hygroma)

In the group of hereditary phakomatoses (e.g., neurofibromatosis, tuberous sclerosis), scanning may be of some value in determining the site and number of cerebral lesions and occasionally in characterizing their extracortical defects (DiChiro, 1962).

Cystic lesions are detectable on the brain scan as areas of decreased or absent activity, even lower than that in normal brain. Table 14-8 lists commonly encountered intracranial cystic lesions. The vertex view is useful for diagnosing these lesions because it compares both cerebral hemispheres in their entirety. In an 18 year old male with generalized seizures, the brain scan revealed nearly completely absent activity in the right cerebrum (Fig. 14-12). Pneumographic studies revealed this to be a porencephalic cyst.

BRAIN TUMORS

Brain tumors account for between 2 and 3 per cent of all neoplasms and occur at all ages, but reach a peak frequency during the fifth decade of life (Fig. 14-13). The gliomas are the commonest tumors (45 per cent), followed by the meningiomas (20 per cent), pituitary adenomas (10 per cent), metastases (10 per cent), and a variety of other tumors (15 per cent) (Table 14-3).

A striking difference is noted in the locations and types of brain tumors in children and adults. In adults, most intracranial tumors are above the tentorium cerebelli, whereas in childhood two thirds are below it. In childhood, there is a high incidence of gliomas. The commonest infratentorial tumors in children are medulloblastoma, cystic astrocytoma, and ependymoma; of the supratentorial tumors, the glioma and craniopharyngioma predominate. The meningioma, glioblastoma, pituitary adenoma, and neurinoma occur almost exclusively in adults (Bailey, 1948).

Brain tumors may be single or multiple; the latter most frequently are metastases. They produce symptoms by expanding, infiltrating, and destroying nervous tissue. Their most common sites of occurrence are listed in Table 14-9.

Detection of intracranial mass lesions by brain scanning has an accuracy greater than 75 per cent (McAfee et al., 1964; Bucy and Ciric, 1965; Mealey et al., 1964). The diagnostic accuracy is greatest in meningioma, glioblastoma, and metastatic carcinoma in that order (Brinkman et al., 1962; Takahashi et al., 1966).

Glioblastoma multiforme is the most malignant of all brain tumors. In a third of the cases the tumor gives an irregular configuration on the scan; how-

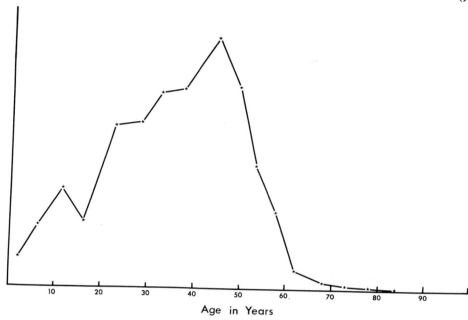

FIGURE 14-13.   Age distribution of brain tumors (modified from Bailey, 1948).

ever, most are seen as localized foci of high activity appearing almost exclusively in the cortical regions. A glioblastoma in a 26 year old mathematician who presented with seizures preceded by visual auras is shown in Figure 14-14. At surgery there was a highly malignant tumor in the left occipitoparietal region.

Meningiomas are found most often in the distribution of the arachnoid granulations. They are highly vascular and characteristically are clearly outlined on the scan. They often cause erosion of the overlying calvaria and hyperostosis. Symptoms are produced by compression of brain tissue and generally disappear rapidly after surgical removal of the tumor. Some of the sites of occurrence of the meningiomas are illustrated in Figure 14-15.

Metastatic carcinoma to the brain is clinically indistinguishable from primary

TABLE 14-9.   RELATIVE FREQUENCY (%) OF COMMON TUMORS AT VARIOUS SITES[*]

	FRONTAL	PARIETAL	TEMPORAL	OCCIPITAL	THIRD VENTRICLE	LATERAL VENTRICLE	REGION OF CHIASMA	UPPER BRAIN STEM	QUADRIGEMINAL PLATE	CEREBELLUM AND FOURTH VENTRICLE	PONTOCEREBELLAR ANGLE	LOWER BRAIN STEM
Astrocytoma	17.4	12.2	11.8	6.6	10.8			10.4	6.1	0.2		22 2
Glioblastoma	19.4	21.8	28.8	25.6				52.9	2.1			
Medulloblastoma									10.1	24.8		
Oligodendroglioma	15.7	8.7	12.4	5.1	3.6	14.5				2.0	0.4	
Ependymoma	2.4	7.5	2.6	6.6	18.0	16.9			12.1	11.1		14.8
Meningioma	30.6	31.3	26.2	27.0		9.7	9 9	1.1		5.3	0.4	3.7
Metastatic	5.4	5.2	2.9	6.6			0.4	5.7		2.5	6.7	3.7
Pituitary adenoma							52 2				1 4	
Pinealoma									26.1			
Neurinoma			0.2								79.2	
Papilloma			0.2		3.6	14.5				2.0		

* Modified from Zülch, 1965.

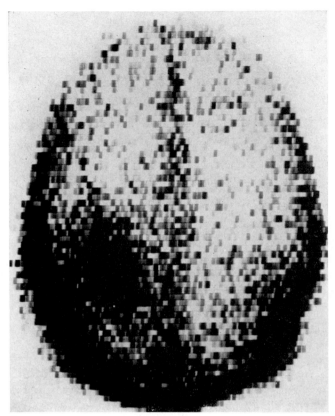

FIGURE 14-14.   Brain scan, vertex view. Glioblastoma multiforme in left occipitoparietal region.

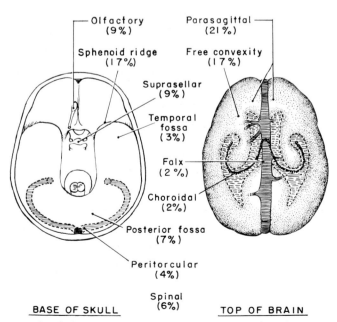

Olfactory
(9%)

Sphenoid ridge
(17%)

Suprasellar
(9%)

Temporal
fossa
(3%)

Falx
(2%)

Choroidal
(2%)

Posterior fossa
(7%)

Peritorcular
(4%)

Parasagittal
(21%)

Free convexity
(17%)

Spinal
(6%)

BASE OF SKULL   TOP OF BRAIN

FIGURE 14-15.   Regional occurrence of meningiomas according to Cushing (313 cases).

tumors. The diagnosis depends on the recognition of a primary tumor elsewhere and is strongly suggested by multiple lesions on the scans as shown in Figure 14-16. These criteria are not absolute, however, as exemplified in the patient in Figure 14-17; this 65 year old female with a history of surgically removed breast carcinoma, hypertension, and atrial fibrillation developed increasing in-

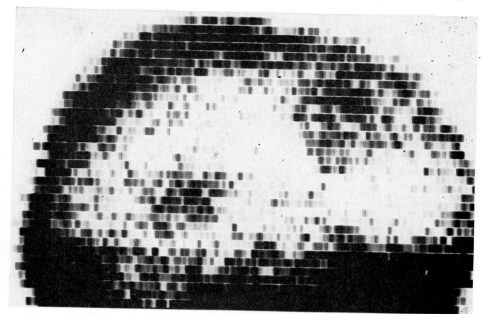

FIGURE 14-16.   Brain scan, lateral view. Multiple foci of activity in a patient with metastatic breast carcinoma.

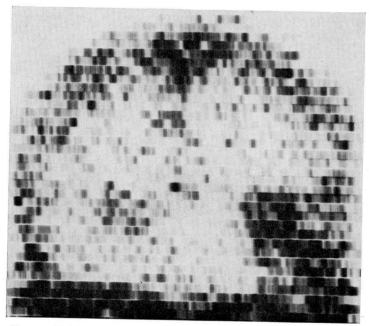

FIGURE 14-17.   Brain scan, anterior view. Multiple cerebral infarcts.

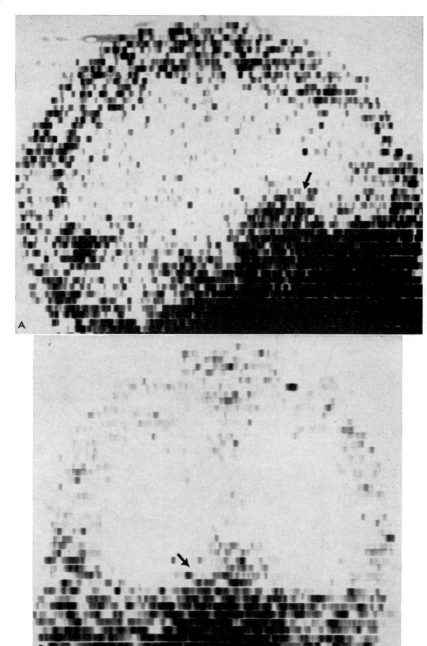

FIGURE 14-18. Brain scan in pituitary adenoma with suprasellar extension. *A,* Lateral view. *B,* Anterior view. Midline mass above nasion.

tracranial pressure. The scan showed multiple cortical lesions suggesting metastatic tumor. At necropsy subarachnoid hemorrhage and multiple hemorrhagic cortical infarcts, but no tumors, were found.

Pituitary adenomas produce signs and symptoms of altered trophic hormone secretion and compression of nervous tissue in the chiasmal region at the base

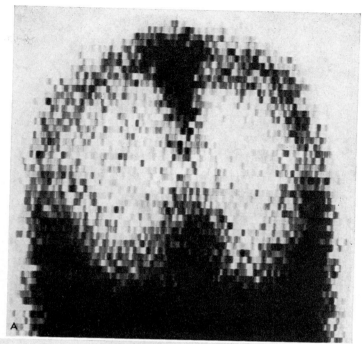

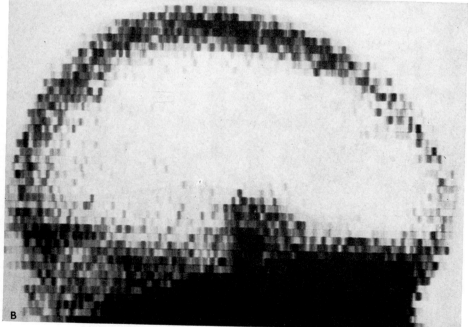

FIGURE 14-19. A and B, Anterior and lateral scans of a boy with a craniopharyngioma showing vertical projection of the tumor from the base on the anterior view and in the region of the sella on the lateral view.

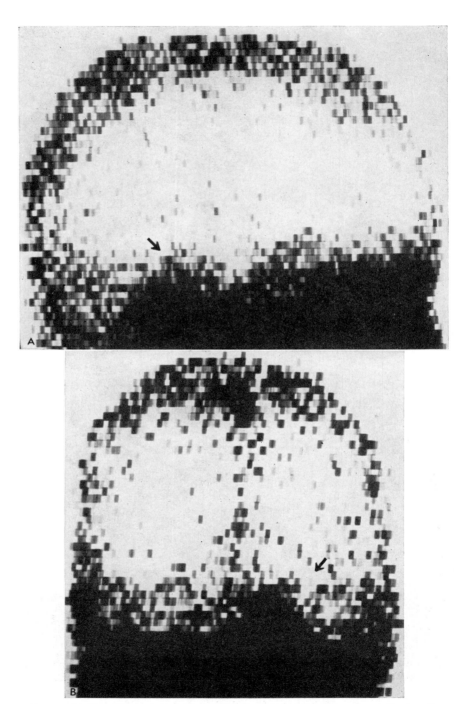

FIGURE 14-20.   Brain scan. *A*, Lateral view. Increased activity above the junction of the lateral sinus and auditory meatus due to acoustic neurinoma. *B*, Posterior view. Tumor seen in the right posterior fossa (in contrast to primary cerebellar tumors, which are midline).

of the brain. On the scan the tumor is seen as an area of increased radioactivity extending vertically from the region of the pituitary sulcus on both lateral views and midline from the nasion in the anterior view (Fig. 14-18).

Craniopharyngiomas most often occur in childhood and adolescence, but occasionally are found in adults. They are usually encapsulated and produce symptoms by expansion in the region of the sella. They develop from embryonic "rests" of the hypophysial duct and can be either a solid tumor or a cyst, both of which may calcify. Figure 14-19 shows the scans obtained in a 9 year old boy with excessive obesity and underdeveloped genitalia, i.e., Frölich's syndrome, who was found at surgery to have a craniopharyngioma.

Of the primary cranial nerve tumors, the eighth cranial nerve is the most often affected, usually at the cerebellopontine angle. Early in the disease an almost classic syndrome of auditory and labyrinthine dysfunction is noted on the side with the lesion, but this specificity is diminished as the disease progresses. The scan usually reveals, on the lateral view, a focus of increased activity in the region of the external auditory meatus and occasionally an asymmetrical focus on the posterior view (Fig. 14-20).

Medulloblastomas and cystic astrocytomas are infratentorial gliomatous

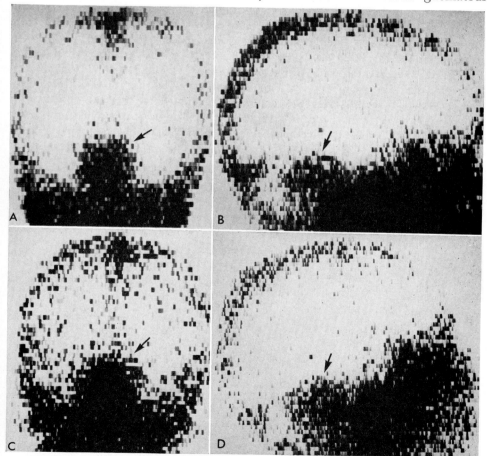

FIGURE 14-21. *A*, Posterior scan after injection of ^{99m}Tc pertechnetate. The lesion indicated by the arrow was a primary cerebellar astrocytoma. *B*, Lateral view of the same patient after injection of ^{99m}Tc pertechnetate. *C*, Posterior scan in the same patient after injection of ^{113m}In chelate. *D*, Lateral scan in the same patient after injection of ^{113m}In chelate.

tumors of childhood and characteristically occur in the vermis region of the cerebellum. Their contiguous expansion generally involves the fourth ventricle and results frequently in internal hydrocephalus. They are seen on the brain scan as highly radioactive midline mass lesions extending superiorly to the torcular on the posterior view and occasionally as a poorly resolved focus of increased activity above the auditory meatus and transverse sinus junction on the lateral views (Fig. 14-21). Many primary cerebellar tumors in adulthood such as hemangioblastomas are also seen as midline lesions extending upward into the tented region created by junction of the falx cerebri and tentorium cerebelli.

TRAUMA

Subdural hematomas, epidural or intracerebral hemorrhages, and cerebral contusions are the most serious complications of trauma to the head. Subdural and epidural hemorrhages, which may be difficult to diagnose on clinical evidence alone, may occasionally be suspected on the basis of an abnormal brain scan. Characteristically they give an asymmetrical crescent-shaped peripheral area of increased activity on the anterior view (Fig. 14-22). The crescentic configuration has also been detected in other conditions (Quinn, 1966). For example, in Figure 14-23 are the scans of a 52 year old female with a history of left radical mastectomy for breast carcinoma, who developed acute headache and vomiting. The scans revealed an asymmetrical left peripheral area of increased activity with the crescentic configuration suggestive of a subdural hemorrhage. At surgery, tumor was found to involve the leptomeninges and inner table of the skull. The involvement of bone rather than the brain itself could

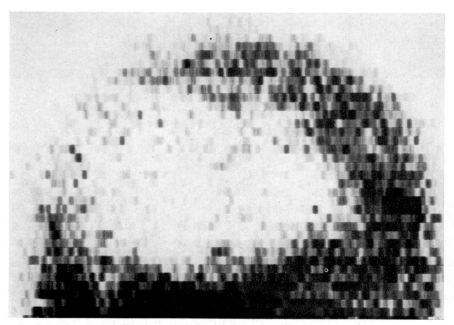

FIGURE 14-22.   Brain scan, anterior view. Subdural hematoma.

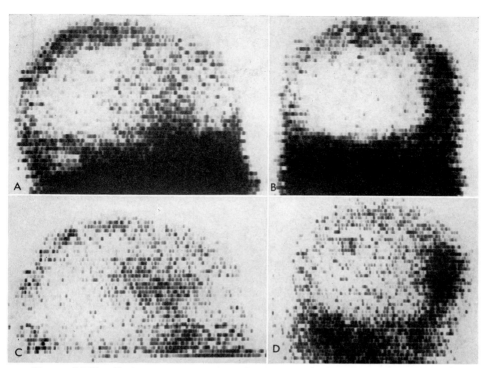

FIGURE 14-23. Brain scan in a patient with metastatic breast carcinoma. A, Lateral view. Increased activity in the frontotemporal area. B, Anterior view. Crescentic lesion in the same patient. C, Lateral and D, Anterior views in the same patient with ^{87m}Sr accumulation in the osseous lesion of the skull.

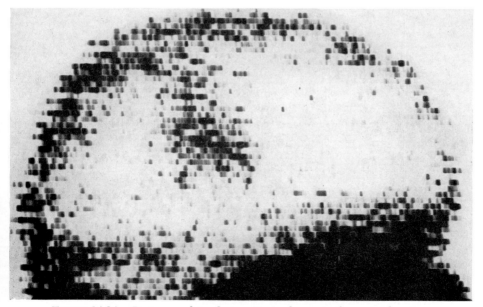

FIGURE 14-24. Brain scan, lateral view. Brain abscess in the parietal region.

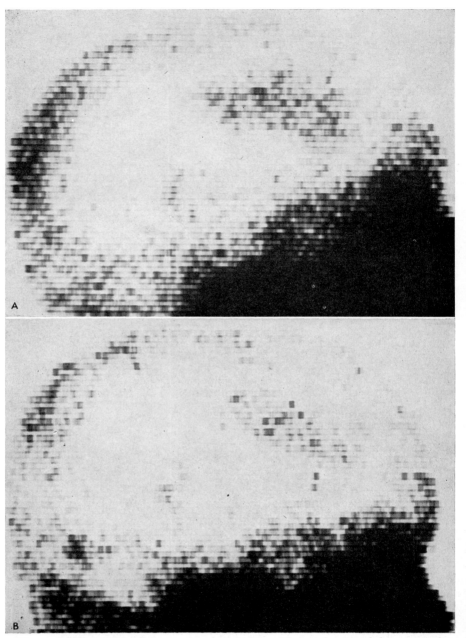

FIGURE 14-25.   Tuberculous meningoencephalitis with ependymitis of the anterior lateral ventricles. A, Right lateral view; B, left lateral view.

be determined by the finding that the calcium analog, strontium-87m, accumulated in the lesion to a greater degree than ^{99m}Tc pertechnetate (Tow and Wagner, 1967).

The accumulation of activity in subdural hematomas is believed to be the result of the tissue reaction to the extravasated blood along the epidural and subdural surfaces (Gilson and Gargano, 1965). This perhaps accounts for the

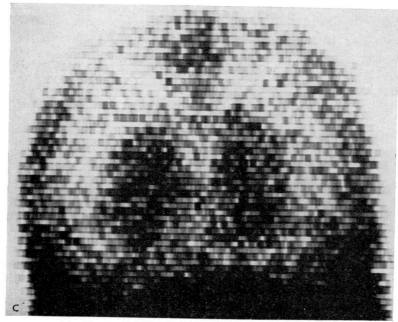

FIGURE 14-25. *Continued. C,* anterior view.

frequent finding of a normal scan early in the disease with a progressive increase in the number of positive scans with time. Bilateral lesions may be symmetrical and are therefore much more difficult to diagnose.

In the study of cerebral contusion, Gilson (1966) noted that the contused area might be seen on the scan as a localized focus of increased activity on the side opposite the direct trauma. The abnormality of the scan disappeared within 6 to 10 weeks.

INFLAMMATORY LESIONS

Positive brain scans from brain abscesses and granulomas may not permit differentiation of these lesions from others. Accumulation of activity within these lesions is quite variable and, as in traumatic vascular lesions, the incidence of positive scans increases with the duration of the disease, presumably because of progressive encapsulation (Overton et al., 1965). Serial brain scanning may be helpful in following the course of therapy. Figure 14-24 is from a patient with rheumatic heart disease, subacute bacterial endocarditis, and septic embolization with subsequent brain abscess. The lesion on the scan almost completely resolved after 10 days of antibiotic therapy.

General inflammation, such as meningoencephalitis, cerebritis, and ependymitis, has infrequently been studied by brain scanning. In certain instances, increased areas of activity are seen on the scan conforming to specific brain structures, presumably because of the uptake of the radiopharmaceutical by the inflammatory tissue. Figure 14-25 shows scans from a patient with tuberculous meningoencephalitis. The scans showed bilateral frontal cortex foci of activity shaped like the anterior horns of the lateral ventricles. At autopsy the patient was found to have ependymitis of the lateral ventricles.

LESIONS OF THE SKULL

Lesions of the calvaria, such as hyperostosis, Paget's disease, osteomyelitis, fibrous dysplasia, and metastatic neoplasia, are usually detectable on radiographs of the skull. With ^{99m}Tc pertechnetate, focal increases of activity in the region of an osseous lesion cannot be differentiated from intracranial lesions (Bollinger et al., 1965). Specific characterization of the type of lesion can occasionally be accomplished by using more than one radiopharmaceutical.

If scans with both ^{99m}Tc pertechnetate and ionic ^{87m}Sr are made, the relative accumulation of the two nuclides can be used to determine the nature of the lesion. If the accumulation of ^{87m}Sr is greater than that of ^{99m}Tc, the lesion is probably in the skull; on the other hand, if ^{99m}Tc activity in the lesion is greater than that of ^{87m}Sr, the lesion is probably not osseous, but in the brain or meninges (Tow and Wagner, 1967).

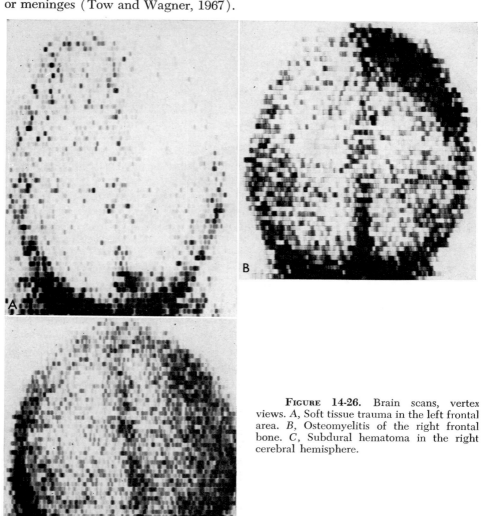

FIGURE 14-26. Brain scans, vertex views. *A,* Soft tissue trauma in the left frontal area. *B,* Osteomyelitis of the right frontal bone. *C,* Subdural hematoma in the right cerebral hemisphere.

Positive brain scans may be obtained for many months after craniotomy.

Figure 14-26 shows the similarity of the appearance of the brain scans in patients with soft tissue trauma, lesions of bone, and subdural hematoma. In interpreting the scan, it is imperative to examine the patient for soft tissue injury, and to look for radiographic abnormalities of the skull. At times, it is helpful to repeat the scan, using ^{87m}Sr.

CEREBROSPINAL FLUID

Intrathecal injection of radioiodinated human serum albumin was first carried out to investigate the rate of formation, flow, and resorption of cerebrospinal fluid. Radioactive tracers have been injected directly into the ventricles for the diagnosis of: spontaneous ventriculostomy; communication between the ventricular system and a porencephalic cyst; the patency of neurosurgical shunts in the treatment of hydrocephalus (Schlesinger et al., 1963); and paranormal cavities (cavum of septum pellucidum, cavum vergae, and cavum of velum interpositum). To localize total or subtotal blocks, the spine is scanned after intrathecal injection of 100 μc. of radioiodinated albumin (Bauer and Yuhl, 1953; Perryman et al., 1958; Bell and Hertsch, 1959; Bell, 1962; Pinto, 1962).

DiChiro injected ^{131}I albumin into the ventricular system and intrathecally to aid in the diagnosis of brain tumor, internal hydrocephalus, and cerebrospinal fluid rhinorrhea (DiChiro et al., 1964). The latter results from abnormal communication between the subarachnoid space and the nasal cavity. Such communications are caused by congenital defects, skull fracture, recent surgery, bone erosion by tumor, infections, and hydrocephalus. The diagnosis of cerebrospinal fluid leakage is often possible on clinical grounds alone, although occasionally the diagnosis of "vasomotor rhinitis" may be made erroneously. After the diagnosis has been made, locating the site of the leakage is a challenging problem. Most often the leaking site is at the base of the anterior fossa, but it may also occur in the middle and posterior fossa. Leaks may occur through the frontal sinus, the lamina cribrosa, or the sphenoidal roof, or through the petrous bone via the middle ear and the eustachian tube. The leak may be on the side opposite the "dripping nostril." The possibility of multiple sites of leakage further complicates the problem. Corrective surgery is necessary if the fistula does not heal spontaneously, since the patient runs the risk of recurrent meningitis.

Radiography, dyes, fluorescent substances, and radioactive tracers have been used to locate the sites of leakage. In some cases, the bone defect may be seen by x-ray examination. Tomography, pneumoencephalography, and subdural pneumography may be helpful. Opaque media have been injected into the subarachnoidal space (Ghouralal et al., 1956; Rockett et al., 1964), the ventricular system, a pneumocephalic cavity (Jungmann and Peyser, 1963), and intranasally (Teng and Edalatpour, 1963). Dyes (indigo carmine and methylene blue) have been introduced within the subarachnoid spaces or intranasally for visual localization of the fistula before or during surgery. Fluorescein has also been used (Kirchner and Proud, 1960). In 1956, radioactive sodium (^{24}Na) was tried (Crow et al., 1956). After injection of the tracer into the cisterna magna, cotton pledgets were placed at the walls and roof of the nose and nasopharynx and at the openings of the eustachian tubes. The cotton pledgets accumulating the highest amount of radioactivity indicated the site of leakage.

The technique of DiChiro and his associates (1964) is as follows: 100 μc. of ^{131}I human serum albumin is introduced intrathecally and the head is scanned serially 1, 3, 6, and 24 hours after injection. Superimposition of the scanning image on the skull x-ray is helpful.

CEREBROVASCULAR DISEASE

In general, disturbance of the cerebral circulation may result from hypoxia, thromboembolism, or hemorrhage. A classification of cerebrovascular disease is given in Table 14-10. In a recent national survey, cerebrovascular accidents (stroke) ranked third as a cause of death, not far behind cancer and far ahead of the fourth-ranking cause, accidents. About 80 per cent of the stroke deaths occurred in people aged 65 years and over, with the largest single number occurring in the 75 to 84 age group.

Some patients with cerebrovascular disease have symptoms that forewarn of a disabling stroke. There may be brief attacks of loss of speech, weakness of limbs, staggering, or loss of consciousness. Because these manifestations lack specificity, ancillary diagnostic tests are necessary for precise diagnosis, which might make it possible to prevent the more serious attack.

THE DIAGNOSTIC PROBLEM

McHenry and Valsamis (1966) have outlined the clinical syndromes produced by occlusion of cerebral arteries (Table 14-11). They emphasized that the overall effects of vessel abnormalities and general reduction of their luminal diameters are more important than the effects of a single lesion in a specific vessel. Cerebral atherosclerosis tends to occur at branchings, bifurcations, and curves in the vessels. Sites of predilection include the carotid sinus in the neck, the internal carotid artery adjacent to the siphon near the origin of the ophthalmic artery, the middle cerebral artery at its first major bifurcation, the vertebral arteries as they enter the cranial cavity, and at their junction to form the basilar artery, the basilar artery 1 cm. above its junction, near the upper basilar bifurcation, the posterior cerebral arteries as they wind around the cerebral peduncle, and the anterior cerebral arteries as they bend posteriorly around the genu of the corpus callosum. Although there are exceptions to these rules, in general these sites are the most severely affected. Atherosclerosis tends to be of about equal severity in the basilar and carotid system.

The role of carotid artery occlusion or stenosis in the production of cerebrovascular insufficiency has recently been emphasized. The frequency of disease of the carotid arteries was pointed out in a study by Samuel (quoted in McHenry and Valsamis, 1966), in which both internal carotid arteries were examined at autopsy in 82 subjects. Seventy-four patients had some degree of atherosclerosis of the carotid arteries and 15 had severe atheroma. Yates and Hutchison (quoted in McHenry and Valsamis, 1966) found diminution of the vascular lumen to one half or less of the normal size in one or more major vessels in the neck in 83

TABLE 14-10. ETIOLOGIES OF CEREBROVASCULAR DISEASE*

Cerebral Hemorrhage
    Atherosclerosis
    Hypertension
    Saccular and mycotic aneurysm
    Angiomatous malformation
    Trauma
    Hemorrhagic disorders
    Anticoagulants
    Hemorrhage into brain tumor
    Arteritis (in pyemia)
Cerebral Infarction
  Thrombotic
    Atherosclerosis
    Infection
    Collagen disease
    Trauma to head and neck
    Uncal herniation
    Dissecting aneurysm cerebral artery
    Blood dyscrasias
    Takayasu (pulseless) disease
    Radiation
    Thromboangiitis obliterans
  Embolic
    From heart (infarcts, arrhythmia, endocarditis, cardiac surgery)
    Atheromatous plaques in aorta or branches
    Paradoxical
    Fat (injuries to long bones)
    Air (decompression sickness)
  Arterial insufficiency
    Carotid stenosis
    Vertebrobasilar stenosis
    Subclavian stenosis
Hypertensive encephalopathy
    Malignant hypertension
    Acute glomerulonephritis
    Eclampsia
    Lead poisoning and other toxins
Venous Thrombosis
    Local infections of ears, sinuses, skin
    Postpartum
    Marasmus
    Polycythemia
    Cardiac decompensation

* Modified from Elliott, 1964.

autopsy cases. Of 22 patients with definite cerebral infarction, only 6 had occlusion of an intracerebral vessel. The possibility of carotid or vertebral artery disease should always be considered in patients with transient attacks of cerebrovascular ischemia. Atherosclerotic changes in the large carotid and vertebral arteries in the neck will reduce the flow of blood to the circle of Willis. Occlusion or stenosis of one carotid or vertebral artery can be compensated by flow in the remaining vessels, and asymptomatic occlusion has occasionally been demonstrated at autopsy. If, however, the overall blood flow to the brain is

TABLE 14-11. CLINICAL SYNDROMES PRODUCED BY OCCLUSION
OF THE CEREBRAL ARTERIES*

ARTERY	REGION SUPPLIED	SYMPTOMS PRODUCED
Internal carotid	Frontal, parietal and temporal areas; caudate and lenticular nuclei; internal capsule and corona radiata; optic nerve and retina.	*Acute:* coma; aphasia (dominant hemisphere); contralateral hemiplegia, hemianesthesia, and homonymous hemianopsia; ipsilateral blindness. *Chronic:* transient attacks of hemiparesis, hemianesthesia, etc., and monocular visual disturbances.
Anterior cerebral	Anterior part of anterior limb of internal capsule; orbital surface and tip of frontal lobe; mesial and parasagittal surface of cerebral hemisphere to parieto-occipital junction; anterior part of caudate nucleus.	Dementia, confusion, or coma; contralateral hemiplegia and cortical sensory loss primarily affecting leg.
Middle cerebral	Convexity of the cerebral hemisphere and its white matter, including lateral orbital frontal region and temporal tip. Perforating branches supply internal capsule, caudate and lenticular nuclei and anterior thalamus.	Syndrome similar to internal carotid occlusion or stenosis except for absence of visual disturbances. *Total infarction:* coma, contralateral facial weakness, hemiplegia, hemianesthesia, and homonymous hemianopsia with aphasia (if dominant hemisphere). *Partial infarction:* usual with partial contralateral involvement: cortical sensory loss and weakness predominantly affect arm rather than leg.
Posterior cerebral	Midbrain, including cerebral peduncles and third nerve; superior cerebellar peduncle; posterior part of thalamus, including lateral geniculate body; posterior part of internal capsule, base and posterior two thirds of temporal lobe, splenium of corpus callosum, and medial surface of occipital lobe.	*Infarction adjacent to or involving subthalamic nucleus:* contralateral hemiballismus resulting from occlusion of perforating thalamic branch. *Occlusion of thalamogeniculate branch with infarction of thalamus and lateral geniculate body:* contralateral hemianopsia and hemianesthesia. *Occlusion of calcarine branches:* homonymous superior quadrantanopsia or hemianopsia. *Occlusion of branch to basis pedunculi:* ipsilateral third nerve palsy and contralateral hemiplegia with or without contralateral tremor.
Basilar	Structures of the posterior fossa (pons, medulla, cerebellum) below bifurcation of basilar into posterior cerebral arteries.	Clinical criteria of disease in basilar system: (1) signs of abnormality involving third to twelfth cranial nerves in any combination—third, sixth, and seventh most commonly, (2) cerebellar dysfunction, and (3) long tract signs, especially corticospinal.
Main trunk	Base and medial parts of tegmentum of midbrain and pons, including corticospinal tracts; corticobulbar tracts; oculomotor, trochlear, abducens, and facial nerves; medial lemnisci.	Stupor or coma; hemiplegia or quadriplegia; dysarthria and dysphagia; pupillary abnormalities; paralysis of gaze or of ocular muscles and face; paresthesia and impaired vibratory and position sense.

TABLE 14-11. (*Continued*)

ARTERY	REGION SUPPLIED	SYMPTOMS PRODUCED
Superior cerebellar	Lateral tegmentum of midbrain and upper pons; superior cerebellum.	Ipsilateral Horner's syndrome and cerebellar ataxia; contralateral loss of pain and temperature.
Middle cerebellar	Anterior and inferior parts of cerebellum; lateral tegmentum of pons and upper medulla.	Ipsilateral cerebellar ataxia and Horner's syndrome; loss of touch, pain, and temperature over face; dizziness and nystagmus; ipsilateral facial paralysis and deafness; contralateral loss of pain over arm, trunk, and leg.
Posterior inferior cerebellar or vertebral	Posterior and inferior parts of cerebellum; lateral tegmentum of medulla, including descending pupillodilator fibers, vestibular nuclei, descending nucleus and tract of trigeminal nerve, and glossopharyngeal and vagus nuclei (nucleus ambiguus); restiform body and dorsal spinocerebellar tract; lateral spinothalamic tract.	Ipsilateral Horner's syndrome; dizziness and nystagmus; ipsilateral loss of pain and temperature senses over face; dysphagia; dysphonia; ipsilateral cerebellar ataxia; contralateral loss of pain and temperature senses over arm, trunk, and leg.

* Modified from McHenry and Valsamis, 1966.

impaired, minor fluctuations in the cerebral perfusion pressure may produce ischemia or infarction.

Stenosis of the left subclavian artery proximal to the origin of the left vertebral artery may result in reversal of blood flow in the left vertebral artery, a condition referred to as the "subclavian steal syndrome." The pressure gradient in the vertebral artery is reversed and diversion of blood flow from the brain results in ischemia.

BRAIN SCANNING IN VASCULAR DISEASE

Serial brain scanning is being used more and more to differentiate between vascular disease and brain tumors. Usually vascular lesions do not alter the blood-brain barrier sufficiently to produce any abnormalities on the scan within the first 2 weeks. According to a recent report (Brown et al., 1966) only 24 of 50 patients with vascular occlusion had a positive brain scan within that period. Fifty-six per cent of the patients with hemorrhagic lesions had positive scans. Of the 32 patients who had a second scan between the third and the eighth week, 50 per cent had abnormal concentrations of radioactivity. In 23 patients whose initial scans were negative, 43 per cent became positive on the second scan. Others have reported similar findings (Morrison et al., 1965; and Overton et al., 1965). Vascularization or hemorrhage into the surrounding brain tissue may be significant factors in producing the positive scan.

Hemorrhage can be localized or extensive and occurs most frequently in hypertension with or without arteriosclerosis. Rarely does intracerebral hemorrhage result without hypertension, trauma, congenital aneurysms, vascular tumors, or blood dyscrasias. Characteristically severe headache followed by vom-

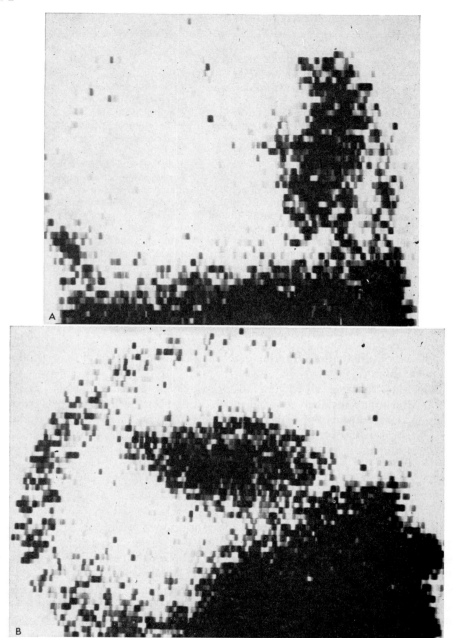

FIGURE 14-27.   Brain scan in cerebral infarct. *A,* Anterior view. *B,* Lateral view.

iting, convulsion, and then unconsciousness is the typical picture, and 60 to 75 per cent of the patients die within the first 24 to 48 hours.

In a study of 2650 necropsies, Moosy (1965) found 142 recent cerebral infarcts, and of these, 55 per cent had demonstrable thrombotic lesions. Cerebral embolism occurs in less than 5 per cent of cerebrovascular lesions and on the scan is indistinguishable from thrombosis. In both instances, the infarcted zone

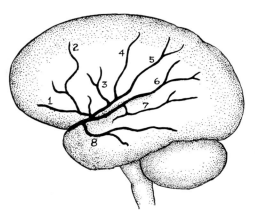

FIGURE 14-28. Distribution of the middle cerebral artery: *1*, orbitofrontal; *2*, prerolandic; *3*, rolandic; *4*, anterior parietal; *5*, posterior parietal; *6*, angular; *7*, posterior temporal; *8*, anterior temporal.

on the scan gives an intense uptake of activity, which is in the distribution of a principal nutrient artery and frequently lies in the periphery of the cortex (Fig. 14-27).

In Moosy's series, 45 per cent of the vascular occlusions were in the middle cerebral artery. In a study of 59 patients, Lascelles and Burrows (1965) concluded that occlusion of the middle cerebral artery could not be differentiated clinically from an occlusion of the internal carotid artery in the neck. Figure 14-28 illustrates the distribution of the branches of the middle cerebral artery.

Positive brain scans are not obtained often enough in cerebrovascular disease for the procedure to be used as a screening test, but a negative scan increases the probability of the patient having a vascular lesion when the diagnosis lies between tumor and vascular disease.

CIRCULATION TIME

The circulation time of the brain has been measured by injection of ^{131}I sodium iodide into the carotid artery with external measurements of radioactivity over the parietal-parasagittal region. The results have been corroborated by rapid serial angiography (Greitz, 1956). With the radiopaque material, the circulation time was taken as the time between the most dense opacification of the carotid siphon to the densest opacification of the parietal parasagittal veins. The radionuclide circulation time was measured from the time of carotid injection to the time of maximum count rate in the parietal parasagittal region. Both the angiographic and the radioactive tracer methods yielded a mean circulation time of about 7 seconds. Circulation time was also measured between the carotid and the region of the confluence of sinuses (torcula); the indicator used was ^{131}I-labeled albumin (Crandall and Cassen, 1958). The carotid-torcula time ranged from 5 to 9 seconds in most patients, and was found to be prolonged in those in whom intracranial pressure was elevated.

Circulation time through the brain has also been measured by rapid injection into a carotid artery followed by serial blood sampling from the jugular vein (Nylin et al., 1960). The circulation time measured from carotid artery peak to jugular activity peak was about 8.5 seconds.

Intravenous techniques are less traumatic than carotid injection although structures other than brain are perfused and a streamed-out bolus enters the brain. In the technique of Oldendorf (1962), a detector is used to monitor the upper half of the head. Iodine-131 hippurate is injected into an antecubital vein while venous return of the arm is obstructed by a cuff. When the cuff is suddenly removed, the distal venous pool collapses and the radionuclide is propelled rapidly into the right heart. About 7 seconds later its leading edge enters the brain. The count rate rises to a peak and falls as the radionuclide leaves the brain. By differentiating the rate meter output electronically, the first derivative (i.e., rate of change) of the tracer content of the brain pool can be obtained. A positive peak in the first derivative curve indicates the entrance of radioactivity into the brain pool, and the later negative peak indicates its exit. The interval between positive and negative peaks is the most common (mode) circulation time through the brain blood pool; this transit time may also be considered to represent the turnover time of the pool, and closely approximates the mean circulation time in the brain (Ljunggren et al., 1961); the normal range is 6 to 11 seconds (Oldendorf and Kitano, 1965).

In another technique, ^{131}I-labeled human serum albumin or chromium-51-labeled erythrocytes are injected intravenously and detectors over the carotid sheath record the radionuclide going to and returning from the brain (Fedoruk and Feindel, 1960; Ljunggren et al., 1961). Normal values are 7 to 11 seconds.

From knowledge of both blood flow through the brain and the circulation time, the volume of the blood pool of the brain may be computed (Nylin et al., 1960). The blood volume of the brain was found to be 2.7 per cent of the total-body blood pool (mean value, 132 ml.). Unfortunately, the procedure is technically complicated since simultaneous samples must be obtained from several great vessels.

DIFFUSIBLE TRACERS

Ingvar and Lassen (1962) measured regional cortical blood flow in a patient undergoing craniotomy for a tumor. Krypton-85, a weak beta-emitter, was dissolved in saline and injected into an internal carotid artery. Uptake and clearance of the radionuclide from the surface of the middle frontal gyrus was recorded by means of a small shielded Geiger-Müller tube mounted 3 mm. from the cortical surface and 5 cm. anterior to the tumor. Average blood flow of the superficial cortical layers (about 1 mm. in depth) calculated from the clearance portion of the curve was 51 and 43 ml./min./100 g.

The recording of beta radiation is of limited usefulness because it requires surgical exposure of the part of the brain in which blood flow is to be determined. This limitation could be overcome by use of a gamma-emitting inert gas such as [79]Kr or [133]Xe.

Because [79]Kr emits gamma-rays that are too energetic to permit precise localization of the area of the brain under study, Glass and Harper (1963) substituted xenon-133, which emits a lower-energy gamma-ray. They dissolved 4 mc. of the radionuclide in 10 ml. of saline for injection into the carotid artery. The clearance of ^{133}Xe from the cerebral cortex was measured with a scintillation detector and focusing collimator. From the initial slopes of clearance, the blood flow was calculated to be 75 ml./min./100 g. at a blood pCO_2 of 20.

Most applications of radioactive tracers to study the cerebral circulation are based on modifications of the Fick principle, and are related to the original nitrous oxide technique (Kety and Schmidt, 1945, 1948a; Scheinberg and Stead, 1949; Kety, 1960). The method of Kety and Schmidt (1948a, b) was the first generally useful technique applicable to man for measurement of cerebral blood flow with reasonable accuracy. The subject breathes a gaseous mixture containing a specified concentration of nitrous oxide, a substance not normally present in blood or brain. After sufficient time for equilibration of gas between jugular venous blood and brain has passed, an indirect measure of the uptake of the gas per unit mass of brain can be obtained from the jugular venous concentration. When this uptake value is divided by the mean difference between the arterial and internal jugular venous concentrations, the mean cerebral blood flow per unit mass of brain is obtained.

Nitrous oxide has the following properties: (1) it is not normally present in blood (or brain); (2) it is chemically inert and is neither utilized by nor produced by the brain; (3) it diffuses through the blood-brain barrier and exchanges between blood and brain tissue; and (4) its concentration in blood is easily measured. The nitrous oxide is administered in low concentrations in inspired air (15 per cent N_2O, 21 per cent O_2, 64 per cent N_2) in a nonrebreathing system. Timed, multiple pairs of arterial and cerebral venous blood samples are drawn at close intervals from the onset of breathing the gas mixture and throughout the ensuing 10 minutes. Arterial blood is obtained from any artery; representative cerebral venous blood is obtained by percutaneous puncture of the superior bulb of the internal jugular vein. The nitrous oxide contents of the blood samples are determined manometrically, and the arterial and cerebral venous concentrations are plotted as a function of time. The integrated arterio-venous difference is determined from these curves.

The quantity of N_2O taken up by the brain cannot be measured directly. However, after the N_2O mixture has been breathed for 10 minutes, the mixed cerebral venous blood and mixed cerebral tissues are approximately in equilibrium with respect to their N_2O concentrations. The brain uptake can then be determined from the cerebral venous concentration since the N_2O in the brain after 10 minutes is then approximately equal to the concentration in the cerebral venous blood.

The mean value for the cerebral blood flow in man by this technique, adjusted to a pCO_2 of 40 mm. Hg (Reivich, 1964), is 52.2 ml./min./100 g.

The principles of the nitrous oxide technique apply to any other freely diffusible, chemically inert tracer that can be assayed in blood. To simplify the assay in blood, radionuclides of krypton or xenon can be substituted for nitrous oxide. The cerebral blood values obtained with [79]Kr as the tracer substance are essentially the same as those found with nitrous oxide. Krypton-79 is inconvenient to use, however, because of its short half-life (34 hours) and the fact that it is produced in a cyclotron.

Krypton-85 is more readily available and has a longer half-life (10 years) (Lassen and Munck, 1955). It emits both beta and gamma radiation, but the incidence of gamma radiation is less than 1 per cent. The beta radiation is usually measured in blood samples.

Krypton-85 is administered in the inspired air in a concentration of 100 μc. per liter either through a closed nonrebreathing system, or a rebreathing system with CO_2 absorption and O_2 replacement. The accuracy of the method is improved by extending the period of breathing and blood sampling from the 10 minutes used in the original nitrous oxide technique to 14 minutes, allowing a closer approach to equilibrium between brain and cerebral venous blood.

In addition to improvement in accuracy and precision, the [85]Kr technique is preferable to the original nitrous oxide technique because of its adaptability to automated analysis of blood samples. The radiation dose to the tracheal epithelium, the tissue receiving the greatest exposure, has been calculated to be about 0.16 rep (Sokoloff, 1964).

In an additional modification of Lassen and Munck's technique, arterial and jugular venous blood were sampled for 14 to 23 minutes following insertion of 19-gauge needles into the superior bulb of the jugular vein and the femoral artery (Alexander et al., 1964).

Albert and associates (1960) modified the Lassen and Munck procedure so that only two arterial (femoral) and six cerebral venous samples (internal jugular bulb) were needed. Good agreement was found with results obtained by their technique in 60 subjects with those found in the same subjects by a modification of the Kety-Schmidt nitrous oxide technique.

Another technique differs from the procedure of Lassen and Munck in that the [85]Kr, in saline solution, is injected into the internal carotid artery (Lassen et al., 1963) and then the rate of clearance of radioactivity over various regions of the cranium is measured for about 10 minutes. This procedure developed out of earlier studies in which Ingvar and Lassen (1962) injected [85]Kr into the carotid artery and measured the rate of clearance from cerebral cortex at craniotomy using a beta counter mounted above exposed tissue. An average perfusion rate of 60 ml./min./100 g. was found in normal persons, and 30 to 40 ml./min./100 g. in patients with cerebrovascular disease.

In a similar procedure, ^{133}Xe has been substituted for [85]Kr to take advantage of its decay by emission of a soft gamma-ray (Glass and Harper, 1963). Because ^{131}I antipyrine washes out of the brain at a rate similar to those of krypton and xenon and is easier to handle than gases, it has been preferred by some investigators (Oldendorf and Kitano, 1964). However, it does not have the advantage of virtually complete exhalation in a single passage through the lung.

Mallett and Veall (1963) administered ^{133}Xe by inhalation. The subjects inhaled air containing [133]Xe (0.5 mc. per liter) in a closed system; measurements were made over a region of the skull midway between the external auditory meatus and the vertex. After 5 minutes' inhalation, the intake of the system was opened to room air, and at the same time the administration of ^{133}Xe, which is rather rapidly eliminated from the bloodstream, was stopped. The decreasing count rate over the skull was recorded for the next 20 minutes. The curve was divided into two exponential components with half-time values of 1.5 and 10 minutes, believed to correspond to disappearance from cortex and white matter, respectively. It was concluded that the half-time of disappearance was inversely related to the perfusion rate (milliliters per minute per 100 g.), and that the latter could be calculated if relative solubilities in blood and brain were known. The solubility of ^{133}Xe in human blood and brain tissues was measured in vitro at 37° C. Brain-blood partition coefficients in the normal hematocrit range were found to be 0.80 and 1.51 for gray and white matter, respectively (Veall and Mallett, 1965).

Using this procedure, Mallett and Veall observed in 39 normal persons that the cerebral blood flow was only 35 ml./min./100 g., which is not in agreement with results obtained by the nitrous oxide procedure or by carotid injection techniques. Recent findings, however, seem to resolve the problem. They suggest that for the clearance of ^{133}Xe three well defined half-times may be recorded. This was noted for the single human subject studied by Johnson and Gollan (1965). These authors speculated that the three half-times may have been the result of different partition coefficients between the blood and various tissues of the head, as well as different parts of the head, but they made no use of the findings in their analysis of the observed curve. Resolution of the discrepancy between results obtained by the ^{133}Xe inhalation technique and those obtained by the nitrous oxide technique, however, may come from observations of Thompson and Obrist (1966). Studies in 16 normal persons by these investigators indicate that in addition to the two components previously associated with gray and white matter, there is a clearly identifiable, slower component detectable by extracranial monitoring for 40 to 60 minutes. The third (slow) component was attributed to extracerebral tissue. Thompson and Obrist subjected their data to a three compartment analysis (corresponding to gray matter, white matter, and extracerebral tissue), with each compartment corrected for recirculation on the basis of arterial or expired air concentration of the radionuclide. The mean values that were obtained for gray matter, white matter, and extracerebral compartments were 77.5 ± 13.1, 24.8 ± 3.7, and 3.3 ± 0.8 ml./min./100 g., respectively, and the "average" cerebral blood flow for the three compartments combined was 56.0 ± 8.8 ml./min./100 g. These "average" flow values obtained are in excellent agreement with the results obtained by carotid injection and by nitrous oxide techniques.

Although at present these techniques are applicable in few medical centers, in view of the widespread research activity in this area it is predictable that within a few years measurement of regional cerebral blood flow will be a widely accepted procedure. Friedberg has pointed out that it is often rewarding to become familiar with at least the principles involved in research developments during their preclinical state in order to facilitate a more profound understanding and a more critical knowledge of their indications, value, and limitations when they become a part of clinical usage. It is likely that in the not too distant future radioisotopes will be applied on a wide scale to the management of patients with cerebrovascular disease.

Finally, as Hoff and Scott have stated, the value of a new technique is measured not only by the success with which it serves the purpose it was devised for, but also by the manner in which it opens new and hitherto unrealized approaches to research.

REFERENCES

Albert, S. N., Albert, C. A., and Fazekas, J. F.: A Rapid and Simple Method for Measuring the Rate of Cerebral Blood Flow in Humans with Krypton. *J. Lab. Clin. Med.* 56:473, 1960.

Alexander, S. C., Wollman, H., Cohen, P. J., Chase, P. E., Melman, E., and Behard, M.: Krypton-85 and Nitrous Oxide Uptake of the Human Brain during Anesthesia. *Anesthesiology* 25:37, 1964.

Ashkenazy, M., Davis, L., and Martin, J.: Evaluation of Technic and Results of Radioactive Diiodofluorescein Test for Localization of Intracranial Lesions. *J. Neurosurg.* 8:300, 1951.

Bailey, P.: Intracranial Tumors. Charles C Thomas, Springfield, Ill., 1948.

Bauer, F. K., and Yuhl, E. T.: Myelography by Means of I-131. The Myeloscintigram. *Neurology (Minneap.)* 3:341, 1953.

Bell, R. L.: Automatic Contour Myelography in Infants. *J. Nucl. Med.* 3:288, 1962.

Bell, R. L., and Hertsch, G. J.: Automatic Contour Scanner for Myelography. *Int. J. Appl. Radiat.* 7:19, 1959.

Blau, M., and Bender, M. A.: Radiomercury (Hg-203) Labeled Neohydrin: A New Agent for Brain Tumor Localization. *J. Nucl. Med.* (Convention Issue) p. 35, 1959.

Bolliger, T. T., Witcofski, R. L., Whitley, J. E., and Maynard, C. D.: Demonstration of Extracranial Neoplasms with Pertechnetate Tc-99m. *J. Nucl. Med.* 6:687, 1965.

Brinkman, C. A., Wegst, A. V., and Kahn, E. A.: Brain Scanning with Mercury-203-Labeled Neohydrin. *J. Neurosurg.* 19:644, 1962.

Brown, A. J., Scheinberg, L. C., and Zingesser, L.: Serial Scanning in Cerebral Infarction. Presented at 18th Annual Meeting of the American Academy of Neurology, Philadelphia, 1966.

Bucy, P. C., and Ciric, I. S.: Brain Scans in Diagnosis of Brain Tumors. *J.A.M.A.* 191:437, 1965.

Cassen, B., Curtis, L., and Reed, C.: Sensitive Directional Gamma-Ray Detector. *Nucleonics* 6:78, 1950.

Crandall, P. H., and Cassen, B.: Methods for the Study of Cerebral Blood Flow Kinetics with Gamma-Emitting Radioisotopes. *Proc. Int. Conf. Peaceful Uses Atomic Energy* 26:186, 1958.

Crow, H. J., Keogh, C., and Northfield, D. W. C.: Localization of Cerebro-Spinal Fluid Fistulae. *Lancet* 2:325, 1956.

Cushing, H., and Eisenhardt, L.: Meningiomas. Charles C Thomas, Springfield, Ill., 1938.

DiChiro, G.: RISA Encephalography and Conventional Neurologic Methods. *Acta Radiol. (Stockholm)* Suppl. 201, 1961.

DiChiro, G.: Anatomy of the Brain and Basic Principles of Brain Scanning. In Kniseley et al. (eds.): Progress in Medical Radioisotope Scanning. U.S. Atomic Energy Commission (TID-7673), 1962.

DiChiro, G., Reames, P. M., and Matthews, W. B.: RISA-Ventriculography and RISA-Cisternography. *Neurology (Minneap.)* 14:185, 1964.

Elliott, F. A.: Clinical Neurology. W. B. Saunders Co., Philadelphia, 1964.

Fedoruk, S., and Feindel, W.: Measurement of Brain Circulation Time by Radioactive Iodinated Albumin. *Canad. J. Surg.* 3:312, 1960.

Ghouralal, S., Myers, P. W., and Campbell, E.: Persistent Cerebrospinal Rhinorrhea Originating in Fracture through Petrous Bone and Cured by Muscle Graft; Report of Case. *J. Neurosurg.* 13:205, 1956.

Gilson, A. J.: Brain Scanning: Localization of Non-neoplastic Intracranial Lesions. In Recent Advances in Nuclear Medicine. Hahnemann Medical College Symposium, 1966, p. 152.

Gilson, A. J., and Gargano, F. P.: Correlation of Brain Scanning and Angiography in Intracranial Trauma. *Amer. J. Roentgen.* 94:819, 1965.

Glass, H. I., and Harper, A. M.: Measurement of Regional Blood Flow in Cerebral Cortex of Man Through Intact Skull. *Brit. Med. J.* 1:593, 1963.

Grant, F. C.: Notes on Series of Brain Tumors. *J.A.M.A.* 153:22, 1953.

Greitz, T.: A Radiologic Study of the Brain Circulation by Rapid Angiography of the Carotid Artery. *Acta Radiol. (Stockholm)* Suppl. 140, 1956.

Harper, P. V., Beck, R., Charleston, D., and Lathrop, K. A.: Optimization of a Scanning Method Using Tc-99m. *Nucleonics* 22:50, 1964.

Hoefer, P. F. A., Schlesinger, E. B., and Pennes, H. H.: Clinical and Electroencephalographic Findings in Large Series of Verified Brain Tumors. *Trans. Amer. Neurol. Ass.* 71:52, 1946.

Holmes, R. A., Herron, C., and Wagner, H. N., Jr.: A Modified Vertex View in Brain Scanning. *Radiology* 88:498, 1967.

Horrax, G.: Benign (Favorable) Types of Brain Tumors: The End Results (up to 20 Years), with Statistics of Mortality and Useful Survival. *New Eng. J. Med.* 250:981, 1954.

Ingvar, D. H., and Lassen, N. A.: Regional Blood Flow of the Cerebral Cortex Determined by Krypton-85. *Acta Physiol. Scand.* 54:325, 1962.

Johnson, A. E., and Gollan, F.: Cerebral Blood Flow Monitoring by External Detection of Inhaled Radioactive Xenon. *J. Nucl. Med.* 6:679, 1965.

Jungmann, A., and Peyser, E.: Roentgen Visualization of Cerebrospinal Fluid Fistula with Contrast Medium. *Radiology* 80:92, 1963.

Kety, S. S.: Theory of Blood-Tissue Exchange and Its Application to Measurement of Blood Flow. *Meth. Med. Res.* 8:223, 1960.

Kety, S. S., and Schmidt, C. F.: The Determination of Cerebral Blood Flow in Man by the Use of Nitrous Oxide in Low Concentrations. *Amer. J. Physiol.* 143:53, 1945.

Kety, S. S., and Schmidt, C. F.: The Nitrous Oxide Method for the Quantitative Determination of Cerebral Blood Flow in Man; Theory, Procedure and Normal Values. *J. Clin. Invest.* 24:476, 1948a.

Kety, S. S., and Schmidt, C. F.: The Effect of Altered Arterial Tensions of Carbon Dioxide and Oxygen on Cerebral Blood Flow and Cerebral Oxygen Consumption of Normal Young Men. *J. Clin. Invest.* 27:484, 1948b.

Kirchner, F. R., and Proud, G. O.: Method for the Identification and Localization of Cerebro-spinal Fluid, Rhinorrhea and Otorrhea. *Laryngoscope* 70:921, 1960.

Lascelles, R. G., and Burrows, E. H.: Occlusion of the Middle Cerebral Artery. *Brain* 88:85, 1965.

Lassen, N. A., Høedt-Rasmussen, K., Sørensen, S. C., Skinhøj, E., Cronquist, S., Bodfors, B., and Ingvar, D. H.: Regional Cerebral Blood Flow in Man Determined by Krypton-85. *Neurology* 13:719 1963.

Lassen, N. A., and Munck, O.: The Cerebral Blood Flow in Man Determined by the Use of Radioactive Krypton. *Acta Physiol. Scand.* 33:30, 1955.

Ljunggren, K., Nylin, G., Berggren, B., Hedlund, S., and Regnström, O.: Observations on the Determination of Blood Passage Times in Brain by Means of Radioactive Erythrocytes and Externally Placed Detectors. *Int. J. Appl. Radiat.* 12:53, 1961.

Long, R. G., McAfee, J. G., and Winkelman, J.: Evaluation of Radioactive Compounds for the External Detection of Cerebral Tumors. *Cancer Res.* 23:98, 1963.

Mallett, B. L., and Veall, N.: Investigation of Cerebral Blood-Flow in Hypertension, Using Radio-active-Xenon Inhalation and Extracranial Recording. *Lancet* 1:1081, 1963.

Matthews, C. M. E., and Mallard, J. R.: Distribution of 99mTc and Tumor-Brain Concentrations in Rats. *J. Nucl. Med.* 6:404, 1965.

Matthews, C. M. E., and Molinaro, G.: A Study of the Relative Value of Radioactive Substances Used for Brain Tumour Localisation and of the Mechanism of Tumour:Brain Concentration. Uptake in Transplantable Fibrosarcoma, Brain, and Other Organs in the Rat. *Brit. J. Exp. Path.* 44:260, 1963.

McAfee, J. G., Fueger, G. F., Stern, H. S., Wagner, H. N., Jr., and Migita, T.: Tc-99m Per-technetate for Brain Scanning. *J. Nucl. Med.* 5:811, 1964.

McHenry, L. C., and Valsamis, M. P.: Pathophysiology of Cerebrovascular Insufficiency. *Amer. Family Physician* 10:38, 1966.

McLaurin, R. L., and Helmer, F. A.: Errors in Diagnosis of Intracranial Tumors. *J..A.M.A.* 180:1011, 1962.

Mealey, J., Dehner, J. R., and Reese, I. C.: Clinical Comparison of Two Agents Used in Brain Scanning. *J.A.M.A.* 189:260, 1964.

Moersch, F. P., Craig, W. M., and Kernohan, J. W.: Tumors of the Brain in Aged Persons. *Arch. Neurol. Psychiat.* 45:235, 1941.

Moore, G. E.: Fluorescein as an Agent in the Differentiation of Normal and Malignant Tissues. *Science* 106:130, 1947.

Moore, G. E.: Diagnosis and Localization of Brain Tumors: A Clinical and Experimental Study Employing Fluorescent and Radioactive Tracer Methods. Charles C Thomas, Springfield, Ill., 1953.

Moosy, J.: Cerebral Infarction and Intracranial Arterial Thrombosis: Necropsy Studies and Clinical Implications. *Trans. Amer. Neurol. Ass.* 90:113, 1965.

Morrison, R. T., Afifi, A. K., Van Allen, M. W., and Evans, T. C.: Scintiencephalography for Detection and Localization of Non-neoplastic Intracranial Lesions. *J. Nucl. Med.* 6:7, 1965.

Mundinger, F.: Radiobismut (Bi206), seine biologischen Grundlagen und Ergebnisse der Lokali-sation und moglichen Artdiagnose intrabranieller raumverdragender Prozesse. Proc. 2nd Int. Cong. Neurol. Surg., 1961, p. 139.

Nylin, G., Silfverskiöld, B. P., Löfstedt, S., Regnström, O., and Hedlund, S.: Studies on Cerebral Blood Flow in Man, Using Radioactive Labelled Erythrocytes. *Brain* 83:293, 1960.

Oldendorf, W. H.: Measurement of the Mean Transit Time of Cerebral Circulation by External Detection of an Intravenously Injected Radioisotope. *J. Nucl. Med.* 3:382, 1962.

Oldendorf, W. H., and Kitano, M.: The Free Passage of I131 Antipyrine Through Brain as an Indication of A-V Shunting. *Neurology* 14:1078, 1964.

Oldendorf, W. H., and Kitano, M.: Isotope Study of Brain Blood Turnover in Vascular Disease. *Arch. Neurol.* 12:30, 1965.

Overton, M. C., Haynie, T. P., and Snodgrass, S. R.: Brain Scans in Nonneoplastic Intracranial Lesions: Scanning with Chlormerodrin Hg 203 and Chlormerodrin Hg 197. *J.A.M.A.* 191: 431, 1965.

Perryman, C. R., Noble, P. R., and Bragdon, F. H.: Myeloscintigraphy—A Useful Procedure for Localization of Spinal Block Lesions. *Amer. J. Roentgen.* 80:104, 1958.

Pinto, F.: Mieloscintilograma. S. Editora Impregrafica Ltda., Rio de Janeiro, 1962.

Planiol, T., and Akerman, M.: Gamma Encephalography in Supratentorial Arteriovenous Aneurysms: Study of 54 Cases. *Presse Méd.* 73:2205, 1965.

Quinn, J. L.: The Crescent Pattern of Increased Activity in Brain Scanning. Scientific exhibit at the 13th Annual Meeting of the Society of Nuclear Medicine, Philadelphia, June, 1966.

Redlich, F. C., Dunsmore, R. H., and Brody, E. B.: Delays and Errors in the Diagnosis of Brain Tumors. *New Eng. J. Med.* 239:945, 1948.

Reivich, M.: Arterial pCO$_2$ and Cerebral Hemodynamics. *Amer. J. Physiol.* 206:25, 1964.

Rockett, F. X., et al.: Pantopaque Visualization of a Congenital Dural Defect of the Internal Auditory Meatus Causing Rhinorrhea. *Amer. J. Roentgen.* 91:640, 1964.

Scheinberg, P., and Stead, E. A.: The Cerebral Blood Flow in Male Subjects as Measured by the Nitrous Oxide Technique, Normal Values for Blood Flow, Oxygen Utilization, Glucose Utilization, and Peripheral Resistance, with Observations on the Effect of Tilting and Anxiety. *J. Clin. Invest.* 28:1163, 1949.

Schlesinger, E. B., Deboves, S., and Stein, B.: A Means of Evaluating the Efficiency of Shunts. Presented at the 31st Annual Meeting of the Harvey Cushing Society, Philadelphia, April, 1963.

Selverstone, B., Sweet, W. H., and Robinson, C. F.: Clinical Use of Radioactive Phosphorus in the Surgery of Brain Tumors. *Ann. Surg.* 130:643, 1949.

Sodee, D. B.: A New Scanning Isotope, Mercury-197—a Preliminary Report. *J. Nucl. Med.* 4:335, 1963.

Sokoloff, L.: Cerebral Blood Flow Measured with Radioisotopes. *In* Kniseley, R. M., and Tauxe, W. N. (eds.): Dynamic Clinical Studies with Radioisotopes. U.S. Atomic Energy Commission (TID-7678), 1964, p. 153.

Sweet, W. H., Mealey, J., Jr., Brownell, G. L., and Aronow, S.: Coincidence Scanning with Positron-Emitting Arsenic or Copper in the Diagnosis of Focal Intracranial Disease. *In* Medical Radioisotope Scanning. International Atomic Energy Agency, Vienna, 1959.

Takahashi, M., Nofal, M. M., and Beierwaltes, W. H.: Correlation of Point Counting after Brain Tumor Scanning with Scan Image and Pathology. Recent Advances in Nuclear Medicine, Hahnemann Medical College Symposium, 1966, p. 163.

Tator, C. H., Morley, T. P., and Olszweski, J.: Study of Factors Responsible for Accumulation of Radioactive Iodinated Human Serum Albumin (RIHSA) by Intracranial Tumors and Other Lesions. *J. Mount Sinai Hosp. N.Y.* 32:527, 1965.

Teng, P., and Edalatpour, N.: Cerebrospinal Fluid Rhinorrhea with Demonstration of Cranio-nasal Fistula with Pantopaque. *Radiology* 81:802, 1963.

Thompson, H. K., Jr., and Obrist, W. D.: Regional Cerebral Blood Flow by Xenon Inhalation. *Clin. Res.* 14:263, 1966 (Abstr.).

Tow, D. E., and Wagner, H. N., Jr.: Scanning for Tumors of Brain and Bone. *J.A.M.A.* 199:104, 1967.

Veall, N., and Mallett, B. L.: The Partition of Trace Amounts of Xenon Between Human Blood and Brain Tissues at 37° C. *Phys. Med Biol.* 10:375, 1965.

Webber, M. M.: Technetium-99m Normal Brain Scans and Their Anatomic Features. *Amer. J. Roentgen.* 94:815, 1965.

Wolff, J.: Transport of Iodide and Other Anions in the Thyroid Gland. *Physiol. Rev.* 44:45, 1964.

Zülch, K. J.: Brain Tumors, Their Biology and Pathology. Ed. 2. Springer Publishing Co., New York, 1965.

CHAPTER XV

THE SKELETON[1]

NORMAN F. MOON

INTRODUCTION

Although it has been known for many years that certain radioactive materials accumulate in the skeleton, it has been only recently that this principle has been put to clinical use. Investigators have used radionuclides to evaluate bone vascularity, investigate metabolic bone diseases, and detect bone tumors. The aim has been to develop simple methods for detection of nonunion of fractures, aseptic necrosis of bone, primary or metastatic bone tumors, and metabolic bone diseases, and possibly for the treatment of neoplastic lesions.

During the period of 1917 to 1925, hundreds of people ingested or inhaled significant amounts of radium, mesothorium, and radiothorium while painting luminous watch dials (Looney, 1954). The radioactive substances concentrated within the skeletal system and eventually led to bone necrosis and osteomyelitis. The deposition was mainly in the mandible, and the disease became known as "radium jaw" (Blum, 1924; Hoffman, 1925). A high incidence (27 per cent) of osteogenic sarcomas in a series of 18 deaths in former dial painters has been reported, and it has been concluded that 0.5 microgram of radium is dangerous (Martland and Humphries, 1929; Martland, 1931). The sarcomas were found to occur in areas of radiation osteitis.

Among the early used bone-seeking radionuclides were oral and parenteral radium chloride in treatment of patients with hypertension, arthritis, gout neuri-

[1] Supported by grants from the University of Michigan Cancer Research Institute (#06090 and #37278) and the Michigan Memorial–Phoenix Project (#37375).

tis, and gout (1915 to 1930), and thorium dioxide (1930 to 1945) in radiographic studies (Looney, 1954). The long-term effects of several radionuclides (^{226}Ra, ^{239}Pu, ^{228}Ra [MsTh$_1$], ^{228}Th [RdTh], and ^{90}Sr) are still being investigated in experimental animals (Dougherty et al., 1962), the aim being to provide information about the maximum permissible levels of these radionuclides.

Bone tissue consists of a combination of organic and inorganic constituents; both are capable of being labeled. The organic matrix consists of osteoid, cells, and ground substance. Radiocerium and radiogallium have been found to deposit in the osteoid tissue; radiosulfur labels the chondroitin sulfuric acid of the ground substance. Bone mineral is a hydroxyapatite crystal; the main constituent is calcium phosphate, although hydroxyl and carbonate ions are also present. Radium, an alkaline-earth metal, exchanges with calcium in bone and remains there because of the low rate of turnover of calcium in mature bone mineral (Rowland, 1960). Several other alkaline-earth radionuclides, including radiostrontium and radiobarium, have also been used to replace calcium within the crystalline lattice.

The original radioisotope tracer investigation of bone was by Chiewitz and Hevesy (1935). They used radiophosphorus (^{32}P), which labels the phosphate moiety of hydroxyapatite. In adult rats, the largest portion of the isotope was found to deposit within the bones.

RADIONUCLIDES USED TO STUDY BONE

BARIUM

Barium-140 emits beta (0.48 Mev.) and gamma (0.306 to 0.540 Mev.) radiation. The half-life is 12.8 days. Bauer and associates (1957) administered intramuscularly 2 to 3 microcuries of ^{140}BaCl$_2$ per kilogram body weight. The bone accretion rate with ^{140}Ba was found to be greater than with ^{45}Ca. The investigators concluded that ^{140}Ba is suitable for use as an indicator of skeletal metabolism in man.

CALCIUM

Calcium-45 is a pure beta-emitter (0.254 Mev.) with a half-life of 164 days. It decays to stable scandium-45, is relatively inexpensive, and is easily obtainable. Pecher (1942) administered radiocalcium intravenously into experimental animals. The highest concentrations of radioactivity were found in areas of new bone formation (roots of teeth, epiphyseal line, or fracture sites). Heaney and Whedon (1958) performed ^{45}Ca tracer studies in adult humans. The normal rate of incorporation into bone was estimated at 9 mg. calcium per kilogram body weight per day.

Calcium-47 is of greater importance in clinical investigation because it is a gamma-emitter and may be detected externally. The half-life is short (4.7 days), and it emits a high-energy gamma-ray (1.31 Mev.), as well as beta-rays and other gamma-rays. Corey and associates (1961b) have described the production of ^{47}Ca by neutron bombardment of ^{46}Ca, a naturally occurring isotope with an abundance of 0.003 per cent. The ^{46}Ca is enriched by electromagnetic separation. After irradiation of $CaCO_3$, the product is dissolved in 0.01N HCl and made up to 20 ml. with 0.9 per cent saline solution and sterilized. The dosages in man range from 20 to 40 microcuries.

CERIUM

The rare-earth elements have been shown to concentrate in the organic or osteoid matrix of forming bone. The elements investigated have been lanthanum, cerium, praseodymium, neodymium, promethium, samarium, and europium (Baserga, 1959). Of this group, a radionuclide of cerium ([144]Ce) has been used most frequently because of its availability and relatively inexpensive cost. Radiocerium has a half-life of 282 days. It emits mainly beta radiation (0.17 and 0.3 Mev.). The isotope has been studied with autoradiographs and is thought to be bound to bone or cartilage when the organic matrix enters the calcifiable state (Asling et al., 1957). The isotope is not recommended for clinical use because it accumulates in the liver and may induce acute liver atrophy (Brues, 1950).

GALLIUM

Radiogallium ([72]Ga) concentrates in the regions of both osteogenic and osteolytic lesions. Dudley and Maddox (1949) found its deposition in osteoid tissues of the rabbit and dog. It is especially concentrated at the epiphyseal junction, in fracture callus, and in osteogenic sarcoma tissue (Dudley et al., 1950). Its concentration in malignant tumors has been reported to be about 20 times that in normal bone (Mulry and Dudley, 1951). Gallium-72 has a half-life of 14.2 hours and emits beta and gamma radiation. External counting techniques with [72]Ga have been used in patients with bone lesions and tumors (Desgrez et al., 1954; Dudley et al., 1956). Van der Werff (1954) did a similar study with nuclides [66]Ga and [67]Ga. Gallium-72 is considered unsuitable for therapeutic use in bone malignancies because of undesirable total-body irradiation even at subtherapeutic dosage levels and because of chemical toxicity (Brucer et al., 1953).

Investigative use of ^{68}Ga, a positron-emitter, has shown promise in human bone scanning. Hayes and associates (1965) have described the preparation of the nuclide from a Brookhaven National Laboratory [68]Ge-^{68}Ga generator. A distinct advantage of this generator system is the long half-life (280 days) of its parent, [68]Ge. The ^{68}Ga decays mainly by positron emission with associated 0.15 Mev. annihilation radiation. Its short half-life of 1.13 hours allows advantages similar to those of ^{18}F and [87m]Sr. Unfortunately, to obtain satisfactory bone scans, stable gallium must be added as a carrier to produce rapid clearance of ^{68}Ga from tissues other than bone.

Ahumada et al. (1965) have used ^{68}Ga citrate in 49 skeletal scans of 41 patients with known or suspected bone lesions. As with other bone scanning agents, it was possible to demonstrate metastatic bone lesions with ^{68}Ga scans before roentgenologic detection (Fig. 15-1). A dosage of 4 mg. per kg. of stable gallium carrier was found to improve the scan. Edwards and associates (1966) have more recently reported 56 ^{68}Ga skeletal scans performed on 46 patients with known or suspected skeletal lesions. In 13 patients, positive findings on

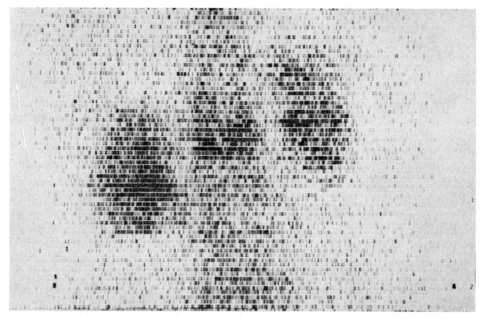

FIGURE 15-1.   Scan of the lumbar vertebrae obtained 30 minutes after an intravenous dose of 6 mc. of ⁶⁸Ga citrate with 2 mg. per kg. carrier. The area of increased radioactivity corresponds to the second lumbar vertebra, which on x-ray was demonstrated to have an osteolytic lesion. (From Ahumada et al., 1965.)

the scans corresponded to known or subsequently demonstrated skeletal lesions. Besides metastatic bone lesions, positive scans were found in fractures, myelofibrosis with osteosclerosis, and inflammatory or degenerative arthritis.

GOLD

Edwards and associates (1964) have used colloidal ¹⁹⁸Au for bone marrow scanning in 29 patients with a variety of bone marrow disorders, including metastatic disease. The dosage range was 1 to 3.5 millicuries, with 2.5 millicuries the most frequently used dosage. The intravenously administered dose gives an absorbed marrow dose of 18 rads. The particles are rapidly removed from the blood stream by the reticuloendothelial cells. Colloidal ¹⁹⁹Au has also been used. The high absorbed radiation dose from both gold nuclides is a serious drawback, although there were no early radiation effects among the patients. The investigators concluded that bone marrow scanning could become a practical clinical procedure.

IODINE

Becchini and associates (1964) have described the use of radioiodinated (¹³¹I) fibrinogen for the investigation of bone tumors. This material was given to 43 patients with diseases of the bones, including 19 with malignant tumors, 13 with benign tumors and dysplastic conditions, and 11 with inflammatory conditions. The dosage was 5 microcuries per kilogram of body weight. Localized concentrations were obtained in 16 of the 19 malignant tumors, in none of the benign or dysplastic conditions, and in 10 of 11 cases of inflammatory processes.

The use of ^{131}I human serum albumin for scanning human tumors has been described (Hisada et al., 1966). The investigators gave 1 millicurie of ^{131}I HSA to 12 patients with tumors. Positive scans were found in a variety of lesions, including an osteolytic femoral metastasis secondary to pulmonary carcinoma and a case of giant cell tumor of the femur. The radiation exposure ($>$ 1 rad) was considered too great for the procedure to be used routinely.

Weiss and associates (1965) have performed scans of joints after the intravenous injection of ^{131}I human serum albumin (I HAS) in patients with rheumatoid arthritis, osteoarthritis, and gout. They found greater localization of the ^{131}I HSA in actively involved joints than in clinically normal joints. The investigators believed that joint scanning and counting may prove to be an objective means for determination of the degree or, in some cases, the type of arthritic activity.

PHOSPHORUS

Phosphorus-32 is a beta-emitter with radiation energy of 1.707 Mev. The half-life is 14.3 days; it decays to stable sulfur-32. The isotope is inexpensive and readily available in the chemical form of $Na_2H^{32}PO_4$. The deposition of this material in normal bone crystal is a function of the alkaline-glycerophosphatase activity (Woodard and Kenney, 1942).

In animal studies, radiophosphorus has been found in increased concentration at a fracture site (Bohr and Sørensen, 1950). Bauer (1954) studied the distribution of ^{32}P in the skeleton as a function of skeletal growth. Armstrong (1955), using ^{32}P tracer techniques in rabbits, observed a slightly greater than 25 per cent turnover in femoral and tibial epiphyses at 50 days. Castle and associates (1964) have found 20.5 per cent skeletal uptake in patients after orally administered radiophosphorus; the intravenously administered radionuclide uptake averaged 32.7 per cent. The ^{32}P uptake in malignant bone tumors has been found to be considerably greater than in benign bone tumors (Justus, 1961).

STRONTIUM

Useful strontium radionuclides include ^{85}Sr, ^{87m}Sr, ^{89}Sr, and ^{90}Sr. Of these, the gamma-emitting nuclides, ^{85}Sr and ^{87m}Sr, are most important as they can be measured by external detectors, such as scanners. Strontium-85 has a half-life of 64 days and decays to stable rubidium-85. It emits a single gamma photon of 0.51 Mev. Following administration, the radiostrontium not excreted becomes fixed to the skeleton. It has been estimated that a 50 microcurie dose of ^{85}Sr delivers 0.326 rad to the total body and 2.28 rads to bone (Fleming et al., 1961).

Charkes and associates (1964) and Meckelnburg (1964) have described the production and use of ^{87m}Sr in scanning techniques. The advantage of ^{87m}Sr over ^{85}Sr is its short half-life (2.8 hours). The radionuclide decays by emission of a single gamma photon of 0.388 Mev. to stable ^{87}Sr. The considerably shorter half-life not only reduces the radiation hazard, but also allows repeated doses at frequent intervals. Strontium-87m may be safely used not only in nonmalig-

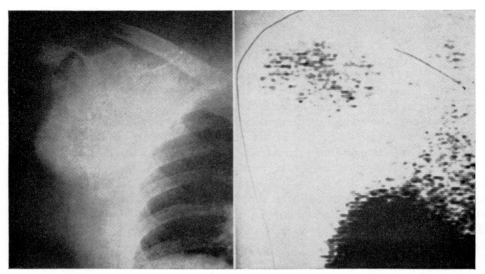

FIGURE 15-2.   Roentgenogram of the right shoulder of a 54 year old man with a rapidly growing chondrosarcoma. The scan was obtained 24 hours after the administration of 150 μc. of ^{75}Se. (From Esteban et al., 1965.)

nant bone disorders, but also in children. The disadvantages of ^{87m}Sr include (1) the short half-life of its yttrium-87 parent; (2) the cost of the generator, which must be renewed every 2 to 3 weeks; and (3) the time-consuming milking and sterilization process in comparison with the ease of handling a multiple dose radiopharmaceutical preparation such as ^{85}Sr nitrate.

Strontium metabolism simulates that of calcium. As an alkaline-earth substitute for calcium in the bone crystal, strontium radionuclides have been used in the clinical investigation of a number of bone disorders. Its use in detection of neoplastic processes will be discussed in detail later in the chapter. Mac-Donald (1960) found the uptake of radiostrontium into cortical bone to be slower in patients with osteoporosis than in normal subjects. Its retention within the skeletal system also is less in these patients (Van Dilla and Arnold, 1956). Cohn and associates (1962) have used whole-body counting techniques to determine the turnover of ^{85}Sr. Increased radiostrontium uptake has been found in infections (Dymling and Wendeberg, 1965), fractures (Wendeberg, 1961), Paget's disease (Klein and Lund, 1964), coxarthrosis (Danielsson et al., 1963), spondylitis (Bauer and Scoccianti, 1961), and various other malignant and non-malignant bone disorders (Rosenthall, 1965).

SULFUR

The use of radiosulfur (^{35}S) in the chemical form of sulfate as a bone-seeking nuclide is limited to lesions of cartilaginous nature; it has been demonstrated by autoradiographic techniques to localize in areas of metabolic synthesis of chondroitin sulfuric acid (Brondolo and Randelli, 1962). Localization is presumably by exchange with sulfate ion within the ground substance of bone. Sulfur-35 is a beta-emitter with an energy of 0.167 Mev. The half-life is 87.1 days, and the nuclide decays to chlorine-35. Radioactive sulfate has been found

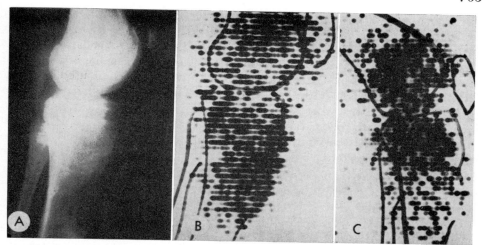

FIGURE 15-3. Fifteen year old white female with a proved poorly differentiated fibrosarcoma. A, Roentgenogram shows the primary lesion in the proximal tibia; B, ^{99m}Tc scan shows uptake in the distal femur and proximal tibia; C, ^{85}Sr scan in the same projection shows a similar pattern of uptake at the knee, but there is relatively less uptake in the tumor. (From Whitley et al., 1966.)

to be selectively retained in chondrosarcoma, chondroma, and normal cartilage, as well as in reparative connective tissue and bone (Gottschalk, 1960).

Radioselenium (^{75}Se) has been used as a substitute for radiosulfur in labeling cartilaginous tumors (Esteban et al., 1965). Selenium-75 has a half-life of 127 days. Scanning techniques may be used since the radionuclide disintegrates by electron capture with a gamma-photon spectrum between 0.136 and 0.280 Mev. Scanning is performed 24 hours after intravenous administration (Fig. 15-2).

TECHNETIUM

Whitley and associates (1966) have performed successful bone scans with technetium-99m. This nuclide is produced in the chemical form of pertechnetate from a ^{99}Mo-^{99m}Tc generator. Twenty-six patients with a variety of proved tumor lesions were given 3 to 5 mc. of ^{99m}Tc pertechnetate intravenously; 17 positive scans were obtained. Of these patients, 2 had metastatic bone lesions, 1 had primary fibrosarcoma of the tibia (Fig. 15-3), 1 had Ewing's sarcoma of the pubis, and 1 had chordoma of the sacrum. Scans were positive in the first 3 and negative in the other 2. Because the half-life is 6 hours, and because of the absence of beta emissions, relatively large doses may be administered and yet the patient's radiation dose is kept to reasonable levels.

DIAGNOSIS OF BONE TUMORS

The gamma-emitting bone-seeking nuclides are used for diagnosis of bone tumors by scanning techniques. Of the various available isotopes, ^{47}Ca, ^{85}Sr, ^{87m}Sr, and ^{18}F appear to be most promising. With beta-emitting nuclides, open biopsies are necessary.

Bauer and Wendeberg (1959) studied the distribution of [47]Ca and [85]Sr in 75 patients. The activity was high over skeletal lesions such as fracture, metastatic cancer, eosinophilic granuloma, chondroma, osteomyelitis, and Paget's disease. The high uptake was interpreted as evidence of an increased rate of turnover of bone tissue. Corey and associates (1961a, b, 1962) used scanning techniques with [47]Ca and [85]Sr. Primary bone tumors and active bone metastases concentrated nuclides to a greater extent than did the corresponding uninvolved bone. The rate of accretion was high in patients with active lesions and normal in those with arrested lesions. Intravenous doses of [47]Ca or [85]Sr were given to 6 patients with suspected bone metastases from carcinoma of the breast. Two patients had increased uptake of radionuclide in painful areas of the thoracic spine, although the roentgenograms revealed no bony lesions. Both patients later were found to have metastatic involvement in these areas.

Brady and associates (1962) gave 40 to 60 microcuries of [47]Ca to nine patients with osteolytic metastatic lesions, and found accumulation in all except two patients. Tamvakopoulos and associates (1963) gave 30 microcuries to patients and followed them for a period of 2 weeks. Radioactivity again was found higher in areas with fractures or bone tumors. Abnormal ratios ranged from 1.2 to 6.0 in metastatic tumor and as high as 16 in certain fractures.

Sargent and associates (1964) studied [47]Ca turnover in patients by means of a whole-body counter. Increased isotope turnover was found in patients with metastatic disease as well as in patients with acromegaly. Cederquist (1964) made similar studies in 16 patients, 8 with various malignant diseases of the skeleton. Intravenous doses of less than 1 microcurie of [85]Sr and [47]Ca were given, and measurements were then made in a whole-body counter. Differences of isotope distribution were determined in normal persons and patients with metastases. The investigator believes that this method may be of differential diagnostic value, as well as useful in the evaluation of therapy.

Treadwell and associates (1942) used radiostrontium for investigation of bone metastases from breast and prostatic carcinoma. The greatest uptake was in growing bone and osteogenic tumor tissue. Gynning, Waldeskog, and associates (1961, 1962) used 50 microcuries of [85]Sr, administered intravenously, in the study of metastatic carcinoma of the breast in 90 patients. The investigators concluded that the procedure is of value in the routine examination of patients with carcinoma of the breast, because metastases were occasionally demonstrated before they were seen on roentgenograms. DeNardo and Volpe (1966) concluded from their series of 164 bone scans that it is particularly useful in the early diagnosis of osteomyelitis and metastases, and in differentiating bone islands from osteoblastic metastases.

Kofman and associates (1963) used a similar technique to evaluate vertebral metastases. A scan of the vertebral column for C7 to L5 was performed one week after the intravenous injection of 20 to 60 microcuries of [85]Sr. Patients with mixed or osteoblastic metastases had greater [85]Sr uptake than normal subjects; those with osteolytic metastases demonstrated normal or increased uptake. Following therapy, changes in [85]Sr uptake could be demonstrated within 1 to 2 weeks.

Simpson and Orange (1965) performed total-body scans with [85]Sr to aid in the diagnosis of metastatic bone disease. Two hundred microcuries of [85]Sr was given to 46 patients who complained of skeletal pain, but whose radiographs were negative. The dose was given intravenously, and the total-body scan was performed 48 hours later. Positive scans were obtained in 34 patients, 20 of whom were subsequently shown to have metastases; 3 did not have skeletal metastases a year or more later; a final evaluation was not possible in the other 11. Twelve patients had negative scans; 3 ultimately developed metastases, 6 did not, and the outcome in the other 3 was inconclusive. When possible, auto-radiographs were performed and it was observed that nuclide deposition occurred in the reactive bone associated with the malignant deposits.

Sklaroff and Charkes (1963 to 1966) have made more than 350 [85]Sr bone scans in cancer patients suspected of having metastatic bone lesions. Their protocol is presented in Table 15-1. In about 21 per cent of their studies, the scan was abnormal despite normal roentgenologic appearance. Positive open biopsy confirmation was obtained in 21 of 26 cases. In 4 cases, positive biopsies were obtained in areas of positive scan but negative roentgenologic evidence of metastases (Fig. 15-4).

Charkes, Sklaroff, and Bierly (1964) used ionic [87m]Sr to detect metastatic bone lesions. They administered [87m]Sr to 16 patients, including 7 with metastatic lesions to bone and 4 with primary bone tumors. Except in 2 patients with eosinophilic granuloma, the scans confirmed the radiographic lesions. These authors concluded that the isotope is useful in detecting metastatic lesions before changes become apparent roentgenologically, in evaluating nonmalignant bone diseases in children, and in following the osteogenic response to therapy of bone diseases.

Blau and associates (1962) introduced ^{18}F for bone scanning to avoid the disadvantages of the other nuclides: the high gamma energy of [47]Ca and the long half-life of [85]Sr. The high specificity of ^{18}F for bone makes it an excellent bone-seeking nuclide. In tracer amounts, the radionuclide either goes to bone or is excreted by the kidneys in approximately equal amounts. The fluoride ion pre-

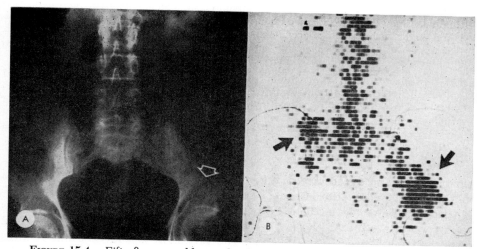

FIGURE 15-4. Fifty-five year old man developed pneumonia and back pain owing to collapse of D5. Carcinoma was suspected but bronchial washings were negative for tumor. A, Bone survey roentgenogram of pelvis was thought to be normal but B, [85]Sr scan revealed "hot spots" in left ilium and right sacroiliac joint (arrows). Biopsy of the left iliac lesion showed anaplastic carcinoma. In retrospect, the "washed-out" appearance above the left acetabulum (arrow) is a radiolucent metastasis. (From Charkes et al., 1966.)

TABLE 15-1. PROTOCOL FOR DETECTION OF OCCULT METASTATIC CARCINOMA
TO BONE BY PHOTOSCANNING WITH ^{85}SR*

1. Purpose: Because calcium content of bone must decrease by 30 to 50 per cent before roentgenographic changes become visible, and because lesions smaller than 1 cm. are difficult to visualize, conventional roentgenographic techniques often fail to detect metastatic cancer in bone. Strontium, which is metabolized by bone in a manner similar to calcium, accumulates in areas of tumor-laden bone in greater concentration than in normal bone, and this can be demonstrated by the photoscanning technique. Strontium-85, a pure gamma-emitter (0.513 Mev.), is well suited for the photoscanning process.

2. Isotope: ^{85}Sr in ionic state.

3. Dose: 100 microcuries I.V. (20 microcuries in children under 20).

4. Time of scanning: Anytime after 1 hour following injection. However, because extra-osseous ^{85}Sr is slowly excreted via urine and feces, a delay of 48 to 72 hours is advisable, if possible.

5. Setting the scanner: Set window to straddle 0.513 Mev. photopeak on pulse-height analyzer. To find appropriate cutoff and contrast factors, place detector (use 19 hole collimator) over a joint being scanned (sacroiliac for pelvis, shoulder for upper chest, knee for leg)—this establishes maximum count rate. To find minimum count rate, place probe over a nonosseous area, such as the loin.

6. Scanning: A line spacing of 0.5 cm. is satisfactory, with scanning speed of 16 to 18 cm./min. since count rate is usually less than 1000 counts/min.

7. Position: When scanning pelvis, patient should be *prone*. In scanning lower extremity it is advisable to include both legs on scan for comparison.

8. Preparation for pelvis and lumbar spine scans: Laxative (e.g., magnesia, 45 ml.) night before scan; high enemas until clear on day of scan; void just before scanning.

9. Localization: Following scanning, two separate marks are made on the skin, and scan is blackened in these areas. Lead shots are then placed on skin marks and a 6 foot *supine* recumbent roentgenogram taken. Scan is then superimposed on roentgenogram, lining up markers as closely as possible. Outline of pelvis, extremity, or skull should be traced on scan with grease pencil for ease of interpretation.

10. Interpretation: Using this method, ^{85}Sr deposition in bone is visualized. Increased strontium deposition is normally noted about certain joints, particularly the sacroiliac articulation, and also in region of acetabula, glenoid fossa, and femoral and tibial condyles. Abnormal ^{85}Sr deposition is engrafted upon this pattern. Normal pattern of ^{85}Sr deposition must be appreciated to correctly interpret the scan.

11. Pitfalls in interpretation: (1) Strontium-85 in colon, particularly in cecum, will be visualized unless patient has been thoroughly prepared with laxative and enemas. (2) Diffuse involvement of all vertebrae may be missed by this method. (3) Increased ^{85}Sr deposition is not specific for tumor.

* Method of N. David Charkes, M.D., and David M. Sklaroff, M.D.

sumably is fixed to the surface of the bone crystal by an exchange with hydroxyl ion, forming a fluorapatite lattice (Posner et al., 1963).

Radiofluorine emits a 0.65 Mev. positron and has a half-life of 109.3 minutes (Armstrong et al., 1958). The estimated dose per millicurie administered is 0.12 rad to the bone (Dworkin et al., 1966). The very short half-life not only reduces the body radiation hazard, but also allows multiple tracer investigations in the same person. On the other hand, because of the short half-life, its clinical use must be close to its source of production.

Of the several methods of radiofluorine production, the most practical method utilizes the bombardment of stable ^{6}Li with a neutron source. The reactions are as follows:

$$^6_3\text{Li} + {_0}\text{n} \rightarrow {^4_2}\text{He} + {^3_1}\text{H} \tag{1}$$

$$^3_1\text{H} + {^{16}_8}\text{O} \rightarrow {_0}\text{n} + {^{18}_9}\text{F} \tag{2}$$

The yield is 2×10^{-5} ^{18}F nuclei per triton produced from the lithium. The radionuclide is carrier free (Bernstein and Katz, 1953). Another method of producing sterile, carrier-free ^{18}F has been described by Nusynowitz and associates (1965).

LaFleur and associates (1966) have modified the method of Bernstein and Katz (1953) in producing radiofluorine suitable for oral or parenteral administration (Table 15-2). On repeated determinations, the level of lithium has ranged from 50 to 70 ppm, and lanthanum has ranged less than 1 to 2 ppm. Both are well below toxic amounts. Tritium contamination has been negligible, and radiosodium amounts to less than 0.05 per cent of activity, well within safe levels. Strict precautions must be observed to minimize radioactive contamination.

Blau and associates (1962) have reported good visualization with ^{18}F scans in 18 patients. Most of these patients had metastatic bone disease, both osteo-

TABLE 15-2. PROTOCOL FOR PRODUCTION OF STERILE RADIOFLUORINE*

1. All chemicals and equipment used in the production of radiofluorine are autoclaved and handled in a sterile manner. Sterile gloves are used during the procedure, and sterile surgical sheets are used to drape a clean radioisotope laboratory space. The laboratory area should have an appropriate hood.

2. Six to 8 g. of $LiNO_3$ is irradiated in an atomic reactor for a period of 3 hours.

3. Under sterile conditions, the irradiated salt is dissolved in distilled water and boiled for 1 minute.

4. The solution is cooled in an ice bath and divided between two 40 ml. centrifuge tubes.

5. About 15 mg. lanthanum perchloride carrier is added to each centrifuge tube; 1 drop of 0.1 per cent phenolphthalein indicator solution is added, and NaOH is added until the solution turns red.

6. The precipitate is centrifuged for about 1 minute.

7. The supernatant is decanted into another 40 ml. centrifuge tube, and the precipitate is dissolved in about 1 ml. 6N HCl.

8. Steps 5 and 6 are repeated, and the second supernatant is discarded.

9. The four lanthanum hydroxide precipitates are combined. The ^{18}F is carried on this precipitate.

10. Sodium hydroxide is added until the solution just turns red.

11. About 1 ml. of hydrochloric acid is then added.

12. The solution is passed through a Bio-rad cation exchange resin AG 50-X8 column, and the eluent is collected.

13. The eluent is made just alkaline with NaOH and evaporated to dryness to remove any remaining tritium.

14. The salts (NaCl and carrier-free Na^{18}F) are dissolved in about 25 ml. of sterile water and filtered through a bacterial filter into a sterile injection bottle. A dosage of 500 to 750 microcuries is appropriate for human scanning techniques.

* Method of Philip D. LaFleur, M.S., of the Michigan Memorial–Phoenix Project.

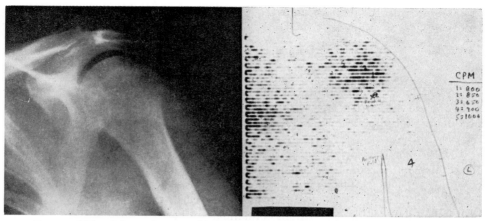

FIGURE 15-5.   Fifty-eight year old white man was seen for painless hematuria 9 months previously. Shortly afterward, a right nephrectomy was performed for renal cell carcinoma. Eight months later, a roentgenogram of the left shoulder demonstrated an osteolytic lesion of the humeral head. Fluorine-18 scan demonstrated heavy uptake in the involved area.

lytic and osteoblastic, although fibrous dysplasia and disuse osteoporosis lesions were also visualized in several patients. Two patients with metastatic bone lesions were found to have uptake of fluoride in areas where no lesions were present roentgenologically.

Dworkin, Moon, and associates (1966) have investigated the experimental and clinical uses of radiofluorine in bone scanning. The nuclide was used in 38 patients with a variety of bone disorders. Positive photoscanning was found in patients with benign bone tumors, malignant bone tumors, metastatic bone lesions (Fig. 15-5), and aseptic necrosis of bone. Patients with rheumatoid spondylitis, Engelmann's disease, and soft tissue sarcomas showed no evidence of increased nuclide uptake. In view of the report of negative ^{85}Sr photoscans in patients with reticulum cell sarcomas (Charkes and Sklaroff, 1964), it is noteworthy that these investigators found positive accumulation of ^{18}F in this disease.

Moon, Dworkin, et al. (1966) administered radiofluorine in doses ranging from 350 to 750 microcuries to their series of 38 patients. Although 750 micro-curies was found ideal for scanning, diagnostic scans were produced at the lower dosages. The radionuclide was given either intravenously or orally. At all dosages, neither adverse symptoms nor signs were noted. Optimal scans are produced beginning 1 hour following nuclide administration.

Van Dyke and associates (1965) have described the use of the positron camera for rapid bone scanning with radiofluorine. These investigators have demonstrated its successful use in cases of Paget's disease, healed fractures (3 years postfracture), and nonunion of fractures (2 to 3 years). The use of the positron camera has also been described by Schaer (1966) in a case of fibrous dysplasia of the skull.

Fluorine-18 and strontium-87m are the best nuclides now available for use in bone scanning. The radiation hazard is less than from routine roentgenographic studies. The isotopes have a high specificity for bone mineral. They decay rapidly, and are rapidly excreted by the kidneys. Although a variety of bone disorders may be successfully diagnosed, the technique is most likely to be useful in the osteogenic series of primary bone tumors. The extent of bone involvement can be assessed since reactive bone formation occurs at the edges of the tumor.

USE OF RADIONUCLIDES IN STUDY OF BONE VIABILITY

Aseptic necrosis or devitalization of bone leads to high morbidity among affected patients, who develop pain, restricted joint motion, and instability. The problem is closely related to nonunion of traumatic fractures, although a similar process called osteochondrosis is occasionally found in certain bones. Both systemic and local factors may lead to a localized form of aseptic necrosis, such as involvement of the femoral head by caisson disease, corticosteroids, and irradiation; in some cases there is no apparent cause (Patterson et al., 1964). Disruption of the blood supply is the usual basis of aseptic necrosis, and the term "avascular necrosis" is preferred by some.

In 1931, Smith-Petersen and associates reported the successful treatment of intracapsular hip fractures by internal fixation. A considerable proportion of the patients had nonunion, presumably with aseptic necrosis of the femoral head. Despite over 30 years of improved surgical techniques, the problem of necrosis of the femoral head following femoral neck fractures remains. For example, follow-up studies of 1485 patients with femoral neck fractures treated by internal fixation were accumulated from 100 orthopedic surgeons and reported by the Fracture Committee of the American Academy of Orthopaedic Surgeons (1939). Of this series, 46 patients developed necrosis of the femoral head and another 127 developed necrosis or absorption of the femoral neck. Such disappointing numbers of patients with necrosis have also been reported in later series.

The clinical diagnosis of aseptic necrosis is usually made by roentgenological studies, although the abnormality may not show for as long as a year after fracture, even though the vascular injury is at the moment of fracture. Because of the increasing number of aged persons in our population, many of whom will sustain hip fractures, there is a need for means of early diagnosis of avascularity, instead of permitting increased morbidity in patients by watchful waiting. Hulth (1965) has summarized various means of viability determination. Included has been a large amount of investigative work performed with radionuclides in the attempt to solve this problem.

Tucker (1950) originally reported the use of radiophosphorus in the diagnosis of avascular necrosis of the femoral head. He gave 150 to 200 microcuries of ^{32}P intravenously to patients before internal fixation of femoral neck fractures. Bone specimens from the greater trochanter and femoral head were removed at the time of surgery. He concluded that satisfactory healing took place when the trochanter-to-head ratio was 3:1, whereas a ratio of 10:1 was evidence of avascular necrosis.

Arden and Veall (1953) used similar investigative techniques in 45 patients. One to two milliliters of sterile isotonic buffered phosphate solution containing approximately 200 microcuries ^{32}P was given 1 hour before hip nailing. Five out of 16 patients had definitely abnormal ratios (7:1 to 30:1). Spurious results occurred because of (1) contamination of the bone specimen by radioactive blood; (2) too long an interval between isotope administration and sample

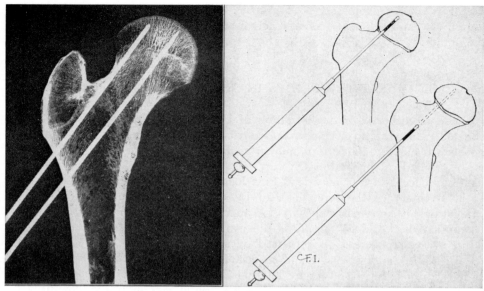

FIGURE 15-6. *Left,* The uptake of the femoral head should be recorded in the area of the superior guide wire. Satisfactory data may also be recorded if the end of the guide wire extends to the subchondral bone plate or penetrates it from 1 to 2 mm. *Right,* The darkened area of the probe is in its sensitive portion. Since the head and trochanteric counts are taken in the same wire track, either count may be repeated if desired. (From Boyd and Calandruccio, 1963.)

removal; (3) variations in samples from different parts of the femoral head; and (4) delay between removal of specimens, since the ^{32}P content of bone steadily rises. In a later report (Arden, 1960), 61 cases were analyzed. These patients were followed at least 2 years. In 50 patients with displaced femoral neck fractures, 28 had low trochanter-to-head ratios, but only 23 (82 per cent) had union of fracture. Primarily because of the technical difficulties and poor clinical correlation, the method was not believed of practical value, a conclusion that Bloch and George (1962) also reached.

In 1955, Boyd and associates reported their clinical study of ^{32}P for determination of femoral head viability in 53 patients. Two microcuries ^{32}P per pound body weight was administered intravenously. The ideal time for measurement was 1 to 1.5 hours after injection. Of various hip problems, higher trochanter-to-head ratios were found in patients with femoral neck fractures (Fig. 15-6). A later report (Boyd and Calandruccio, 1963) was made upon 2 year follow-up of 95 patients with displaced femoral neck fractures. The critical ratio of trochanter-to-head was 4.0. Of the 43 patients with ratios less than 4.0, 33 (about 75 per cent) healed well; avascular necrosis developed in 10. Of the 52 patients with ratios more than 4.0, 13 healed well, but 39 (about 75 per cent) developed avascular necrosis. The authors believed that radiophosphorus uptake studies were of prognostic value in two thirds of patients with displaced fractures of the neck of the femur.

Stein and associates (1956) have carried out a similar study. More recently (1963) they studied the circulation of the femoral head in dogs. Radiophosphorus-labeled diisopropyl fluorophosphonate (DF^{32}P) was given to adult mongrel dogs. Isotope uptake was measured by a fixed Robinson-Selverstone probe, and autoradiographs of the control and treated hips were compared. The surgery consisted of (1) total capsulotomy of the hip; (2) capsulotomy and section of the ligamentum teres; and (3) capsulotomy and femoral neck transection. In other dogs the hip was not operated on. Dogs with total capsulotomy and sectioning of ligamentum teres had a decrease in circulation. There was a severe impairment of circulation in dogs subjected to total capsulotomy and femoral neck section.

Laing and associates (1957) concluded that studies of ^{32}P uptake provide an index of the availability of radiophosphorus to the bone crystal rather than an indication of bone viability. After experimental study of ^{32}P uptake in rabbits, the authors concluded that the vascularity of the femoral head is particularly difficult to evaluate accurately.

Massie (1964) has developed a fenestrated sliding nail-plate to follow vascularity in the femoral head after internal fixation of intracapsular fractures during the convalescent period. The patient's red blood cells are tagged with ^{32}P before internal fixation. Within 45 minutes, readings can be taken in the femoral head and neck by a detector accurately placed in an appropriate fenestration. Repeat percutaneous readings are taken after 3 days, 1 week, 2 weeks, and so on until the head-to-neck ratio returns to normal or shows a definite plateau. Fifty-nine patients with intracapsular femoral neck fracture were studied. Forty-six had displaced fractures and 13 undisplaced. In none of the patients was there a vascular reduction of the femoral head of greater than 90 per cent at surgery. In many cases, vascular impairment greater than 50 per cent at surgery returned to a normal reading in less than 1 week. Venous engorgement around the hip rather than an arterial ischemia was suggested. Avascular necrosis developed in 18 per cent of the 59 patients. Twenty-seven per cent with consistently normal readings had no necrosis; 45 per cent with eventual return of the readings to normal had 14 per cent necrosis. Of 34 patients whose fractures healed in less than 4 months there was 3 per cent necrosis; of 9 patients with delayed union there was 33 per cent necrosis; and all 3 patients with nonunion developed avascular necrosis. It was concluded that the fate of the femoral head can be predicted accurately by repeated readings within the first month after surgery.

Laing and Ferguson (1958, 1959a) developed a ^{24}Na clearance method for the determination of bone vascularity. They studied nine patients with femoral neck fractures, five with hip dislocations or fracture-dislocations, and one with spontaneous aseptic necrosis. At time of surgery, 5 to 6 microcuries ^{24}Na in about 0.1 ml. ionic solution was injected into the femoral head by a special syringe. The syringe was placed tightly within a previously drilled hole. Care was taken to prevent leakage. A scintillation detector was placed over the hip joint and counts obtained every minute for 10 minutes. The investigators concluded that ^{24}Na clearance from the superior portion of the head is of prognostic value. In two patients with roentgenologic evidence of aseptic necrosis of the femoral head, no clearance was obtained.

Later, these same investigators (1959b) found clearance technique with ^{131}I to be superior to ^{24}Na. Using a technique similar to that described with ^{24}Na, they studied 45 patients. Fifteen were diagnosed as having avascular necrosis from the clearance data. On follow-up study of 11 of these patients, all had pathological and radiological evidence of avascularity. Normally, the vascular femoral heads showed 80 per cent isotope clearance in 10 minutes; low clearance rates were less than 7 per cent.

Johansson (1962, 1964) also has used ^{131}I for prognostic assessment of femoral neck fractures. At the time of surgery, a dosage of 15 to 25 microcuries in 1.5 ml. saline is injected into the femoral neck by a cannula, and a scintillation counter is placed over the precordium. Comparison is made with another dosage injection into the trochanteric region. A steep, pronounced increase in counts indicates a functioning circulation; a slow and insignificant increase denotes avascularity of the femoral head. In a series of 129 cases of intracapsular femoral neck fracture, the test has been found of prognostic value in over 80 per cent of those followed.

Holmquist and Alffram (1965) performed similar ^{131}I studies on 32 patients with cervical fractures of the femur. Twenty-five patients were followed for more than 30 months. In 21 of these 25, the prognosis regarding femoral head survival was accurately predicted.

USE OF RADIONUCLIDES IN THERAPY OF MALIGNANT BONE LESIONS

At the present time, radionuclides are of limited value in the treatment of malignant bone lesions. The greatest hazard is the associated irradiation of the bone marrow and hematopoietic system. Chemical toxicity is also a hazard. The radionuclide must have a very high specificity for tumor tissue or reactive bone formation, a low specificity for other tissues, a low elemental toxicity, and a long enough half-life to concentrate within the tumor, yet short enough to diminish the total body radiation hazard; it must also be readily available and within reasonable cost. Radionuclides should be considered only after external radiation therapy proves ineffective.

REFERENCES

Ahumada, J., Hayes, R. L., Tanida, R., and Edwards, C. L.: Gallium-68 Citrate in Bone Scanning. ORINS-53, Oak Ridge, 1965, pp. 85–90.
Arden, G. P.: Radioactive Isotopes in Fractures of the Neck of the Femur. *J. Bone Joint Surg.* 42B:21, 1960.
Arden, G. P., and Veall, N.: The Use of Radioactive Phosphorus in Early Detection of Avascular Necrosis in the Femoral Head in Fractured Neck of Femur. *Proc. Roy. Soc. Med.* 46:344, 1953.
Armstrong, W. D.: Radiotracer Studies of Hard Tissues. *Ann. N.Y. Acad. Sci.* 60:670, 1955.
Armstrong, W. D., Singer, L., and Carlson, C.: The Half-life of Radioactive Fluoride. *J. Dent. Res.* 37:69, 1958.
Asling, C. W., Johnston, M. E., Durbin, P. W., and Hamilton, J. G.: Localization of Cerium-144 in the Skeletal Tissues of Fetal Rats. UCRL-8024, Biology and Medicine. U. S. Atomic Energy Commission, 1957, pp. 1–28.
Baserga, R.: Radioactive Isotopes in Orthopaedics. *In* Turek, S. L.: Orthopaedics: Principles and Their Application. J. B. Lippincott Co., Philadelphia, 1959, pp. 843–854.
Bauer, G. C. H.: The Importance of Bone Growth as a Factor in the Redistribution of Bone Salt. II. Redistribution of Radio-active Phosphorus in the Skeleton of Rats. *J. Bone Joint Surg.* 36A:381, 1954.
Bauer, G. C. H., Carlsson, A., and Lindquist, B.: Metabolism of Ba^{140} in Man. *Acta Orthop. Scand.* 26:241, 1957.

Bauer, G. C. H., and Scoccianti, P.: Uptake of Sr[85] in Non-malignant Vertebral Lesions in Man. *Acta Orthop. Scand.* 31:90, 1961.

Bauer, G. C. H., and Wendeberg, B.: External Counting of Ca[47] and Sr[85] in Studies of Localized Skeletal Lesions in Man. *J. Bone Joint Surg.* 41B:558, 1959.

Becchini, M. F., Pietrabissa, G., and Riccioni, N.: L'impiego del radio-fibrinogeno nella diagnosi dei tumori ossei. *Minerva Nucl.* 8:351, 1964.

Bernstein, R. B., and Katz, J. J.: Fluorine-18: Preparation, Properties, Uses. *Nucleonics* 11:46, 1953.

Blau, M., Nagler, W., and Bender, M. A.: Fluorine-18: a New Isotope for Bone Scanning. *J. Nucl. Med.* 3:332, 1962.

Bloch, B., and George, E. P.: The Use of Radiophosphorus in Fractures of the Neck of the Femur. *Med. J. Aust.* 2:463, 1962.

Blum, T.: Osteomyelitis of the Mandible and Maxilla. *J. Amer. Dent. Ass.* 11:802, 1924.

Bohr, H., and Sørensen, A. H.: Study of Fracture Healing by Means of Radio-active Tracers. *J. Bone Joint Surg.* 32A:567, 1950.

Boyd, H. B., and Calandruccio, R. A.: Further Observations on the Use of Radioactive Phosphorus (P[32]) to Determine the Viability of the Head of the Femur. *J. Bone Joint Surg.* 45A:445, 1963.

Boyd, H. B., Zilversmit, D. B., and Calandruccio, R. A.: The Use of Radio-Active Phosphorus (P[32]) to Determine the Viability of the Head of the Femur. *J. Bone Joint Surg.* 37A:260, 1955.

Brady, L. W., Croll, M. N., Stanton, L., Hyman, D., and Rubins, S.: Evaluation of Calcium-47 in Normal Man and Its Use in the Evaluation of Bone Healing Following Radiation Therapy in Metastatic Disease. *Radiology* 78:286, 1962.

Brondolo, W., and Randelli, G.: La distribuzione del radioisotopo S[35] nelle ossa lunghe di ratti albini. *Arch. Ortop.* 75:1414, 1962.

Brucer, M., Andrews, G. A., and Bruner, H. D.: A Study of Gallium[72]: Summary and Conclusions. *Radiology* 61:534, 1953.

Brues, A. M.: Isotopes: Radioactive; Toxicity. *In* Glasser, O.: Medical Physics. Vol. 2. Year Book Medical Publishers, Chicago, 1950, pp. 467–471.

Castle, J. N., Scott, K. G., and Reilly, W. A.: The Skeletal Uptake of Radiophosphorus (P[32]). *Amer. J. Roentgen.* 91:1128, 1964.

Cederquist, E.: Short-term Kinetic Studies of Sr[85] and Ca[47] by Whole Body Counting in Malignant Diseases of the Skeleton. *Acta Radiol.* 2:42, 1964.

Charkes, N. D., and Sklaroff, D. M.: Early Diagnosis of Metastatic Bone Cancer by Photoscanning with Strontium-85. *J. Nucl. Med.* 5:168, 1964.

Charkes, N. D., and Sklaroff, D. M.: Detection of Occult Metastases to Bone by Photoscanning with Radioisotopes of Strontium. *Progr. Clin. Cancer* 1:235, 1965a.

Charkes, N. D., Sklaroff, D. M.: The Radioactive Strontium Photoscan as a Diagnostic Aid in Primary and Metastatic Cancer in Bone. *Radiol. Clin. N. Amer.* 3:499, 1965b.

Charkes, N. D., Sklaroff, D. M., and Bierly, J.: Detection of Metastatic Cancer to Bone by Scintiscanning with Strontium 87m. *Amer. J. Roentgen.* 91:1121, 1964.

Charkes, N. D., Sklaroff, D. M., and Young, I.: A Critical Analysis of Strontium Bone Scanning for Detection of Metastatic Cancer. *Amer. J. Roentgen.* 96:647, 1966.

Chiewitz, O., and Hevesy, G.: Radioactive Indicators in the Study of Phosphorus Metabolism in Rats. *Nature* 136:754, 1935.

Cohn, S. H., Spencer, H., Samachson, J., and Robertson, J. S.: The Turnover of Strontium-85 in Man as Determined by Whole-body Counting. *Radiat Res.* 17:173, 1962.

Corey, K. R., Kenny, P., Greenberg, E., and Laughlin, J. S.: Detection of Bone Metastases in Scanning Studies with Calcium-47 and Strontium-85. *J. Nucl. Med.* 3:454, 1962.

Corey, K. R., Kenny, P., Greenberg, E., Laughlin, J. S., and Ray, B. S.: Diagnostic Applications of Ca[47] and Sr[85] to Tumors Involving Bone. *J. Nucl. Med.* 2:119, 1961a.

Corey, K. R., Kenny, P., Greenberg, E., Pazianos, A., Pearson, O. H., and Laughlin, J. S.: The Use of Calcium[47] in Diagnostic Studies of Patients with Bone Lesions. *Amer. J. Roentgen.* 85:955, 1961b.

Danielsson, L. G., Dymling, J.-F., Heripret, G.: Coxarthrosis in Man Studied with External Counting of Sr[85] and Ca[47]. *Clin. Orthop.* 31:184, 1963.

Desgrez, H., Guerin, R.-A., and Guerin, M.-T.: Le test au 72 gallium dans les tumeurs malignes des os. *Presse Med.* 62:997, 1954.

DeNardo, G. L., and Volpe, J. A.: Detection of Bone Lesions with Strontium-85 Scintiscan. *J. Nucl. Med.* 7:219, 1966.

Dougherty, T. F., Stover, B. J., Dougherty, J. H., Jee, W. S. S., Mays, C. W., Rehfeld, C. E., Christensen, W. R., and Goldthorpe, H. C.: Studies of the Biological Effects of Ra[226], Pu[239], Ra[228] (MsTh$_1$), Th[228] (RdTh), and Sr[90] in Adult Beagles. *Radiat. Res.* 17:625, 1962.

Dudley, H. C., Imirie, G. W., Jr., and Istock, J. T.: Deposition of Radiogallium (Ga⁷²) in Proliferating Tissues. *Radiology* 55:571, 1950.

Dudley, H. C., and Maddox, G. E.: Deposition of Radiogallium (Ga⁷²) in Skeletal Tissues. *J. Pharmacol. Exp. Ther.* 96:224, 1949.

Dudley, H. C., Markowitz, H. A., and Mitchell, T. G.: Studies of the Localization of Radioactive Gallium (Ga⁷²) in Bone Lesions. *J. Bone Joint Surg.* 38A:627, 1956.

Dworkin, H. J., Moon, N. F., Lessard, R. J., and LaFleur, P.: A Study of the Metabolism of ¹⁸F in Dogs and Its Suitability for Bone Scanning. *J. Nucl. Med.* (in press).

Dymling, J.-F., and Wendeberg, B.: External Counting of ⁸⁵Sr and ⁴⁷Ca in Localized Bone Infections. *Acta Orthop. Scand.* 36:8, 1965.

Edwards, C. L., Andrews, G. A., Sitterson, B. W., and Kniseley, R. M.: Clinical Bone Marrow Scanning with Radioisotopes. *Blood* 23:741, 1964.

Edwards, C. L., Hayes, R., Ahumada, J., and Kniseley, R. M.: Gallium-68 Citrate: a Clinically Useful Skeletal Scanning Agent. *J. Nucl. Med.* (in press).

Esteban, J., Lasa, D., and Perez-Modrego, S.: Detection of Cartilaginous Tumors with Selenium 75. *Radiology* 85:149, 1965.

Fleming, W. H., McIlraith, J. D., and King, E. R.: Photoscanning of Bone Lesions Utilizing Strontium 85. *Radiology* 77:635, 1961.

Fracture Committee of American Academy of Orthopaedic Surgeons: Treatment of Fractures of the Neck of the Femur by Internal Fixation. *J. Bone Joint Surg.* 21:483, 1939.

Gottschalk, R. G.: Radioactive Sulfur in Chondrosarcomata. *J. Bone Joint Surg.* 42A:1239, 1960.

Gynning, I., Langeland, P., Lindberg, S., and Waldeskog, B.: Localization with Sr⁸⁵ of Spinal Metastases in Mammary Cancer and Changes in Uptake after Hormone and Roentgen Therapy. A Preliminary Report. *Acta Radiol.* 55:119, 1961.

Hayes, R. L.: Radioisotopes of Gallium. *In* Andrews, G. A., Kniseley, J. W., and Wagner, H. N., Jr.: Radioactive Pharmaceuticals. U.S. Atomic Energy Commission, 1966.

Hayes, R. L., Carlton, J. E., and Byrd, B. L.: Bone Scanning with Gallium-68: a Carrier Effect. *J. Nucl. Med.* 6:605, 1965.

Heaney, R. P., and Whedon, G. D.: Radiocalcium Studies of Bone Formation Rate in Human Metabolic Bone Disease. *J. Clin. Endocr.* 18:1246, 1958.

Hisada, K., Hiraki, T., Ohba, S.: Positive Delineation of Human Tumors with ¹³¹I Human Serum Albumin. *J. Nucl. Med.* 7:41, 1966.

Hoffman, F. L.: Radium (Mesothorium) Necrosis. *J.A.M.A.* 85:961, 1925.

Holmquist, B., and Alffram, P.-A.: Prediction of Avascular Necrosis Following Cervical Fracture of the Femur Based on Clearance of Radioactive Iodine from the Head of the Femur. *Acta Orthop. Scand.* 36:62, 1965.

Hulth, A.: Prediction of the Viability of the Femoral Head in Femoral Neck Fractures: a Survey of Different Predicting Methods. *Acta Chir. Scand.* 129:72, 1965.

Johansson, S. H.: Prognostic Assessment in Fractured Neck of Femur Using I¹³¹ and Venography. *Acta Chir. Scand.* 123:298, 1962.

Johansson, S. H.: The Prognostic Value of the Radio-iodine Test in Femoral Neck Fractures. *Acta Soc. Med. Upsal.* 69:64, 1964.

Justus, G.: P³² in der Diagnose der Knochentumoren. *Zbl. Chir.* 86:2298, 1961.

Klein, E. W., and Lund, R. R.: Strontium 85 Photoscanning in Paget's Disease with Comments on Several Other Skeletal Problems. *Amer. J. Roentgen.* 92:195, 1964.

Kofman, S., Sky-Peck, H. H., Thibaudeau, Y., Ray, R. D., and Taylor, S. G.: The Use of Strontium-85 in the Evaluation of Bone Metastases. A Preliminary Report. *J. Nucl. Med.* 4:9, 1963.

LaFleur, P. D., Moon, N. F., and Dworkin, H. J.: Production of Sterile Low Tritium ¹⁸F. *J. Nucl. Med.* (submitted for publication).

Laing, P. G., and Ferguson, A. B., Jr.: Sodium-24 as an Indicator of the Blood Supply of Bone. *Nature* 182:1442, 1958.

Laing, P. G., and Ferguson, A. B., Jr.: Radiosodium Clearance Rates as Indicators of Femoral-
head Vascularity. *J. Bone Joint. Surg.* 41A:1409, 1959a.

Laing, P. G., and Ferguson, A. B., Jr.: Iodine-131 Clearance-rates as an Indication of the Blood Supply of Bone. *Nature* 183:1595, 1959b.

Laing, P. G., Ferguson, A. B., Jr., Vaughan, L., and Grebner, M.: Use of Radiophosphorus for Bone Vascularity Determinations. *Arch. Surg.* 75:31, 1957.

Looney, W. B.: The Initial Medical and Industrial Use of Radioactive Materials (1915–1940). *Amer. J. Roentgen.* 72:838, 1954.

MacDonald, N. S.: The Radioisotope Osteogram-kinetic Studies of Skeletal Disorders in Humans. *Clin. Orthop.* 17:154, 1960.

Martland, H. S.: The Occurrence of Malignancy in Radioactive Persons. A General Review of Data Gathered in the Study of the Radium Dial Painters, with Special Reference to the Occurrence of Osteogenic Sarcoma and the Inter-relationship of Certain Blood Diseases. *Amer. J. Cancer* 15:2435, 1931.

Martland, H. S., and Humphries, R. E.: Osteogenic Sarcoma in Dial Painters Using Luminous Paint. *Arch. Path.* 7:406, 1929.

Massie, W. K.: Fractures of the Hip. *J. Bone Joint Surg.* 46A:658, 1964.

Meckelnburg, R. L.: Clinical Value of Generator Produced 87-M Strontium. *J. Nucl. Med.* 5:929, 1964.

Moon, N. F., Dworkin, H. J., and LaFleur, P. D.: The Clinical Use of Radiofluorine in Bone Photoscanning. *J.A.M.A.* (submitted for publication).

Mulry, W. C., and Dudley, H. C.: Studies of Radiogallium as a Diagnostic Agent in Bone Tumors. *J. Lab. Clin. Med.* 37:239, 1951.

Nusynowitz, M. L., Feldman, M. H., and Maier, J. G.: A Simple Method of Producing ^{18}F Fluoride for the Study of Bone Disease. *J. Nucl. Med.* 6:473, 1965.

Patterson, R. J., Bickel, W. H., and Dahlin, D. C.: Idiopathic Avascular Necrosis of the Head of the Femur. *J. Bone Joint Surg.* 46A:267, 1964.

Pecher, C.: Biological Investigations with Radioactive Calcium and Strontium. *Univ. Calif. Publ. Pharmacol.* 2:117, 1942.

Posner, A. S., Eanes, E. D., Harper, R. A., and Zipkin, I.: X-ray Diffraction Analysis of the Effect of Fluoride on Human Bone Apatite. *Arch. Oral Biol.* 8:549, 1963.

Rosenthall, L.: The Role of Strontium 85 in the Detection of Bone Disease. *Radiology* 84:75, 1965.

Rowland, R. E.: The Deposition and the Removal of Radium in Bone by a Long-term Exchange Process. *Clin. Orthop.* 17:146, 1960.

Sargent, T., Linfoot, J. A., Stauffer, H., and Lawrence, J. H.: Use of a Whole Body Counter in Turnover Studies with Ca^{47}. *J. Nucl. Med.* 5:407, 1964.

Schaer, L. R.: Supraorbital Fibrous Dysplasia Demonstrated by Fluorine-18 and the Scintillation (Positron) Camera. *Radiology* 86:506, 1966.

Simpson, W. J., and Orange, R. P.: Total Body Scanning with Strontium-85 in the Diagnosis of Metastatic Bone Disease. *Canad. Med. Ass. J.* 93:1237, 1965.

Sklaroff, D. M., and Charkes, N. D.: Studies of Metastatic Bone Lesions with Strontium 85. *Radiology* 80:270, 1963.

Sklaroff, D. M., and Charkes, N. D.: Diagnosis of Bone Metastasis by Photoscanning with Strontium 85. *J.A.M.A.* 188:1, 1964.

Smith-Petersen, M. N., Cave, E. F., and Vangorder, G. W.: Intracapsular Fractures of the Neck of the Femur. *Arch. Surg.* 23:715, 1931.

Stein, I., Beller, M. L., and Nedwich, A.: Circulation of the Femoral Head (an End Organ) in Dogs. *J. Trauma* 3:534, 1963.

Stein, I., Serber, W., and Beller, M.: Determination of Radioactive Phosphorus Pickup in the Upper Femur. *J. Bone Joint Surg.* 38A:943, 1956.

Tamvakopoulos, S. K., Collins, J. J., Jr., Banks, H. H., Wilson, R. E., and Moore, F. D.: Studies of Bone Disease Using Calcium-47. *Surg. Forum* 14:458, 1963.

Treadwell, A. de G., Low-Beer, B. V. A., Friedell, H. L., and Lawrence, J. H.: Metabolic Studies on Neoplasm on Bone with the Aid of Radioactive Strontium. *Amer. J. Med. Sc.* 204:521, 1942.

Tucker, F. R.: The Use of Radioactive Phosphorus in the Diagnosis of Avascular Necrosis of the Femoral Head. *J. Bone Joint Surg.* 32B:100, 1950.

Van der Werff, J. T.: Clinical Investigations on the Use of Radioactive Gallium (Ga^{65} and Ga^{67}) in Bone Diseases. *Acta Radiol.* 41:343, 1954.

Van Dilla, M. A., and Arnold, J. S.: Strontium^{85} Tracer Studies in Humans. *Int. J. Appl. Radiat.* 1:129, 1956.

Van Dyke, D., Anger, H. O., Yano, Y., and Bozzini, C.: Bone Blood Flow Shown with F^{18} and the Positron Camera. *Amer. J. Physiol.* 209:65, 1965.

Waldeskog, B., Gynning, I., and Langland, P.: Localization with Sr^{85} of Spinal Metastases in Mammary Cancer and Changes in Uptake after Hormone and Roentgen Therapy. Technical Reports Series No. 10, International Atomic Energy Agency, Vienna, 1962, pp. 104–106.

Weiss, T. E., Maxfield, W. S., Murison, P. J., and Hidalgo, J. U.: Iodinated Human Serum Albumin (I^{131}) Localization Studies of Rheumatoid Arthritis Joints by Scintillation Scanning (Preliminary Report). *Arthritis & Rheum.* 8:976, 1965.

Wendeberg, B.: Mineral Metabolism of Fractures of the Tibia in Man Studied with External Counting of Sr^{85}. *Acta Orthop. Scand. Suppl.*, 52:1, 1961.

Whitley, J. E., Witcofski, R. L., Bolliger, T. T., and Maynard, C. D.: Tc^{99m} in the Visualization of Neoplasm Outside the Brain. *Amer. J. Roentgen.* 96:706, 1966.

Woodard, H. Q., and Kenney, J. M.: The Relation of Phosphatase Activity in Bone Tumors to the Deposition of Radioactive Phosphorus. *Amer. J. Roentgen.* 47:227, 1942.

XVI

RADIATION INJURY

TIMOTHY MERZ

The effects of a given dose of electromagnetic or particulate radiation, regardless of the source, can be assayed during a time period beginning immediately following insult, and stretching into generations of cells and organisms.

The kind of damage observed is not peculiar to radiation injury, nor does it change qualitatively in relation to amount (dose). The changes can be seen only as shifts in the frequency of the occurrence of any event; the higher the dose, the more frequent the event. There is still no documented threshold below which any biological response to radiation has been shown not to occur.

The sequence of events extends directly from the absorption of energy and the production of active radicals (HO_2 and OH, produced in water and organic radicals) to the initial biological damage (Lea, 1962). The consequences of that damage range from total recovery to cell death and include such effects as the production of tumors and mongoloid offspring.

Radiation damage can be modified, with a resultant increase or decrease in response at the time of energy absorption, at the time of the production of radicals, or at any stage in the biological sequence of events.

A discussion of the absorption and distribution of energy in tissue as a result of ionizing radiation, though relevant, is not directly pertinent to this discussion of the biological consequences of the complex physical and chemical events that precede them. Suffice it to say that when an incident particle transfers sufficient energy to produce an active radical in a critical area, it precipitates a series of events leading to the biological changes to be discussed in this chapter.

It is obvious that a complete presentation of the deleterious biological effects of radiation within the limits of this chapter is an impossibility, and unfortunately there is a paucity of good texts to rely on for reference material. There is, however, an extensive literature into which one can delve for help and all useful reviews as well as investigative studies are listed in the bibliography.

THE TARGET

Perhaps the best beginning for any understanding of the effect of radiation on living systems is the identification of the critical target or site of damage. The possibilities are numerous. Clearly the sensitive area must be cellular in most living systems, since the unit of structure is the cell, except, of course, in acellular systems such as viruses. The target in viruses must of necessity be genetic since the particle consists of DNA (in some cases RNA) and a protein coat, which is not involved in intracellular viral activity. In cellular and multicellular organisms one must consider not only the genetic material organized as chromosomes, but also the membrane systems and the other organelles lying in the cytoplasm. The list is rather imposing: (1) the nucleus, consisting of genetic material (DNA, RNA, histone, and other proteins, plus a considerable number of metallic elements) organized as chromosomes; (2) the nuclear membrane; (3) the endoplasmic reticulum; (4) the Golgi apparatus; (5) the ribosomes; (6) the lysosomes; (7) the mitochondria; and (8) the plasma membrane. A diagrammatic representation of these cell components can be seen in Figure 16-1.

At present there exist two widely divergent points of view about the site of damage. There is nearly universal agreement by radiation biologists that the sensitive target of radiation insult is in the nucleus. A small group of workers have sought to explain cellular damage by the "enzyme release" hypothesis (Bacq and Alexander, 1961) which implicates proteolytic enzymes from lysosomes (whose membranes have been ruptured) in intracellular degradation and subsequent death. Anna Goldfeder (1964) has demonstrated with electron micrographs that radiation does in fact damage many of the various cellular membrane systems responsible at least in part for cellular integrity. The proof, however, does not lie simply in the observation of damaged structures but in the ability or inability of the membrane to recover from such damage when it is produced by treatment with ionizing radiation.

The evidence supporting the idea that the site of radiation damage is the chromosome is overwhelming at present (Gray, 1957). Historically, Koernicke in 1905 observed that radiation induces structural changes in chromosomes. In addition, the genetic effects of irradiation have been chronicled since Muller's discovery in 1927. One of the most convincing series of experiments are those by von Borstel and Rogers (1958) and Rogers and von Borstel (1957) using alpha particles and *Habrobracon* (a parasitic wasp) eggs. These eggs have nuclei situated at the surface, enabling the experimenters to direct radiation at either the nucleus or cytoplasm. The resulting comparison showed that a single alpha particle passing through the nucleus was lethal to the egg. A total of 16 × 10^6 alpha particles passing through the cytoplasm was lethal to only 50 per

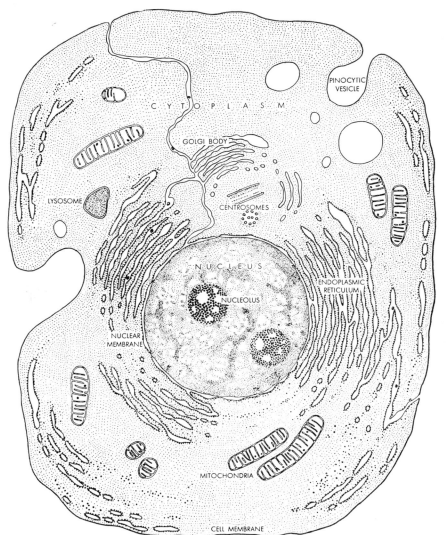

FIGURE 16-1. Diagram of a typical cell. The dots lining the endoplasmic reticulum represent ribosomes. (From "The Living Cell" by Jean Brachet. Copyright © 1961 by Scientific American, Inc. All rights reserved.)

cent of the eggs. The fact that DNA base analogs, which are exclusively incorporated into DNA, increase the damage in cells exposed to radiation (Kihlman, 1962, 1966) is further evidence of the importance of the nucleus in the response to radiation. In addition, all of the work with ultraviolet radiation indicates that the site of the lesions induced by ultraviolet radiation and the site of reactivation of the lesions is exclusively nuclear DNA (Zelle and Hollaender, 1955; Rupert, 1960; Setlow and Setlow, 1963; Howard-Flanders et al., 1964). Further evidence is provided by Sparrow (1964), whose recent work has demonstrated that radio-sensitivity is unalterably tied to nuclear volume and more particularly to chromosome volume. The number of experiments performed to define the sensitive target of radiation is very large and the results are so constant as to leave few, if any, doubts (Davies and Evans, 1966). That there exists some meaningful relationship between the cytoplasm and radiation response is by no means to be denied, but that that relationship is not nearly so meaningful as that between the nucleus and radiation response is an established fact. It is hardly surprising that the cell cannot easily survive alterations in its nucleus, which is the directive center of cell synthesis, as well as the source of ribosomal structural RNA (Brown, 1966; Ritossa, 1965).

Since the genetic material and that region responsible for the production of ribosomal structural RNA are structured as chromosomes, it follows logically that alterations of chromosome structure and integrity are a good measure of damage induced by radiation (Evans, 1962). Lethality, though conclusive, is not a useful end point to assay, because it is not sufficiently informative.

THE EFFECT OF CELL CYCLE IN SOMATIC CELLS

One of the most important variables bearing on radiation injury to cells, tissues, organs, and organisms is the state of the cell itself. The cell cycle, or specifically the state of the chromosomes, determines, in large part, the response of the chromosome to damage inflicted by radiation.

In early development all cells are dividing. During and after the process of differentiation, cells are of two kinds: dividing or potentially dividing, and nondividing.

The cycle of the proliferating somatic cell has been divided into four stages by Howard and Pelc (1953). Figure 16-2 is a diagrammatic representation of these stages. First is the actual division sequence of mitoses, labeled the D or M phase. Second is the stage of interphase concerned with general synthesis that precedes chromosomal replication. This second stage has been labeled the G_1 phase. The stage during which the genetic material is replicated is termed the S phase and is so named for the synthesis of DNA, which is marked and defined by the uptake of tritiated (^{3}H) thymidine, a base specifically incorporated into DNA. It should be understood that the time period covering S begins at the

FIGURE 16-2. Stages in the life cycle of proliferating cells. D, Division or mitotic (M) stage including prophase to telophase; G_1, gap in time between mitosis and S, the synthetic stage defined by the incorporation of thymidine into DNA; G_2, subsequent gap between S and the following mitosis. The outer circle is representative of cells of man and hamster in culture, broad bean root-tip cells, and grasshopper spermatagonia and spermatocytes. S is one third of the total cycle. The middle circle in which S occupies nearly the entire interphase is representative of *Tetrahymena* and grasshopper neuroblasts. The inner circle is a representation of the sea urchin cell cycle in which there is no G_1 and a long G_2. (From Swanson, C. P., Merz, T., and Young, W. J.: Cytogenetics. Prentice-Hall, Inc., Englewood Cliffs, N. J., 1967.)

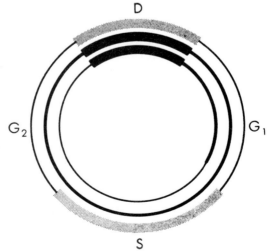

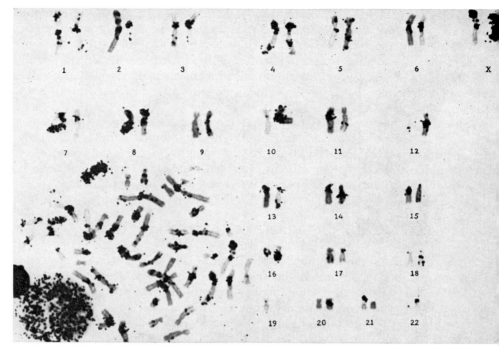

FIGURE 16-3. Autoradiograph of human chromosomes of cultured lymphocytes illustrating the asynchrony of various chromosomes and chromosome segments late in the S stage. (From German, J. L., 3rd: *Trans. N. Y. Acad. Sci.* 24:395, 1962).

moment of the first uptake of thymidine ^{3}H and ceases when no more is incorporated. The S stage is, then, a *cellular* event as it is measured, but in relation to each chromosome it is a much shorter event. Each set of chromosomes has a particular synthesis sequence in relation to other chromosomes and in many instances certain segments of given chromosomes synthesize their DNA at times that differ from the time of synthesis of other segments in the same chromosome (German, 1962) (Fig. 16-3). The stage following the uptake of thymidine ^{3}H is termed G_2 and it is the period of time that follows S and precedes M (mitosis). It is clear that operationally these stages are related to only one activity in interphase, S (the synthesis of DNA). The relationship of these stages to the effects of radiation is examined in a following section.

Perhaps the greatest resistance to lethal damage by radiation is exhibited by cells that are not dividing. The one exception to this rule is the lymphocyte, which is recognized as being exceedingly sensitive to small amounts of radiation in the nondividing state. For the most part, however, a cell can sustain considerably more damage and survive if it does not divide. Division will result in the expression of that damage as chromosomal aberrations which may well be responsible for most radiation-induced lethality in a population of proliferating cells.

Before we consider chromosomal aberrations and subsequent cell death it should be noted that observations of damage actually include three inseparable events: damage, repair, and the expression of the remaining damage. The extent of the damage is, therefore, of no more significance than is the extent of the repair.

Structural alterations of chromosomal material are of two main types (Fig. 16-4). Chromosomes in G_1 stage cells sustain *chromosome-type* aberrations in which the entire chromosome is broken as a unit. The chromosomal DNA is not replicated at this stage, the bipartite structure of the chromosome (sister-chromatids) is not observable, and it responds functionally as a single unit. Cells in the S or G_2 stages yield *chromatid-type* aberrations in which the sister-chromatids are the functional units of breakage and repair. A third type of structural alteration occurs in cells that have entered M, mitosis, and are in prophase (Hsu, Dewey, and Humphrey, 1962). In prophase a subchromatid structure is involved, resulting in what are termed half-chromatid aberrations. The time sequences of the cell cycle are such that cells spend much less time in the prophase configuration than in G_1, S or G_2 and consequently this stage is not as great a contributor to lethal events as the others.

The consequences of a simple deleted piece of chromosomal material is quite different for each type. Since the chromosome-type aberration involves both chromatids, both daughter cells will be deficient in genetic material. A chromatid-type deletion involving only one chromatid will involve only one of the two cells resulting from the division. Likewise a half-chromatid deletion is effective only in the subsequent division and, therefore, involves only one of four cells.

More important than the consequences of a single event being realized as a chromosome, chromatid or half-chromatid aberration is the total amount of damage sustained from an exposure at any given stage.

Classically, cells in G_1 are considered to be in the most resistant configura-

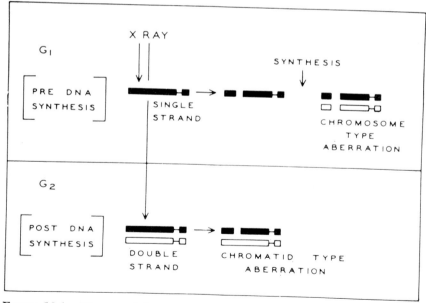

FIGURE 16-4.   Diagram of the two types of chromosomal aberrations induced at different times in the cell cycle. The type of aberration, chromosome or chromatid, depends on the time in relation to DNA synthesis (S) when the radiation-induced break occurs.

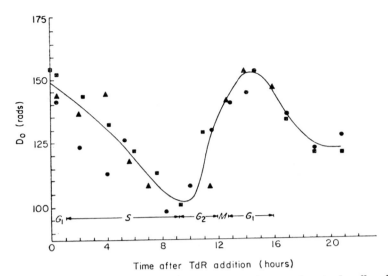

Time after TdR addition (hours)

FIGURE 16-5. Radiation survival measurements using synchronized cell cultures and measuring survival as a function of age in the cell cycle. The cells are synchronized by the use of ³H thymidine at high doses which effectively kills all cells not in G_1 at the end of 6 hours. Survival has been measured as a function of D_0. The abscissa is time after addition of cold thymidine. Sixteen to 20 hours is about one generation. (From Whitmore, G. F., Gulyas, S., and Botond, J.: Cellular Radiation Biology. Williams and Wilkins Co., Baltimore, 1965.)

tion. Sensitivity, measured by the production of chromosome aberrations, increases considerably as cells approach and enter G_2 (Hsu, Dewey, and Humphrey, 1962). Figure 16-5 indicates this changing sensitivity assayed by survival. This picture is not so clear when sensitivity is measured by the loss of the cells' reproductive integrity (Davies and Evans, 1966), although in general it is reasonable to describe changing sensitivity as a process correlating with the cells' continuing preparation for the division sequence. It is possible, however, that the S stage is the most resistant stage of all of the predivision stages. Resistance is conferred, then, on those cells not preparing for division and on those cells with a repair system adequate to contend with the damage inflicted.

THE EFFECT OF CELL CYCLE IN GERM CELLS

Germ cells are a somewhat different matter. It has been clearly demonstrated that spermatogonia are sensitive to extremely low doses of radiation (Oakberg, 1962), exhibiting lethal responses to as little as 3 rads of x-rays. The main decrease in the population of early spermatogonial cells seems to occur before mitotic division, in what may appear to be very early prophase or the preceding interphase, and, unlike the later gonial stages, does not seem to involve the loss of chromosomal material via aberrations and division.

According to Russell, the sensitivity of oogonia seems to be associated with mitosis. It should be remembered that sublethal, as well as lethal, genetic alterations occur at these stages, whether observable as structural alterations or not.

Spermatocytes, unlike spermatogonial cells, are not eliminated by relatively low doses of radiation (25 to 100 rads). They persist and result in a lower sperm count as well as a lowered production of viable offspring. Spermatids as well as spermatozoa show chromosomal aberrations after radiation exposure and contribute to loss of fertility and an increased mutation rate, the extent depending on the dose.

It might be well to mention at this time that an increase in viability as a consequence of increased protection or recovery following damage is not necessarily paralleled by a decrease in mutation rate. Increasing viability of individuals that normally would die at higher doses of radiation results in the survival, in a population, of a number of individuals exposed to a dose just above what would otherwise be the threshold of lethality. The retention of this group is in effect the retention of a high incidence of mutations, which may more than offset the decrease in mutations that is a consequence of protection or recovery for the other individuals that have incurred sublethal damage.

Oocytes, in contradistinction to spermatocytes, have been shown to be immediately sensitive to doses as low as 10 to 20 R (Oakberg, 1962; Peters, 1961; Peters and Borum, 1961; Peters and Levy, 1964). This results in a greatly decreased fertility, or, at reasonably high doses, even complete sterility.

THE EFFECT OF INTRACELLULAR RADIATION

The difference in effect of radiation sources at varying biological sites is related to both the response of those sites to radiation and their importance in the maintenance of the integrity of the organ and the organism. This is a large part of the explanation of the RBE (relative biological effectiveness) of any given radioactive isotope; the other important factors are biological half-life (incorporation versus excretion and radioactive decay or half-life) and the quality of the radiation.

Cells that are particularly responsive to radiation, such as lymphocytes and progenitor cells of the bone marrow, whose existence is a necessity for the life of the individual, can be irradiated lethally by what amounts to low total-body doses of radiation because they are localized in critical areas. The same is true for any dividing tissue exposed to a labeled compound such as tritiated thymidine, which becomes a part of the genetic material as DNA replication proceeds (Bender, Gooch, and Prescott, 1962). What is even more important, perhaps, is the increase in chromosome breakage or mutation rate induced by radioactive compounds incorporated in or near the nuclei of germ or somatic cells. The danger in these cases is not limited to the fatal doses for critical cells but can also be directly related to surviving but altered cells whose effects will be expressed in later generations of cells (tumor induction) or individuals (congenital defects).

Mutations and chromosome aberrations in high frequency are obvious results of incorporation into genetic material of tritiated base analogs. Tritium β-rays have very high linear energy transfer (LET)—and concomitantly no penetrating ability—and as a result are likely to produce more damage to genetic material per unit dose than might be expected, especially when one considers the localization of such compounds and the long half-life (12.5 years) of tritium (Wimber, 1964; Cairns, 1961). One can expect then to see marrow and circulating leukocyte depression, or germ cell alterations from doses as low as 10 μc. in mice (Cronkite, Fliedner, Killman, and Rubini, 1962). Damage to marrow cells has been documented in 300 g. rats for as long as 30 days with as little as a 25 μc dose of calcium-45 (Barranco, Beers, and Merz, 1967).

INTENSITY

One of the more perplexing aspects of the biological effects of radiation continues to be the influence of dose rate on the consequences of radiation exposure. It is important to note that dose rate does not apply exclusively to doses received from external sources. It is equally applicable to radiation from internal emitters.

The effect of altering the intensity is clearly one of altering the amount of damage done at any one period of time. Within biomedical dose ranges, increasing or decreasing the rate at which radiation impinges upon cells will increase or decrease the amount of primary response per unit time. Assuming everything else to be equal, one might expect that the only effect of reduced dose rates would be a lengthening of the period of time over which damage occurs. This is not the case. There are two factors that make the picture somewhat more complicated. First, if the dose rate is low enough the process of recovery can take place. This replenishes the cell population lost through incurred damage with cells that are provided by the division of normal, undamaged cells. Second, repair of damage within the nuclei of injured cells (a known and

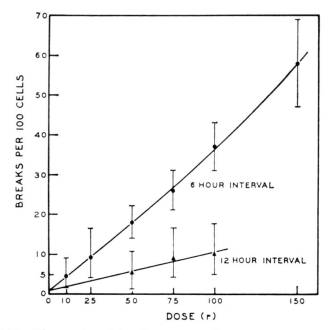

FIGURE 16-6. The number of breaks per 100 cells represented as a response to dose variation at two different intensities. The upper curve is the result of giving each dose over a 6 hour interval and the lower curve is the result of giving each dose over a 12 hour interval. The material is the corneal epithelium of the Chinese hamster in tissue culture. (From Brewen, J. G.: Science 138:820, 1962.)

TABLE 16-1. NUMBER OF RADIATION-INDUCED MUTATIONS AT SPECIFIC LOCI IN MOUSE SPERMATOGONIA AT VARIOUS DOSE RATES (NUMBERS OF MUTANTS ARE GIVEN FOR 90 R/MIN. AND 9 R/MIN.)*

DOSE RATE (R/min.)	RADIATION	LOCUS								
		a	b	c	p	d	se	dse	s	TOTAL
90	X	2	32	15	22	24	2	—	69	166
9	„	1	1	3	7	3	—	1	10	26

* From Russell, W. L.: The Nature of the Dose-Rate Effects of Radiation on Mutation in Mice. *Japan. J. Genetics* Suppl. 40:132, 1966.

measurable phenomenon) reduces the total amount of damage that exists within the cell at any given moment during exposure. Both processes operating simultaneously produce a picture that is classically considered radioresistance. Perhaps the best example of this is Brewen's study (1962) utilizing the corneal epithelium of the Chinese hamster, with dose rates of 2 R/min., 60 R/min., and 600 R/min. of x-rays. As is seen in Figure 16-6, the amount of damage, as assayed by chromosomal (chromatid) aberrations, depends not only on the dose, but on the rate as well. It should not be concluded that less damage is incurred at the lower rates since initial damage cannot be observed. It should be interpreted as indicating that at the higher rates more alterations remain unrepaired and available for assay by the observer.

Russell's work (1966) using mutation frequency in mice as an indication of the effect of lowering the dose rate would also seem to demonstrate the increased influence of repaired nucleic acid lesions on the final result. This is clearly seen in Table 16-1.

Hornsey (1965), also using mice, has demonstrated the same phenomena at different but high dose rates. She assayed the changing result by measuring the L.D.$_{50}$ at 4 days. It is evident that even at high dose rates the effect of variation in intensity is noticeable.

In essence, then, the effect of varying the intensity is directly and unalterably linked to the phenomena of repair. The decrease in final observed damage is not related simply to a decrease in effect per unit time but to a unit time in which initial damage can be repaired before subsequent damage occurs.

DOSE EFFECTS

The effect of altering the dose can be viewed more than one way, depending largely on the resolution of the assay system one uses as a lens. The two basic assay methods are primary genetic damage, and lethal damage or loss of reproductive integrity. The two methods give somewhat different results. Clearly the most sensitive of these techniques is to measure primary alterations that are unrepaired (chromosomal aberrations and mutations) instead of their result (death or loss of reproductive integrity).

There is very little mystery about the relationship of high doses, delivered as a single burst, to biological response. It appears linear, an increase in dose being seen as a linear increase in effect. Except in so far as therapy is concerned,

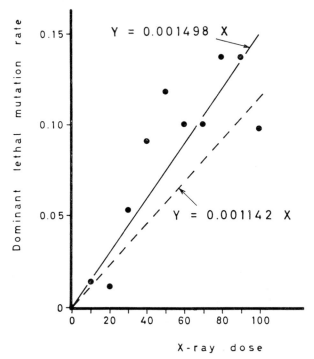

FIGURE 16-7. The dominant lethal mutation rate in mouse spermatozoa in response to doses from 10 to 100 R. The solid line indicates the regression coefficient from the most recent published results, the dotted line from previous experiments. Earlier experiments had shown the same linearity from 1500 R down to 100 R. (From Leonard, A., and Deknudt, G.: *Mutation Res.* 4:234, 1967.)

the most interesting and significant results are seen after very low doses, and in fact one of the major questions still remains: is there a threshold below which there is no biological response? The answer continues to be negative.

Recent data, based on techniques that measure the alterations in genetic material, indicate that there is no threshold below which there is no measurable change. Glass (1965), measuring mutations resulting in altered body bristle of the fruit fly, *Drosophila melanogaster* (animals that can withstand more than an order of magnitude more radiation than humans), was able to demonstrate that the radiation-induced mutation rate was linear down to 5 R. Leonard and Deknudt (1967) have demonstrated the same thing down to 10 R for dominant lethals in mice (Fig. 16-7). Steffensen (1964) has demonstrated the same lack of threshold in *Tradescantia* by measuring micronuclei (acentric fragments of broken chromosomal strands) produced spontaneously and by doses of x-ray ranging from 0.3 R to 6.0 R. The response remains linear to the origin (Fig. 16-8). Schmickel's (1967) work indicates that increases in aberrant chromosomes from human lymphocytes irradiated *in vivo* are obvious after doses as low as 5.0 R delivered dose and reach the 3.3 per cent level at 48 R delivered dose. Suffice it to say that if there is a level of absorbed radiation dose below which there is no apparent biological alteration observed, it is a diminishingly small dose and the observed lack of changes simply reflects our rather gross assay systems. High

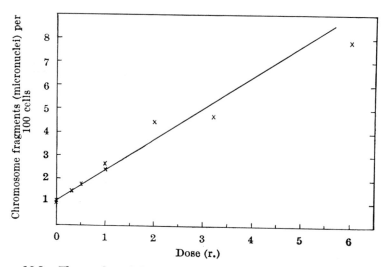

FIGURE 16-8. The number of chromosome fragments measured as micronuclei after doses of x-ray as small as 0.3 R. The origin is the spontaneous level of fragments which is below 1 per 100 cells. A dose of 0.3 R results in a 50 per cent increase. The dose response curve is essentially linear, no threshold being discernible. (From Steffensen, D.: *Nature* 201:205, 1964.)

dose levels, in the 400 rad to 800 rad range, delivered as a single total-body dose, are usually lethal for humans.

DOSE FRACTIONATION

A most significant influence on the biological effects of any radiation exposure is that created by dividing the dose into fractions delivered at intervals separated by significant time periods. The greatest effect can be correlated with an interval approaching the time necessary for the previously exposed cells to repair the incurred damage and repopulate the tissue (recovery). When concerned only with cell survival the interval need be only as long as the repair time for any single cell (according to Merz and Prempree [1966], most are approximately the same). Cell survival is not enough for certain replacement tissues such as marrow, gut epithelial lining, and skin, which must continually proliferate to keep pace with the cell loss occurring naturally. Simply surviving radiation exposure will result in absence of critical cell populations and the subsequent death of the organism.

Repair of damage to chromosomes and the demonstration of a limited time period during which repair must be accomplished or fail is credited to Wolff and Luippold (1955). They showed that repair is probably an enzymatic process (since substantiated by investigations of ultraviolet repair systems [Rupert, 1960; Howard-Flanders et al., 1964]) that, at least for ionizing radiation-induced damage *in vivo*, requires the production of energy, ATP. If metabolism is interrupted significantly, repair concomitantly suffers the same interruption. Wolff also demonstrated that at least part of the mechanism responsible for repair can also be damaged by radiation and, therefore, the time necessary for repair

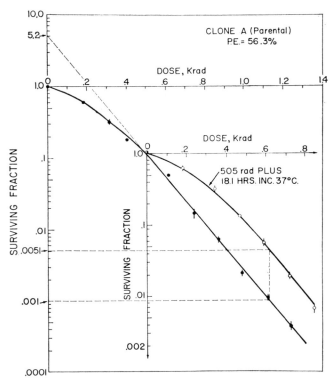

FIGURE 16-9. A dose response curve for Chinese hamster cells in culture. The response is measured as the surviving fraction and plotted on the ordinate as the log of that number. The abscissa shows the varying doses in K rad. The initial slope is a shoulder, which represents repair of sublethal damage. The inner graph represents an initial dose of 505 rads and an 18.1 hour recovery period, and then a new dose response curve whose initial slope is once again a shoulder, indicating a return to the original state of repairability. (From Elkind, M. M., and Sutton, H.: *Radiat. Res.* 13:556, 1960.)

included that required for the repair system to accomplish its own recovery and subsequently to restore broken chromosomal strands. The demonstration of a repair system was accomplished by separating a dose into two fractions which were delivered at ever increasing time intervals until repair of damage inflicted by the first x-ray dose had been completed and the broken strands were no longer available to rejoin with the broken strands produced by the second treatment. The assay system consisted of measuring a change in the frequency of observed exchanges ("illegitimate reunion") from an exponential to an additive response relationship.

Since that first demonstration, much more sophisticated studies of repair have shown the same kind of process occurring in many biological systems, including mammalian cells (Whitmore, 1967; Elkind, 1960). Figures 16-9 and 16-10 show the results of Elkind's rather elegant studies of repair. It is evident in the results shown in Figure 16-10 that the cells can repair damage between radiation exposures and in addition that there is a critical time after repair has been initiated when the cells seem considerably more susceptible to the effects of the second dose. This is most reasonably explained by a combination of two known effects. First, the cells are inhibited mitotically and, therefore, cycled

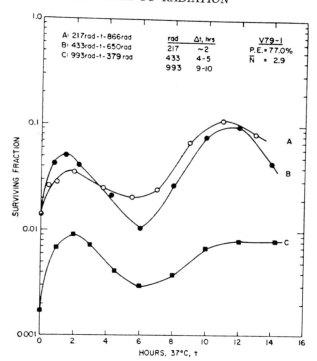

FIGURE 16-10. Fractionation curves of two doses of 55 kv. x-rays given to V 79-1 Chinese hamster cells in culture. The total doses in curves A and B are the same. The first doses differ, A being 217 rads and B 433 rads. Curve C represents a first dose of 993 rads and a higher total dose. P.E., Plating efficiency; N, mean cell multiplicating at first exposure; Δt, estimate of delay of division induced by the first doses. The time between the two dose fractions is shown on the abscissa. Repair is induced by the change in the log surviving fraction shown on the ordinate. (Elkind, M. M., and Sinclair, W. K.: *In* Current Topics in Radiation Research. Ebert, M., and Howard, A. (eds.) North Holland Publishing Co., Amsterdam, 1965.)

almost synchronously in the first postirradiation division. Second, the stage G_2 is not only more sensitive than other preceding stages to damage by radiation, but also it is the stage in which most cells are held as a result of the radiation-induced mitotic inhibition.

In spite of the fact that an active and significantly effective repair system is operating to limit final damage and return the cells to their previous state of resistance and function, some damage does remain. It is this damage that remains as sublethal in many cells and contributes to the effects that are seen to be accumulative with subsequent exposures to radiation.

Damage, then, can be and is normally repaired effectively by systems operating within the cell, but all damage is not completely repaired and accumulates from exposure to exposure.

MODIFICATION OF THE RESPONSE TO RADIATION

There are several means by which radiation responses can be changed. I have pointed out several of these previously (e.g., dose fractionation and intensity), but there are others that should be mentioned here even though they have been covered elsewhere in this volume.

The concept of radiation quality is an important one; it has been extensively studied and is presently well understood. It can be expressed simply as follows: the higher the linear energy transfer (LET), the greater the effect. It is also true that the higher the LET, the less the effect of any modification of response. That is, the higher the dose, the greater the effect, and the more difficult the modification. In a very real sense, then, LET is related to the differences that may exist between delivered dose (R) and absorbed dose (rad). All other relationships explained in this chapter remain the same.

The understanding of the meaning of RBE (relative biological effectiveness) requires more parts, but it is equally simple. The biological effect of any radiation exposure is a function of its quality (LET), how it is delivered (intensity), and how much is delivered (dose). To know the RBE of a given radiation exposure, one must know only the quality of the particle, how it is administered—pulsed or as a single bolus—and how long it is present, which is its biological half-life, a combination of its physical half-life and its excretion rate. To these facts should be added a knowledge of the localization of the radioactive substance in specific tissues, the response of the particular tissue to radiation, and the critical nature of the tissue in relationship to the survival of the individual.

ENVIRONMENTAL EFFECTS ON RADIATION RESPONSE

One of the most familiar environmental factors known to enhance radiation response is the high-oxygen-tension environment. The results of the studies of Deschner and Gray (1959) are shown in Figure 16-11. High oxygen tension merits intensive study as an adjuvant to therapy in the treatment of tumors because of the dramatic differences in response between oxygenated

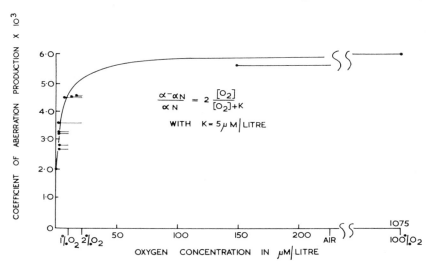

$$\frac{\alpha - \alpha_N}{\alpha_N} = 2 \frac{[O_2]}{[O_2] + K}$$

$$\text{WITH} \quad K = 5\mu M/\text{LITRE}$$

FIGURE 16-11. The change in frequency of chromosome aberrations measured by the coefficient of aberration production $\times 10^3$ as a result of varying the oxygen concentration. An increase from anoxia to 1 per cent O_2 (μM./liter) results in a doubled response which is at the same time nearly the maximum, a level achieved at normal air concentrations. (Deschner, E. E., and Gray, L. H.: Radiat. Res. 11:115, 1959.)

and mildly hypoxic tissues. Even those changes in respiration induced by sedation are sufficient to decrease tissue responses (Brewen and Merz). The results of changes in oxygen concentration are of two types. First, the radical formation increases as oxygen concentration increases; therefore, damage increases with increasing oxygen concentration. This enhancement decreases as the LET of the radiation increases (the higher the LET, the lower the modification). Second, as oxygen concentrations become diminishingly low, oxidative phosphorylation decreases, ATP production decreases, and repair activity is affected. The oxygen effect is the sum of increase in damage minus repair activity.

This summation can become rather complex in radiotherapy. It is known that in relatively large tumors there are areas of hypoxia in which cells suffer less damage than those in well oxygenated portions. According to what has just been stated, it would follow that cells that are hypoxic would also have a markedly reduced repair ability, but many tumor cells are able to derive their energy in the absence of active oxidative phosphorylation and, therefore, may still have operable repair systems. What more likely candidate for a classically radioresistant cell than this—lower initial damage due to hypoxia and at the same time a working repair system. In addition, the tumor has no group of cells that is critical for its survival; almost any cell is as good as any other to rebuild the population from a minimal number.

It might be well to add here that many of the chemicals that enhance the biological effectiveness of radiation may do so by altering the repair between radiation exposures. It is wise always to keep in mind the effects of the overall general condition of the organism and the effect of previous treatment on the repair ability when evaluating the probable response of cells or tissues to given dose of radiation.

Chemical protection by single and combination treatments with a variety of agents has aroused interest but is of little practical value at present. The agents are relatively toxic themselves and have not yet been shown to be uniformly effective except at nearly lethal dose levels. The effect of most of these agents has been explained generally in three ways: (1) by their possible effect on intracellular oxygen concentration; (2) by the hypothesis that they act as a dilutant for sensitive chemical bonds (S-H), as a sort of radical sponge; and (3), by theorizing that they contribute a proton to disrupted bonds, thereby effecting chemical repair. The evidence for these theories is incomplete.

In addition to other known modifications of radiation response there is that of the interaction of chromosomal breaks produced by radiation and those produced by radiomimetic agents (Merz, Swanson, and Cohn, 1961). Radiomimetic agents are compounds which induce damage to genetic material that is observably indistinguishable from damage done by radiation. This is an ever increasing number of agents which now includes viruses (Nichols, 1965). A radiomimetic drug (nitrogen mustard, betapropiolactone, caffeine, etc.) that induces chromosomal breaks that interact with those induced by x-ray results in a synergistic effect, an effect greater than the addition of the effects of the two treatments. The response is exactly the same as giving two or more fractionated doses of radiation. Even the relationship of the time intervals between treatments to repair remains the same although absolute repair time of damage done by some chemicals is apparently different from that of x-ray-induced damage.

LATE OR DELAYED EFFECTS

The delayed effect of sublethal irradiation of animals on subsequent lifespan, the induction of disease, not to mention embryological development (Rugh, 1963), is the subject of an increasing number of investigations. Although the data, which may take several generations of animals to collect, is still sparse, the direction is clear. The arguments about threshold are being resolved in the same way and with the same results as those recently demonstrated in acute radiation response studies.

Curtis (1967) has summarized the dose-effect relationship as follows: (1) The occurrence of degenerative diseases in animals increases as the dose of radiation increases. (2) Damage induced by x-rays and γ-rays is reparable. (3) Damage induced by densely ionizing (high LET) radiation is not repaired.

Delayed effects following exposure to radiation also vary according to the dose rate, at least to some extent. Low chronic doses of x-rays and γ-rays seem to result in less observed damage at later periods than large single doses (Curtis, 1967). This does not seem to be the case for high-LET radiation in which no differences are discernible. The difference is again probably due to the lack of repair exhibited by cells irradiated by high LET radiation.

The life-shortening effects of radiation are being intensively investigated. The studies of Lindop and Rotblot (1961) indicated that death from all causes occurred at an earlier age in irradiated animals than in control animals although the decrease in age of onset was different for different diseases, being more striking for neoplastic disease in most instances.

E. B. Lewis (1963) observed a dramatic increase in the occurrence of leukemia, multiple myeloma, and aplastic anemia in radiologists (Table 16-2). Other later evidence tends to corroborate these findings (Warren, 1956; Warren

TABLE 16-2. MORTALITY AMONG RADIOLOGISTS: DEATHS ATTRIBUTED TO CANCERS OF THE LYMPHATIC AND BLOOD-FORMING TISSUES AND FROM APLASTIC ANEMIA*

INTER-NATIONAL CODE RUBRIC	PRINCIPAL DISEASE	NUMBER OF DEATHS		p†	MORTALITY RATIO (M.R.)	95% CONFIDENCE M.R.
		OBSERVED	EXPECTED			
200	Lymphosarcoma	4‡	2.4	>.05	1.7	0.5 to 4.3
201	Hodgkin's disease	1	1.6	>.05	0.6	0.02 to 3.5
202, 205	Lymphoblastoma	1	0.38	>.05	2.6	0.07 to 14.6
203	Multiple myeloma	5	1.01	.004	5.0	1.6 to 11.6
204	Leukemia	12	4.02	.001	3.0	1.5 to 5.2
292.4	Aplastic anemia	4	0.23	.0001	17.0	4.7 to 44.5

* From Lewis, E. B.: Leukemia, Multiple Myeloma, and Aplastic Anemia in American Radiologists. *Science* 142:1492–1494, 1963. Copyright 1963 by the American Association for the Advancement of Science. Only deaths occurring between the ages of 35 and 74, inclusive, in the 14 year period, 1948–1961, are included.

† Probability that the observed number of deaths, or a larger number, would occur by chance.

‡ Includes two deaths from lymphosarcoma, one from reticulum cell sarcoma, and one from malignant lymphoma.

and Lombard, 1966). (It is of interest to note the high correlation between a certain form of chronic granulocytic leukemia and a deleted piece of a 21 chromosome in humans, called the Philadelphia chromosome.)

A study in mortality and causes of death in a population of x-ray technicians in Japan (Takashi and Kihachiro, 1967) indicated that the age-corrected death from all causes is higher in these individuals and that the life expectancy at 20 years was 5 years shorter in this group than in other technical workers.

Studies by Shellabarger and Schmidt (1967) relating the incidence of mammary tumors to dose of partial-body irradiation of rats showed a linear relationship from 222 R to 888 R.

Studies of populations in Hiroshima and Nagasaki at the time of the atomic bomb explosions (Neel and Schull, 1962) listed increases in mongolism among other effects. This is mentioned here because it is easy to relate this condition (of trisomy) to radiation-induced chromosomal exchange.

Even shifts in sex ratio of offspring of irradiated men and women have been recorded (Lejeune, Turpin and Rethore, 1960) and tend to implicate induced changes in genetic material which are expressed at a time somewhat removed from exposure to radiation.

Studies of delayed effects are really just beginning to bear fruit, but the directions of these early studies are of great significance both to those who are exposed intentionally after calculated risks are weighed and to those who are exposed unintentionally but avoidably to changes that are realized many years after they are begun.

REFERENCES

Bacq, Z. M., and Alexander, P.: Fundamentals of Radiobiology. Pergamon Press, London, 1961.

Barranco, S. C., Beers, R. F., and Merz, T.: Unpublished Data.

Bender, M. A., Gooch, P. C., and Prescott, D. M.: Aberrations Induced in Human Leukocyte Chromosomes by H^3 Labeled Nucleosides. *Cytogenetics* 1:65, 1962.

Brewen, J. G.: X-Ray-Induced Chromosome Aberrations in the Corneal Epithelium of the Chinese Hamster. *Science* 138:820, 1962.

Brewen, J. G., and Merz, T.: Unpublished Observations.

Brown, D.: The Nucleolus and Synthesis of Ribosomal RNA during Oogenesis and Embryogenesis of Xenopus Laevis. *Nat. Cancer Inst. Monogr.* 23:297, 1966.

Cairns, J.: An Estimate of the Length of the DNA Molecule of T2 Bacteriophage by Autoradiography. *J. Molec. Biol.* 3:756, 1961.

Cronkite, E. P., Fliedner, T. M., Killman, S. A., and Rubini, J. R.: Tritium in the Physical and Biological Sciences. Vol. 2. International Atomic Energy Agency, Vienna, 1962, p. 190.

Curtis, H. J.: Biological Mechanisms of Delayed Radiation Damage in Mammals. *In* Ebert, M., and Howard, A.: Current Topics in Radiation Research. Vol. 3. Humanities Press, Inc., New York, 1967, p. 121.

Davies, D. R., and Evans, H. J.: The Role of Genetic Damage in Radiation-Induced Cell Lethality. *In* Augenstein, L., et al. (eds.): Advances in Radiation Biology. Vol. 2. Academic Press, New York, 1966, p. 243.

Deschner, E. E., and Gray, L. H.: Influence of Oxygen Tension on X-Ray-Induced Chromosomal Damage in Ehrlich Ascites Tumor Cells Irradiated *in vitro* and *in vivo*. *Radiat. Res.* 11:115, 1959.

Elkind, M. M., and Sutton, H.: Radiation Response of Mammalian Cells Grown in Culture. I. Repair of X-Ray Damage in Surviving Chinese Hamster Cells. *Radiat. Res.* 13:556, 1960.

Evans, H. J.: Chromosome Aberrations Induced by Ionizing Radiation. *Int. Rev. Cytol.* 13:221, 1962.

German, J. L., 3rd: DNA Synthesis in Human Chromosomes. *Trans. N. Y. Acad. Sci.* 24:395, 1962.

Glass, B.: Personal Communication, 1965.

Goldfeder, A.: The Integrity of Cytoplasmic Ultrastructures: A Factor in Cellular Radiosensitivity. Cellular Radiation Biology. 18th Symposium on Fundamental Cancer Research. Williams and Wilkins Co., Baltimore, 1964, p. 539.

Gray, L. H.: Ciba Foundation Symposium on Ionizing Radiation and Cell Metabolism. Little, Brown & Co., Boston, 1957, p. 255.

Hornsey, S.: The Effect of Fractionation on Four Day Survival of Mice after Whole-Body Neutron Irradiation. *Brit. J. Radiol.* 38:878, 1965.

Howard, A., and Pelc, S.: Synthesis of DNA in Normal and Irradiated Cells and Its Relation to Chromosome Breakage. *Heredity* 6:261, 1953.

Howard-Flanders, P., Simson, E., and Theriot, L.: The Excision of Thymine Dimers from DNA, Filament Formation and Sensitivity to Ultra-Violet Light in *E. coli* K-12. *Mutat. Res.* 1:219, 1964.

Hsu, T. C., Dewey, W. C., and Humphrey, R. M.: Radiosensitivity of Cells of Chinese Hamster *in vitro* in Relation to the Cell Cycle. *Exp. Cell Res.* 27:441, 1962.

Kihlman, B. A.: Different Effects of 5-Fluorodeoxyuridine and 5-Bromodeoxyuridine on the Frequencies of Chromatid Aberrations Obtained in Vicia faba after Irradiation with X-Rays. *Exp. Cell Res.* 27:604, 1962.

Kihlman, B. A.: Actions of Chemicals on Dividing Cells. Prentice-Hall, Inc., Englewood Cliffs, N. J., 1966.

Koernicke, M.: *Ber. Deutsch. Botan. Ges.* 23:405, 1905.

Lea, D. E. A.: Actions of Radiations on Living Cells. Ed. 2. Cambridge University Press, New York, 1962.

Lejeune, J., Turpin, R., and Rethore, M. O.: Les enfants nés de parents irradiés (cas particulier de la sex ratio). IX Congr. Intern. de radiol., Munich. 1089–1095, 1959.

Leonard, A., and Deknudt, G.: The Rate of Dominant Lethals after Low X-Ray Doses Given to Mouse Spermatozoa. *Mutat. Res.* 4:234, 1967.

Lewis, E. B.: Leukemia, Multiple Myeloma, and Aplastic Anemia in American Radiologists. *Science* 142:1492, 1963.

Lindop, P., and Rotblot, J.: Shortening-of-Life in Causes of Death in Mice Exposed to Single Whole-Body Dose of Radiation. *Nature* 189:645, 1961.

Merz, T., and Prempree, T.: Chromosomal Repair Time at Different Stages of Mitotic Interphase in Human Lymphocytes. International Congress of Radiation Research, 1966.

Merz, T., Swanson, C. P., and Cohn, N. S.: Interaction of Chromatid Breaks Produced by X-Rays and Radiomimetic Compounds. *Science* 133:703, 1961.

Muller, H. J.: Artificial Transmutation of the Gene. *Science* 66:84, 1927.

Neel, J. V., and Schull, W. J.: Genetic Effects of the Atomic Bomb. *Acta Radiol.* 58:385, 1962.

Nichols, W.: Chromosome Damage Associated with the Measles Virus *in vitro*. *Heredity* 54:101, 1965.

Oakberg, E. F.: Gamma-ray Sensitivity of Oocytes of Immature Mice. *Proc. Soc. Exper. Biol. Med.* 109:763, 1962a.

Oakberg, E. F.: The Effect of Low Radiation Doses on Spermatogonia and Oocytes of the Mouse. *Strahlentherapie* 51:103, 1962b.

Peters, H.: Radiation Sensitivity of Oocytes at Different Stages of Development in the Immature Mouse. *Radiat. Res.* 15:582, 1961.

Peters, H., and Levy, E.: Effect of Irradiation in Infancy on the Mouse Ovary. A Quantitative Study of Oocyte Sensitivity. *J. Reprod. Fertil.* 7:37, 1964.

Peters, H., and Borum, V.: The Development of Mouse Ovaries after Low-Dose Irradiation at Birth. *Internat. J. Radiat. Biol.* 3:1, 1961.

Ritossa, F.: Localization of DNA Complementary to Ribosomal RNA in the Nucleolus Organizer Region of Droscphila melanogaster. *Proc. Nat. Acad. Sci.* 53:737, 1965.

Rogers, R. W., and von Borstel, R. C.: Alpha-Particle Bombardment of the Habrobracon Egg. I. Sensitivity of the Nucleus. *Radiat. Res.* 7:484, 1957.

Rugh, R.: The Impact of Ionizing Radiations on the Embryo and Fetus. *Amer. J. Roentgen.* 89:182, 1963.

Rupert, C. S.: Photoreactivation of Transforming DNA by an Enzyme from Bakers' Yeast. *J. Gen. Physiol.* 43:573, 1960.

Russell, W.: The Nature of the Dose-Rate Effects of Radation on Mutation in Mice. *Japan. J. Genetics* Suppl. 40:132, 1966

Schmickel, R.: Chromosome Aberrations in Leukocytes Exposed *in vitro* to Diagnostic Levels of X-Rays. *Amer. J. Hum. Genet.* 19:1, 1967.

Setlow, J. K., and Setlow, R. B.: Nature of the Photoreactive Ultra-Violet Lesion in Deoxy-ribonucleic Acid. *Nature* 197:560, 1963.

Shellabarger, C., and Schmidt, R.: Mammary Neoplasia in the Rat as Related to Dose of Partial-Body Irradiation. *Radiat. Res.* 30:497, 1967.

Sparrow, A. H.: Relationship between Chromosome Volume and Radiosensitivity in Plant Cells. Cellular Radiation Biology. 18th Symposium on Fundamental Cancer Research. Williams and Wilkins Co., Baltimore, 1964, p. 199.

Steffensen, D.: Chromosome Aberrations Arising Spontaneously and Induced in Meiotic Cells at Low Levels of Radiation in Tradescantia. *Nature* 201:205, 1964.

Takashi, K., and Kihachiro, K.: *Indust. Med. & Surg.* 44:135, 1967.

von Borstel, R. C., and Rogers, R. W.: Alpha-Particle Bombardment of the Habrobracon Egg. II. Response of the Cytoplasm. *Radiat. Res.* 8:248, 1958.

Warren, S.: Leukemic Deaths—Radiologists. *J.A.M.A.* 162:464, 1956.

Warren, S., and Lombard, O. M.: Leukemic Deaths—Radiologists. *Arch. Environ. Health* 13:415, 1966.

Whitmore, G.: Studies on Recovery Process in Mouse L Cells. *Nat. Cancer Inst. Monogr.* 24:141, 1967.

Wimber, D. E.: Effects of Intracellular Irradiation with Tritium. *In* Augenstein, L., et al., (eds.): Advances in Radiation Biology. Vol. 1. Academic Press, New York, 1964, p. 85.

Wolff, S., and Luippold, H.: Metabolism and Chromosome Break Rejoining. *Science* 122:231, 1955.

Zelle, M. R., and Hollaender, A.: *In* Hollaender, A. (ed.): Radiation Biology. Vol. 2. McGraw-Hill Book Co., New York, 1955, p. 365.

XVII

RADIATION DOSIMETRY

EDWARD M. SMiTH

GORDON L. BROWNELL

WILLIAM H. ELLETT

INTRODUCTION

To evaluate the potential toxic effects of medically useful radioactive materials, we must first estimate the radiation absorbed by the patient during the procedure. The quantity of energy deposited in tissue is referred to as the *absorbed dose*. It is a measure of the potential risk to the patient, which must be weighed against the probable gains from the procedure. Calculation of absorbed dose should be made for medical uses of radioactive pharmaceuticals, for evaluation of chronic environmental exposure, and in cases of accidents involving radioactive materials.

Factors that affect the absorbed dose include: the activity of the administered radiopharmaceutical, its chemical and physical state, the route of administration, and the energy released per disintegration. The metabolic fate of radiopharmaceuticals is variable and sometimes must be evaluated with only limited data from animals and patients. The location, mass, and shape of the organ also affect the radiation hazard. Usually only the *average* absorbed dose for the organ as a whole can be calculated, even though the concentration of the radionuclide may be very high in certain parts of the organ. If we know that a radiopharmaceutical concentrates in a particular part of an organ—e.g., chlormerodrin in the renal cortex—the absorbed dose should be calculated for that part.

The absorbed dose should be calculated for the group of organs that are irradiated for the longest period of time or have the highest concentration of the radiopharmaceutical. It is customary to calculate the total body dose; however, in many instances the absorbed dose to an individual organ will be higher. The gonadal dose should always be evaluated.

Because of the many factors that must be taken into consideration, dosage calculations cannot be entirely accurate. The calculated dose is only an estimate and it is advisable to determine upper and lower values based on the best available data.

UNITS AND REGULATIONS

UNITS

In Report 10a, Radiation Quantities and Units (International Commission on Radiological Units, 1962), the following definitions are recommended:

rad = the unit of absorbed dose. The absorbed dose (D) is the energy deposited by ionizing radiation in matter. One rad equals 100 ergs per gram of matter.

curie = the unit of activity. One curie (c.) is equal to 3.7×10^{10} disintegrations per second.

The biological effects of ionizing radiation depend on the energy absorbed and various modifying factors. The *dose equivalent* unit is the "rem;" the dose in rems is equal to the absorbed dose in rads multiplied by the modifying factors related to the tissue sensitivity. The use of this unit is described in the Report of the *Relative Biological Effectiveness* (RBE) Committee (ICRP and ICRU, 1963). The dose equivalent in rems and the absorbed dose in rads are numerically identical for most clinically useful radionuclides.

MAXIMUM PERMISSIBLE DOSE

The maximum permissible dose (MPD), originally developed as a guideline for occupational exposure, may be used to evaluate the significance of the absorbed dose in diagnostic procedures. In designating the MPD, organs of the body are divided into four groups. All organs within each group have the same maximum permissible dose. The MPDs of the four groups of organs are (ICRP, 1964, 1966):

Gonads, red bone marrow, and whole body: 5 rems in a year
Skin, thyroid, and bone: 30 rems in a year
Hands and forearms: 75 rems in a year
All other organs: 15 rems in a year
One half the annual limit is permitted within a period of 3 months.

EQUATIONS FOR CALCULATING ABSORBED DOSE[1]

The classic equations for computing absorbed dose can be represented as follows:

---

[1] The mathematical formalism used in this chapter is based, in part, on a manuscript entitled "A Formalism for Calculation of Absorbed Dose from Radionuclides" (Loevinger and Berman, 1967) and was adopted by the *ad hoc* Committee on Medical Internal Radiation Dose (MIRD) of the Society of Nuclear Medicine. This material will be published in the Journal of Nuclear Medicine as MIRD pamphlet No. 1, "A Schema for Absorbed Dose Calculations for Biologically Distributed Radionuclides."

$$D = (51.2\, \overline{E}_\beta + 0.024\, \Gamma\, \overline{g}) \int_{t_1}^{t_2} C\, dt$$

where $\overline{E}_\beta$ = average energy in million electron volts per disintegration of all locally absorbed radiation including beta particles, conversion electrons, Auger electrons, and photons of 11.3 kev. or less.

             Γ = the specific gamma-ray constant, roentgens per hour per millicurie at 1 cm.

             $\overline{g}$ = the average geometrical factor for the absorber.

$\int_{t_1}^{t_2} C\, dt$ = the cumulative concentration of the isotope in the absorber, microcurie-days per gram.

Nonpenetrating radiation includes beta particles, conversion electrons, Auger electrons, and low energy photons, equal to or less than 11.3 kev. The energy of these radiations is assumed to be completely absorbed within the organ in which it is released. Penetrating radiation consists of electromagnetic radiation with energy greater than 11.3 kev. Absorption of penetration radiation is usually calculated by use of an "effective" exponential absorption coefficient. The equations just given are not valid for penetrating radiation below 100 kev. (Quimby, 1963). The general limitations of these equations have been reviewed by Smith (1966).

The method used to calculate absorbed dose should be simple yet flexible and applicable to any type of radiation, eliminating the dichotomy of penetrating and nonpenetrating radiations. In addition, the method should not contain unnecessary or hidden assumptions, nor need it be limited to previously established methods of calculating absorbed dose. The equations presented in this chapter fulfill these requirements.

The general equation for the calculation of the average absorbed dose is:

$$\overline{D}(v{\leftarrow}r) = \frac{\tilde{A}_r}{m_v} \sum_i \Delta_i\, \phi_i\, (v{\leftarrow}r) \qquad\qquad \text{rad} \qquad\qquad (1)$$

where

$\overline{D}(v{\leftarrow}r)$ = average absorbed dose to the volume, v, from the source, r. The source may be a point, line, surface, or volume.

$\tilde{A}_r$ = cumulative activity of the region, r, in microcurie-hours.

m_v = mass of volume, v, in grams.

Δ_i = equilibrium absorbed dose constant for radiations of type i = 1, 2, 3 . . . with a fractional frequency n_i per disintegration, and a mean energy, $n_i\overline{E}_i$, in million electron volts per disintegration.

Δ_i = $2.13 n_i\, \overline{E}_i\, \dfrac{\text{g.-rads}}{\mu\text{c.-hr.}}$

$\phi_i(v{\leftarrow}r)$ = absorbed fraction (dimensionless) for the ith type of radiation.

$\phi_i(v{\leftarrow}r)$ = $\dfrac{\text{energy from the } i^{th} \text{ type of radiation in source, r, absorbed in target volume, v}}{\text{energy of the } i^{th} \text{ type of radiation emitted by source region, r.}}$

In the case of self-irradiation, equation 1 becomes:

$$\overline{D}(v{\leftrightarrow}v) = \tilde{C}_v \sum_i \Delta_i\, \phi_i\, (v{\leftrightarrow}v) \qquad\qquad \text{rad} \qquad\qquad (2)$$

where

$\overline{D}(v \leftrightarrow v)$ = mean absorbed dose (rad) the target volume, v, receives from the source distributed within the target volume, v.

$\tilde{C}_v$ = cumulated concentration of activity in volume, v, in $\dfrac{\mu c.\text{-hr.}}{g.}$

$\phi_i(v \leftrightarrow v)$ = $\dfrac{\text{energy from the } i^{th} \text{ type of radiation in the source v absorbed in volume, v.}}{\text{energy of the } i^{th} \text{ type of radiation emitted by the source volume, v.}}$

Equations 1 and 2 apply to all radiations for which the absorbed fraction can be calculated or determined. The equations may be changed from absorbed dose to absorbed dose rate by changing the cumulative activity, $\tilde{A}$, and the cumulative concentration, $\tilde{C}$, to the instantaneous activity, A, and instantaneous concentration, C, at the time for which the dose rate is to be calculated.

To summarize, the calculation of absorbed dose by this method requires knowledge of: (1) the activity and the time during which the target is exposed to this activity, given by A or $\tilde{C}$; (2) the energy of the various radiations emitted by the nuclide, given by Δ_i; and (3) the fraction of the energy of each of the radiations absorbed by the target, given by ϕ_i.

One of the components, Δ_i, is a constant characteristic of each nuclide. A Δ_i for each radiation emitted by the nuclide can be determined with precision from knowledge of the decay scheme. Once computed, the Δ_i's characteristic of a given nuclide are applicable to all cases. In the section that follows, methods will be presented for computing each of the three components of the basic absorbed dose equations.

TABLE 17-1. SYMBOLS AND UNITS FOR THE ABSORBED DOSE AND ABSORBED DOSE RATE SYSTEMS

QUANTITY	SYMBOL	UNITS
Equilibrium absorbed dose constant	Δ	$\dfrac{g.\text{-rad}}{\mu c.\text{-hr.}}$
Absorbed dose	D	rad
Cumulated activity	$\tilde{A}$	$\mu c.\text{-hr.}$
Cumulated concentration	$\tilde{C}$	$\dfrac{\mu c.\text{-hr.}}{g.}$
Absorbed dose rate	R	$\dfrac{rad}{hr.}$
Activity	A	$\mu c.$
Concentration	C	$\dfrac{\mu c.}{g.}$

A bar over a quantity denotes a mean value, e.g., $\overline{D}$ rad. A tilde over a symbol denotes a time integral, e.g., $\tilde{A}$ $\mu c.$-hr.

DATA REQUIRED FOR ABSORBED DOSE CALCULATIONS

Concentration of Activity as a Function of Time

Tissue distribution data

The concentration of the administered radionuclide in various organs, tissues, and body compartments must be determined as a function of time. This is obtained from sampling of blood, urine, and feces, from external counting, and from tissues removed at operation or autopsy. Data in man may be supplemented by that from several species of experimental animals.

If the radiopharmaceutical concentrates in one or more organs, external counting techniques can be employed to determine how much of the material is retained and for how long. Organ phantoms may be useful for this. When feasible, autopsy and biopsy samples should be obtained to determine the concentration of the radiopharmaceutical in the organs.

Urine and fecal collections may present a problem in long-term studies, but this can be solved by the use of a whole body counter. The fraction of the administered activity retained by the patient is determined rather than that excreted. Urine and fecal samples should be correlated with the results obtained in the whole-body counter. Blood specimens should be taken periodically during the whole-body counting procedure.

The standard used to evaluate the activity in a tissue sample should be measured as precisely as possible in relation to the injected activity. If possible, the same syringe and needle should be used for preparation of dose and standard. Tissue samples should be small to minimize differences in counting efficiency due to variable absorption and geometry. Alternatively, the samples can be dissolved in concentrated nitric acid and brought to uniform volume. Nitric acid will dissolve all tissues except fat, which can be dissolved in isoamyl alcohol.

Organ mass and shape

External counting techniques must often be used to determine the amount of the radionuclide in an organ. The mass of the organ must be known for calculation of concentrations. Mass may be estimated on the basis of scanning, radiography, physical examination, or other data. Values of organ mass of a 70 kg. average of "standard" man are given in Table 17-2 (ICRP, 1960). Recently, Cook and Snyder (1965) have pointed out the limitations in the use of a standard man, and the ICRP has a task group revising the data characterizing standard man.

In calculating absorbed dose, it is often assumed that organs are spherical in shape and of unit density. These assumptions usually lead to overestimation of the absorbed dose since a sphere is the shape that results in the greatest absorption of self-contained radiation. Most organs are not spherical and therefore absorb somewhat less radiation than a mass-equivalent sphere. The error introduced by assuming that the organ is a sphere is not often serious because the estimate of dose is on the higher side. In cases in which the error is large,

TABLE 17-2. ORGANS OF STANDARD MAN. MASS AND EFFECTIVE RADIUS OF ORGANS OF THE ADULT HUMAN BODY*

	MASS, m (g.)	PER CENT OF TOTAL BODY*	EFFECTIVE RADIUS, X (cm.)
Total body†	70,000	100	30
Muscle	30,000	43	30
Skin and subcutaneous tissue‡	6100	8.7	0.1
Fat	10,000	14	20
Skeleton			
Without bone marrow	7000	10	5
Red marrow	1500	2.1	
Yellow marrow	1500	2.1	
Blood	5400	7.7	
Gastrointestinal tract†	2000	2.9	30
Contents of GI tract			
Lower large intestine	150		5
Stomach	250		10
Small intestine	1100		30
Upper large intestine	135		5
Liver	1700	2.4	10
Brain	1500	2.1	15
Lungs (2)	1000	1.4	10
Lymphoid tissue	700	1.0	
Kidneys (2)	300	0.43	7
Heart	300	0.43	7
Spleen	150	0.21	7
Urinary bladder	150	0.21	
Pancreas	70	0.10	5
Salivary glands (6)	50	0.071	
Testes (2)	40	0.057	3
Spinal cord	30	0.043	1
Eyes (2)	30	0.043	0.25
Thyroid gland	20	0.029	3
Teeth	20	0.029	
Prostate gland	20	0.029	3
Adrenal glands or suprarenal (2)	20	0.029	3
Thymus	10	0.014	
Ovaries (2)	8	0.011	3
Hypophysis (pituitary)	0.6	8.6×10^{-6}	0.5
Pineal gland	0.2	2.9×10^{-6}	0.04
Parathyroids (4)	0.15	2.1×10^{-6}	0.06
Miscellaneous (blood vessels, cartilage, nerves, etc.)	390	0.56	

* From International Commission on Radiation Protection, Committee II, 1959: Permissible Dose for Internal Radiation. *Health Phys.* 3:1, 1960.

† Does not include contents of the gastrointestinal tract.

‡ The mass of the skin alone is taken to be 2000 grams.

as, for example, in computing whole-body dose, a more realistic geometrical model, such as an ellipsoid or a right cylinder, will yield a more accurate result.

BIOLOGICAL, PHYSICAL, AND EFFECTIVE HALF-LIFE

The quantity of a radionuclide that remains in an organ can often be represented by a single exponential function of time or as a sum of several independent exponentials. Since the sum of several independent exponentials is also exponential, the combined rate of elimination, due to both biological and physical processes, can also be described by an exponential function.

If a radionuclide is eliminated from an organ by biological processes with a fractional clearance, λ_1, in units of reciprocal time, and simultaneously disappears as a result of physical decay at a rate given by the physical decay constant, λ, in the same units, then the effective decay constant, λ_{eff}, due to both processes is:

$$\lambda_{eff} = \lambda_1 + \lambda$$

Physical decay of a radionuclide can be represented by:

$$A_t = A_o \, e^{-\lambda t}$$

where A_t is the activity of the radionuclide at any time, t, and the initial activity at $t = 0$ is A_o, which is decaying at a rate given by λ. When the activity of the radionuclide has decreased to one half the initial value and T is the physical half-life of the radionuclide, then,

$$A_t/A_o = 0.5 \text{ and } 0.500 = e^{-\lambda T}$$

Inverting and taking the natural logarithm of both sides of this equation:

$$0.693 = \lambda T$$

and

$$\lambda = \frac{0.693}{T}$$

When a single exponential describes the rate of biological elimination from an organ, a similar expression may be written for λ_1

$$\lambda_1 = \frac{0.693}{T_1}$$

where T_1 is the biological half-life. The effective rate constant, λ_{1eff}, is:

$$\lambda_{1eff} = \frac{0.693}{T_{1eff}}$$

where T_{1eff} is the effective half-life of the radionuclide in the organ. Thus:

$$\frac{0.693}{T_{1eff}} = \frac{0.693}{T} + \frac{0.693}{T_1}$$

solving for T_{1eff}

$$T_{1eff} = \frac{T \times T_1}{T + T_1} \tag{3}$$

The effective half-life is always less than both the physical half-life and biological half-life.

EXAMPLE 1. The biological half-life of iodide in the thyroid of a patient is approximately 25 days. The physical half-life of ^{132}I is 2.3 hours and the physical half-life of ^{125}I is 60 days. Calculate the effective half-life for both cases:

$$^{132}\text{I} \qquad T = 0.096 \text{ d.} \qquad T_1 = 25 \text{ d.}$$

$$T_{1\text{eff}} = \frac{0.096 \times 25}{0.096 + 25} = 0.096 \text{ d.}$$

$$^{125}\text{I} \qquad T = 60 \text{ d.} \qquad T_1 = 25 \text{ d.}$$

$$T_{1\text{eff}} = \frac{60 \times 25}{60 + 25} = 17.6 \text{ d.}$$

In the case of ^{132}I the effective half-life is determined primarily by the physical decay of ^{132}I; for ^{125}I, by the rate of biological elimination from the thyroid.

In many instances, two or more equations are required to describe biological elimination of a radionuclide. A plot of the log concentration of the radionuclide versus time can be resolved into two or more components in such cases. The biological half-life of each component can then be determined directly (Chapter III). Figure 17-1 illustrates graphic determination of the components of a biological elimination curve. The straight portion of the blood activity curve (A) is extrapolated to zero time. The extrapolated curve (B) is then subtracted, point by point, from the original curve (A). The straight portion of the resultant curve (C) is then extrapolated to zero time. The process is repeated until the original curve is resolved into its components.

When the last measurement was made in the experiment depicted in Figure 17-1, the fraction of the administered activity in the blood was 0.135. We cannot be certain that the activity remaining in the organ will disappear at the same rate as during the first 17 days. Therefore it is safer to assume that the activity remaining in the organ will decrease at a rate equal only to the decay constant of the radionuclide.

CALCULATIONS

The absorbed dose is determined from the cumulated activity, $\tilde{A}$, and the cumulated concentration, $\tilde{C}$, by using the equations that follow. A set of equations for calculation of the absorbed dose rate from the activity, A, and the concentration, C, may be derived by appropriate changes in units.

The purpose of the expressions A and C is to permit calculation of the absorbed dose, and they should not be interpreted as definitive evidence of physiological mechanisms.

General Equations for Cumulated Activity and Concentration. The general equation for the cumulated activity, $\tilde{A}$, is:

$$\tilde{A} = \int_{t_1}^{t_2} A(t)dt \qquad \mu\text{c.-hr.} \tag{4}$$

where $A(t) =$ the activity, in μc., irradiating the tissue at any time, t, in hours.

t_1 and $t_2 =$ the time interval (in hours) for which the absorbed dose is being calculated; $0 \leq t_1 < t_2$ and $t_1 < t_2 \leq \infty$.

The generalized equation for the cumulated concentration, $\tilde{C}$, is:

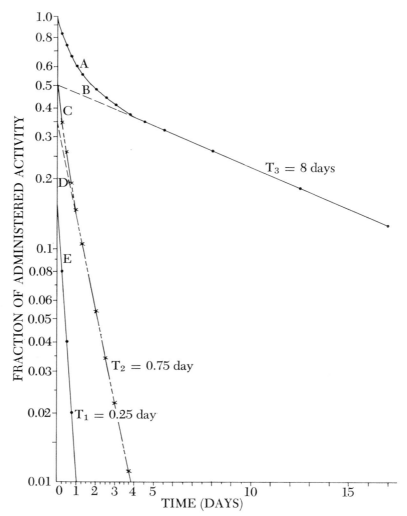

FIGURE 17-1. Graphic determination of the half-life of the components of a complex blood disappearance curve. The data have been corrected for physical decay.

$$\tilde{C} = \int_{t_1}^{t_2} C(t)dt \qquad \frac{\mu c.\text{-hr.}}{g.} \qquad (5)$$

where $C(t)$ = the concentration, in $\mu c./g.$, of the radionuclide in the tissue at any time, t, in hours, for which the absorbed dose is being calculated.

t_1 and t_2 = the time interval (in hours) for which the absorbed dose is being calculated; $0 \leq t_1 < t_2$ and $t_1 < t_2 \leq \infty$.

The expressions $A(t)$ and $C(t)$ often consist of one or more exponentials; therefore,

$$A(t) = \sum A_j(0)e^{-\lambda_{jeff}t}$$

and

$$\lambda_{eff} = \frac{0.693}{T_{eff}}$$

then

$$A(t) = \sum_j A_j(0)e^{-0.693t/T_{jeff}} \qquad \mu c. \qquad (6)$$

$$C(t) = \sum_j C_j(0)e^{-0.693t/T_{jeff}} \qquad \frac{\mu c.}{g.} \qquad (7)$$

where $A_j(0)$ = the initial activity, in $\mu c.$, in the tissue for the jth component
of the disappearance curve.

T_{jeff} = the effective half-life, in hours, of the jth component of the disappearance curve for a given organ.

$C_j(0)$ = the initial concentration, in $\mu c./g.$, in the tissue for the disappearance curve.

If $A(t)$ and $C(t)$ cannot be fitted by a series of exponentials, or by a power function, they may be determined by graphical integration.

Integrated Equations for Any Time Interval. The integrated forms of
equations 4 and 5 are:

$$\tilde{A} = 1.44 \sum_j A_j(0) T_{jeff} (e^{-0.693t_1/T_{jeff}} - e^{-0.693t_2/T_{jeff}}) \ \mu c.\text{-hr.} \qquad (8)$$

$$\tilde{C} = 1.44 \sum_j C_j(0) T_{jeff} (e^{-0.693t_1/T_{jeff}} - e^{-0.693t_2/T_{jeff}}) \ \frac{\mu c.\text{-hr.}}{g.} \qquad (9)$$

$\acute{A}$ and $\tilde{C}$ may be calculated for any time interval from t_1 to t_2. When using these
equations, we assume that the time during which the radioactivity is accumu-
lated by the tissue is negligible compared to the time during which it is
eliminated.

EXAMPLE 2. Calculate the cumulated concentration in the blood ($\tilde{C}$) between the second and fourth day from the data of Figure 17-1. The blood mass
is assumed to be 5400 g.; the patient received an injection of 100 $\mu c.$ of a radiopharmaceutical labeled with ^{131}I with a physical half-life of 8.05 days. From
Figure 17-1, we note that

$$C_1(0) = 0.16 \times \frac{100}{5400} = 0.0030 \ \mu c/g.$$

$$C_2(0) = 0.34 \times \frac{100}{5400} = 0.0063 \ \mu c./g.$$

$$C_3(0) = 0.50 \times \frac{100}{5400} = 0.0093 \ \mu c./g.$$

$$T_1 = 0.25 \text{ d.}; \ T_{1eff} = \frac{8.05 \times 0.25}{8.05 + 0.25} = 0.24 \text{ d.} \times 24 \text{ hr./d.} = 5.8 \text{ hr.}$$

$$T_2 = 0.75 \text{ d.}; \ T_{2eff} = \frac{8.05 \times 0.75}{8.05 + 0.75} = 0.69 \text{ d.} \times 24 \text{ hr./d.} = 17 \text{ hr.}$$

$$T_3 = 8 \text{ d.}; \quad T_{3eff} = \frac{8.05 \times 8}{8.05 + 8} = 4 \text{ d.} \times 24 \text{ hr./d.} = 96 \text{ hr.}$$

$$t_1 = 2 \text{ d.} \quad t_2 = 4 \text{ d.}$$

Substituting into equation 7,

$$\tilde{C} = 1.44 \sum_{j=3}^{j=1} [(0.0030 \times 5.8)(e^{-0.693\times4/0.24} - e^{-0.693\times2/0.24})]$$

$$+ [(0.0063 \times 17)(e^{-0.693\times4/0.69} - e^{-0.693\times2/0.69})]$$
$$+ [(0.0093 \times 96)(e^{-0.693\times4/4} - e^{-0.693\times2/4})]$$
$$= 1.44\ (5.22 \times 10^{-5} + 12.4 \times 10^{-3} + 185 \times 10^{-3})$$

$$\tilde{C} = 0.285\ \frac{\mu c.\text{-hr.}}{g.}$$

Equations for Complete Elimination of the Radionuclide. To determine the absorbed dose over the entire period during which the radionuclide is present, it is necessary to determine $\tilde{A}$ and $\tilde{C}$ from time $t_1 = 0$ to time $t_2 = $ infinity. When integrated between these limits, equations 4 and 5 become:

$$\tilde{A} = \int_o^\infty A(t)dt = 1.44 \sum A_j(0)\ T_{jeff} \qquad \mu c.\text{-hr.} \qquad (10)$$

$$\tilde{C} = \int_o^\infty C(t)dt = 1.44 \sum_j C_j(0)\ T_{jeff} \qquad \frac{\mu c.\text{-hr.}}{g.} \qquad (11)$$

These are maximum values for $\tilde{A}$ and $\tilde{C}$, and assume instantaneous uptake of the radionuclide. We sometimes assume that the slope of the last component of the curve describes the rate of elimination after the last measurement is made. It is better to use the physical half-life of the radionuclide rather than the extrapolated effective half-life for the time after the last datum point on the radionuclide disappearance curve. If this is done, equations 10 and 11 become:

$$\tilde{A} = 1.44 \sum_{j=1}^{j=n-1} A_j(0)T_{jeff} + 1.44A_n(0)\ T_{neff}\ (1 - e^{-0.693t*/T_{neff}})$$

$$+ 1.44\ A_n\ (t*)\ T\ (e^{-0.693t*/T}) \qquad \mu c.\text{-hr.} \quad (12)$$

$$\tilde{C} = 1.44 \sum_{j=1}^{=n-1} C_j(0)T_{jeff} + 1.44\ C_n(0)\ T_{neff}\ (1 - e^{-0.693t*/T_{neff}})$$

$$+ 1.44\ C_n\ (t*)\ T\ (e^{-0.693t*/T}) \qquad \frac{\mu c.\text{-hr.}}{g.} \quad (13)$$

where $A_n(0)$ = the initial activity, in $\mu c.$, in the tissue for the longest-lived component of the disappearance curve.

$A_n(t*)$ = the activity, in $\mu c.$, in the tissue for the longest-lived component of the disappearance curve at time, $t*$, when the last datum point was determined.

T_{neff} = the effective half-life, in hours, of the longest-lived component of the disappearance curve for a given organ.

$t*$ = the time, in hours, after the activity was administered, to the time that the last datum point on the disappearance curve was determined.

T = the physical half-life, in hours, of the radionuclide.

$C_n(0)$ = the initial concentration, in $\mu c./g.$, in the tissue for the longest-lived component of the disappearance curve.

$C_n(t^*)$ = the concentration, in μc./g., in the tissue for the longest-lived component of the disappearance curve at time, t^*, when the last datum point was determined.

EXAMPLE 3. Use the data from example 2 and calculate $\tilde{C}$ for complete elimination of the radionuclide from the blood under the following conditions: (1) The 8 day biological half-life accurately predicts the elimination of ^{131}I from the blood beyond day 17 when the last measurement was made. (2) The 8 day biological half-life does not accurately predict the elimination of ^{131}I from the blood beyond day 17, and the ^{131}I remaining in the blood at this time can only be considered to be eliminated by physical decay.

$$C_1(0) = 0.0030 \ \mu\text{c./g.} \qquad T_{1\text{eff}} = 5.8 \text{ hr.}$$
$$C_2(0) = 0.0063 \ \mu\text{c./g.} \qquad T_{2\text{eff}} = 17 \text{ hr.}$$
$$C_3(0) = 0.0093 \ \mu\text{c./g.} \qquad T_{3\text{eff}} = 4 \text{ d.} = 96 \text{ hr.}$$
$$C_3(t^*) = 0.0025 \ \mu\text{c./g.} \qquad t^* = 17 \text{ d.} = 408 \text{ hr.}$$
$$\qquad\qquad\qquad\qquad\qquad\qquad\quad T = 8.05 \text{ d.} = 193 \text{ hr.}$$

(1) Substituting into equation 11,

$$\tilde{C} = 1.44 \ [(0.0030 \times 5.8) + (0.0063 \times 17) + (0.0093 \times 96)]$$

$$\tilde{C} = \frac{1.47 \ \mu\text{c.-hr.}}{\text{g.}}$$

(2) Substituting into equation 13,

$$\tilde{C} = 1.44 \ [(0.0030 \times 5.8) + (0.0063 \times 17)]$$
$$+ \ (1.44 \times 0.0093 \times 96)(1 - e^{-0.693 \times 17/4})$$
$$+ \ (1.44 \times 0.0025 \times 193) \ e^{-0.693 \times 17/8.05}$$

$$\tilde{C} = 1.55 \ \frac{\mu\text{c.-hr.}}{\text{g.}}$$

The true value for $\tilde{C}$ in example 3 lies somewhere between 1.47 and 1.55 μc.-hr./g., but since measurements were not made beyond 17 days, the more conservative value must be used. The true value can only be determined by following the disappearance curve for a longer period of time. If ^{125}I, with a physical half-life of 60 days, was the radionuclide under consideration in example 3, the values for $\tilde{C}$ would be 6.65 and 7.35. For 8 day ^{131}I, $\tilde{C}$ is increased by 1.05; for long-lived ^{125}I, $\tilde{C}$ is increased by 1.11. It is apparent that when long-lived radionuclides are used, the disappearance curves must be followed for longer periods of time. If this is not done, the quantity of activity that can be administered to a patient may be limited because of insufficient distribution data, forcing one to make an unrealistically high estimate of the absorbed dose.

Equations To Be Used When the Amount of Time Required for Uptake Is Significant. An error may be introduced into the calculated value of $\tilde{A}$ or $\tilde{C}$ if one assumes instantaneous uptake of the radionuclide by the tissue. When the physical half-life of the radionuclide is comparable to the biological half-time for uptake, the error due to this assumption is especially great (Loevinger et al., 1956a). If a short-lived radionuclide is used, we will overestimate the absorbed dose unless the physical decay of the short-lived radionuclide is taken into account during the uptake period. This consideration is becoming more important in nuclear medicine with the increasing use of short-lived radionuclides such as iodine-132, strontium-87m, technetium-99m, and gallium-68.

The concentration of the radionuclide at any time during the period of uptake is given by:

$$C(t) = C(0)(e^{-0.693t/T_{eff}} - e^{-0.693t/T_{up}}) \qquad \frac{\mu c.}{g.}$$

where $C(t)$ = concentration, in μc./g., in the tissue at time, t.

$C(0)$ = maximum concentration, in μc./g., in the tissue if there were instantaneous uptake, i.e. T_{up} = 0, or $C(0)$ would be approached asymptotically if there were no elimination from the tissue, i.e., $T_{eff} \rightarrow \infty$.

T_{up} = effective half-time, in hours, for uptake in the tissue.

$$= \frac{T \times T_{bu}}{T + T_{bu}}$$

T_{bu} = biological half-time, in hours, for uptake in the tissue.

To evaluate $C(0)$, one extrapolates back to time t = 0, on the curve describing the exponential elimination of the radionuclide.

Thus to evaluate $\tilde{A}$ and $\tilde{C}$ for complete elimination of the radionuclide when the initial uptake period must be considered (see Loevinger et al., 1956a for derivation), we use the following equations:

$$\tilde{A} = 1.44 \, A(0) \, [T_{eff} - T_{up}] \quad \mu c.\text{-hr.} \tag{14}$$

$$\tilde{C} = 1.44 \, C(0) \, [T_{eff} - T_{up}] \quad \frac{\mu c.\text{-hr.}}{g.} \tag{15}$$

By rearranging equation 15,

$$\tilde{C} = 1.44C \, (0) \, T_{eff} \left(1 - \frac{T_{up}}{T_{eff}}\right)$$

As a rule of thumb, if T_{eff} is at least 20 times greater than T_{up}, T_{up} can be neglected in absorbed dose calculations since the error would be 5 per cent or less.

EXAMPLE 4. Calculate $\tilde{C}$ for a thyroid gland where T_{bu} is 5 hours, T_1 (biol. excretion) is 50 days, and the initial concentration of radioactive iodine is 1 μc./g. Calculate for ^{131}I, T = 8.05 days, for the following conditions: (1) assuming instantaneous uptake of the radionuclide by the thyroid and complete elimination; and (2) repeat the calculations, taking into account the period of initial uptake.

$$T = 8.05 \text{ d.} \times 24 \text{ hr./d.} = 193 \text{ hr.}$$

$$T_{up} = \frac{T \times T_{bu}}{T + T_{bu}} = \frac{193 \times 5}{193 + 5} = 4.9 \text{ hr.}$$

$$T_{eff} = \frac{T \times T_1}{T + T_1} = \frac{8.05 \times 50}{8.05 + 50} = 6.95 \text{ d.} = 167 \text{ hr.}$$

(1) Substitute into equation 11,

$$\tilde{C} = 1.44 \times 1 \times 167 = 240 \, \frac{\mu c.\text{-hr.}}{g.}$$

(2) Substitute into equation 15,

$$\tilde{C} = 1.44 \times 1 \; [167 - 4.9] = 234 \; \frac{\mu c.\text{-hr.}}{g.}$$

In the case of ^{132}I,

$$T = 2.33 \text{ hr.}$$

$$T_{up} = \frac{2.33 \times 5}{2.33 + 5} = 1.59 \text{ hr.}$$

$$T_{eff} = \frac{2.33 \times (50 \times 24)}{2.33 + (50 \times 24)} = 2.32 \text{ hr.}$$

(1) Substitute into equation 11,

$$\tilde{C} = 1.44 \times 1 \times 2.33 = 3.36 \; \frac{\mu c.\text{-hr.}}{g.}$$

(2) Substitute into equation 15,

$$\tilde{C} = 1.44 \times 1 \; [2.33 - 1.59] = 1.07 \; \frac{\mu c.\text{-hr.}}{g.}$$

One can readily see that the initial uptake period could have been neglected for ^{131}I. However, for ^{132}I, one would have overestimated $\tilde{C}$ by a factor of 3, if the initial uptake period had not been considered in the calculation of $\tilde{C}$.

Equations To Be Used When Only Limited Tissue Distribution Data Are Available. At times, we must evaluate $\tilde{A}$ or $\tilde{C}$ from limited distribution data when simple exponential functions do not describe elimination of the radionuclide. In such cases, $\tilde{A}$ or $\tilde{C}$ can be approximated by graphic integration of the concentration or activity versus time curves. The activity remaining in the tissue after the last observation is assumed to be eliminated at a rate equal to the decay constant of the radionuclide. Equations 16 and 17 are used to make these calculations.

$$\tilde{A} = \sum_{j=1}^{j=n-1} (A_j - A_{j+1}) \left[T_j + \left(\frac{T_{j+1} - T_j}{2} \right) \right] + A_n T_n + .44 \, A_n T \qquad \mu c.\text{-hr.} \quad (16)$$

$$\tilde{C} = \sum_{j=1}^{j=n-1} (C_j - C_{j+1}) \left[T_j + \left(\frac{T_{j+1} - T_j}{2} \right) \right] + C_n T_n + 1.44 \, C_n T \qquad \frac{\mu c.\text{-hr.}}{g.} \quad (17)$$

where A_j = activity, in $\mu c.$, irradiating the tissue at the jth observation made at time T_j, in hours.

A_{j+1} = activity, in $\mu c.$, irradiating the tissue at the $j + 1^{th}$ observation made at time T_{j+1}, in hours.

A_n = activity, in $\mu c.$, irradiating the tissue when the last observation was made, $j = n$, at time, T_n, in hours.

C_j = concentration, in $\mu c./g.$, in the tissue at the jth observation made at time T_j, in hours.

C_{j+1} = concentration, in $\mu c./g.$, in the tissue at the $j + 1^{th}$ observation made at time T_{j+1}, in hours.

C_n = concentration, in $\mu c./g.$, in the tissue when the last observation was made, j = n, at time T_n, in hours.

Equations 16 and 17 will tend to overestimate $\tilde{A}$ and $\tilde{C}$ by 5 to 10 per cent.

EXAMPLE 5. Calculate $\tilde{C}$ for the kidneys based on the following limited data for a ^{99m}Tc-labeled compound.

Observation, j	1	2	3	4	5
T_j (hours)	0	1	2	4	8
C_j ($\mu c./g.$)	10	5.75	3.55	1.75	0.70

T = 6 hr.

n = 5

C_n = 0.70 $\mu c./g.$

T_n = 8 hr.

Substituting into equation 17,

$$\tilde{C} = \sum_{i=1}^{j=4}\left\{(10 - 5.75)\left[0 + \left(\frac{1-0}{2}\right)\right] + (5.75 - 3.55)\left[1 + \left(\frac{2-1}{2}\right)\right]\right.$$

$$\left. + (3.55 - 1.75)\left[2 + \left(\frac{4-2}{2}\right)\right] + (1.75 - 0.70)\left[4 + \left(\frac{8-4}{2}\right)\right]\right\}$$

$$ + (0.70 \times 8) + (1.44 \times 0.70 \times 6)$$

$$= \sum_{j=1}^{j=4}(2.13 + 3.30 + 5.40 + 6.30) + 5.60 + 6.04$$

$$\tilde{C} = 28.8 \; \frac{\mu c.\text{-hr.}}{g.}$$

EQUILIBRIUM ABSORBED DOSE CONSTANT

The equilibrium absorbed dose constant, Δ, is the total energy emitted by a radionuclide per disintegration. Then

$$\Delta = \sum_i \Delta_i = \sum_i n_i \bar{E}_i \; \frac{\text{Mev.}}{\text{disint.}}$$

where Δ_i = equilibrium absorbed dose constant for the ith type of radiation emitted by the radionuclide.

n_i = fractional frequency of the ith type of radiation, e.g., gamma-rays, x-rays, conversion electrons, beta particles, emitted per disintegration.

$\bar{E}_i$ = energy of the ith type of radiation, Mev.

$n_i \bar{E}_i$ = mean energy, Mev./disint., for the ith type of radiation.

The equilibrium absorbed dose constant, Δ, represents the amount of energy that would be deposited in an absorber if absorption were complete. It is necessary to compute Δ_i separately for each type and energy of radiation emitted by the nuclide since ϕ, the absorbed fraction, depends upon both these factors. Δ_i may be expressed in other more convenient units.

$$\Delta_i = n_i\overline{E}_i \frac{\text{Mev.}}{\text{disint.}} \times 1.6 \times 10^{-6} \frac{\text{ergs}}{\text{Mev.}} \times 3.7 \times 10^4 \frac{\text{disint./sec.}}{\mu c.} \times 3600 \frac{\text{sec.}}{\text{hr.}}$$

$$\times 10^{-2} \frac{\text{rads}}{\text{g.-ergs}}$$

$$\Delta_i = 2.13 \ n_i E_i \frac{\text{g.-rads}}{\mu c.\text{-hr.}} \tag{18}$$

or:

$$\Delta_i = 2.13 \ n_i\overline{E}_i \frac{\text{g.-rads}}{\mu c.\text{-hr.}} \times \frac{24 \ \text{hr.}}{\text{d.}}$$

$$\Delta_i = 51.12 \ n_i\overline{E}_i \frac{\text{g.-rads}}{\mu c.\text{-d.}}$$

The determination of n_i and $\overline{E}_i$ for various modes of decay is considered in the following section.

ENERGY AND FRACTIONAL FREQUENCY OF ELECTROMAGNETIC AND PARTICULATE RADIATIONS

BETA MINUS AND BETA PLUS PARTICLES

We have seen in Chapter IV that the energies of beta particles range from a maximum value, characteristic of the particular radionuclide, through a continuous spectrum of lower energies. Usually we can find this mean value $\overline{E}$ in a table, once the correct values are obtained, the equilibrium absorbed dose constant may be calculated using equation 18.

$$\Delta_i = 2.13 \ n_i\overline{E}_i \frac{\text{g.-rad}}{\mu c.\text{-hr.}}$$

where $\qquad\qquad n_i\overline{E}_i = n_\beta{}^-\overline{E}_\beta{}^- \text{ or } n_\beta{}^+\overline{E}_\beta{}^+$

If values of $n_\beta{}^-{}_\beta\overline{E}_\beta{}^-$ or $n_\beta{}^+\overline{E}_\beta{}^+$ cannot be obtained, $\overline{E}_\beta$ can be obtained from empirical equations suggested by the ICRP (1960). Results are, in most cases, accurate to within 5 per cent (Morgan, 1950).

For beta minus particles:

$$n_i\overline{E}_i = n_\beta{}^-\overline{E}_\beta{}^- = 0.33 \ E_o n_i \left(1 - \frac{Z^{\frac{1}{2}}}{50}\right)\left(1 + \frac{E_o^{\frac{1}{2}}}{4}\right)\frac{\text{Mev.}}{\text{disint.}} \tag{19}$$

For beta plus particles:

$$n_i\overline{E}_i = n_\beta{}^+\overline{E}_\beta{}^+ = 0.33 \ E_o n_i \left(1 + \frac{E_o^{\frac{1}{2}}}{4}\right)\frac{\text{Mev.}}{\text{disint.}} \tag{20}$$

where Z = atomic number

n_i = fractional frequency of the type of decay per disintegration

E_o = maximum beta particle energy (Mev.)

Although equations 19 and 20 are applicable to most cases of beta decay, in some cases the beta particle spectrum has an atypical shape that results in a significant error in the calculated values. For example, $n_\beta^- E_\beta^-$ for strontium-90 will be underestimated by 17 per cent and bismuth-210 (RaE) will be overestimated by 23 per cent (Loevinger et al., 1956a) if equation 19 is used.

Whenever a radionuclide decays by beta plus emission, two 0.51 Mev. photons are produced as a result of the annihilation process (Chapter IV). The equilibrium absorbed dose constant for the annihilation radiation is calculated as follows:

$$\Delta_{\text{annihilation}} = 2.13 \times 2 \; n_\beta^+ E_{0.51}$$

where 2 = annihilation photon yield per positron emitted.

n_β^+ = fractional frequency per disintegration for positron emission.

$E_{0.51}$ = 0.51 Mev.

ELECTRON CAPTURE

When a radionuclide decays by electron capture, a vacancy is created in an orbital electron shell, which is filled almost immediately by an electron from an outer orbit. For example, following K electron capture, the vacancy will be filled by an electron from the L-, M-, N-, or O-shell. When an electron from an outer shell fills the vacancy created by electron capture, an x-ray that is characteristic of the *daughter* nuclide is emitted. When a K vacancy is filled by an L electron, the characteristic radiation is called a K_α x-ray, the energy of which is equal to the binding energy of the K electron, E_K, le 's the average binding energy of the L_{II} and L_{III} electrons, $E_{L_{II\text{-}III}}$. A K_β x-ray results if the vacancy created by K electron capture is filled by an M electron. Similarly, L x-rays result from vacancies in the L shell filled by M or N electrons.

The characteristic x-ray may escape from the atom in which it originated or it may interact with one of the remaining orbital electrons, ejecting the electron from the atom. An electron released by this phenomenon is known as an Auger electron. Auger electrons are monochromatic and have energy equal to the characteristic x-ray minus their binding energy.

The "fluorescent yield," denoted by ω, is the fraction of shell vacancies that result in x-rays escaping from the atom, and $(1 - \omega)$ is the fraction resulting in Auger electrons. Only ω_K, the K-shell fluorescent yield, need be considered. Ninety-five per cent or more of the energy of L or less energetic x-rays from elements with atomic number less than 82 is deposited in tissue within 1 cm. of their origin. Values for ω_K are included in the Appendix.

Previous authors (Loevinger et al., 1956a) assumed that all K x-rays were K_α. It is more accurate to use the actual yields of K_α and K_β. This is particularly important in nuclides of high atomic number, since K x-rays constitute a major part of the photon yield. L x-rays contribute a large share of the energy deposited near the atom which has undergone electron capture.

In decay by electron capture, the energy per disintegration is designated as $n_\epsilon \bar{E}_\epsilon$. The component of $n_\epsilon \bar{E}_\epsilon$ caused by the L and M vacancies resulting from the production of K x-rays is given by:

$$n_{\epsilon_K} \omega_K \left[\left(\frac{K_\alpha}{K_\alpha + K_\beta} \right) E_{L_{II\text{-}III}} + \left(\frac{K_\beta}{K_\alpha + K_\beta} \right) E_{M_{II\text{-}III}} \right] \text{ Mev./disint.} \quad (21a)$$

where n_{ϵ_K} = fractional frequency of K electron capture per disintegration.

$E_{L_{II-III}}$ = average binding energy of L_{II} and L_{III} electrons (Mev.).

$E_{M_{II-III}}$ = average binding energy of M_{II} and M_{III} electrons (Mev.).

$\dfrac{K_\alpha}{K_\alpha + K_\beta}$ = relative abundance of K_α x-rays.

$\dfrac{K_\beta}{K_\alpha + K_\beta}$ = relative abundance of K_β x-rays.

The values of 0.75 and 0.25 may be used for $\dfrac{K_\alpha}{K_\alpha + K_\beta}$ and $\dfrac{K_\beta}{K_\alpha + K_\beta}$ respectively, with reasonable accuracy for nuclides with atomic numbers between 35 and 82. (More accurate values may be found in *Nuclear Spectroscopy Tables*, page 81 [Wapstra et al., 1959].) Equation 21a includes all Auger electrons except K Auger electrons since the *binding energies* of the L and M electrons were used.

The energy released in association with Auger electrons includes electrons released by K, L, or M x-rays, and is given by:

$$n_{\epsilon_K} (1 - \omega_K) E_K \text{ Mev./disint.} \tag{21b}$$

Electron capture from the L_I, L_{II}, and M_T-shells can also occur. This is discussed in detail by Smith, Harris and Rohrer (1965). The energy from L_I, L_{II} and M_I electron capture is given by:

$$n_{\epsilon_{L_I}} E_{L_I} + n_{\epsilon_{L_{II}}} E_{L_{II}} + n_{\epsilon_{M_I}} E_{M_I} \text{ Mev./disint.} \tag{21c}$$

where $n_{\epsilon_{L_I}}$, $n_{\epsilon_{L_{II}}}$, and $n_{\epsilon_{M_I}}$ = fractional frequency of L_I, L_{II}, and M_I electron capture per disintegration, respectively.

E_{L_I}, $E_{L_{II}}$, and E_{M_I} = binding energies of the L_I, L_{II}, and M_I electrons, respectively.

The fractions n_{ϵ_K}, $n_{\epsilon_{L_I}}$, $n_{\epsilon_{L_{II}}}$ and $n_{\epsilon_{M_I}}$ may be determined from K/L/M (sometimes denoted as e_L/e_K and e_M/e_L) capture ratios. These ratios are listed in the Nuclear Data Sheets. When sufficient nuclear energy is available, positron emission competes with electron capture as a mode of decay. Therefore, we must take into account the branching ratio between electron capture and positron emission in calculating n_ϵ.

By combining equations 21a, 21b, and 21c, one may obtain $n_\epsilon \bar{E}_\epsilon$ for electron capture.

$$n_\epsilon \bar{E}_\epsilon = n_{\epsilon_K} \omega_K \left[\left(\frac{K_\alpha}{K_\alpha + K_\beta} \right) E_{L_{II-III}} + \left(\frac{K_\beta}{K_\alpha + K_\beta} \right) E_{M_{II-III}} \right]$$
$$+ n_{\epsilon_K}(1 - \omega_K)E_K + n_{\epsilon_{L_I}}E_{L_I} + n_{\epsilon_{L_{II}}}E_{L_{II}} + n_{\epsilon_{M_I}}E_{M_I} \text{ Mev./disint.} \tag{21d}$$

Some radionuclides decay by electron capture to more than one energy state, which is indicated in the capture branching ratios; each transition should be calculated separately. Then:

$$n_\epsilon \bar{E}_\epsilon = n_{\epsilon 1} \bar{E}_{\epsilon 1} + n_{\epsilon 2} \bar{E}_{\epsilon 2} + \ldots$$

Once $n_\epsilon \bar{E}_\epsilon$ has been calculated for a radionuclide that decays by electron capture, the equilibrium absorbed dose constant for electron capture, Δ_ϵ, may be calculated using equation 18.

EXAMPLE 6. Calculate Δ_ϵ for $^{131}_{55}\text{Cs}$ which decays 100 per cent of the time by electron capture to $^{131}_{54}\text{Xe}$ and $e_L/e_K = 0.153$. From the Appendix, ω_K for Xe $= 0.87$.

Electron binding energies for xenon are:

$$E_K = 0.0346 \text{ Mev.}$$

$$E_{L_1} = 0.00545 \text{ Mev.}$$

$$E_{L_{II-III}} = 0.00494 \text{ Mev.}$$

$$E_{M_{II \; III}} = 0.00096 \text{ Mev.}$$

$$e_L + e_K = 1 \quad e_L/e_K = 0.153$$

$$e_L = 0.133 = n_{eL} \quad e_K = 0.867 = n_{eK}$$

Substituting into equation 21,

$$n_\epsilon \, \bar{E}_\epsilon = (0.867 \times 0.87) \, [(0.75 \times 0.00494) + (0.25 \times 0.00096)]$$
$$+ \, 0.867 \, (1 - 0.87) \, 0.0346 + (0.133 \times 0.00545)$$

$$n_\epsilon \, \bar{E}_\epsilon = 0.0076 \text{ Mev./disint.}$$

Substituting into equation 18,

$$\Delta_\epsilon = 2.13 \times 0.0076$$

$$\Delta_\epsilon = 0.0162 \, \frac{\text{g.-rads}}{\mu\text{c.-hr.}}$$

INTERNAL CONVERSION

When a radionuclide decays by β^-, β^+ emission or by electron capture, the resulting daughter nuclide may be left in an excited state. The transition from the excited state to the ground state of the daughter nuclide is accompanied by either the emission of a gamma-ray or transfer of the excitation energy to an orbital electron, which is then called a conversion electron. The process is known as internal conversion (Chapter IV). Monoenergetic conversion electrons are ejected with kinetic energy equal to that of the unconverted gamma-rays, minus the binding energy of the ejected electron.

Gamma-ray emission and internal conversion are competitive processes. The relative occurrence of these two processes is given by the internal conversion coefficient, α, which is the ratio of the number of conversion electrons, N_e, emitted to the number of gamma-rays emitted, N.

$$\alpha = \frac{N_e}{N_\gamma}$$

Internal conversion is most probable in the innermost electron shells, K, L, M. There will be an internal conversion coefficient for each electron shell.

$$\alpha_{\text{total}} = \alpha_t = \alpha_K + \alpha_L + \alpha_M + \ldots$$

Vacancies in the shells caused by internal conversion are filled by electrons from outer orbits, resulting in characteristic x-rays and Auger electrons. In the Nuclear Data Sheets α_t is given as α.

The number of K, L, M . . . conversion electrons arising from a photon of energy, E_γ, per disintegration will be described as N_{eK}, N_{eL}, N_{eM} . . ., respectively.

and

$$N_{eK} = \frac{\alpha_K}{1 + \alpha_t} \qquad N_{eL} = \frac{\alpha_L}{1 + \alpha_t} \qquad N_{eM} = \frac{\alpha_M}{1 + \alpha_t}$$

where α_K, α_L, and α_M are the internal conversion ratios for the K, L, and M electron shells, respectively. In many instances, the Nuclear Data Sheets give α_K or α_t, and the K/L/M/N ratio, i.e., the numerical ratio of K conversion electrons to L conversion electrons to M conversion electrons. These data are sufficient to calculate N_e.

In internal conversion, the energy per disintegration deposited in the vicinity of the nuclide is designated as $n_e \bar{E}_e$. The following equation gives the components of $n_e \bar{E}_e$:

$$n_e \bar{E}_e = f_\gamma N_{eK} (E_\gamma - E_K) + f_\gamma N_{eL} E_\gamma + f_\gamma N_{eM} E_\gamma + f_\gamma N_{eK} (1 - \omega_K) E_K$$
$$+ f_\gamma N_{eK} \omega_K \left[\left(\frac{K_\alpha}{K_\alpha + K_\beta} \right) E_{LII\text{-}III} + \left(\frac{K_\beta}{K_\alpha + K_\beta} \right) E_{MII\text{-}III} \right]$$

where f_γ is the fractional frequency of the disintegrations that give rise to a photon of energy E_γ. (This is the fractional frequency before the photon has been corrected for internal conversion.) The terms on the first line of the equation give the direct contribution from the conversion electrons from the K-, L-, and M-shells, respectively. The term on the second line gives the contribution from K Auger electrons following conversion in the K electron shells. The last term states the contribution from L and lower-order x-rays and Auger electrons from K x-ray emission following K internal conversion.

The equation for $n_e \bar{E}_e$ may be simplified by combining terms to:

$$n_e \bar{E}_e = f_\gamma N_{eK} \left[E_\gamma - \omega_K E_K + \omega_K \left\{ \left(\frac{K_\alpha}{K_\alpha + K_\beta} \right) E_{LII\text{-}III} + \left(\frac{K_\beta}{K_\alpha + K_\beta} \right) E_{MII\text{-}III} \right\} \right]$$
$$+ f_\gamma E_\gamma (N_{eL} + N_{eM} + \ldots) \quad \text{Mev./disint.} \quad (22)$$

The effects of internal conversion of gamma-rays of different energy in the same or competitive decay processes are summed. Then,

$$n_e \bar{E}_e = n_{e_1} \bar{E}_{e_1} + n_{e_2} \bar{E}_{e_2} \ldots$$

CHARACTERISTIC X-RAYS

Characteristic x-rays are produced as a result of electron capture and internal conversion of photons. The fractional frequency of K_α and K_β x-rays is calculated from the expressions for electron capture and internal conversion. We calculate the fractional frequency of K_α and K_β x-rays only because the energy of L and lower-order x-rays is included in the expressions for electron capture and internal conversion.

The K_α and K_β x-ray yield resulting from decay by electron capture and internal conversion of photons is given by:

$$n_{K_\alpha} = \omega_K \left(\frac{K_\alpha}{K_\alpha + K_\beta} \right) \left[\sum_i n_{\epsilon K_i} + \sum f_{\gamma j} N_{eK_j} \right] \qquad \frac{\text{number}}{\text{disint.}} \qquad (23a)$$

$$n_{K_\beta} = \omega_K \left(\frac{K_\beta}{K_\alpha + K_\beta} \right) \left[\sum_i n_{\epsilon K_i} + \sum f_{\gamma j} N_{eK_j} \right] \qquad \frac{\text{number}}{\text{disint.}} \qquad (23b)$$

where n_{K_α} = fractional frequency of K_α x-rays emitted per disintegration.

n_{K_β} = fractional frequency of K_β x-rays emitted per disintegration.

$n_{\epsilon K_i}$ = fractional frequency of K electron capture per disintegration to the ith energy level.

f_{γ_j} = fractional frequency of the disintegrations that give rise to a photon of energy, E_{γ_j}. (This is the fractional frequency before the photon yield has been corrected for internal conversion.)

N_{eK_j} = number of K conversion electrons arising from the conversion of a photon of energy E_{γ_j} per disintegration.

GAMMA-RAYS

The fractional frequency of unconverted photons, that is, the proportion of the photons that are not internally converted, may be calculated from the following equation:

$$n_{\gamma_i} = f_{\gamma_i} \left(\frac{1}{1 + \alpha_{t_i}} \right) \qquad \frac{\text{number}}{\text{disint.}} \tag{24}$$

where $n_{\gamma i}$ = fractional frequency of unconverted gamma-rays per disintegration of energy, $E_{\gamma i}$.

$f_{\gamma i}$ = fractional frequency of gamma-rays per disintegration of energy, $E_{\gamma i}$ (fractional frequency not corrected for internal conversion).

$\alpha_{t i}$ = total internal conversion coefficient for gamma-ray of energy, $E_{\gamma i}$.

EXAMPLE 7. Calculate Δ_e, Δ_{K_α}, Δ_{K_β} and Δ_γ for ^{99m}Tc. The decay scheme is shown in Figure 17-2, along with the conversion coefficients and branching ratios.

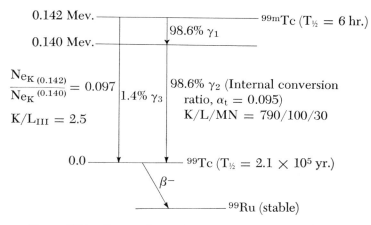

FIGURE 17-2. Decay scheme of technetium-99m (Smith, 1965).

$$\omega_K \text{ for Tc} = 0.76$$

$$E_K = 0.0211 \text{ Mev.}$$

$$E_{L_{II}\text{-}III} = 0.0027 \text{ Mev.}$$

$$E_{M_{II}\text{-}III} = 0.0004 \text{ Mev.}$$

From Smith (1965),

$$\frac{K_\alpha}{K_\alpha + K_\beta} = 0.815 \qquad \frac{K_\beta}{K_\alpha + K_\beta} = 0.185$$

1. For the 0.140 Mev. gamma-ray, γ_2,

$$N_{et} = \frac{\alpha_t}{1 + \alpha_t} = \frac{0.095}{1 + 0.095} = 0.0868$$

$$N_{eK} = \left(\frac{790}{790 + 100 + 30}\right) N_{et} = 0.0746$$

$$N_{eL} + N_{eM} = N_{et} - N_{eK} = 0.0122$$

Substituting into equation 22,

$$n_{e2}\bar{E}_{e2} = (0.986 \times 0.0746)[0.140 - (0.76 \times 0.0211) + 0.76\{(0.815 \times 0.0027)$$
$$+ (0.185 \times 0.0004)\}] + (0.986 \times 0.140 \times 0.0122)$$

$$n_{e2}\bar{E}_{e2} = 0.0109 \text{ Mev./disint.}$$

Substituting into equation 24,

$$n_{\gamma 2} = 0.986 \left(\frac{1}{1 + 0.095}\right) = 0.900 \text{ gamma-rays/disint.}$$

2. For the 0.142 Mev. gamma-ray, γ_3,

$$N_{eK3} = 0.097 \, N_{eK2} = 0.00724$$

$$N_{eL_{III}} = N_{eK3/2.5} = 0.00229$$

Substituting into equation 22,

$$n_{e3}\bar{E}_{e3} = 0.0013 \text{ Mev./disint.}$$

Substituting into equation 24,

$$n_{\gamma 3} = 0.004 \text{ gamma-rays/disint.}$$

3. For the 0.002 Mev. gamma-ray, γ_1,

$$n_{\gamma 1} = 0.986 \text{ gamma-rays/disint.}$$

4. For K_α x-rays, substituting into equation 23a,

$$n_{K\alpha} = (0.76 \times 0.815) \sum (0.986 \times 0.0746) + (0.014 \times 0.00724)$$

$$n_{K\alpha} = 0.0455 \, K_\alpha \text{ x-rays/disint.}$$

5. For K_β x-rays, substituting into equation 23b,

$$n_{K\beta} = (0.76 \times 0.185) \sum (0.968 \times 0.0746) + (0.014 \times 0.00724)$$

$$n_{K\beta} = 0.0103 \, K_\beta \text{ x-rays/disint.}$$

TYPE OF RADIATION	FRACT. FREQ./DISINT. (not corrected for internal conversion) f_i	FRACT. FREQ./DISINT. (corrected for internal conversion) n_i	MEAN ENERGY $\overline{E}_i$ (Mev.)	$n_i\overline{E}_i$ Mev. disint.	Δ_i g.-rads μc.-hr.
Internal Con. of γ_2	—	—	—	0.0109	0.0232
Internal Con. of γ_3	—	—	—	0.0013	0.00277
γ_1	0.986	0.986	0.002	0.00197	0.00420
γ_2	0.986	0.900	0.140	0.126	0.268
γ_3	0.014	0.004	0.142	0.00057	0.00122
K_α x-ray	0.0455	0.0455	0.0183*	0.00083	0.00177
K_β x-ray	0.0103	0.0103	0.0206*	0.00021	0.00045

* From Appendix

METHODS OF COMPUTING ABSORBED FRACTION

PHOTONS

The Monte Carlo Method. The term "absorbed fraction" was originally applied by Ellett, Callahan, and Brownell (1964, 1965) to calculations made using the Monte Carlo method. This method uses a computer to track an emitted photon through an infinite absorber of tissue equivalent material. The energy lost in each interaction and the spatial coordinates of the point at which the interaction occurs is recorded on magnetic tape. The process is repeated 40,000 to 60,000 times for a photon of a given energy to obtain a complete three-dimensional picture of the energy deposition within the infinite absorber. If the computer is then informed of the spatial coordinates of the surface of any finite absorber, the energy deposition within those coordinates can be retrieved from the tape and the average absorbed energy calculated. Figure 17-3 illustrates schematically how this is done.

Photon E_1 in Figure 17-3 is shown undergoing a Compton interaction (C). It changes direction and deposits energy, ΔE_1, near the site of the Compton interaction. The distance traveled by the photon before an interaction occurs, the type of interaction, the scattering angle, and thus ΔE_1 depend on the original energy of the photon, and the photoelectric and Compton interaction cross sections. After the first interaction, the energy of the scattered photon is equal to $E_1 - \Delta E_1$. The probability of the next interaction is determined by the energy and interaction cross sections for the scattered photon. This process is repeated until the photon is absorbed in a photoelectric interaction or until it is degraded in energy to 10 kev. or less. A photon with this energy is assumed to be absorbed photoelectrically in the next interaction.

Consider the region bounded by the ellipse labeled (1) in Figure 17-3. All three photons originate at the center with the same initial energy E. Photon E_1, undergoes two Compton interactions with a transfer of energy to ΔE_1 and $\Delta E'_1$; it then escapes from the geometrical region of interest. Photon E_2 undergoes a photoelectric interaction (PE), and deposits all its energy in this first interaction. Photon E_3 deposits all its energy in the geometrical region of interest by undergoing a Compton interaction and then a terminal photoelectric interaction. The absorbed fraction, $\phi(v \leftarrow r)$, under these conditions is given by:

$$\phi(v \leftarrow r) = \frac{\Delta E_1 + \Delta E_1' + E_2 + \Delta E_3 + \Delta E_3'}{E_1 + E_2 + E_3}$$

since

$$E = E_1 = E_2 = E_3$$

and

$$E_3 = \Delta E_3 + \Delta E_3'$$

then

$$\phi(v \leftarrow r) = \frac{\Delta E_1 + \Delta E_1' + 2E}{3E}$$

Consider the region bounded by the ellipse labeled (2). Photon E_1 deposits energy ΔE_1 in region (2) and photon E_2 deposits energy E in region (2). Photon E_3 deposits no energy in region (2). The energy from photon E_3 that is deposited in region (2) results from its being scattered back from a point beyond region (2); therefore, $\Delta E_3'$ should not be included in the energy deposited in region (2) since this would not occur if the organ were bounded only by the smaller ellipse. We do this since we wish to use the interaction data evaluated for a phantom of infinite size when we evaluate the absorbed fraction for a *finite*-sized organ. The absorbed fraction for region (2) is taken to be:

$$\phi(v \leftarrow r) = \frac{\Delta E_1 + E}{3E}$$

The mass of the organ affects the absorbed fraction: the greater the mass.

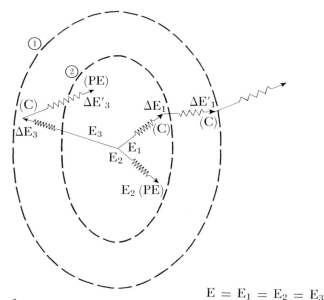

For ellipse 1:

$$\phi_i(v \leftarrow r) = \frac{\Delta E_1 + \Delta E_1' + E_2 + E_3}{E_1 + E_2 + E_3} = \frac{\Delta E_1 + \Delta E_1' + 2E}{3E}$$

For ellipse 2:

$$\phi_i(v \leftarrow r) = \frac{\Delta E_1 + E_2}{E_1 + E_2 + E_3} = \frac{\Delta E_1 + E_2}{3E}$$

$$\phi_i = f(E_\gamma, \text{mass, shape, radionuclide distribution})$$

FIGURE 17-3.   Monte Carlo method for calculating the absorbed fraction.

TABLE 17-3. COMPARISON OF THE ABSORBED FRACTION FOR PHANTOMS OF EQUAL MASS, BUT DIFFERENT SHAPE AND SOURCE DISTRIBUTION. PHOTON ENERGY 0.662 MEV.

PHANTOM MASS (kg.)	CENTRAL POINT SOURCE			UNIFORM SOURCE DISTRIBUTION		
	ELLIPSOID	ELLIPTICAL CYLINDER	SPHERE	ELLIPSOID	ELLIPTICAL CYLINDER	SPHERE
17.7	0.333	0.337	0.457	0.248	0.254	0.343
32.5	0.392	0.397	0.538	0.291	0.303	0.398
50.1	0.437	0.442	0.600	0.325	0.329	0.437
70.0	0.475	0.481	0.651	0.348	0.361	0.469
92.0	0.508	0.513	0.693	0.368	0.385	0.492

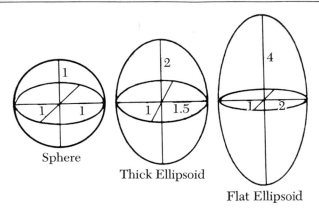

FIGURE 17-4.   Models for organs of various shapes (Ellett et al., 1964).

the larger the absorbed fraction (Table 17-3). For phantoms of equal mass, but different shapes, the sphere has the highest absorbed fraction (Table 17-3). Many organs are not spherical and so absorb significantly less radiation than a mass equivalent sphere. The assumed shape that best fits the real case should be chosen. Whole-body radiation in man is best calculated using as a model an elliptical cylinder (ratio of axes: 1/1.8/6.19) or an ellipsoid (ratio of axes: 1/1.8/9.27) (Table 17-3). Values of the absorbed fraction for point and distributed sources for these and other geometrical models (Figure 17-4) of various masses have been calculated (Ellett et al., 1964, 1965; Reddy et al., 1967; Brownell et al., 1967). Tables of these values may be found in the Appendix.

The dependence of the absorbed fraction on photon energy is shown in Figure 17-5. In all cases, the dependence is marked at photon energies below 100 kev. In large absorbers, the dependence extends to higher energies as well. At low photon energies, where photoelectric absorption predominates, the absorbed fraction approaches unity.

The absorbed fraction for a uniform distribution of a radionuclide varies between two thirds and three quarters of the absorbed fraction for a central point source distribution depending upon photon energy, phantom mass, and shape (Table 17-3 and tables in the Appendix). The absorbed dose calculated for a central point source represents the maximal absorbed dose; the absorbed dose for a uniformly distributed source is the average absorbed dose. Through the use of the dose reciprocity theorem (see p. 776), the central point source calculation can be used to find the dose at points along the central axis of the body (e.g., the gonadal absorbed dose) from activity uniformly distributed in the body.

The amount of radiation escaping from a phantom is a function of the shape and mass of the phantom, and of the position of the source. The effect of source position in elliptical cylinders is shown in Table 17-4. It is seen that for sources within the body, the absorbed fraction is relatively independent of source position along the central axis. The error in using the absorbed fraction for a central point source to compute the absorbed dose to the total body from such eccentric source positions as the vagina is of the order of 10 per cent. The absorbed fraction for sources not on the central axis is slightly lower than those for a central point source. The variation in the absorbed fraction with the average radius of an ellipse is almost linear (± 5 per cent). Thus the loss in absorbed dose due to increased escape of photons through the side closest to the source is largely compensated by increased absorption in the opposite direction.

Sources located on the end plane of an elliptical cylinder emit only half of their photons into the phantom, with the result that the absorbed fraction is less than half of what it is for a central point source (Table 17-5). When the phantom is sufficiently elongated, the height being twice the major diameter (e.g., the elliptical cylinders in Table 17-4), the absorbed fraction is practically independent of phantom height. Thus, the difference between the absorbed fraction for an end source and the absorbed fraction for a central point source divided

TABLE 17-4. ABSORBED FRACTIONS FOR POINT SOURCES LOCATED ON THE AXIS OF AN ELLIPTICAL CYLINDER AT DISTANCES $\frac{1}{2}$, $\frac{1}{6}$, AND $\frac{1}{12}$ THE HEIGHT OF THE CYLINDER*

MASS (kg.)	$E_\gamma = 0.080$ Mev. SOURCE DISTANCE			$E_\gamma = 0.662$ Mev. SOURCE DISTANCE			$E_\gamma = 2.75$ Mev. SOURCE DISTANCE		
	1/2	1/6	1/12	1/2	1/6	1/12	1/2	1/6	1/12
2	0.169	0.161	0.152	0.179	0.168	0.153	0.127	0.118	0.108
4	0.217	0.208	0.191	0.219	0.208	0.190	0.157	0.147	0.136
6	0.253	0.243	0.222	0.247	0.234	0.215	0.178	0.167	0.155
8	0.283	0.273	0.248	0.268	0.254	0.234	0.194	0.183	0.169
10	0.308	0.298	0.270	0.285	0.271	0.250	0.207	0.196	0.182
20	0.397	0.387	0.351	0.346	0.328	0.304	0.255	0.242	0.224
30	0.456	0.446	0.400	0.385	0.366	0.340	0.287	0.273	0.253
40	0.501	0.491	0.451	0.415	0.396	0.368	0.311	0.297	0.276
50	0.537	0.528	0.487	0.439	0.420	0.390	0.331	0.317	0.294
60	0.567	0.559	0.517	0.460	0.441	0.409	0.348	0.334	0.310
70	0.593	0.585	0.543	0.477	0.459	0.426	0.362	0.349	0.323
80	0.616	0.608	0.566	0.493	0.475	0.441	0.375	0.362	0.336
90	0.636	0.629	0.587	0.507	0.489	0.455	0.386	0.374	0.347
100	0.654	0.647	0.605	0.520	0.502	0.467	0.397	0.384	0.357
120	0.685	0.679	0.637	0.543	0.525	0.489	0.416	0.403	0.374
140	0.710	0.705	0.664	0.562	0.545	0.508	0.432	0.419	0.390
160	0.731	0.727	0.687	0.580	0.563	0.525	0.446	0.434	0.404
180	0.750	0.746	0.706	0.595	0.579	0.541	0.458	0.446	0.416
200	0.765	0.762	0.723	0.610	0.593	0.555	0.470	0.458	0.428

* From Brownell et al., 1967.

TABLE 17-5. ABSORBED FRACTIONS FOR AN AXIAL POINT SOURCE ON THE END OF
AN ELLIPTICAL CYLINDER AND THE FRACTION OF THE EMITTED SOURCE
ENERGY BACKSCATTERED FROM THE PHANTOM*

MASS (kg.)	E_γ = 0.080 Mev.		E_γ = 0.662 Mev.		E_γ = 2.75 Mev.	
	END	ESCAPE	END	ESCAPE	END	ESCAPE
2	0.071	0.013	0.088	0.002	0.064	—
4	0.088	0.021	0.018	0.003	0.079	—
6	0.100	0.027	0.121	0.005	0.090	—
8	0.110	0.032	0.130	0.006	0.097	—
10	0.118	0.037	0.138	0.006	0.104	—
20	0.145	0.054	0.165	0.010	0.127	—
30	0.162	0.066	0.182	0.012	0.142	—
40	0.174	0.076	0.195	0.014	0.154	0.001
50	0.184	0.084	0.205	0.016	0.163	0.001
60	0.193	0.091	0.214	0.018	0.172	0.002
70	0.200	0.097	0.222	0.019	0.178	0.002
80	0.206	0.102	0.228	0.021	0.185	0.002
90	p.211	0.107	0.234	0.022	0.190	0.003
100	0.216	0.112	0.293	0.023	0.195	0.003
120	0.224	0.119	0.249	0.025	0.204	0.004
140	0.231	0.125	0.257	0.027	0.212	0.004
160	0.236	0.130	0.264	0.029	0.218	0.005
180	0.241	0.135	0.270	0.030	0.224	0.005
200	0.244	0.139	0.275	0.031	0.229	0.006

* From Brownell et al., 1967.

TABLE 17-6. INCREASE OF ABSORBED FRACTION IN A CENTRAL ORGAN DUE TO
BACKSCATTER RADIATION ORIGINATING IN A 70 KG. PHANTOM SURROUNDING
THE ORGAN*
(Energies in Mev.)

0.020	0.030	0.040	0.060	0.080	0.100	0.160	0.364	0.662	1.460	2.75
1.01	1.08	1.19	1.24	1.28	1.26	1.17	1.05	1.04	1.02	1.01

* From Brownell et al., 1967.

by 2 is due to backscatter escape from the phantom. For example, the absorbed
fraction for a 662 kev. central point source in a 70 kg. phantom (elliptical cylinder) is 0.481. For an end source the absorbed fraction is 0.221 and the escape
is 0.020 (Table 17-5). In this case, the absorbed fraction is reduced by approximately 8 per cent because of backscatter escape from the phantom. From Table
17-5 it is seen that the backscatter component is most important for low-energy
photons and the larger phantom masses.

In addition to self-irradiation, organs within the thorax and abdomen receive
additional irradiation from the backscatter of photons distributed throughout the
body and from photons originating within the organs themselves. The backscatter
to a central region within a 70 kg. man has been calculated (Table 17-6). If the
radioactivity is confined to a region such as the head, where backscatter is less,
the use of this factor would not be justified.

The absorbed fraction determined by the method of Ellett and his co-workers has been confirmed by Snyder and Ford (Snyder, 1965) who also use the

Monte Carlo method. Their approach to the problem allows more freedom to specify the size and shape of phantoms, source, and target regions. As an example of this flexibility, Snyder and Ford were able to calculate the absorbed dose to the ovaries from ^{203}Hg contained in the cortex of the kidney.

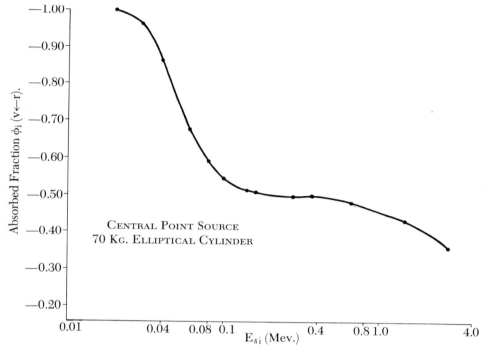

FIGURE 17-5. Absorbed fraction as a function of initial gamma-ray energy (Ellett et al., 1964; Reddy et al., 1967).

Geometrical Factors. The geometry factor, g_p or $\bar{g}$, has been used in calculations of radiation dose for many years, and a number of tables of values have been published. In cases in which the absorbed fraction has not yet been calculated by the Monte Carlo method, a "pseudo" absorbed fraction can be calculated. The geometry factors are defined as follows:

$$g_p = g(p \leftarrow v) = \int_v \frac{e^{-\mu_{eff}x}}{x^2} \, dv \qquad \text{cm.}$$

$$\bar{g} = g(v \leftrightarrow v) = \frac{1}{v} \int_v g_p dv \qquad \text{cm.}$$

where $e^{-\mu_{eff}x}$ = the tissue attenuation of the photons originating from the elemental volume, dv, and incident on p.

$\frac{1}{x^2}$ = the inverse-square law diminution of the radiation field emanating from dv and incident on p.

The "effective" tissue absorption coefficient, μ_{eff}, which is a function of the distance from the point source, is usually taken to be 0.028 cm.$^{-1}$. Thus these calculations are valid only to the extent that this value is an adequate representation of the distribution of absorbed energy around a point source.

The average geometrical factor, g, can be approximated for spheres of unit density with a radius, R, less than 10 cm. (Loevinger et al., 1956a) by:

$$\bar{g} = 3\pi R \qquad\qquad cm.$$

The method of calculating g_p for a specified point that is inside, on the surface, or outside a sphere has been described by Loevinger et al. (1956a).

Values of g for cylinders containing a uniform distribution of a gamma-emitting radionuclide have been calculated by Focht and her co-workers (1965) (Tables of $\bar{g}$ are given in the Appendix). The values calculated by Focht are revisions of previously published figures (Glasser et al., 1961; Loevinger et al., 1956a; Quimby, 1963) that were initially calculated for a point source at the end of a cylinder rather than for a uniform distribution.

Values of g_p for the central axis of a "standard" human body are given in Figure 17-6. These values are useful in approximating the absorbed dose that an organ such as the thyroid, ovary, or testicle receives from a radionuclide uniformly distributed within the body. The absorbed dose calculated with $\bar{g}$ gives an average value; values calculated with g_p give the maximal absorbed dose.

The following relationship converts values of g_p and g into values of the "pseudo" absorbed fraction (Loevinger, 1966):

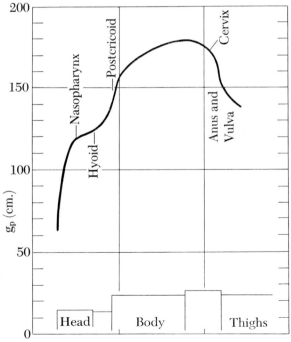

FIGURE 17-6. Geometry factor, g_p, for points along the central axis of a human body containing a uniform distribution of a gamma-ray emitting radionuclide (Bush, 1949; Loevinger, 1956a).

$$\phi^{*}{}_{iph} (v \leftarrow r) = \frac{(\mu_{en})_i}{4\pi} g (r \leftarrow v)$$

and

$$r = p \text{ or } v$$

$$g (p \leftarrow v) = g_p \quad g (v \leftrightarrow v) = \bar{g} \tag{25}$$

where $(\mu_{en})_i$ is the energy absorption coefficient, in $cm.^{-1}$, for the initial photon energy, E_{oi}, in Mev. (The Appendix contains a table of values of μ_{en} for various tissues.)

The values for the absorbed fraction calculated by equation 25 carry only the degree of validity attached to the original g_p or g values. Quimby (1963) has stated that the use of g_p or g is valid only with photon energies between 0.1 to 2.0 Mev.—in other words, when the effective absorption coefficient is essentially constant. This was to be expected since the geometrical factors were originally developed for photon energies in the range of those from radium (above 200 kev.). At low energies a larger value of μ_{eff} should be used in calculating $\bar{g}$, and multiple interactions must be considered in the case of larger phantoms. Even at photon energies greater than 100 kev., the use of geometrical factors leads to underestimation of the absorbed dose. This is due in part to the fact that the original calculations on which $\bar{g}$ was based tended to neglect backscatter. Ellett and his co-workers (1964, 1965) and Smith (1965, 1966) showed the advantage of the absorbed fraction method of calculation of the absorbed dose, compared to the method using the geometrical factor.

Nonpenetrating radiation

Nonpenetrating radiation includes both charged particles and low-energy photons in which 95 per cent or more of the particle or photon's energy is transferred to the volume in which it originated, that is, $v_1 = v_1$.

$$\phi_{n-p} (v_1 \leftrightarrow v_1) = 1 \qquad\qquad v_1 = v_1 \tag{26a}$$

$$\phi_{n-p} (v_i \leftarrow v_2) = 0 \qquad\qquad v_1 \neq v_2 \tag{26b}$$

Equation 26a states that if the radiation is nonpenetrating and is in the target volume, $v_1 = v_1$, the absorbed fraction is unity. On the other hand, equation 26b states that if the radiation is nonpenetrating and is not located in the target volume, v, the absorbed fraction is zero.

In many instances the biological target, e.g., the organ, will be 1 cm. in radius or larger. For this situation, all charged particles from radionuclides, and all photons with an energy less than or equal to 11.3 kev. are considered nonpenetrating. In some instances, the biological target will be less than 1 cm. in radius, and the distance required for each type of radiation to deposit 95 per cent of its energy must be determined before the radiation can be classified as nonpenetrating. All radiations that can be defined as nonpenetrating for a particular situation can be lumped together into one equilibrium absorbed dose constant for nonpenetrating radiation, Δ_{n-p}, and treated jointly in the absorbed dose calculation.

ASSUMPTIONS, UNCERTAINTIES, AND LIMITATIONS

ASSAY OF THE ADMINISTERED RADIOPHARMACEUTICAL

To calculate the absorbed dose that a patient receives from a radiopharmaceutical, we must know its identity, activity, and metabolism.

Quantification of the Administered Activity. To determine activity, we need to know the decay scheme and fractional frequency of photons emitted per disintegration. If the photon yield for a radionuclide is not known accurately, it is impossible to carry out a reliable assay. This is an important problem when decay is by electron capture and isomeric transition, since in these cases determination of photon yield is difficult.

Radionuclidic Purity. Radionuclidic purity is defined as the fraction of the total activity that is present as the stated radionuclide. If there are radionuclidic impurities, these must be taken into account in calculating the absorbed dose. Usually, daughter radionuclides are not included in the statement of radionuclidic purity, and their activity must be calculated by the user. The contribution from daughter radionuclides must be included in the absorbed dose calculations.

As described in Chapter VI, radionuclidic impurities are frequently isotopes of the product radionuclide, for example, calcium-45 in calcium-47, mercury-203 in mercury-197, and iodine-126 in iodine-125.

Radiochemical Purity. As already defined in Chapter VI, radiochemical purity is the fraction of the radionuclide present in the stated chemical form. For example, if a preparation of L-triiodothyronine-^{131}I is said to be 99 per cent radiochemically pure, we mean that 99 per cent of the ^{131}I present is in the chemical form of L-triiodothyronine. Absorbed dose calculations based on the metabolism of a particular chemical form will be in error if there are radiochemical impurities that are metabolized differently. The topic of radiochemical purity is discussed in detail by Bayly (1966), Briner (1966), Charlton (1966), and Cohen (1966).

An example of a radiochemical impurity is free iodide in iodinated compounds; this could lead to an unexpectedly high absorbed dose to the thyroid. Another example of an impurity is the presence of variable particle size in macroaggregated albumin. This would result in some of the particles being taken up by the liver instead of being retained in the lungs. As a result, absorbed dose to the liver would be higher than expected. Radiochemical impurities may form during storage of the radiopharmaceutical, possibly as a result of self-irradiation.

When a radiopharmaceutical has a short effective half-life, it is often possible to administer millicurie amounts without an excessive absorbed dose. A short effective half-life is the result of either a short physical half-life or a short biological half-life or both, and the effect of radiochemical and radionuclidic impurities depends somewhat upon which mode of elimination predominates. If prompt biological decay is depended upon to limit the dose, any impurity having a longer biological half-life can increase the absorbed dose by prolonging the exposure. Both radiochemical and radionuclidic impurities could have this effect. When physical decay predominates, only a radionuclidic impurity could seriously prolong the exposure. In either case, a radiochemical impurity could deliver the dose to an unexpected target organ, perhaps one that is more radio-sensitive, or cause the nuclide to reach an unexpectedly high concentration in the intended target or elsewhere.

Nonhomogeneous distribution of activity

The calculation of the absorbed dose for nonpenetrating radiation is based on two assumptions: (1) the radionuclide is uniformly distributed in a tissue of uniform composition; and (2) the range of the beta particle is small compared to the dimensions of the tissue in which the radionuclide is distributed. If the second assumption is not valid, the radiation is improperly classified as non-penetrating.

These assumptions lead to a number of problems. For example, chlormero-drin (Neohydrin) labeled with ^{203}Hg or ^{197}Hg concentrates almost exclusively in the renal cortex (Greif et al., 1956; Raynaud et al., 1963) rather than being distributed uniformly in the kidney. If we assume that the radioactive material is uniformly distributed, we underestimate the absorbed dose by a factor of about 2.

A similar problem concerns radioiodine in the thyroid. Anspaugh (1965) has shown that in the normal human thyroid gland, the absorbed dose is homo-geneous even though the distribution of ^{131}I is not. In the case of ^{125}I, however, the distribution of the absorbed dose in the normal thyroid is not homogeneous because of the low energy of the ^{125}I radiations.

Another example of nonhomogeneous distribution of a radiopharmaceutical is that of macroaggregates of human serum albumin (MAA) in the lung. Tow and his associates (1966) have made some detailed absorbed dose calculations based on the experimental distribution of the albumin particles in the lungs. They found that if a homogeneous distribution of MAA in the lungs is assumed, the average absorbed dose in the lung is 1.2 to 1.8 rads for 300 μc. of ^{131}I as MAA. However, if a more realistic volume of distribution is assumed, namely, the capillary bed of the lungs, the average local absorbed dose is 4.6 to 6.6 rads. The absorbed dose received by the capillary epithelium adjacent to the particle is several orders of magnitude greater than the average absorbed dose.

Calculation of the absorbed dose at the cellular level may be of questionable value unless due consideration is given to the location of the labeled compound in the cell, the biochemistry of the labeled compound, the location of the radio-nuclide in the compound, and the nuclear characteristics of the radionuclide. Effects such as bond rupture resulting from nuclear recoil after beta emission, the chemical implication of nuclear transmutation on the functional integrity of the molecule, and the spatial distribution of the absorbed energy cannot be evaluated if only the integrated absorbed dose (equations 1 and 2) is con-sidered. Koch (1965) has discussed some of these factors, and has investigated the importance of the cellular distribution of tritiated compounds with respect to the different degrees of irradiation of the deoxyribonucleic acid of the cell by various tritiated compounds. Stewart (1964), Robertson (in press), and Koch (1965) have presented and summarized methods of calculating the spatial dis-tribution of the absorbed dose resulting from a point source of tritium. From a study of available data Bond and Feinendegen (1966) have shown that the degree of early somatic biological effect from intranuclear tritium is that antici-

TABLE 17-7. ABSORBED DOSE FROM THE ORAL ADMINISTRATION OF RADIOACTIVE IODIDE FOR DIAGNOSTIC TESTS AT VARIOUS AGES*

ORGAN	RADIONUCLIDE	NEWBORN	1 YEAR	5 YEARS	10 YEARS	15 YEARS	STANDARD MAN
		Absorbed dose in mrads/μc. administered					
Whole body	Na^{131}I	10.	2.0	1.3	0.81	0.53	0.45
	Na^{125}I	9.4	1.6	1.0	0.67	0.44	0.39
	Na^{132}I	1.1	0.44	0.27	0.17	0.11	0.09
		Absorbed dose in rads/μc. administered					
Thyroid	Na^{131}I	32.	10.0	4.3	3.1	1.7	1.3
	Na^{125}I	19.	6.2	2.6	1.8	1.0	0.82
	Na^{132}I	1.2	0.4	0.17	0.12	0.07	0.05

* From Kereiakes, J. G., Seltzer, R. A., Blackburn, B., and Saenger, E. L.: Radionuclide Doses to Infants and Children: A Plea for a Standard Child. *Health Phys.* 11:999, 1965.

TABLE 17-8. BODY WEIGHTS, ORGAN WEIGHTS (STUART, 1959), AND CALCULATED GEOMETRICAL FACTORS (KEREIAKES ET AL., 1965) FOR VARIOUS AGES

		NEWBORN	1 YEAR	5 YEARS	10 YEARS	15 YEARS	STANDARD MAN
Whole body	wt. (g.)	3540	12,100	20,300	33,500	55,000	70,000
	ht. (cm.)	50	75	108	139	166	170
	$\bar{g}$ (cm.)	64	89	94	102	112	126
Thyroid	wt. (g.)	1.9	2.5	6.1	8.7	15.8	20.0
	$\bar{g}$ (cm.)	7.0	8.0	11.0	12.0	14.0	15.0
	g_P (cm.)	71.0	99	104	113	124	140
Kidney	wt. (g.)	23	72	112	187	247	300
	$\bar{g}$ (cm.)	16	22	25	30	33	35
	g_P (cm.)	92	127	134	146	160	180
Liver	wt. (g.)	136	333	591	918	1289	1700
	$\bar{g}$ (cm.)	27	36	44	50	55	59
	g_P (c.)	92	127	134	146	160	180
Spleen	wt. (g.)	9.4	31	54	101	138	150
	$\bar{g}$ (cm.)	12	17	20	25	28	29
	g_P (cm.)	92	127	134	146	160	180

pated on the basis of the calculated average absorbed dose to the cell nucleus, at least down to absorbed doses of 5 rads or less. This result indicates that the absorbed dose concept holds down to the order of 10^{-11} g. or less, and somatic effects can be predicted on this basis.

EFFECT OF AGE ON ABSORBED DOSE

Organ mass, size, and metabolic activity change as the newborn matures to adulthood. These factors have a marked effect on the absorbed dose (Kereiakes et al., 1965; Seltzer et al., 1964). Table 17-7 summarizes the variation with age of absorbed dose for radioactive iodine. The thyroid of an infant receives an absorbed dose 25 times greater than the thyroid of an adult for equal activity administered. (The original article should be consulted for the assumptions and method of calculating the absorbed dose before these values are used.)

Table 17-8 summarizes the variability of organ weight with age (Stuart and Stevenson, 1959), and the corresponding calculated values for the geometrical factors (Kereiakes et al., 1965).

PHARMACOLOGICAL REDUCTION OF ABSORBED DOSE

The reduction of the concentration of the radiopharmaceutical in a non-target tissue may be accomplished by giving a large quantity of a nonradioactive isotope(s) of the radioactive isotope that the tissue normally concentrates. An example is the administration of iodide to decrease the thyroidal uptake of radioactive isotopes of iodine, when these isotopes are being utilized for studies other than the thyroid. The thyroidal uptake can be reduced from a normal uptake of 20 to 30 per cent to 3 to 5 per cent (Cuddihy, 1966; Saxena et al., 1962). Normally 100 to 200 mg. of stable iodide (Lugol's solution) is administered several hours before the radiopharmaceutical containing ^{125}I or ^{131}I is administered.

Another example of isotopic dilution is the use of nonradioactive Mercuhydrin to reduce the renal retention of ^{203}Hg- or ^{197}Hg-labeled Neohydrin (chlormerodrin) for brain scanning. One milliliter of Mercuhydrin administered 24 hours before the labeled Neohydrin will reduce the fraction of labeled Neohydrin retained by the kidneys by one third to one half (McAfee and Blau, 1966). There is no effect on the rate at which the material is eliminated by the kidneys.

One can also use an agent which is not chemically identical to the radiopharmaceutical as long as it is handled biologically by the tissue in a similar fashion so as to dilute the radioactive agent. This is known as nonisotopic dilution. An example would be the use of iodide to reduce the uptake of ^{99m}Tc by the thyroid.

OTHER CONSIDERATIONS

The pathological state of a patient may drastically change the expected biological distribution of the radiopharmaceutical and therefore the absorbed dose. Wagner (1963) has discussed this problem with respect to Neohydrin in patients with renal insufficiency, and Smith (1965) has discussed it with respect to intravenously administered colloidal particles in patients with hepatic disease.

The biological distribution of a radiopharmaceutical as well as its effective half-life may be significantly different for diagnostic and therapeutic levels of the same radiopharmaceutical. A diagnostic study employing 5 μc. of ^{131}I in an adult would not affect the normal function of the thyroid, but a 5 mc. dose would. The effective half-life of ^{131}I and its percentage uptake may be significantly altered at therapeutic levels compared to diagnostic.

The specific activity of a radiopharmaceutical may significantly alter its biological distribution. For example, a higher percentage incorporation of chromium-51 or iron-59 into red cells is found when high-specific-activity chromium-51 or iron-59 is used.

DOSE RECIPROCITY THEOREM—CALCULATION
OF THE REVERSE ABSORBED DOSE

GORDON L. BROWNELL
WILLIAM H. ELLETT

The dose reciprocity theorem (Mayneord, 1945) states that the absorbed dose delivered to a point from a uniform volume distribution of activity is equal to the average absorbed dose delivered to that volume by the same amount of activity concentrated at that point. Loevinger, Japha, and Brownell (1956b) have restated the dose reciprocity theorem for three generalized geometrical situations: (1) Two sources containing the same total amount of activity deliver to each other the same *average* absorbed dose, irrespective of size, shape, or distance. (2) Two sources with the same concentration of activity deliver to each other the same *total* (integral) absorbed dose, irrespective of size, shape, or distance. (3) The *average* absorbed dose delivered to a given volume by a given amount of activity at some fixed point equals the absorbed dose *at that point* due to the same amount of activity distributed uniformly inside the specified volume. The third situation is of prime importance in the evaluation of the absorbed dose to the total body when a radiopharmaceutical concentrates in a few organs.

The dose reciprocity theorem is exact in an infinite homogeneous medium and is approximately correct in any medium in which boundary effects can be neglected and no marked discontinuities in absorption properties are encountered. The reciprocity theorem gives quite accurate values, particularly in tissue-like media.

In Figure 17-7, the volume, v, represents a large homogeneous medium of density, ρ, within which is defined v_1, and a point, p, of cumulative activity, $\tilde{A}$. The point source function is defined as $J(x)$ and can be of any form as long as it accurately predicts the absorbed dose rate at a distance, x, from a point source.

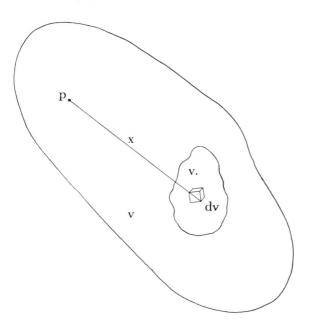

FIGURE 17-7.

The integral absorbed dose, Σ, in g.-rads, received by v_1 from the point source, p, of cumulated activity, $\tilde{A}_p$, is given by:

$$\Sigma = \int_{v_1} \rho \tilde{A}_p\, J(x)\, dv_1 \qquad \text{g.-rad}$$

and the average absorbed dose, $\overline{D}_{v_1 \leftarrow p}$, received by v_1 from p is:

$$\overline{D}_{v_1 \leftarrow p} = \sum_{m_{v_1}} = \frac{\rho \tilde{A}_p}{m_{v_1}} \int_v J(x) dv_1 \qquad \text{rad}$$

Alternatively, the absorbed dose at p from v_1, $D_{p \leftarrow v_1}$, assuming that $\tilde{A}_p$ is distributed uniformly throughout v_1, that is, $\tilde{C}_v = \dfrac{\tilde{A}_v}{m_v}$ and $\tilde{A}_p = \tilde{A}_v$, is:

$$D_{p \leftarrow v_1} \int_{v_1} J(x) dv_1 \qquad \text{rad}$$

or

$$\overline{D}_{v_1 \leftarrow p} = D_{p \leftarrow v_1}$$

which is the usual statement of the dose reciprocity theorem, i.e., the third geometrical situation as stated by Loevinger and his associates.

The usefulness of the dose reciprocity theorem is that calculations of the average absorbed dose from point sources can be directly converted to absorbed dose at a point from a volume distribution. If a second volume distribution is considered as a series of points, an equivalent statement can be made concerning two uniform volume distributions in a large homogeneous region; i.e., the average absorbed dose to volume 1 from a uniform activity distribution in volume 2 is equal to the average dose to volume 2 from a uniform activity distribution in volume 1 for equal activity concentrations.

The reciprocity theorem is amenable to direct experimental or computational verification. Using exact scattering calculations, Ellett, Callahan, and Brownell (1965) have shown that the reciprocity theorem holds for the case of 2200 cc. centrally located within a 70 kg. phantom, and it is expected that for most regions of activity within the trunk its use should give quite acceptable results.

EXAMPLE 8.   Calculate the maximum absorbed dose rate from a uniform concentration of 10^{-9} curies per gram of cesium-137 in a 70 kg. unit density ellipsoidal phantom. The maximal absorbed dose is at the center of the phantom. If all the activity were concentrated at this point, the source strength, A, would be:

$$A = (70 \times 10^3 \text{ g.}) (10^{-9} \text{ curies/g.}) = 70\ \mu c.$$

The average absorbed dose rate, $\overline{R}_{v_1 \leftarrow p}$ to the phantom from a *central point source of this activity*, would be, from equation 1 and the tables of absorbed fractions in the Appendix,

$$\overline{R}_{v_1 \leftarrow p} = \frac{A_v \rho}{m_v} \Delta \phi(v \leftarrow p)$$

$$= \frac{70 \times 1}{70 \times 10^3} \times 11.8 \times 10^{-1} \times 0.48$$

$$\overline{R}_{v_1 \leftarrow p} = 0.566 \text{ mrad/hr.}$$

Since $\overline{R}_{v_1 \leftarrow p} = R_{p \leftarrow v}$, the absorbed dose rate at the center of a 70 kg. volume containing a uniform concentration of 1 $\mu c./g.$ will be 0.566 mrad/hr.

Alternatively, the average absorbed dose rate in the phantom from a uniform concentration of activity can be obtained from the absorbed fraction for a *uniform concentration* of activity in an ellipsoidal phantom (equation 2 and tables of absorbed fractions in the appendix).

$$\overline{R}_{v \leftarrow v} = C_v \Delta \phi (v \leftarrow v)$$

$$= 1 \times 10^{-3} \times 11.8 \times 0.35$$

$$\overline{R}_{v \leftarrow v} = 0.414 \text{ mrad/hr.}$$

EXAMPLE OF ABSORBED DOSE CALCULATIONS FOR MACROAGGREGATED ALBUMIN (MAA)

The following calculations are based on the assumptions and biological data for MAA in man given by Tow and his associates (1966). All calculations are based on an administered activity of 300 μc. of ^{131}I as MAA. The physical half-life of ^{131}I is 8.05 days.

TYPE OF RADIATION	$\overline{E}_i$ Mev.	n_i fraction disint.	$n_i \overline{E}_i$ Mev. disint.	$\Delta_i = 2.13 \, n_i \overline{E}_i$ g.-rads μc.-hr.
β	—	—	0.188	0.400
x, K	≈ 0.03	0.05	0.0015	0.00320
γ	0.080	0.02	0.0016	0.00341
γ	0.284	0.06	0.0170	0.0363
γ	0.364	0.79	0.288	0.613
γ	0.638	0.09	0.0574	0.122
γ	0.724	0.03	0.0217	0.0463

TOTAL BODY

The total-body absorbed dose calculation for a standard 70 kg. man was based on measurement of urinary and fecal excretion for a period of 30 days in three normal volunteers who had received ^{125}I MAA. The use of ^{125}I (T = 60 days) made possible the extended excretion studies necessary to account for all of the injected activity. For the total-body absorbed dose calculation a uniform distribution of activity in the total body of a standard man was assumed. Eighty-seven per cent of the activity was excreted with a $T_{eff} = 0.47$ days and the remainder with a $T_{eff} = 4.65$ days. Two per cent of the activity was unaccounted for in the excreta when the last measurement was made at 30 days.

$$C_1(0) = 0.87 \times \frac{300}{70,000} = 0.00373 \frac{\mu c.}{g.} \qquad T_1 = 0.50 \text{ d.} \qquad T_{1eff} = 0.47 \text{ d.}$$

$$C_2(0) = 0.13 \times \frac{300}{70,000} = 0.000557 \frac{\mu c.}{g.} \qquad T_2 = 11.0 \text{ d.} \qquad T_{2eff} = 4.65 \text{ d.}$$

$$C_2(t^*) = 0.02 \times \frac{300}{70,000} = 0.0000857 \frac{\mu c.}{g.} \qquad t^* = 30 \text{ d.} \qquad n = 2$$

Substituting into equation 13,

$$\tilde{C}_v = 1.44 \sum_{j=1}^{j=n-1} C_j(0)T_{jeff} + 1.44C_n(0)T_{neff}(1 - e^{-0.693t*/T_{eff}})$$

$$+ 1.44\ C_n(t^*)T(e^{-0.693t*/T})$$

$$= (1.44 \times 0.00373 \times 0.47) + [(1.44 \times 0.000557 \times 4.65)(1 - e^{-0.693\times30/4.65})]$$
$$+ [(1.44 \times 0.0000857 \times 8.05)(e^{-0.693\times30/8.05})]$$

$$\tilde{C}_v = 0.00628 \frac{\mu c.-d.}{g.}$$

If we assumed that the value for T_2 was valid to $t = \infty$, and did not use T, the physical half-life, after the last measurement at $t = 30$ days, $\tilde{C}_v$ would be, using equation 11,

$$\tilde{C}_v = 1.44 \sum_j C_j(0)T_{jeff}$$

$$= 1.44[(0.00373 \times 0.47) + (0.000557 \times 4.65)]$$

$$\tilde{C}_v = 0.00625 \frac{\mu c.-d.}{g.}$$

The difference in $\tilde{C}_v$ using the two methods is negligible, but the former method (equation 13) is preferred if measurements are not continued until all of the administered dose can be accounted for or complete decay can be assumed. The difference in $\tilde{C}_v$ as calculated by equations 11 and 13 is not always negligible as will be demonstrated shortly. This consideration becomes increasingly important when long-lived radionuclides are used.

TYPE OF RADIATION	$\bar{E}_i$	Δ_i	ϕ_i FOR 70 kg. ELLIPSOID (UNIFORM DISTRIBUTION)	$\Delta_i\phi_i$
β	—	0.400	1.00	0.400
x, K	≈ 0.03	0.00320	0.753	0.00241
γ	0.080	0.00341	0.375	0.00127
γ	0.284	0.0363	0.344	
γ	0.364	0.613	0.345	
γ	0.638	0.122	0.346 } 0.345	} 0.282
γ	0.724	0.0463	0.346	

$$\sum \Delta_i\phi_i = 0.686$$

Substituting into equation 2 and multiplying by 24 hours/day to convert units of $\tilde{C}_v$ from $\frac{\mu c.-d.}{g.}$ to $\frac{\mu c.-hr.}{g.}$

$$\bar{D}_\infty(v \leftrightarrow v) \approx 24\tilde{C}_v \sum_i \Delta_i\phi_i\ (v \leftrightarrow v) \qquad \text{rad}$$

$$\bar{D}_\infty(v \leftrightarrow v) = 24 \times 0.00628 \times 0.686$$

$$\bar{D}_\infty(v \leftrightarrow v) = 0.103 \text{ rad} \qquad \text{total-body absorbed dose}$$

BLOOD

The blood absorbed dose calculation was based on serial blood measurements made on four normal volunteers over a period of 4 days. The initial concentration was 0.013 ± 0.005 μc./g. of whole blood. The effective half-life was 1.85 days. The concentration was 0.00405 ± 0.00096 μc./g. on the fourth day when the last measurement was made.

$$C_1(0) = 0.013 \; \mu\text{c./g.} \qquad T_1 = 2.4 \text{ d.} \qquad T_{1\text{eff}} = 1.85 \text{ d.}$$
$$C_1(t^*) = 0.00405 \; \mu\text{c./g.} \qquad t^* = 4 \text{ d.} \qquad n = 1$$

Substituting in equation 13,

$$\tilde{C}_v = (1.44 \times 0.013 \times 1.85)(1 - e^{-0.693 \times 4/1.85})$$
$$+ (1.44 \times 0.00405 \times 8.05)(e^{-0.693 \times 4/8.05})$$

$$\tilde{C}_v = 0.0603 \; \frac{\mu\text{c.-d.}}{\text{g.}}$$

If we assume T_1 valid to $t = \infty$ as we did for the total-body absorbed dose, then, substituting into equation 11,

$$\tilde{C}_v = 1.44 \times 0.013 \times 1.85$$

$$\tilde{C}_v = 0.0346 \; \frac{\mu\text{c.-d.}}{\text{g.}}$$

In this case, there is a difference of 1.7 between the results calculated by equations 11 and 13. The true value lies somewhere between these values. A cautious approach is to use 0.0603 μc.-d./g., but it is better to state the range of values. The range of values for $\tilde{C}_v$ for blood could be decreased if blood samples had been taken for a longer period of time. The lower value is more consistent with the urinary and fecal excretion data.

If we assume that the nonpenetrating beta radiation is completely absorbed in the blood, then $\phi_\beta = \phi_{np} = 1.0$. This is a conservative estimate for ϕ_β, since a certain fraction of the particulate energy is not deposited in the blood. Ideally one would like to divide the vascular system into two or three subsystems, assign an effective diameter to each, and then determine the absorbed fraction for that effective diameter. Since the blood pool can be considered to be uniformly distributed throughout the body, we use the total-body distribution data and values of ϕ_i to calculate the absorbed dose resulting from penetrating radiations. Substituting into equation 2 for the penetrating and nonpenetrating cases and multiplying by 24,

Penetrating:

$$\overline{D}_\infty(v \leftrightarrow v) = (24 \times 0.00628)(0.686 - 0.400)$$
$$\overline{D}_\infty(v \leftrightarrow v) = 0.043 \qquad \text{rad}$$

Nonpenetrating (based on equation 11):

$$\overline{D}_\infty(v \leftrightarrow v) = 24 \times 0.0346 \times 0.400$$
$$\overline{D}_\infty(v \leftrightarrow v) = 0.33 \qquad \text{rad}$$

(based on equation 13):

$$\overline{D}_\infty(v \leftrightarrow v) = 24 \times 0.0603 \times 0.400$$
$$\overline{D}_\infty(v \leftrightarrow v) = 0.58 \qquad \text{rad}$$

The estimate of $\overline{D}_\infty(v \leftrightarrow v)$ for blood lies somewhere between 0.37 and 0.62 rad. If ^{131}I levels in blood had been determined for a longer period of time, this wide range in $\overline{D}_\infty(v \leftrightarrow v)$ could have been markedly reduced.

GONADAL

In males, the penetrating radiation component of the absorbed dose to the gonads is essentially the same as the penetrating radiation component of the total-body absorbed dose. In calculating the female gonadal absorbed dose, the contribution from backscattered radiation must be taken into account since the ovaries are centrally located. This will add about 5 per cent to the absorbed dose.

Since iodide does not concentrate in the ovaries, the absorbed dose resulting from nonpenetrating radiation lies between the value for the total body and that for blood. The exact value depends on blood flow to the gonads and the diameter and wall thickness of the blood vessels of the gonads.

LIVER

The liver absorbed dose calculation was based on external counting for a period of 24 days over the livers of seven normal volunteers who had received MAA. Approximately 20 per cent of the MAA went to the liver and spleen, and was assumed to be uniformily distributed. The liver was considered to be a 1.7 kg. flat ellipsoid. The mass of the liver and spleen is assumed to be 1850 g.

$$C_1(0) = 0.60 \times 0.20 \times \frac{300}{1850} = 0.0195 \qquad T_1 = 0.0208 \text{ d.} \qquad T_{1eff} = 0.0207 \text{ d.}$$

$$C_2(0) = 0.30 \times 0.20 \times \frac{300}{1850} = 0.00973 \qquad T_2 = 0.375 \text{ d.} \qquad T_{2eff} = 0.363 \text{ d.}$$

$$C_3(0) = 0.10 \times 0.20 \times \frac{300}{1850} = 0.00324 \qquad T_3 = 11 \text{ d.} \qquad T_{3eff} = 4.65 \text{ d.}$$

Substituting into equation 11,

$$\tilde{C}_v = 1.44 \, [(0.0195 \times 0.0207) + (0.00973 \times 0.363) + (0.00324 \times 4.65)]$$

$$\tilde{C}_v = 0.0274 \, \frac{\mu c.\text{-}d.}{g.}$$

TYPE OF RADIATION	$\bar{E}_i$	Δ_i	ϕ_i FOR 1.7 kg. FLAT ELLIPSOID (UNIFORM DISTRIBUTION)	$\Delta_i\phi_i$
β	—	0.400	1.00	0.400
x, K	≈ 0.03	0.00320	0.534	0.00171
γ	0.080	0.00341	0.166	
γ	0.284	0.0363	0.167	
γ	0.364	0.613	0.167 } 0.167	} 0.137
γ	0.638	0.122	0.167	
γ	0.724	0.0463	0.167	

$$\sum_i \Delta_i\phi_i = 0.539$$

Substituting into equation 2 and multiplying by 24,

$$\overline{D}_\infty(v \leftrightarrow v) = 24 \times 0.0274 \times 0.539$$

$$\overline{D}_\infty(v \leftrightarrow v) = 0.354 \quad \text{rad}$$

To 0.354 rad we must add a certain fraction of the absorbed dose to the total body resulting from penetrating radiations since these radiations are also irradiating the liver. To be conservative, we will assume 80 per cent of this value

$$\overline{D}_\infty(v_{Li} \leftarrow v_{TB}) = 0.80\ \overline{D}_\infty\ \text{(total-body penetrating)} = 0.043\ \text{rad}$$

Then the total absorbed dose to the liver is 0.397 rad.

LUNGS

The average lung absorbed dose calculation was based on external counting over the lungs of nine normal persons for a period of 4 days. It was assumed that 80 per cent of the MAA was trapped in the capillary bed of the lung and disappeared with an effective half-life of 0.29 ± 0.06 day. There was a long-lived component that consisted of approximately 1 per cent of the administered activity and was attributed to the ^{131}I activity in blood. The lungs were assumed to weigh 1000 g. and to have a density of 0.3 g./cm.[3]

$$C_1(0) = 0.80 \times \frac{300}{1000} = 0.24 \qquad T_1 = 0.31\ \text{d.} \qquad T_{1eff} = 0.29\ \text{d.}$$

Substituting into equation 11,

$$\tilde{C}_v = 1.44 \times 0.24 \times 0.29 = 0.100\ \frac{\mu c.\text{-}d.}{g.}$$

Since the Monte Carlo calculations for the absorbed fraction are for a tissue volume of arbitrary density, we may use these results for lung tissue even though the density is 0.3 g./cm.[3]. The lungs can be represented by a 1000 g. thick ellipsoid (Fig. 17.4).

TYPE OF RADIATION	$\overline{E}_i$	Δ_i	ϕ_i FOR 1000 g. THICK ELLIPSOID (UNIFORM DISTRIBUTION)	$\Delta_i\phi_i$
β	—	0.400	1.00	0.400
x, K	≈ 0.03	0.00320	0.486	0.00156
γ	0.080	0.00341	0.138	0.00047
γ	0.284	0.0363	0.144 ⎫	⎫
γ	0.364	0.613	0.144 ⎬ 0.145	⎬ 0.119
γ	0.638	0.122	0.146 ⎭	⎭
γ	0.724	0.0463	0.146	

$$\sum_i \Delta_i\phi_i = 0.521$$

Substituting into equation 2 and multiplying by 24

$$\overline{D}_\infty(v \leftrightarrow v) = 24 \times 0.100 \times 0.521$$

$$\overline{D}_\infty(v \leftrightarrow v) = 1.25\ \text{rad}$$

The above value for the absorbed dose to the lung includes only the activity in the lung; to this we must add the absorbed dose to blood resulting from nonpenetrating radiation as well as the long-lived component of the total-body absorbed dose resulting from penetrating radiation. This is calculated as follows:

$$\overline{D}_\infty(v_{Lu} \leftarrow v_B) = 24 \ \tilde{C}_v \ \Delta_\beta\phi_\beta(v \leftarrow v)$$

$$= 24 \times 0.0603 \times 0.400$$

$$\overline{D}_\infty(v_{Lu} \leftarrow v_B) = 0.58 \quad rad$$

Total body to lung

$$\overline{D}_\infty(v_{Lu} \leftarrow v_{TB}) = 24 \times 1.44 [C_2(0) \times T_{2eff}] \sum \Delta_i \phi_{iph}$$

$$= 24 \times 1.44 \times 0.000557 \times 4.65 \times 0.286$$

$$\overline{D}_\infty(v_{Lu} \leftarrow v_{TB}) = 0.0256 \quad rad$$

Then the total average lung absorbed dose is:

$$\overline{D}_\infty = 1.25 + 0.58 + 0.03$$

$$\overline{D}_\infty = 1.9 \quad rad$$

REFERENCES

Anspaugh, L. R.: Special Problems of Thyroid Dosimetry—Considerations of I-131 Dose as a Function of Gross Size and Inhomogeneous Distribution. UCRL-12492, Lawrence Radiation Laboratory, March 25, 1965.

Bayly, R. J.: Labeled Compounds in Medical Diagnosis. *Nucleonics* 24:46, 1966.

Bond, V. P., and Feinendegen, L. E.: Intranuclear H-3 Thymidine: Dosimetric, Radiobiological and Radiation Protection Aspects. *Health Phys.* 12:1007, 1966.

Briner, W. H.: Quality Control, Pyrogen Testing, and Sterilization of Radioactive Pharmaceuticals. *In* Radioactive Pharmaceuticals. CONF-651111, U.S. Department of Commerce, Springfield, Va., 1966, p. 93.

Brownell, G. L., Ellett, W. H., and Reddy, A. R.: Absorbed Fractions and Specific Absorbed Fractions for Photons. MIRD Pamphlet No. 3. *J. Nucl. Med.* (to be published).

Bush, F.: The Integral Dose Received From a Uniformly Distributed Radioactive Isotope. *Brit. J. Radiol.* 22:96, 1949.

Charlton, J. C.: Problems Characteristic of Radioactive Pharmaceuticals. *In* Radioactive Pharmaceuticals. CONF-651111, U.S. Department of Commerce, Springfield, Va., 1966, p. 33.

Cohen, Y.: Chemical and Radiochemical Purity of Radioactive Pharmaceuticals Related to Their Biological Behavior. *In* Radioactive Pharmaceuticals, CONF-651111, U.S. Department of Commerce, Springfield, Va., 1966, p. 67.

Cook, M. J., and Snyder, W. S.: Estimation of Population Exposure. *Health Phys.* 11:810, 1965.

Corey, K. R., Rothschild, E. O., Weber, D. A., and Meyers, W. P.: The Turnover of Se-75 in Patients Injected with Labeled Selenomethionine. *J. Nucl. Med.* 6:338, 1965.

Cuddihy, R. G.: Thyroidal Iodine-131 Uptake, Turnover and Blocking in Adults and Adolescents. *Health Phys.* 12:1021, 1966.

Ellett, W. H., Callahan, A. B., and Brownell, G. L.: Gamma-Ray Dosimetry of Internal Emitters. I. Monte Carlo Calculations of Absorbed Dose from Point Sources. *Brit. J. Radiol.* 37:45, 1964.

Ellett, W. H., Callahan, A. B., and Brownell, G. L.: Gamma-Ray Dosimetry of Internal Emitters. II. Monte Carlo Calculations of Absorbed Dose from Uniform Sources. *Brit. J. Radiol.* 38:541, 1965.

Fine, S., and Hendee, C. F.: Energies of X-Ray K and L Emission Lines and Critical Absorption Edges for All the Elements. *In* The Encyclopedia of X-Rays and Gamma-Rays. Reinhold Pub. Corp., New York, 1963, p. 334.

Fink, R. W., Jopson, R. C., Mark, H., and Swift, C. D.: Atomic Fluorescent Yields. *Rev. Mod. Physics* 38:513, 1966.

Focht, E. F., Quimby, E. H., and Gershowitz, M.: Revised Average Geometric Factors for Cylinders in Isotope Dosage. *Radiology* 85:151, 1965.

Glasser, O., et al.: Physical Foundation of Radiology. Paul B. Hoeber, Inc., New York, 1961, p. 376.

Gray, P. R.: *Phys. Rev.* 101:1306, 1956.

Greif, R. L., Sullivan, W. J., Jacobs, G. S., and Pitts, R. F.: Distribution of Radiomercury Administered as Labelled Chlormerodrin (Neohydrin) in the Kidneys of Rats and Dogs. *J. Clin. Invest.* 35:38, 1956.

Hill, R. D., Church, E. L., and Mihelich, J. W.: The Determination of Gamma-Ray Energies from Beta-Ray Spectroscopy and a Table of Critical X-Ray Absorption Energies. *Rev. Sci. Instr.* 23:523, 1952.

International Commission on Radiological Protection: Recommendations of the International Commission on Radiological Protection. Publication 6. Pergamon Press, New York, 1964.

International Commission on Radiological Protection: Recommendation of the International Commission on Radiological Protection. Publication 9. Pergamon Press, New York, 1966.

International Commission on Radiological Protection, Committee II. 1959: Permissible Dose for Internal Radiation. *Health Phys.* 3:1, 1960.

International Commission on Radiological Protection and International Commission on Radiological Units and Measurements: Report of the RBE Committee. *Health Phys.* 9:357, 1963.

International Commission on Radiological Units and Measurements: Report 10a, Radiation Quantities and Units. NBS Handbook 84, U.S. Government Printing Office, Washington, D.C., 1962.

Kereiakes, J. G., Seltzer, R. A., Blackburn, B., and Saenger, E. L.: Radionuclide Doses to Infants and Children: A Plea for a Standard Child. *Health Phys.* 11:999, 1965.

Koch, A. L.: A Distributional Basis for the Variation in Killing Efficiencies by Different Tritiated Compounds Incorporated into Escherichia Coli. *Radiat. Res.* 24:398, 1965.

Loevinger, R.: Average Energy of Allowed Beta-Particle Spectra. *Phys. Biol. Med.,* 1:330, 1957.

Loevinger, R., Holt, J. G., and Hine, G. J.: Internally Administered Radioisotopes. *In* Hine, G. J., and Brownell, G. L. (eds.): Radiation Dosimetry. Chapter 17. Academic Press, New York, 1956a.

Loevinger, R., Japha, E. M., and Brownell, G. L.: Discrete Radioisotope Sources. *In* Hine, G. J., and Brownell, G. L. (eds.): Radiation Dosimetry. Chapter 16. Academic Press, New York, 1956.

Lyon, W. S., Reynolds, S. A., and Wyatt, E. I.: Methods for Assay of Radioisotopes. *Nucleonics* 24:116, 1966.

Mayneord, W. V.: Energy Absorption. IV. The Mathematical Theory of Integral Dose in Radium Therapy. *Brit. J. Radiol.* 18:12, 1945.

McAfee, J. G., and Blau, M.: Comments on Available Hg-203 Chlormerodrin Biological Distribution Data. Report to the MIRD Committee, June 16, 1966.

McAfee, J. G., Fueger, C. F., Stern, H. S., Wagner, H. N., Jr., and Migita, T.: Tc-99m Pertechnetate for Brain Scanning. *J. Nucl. Med.* 5:811, 1964.

Morgan, K. Z.: Health Control and Nuclear Research. Chapter VI. Oak Ridge National Laboratory, unpublished data (1950).

Quimby, E. H.: Dosage Calculations for Radioactive Isotopes. *In* Quimby, E. H., and Feitelberg, S. (eds.): Radioactive Isotopes in Medicine and Biology—Basic Physics and Instrumentation. Lea and Febiger, Philadelphia, 1963.

Raynaud, C., Desgrez, A., and Kellershohn, C.: Exploration rénale à l'aide de la néohydrine et du bichlorure de mercure marqués aux mercures radioactifs Hg-197 et Hg-203. *Sonderbaude Zur Strahlentherapie* 53:318, 1963.

Reddy, A. R., Ellett, W. H., and Brownell, G. L.: Gamma-Ray Dosimetry of Internal Emitters. III. Monte Carlo Calculations of Absorbed Dose for Low-Energy Gamma-Rays. *Brit. J. Radiol.* 42:512, 1967.

Robertson, J. S.: Computer Applications in Nuclear Medicine. *J. Chron. Dis.* Symposium Issue—Computers in Medicine (In press).

Saxena, K. M., Chapman, E. M., and Pryles, C. V.: Minimal Dosage of Iodide Required to Suppress Uptake of I-131 by Normal Thyroid. *Science* 138:430, 1962.

Seltzer, R. A., Kereiakes, J. G., and Saenger, E. L.: Radiation Exposure from Radioisotopes in Pediatrics. *New England J. Med.* 271:84, 1964.

Smith, E. M.: Internal Dose Calculations for Tc-99m. *J. Nucl. Med.* 6:231, 1965.

Smith, E. M.: Calculating Absorbed Doses from Radiopharmaceuticals. *Nucleonics* 24: 1966.

Smith, E. M., Harris, C. C., and Rohrer, R. H.: Calculation of Local Energy Deposition Due to Electron Capture and Internal Conversion. *J. Nucl. Med.* 7:23, 1965.

Snyder, W. S.: Personal Communications and Unpublished Data, 1965.

Snyder, W. S., and Ford, M. R.: A Monte-Carlo Code for Estimation of Dose from Gamma-Ray Sources. *Health Phys.* 11:838 (1965) and ORNL-3849.

Stewart, F. S.: The Calculation of Radiation Dose from Distributed Sources of Tritium. *Int. J. Radiat. Biol.* 8:545, 1964.

Stuart, H. C., and Stevenson, S. S.: General Factors in the Care and Evaluation of Children, Physical Growth and Development. *In* Nelson, W. E. (ed.): Textbook of Pediatrics. Ed. 7 W. B. Saunders Co., Philadelphia, 1959, p. 12.

Tow, D. E., Wagner, H. N., Jr., Lopez-Majano, V., Smith, E. M., and Migita, T.: Validity of Measuring Regional Pulmonary Arterial Blood Flow with Macro-aggregates of Human Serum Albumin. *Amer. J. Roentgen.* 96:664, 1966.

Wagner, H. N., Jr.: Radioactive Pharmaceuticals. *Clin. Pharm. & Ther.* 4:351, 1963.

Wapstra, A. H., Nijh, G. J., and Van Lieshout, R.: Nuclear Spectroscopy Tables. Interscience Publishers, Inc., New York, 1959.

XVIII

PRINCIPLES OF
RADIATION SAFETY

RALPH PENNER

The scope of the radiation protection program necessary for a clinical or research facility for handling radioactivity is quite variable and may range from an extremely simple to a very elaborate program. Code of Federal Regulations, Title 10, Part 30, dictates various requirements, but does not specify any particular methods to meet these requirements. The person seeking a license must state in his application what type of program he is going to initiate and what records he will keep. If the program passes the scrutiny of the Atomic Energy Commission or the responsible agents of those states that have assumed licensing and regulation, the protection program becomes, in essence, a part of the requirements associated with the license. The purpose of this chapter is to outline an adequate and complete, but not unduly restrictive, program. A frequent error is to undertake a program that is designed for particular needs and not general enough to be applied to future needs.

TYPES OF HUMAN-USE LICENSES

GENERAL LICENSES

A physician may obtain a general license for the use of radioisotopes provided they are in capsules, disposable syringes, or other forms of prepackaged individual doses. The isotopes that can be used under this license are limited both in number and in usage, and also in total quantity on hand. The storage and handling is specified in Human Uses of Byproduct Material, Part 35:31, General License for Medical Use of Certain Quantities of Byproduct Material. Applications for a general license are made on Atomic Energy Commission form 482.

SPECIFIC LICENSES ISSUED TO PHYSICIANS FOR THEIR PRIVATE PRACTICE

This type of license is usually issued for an office-type practice, but may also be used by a physician in a hospital if he conducts a private practice there, provided the hospital itself is unlicensed. The license specifically names the user and the isotopes that can be used, but does not provide for training. Other physicians cannot use isotopes under this license. The use of isotopes is limited to well established uses of byproduct material. The requirements for this license are cited in Code of Federal Regulations, Section 30:24(b), Title 10, Part 30.

SPECIFIC LICENSES ISSUED TO MEDICAL INSTITUTIONS

This type of license is issued to institutions and specifies the physicians who can use isotopes as well as the particular studies that may be performed. The institution that obtains this type of license must have a radioisotope committee to evaluate all proposals for research, diagnostic, and therapeutic uses of radioisotopes within the institution. The physician users may be named specifically on the institution license, but must conduct their programs under the guidance of the isotope committee. The designation of the users of radioactive isotopes at the hospital or clinic can be made in several ways. An individual user or several users can be named in the license as being approved for one, several, or all of the isotopes listed on the license. This method is simple, but has drawbacks. If the authorized user is absent from the hospital, the isotopes cannot be used and the license is essentially invalid until the authorized user returns. An alternative method is to have the radioisotope committee function as a governing body for approval of users as well as proposed uses of authorized isotopes. Physicians may be trained in radioisotope methods under this type of license.

BROAD MEDICAL LICENSES ISSUED TO INSTITUTIONS

To obtain this type of license, the institution must have had experience under a specific institutional license and be engaged in medical research. The program of this license is completely controlled by the isotope committee, which approves the users of isotopes as well as the proposed uses. A formal and detailed protection program is required. Provisions for insuring purity and sterility of isotope preparations as well as for calibration of activity are required for those isotopes not supplied by a licensed drug manufacturer.

LARGE SEALED-SOURCE LICENSES

Teletherapy units and other large quantities of radioactivity in sealed form are separately licensed and not included with other human-use licenses.

TRAINING REQUIREMENTS FOR USERS

The basic training for users of isotopes includes a minimum of 30 hours of instruction in the principles and practice of radiological protection, measurements of radioactivity, and standardization, handling, and monitoring techniques. The user must be able to compute dosage and calculate results, know the biological effects of radiation, and have practical experience with the isotopes that he wishes to use. This must include five cases that he has managed completely for each isotope and procedure. In certain instances, the number of required cases may vary. For scans, three cases are usually required, the same number as for the therapeutic administration of unsealed isotopes. To use sealed isotopes therapeutically, three years of experience in therapy is required, preferably in a radiation therapy department.

In the case of research, familiarity with both the isotope and the technique to be used is mandatory, together with significant experience with other isotopes. The use of isotopes in human research requires that dosage be kept as low as possible and that the dose to the critical organ and whole body be calculated. If previous work with this isotope in man has not been done, animal investigation is required before use in man.

Training of the user should be submitted on A.E.C. form 313a, page 3, or on an appropriate state licensing form. This should be done even if the approval is given by the isotope committee rather than by the A.E.C. or state.

If the isotope committee is to control the program, the training and experience of the members of the committee must be given in the license application. Details about training, including dates, institutions, and degrees held, should be listed, as well as specialty board certification, postgraduate studies, and experience in dealing with radioactive isotopes. The training and experience of the committee members should not be limited to the radioisotope field, since some members of the committee may have had specialized training in other areas of medicine, such as hematology.

PROTECTION PROGRAM

Enforcement of the radiation protection program is a joint responsibility of several persons except in the case of the private physician license, in which case sole responsibility is placed upon the user. In the case of institutional licenses, the responsibility is shared by the radiation protection officer and the users. The isotope committee is responsible for the entire program but is not physically involved in the protection aspects. The committee must be certain that no one is overexposed to external radiation or receives a harmful internal dose of a radioactive isotope.

Certain controls are required for personnel protection: shielding, signs and labels, monitoring of both personnel and areas, and disposal of radioactive wastes.

SHIELDING

If the program is small, frequently a few lead bricks will provide adequate shielding so that radiation levels will be well under acceptable occupational levels of 2 milliroentgens per hour. With increased quantities of radioactive material on hand, there will be increased shielding requirements, particularly since workers may have to spend more time locating the desired isotope in the storage area. Rotating storage vaults encased by lead have been used to facilitate the obtaining of a particular isotope with a minimum of radiation exposure.

SIGNS

Four types of signs are approved for use in radiation work. All are yellow and magenta and contain the three bladed propeller. The wording of the signs must be either *radioactive material, radiation area, high radiation area,* or *airborne radiation area.* There is confusion in Part 30 of the Code of Federal Regulations in the delineation of *radiation areas* and *restricted areas.* A *restricted area* is interpreted to be an area in which a person might receive radiation in excess of 2 mr. per hour if he were continually present, and it is controlled by the license. At the level of 5 mr., *radiation area* signs must be posted. One might be in a restricted area without being aware of it, since signs are not required. It is sometimes useful to post signs stating *unauthorized persons prohibited* at the entrance to areas in which the radiation level is over 2 mr., but less than 5 mr. per hour. The limits of a *radiation area* must be posted clearly with the appropriate sign. A *high radiation area* starts at 100 mr. per hour and should be delineated by appropriate signs. In general, rooms containing radioactive materials in amounts required for medical work must be posted with the sign *radiation material* in addition to the others. All containers in the storage area must be labeled to indicate the isotope, the amount of activity, and the date of assay. An approved label must indicate that it is *radioactive material.* Only occasionally are the signs *caution: airborne radioactivity area* used in medical work; these signs should be used only if radioactive gases, mists, or vapors escape to the atmosphere.

MONITORING

Three types of monitoring are used routinely: personnel monitoring and two types of area monitoring, one for radiation levels and the other for radiation contamination. Personnel monitoring may be by film badge, which has the advantage of providing a permanent record of the exposure received, or by a radiation dosimeter, usually direct-reading. In high radiation areas, both types should be worn to give an immediate and permanent indication of dose. It is advisable to use wrist or finger film badges in laboratory experiments in which various manipulations are necessary. Permanent records of radiation exposures to radiation workers are required. A monitored radiation worker is defined as one who is potentially exposed to radiation levels in excess of 1.25 roentgens per year. Visitors may or may not be monitored, depending upon the estimated dosage that they might receive.

Areas are monitored for radiation levels and contamination with a survey instrument which may be of the Geiger-Müller or ionization chamber type. The instrument must be able to detect 0.01 mr. per hour and should be limited to 0.5 mr. per hour at full-scale detection on the lowest setting. Since some survey meters contain calibration sources, it is important to check these periodically for leaks and maintain appropriate records. The instrument must have the ability to detect both beta and gamma radiation. If the isotope program is limited to commercially produced precalibrated doses of radioactive materials, this instrument will be sufficient. If solutions are handled before administration, wipe testing for detection of removable activity in the area should also be performed. Storage and preparation areas should be monitored with the survey instrument to establish radiation levels and to detect radioactivity that may have been spilled. The radiation level of the storage area should be checked after storage of each new shipment and the work areas and floors monitored for contamination at least weekly. If contamination of floors or bench tops is found, an extensive survey should be conducted to determine whether activity has been tracked into surrounding areas or transferred to the clothing of the persons working in the area. If evidence of a spread of contamination is detected, immediate action must be taken to close off the contaminated area to prevent further spread. The area must then be decontaminated.

Monitoring of the area by wiping is used to detect removable contamination. Areas that may be contaminated are wiped with filter paper or with damp or dry cloth patches, which are then counted with an appropriate detector. Normally, an area of approximately 100 sq. cm. is wiped at a time. Before use, the wiping material should be cut to fit the sample holder. The quantity of contaminant that can be removed is dependent upon the nature of the material spilled and the porosity of the surface wiped. Thus, the decision as to whether significant contamination has occurred should be based not only on the results of the wiping, but also upon the best estimate of how much radioactive material is fixed to the surface. Direct measurement of the surface, followed by scrubbing and remonitoring with a survey meter, may also be used as an indication of removable activity. Wipe surveying cannot be surpassed for its simplicity, however. If tritium compounds have been used, assay of the urine of the workers is the method of choice in monitoring for contamination.

CALIBRATION OF INSTRUMENTS

The calibration of survey instruments requires at least a two point calibration of each scale and a determination of the linearity of response of the instrument. This calibration must be carried out at least every 3 months and after change of batteries or maintenance. A check of the operating response of the instrument should be made against a reference source before each survey. This reference check is not a substitute for calibration but an indication that the calibration data are still valid.

EQUIPMENT

The laboratory area should be designed so that in the event of a spill or other accident, decontamination can be accomplished with a minimum of effort and expense. Use of a waxed vinyl floor gives a rather impervious surface. If tile is used, a waterproof barrier beneath the tile will prevent spread of radioactivity into the subfloor area. The work benches should be of stainless steel or other resistant material and they should not have sharp corners or projections that are difficult to decontaminate. Stainless steel trays with raised edges should be provided at work areas. Absorbent paper should be placed in the trays to absorb spilled liquids. One or more sinks for cleaning contaminated glassware should be provided. If a large quantity of liquid wastes is to be disposed of, a holding tank may be provided for one or more sinks for temporary storage of liquids. The walls in the work area should also be of a smooth impervious material. If procedures such as radioactive labeling are performed with possible release of radioactivity, a radiochemical fume hood should be provided. This should be equipped with absolute filters and should have an airflow of 150 lineal feet per minute across the face of the open hood. Remote pipetting equipment is desirable if high levels of radioactivity are used, and remote handling equipment is required in some cases. Lead shields and blocks are nearly always necessary. The storage area for isotopes should be locked for security purposes. If large quantities are to be stored, exhaust ventilation of the storage area is desirable. Shelves in the storage area should be lined with absorbent paper if liquids are stored.

If several different areas are used, portable survey meters should be provided for each area in case of a spill or other emergency. A supply of decontamination solutions for personnel decontamination should also be readily available. If large amounts of liquid radioactivity are used, an emergency shower may be advisable.

SEALED SOURCES

Sealed sources, such as beta applicators containing ^{90}Sr, cobalt needles, teletherapy sources, and calibration sources other than naturally occurring radioactive materials, must be wipe tested for leakage at least every 6 months. Activity should be determined on an instrument capable of detecting 0.005 μc. of activity. If there is evidence of leakage over this amount, the source should be withdrawn from use and be disposed of or returned to the manufacturer for repair. In the case of high-level sources, such as in teletherapy, the source need not be wiped, but the surface most accessible and nearest to the source should be wiped to determine leakage.

WASTE DISPOSAL

Disposal of unused radioactive material or contaminated items may be accomplished in one of several ways. If there is a large quantity of radioactive waste, it may be best to utilize the services of a licensed commercial disposal facility. Waste material is packaged in drums for shipping. If liquid material is included, an absorbing agent must be added to prevent leakage. Information about allowable radiation levels and labeling is given in Interstate Commerce Commission Regulation Title 49, Parts 71 to 78 of the Code of Federal Regulations. These regulations are also contained in Tariff No. 13 of the Bureau of Explosives of the American Association of Railroads and in supplements of Tariff No. 8 of Motor Carriers' Explosive and Dangerous Articles.

Waste disposal may be accomplished by other methods when the quantity to be disposed of is not large. Radioactive materials may be stored and allowed to decay. Normally, a period of 10 half-lives is sufficient (except in the case of high levels, such as therapeutic doses) to permit sufficient decay to meet the requirements for disposal through the sanitary sewers in the case of liquids. Records of the quantities so disposed must be maintained. Solid wastes, such as animal carcasses and excreta, may be buried if the activity does not exceed 1000 times the amount specified in Appendix C, Part 20, Code of Federal Regulations. Burial must be at a minimum depth of 4 feet, successive burials must be separated by a distance of 6 feet, and not more than 12 burials a year may be performed. Incineration of radioactive materials is not permitted without a special amendment to the license permitting incineration; this requires a computation including the quantity of radioactivity relative to the total amount of material burned and the volume of airflow through the stack, stack height, and dispersion characteristics under adverse conditions. One must be certain that significant concentrations are not released into the surrounding environment.

Administrative procedures

The protection program must provide written instructions to nurses and other supportive personnel involved in the care of patients receiving therapeutic radioactive materials. This must be done for each therapeutic isotope used. Information must include the person who is to be notified and what action is to be taken in case of emergency. Proper handling of the body of a deceased person containing therapeutic quantities of isotopes must be described.

Duties of the isotope committee must be described in detail and issued at the same time as administrative orders appointing the members. The duties of the radiation protection officer should be clearly stated and should have the approval of the isotope committee. A form used for submitting proposals to the committee for uses of isotopes should be provided, and must include all necessary information.

Records

Records may be kept on index cards, loose leaf files, or in bound ledgers, provided the data are readily usable. A license violation often occurs or an isotope may be ordered in excess if records are poorly organized. The most essential record is the inventory of the isotopes. Usually, an inventory sheet is kept for each shipment and the amounts used are progressively subtracted from the total. One difficulty is that if several shipments of the same nuclide have been received, it may be difficult to determine the total quantity of each isotope on hand. Therefore, the total quantity of each nuclide must also be kept. Regardless of the system used, it must be kept current. Removal of pages to a storage or depleted file when the supply of the isotope is exhausted or is being held for decay will keep the active files from becoming too bulky.

Personnel exposure records are kept on A.E.C. form 5; a compilation of the past history of each worker's exposure is maintained on A.E.C. form 4. A periodic review of these exposure records may indicate potential problem areas. A constantly increasing exposure or high exposures that cannot be explained may indicate carelessness of the worker or an unsuspected radiation hazard within the lab.

If sealed sources are used, a record of the sources, the date of wipe tests, the person performing the tests, and the results stated in microcuries of removable activity should be maintained.

SURVEY INSTRUMENT CALIBRATION RECORDS

These are usually combined with the maintenance records on the instruments. A label pasted on the instrument indicating the date of the last calibration may be sufficient. If several instruments are used, the label method has the pitfall that the date of the required calibration of the survey instruments throughout the facility might be overlooked.

WASTE DISPOSAL RECORDS

Any radioactive material disposed of through the sanitary sewer or by burial should be carefully recorded in the waste disposal record. The method of disposal should be indicated, since Part 30, Title 10, Code of Federal Regulations limits the quantity that can be disposed of by these methods: not over 1 curie per year, and not over 10 times the quantities in Appendix C of the regulations through the sanitary sewer, or 1000 times the quantities in Appendix C by burial. The dilution factor used during sewage disposal must be recorded to insure that concentrations have not exceeded limits specified in Appendix B, Table I, Column 2, of Part 30.

MEDICAL EXAMINATIONS OF RADIATION WORKERS

A thorough medical history and examination is desirable before employment of a person in radiation work. With some types of exposure, certain studies must be added to the basic examination, which includes a medical history, a physical examination and laboratory studies.

Medical History. A complete medical history should be obtained. Special attention should be paid to the following areas:

Is there a higher than normal familial occurrence of malignant disease, especially the leukemias? Has there been evidence of an increased incidence of the nonmalignant blood dyscrasias?

Has there been a family history of developmental abnormalities (i.e., congenital heart disease, ectodermal anomalies, or neurological disease)? This information may help establish the possibility that subsequent diseases in the applicant or his children may have been familial rather than radiation-induced.

Information should be obtained as to the worker's past radiation exposure, both occupational and medical. Accidental occupational exposure should be well documented, as well as any radiation therapy. If therapy has been administered, a detailed history as to location, area, and dosage should be recorded. A history of diagnostic radiographic procedures should also be recorded with an estimate of the areas involved and dosage.

Marital status should be recorded. Does the applicant have any children? Are children desired? Are there sterility problems present?

Physical Examination and Laboratory Studies. The physical examination should be complete, and attention should be directed to any evidence of abnormalities of neuromuscular coordination or other physical handicaps that might impair the worker's ability. The skin should be evaluated for evidence of atrophy, telangiectasis, or early malignancy. The applicant's visual acuity and coordination should be evaluated.

Laboratory studies should include a determination of hemoglobin or hematocrit, and a platelet count. At least three periodic white blood counts and differentials are desired to establish a baseline if the possibility of an occupational overexposure is present.

Other precautions are sometimes necessary. If the person is to work with unsealed radioactive materials, the presence of a chronic dermatological condition should be disqualifying, since decontamination procedures are likely to aggravate the condition as well as make decontamination difficult.

Periodic physical examinations should be performed. At the time of the examination the record of exposure to ionizing radiation as well as bioassay reports such as measurements of urinary tritium should be reviewed. Laboratory procedures should include hematocrit or hemoglobin, white count, and differential count. Only one determination is required unless the results are abnormal or significantly changed from the baseline study.

MEDICAL EVALUATION OF AN ACCIDENTAL EXPOSURE

A radiation worker is unlikely to be exposed to significant external radiation in a medical isotope facility unless sealed sources, such as teletherapy sources, are used. If such exposure occurs, the evaluation of the person can be considered in three categories: (1) Are there clinical symptoms? If no nausea or vomiting existed after the exposure, it can be assumed that the exposure was less than 150 rem and probably less than 100 rem. (2) What was the exposure recorded by the dosimeter? This may not always indicate the total body exposure, since the dosimeter may have been shielded by the body or may not have been in the beam of radiation. (3) Has there been a change in the blood elements? Failure to detect changes in the numbers and morphology of the circulating white blood cells in studies at weekly intervals for 4 weeks indicates a total whole-body dose below 5 rem. With these three parameters, one can estimate how much radiation the worker received. Details of the exposure and medical evaluation should be entered into his records.

Internal contamination may occur through lacerations, inhalations, or ingestion. If the total amount of radioactivity involved in an accident was of the order of a *therapeutic dose* or greater, immediate evaluation of the person for possible internal contamination is required. Evidence of radioactivity about the mouth and nares or radioactive matter in a wound indicates probable internal contamination. It may be advisable to attempt to block the critical organ. Attempts to hasten excretion may be attempted if counting of the critical organ, in the case of gamma emitters, indicates relatively high levels of activity. For beta emitters such as ^{90}Sr, ^{3}H, and ^{32}P, urinalysis for activity should be performed. Carbon-14 may appear either in the expired air as carbon dioxide or in the urine, depending upon the nature of the tagged material.

GENERAL SAFETY

Occasionally so much stress is placed upon radiation hazards that general safety rules are overlooked. Accidents have occurred and will occur in the future because of lack of observance of general rules of safety. Care should be taken to assure that all electrical equipment is grounded, that volatile flammables are not used near open flames or sparks, that compressed gas cylinders are secure, and that housekeeping in general is satisfactory. A fire and emergency plan is mandatory and drills should be conducted periodically. Emergency equipment should be available and should be maintained in good working order. The fire department should be kept aware of the nature of the materials in the laboratory or storage area and of radiation hazards, if any, involved, in case they are called to fight a fire.

REFERENCES

Atomic Energy Commission Licensing Guide: The Licensing Requirements for the Medical Use of Byproduct Material (Radioisotopes). Atomic Energy Commission, Division of Licensing and Regulation, July, 1963.

Atomic Energy Commission Licensing Guide: A Guide for the Preparation of Applications for the Medical Use of Radioisotopes. Atomic Energy Commission, Division of Materials Licensing, March, 1965.

Atomic Energy Commission Rules and Regulations. Title 10. Atomic Energy. Part 30. Rules of General Applicability to Licensing of Byproduct Material. June, 1965.

Manual on Use of Radioisotopes in Hospitals. American Hospital Association, Chicago, Ill., 1958.

Maximum Permissible Amounts of Radioisotopes in the Human Body and Maximum Permissible Concentrations in Air, Water. National Committee on Radiation Protection[3], NBS Handbook 52, 1953.

Maximum Permissible Body Burdens and Maximum Permissible Concentrations of Radionuclides in Air and Water for Occupational Exposure. National Committee on Radiation Protection and Measurements[3], NBS Handbook 69, 1959.

Protection Against Radiations from Sealed Gamma Sources. National Committee on Radiation Protection and Measurements[3], NBS Handbook 73, 1960.

Safe Handling of Bodies Containing Radioactive Isotopes. National Committee on Radiation and Protection and Measurements[3], NBS Handbook 65, 1958.

Safe Handling of Radioactive Materials. National Committee of Radiation Protection and Measurements[3], NBS Handbook 92, 1964.

CHAPTER XIX

IN VITRO TESTS

SHIGEKOTO KAIHARA

HENRY N. WAGNER, Jr.

At present, when we measure a body function as an aid to diagnosis or in the course of a physiological investigation, if a radioactive tracer is used, usually it is administered by mouth or by injection to the patient under study. Sometimes, however, the tracers are used in *in vitro* procedures, more and more of which are coming into routine use in medical diagnosis. Carbon-14 and tritium have been widely used in biochemical research, because of the large numbers of chemicals of biological importance that can be labeled with these nuclides. Unfortunately, these nuclides are not useful for external detection and have been rather neglected in nuclear medicine.

Bayly (1966) has pointed out that many techniques used in biochemical research could be applied to clinical diagnosis, if sufficient developmental work were carried out. This is particularly true in the diagnosis of metabolic diseases.

The use of radioisotopes in *in vitro* tests can be divided into two main categories: evaluation of biochemical reactions in isolated tissues and assay of biological substances.

BIOCHEMICAL REACTIONS IN BLOOD
OR BIOPSY SPECIMENS

One of the most important advances in medical diagnosis was made with the introduction and development of tissue biopsies, such as those of the liver and kidney. These procedures provided information of the type that formerly could be obtained only at postmortem examination and that was useful in categorizing diseases into classic histopathological categories. With proper care these bits of tissue could continue to carry out some of the same functions that they performed within the living body, yet little was done in the way of measurement of biochemical reactions within biopsy specimens prior to the use of radioactive tracers. Usual chemical methods were too insensitive to be used with the small amounts of tissue that were obtained, but radioactive tracer techniques provided a sensitivity, specificity, and technical ease that resulted in a new look at the problem.

For example, one simple way to assess biochemical reactions in isolated tissues is to measure $^{14}CO_2$ liberated when tissues are incubated with certain ^{14}C-labeled substrates. By incubating tissue with an appropriate substrate it is possible to measure quantitatively the ability of the tissue to metabolize the substrate. This technique is commonly used in biochemistry and is now being used more and more in clinical tests.

In 1961, Snyder and Godfrey used a Warburg flask as the reaction chamber for incubation of tissues with ^{14}C-labeled substrate; the liberated $^{14}CO_2$ was measured by means of a liquid scintillation counter. Weinberg (1961) used a 25 ml. Erlenmeyer flask sealed with rubber stoppers from which were suspended glass wells. Keen et al. (1963) modified the method so that it could be used with as much as 30 mg. and as little as a few micrograms of tissue. Chiriboga (1962) and Buhler (1962) used filter paper wet with potassium hydroxide or sodium hydroxide as a trapping agent for carbon dioxide. In their technique, the paper strip containing the ^{14}C was dropped into the liquid scintillation media and the radioactivity determined. In another modification, Saba and DiLuzio (1966) used a 50 ml. Erlenmeyer flask as the reaction chamber to which was attached a liquid scintillation vial as shown in Figure 19-1. Liberated carbon dioxide was trapped on Whatman No. 40 filter paper (approximately 1.5 by 4.0 in. in size) that was soaked with 0.6 ml. of 10 per cent potassium hydroxide and placed inside the collection vial. With this technique, it is not necessary to transfer the trapped carbon dioxide to the counting vial; serial collections of carbon dioxide from the same sample are possible. It is important to be sure that the radioactive substrates do not contaminate the collection system. At times, volatile compounds result in ^{14}C being absorbed by alkali, or quenching agents may be absorbed and create problems. When Hyamine is used it may result in a vapor that may be poisonous to the tissue in the reaction chamber; it is therefore better to add the Hyamine after the reaction has taken place, rather than before.

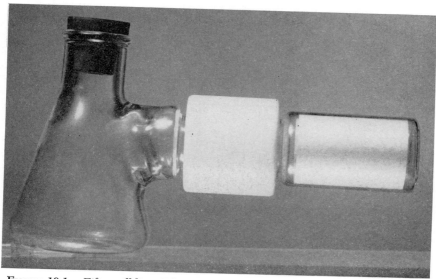

FIGURE 19-1. Fifty milliliter Erlenmeyer flask to which a liquid scintillation vial is attached. Liberated $^{14}CO_2$ is trapped on filter paper in the vial soaked with potassium hydroxide.

GALACTOSEMIA

One use of this technique has been in the diagnosis of congenital galactosemia (Weinberg, 1961). This disease is a hereditary disorder in which galactose-1-phosphate uridyl transferase (GPUT) is absent. This enzyme, ordinarily present in erythrocytes, is essential for the oxidation of galactose to carbon dioxide. If blood is incubated with tracer amounts of galactose-1-^{14}C, the release of carbon dioxide is dependent on the presence of GPUT. The results obtained by Weinberg are shown in Table 19-1. Differentiation of the patients from normal persons is clear-cut. Since the test is very simple and rapid, it is a useful screening test for galactosemia in infancy. The lack of GPUT can also be shown in liver tissue obtained by biopsy (Keen et al., 1963).

TABLE 19-1. GALACTOSE-1-^{14}C OXIDATION BY BLOOD FROM GALACTOSEMIC AND NONGALACTOSEMIC INDIVIDUALS*

SUBJECT	NUMBER	AGE	$^{14}CO_2$ COUNTS/MIN./ 2 ML. WHOLE BLOOD/ 1.5 HR.
Normal	7	18–29	18,550–35,900
Nongalactosemic children on galactose-free diet for milk allergy	2	1	18,900–29,000
Galactosemic children	5	6–13	0–73
Baby B (normal family history)		cord	39,000
Baby R (galactosemic sibling)		cord	37,500
Galactosemic adult	1	28	477

* From Weinberg, A. N.: Detection of Congenital Galactosemia and the Carrier State Using Galactose C^{14} and Blood Cells. *Metabolism* 10:728–734, 1961. Used by permission.

TABLE 19-2.   INCREASE IN PERCENTAGE OF $^{14}CO_2$ PRODUCED BY BLOOD
FOLLOWING TREATMENT OF THYROTOXICOSIS WITH RADIOACTIVE IODINE*

SUBJECTS		PERCENTAGE OF $^{14}CO_2$ PRODUCED FROM 5 μc. OF GLUCOSE-1-^{14}C		
Time after treatment			6 weeks	12 weeks
Thyrotoxicosis	1	4.8	6.1	8.2
	2	4.4	6.6	—
	3	4.6	6.7	8.4
	4	5.3	7.1	—
	5	2.0	4.0	—
	6	8.9	7.8	7.1
Normal (12)		10 ± 0.4		

* From Johnson, P. C., and Redding, T. R.: Glucose-1-C-14 Oxidation by Blood: A Potential Test for Tissue Effects of Thyrotoxicosis. *J. Nucl. Med.* 4:393, 1963.

THYROID DISEASE

Another example of the use of this principle is the study of Johnson and Redding (1963), who found that increased levels of thyroid hormone suppress the initial oxidation of glucose via the hexose monophosphate shunt in erythrocytes. Oxidation of glucose via this pathway can be measured by determining the rate of production of $^{14}CO_2$ from glucose-1-^{14}C. Johnson and Redding incubated 5 ml. of heparinized blood in a Warburg flask together with 5μc. of glucose-1-^{14}C and measured the liberated $^{14}CO_2$ by means of a liquid scintillation counter. Table 19-2 summarizes the results. Blood from thyrotoxic patients oxidized glucose-1-^{14}C at a slower rate than blood from normal persons, and the depression of glucose oxidation tended toward normal as clinical thyrotoxicosis subsided. In experiments in rats, similar changes could be produced by administration of thyroxine or thyroid-stimulating hormone (TSH). The investigators proposed that this method might be used to estimate tissue levels of thyroid hormone activity. Keen et al. (1963) suggested that this principle might be used to assay the TSH level of serum, but this has not yet been accomplished. The same principle has been used for the diagnosis of congenital intolerance to fructose (Milaud, 1963).

PHENYLKETONURIA

Metabolites other than carbon dioxide have been determined in biopsied specimens although the methods are somewhat more complicated. One example is the study of phenylalanine metabolism. Jervis (1953) studied pieces of liver from a phenylketonuric patient and found a deficiency of the enzyme phenylalanine hydroxylase. Hsia (1966) incubated DL-phenylalanine-^{14}C with liver biopsy specimens from normal persons and from phenylketonuric patients; in the latter, phenylalanine was not converted to tyrosine. In the diagnosis of phenylketonuria, the radioactive tracer method has not been widely used, since the use of ferric chloride solution is much simpler. Hsia (1966) has suggested that hyperphenylalanemia may result from causes other than phenylketonuria. There fore the direct assay of the specific enzyme activity of the liver obtained by needle biopsy may be useful in distinguishing true phenylketonuria from other causes of hyperphenylalanemia.

CELIAC DISEASE

The metabolic activity of biopsy specimens of human intestinal mucosa in celiac disease was studied by Dawson and Isselbacher (1960). This study was extended by Brice and his co-workers (1965) and Parkins (1966), who agree that in celiac disease the ability of intestinal mucosa to esterify palmitate-1-^{14}C to ^{14}C-labeled glyceride is decreased. This finding was of possible importance in our understanding of pathogenesis of celiac disease and also in its diagnosis.

It is predictable that there will be more studies of this type in the future. Using human liver homogenates obtained by biopsy, Ekdahl and his co-workers (1965) studied conjugation of ^{14}C-labeled cholic acid and suggested its possible use as a liver function test. In leukocytes the metabolism of glucose is stimulated during phagocytosis. By measuring stimulated CO_2 production from glucose-^{14}C, the measurement of phagocytic activity may be possible.

ASSAY OF BIOLOGICAL MATERIALS

SATURATION ANALYSIS

Several substances of biological importance have been assayed with great sensitivity by means of the principle known as saturation analysis. Several are outlined in Table 19-3. The term "saturation analysis" was first used for this assay by Barakat and Ekins (1961). The same general principles apply to analysis of all substances: (1) the substance to be assayed must be available in radioactive form; (2) an agent must be available that will bind the substance being assayed; and (3) a means must be available for separating the free and the bound form of the unknown substance.

The schematic representation of the method is illustrated in Figure 19-2. In essence, the radioactive form of the substance is added to the substance under investigation, which is present in an unknown quantity. The radioactive and stable forms of the substance are completely mixed and then reacted with the proper amounts of the binding agent. The degree of binding of the radioactivity to the binding agent is a function of the total quantity of the unknown present originally. From the measurement of the ratio of the bound to the free radioactivity, the amount of the unknown originally present can be calculated.

The widest application of the technique has been in the field of radioimmunoassay of various hormones, originated by Berson and Yalow (1958). In radioimmunoassay the binding agent is the specific antibody to each hormone; the method of separation was first based on the fact that free and bound hormones

TABLE 19-3. ASSAY OF BIOLOGICAL SUBSTANCES BY SATURATION ANALYSIS*

SUBSTANCE	RADIOACTIVE SUBSTANCE	BINDER	METHOD OF SEPARATION	REPORTED BY
Cyanocobalamine	^{57}Co cyanocobalamine	Intrinsic factor	Dialysis	Barakat and Ekins, 1961
Cyanocobalamine	^{57}Co cyanocobalamine	Intrinsic factor	Bound vitamin B_{12} removed by protein precipitation	Rothenberg, 1963
Cyanocobalamine	^{57}Co cyanocobalamine	Intrinsic factor	Free vitamin B_{12} removed by albumin-coated charcoal	Lau et al., 1965
Insulin	^{131}I insulin	Antibody to insulin	Electrophoresis	Berson and Yalow, 1958
Insulin	^{131}I insulin	Antibody to insulin	Free insulin removed by dextran-coated charcoal	Herbert et al., 1965
Growth hormone	^{131}I growth hormone	Antibody to growth hormone	Electrophoresis	Hunter and Greenwood, 1962
Parathyroid hormone	^{131}I parathyroid hormone	Antibody to hormone	Electrophoresis	Berson et al., 1964
Glucagon	^{131}I glucagon	Antibody to glucagon	Electrophoresis	Unger et al., 1959
Serum iron-binding capacity	^{59}Fe	Serum globulin	Free iron removed as insoluble salt	Feinstein et al., 1952
Serum iron-binding capacity	^{59}Fe	Serum globulin	Free iron removed by resin	Bothwell et al., 1957
Serum iron-binding capacity	^{59}Fe	Serum globulin	Free iron removed by coated charcoal	Herbert et al., 1966
Triiodothyronine-binding capacity	^{131}I triiodothyronine	Serum globulin	Erythrocytes	Hamolsky et al., 1959
Triiodothyronine-binding capacity	^{131}I triiodothyronine	Serum globulin	Free thyronine removed by resin	Sterling and Tabchnick, 1961
Triiodothyronine-binding capacity	^{131}I triiodothyronine	Serum albumin	Free thyronine removed by albumin-coated charcoal	Herbert et al., 1965
Corticosteroids	4-^{14}C cortisol	Corticosteroid-binding globulin	Dextran-coated charcoal	Nugent and Mayes, 1966

* For radioimmunoassay see Chapter VIII.

show different electrophoretic mobility. The method was devised to assay insulin and has now been extended to glucagon, parathyroid hormone, ACTH, and gonadotropic hormones. These techniques have been discussed in Chapter VIII.

VITAMIN B_{12} ASSAY

Saturation analysis has also been applied to the assay of vitamin B_{12}. This vitamin combines stoichiometrically with intrinsic factor. If free vitamin B_{12} and labeled vitamin B_{12} are present together with intrinsic factor, the unlabeled and labeled vitamin B_{12} compete for the binding sites of intrinsic factor. The greater the quantity of unlabeled vitamin B_{12}, the less will be the binding of labeled vitamin B_{12} to intrinsic factor. This makes possible assay of vitamin B_{12}.

At first, electrophoresis was used to separate free and bound vitamin B_{12}, because of the observation that free vitamin B_{12} has no electrophoretic mobility whereas the vitamin bound to intrinsic factor migrates toward the anode. This technique proved difficult because of the low concentration of the vitamin in serum. To overcome the problem of low counting rates, Rothenberg (1963) used a barium hydroxide–zinc sulfate protein precipitation to separate free vitamin B_{12} from the vitamin B_{12} bound by intrinsic factor. With this method, only protein-bound vitamin B_{12} is precipitated, leaving unbound vitamin B_{12} in solution. The serum vitamin B_{12} concentration in normal persons was 160 to 800 $\mu\mu$g. per ml., and in patients with vitamin B_{12} deficiency and megaloblastic anemia, 4 to 70 $\mu\mu$g.

The technique has been further simplified by the use of protein-coated charcoal to adsorb free vitamin B_{12} and separate it from the bound vitamin. Gottlieb

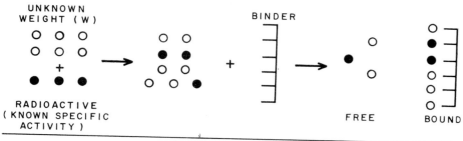

FIGURE 19-2.   Principle of saturation analysis. (Modified from Bayly.)

et al. (1965) found that uncoated charcoal adsorbs both free and protein-bound vitamin B_{12}, but that charcoal precoated by mixing with saturating quantities of albumin adsorbs only free vitamin B_{12}. The mechanism is believed to be that small molecules, such as vitamin B_{12}, pass through the protein coating, but that large molecules cannot.

The technique was applied to the measurement of serum vitamin B_{12} by Lau et al. (1965), who found the method to be simple, rapid, and reproducible. Presumably the protein-coated charcoal method could be applied to other assay procedures, provided: (1) the substance is adsorbed by charcoal when in the free form; and (2) a binding agent exists whose molecular weight and configuration is such that only the free substance will be adsorbed by appropriately coated charcoal. This method of separation has been applied to the assay of serum insulin, serum iron-binding capacity, and serum triiodothyronine.

Unsaturated Iron-Binding Capacity

The plasma iron-binding protein (siderophilin, transferrin), a globulin with a molecule weight of about 90,000 is capable of binding two atoms of iron, and is normally about one third saturated with iron. Knowledge of both the level of saturation of the iron-binding protein and the unsaturated iron-binding capacity (UIBC) of plasma is useful in the diagnosis of certain metabolic disorders and important in reflecting the transport and storage of iron. A number of methods have been used to determine the UIBC, including spectrophotometric, immunological and radioactive tracer techniques. Iron is bound to a plasma protein; therefore, whenever additional iron is added, it will be protein-bound in an amount proportional to the amount of unbound protein. If we can measure the ratio of free and bound iron, we can measure the UIBC. The only difference between this technique and the hormone immunoassay or vitamin B_{12}–intrinsic factor assay is that the binding substance preexists in serum and already contains the substance of interest in a bound form.

Use of radioactive iron in the measurement of UIBC was introduced by Feinstein and co-workers (1952). An excess of radioiron ^{59}Fe was added to the serum; neutralized ammonium sulfate was added to precipitate the protein-bound radioactive iron; and the remaining free radioactive iron was determined. Coprecipitation of free radioiron led to falsely high results. Bothwell and co-workers (1959) used an iron-free anion exchange resin (Amberlite IRA-401). The method was modified by the use of a polyether foam sponge in which a finely divided strongly basic anion exchange resin (Amberlite IRA-400 type, chloride form) was embedded. This system is now available commercially. Herbert and co-workers (1966) used hemoglobin-coated charcoal in the measurement of UIBC. After incubation of serum with ionic ^{59}Fe, 2 ml. of hemoglobin-coated charcoal was added in order to separate free iron. The radioactivity of the supernatant was then determined.

TRIIODOTHYRONINE-BINDING CAPACITY

This test is routinely used in many laboratories. It is based on the observation of Hamolsky et al. (1957, 1959) that red cells from hyperthyroid patients bind more ^{131}I triiodothyronine than do those from normal persons when incubated in the presence of the patient's plasma. Thyroxine is bound primarily to a plasma protein that migrates electrophorectically at pH 8.6 between the alpha$_1$ and alpha$_2$ globulins. Triiodothyronine is bound less completely and less firmly to this protein. Small amounts of thyroxine are also bound to albumin, which serves as a secondary carrier, particularly when plasma thyroxine levels are increased. As more thyroxine is added to plasma, the binding sites of the globulin are more fully occupied and additional thyroxine then spills over to be bound by albumin. It has been postulated that the distribution of thyroid hormones between plasma and the cells of the body is dependent upon the relative binding affinities of plasma proteins and the proteins of cells.

When red blood cells are incubated with ^{131}I-labeled triiodothyronine, the binding of triiodothyronine by the red cells amounts to about 10 to 17 per cent of the total radioactivity in euthyroid persons and 16 to 34 per cent in hyperthyroid persons. The mechanism of the increased binding by the red cells of hyperthyroid patients is that fewer binding sites are available to the labeled triiodothyronine. Sterling and Tabchnick (1961) used ion exchange resins instead of red blood cells and established the basis for an even simpler *in vitro* test of thyroid function, which is now available commercially and has been described in Chapter VII.

This test is another example of the use of the principle of saturation analysis: the *binder* is thyroxine-binding globulin and the method of separation is the use of erythrocytes or resin.

CORTICOSTEROIDS

Nugent and Mayes (1966) reported measurement of plasma corticosteroids using corticosteroid-binding globulin (CBG) and dextran-coated charcoal. As a source of CBG, they used human plasma with low corticosteroid concentration. The concentration of CBG was adjusted so that in the presence of labeled corticosteroids most of the labeled material was bound to CBG. Corticosteroids in plasma were extracted with methylene chloride and were added to the CBG with 4-^{14}C cortisol. Free and bound corticosteroids were separated by means of coated charcoal. The results agreed closely with results obtained with a chromatographic-fluorometric technique.

DOUBLE ISOTOPE DERIVATIVE ANALYSIS

This technique is a combination of isotope dilution analysis and isotope derivative analysis (Keston et al., 1946) and has been used successfully in the assay of steroid hormones. Table 19-4 outlines the uses of this technique in the assay of various substances.

Dilution analysis makes possible quantitative assay without quantitative recovery of the substance of interest. We simply calculate the recovery after the process of purification and make the appropriate correction. One radionuclide is used to correct the yield of each sample; another is used for the quantification of the amount of the substance present by making chemical derivatives of the compound of interest. This use of two radionuclides is referred to as double isotope derivative analysis, and its principle is outlined in Figure 19-3.

To a compound of unknown weight (W) with molecular weight (M), the same radioactive compound with known weight (W') and activity (P) is added. The radioactivity serves as a correction for yield after purification. After partial purification, an excess of a radioactive reagent is reacted to form a derivative of the compound. Since the molar specific activity of this reagent and the stoichiometric relationships are known, by measuring the radioactivity of the second radioisotope, we determine the amount of the unknown substance that was present. A final correction is made for the losses during processing.

ALDOSTERONE

The first successful use of this principle was by Kliman and Peterson (1960) in the assay of aldosterone. Dried extracts of plasma or urine were acetylated with tritium-labeled acetic anhydride in benzene in the presence of pyridine to convert aldosterone quantitatively to the tritium-labeled diacetate. A measured amount of aldosterone-diacetate-^{14}C was added to each sample and the double-

TABLE 19-4. DOUBLE ISOTOPE DERIVATIVE ANALYSIS IN THE ASSAY OF VARIOUS SUBSTANCES

SUBSTANCE	LABELED SUBSTANCE	DERIVATIVE FORMATION
Aldosterone	[14]C aldosterone	Acetylation with ^{3}H acetic anhydride
Testosterone	[3]H testosterone	Formation of semicarbazone with ^{35}S semicarbazide
Digitoxin	[3]H digitoxin	Acetylation with ^{3}H acetic anhydride
Thyroxine	[131]I thyroxine or (1-^{14}C) acetyl-DL-thyroxine	Acetylation with ^{3}H acetic anhydride

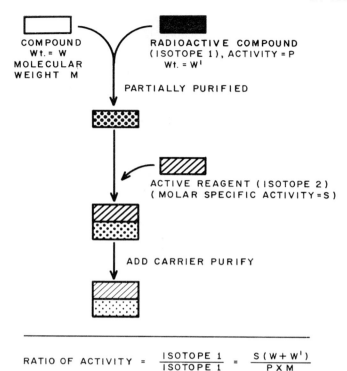

$$\text{RATIO OF ACTIVITY} = \frac{\text{ISOTOPE 1}}{\text{ISOTOPE 1}} = \frac{S(W+W')}{P \times M}$$

FIGURE 19-3.   Principle of isotope dilution derivative analysis. (From Bayly, 1966.)

labeled steroid identified and purified by paper chromatography. The samples were treated with 0.5 per cent chromic acid in glacial acetic acid to form a monoacetate oxidation product; this was subjected to a final chromatography to separate aldosterone from other tritium-labeled materials. The tritium and ^{14}C content of the purified steroid hormone were assayed in a liquid scintillation counter. The amount of aldosterone present in the original extract was calculated by determining the amount of ^{14}C indicator lost during the purification, the yield of tritium radioactivity, and the specific radioactivity of the tritium-labeled acetic anhydride. This method can be used to measure as little as 0.01 $\mu g.$ of aldosterone.

TESTOSTERONE

The same principle was employed by Riondel et al. (1963), who used sulfur-35 thiosemicarbazide in the assay of testosterone. Thiosemicarbazide reacts quantitatively with ketonic steroids to form thiosemicarbazone, which can be mapped chromatographically on the paper systems used for steroids. About 100 $\mu c.$ per mM. of ^{35}S thiosemicarbazide was used to make derivatives and 1,2-^3H testosterone (137 $\mu c.$ per $\mu g.$) to measure recovery. Purification was obtained by silica-gel thin-layer chromatography or paper chromatography. The precision and accuracy of the method was 6 per cent. Plasma levels of testosterone in 11

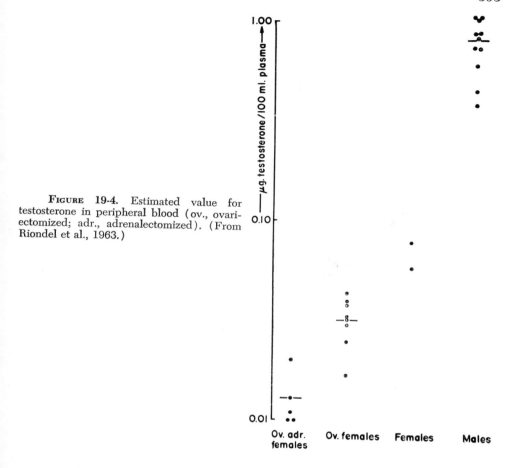

FIGURE 19-4. Estimated value for testosterone in peripheral blood (ov., ovariectomized; adr., adrenalectomized). (From Riondel et al., 1963.)

normal males were 0.80 ± 0.25 μg. per 100 ml., and in normal women during the progestational phase of the menstrual cycle, 0.059 and 0.079 μg. per 100 ml. (Fig. 19-4).

DIGITOXIN

Lukas and Peterson (1966) extended the technique to the assay of digitoxin in biological samples. Tritium-labeled digitoxin of high specific activity was added to the sample at the beginning of the analysis. Digitoxin was extracted from the sample and converted to digitoxin triacetate-1-^{14}C, which was isolated and purified. The amount of ^{14}C in the pure derivative is related stoichiometrically to the digitoxin content. The ratio of tritium added to tritium recovered was used to correct for losses of digitoxin during analysis. Lukas and Peterson reported that 0.01 μg. of the glycoside could be detected with an accuracy of 101 ± 3 per cent (mean ± S.E.) in the assay of 0.01 to 0.2 μg. in plasma. Assay of plasma thyroxine or other related compounds using double isotope dilution derivative methods was also reported by Whitehead and Beale (1959) and Beale and Whitehead (1960).

BIOASSAY USING RADIOACTIVE MATERIALS

If a radioactive reactant is added to an isolated tissue under standardized conditions, reactions that occur can be measured with precision. The technique can be called *radiobioassay*. Although the possibilities of the method are great, the method has been used only to a limited extent.

One application has been the assay of insulin-like activity. Measurement

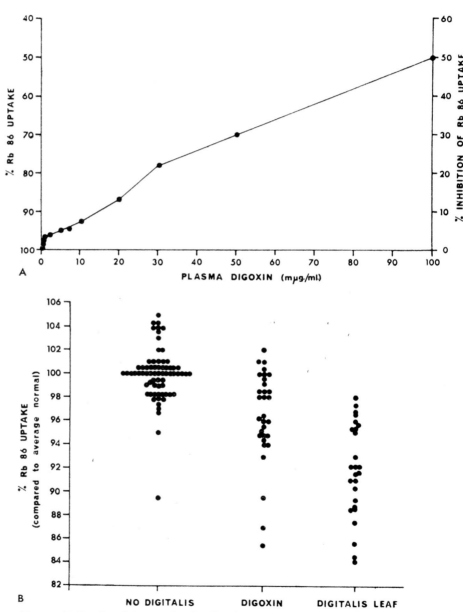

FIGURE 19-5. *A*, Inhibition of red cell Rb-86 uptake by plasma digoxin. *B*, Comparative red cell Rb-86 uptakes of three groups of patients, with the average uptake of those patients not on digitalis taken as 100 per cent. (From Lowenstein, 1965.)

was made of the metabolism of glucose-1-^{14}C to $^{14}CO_2$ by the epididymal fat pad of the rat and the effect of insulin on this system was determined. This technique has been discussed in Chapter VIII.

The assay of intrinsic factor (Sullivan et al., 1963) is based on the finding that the uptake of vitamin B_{12} by rat liver slices is enhanced by intrinsic factor. Sullivan and his co-workers modified the method by using homogenized guinea pig intestinal mucosa and circumvented the variation associated with the use of rat liver or guinea pig ileum sacs.

Another example is the measurement of the serum level of digitalis (Lowenstein, 1965). Schatzmann (1953) observed that extremely small concentrations of cardiac glycosides inhibit the uptake of radioactive potassium by human red cells. Using rubidium-86, Lowenstein standardized this system for the measurement of the serum level of digitalis glycosides. Standard O-type, Rh-positive red blood cells were incubated with ^{86}Rb solution and the percentage uptake of radioactivity was measured. The inhibition of ^{86}Rb uptake correlated well with the plasma digoxin level between 0.05 to 100 mμg. per ml. The lower limit of detection was 1 mμg. per ml. Patients receiving digitalis leaf had much higher circulating levels than did patients on digoxin (average value 9.5 mμg. per ml. of digoxin equivalent for digitalis leaf, 0.05 mμg. per ml. for digoxin). Patients with digitalis overdosage averaged 6 mμg. per ml. (Fig. 19-5).

ENZYME ACTIVITY OF BIOLOGICAL SAMPLES

Estimations of the enzyme content of biological fluids have proved to be of considerable value for medical diagnosis; a few, such as GOT, GPT, or alkaline phosphatase, are employed as routine tests.

The use of radioactive tracers may provide simpler and more specific and sensitive methods of assay. Labeled compounds can be used as substrates and, after incubation with the enzyme, the amount of unreacted substrate or its end products can be measured. It is necessary to separate the substrate from the end product and to determine the radioactivity of either. At times, the separation is a problem of considerable magnitude.

Ingenious methods have been reported, some of which are summarized in Table 19-5. One example is the radioisotopic assay of monoamine oxidase (Otsuka and Kobayashi, 1964). Many methods have been used to carry out this assay, based on the disappearance of substrate, consumption of oxygen, produc-

TABLE 19-5. EXAMPLES OF RADIOISOTOPIC ENZYME ASSAY

ENZYME	SUBSTRATE	METABOLITE	METHOD OF SEPARATION
Monoamine oxidase	^{14}C tyramine	Hydroxyphenyl acetaldehyde	Extraction into scintillator (anisole) and aqueous phase frozen for separation
Choline esterase	Acetylcholine-carboxyl-^{14}C	Choline Acetic acid	Acetic acid volatilized
Ornithine carbamoyl transferase	L-Citrulline-carbamoyl-^{14}C	$^{14}CO_2 + NH_3$ + ornithine	$^{14}CO_2$ trapped for counting
Arginase	L-Arginine-guanido-^{14}C	Urea-^{14}	Urea is decomposed by urease and $^{14}CO_2$ is counted

tion of ammonia, or production of peroxide, but none has been adopted for use with a large number of samples. Otsuka and Kobayashi incubated ^{14}C tyramine with enzymes and selectively extracted a metabolite by means of anisole at pH 3. Since anisole can be used as a solvent for liquid scintillation counting, these investigators dissolved scintillation phosphors in the anisole. After freezing, both the anisole containing phosphor and that containing the radioactivity were transferred to a counting vial for assay in a liquid scintillation counter. As little as 2 mμg. of tyramine could be detected and monoamine oxidase activity was detectable in human plasma. The extraction of metabolite by means of the liquid scintillator and the separation from the aqueous phase by freezing made the procedure simple and readily applicable.

Another use of this principle is measurement of ornithine carbamoyl trans-ferase (OCT) activity using L-citrulline (Reichard, 1962). In this system one of the end products is $^{14}CO_2$, which is easily trapped and whose radioactivity is easy to measure. Serum OCT levels have been reported to be of diagnostic significance in liver disease. Arginase is another specific enzyme for the liver and can be measured by the same technique. An end product, urea, is decomposed to CO_2 by urease, and liberated $^{14}CO_2$ is measured. With this method there is no interference by the urea physiologically present, and the assay of serum arginase is easily performed.

Another example is measurement of the enzyme choline esterase using acetylcholine-carboxyl-[14]C (Winteringham and Disney, 1964). In this system, acetic acid is the end product and can be volatilized at the end of reaction. From the amount of residual activity, enzyme activity can be determined.

Many other systems are available in which chromatography is employed for the separation of substrates and metabolites. Details of the technique are given by Mudd et al. (1964), Ng et al., (1964), and Reed (1966).

RADIOMETRIC ANALYTICAL METHODS

The use of labeled compounds is often helpful in the assay of unlabeled compounds. Measurements of cholesterol is one example. In the past, the assay of cholesterol has been based chiefly on spectrophotometry and its accuracy has not been adequate for biological work. The use of ^3H digitonin provides a more accurate method of assay. If an excess amount of ^3H digitonin is added to a solution containing cholesterol, it forms insoluble cholestal digitonin stoichiometrically; from the resultant ^3H activity in the supernatant, it is possible to calculate the cholesterol in the original solution (Morris, 1965).

Chiriboga and Roy (1962) reported measuring trace amounts of calcium, using oxalic acid-[14]C. The insoluble salt, calcium oxalate, was precipitated on filter paper and its radioactivity was counted. With this type of assay, it may be possible to measure trace amounts of other alkaline earth metals.

REFERENCES

Allen, R. J., Heffelfinger, K. E., Masotti, R. E., and Tsau, M. W.: Phenylalanine Hydroxylase Activity in Newborn Infants. *Pediatrics* 33:512, 1964.

Barakat, R. M., and Ekins, R. P.: Assay of Vitamin B12 in Blood. A Simple Method. *Lancet* 2:25, 1961.

Bayly, R. J.: Labeled Compounds in Medical Diagnosis. *Nucleonics* 24:46, 1966.

Beale, D., and Whitehead, J. K.: A Preliminary Investigation of the Levels of 3-Monoiodotyrosine and 3,5-Diiodotyrosine in Human Blood Plasma Using Double Isotope Dilution Technique. *Clin. Chim. Acta* 5:150, 1960.

Berson, S. A., and Yalow, R. S.: Isotope Tracers in the Study of Diabetes. *Advances Biol. & Med. Phys.* 6:349, 1958.

Berson, S. A., Yalow, R. S., Glick, S. M., and Roth, J.: Immunoassay of Protein and Peptide Hormones. *Metabolism* 13:1135, 1964.

Bothwell, T. H., Jacobs, P., and Kamener, R.: The Determination of the Unsaturated Iron Binding Capacity of Serum Using Radioactive Iron. *S. Afr. J. Med. Sci.* 24:93, 1959.

Brice, R. S., Jr., Owen, E. E., and Tyor, M. P.: Aminoacid Uptake and Fatty Acid Esterification by Intestinal Mucosa from Patients with Whipple's Disease and Non-tropical Sprue. *Gastroenterology* 48:584, 1965.

Buhler, D. R.: A Simple Scintillation Counting Technique for Analyzing $^{14}CO_2$ in a Warburg Flask. *Anal. Biochem.* 4:413, 1962.

Chiriboga, J.: Radiometric Analysis of Metals Using Chelates Labeled with Carbon-14 and Liquid Scintillation Counting Procedure. *Anal. Chem.* 34:1843, 1962.

Chiriboga, J., and Roy, D. N.: Rapid Method for Determination of Decarboxylation of Compounds Labelled with C-14. *Nature* 193:684, 1962.

Dawson, A. M., and Isselbacher, K. J.: The Esterification of Palmitate-1-C^{14} by Homogenate of Intestinal Mucosa. *J. Clin. Invest.* 39:150, 1960.

Ekdahl, P. H., Gottfries, A., and Scherstein, T.: Conjugation of C^{14} Labeled Cholic Acid in Human Liver Homogenates as a Test of Liver Function. *Advances Tracer Meth.* 3:313, 1966.

Ekins, R. P., and Sgherzi, A. M.: Microassay of Vitamin B12 in Human Plasma by the Saturation Assay Technique. *In* Symposium on Radiochemical Methods of Analysis. Vol. 2. International Atomic Energy Agency, Vienna, 1965, p. 239.

Feinstein, A. R., Bethard, W. F., and McCarthy, J. D.: A New Method, Using Radioiron, for Determining the Iron-Binding Capacity of Human Serum. *J. Lab. Clin. Med.* 42:907, 1952.

Gottlieb, C., Lau, K., Wasserman, L. R., and Herbert, V.: Rapid Charcoal Assay for Intrinsic Factor, Gastric Juice, Unsaturated Vitamin B12 Capacity, Antibody to IF and Serum Vitamin B12 Unsaturated Capacity. *Blood* 25:875, 1965.

Hales, C. N., and Randle, P. J.: Immunoassay of Insulin with Insulin-Antibody Precipitate. *Biochem. J.* 88:137, 1963.

Hamolsky, M. W., Golodetz, A., and Freedberg, A. S.: The Plasma Protein Thyroid Hormone Complex in Man. III. Further Studies on the Use of the In Vitro Blood Cell Uptake of I-131 Labeled Triiodothyronine as a Diagnostic Test of Thyroid Function. *J. Clin. Endocr.* 19:103, 1959.

Hamolsky, M. W., Stein, M., and Freedberg, A. S.: Thyroid Hormone–Plasma Protein Complex in Man. II. A New In Vitro Method for Study of Uptake of Labelled Hormonal Components by Human Erythrocytes *J. Clin. Endocr.* 17:33, 1957.

Herbert, V., Gottlieb, C. W., Lau, K., Fisher, M., Gervitz, N. R., and Wasserman, L. R.: Coated Charcoal Assay of Unsaturated Iron-Binding Capacity. *J. Lab. Clin. Med.* 67:855, 1966.

Herbert, V., Gottlieb, C. W., Lau, K. B., Gilbert, P., and Silver, S.: Adsorption of I-131 Triiodothyronine (T_3) from Serum by Charcoal as an In Vitro Test of Thyroid Function. *J. Lab. Clin. Med.* 66:814, 1965.

Herbert, V., Lau, K. B., Gottlieb, C. W., and Bleicher, S. J.: Coated Charcoal Immunoassay of Insulin. *J. Clin. Endocr.* 25:1375, 1965.

Hsia, D. Y.: Phenylketonuria: A Study of Human Biochemical Genetics. *Pediatrics* 38:173, 1966.

Hunter, W. M., and Greenwood, F. C.: Radioimmunoelectrophoretic Assay for Human Growth Hormone. *Acta Endocrinol.* Suppl. 67:59, 1962.

Jervis, G. A.: Phenylpyruvic Oligophrenia: Deficiency of Phenylalanine-Oxidizing System. *Proc. Soc. Exp. Biol. Med.* 82:514, 1953.

Johnson, P. C., and Redding, T. R.: Glucose-1-C-14 Oxidation by Blood: A Potential Test for Tissue Effects of Thyrotoxicosis. *J. Nucl. Med.* 4:393, 1963.

Keen, H., Field, J. B., and Pastan, I. H.: Simple Method for In Vitro Metabolic Studies Using Small Volumes of Tissue and Medium. *Metabolism* 12:143, 1963.

Keston, A. S., Udenfriend, S., and Cannan, R. K.: Microanalysis of Mixtures (Amino Acids) in the Form of Isotopic Derivatives. *J. Amer. Chem. Soc.* 68:1390, 1946.

Kliman, B., and Peterson, R. E.: Double Isotope Derivative Assay of Aldosterone in Biological Extracts. *J. Biol. Chem.* 235:1639, 1960.

Lau, K., Gottlieb, C., Wasserman, L. R., and Herbert, V.: Measurement of Serum Vitamin B12 Level Using Radioisotope Dilution and Coated Charcoal. *Blood* 26:202, 1965.

London, M., Marymont, J. H., and Fuld, J.: A Microdiffusion Test for Congenital Galactosemia Utilizing Galactose-1-C14. *Pediatrics* 33:421, 1964.

Lowenstein, J. M.: A Method for Measuring Plasma Levels of Digitalis Glycosides. *Circulation* 31:228, 1965.

Lukas, D. S., and Peterson, R. E.: Double Isotope Dilution Derivative Assay of Digitoxin in Plasma, Urine and Stool of Patients Maintained on the Drug. *J. Clin. Invest.* 45:782, 1966.

Milaud, G.: Technique nouvelle de mise en évidence d'erreurs congénitales du metabolisme chez l'homme. *Arq. Brasil Endocr.* 13:49, 1963.

Morris, M. D.: Measurement of 3-b-Hydroxy-Steroles by Tritiated Digitonine. *Anal. Biochem.* 11:402, 1965.

Mudd, S. H., Finkelstein, J. D., Irreverre, F., and Laster, L.: Homocystinuria—an Enzymatic Defect. *Science* 143:1443, 1964.

Ng, W. G., Bergren, W. R., and Donnell, G. N.: Galactose-1-Phosphate Uridyltransferase Assay by Use of Radioactive Galactose-1-Phosphate. *Clin. Chim. Acta* 10:337, 1964.

Nugent, C. A., and Mayes, R. M.: Plasma Corticosteroids Determined by Use of Corticosteroid Binding Globulin and Dextran-Coated Charcoal. *J. Clin. Endocr.* 26:125, 1966.

Otsuka, S., and Kobayashi, Y.: A Radioisotopic Assay for Monamine Oxidase Determination in Human Plasma. *Biochem. Pharmacol.* 13:995, 1964.

Parkins, R. A.: The Metabolic Activity of Human Small Intestinal Biopsies in Health and Celiac Sprue. The effect of wheat gliadin. *Gastroenterology* 51:345, 1966.

Reed, R. J.: Methodology of Radioactive Tracer Enzyme Assays. Presented at the 11th Symposium on Advances in Tracer Methodology, Boston, 1966.

Reichard, H.: Determination of Ornithine Carbamoyl Transferase in Serum—a Rapid Method. *J. Lab. Clin. Med.* 63:1061, 1962.

Reichard, H.: Ornithine Carbamoyl Transferase Activity in Man. *Acta Med. Scand.* 172:723, 1962.

Riondel, A., Tail, J. F., Gut, M., Tail, S. A. S., Joachim, E., and Little, B.: Estimation of Testosterone in Human Peripheral Blood Using S-35 Thiosemicarbazide. *J. Clin. Endocr.* 23:620, 1963.

Rothenberg, S. P.: Radioassay of Serum Vitamin B_{12} by Quantitating the Competition between Co-57 B_{12} and Unlabeled B_{12} for the Binding Sites of Intrinsic Factor. *J. Clin. Invest.* 42:1391, 1963.

Saba, T. M., and DiLuzio, N. R.: Method for Collection and Determination of $^{14}CO_2$ for In Vitro Metabolic Studies. *J. Lipid Res.* 7:566, 1966.

Schalch, D. S., and Parker, M. L.: Sensitive Double Antibody Immunoassay for Human Growth Hormone in Plasma. *Nature* 203:1141, 1964.

Schatzmann, H. J.: Herzglykoside als Hemmstoffe für den aktiven Kalium- und Natriumtransport durch die Erythrocytenmembran. *Helv. Physiol. & Pharmacol. Acta* 11:344, 1953.

Snyder, F., and Godfrey, P. J.: Collecting $^{14}CO_2$ in a Warburg Flask for Subsequent Scintillation Counting. *J. Lipid Res.* 2:195, 1961.

Spear, P. W., and Sass, M. D.: Some Current Concepts of Red Cell Metabolism. *Metabolism* 13:911, 1964.

Sterling, K., and Tabchnick, M.: Resin Uptake of I-131 Triiodothyronine as a Test of Thyroid Function. *J. Clin. Endocr.* 21:456, 1961.

Sullivan, L. W., Herbert, V., and Castle, W. B.: In Vitro Assay for Human Intrinsic Factor. *J. Clin. Invest.* 42:1443, 1963.

Tauxe, W. N.: A Rapid Radioactive Method for the Determination of the Serum Iron Binding Capacity. *Amer. J. Clin. Path.* 35:403, 1961.

Unger, R. H., Eisentraut, A. M., McCall, M. S., Keller, S., Lang, H. C., and Madison, L. L.: Glucagon Antibodies and Their Use for an Immunoassay for Glucagon. *Proc. Soc. Exp. Biol. & Med.* 102:621, 1959.

Weinberg, A. N.: Detection of Congenital Galactosemia and the Carrier State Using Galactose C14 and Blood Cells. *Metabolism* 10:728, 1961.

Whitehead, J. K., and Beale, D.: The Determination of Thyroxine Levels in Human Plasma by Double Isotope-Dilution Technique. *Clin. Chim. Acta* 4:710, 1959.

Wilde, C. E., Orr, A. H., and Bagshave, K. D.: Radioimmunoassay for Human Chorionic Gonadotrophin. *Nature* 205:191, 1965.

Winteringham, F. P. W., and Disney, R. W.: Radiometric Study of Cholinesterase and Its Inhibition. *Biochem. J.* 91:506, 1964.

Yalow, R. S., and Berson, S. A.: Assay of Plasma Insulin in Human Subjects by Immunological Methods. *Nature* 184:1648, 1959.

CHAPTER XX

ACTIVATION ANALYSIS

HENRY H. KRAMER

WERNER H. WAHL

INTRODUCTION

Neutron activation analysis is one of the most sensitive and most accurate methods for the determination of trace elements in biological materials. As many as 70 elements can be measured in the range of 10^{-6} to 10^{-12} g. with relative freedom from reagent blanks. The principles upon which activation analysis is based are fundamental to the physical basis of nuclear medicine. Therefore the time spent in achieving an understanding of all aspects of activation analysis is well worthwhile.

In a typical activation analysis, the sample to be analyzed is exposed to an intense beam of neutrons which interact with the nuclei of the atoms in the sample to produce radioactive and stable isotopes. The sample is left in the neutron flux (e.g., a nuclear reactor) long enough to produce a measurable amount of the radionuclide, which is subsequently used to quantify the amount of the original element present. After irradiation, the sample is removed from the reactor and the radiations of certain of the radioactive elements produced are isolated from other radionuclides by instrumental means, chemical methods, or physical methods, or by differences in the rate of decay. Each radioactive isotope is uniquely characterized by its rate of decay and the type of radiations emitted; therefore, positive identification and quantitative measurement of the radionuclide is possible. The amount of an element in a sample can be determined directly from the radioactivity measurement because the induced radioactivity is directly proportional to the number of atoms of the stable isotope in the original sample and to the neutron flux that interacts with the stable nuclei. The technique permits quantitative elemental analyses with a precision and accuracy of about ± 2 per cent, although the commonly attained precision and accuracy are in the range of ± 5 to 10 per cent.

GENERAL PRINCIPLES

NEUTRON REACTIONS

A neutron-induced reaction can occur when a neutron comes close enough to a nucleus to unite with it, forming a new compound nucleus. This compound nucleus, excited by both the kinetic and binding energy of the neutron with the nucleus, almost instantaneously reverts to a more stable state by emitting radiation, which produces either stable or radioactive nuclides. The radioactive nuclides are used as the analytical indicators of the elements in the sample. Examples of several nuclear transformations of this type are illustrated in Table 20-1 and Figure 20-1. The nucleon interactions are abbreviated as follows:

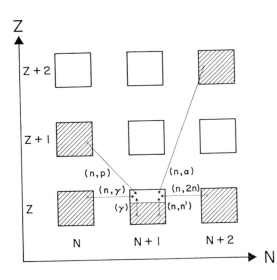

FIGURE 20-1. Typical neutron reactions in a reactor.

TABLE 20-1. TYPES OF NEUTRON NUCLEUS REACTIONS

TYPE	NUCLIDE		COMPOUND NUCLEUS		EMISSION		PRODUCT
n,γ	$^{37}Cl + n$	→	^{38}Cl	→	γ	+	^{38}Cl
n,n'	$^{115}In + n$	→	^{116}In	→	n'	+	^{115m}In
n,p	$^{58}Ni + n$	→	^{59}Ni	→	p	+	^{58}Co
n,α	$^{35}Cl + n$	→	^{36}Cl	→	α	+	^{32}P
$n,$fission	$^{235}U + n$	→	^{236}U	→	Fission products		

^{37}Cl(n,γ)^{38}Cl, ^{115}In(n,n')^{115m}In, ^{58}Ni(n,p)^{58}Co, ^{35}Cl(n,α)^{32}P, and ^{235}U(n,f)FP. The terms in parentheses describe the incident and emitted particles, respectively.

The probability that a nuclear interaction will lead to a particular nuclear species is expressed in terms of its *cross section*. The unit of cross section is the barn (1×10^{-24} cm.^{2}), which is the order of magnitude of the cross sectional area of nuclei. When a beam of neutrons is incident upon a sample, some of the neutrons pass through the sample and are unaffected; some are absorbed and some are scattered from the neutron beam. The fractional decrease in intensity ($-dI/I$) of the neutron beam passing through a thin layer of sample is equal to $\sigma_t$ndx, where σ_t is the total cross section of each nucleus and n is the number of nuclei in the layer dx. Hence, the intensity I of the neutron beam after it has passed through a sample of thickness x is expressed as:

$$I = I_0 e^{-\sigma_t nx}$$

The total cross section per nucleus can be calculated from the results of transmission measurements. This total cross section is the *sum* of the cross sections for all the absorption and scattering interactions. A summary of these processes is shown in Table 20-2 (Taylor and Havens, 1956). The most important interaction in neutron activation analysis is that which produces a radionuclide. The cross section for this type of interaction is commonly called the *activation cross section*. Since activation is only one of the absorption processes, the total absorption cross section is not the same as the activation cross section.

The total cross section of a given isotope depends upon the energy (or velocity) of the incident neutron (Hughes and Harvey, 1958). At very high neutron energies (above 100 kev.) the effective total cross section is roughly twice the geometric size of the nucleus. The principal interaction processes in this high energy region result in the emission of nuclear particles, e.g., (n,n'), (n,2n), (n,p), and (n,α) reactions. As the energy (E) of the neutrons decreases, the cross section increases approximately as $1/\sqrt{E}$, or as $1/v$, since $E = kv^2$ (v = velocity of the neutron). In the range of neutron energies from 1 e.v. to 10 kev., the total cross section usually shows a marked increase because of resonance absorption and resonance scattering. One or more of these resonances exist for most nuclei, and they are characteristic for each nuclear species. At neutron energies below the lowest energy resonance, but higher than those involved in crystal diffraction, the total cross section varies as $1/v$. In this region (<1 e.v.) the scattering cross section is essentially constant; hence, the absorp-

TABLE 20-2. TYPES OF NEUTRON INTERACTIONS

σ_t	=	Σ^{σ_a}	+	Σ^{σ_s}

Absorption Processes	*Scattering Processes*
n,γ	Elastic nuclear scattering
n,p	Inelastic nuclear scattering
n,α	Resonant nuclear scattering
n,d	Coherent crystal (diffraction)
n,2n	Ferromagnetic scattering
n,np	Paramagnetic scattering
n,fission	Inelastic molecular scattering
	Neutron-electron scattering

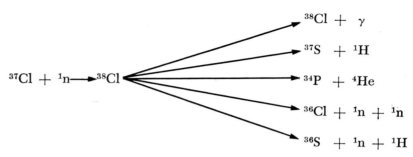

FIGURE 20-2. Neutron absorption process of chlorine-37.

tion cross section (and activation cross section) varies as $1/v$. In this energy region, the principal activation process is the (n,γ) reaction, which is called radiative neutron capture because the gamma-ray is emitted from the compound nucleus shortly after it is formed. When the energy of the neutron is decreased to the point at which the associated wavelength is of the order of the distance between atoms in crystals, diffraction effects occur.

The type of interaction between the neutron and the nucleus depends primarily upon the nuclide involved and the energy of the absorbed neutron (Hughes, 1953). For example, the absorption of a neutron by chlorine-37 may give rise to an (n,γ), (n,p), (n,α), or $(n,$ multiple particle$)$ reaction (Fig. 20-2). In general, the different types of reactions have been listed in order of increasing neutron energy; however, for each system there is a set of competitive nuclear reactions, one of which will be most prominent for a given neutron energy. The most common reaction with thermal neutrons is the (n,γ) reaction, which involves the capture of a neutron by a stable nucleus to produce a radioisotope of the original element.

PRODUCTION OF A RADIONUCLIDE

When nuclei of any stable isotope are exposed to neutrons or any other particle, the resulting nuclear reaction may be represented by $A \xrightarrow{\sigma} B \xrightarrow{\lambda} C$. The stable isotope A with activation cross section σ interacts with neutrons to form radionuclide B, which decays with its characteristic decay constant λ to the nuclide C.

The rate of formation of a radionuclide is given by:

$$\frac{dN^*}{dt} = \dot{N}\phi\sigma \tag{1}$$

The rate of decay is given by:

$$-\frac{dN^*}{dt} = \lambda N^* \tag{2}$$

The net rate of change in the number of radioactive nuclei is given by combining the two equations together with the relation $\dot{N} = N - N^*$:

$$\frac{dN^*}{dt} = \dot{N}\phi\sigma - \lambda N^* = N\phi\sigma - N^*(\phi\sigma + \lambda) \tag{3}$$

where ϕ = neutron flux (neutrons/cm.²/sec.)
σ = activation cross section (10^{-24} cm.²/atom)
N = number of target atoms of isotope A before irradiation
$\dot{N}$ = number of target atoms of isotope A at any time t
N^* = the number of radioactive nuclei B
λ = the decay constant of radionuclide B
t = irradiation period

and

$$N = \frac{w}{A} \times F \times Av$$

where A = the atomic weight of the element
w = weight of element in sample (grams)
F = the fractional abundance of the isotope undergoing reaction
Av = Avogadro's number

The solution of equation 3 may be simplified by considering N to be a constant[1] because N^* is very small compared to N, and by letting $x = N\phi\sigma - N^*(\phi\sigma + \lambda)$ (Taylor and Havens, 1956). Hence, from equation 3:

$$\frac{dN^*}{dt} = x \tag{4}$$

and from the definition of x:

$$dx = -(\phi\sigma + \lambda)dN^* \tag{5}$$

Combining equations 4 and 5, rearranging terms, integrating, and solving for N^* gives

$$N^* = \frac{N\phi\sigma\,[1 - e^{-(\phi\sigma + \lambda)t}]}{(\phi\sigma + \lambda)} \tag{6}$$

In essentially all cases in activation analysis $\phi\sigma \ll \lambda$ and equation 6 reduces to

$$N^* = \frac{N\phi\sigma\,(1 - e^{-\lambda t})}{\lambda} \tag{7}$$

When $t \ll 1/\lambda$ or $t \ll 1/(\phi\sigma + \lambda)$, both equations 6 and 7 reduce to equation 8.

$$N^* = \frac{N\phi\sigma\lambda t}{\lambda} \tag{8}$$

When the time of irradiation is very long compared to the half-life, or large with respect to $1/\lambda$,

$$N^* = \frac{N\phi\sigma}{\lambda} \tag{9}$$

The activity A in terms of disintegrations per second of the radioactive atoms N^* present after an irradiation time t is λN^*; therefore

---

[1] In the derivation of the activation equation, it was assumed that the number of target atoms N was not significantly decreased during the irradiation period. This is true in the usual case. However, a correction is needed for isotopes that have a large activation cross section and are irradiated for long periods in a very high flux (Rubinson, 1949).

$$A = \lambda N^* = N\phi\sigma \left(1 - e^{-\lambda t}\right) \tag{10}$$

The half-life, $T_{\frac{1}{2}}$, is related to the decay constant, λ, by $\lambda = \ln 2/T$, or $0.693/T_{\frac{1}{2}}$. Hence, equation 10 may be rewritten

$$A = N\phi\sigma \left(1 - e^{-0.693t/T_{\frac{1}{2}}}\right) = N\phi\sigma S \tag{11}$$

The term $\left(1 - e^{-0.693/T_{\frac{1}{2}}}\right)$ is called the *saturation factor, S*. For a time of irradiation equal to the half-life, the activity produced is one half the maximum activity produced at saturation. When the irradiation period is equal to 10 half-lives, the saturation factor becomes 0.999. The *saturation factor* as a function of the number of half-lives of irradiation is shown in Figure 20-3.

As soon as the sample is removed from the irradiation source, each radio-nuclide in the sample decays at the rate expressed by equation 2:

$$\frac{dN^*}{dt} = -\lambda N^* \tag{2}$$

Integrating this equation gives

$$\ln N^* = -\lambda t_d + a \tag{12}$$

where a is the constant of integration and t_d is the decay period. At $t_d = 0$, $a = \ln N_0^*$; where N_0^* is the number of radioactive atoms at the end of the irradiation period. Thus equation 12 reduces to:

$$N^* = N_0^* e^{-\lambda t_d} \tag{13}$$

The activity of a given radioactive species at any time after bombardment is:

$$A = N\phi\sigma SD \tag{14}$$

where $D = e^{-\lambda t_d}$, an expression commonly called the decay factor.

Equation 14, which is commonly called the activation equation, is applicable only in the cases in which isotope A is transmuted to radionuclide B, which decays to the stable isotope C. This process, which is represented by $A \xrightarrow{n} B \xrightarrow{\lambda} C$, is the most common one in radioisotope production. However, several cases arise

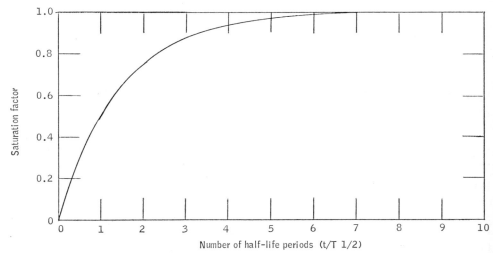

FIGURE 20-3. Growth of activity during irradiation.

in which isotope C is also radioactive, and it may be the more important isotope, e.g., tellurium-130—$\xrightarrow{n}$tellurium-131—$\xrightarrow{\lambda}$iodine-131. This type of process is represented by A—$\xrightarrow{\lambda}$B—$\xrightarrow{\lambda_2}$C—$\xrightarrow{\lambda_2}$D. In such cases, the activity of C present in an irradiated sample at any time after bombardment is represented by

$$A_C = \sigma\phi N \left\{ \frac{\lambda_2}{\lambda_2 - \lambda_1} S_B(D_B - D_C) + D_C \left[S_C + \frac{\lambda_2}{\lambda_1 - \lambda_2} (S_C - S_B) \right] \right\} \quad (15)$$

where subscripts B and C identify the saturation (S) and decay factors (D) for radionuclides B and C, respectively (Crouthamel, 1960). The equation is true only if none of the nuclides A, B, or C are appreciably decreased by interactions with neutrons during the bombardment and if no appreciable amounts of B or C are present at the start of the bombardment.

Radioactive nuclei can also undergo subsequent nuclear reactions. In the development of the activation equation, it was assumed that few of the radioactive atoms produced by activation undergo these reactions. When second order reactions are significant, the rate of disappearance of a radionuclide should be represented by the more complex rate expression:

$$-\frac{dN^*}{dt} = N^*(\lambda + \phi\sigma^*) \quad (16)$$

where σ^* is the activation or absorption cross section for the radioisotope N^*. The number of radioactive nuclei produced after an irradiation time t is:

$$N^* = \frac{N\phi\sigma \left[1 - e^{-(\phi\sigma + \lambda + \phi\sigma^*)t} \right]}{(\phi\sigma + \lambda + \phi\sigma^*)} \quad (17)$$

An example is the conversion of gold-198 to gold-199. When gold (^{197}Au) is irradiated with neutrons, 2.7 day ^{198}Au is formed. Although the number of ^{198}Au atoms formed is small, their high activation cross section (35,000 barns) will result in a loss of almost 50 per cent of the ^{198}Au atoms at a flux of 1×10^{14} neutrons/cm.^{2}/sec. at saturation.

The radionuclide (N^{**}) formed by the secondary activation must be considered in the measurement of the activity of the primary product. The activity of the secondary product N^{**} is calculated by the same method as that of the primary product N^*.

QUANTITATIVE ELEMENTAL ANALYSIS

Once radioactivity has been induced and the radiations of the radionuclide of interest have been isolated, quantitative measurements can be made. In principle, the activation technique is an absolute method of analysis; the weight of an element can be determined directly from the measured activity and a knowledge of the nuclear constants and experimental conditions. However, the absolute method is almost never used because of the difficulties associated with making absolute measurements. Instead, a comparative method is almost always used. In this method, a known amount of the element to be determined is irradiated, processed, and counted in the exact same way as the sample being analyzed. The activity of the analytical indicator induced in the sample is then compared with the activity induced in the comparator.

Since the samples and comparator are counted the same way, the counting variables are the same, and, consequently, the following relationship is true

$$\frac{A_s}{A_c} = \frac{C_s}{C_c} \tag{18}$$

where A and C are the activity (disintegrations per second) and count rate (counts per unit time), respectively, and the subscripts s and c designate the sample and comparator, respectively.

Since the sample and comparator are irradiated in the same irradiation zone and usually for the same period of time, most of the factors that give rise to inaccuracies in the absolute method are eliminated by comparing the count rate of the radioactive analytical indicator directly with that of the comparator. This comparison is shown in equation 19.[2]

$$\frac{C_s}{C_c} = \frac{W_s D_s}{W_c D_c} \tag{19}$$

In those cases in which the decay and counting periods are the same for the sample and comparator, in addition to the irradiation period, the ratio of the activities is directly proportional to the weight as shown in equation 20.

$$\frac{C_s}{C_c} = \frac{W_s}{W_c} \tag{20}$$

This expression can be rearranged in terms of the unknown weight of the element in the sample.

$$W_s = \frac{C_s W_c}{C_c} \tag{21}$$

SEPARATION OF RADIONUCLIDES

The amount of radioactivity produced in a neutron-irradiated sample is influenced by those factors that are fixed for any one element, such as the cross section, decay constant, and isotopic abundance, and those which may be varied by the analyst, such as the irradiation time, sample size, and flux. The analyst normally selects the experimental conditions to produce a measurable amount of the desired analytical indicator. However, if several different elements are present in the irradiated sample, a large number of different radioactive species may be formed. The analyst is confronted with the problem of measuring the activity of the analytical indicator in the presence of all the other induced radionuclides. He has at his disposal a number of methods that can be used to isolate the radiations of the radionuclide of interest from all the others in the activated sample. Essentially all the methods can be listed under four categories: time, instrumental, chemical, and computer.

The *time* method of isolation is almost unique to the neutron activation technique. It is often possible to maximize or minimize the activity of almost any radionuclide with respect to another radionuclide present in an activated

---

[2] If the isotope abundance is the same for sample and comparator, it also is eliminated from the equation.

sample by the proper choice of irradiation and decay time periods. The ability to discriminate in this manner depends primarily on the differences in the half-lives of the radionuclides in the samples.

Analysis of the type of decay by *instrumental* methods is another useful analytical tool. Although the beta particles emitted by each radionuclide have a characteristic maximum energy, the beta-ray energy spectrum is a continuum extending over a wide range of energies. Consequently, the beta particles are seldom used for analysis unless the radionuclide emits only beta-rays or unless it can be isolated in a radiochemically pure state. In contrast, gamma-rays are emitted with discrete energies that can be resolved by gamma-ray detection methods, which permit simultaneous analysis of a number of radionuclides in the sample. However, there are situations in which several radionuclides in the sample will emit gamma-rays of similar energy. When the analyst is confronted with this situation, or with a situation in which the radionuclides of interest cannot be distinguished from emissions of other radionuclides in the sample, he must resort to the other methods of isolation, i.e., computer and chemical methods.

There are several different *computer* methods that are applied in unraveling complex gamma-ray spectra, e.g., least squares, multiple regression, linear programming, machine stripping, and stepwise fitting (Table 20-3) (Applications of Computers to Nuclear and Radiochemistry, 1962). Least squares and multiple regression techniques are mathematically based; whereas machine stripping and stepwise fitting are techniques that are machine oriented, i.e., use the rapid calculation ability of a computer to do simple additions and subtractions. Linear programming is a technique that was originally machine oriented, but lately has been studied from a purely mathematical basis.

Each computer method requires that the sample spectra and the standard spectra be obtained under exactly the same instrumental and detection conditions. If the standard spectra were added together in the proportions contained in the sample, the resultant spectrum should be identical to that obtained from the sample. It must be pointed out, however, that computer methods are applicable only in unraveling spectra of radionuclides whose activity is greater than the

TABLE 20-3. COMPUTER TECHNIQUES USED TO UNRAVEL
COMPLEX GAMMA-RAY SPECTRA

TECHNIQUE	DESCRIPTION
Least squares	A technique that calculates the amount of each component that produces the least sum of the squares of the residuals between the unknown spectrum and the calculated composite of the standard components.
Linear programming	A technique that assumes there is a best linear solution of a combination of known spectra which conforms exactly to the sample spectrum. The computer calculates, at very high speed, every solution and selects the best.
Machine stripping	A simple subtraction technique in which known spectra are subtracted from the sample spectrum until the resultant spectrum appears to be the same as background.
Multiple regression	A combination of machine stripping and least squares methods.
Stepwise fitting	A simple addition technique in which known spectra are added in small increments until the composite spectrum fits the sample spectrum.

TABLE 20-4. CHARACTERISTICS OF CHEMICAL SEPARATION TECHNIQUES

METHOD	MINIMUM SEPARATION TIME (minutes)	COMMENTS
Precipitation	1	Has general applicability; however, all precipitates tend to absorb other elements. Usually more than one precipitation step is necessary to obtain radiochemical purity.
Solvent extraction	1	Perhaps the quickest and cleanest method of separation.
Ion exchange	20	Excellent method for separation. However, carriers are normally not used; consequently, determination of the efficiency of separation is difficult.
Electro-deposition	30	Specific for only a few elements. Holds promise for preirradiation chemical separation of certain elements.
Volatilization	5	Usually restricted to nonmetals and a few metals which form volatile covalent compounds.

statistical fluctuations associated with the emissions of the other radionuclides present in the sample. The requirements for usage of the computer to unravel complex gamma-ray spectra are stringent, but they can be met. Many laboratories are using these techniques for routine quantitative analyses of samples of known elemental content.

Chemical methods can also be used to isolate the analytical indicator (Subcommittee on Radiochemistry, 1960). Even though the element of interest (or analytical indicator) is present in extremely low concentrations, the chemical methods are the same as those used in general quantitative analyses. After the sample has been irradiated, a known amount of the stable element of the analytical indicator is added to the sample as a carrier. The addition of a known weight of the nonradioactive chemical carrier permits the efficiency of the chemical separation to be determined. Thus, the chemical separations need *not* be quantitative because the radioactivity measurements can be corrected by the known efficiency of the chemical processing. A brief outline of the chemical methods used in neutron activation analysis is presented in Table 20-4. The methods are listed in order of decreasing usage.

NEUTRON SOURCES

NUCLEAR REACTORS

The nuclear reactors are the most important sources of neutrons for activation analysis. The neutron fluxes available in a nuclear reactor range from 10^{11} to 10^{14} neutrons/cm.^{2}/sec. and permit elemental analyses for most of the elements, in the 10^{-12} to 10^{-6} g. range, the range of importance for trace element analysis of biological samples.

When a uranium-235 nucleus undergoes fission, an average of 2.5 neutrons are emitted per disintegration. The energy spectrum of the fission neutrons extends up to 20 Mev., with a maximum yield at about 1.5 Mev. The fission neutrons undergo collision with a moderator, such as water, deuterium oxide, beryllium, or graphite, and lose energy in the process. Some of these slowed neutrons are consumed to maintain the chain reaction of the pile; part of the surplus is available for neutron activation analysis. The neutrons most useful for activation analysis are those in thermal equilibrium with the surroundings, i.e., the thermal neutrons. Their energy spectrum approximates a Maxwellian distribution with a maximum at 0.025 e.v. and a high-energy tail extending to about 0.4 e.v. Advantage is sometimes taken of the higher-energy neutrons in the fission spectrum in inducing fast neutron reactions, although more generally these reactions have to be considered as potential interferences in normal thermal neutron activation analyses.

NEUTRON GENERATORS

Cyclotrons, linear accelerators, Van de Graaff generators, Cockcroft-Walton generators, and synchrotrons can also produce neutrons for activation analysis. The various bombarding particles (protons, deuterons, and helium nuclei), target materials and nuclear reactions involved in the production of neutrons are summarized in Table 20-5.

The output of a neutron generator is normally expressed by the number of neutrons per second emitted from the target, whereas in activation analysis, we are interested primarily in the number of neutrons per square centimeter per second at the sample irradiation position. Since the target is essentially a point source that emits neutrons isotropically, the useful flux at the sample is about 100 times less than the total neutron production rate. Typical fluxes available from neutron generators range from 10^5 to 10^9 neutrons/cm.²/sec. The low flux of these machines has been a major limitation. For example, in trace element analyses, typical detection sensitivities for most elements is 1 mg. or higher at fluxes of 10^8 neutrons/cm.²/sec.

In some cases, the neutrons produced by generators are essentially mono-

TABLE 20-5.   ACCELERATOR NEUTRON SOURCES

ACCELERATING PARTICLE	TARGET MATERIAL	NEUTRON PRODUCING REACTION	NEUTRON ENERGY	TYPE OF GENERATOR *
Electrons (>1.7 Mev.)	Gold	(a) $\beta\rightarrow$bremsstrahlung (b) thin $^9Be(\gamma,n)^8Be$	100 kev.	VdG
Protons	Tritium	$T(p,n)^3He$	64 kev.	Cycl
	Lithium	$^7Li(p,n)^7Be$	30 kev.	Cycl
Deuterons	Deuterium	$D(d,n)^3He$	2.4 Mev.	C-W, VdG, Cycl
	Tritium	$T(d,n)^4He$	14 Mev.	C-W, VdG, Cycl
	Carbon	$^{12}C(d,n)^{13}N$	3.4 kev.	Cycl
Helium nuclei	Beryllium	$^9Be(\alpha,n)^{12}C$	5.3 Mev.	Cycl
	Carbon	$^{13}C(\alpha,n)^{16}O$	2.1 Mev.	Cycl

* VdG = Van de Graaff; C-W = Cockcroft-Walton; Cycl = Cyclotron.

TABLE 20-6.   TYPICAL ISOTOPIC SOURCES

RADIONUCLIDE	TARGET MATERIAL	NEUTRON PRODUCING REACTION	APPROXIMATE NEUTRON YIELD (n/sec. curie)
Antimony-124	Beryllium	$^9Be(\gamma,n)^8Be$	2×10^6
Sodium-24	Deuterium	$^2H(\gamma,n)^1H$	4×10^6
Yttrium-88	Beryllium	$^9Be(\gamma,n)^8Be$	2×10^6
Radium-226	Beryllium	$^9Be(\alpha,n)^{12}C$	1×10^7
Radium-226	Boron	$^{11}B(\alpha,n)^{14}N$	5×10^6
Polonium-210	Beryllium	$^9Be(\alpha,n)^{12}C$	3×10^6
Plutonium-239	Beryllium	$^9Be(\alpha,n)^{12}C$	2×10^6
Americium-241	Beryllium	$^9Be(\alpha,n)^{12}C$	2×10^6

energetic and can be used in high-energy neutron activation analysis of elements of low atomic number (6 to 15) without interference from other interactions. At higher atomic numbers, the cross sections for low-energy neutron interactions are about 100 times greater than those for high-energy neutron interactions; consequently, most neutron-generator applications require thermalization of the neutrons for maximum sensitivity.

ISOTOPIC SOURCES

Isotopic sources produce neutrons as a result of the interaction between the radiations from a radioactive isotope and a suitable target material. These reactions occur when the binding energy of one of the neutrons in the nucleus is low, e.g., in some of the low atomic number elements, such as deuterium through fluorine. Isotopic neutron sources fall into two classes: photoneutron sources (neutrons produced by gamma-ray interactions) and alpha-neutron sources (neutrons produced by alpha-particle interactions). Examples of these sources are given in Table 20-6. As in the case of neutrons produced by generators, neutrons emitted from isotopic sources have rather high energies ($>$10 kev.), but, unlike them, they usually have a broad range of energies. Consequently, neutrons from isotopic sources must be thermalized to be useful for activation analyses. The low neutron yield (rarely exceeding 10^6 neutrons/cm.^{2}/sec.) makes isotopic sources impractical for trace element analysis by the neutron activation technique.

RADIONUCLIDE DETECTION METHODS IN ACTIVATION ANALYSIS

MODES OF DECAY

If several different elements are present in the irradiated sample, a number of different radionuclides may be produced. Consequently, it is usually necessary to measure the activity of a particular radionuclide in the presence of the others.

At present, 1095 radioactive nuclides can be artificially produced, and 66 occur naturally. No two of these 1161 radioactive species have the same decay characteristics, i.e., both the same rate of decay and mode of decay.

The most common modes of radioactive decay are by the emission of alpha particles, gamma-rays and by the process of beta decay. Emission of alpha particles is found among the higher atomic weight nuclides whereas beta decay is common throughout the whole periodic table. There are three different processes of beta decay: (1) negatron emission; (2) positron emission; and (3) electron or K capture, in which an orbital electron is incorporated into the nucleus. In all three beta-decay processes, the atomic mass remains essentially constant while the atomic number changes, whereas both the atomic mass and atomic number change in an alpha-decay process. The process of alpha or beta decay often leaves the resultant nucleus in an excited state, which in turn results in the emission of gamma radiation. In some cases, the excited state may persist for periods from fractions of a second to years, before the return to a ground state. This type of decay is called isomeric transition.

An accepted way of symbolizing decay processes is shown in Figure 20-4. By convention, the negatron emission is designated by an arrow pointed downward to the right, indicating a decrease in the energy state of the excited nucleus and the formation of a nucleus of higher atomic number. An arrow pointing down and to the left represents positron decay or an electron-capture process that produces a nucleus of a lower atomic number. A vertical arrow, pointing down, signifies a gamma-ray emission that is the result of an excited nucleus decaying to the ground state of the same isotope.

GAMMA-RAY SCINTILLATION SPECTROMETRY

Gamma-ray scintillation spectrometry is based on the interaction of gamma-rays with a material that responds to the interaction by emitting photons of visible light, whose intensity is directly proportional to the energy of the

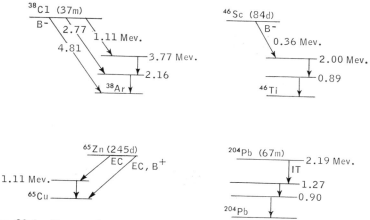

FIGURE 20-4. Decay scheme. IT, Isomeric transition; B⁻, negatron decay; B⁺, positron decay; EC, electron capture.

absorbed gamma ray (Crouthamel, 1960). The process has been described in Chapter V. In essence, a gamma-ray scintillation spectrometer consists of a photomultiplier to detect the light emissions and convert them into electronic pulses, and a differential (multichannel) pulse-height analyzer, which sorts the electronic pulses from the photomultiplier into groups according to their amplitude. The pulse-height analyzer also counts the number of pulses in each amplitude group during a given counting period. The result is a recording of the energy spectral distribution of the gamma-rays emitted by the radionuclides in the sample, that is, a scan of the differential counting rate vs. the energies of the gamma-rays.

The characteristic components of a gamma-ray spectrum are due to the ways gamma-rays interact with matter. In the energy range from a few electron volts to about 5 million, gamma-rays interact with matter primarily in three ways: photoelectric effect, Compton effect, and pair production. In the photoelectric effect, the gamma-ray transfers all its energy to a bound orbital electron, detaching it completely from its atom and giving it kinetic energy almost equal to that of the original gamma-ray. These electrons then lose their energy by ionization and excitation, giving rise to scintillations within the detector. The interactions occur so quickly compared with the response time of the detection apparatus that the output of the photomultiplier is a single electronic pulse whose amplitude represents the sum of all the scintillations caused by a single gamma-ray interaction. This results in a peaked response in the pulse-height spectrum, commonly called the photoelectric peak, that corresponds to the energy of the gamma-ray emitted in the decay of a radionuclide.

In a NaI(Tl) scintillation detector, the photoelectric effect is the primary mode of gamma-ray interaction up to an energy of 300 kev. At higher energies, the Compton effect becomes more important. In the Compton effect, a gamma-ray transfers only part of its energy to an orbital electron, which is ejected from the atom and becomes deexcited in the same manner as the photoelectric electron. The degraded gamma-ray may undergo other interactions or may escape the detector. The loss of the degraded gamma-ray gives rise to a continuum in the recorded gamma-ray spectrum whose maximum energy is less than that of the photopeak.

A gamma-ray that has an energy exceeding 1.02 Mev. may be totally annihilated by the Coulomb field of a nucleus to produce a positron-negatron pair (pair production) with total kinetic energy equal to the energy of the interacting gamma-ray minus 1.02 Mev., the mass energy equivalent of the pair. As in the photoelectric effect and Compton effect, these electrons lose energy by ionization and excitation, giving rise to scintillations in the detector. When the positron is slowed to thermal energies, it then combines (annihilates) with a negatron to produce two 0.51 Mev. gamma-rays, which then may undergo photoelectric or Compton interaction in the detector or may escape the detector. Pair-production interaction gives rise to several characteristic peaks in the recorded gamma-ray spectrum.

A gamma-ray may lose all its energy within the detector by a single photoelectric event or by combination of all three primary interactions. These interactions occur essentially simultaneously and can result in a detector response equal to that obtained from a photoelectric effect. Thus, the multiple interaction cannot be distinguished from a photoelectric interaction and gives the desired result of increasing the number of pulses having photopeak amplitudes.

Beta-Ray Gas Detectors

The beta-ray detectors used in activation analyses are usually gas-filled or gas-flow proportional counters or Geiger counters. The basic design consists of two electrodes and a gas that undergoes ionization when an interaction with radiation occurs. When the electrodes are separated by a potential difference, the ionized particles and electrons are attracted to the electrodes of opposite polarity. Once the ions in the gas are neutralized by the electrodes, the current flow ceases until another ionizing event occurs. If the voltage potential across the electrodes is small, as in an *ionization chamber,* the radiation produces only primary ionization, and the output pulse is proportional to the energy of the beta-ray. The voltage of the electrodes can be increased to an extent that the primary ions are accelerated and produce secondary ionization which remains proportional to the radiation energy. This type of counter is called a *proportional counter.* If the voltage is raised even higher, a point will be reached at which one primary ion will produce secondary ionization throughout the tube. The resultant output pulse is of constant amplitude independent of the energy of the ionizing radiation. When this occurs, the detector is called a *Geiger counter.*

A summary of the characteristics of gas-filled beta-particle detectors is given in Table 20-7. A Geiger counter has the advantage of requiring less amplification of the detector signal in order to trigger a counting device. On the other hand, the proportional counter can count higher activity samples with little or no correction needed for the dead time of the detector and can distinguish between beta-rays of different energies.

Solid-State Detectors

A solid-state radiation detector is an ionization chamber in which the gas has been replaced with a semiconducting solid (Dearnaley and Northrop, 1963). This type of detector has had limited use in activation analyses because the detection efficiency is several orders of magnitude lower than that of the NaI(Tl) scintillation detectors, resulting in a diminished sensitivity for the analysis.

TABLE 20-7. CHARACTERISTICS OF GAS-FILLED DETECTORS

DETECTOR	DETECTOR MULTIPLICATION	OUTPUT SIGNAL (volts)	RESOLVING TIME (seconds)
Ionization chamber	1	10^{-6}–10^{-3}	10^{-6}
Proportional counter	10^2–10^4	10^{-4}–1	10^{-6}
Geiger counter	10^7	0.1–10	10^{-4}–10^{-3}

TABLE 20-8. CONCENTRATIONS OF ELEMENTS IN BIOLOGICAL SUBSTANCES

PPM*	BLOOD	URINE	TISSUE
>1000	Cl, K, Na	Cl, K, Na, P, S	Cl, K, Na, P, S
> 100	Fe, P, S	Ca, Mg	Ca, Mg
> 10	Mg, Ca		Fe, Zn
> 1	Br, Cu, Rb, Si, Zn	Br, Rb	Br, Cu, Rb
< 1		All other elements	

* Parts per million.

However, semiconductor devices have much higher resolving power than the NaI(Tl) detectors, and can be used advantageously when the energies cannot be resolved by gamma-ray scintillation spectrometry.

MAJOR PROBLEMS IN THE ANALYSIS OF THE TRACE ELEMENT CONTENT OF BIOLOGICAL TISSUES

Biological substances are composed chiefly of hydrogen, nitrogen, oxygen, and carbon. None of these elements is readily activated by thermal neutrons and, consequently, they do not interfere with the assay of trace elements. Only about a dozen other elements (Table 20-8) are present in concentrations that exceed 1 ppm. The other elements are normally present in concentrations of less than 1 ppm. Because of the extremely low concentrations of most elements, there are two major problems in the assay of elements in biological tissues and fluids: activation of other trace elemental constituents and contamination. The radioactivity produced by the activation of the other elements often masks that produced by the trace element of interest. Therefore the analyst must isolate chemically the element of interest.

A more serious problem is contamination. With biological tissues and fluids, the problem is greater than with inert matrices, since an inert sample is often much larger and can be cleaned. When dealing with biological samples, especially from man, we must be concerned with: the antiseptic used for topical cleansing, the method used to sterilize sampling equipment, the sample storage vessels, and equipment and reagents used to prepare the sample for analysis (Table 20-9).

As illustrated in Table 20-9, one of the best ways to reduce possible contamination is to avoid contact with metal. Whenever possible, we use dust-free plastic ware cleaned with nitric acid, deionized water, and ethyl alcohol. Stainless steel can also be used, but knives and scissors, although labeled stainless steel, are often plated with zinc, nickel, or chromium. It is helpful to use plastic, aluminum, or platinum needles. Usually it is not the stainless steel needle that contaminates samples but the hubs or shanks, which are constructed of brass plated with nickel or chromium.

Two major sources of contamination are the autoclave and the drying oven. The autoclave may contaminate instruments with trace amounts of metals from the soldered joints in the autoclave and from the water used to produce the steam. All sampling tools should be sterilized with ethylene oxide and stored in plastic wrappers. Drying ovens are notorious for coating samples with a film of

TABLE 20-9. MAJOR SOURCES OF ELEMENTAL CONTAMINATION OF BIOLOGICAL SAMPLES

SOURCES OF CONTAMINATION	OBSERVED ELEMENTAL CONTAMINATION	BEST CHOICE(s) *
Antiseptic	I, Hg, Mn, As	Ethyl alcohol
Metal needles with hubs	Ni, Cr, Zn, Mn, Cu, Cd, Ag	Platinum; stainless steel needles without hubs
Metal syringes	Ni, Cr, Zn, Mn, Cu, Fe	Plastic
Metal storage vessels	Many!	Plastic
Metal-plated knives and scissors	Zn, Ni, Cr	Plastic; stainless steel
Autoclave	Pb, Ag, Cd, As, Cu, Mn	Sterilization by ethylene oxide
Drying ovens	Many!	Infrared lamp
Reagents	Many!	None

* In order of decreasing preference.

"dust" that is vaporized from the heating elements and insulation. All samples should be dried in a properly closed system with either vacuum or infrared lamps.

Other major sources of contamination are reagents used in the analysis. Since all reagents contain trace amounts of many elements that are virtually impossible to remove, this source of contamination has been termed *reagent blank* —a necessary evil in virtually all microelemental analytical methods *except* neutron activation analysis. Since no reagents come in contact with the sample until after it has been activated, they cannot contaminate an activated sample with radioactivity.

BIOMEDICAL APPLICATIONS

It is clear that trace elements play an important role in human physiology. Underwood (1962) has reviewed the role of some 20 trace elements from the point of view of human and animal nutrition. Deficiency diseases can be caused by a lack of essential trace elements, and high dietary concentrations can be toxic. The role of trace elements in biology has been discussed in monographs by Comar and Bronner (1964) and by Schütte (1964).

Detailed studies of trace elements in normal human tissue from widely diverse geographic origins have been carried out by Tipton and co-workers (1965), and Schroeder and Balassa (1966) have examined the role of certain abnormal trace elements in man.

Investigations have been limited by the analytical methods used, which have included emission spectroscopy, flame spectrophotometry, and atomic absorption. Neutron activation analysis, because of its exceptionally high detection sensitivity for many elements (Table 20-10), has helped to extend knowledge of the metabolic behavior of trace elements in the human body.

Table 20-10 indicates the potential value of neutron activation analysis. In general, the observed concentrations are above the limit of sensitivity. As stated, these are not the ultimate limits of sensitivity, but have been determined under specific experimental conditions. In most cases, the listed sensitivities could be improved upon by several orders of magnitude.

TABLE 20-10. NEUTRON ACTIVATION ANALYSIS OF TISSUE

ELEMENT DETERMINED	CONCENTRATIONS OBSERVED (ppm)	LIMIT OF SENSITIVITY (ppm)
Antimony	0.01 –10	0.005
Arsenic	0.005–1	0.001
Bromine	1–10	0.001
Cadmium	1–5	0.01
Cesium	1–10	0.05
Cobalt	0.1 –1	0.05
Copper	0.1 –700	0.01
Gold	0.01 –1	0.002
Iodine	1–10	0.05
Molybdenum	0.2 –2	0.2
Nickel	0.5 –2	0.1
Potassium	100–1000	0.02
Rubidium	10–100	0.1
Selenium	0.001–10	0.001
Silver	0.1 –1	0.1
Strontium	1–300	0.5
Tellurium	10–100	0.2
Vanadium	0.001-0.5	0.001
Zinc	1–1000	0.02
Zirconium	1–10	0.2

A few specific examples will be outlined to illustrate the principles of the technique; other examples are given by Comar (1966), Lenihan (1965a, b), Loveridge and Smales (1957), and Smith (1964).

THYROID UPTAKE OF IODIDE

One of the early applications of neutron activation analysis to a biomedical problem was the determination of the stable iodide uptake of the thyroid by Wagner and co-workers (1961). The usual radioactive iodine thyroid uptake test does not give a quantitative measure of the stable inorganic iodide being accumulated by the gland; occasionally a high radioiodine uptake can be attributed to a small extrathyroidal iodide pool.

In these studies, carrier-free tracer doses of iodine-131 or iodine-132 were administered by either oral or intravenous routes to fasting patients, and the thyroid uptake was measured after 2 hours. After the thyroid measurements, a urine specimen was obtained and both the radioactive and stable iodine contents were measured. The determination of stable iodide was carried out by a neutron activation technique that included absorbing urinary iodine on an anionic exchange resin that allowed sodium and other cations to pass. The chloride on the resin column was then preferentially eluted with ammonium thiocyanate solution. The fractional amount of iodine absorbed on the resin was easily determined in each sample from direct radiometric measurements of the ^{131}I or [132]I already in the urine from the administered radioiodine dose. After the radioiodine had decayed sufficiently, the resin columns were activated at a thermal neutron flux of 2×10^8 neutrons/cm.^{2}/sec. After activation, the iodine in the sample was determined by measuring the induced [128]I activity by gamma-ray scintillation spectrometry. From the radioiodine uptake and the ratio of radio-active to stable iodine in the urine, the uptake of stable iodide by the thyroid was readily calculable.

CYSTIC FIBROSIS

Patients with cystic fibrosis were found to have higher sodium contents in their sweat, hair, and nails than normal controls in studies by Kopito and Shwachman and their co-workers (1964, 1965). Using neutron activation analysis, Babb et al. (1966) at the University of Washington confirmed the observation of Kopito et al. that nail analysis is a reliable diagnostic tool for cystic fibrosis. In these studies, nail clippings from the fingers and toes of 35 cystic fibrosis patients and from 27 healthy children, all under 17 years of age, were irradiated in a thermal neutron flux of 10^{11} neutrons/cm.^{2}/sec. These samples and standards were analyzed for sodium-24, the analytical indicator for sodium, with a 3 in. by 3 in. NaI(Tl) detector to determine the 2.75 Mev. gamma-ray photopeak area. By this method, the sodium content of these samples was determined rapidly by purely instrumental means. On the basis of their results, total sodium values less than 55 mEq./kg. nails indicate the absence of cystic fibrosis, whereas values higher than 85 mEq./kg. nails indicate cystic fibrosis on the basis of clinical evaluation.

Although this test will probably not replace the usual sweat test, it does have value because smaller samples are required for neutron activation analysis than for conventional chemical methods; patients in remote locations who cannot obtain a reliable sweat test can send nail clippings for a neutron activation analysis determination; and the procedure may be used as a supporting or confirmatory test. Further, this test is amenable to mass screening.

In vivo STABLE ISOTOPIC TRACER STUDIES

These studies comprise a whole new area of biological tracer studies. In some cases, *radioactive* tracers cannot be used for diagnostic studies of body functions, such as in newborn infants or pregnant women, or when suitable radioactive isotopes are not available. The use of a highly enriched sample of an isotope of low natural abundance as a biological tracer differs from the use of a radioactive isotopic tracer mainly in its mode of detection: the radioactive isotope tracer can be detected *in vivo* by external radiation detectors if the emitted radiations are sufficiently energetic to penetrate tissue; the stable tracer is detected in a sample (e.g., urine or serum) that has been removed from the patient.

Since neutron activation is essentially an isotopic method of analysis, i.e., the bombarding neutrons interact with the isotopes of an element to give rise to a unique product for each isotope, it is the analytical method of choice in tracer studies involving enriched stable isotopes. This field has been reviewed by Wahl and co-workers (1965). The method involves administration of the stable tracer (orally or by injection) with the analysis of samples of plasma or urine by neutron activation analysis.

One of the early studies was the determination of plasma iron clearance by Lowman and Krivit (1962, 1963). In their *in vivo* studies, the ^{58}Fe tracer added approximately 0.05 μg. of ^{58}Fe to each milliliter of circulating plasma, which is about 10 to 20 times the concentration of this isotope normally present in the circulating plasma. The total stable iron concentration, however, was increased by only a few per cent. Radioactive ^{59}Fe was administered simultaneously as ferrous citrate in a dose of 5 μc. Blood samples were obtained before the iron injection and 10, 30, 60, 90, 120, and 180 minutes later. The samples were centrifuged and 2 ml. aliquots of plasma were pipeted into counting vials. Plasma-clearance curves of the ^{59}Fe were obtained from the measured counting rates.

One milliliter aliquots of plasma samples were activated by thermal neutrons, and the ^{58}Fe was quantified by measurement of the 1.28 Mev. gamma-ray photopeak of ^{59}Fe, which was produced by the (n,γ) reaction of ^{58}Fe. The ^{59}Fe count rate in the activated preinjection samples was subtracted from each of the postinjection samples. This blank correction was necessary because of the small amount of naturally occurring ^{58}Fe. Interference from simultaneously injected ^{59}Fe was shown to be negligible by counts of 1 ml. aliquots of the original serum samples made before irradiation.

The iron plasma clearance curves were nearly identical for both tracers, stable ^{58}Fe and radioactive ^{59}Fe. These results confirm that ^{58}Fe is cleared and handled by the body in the same manner as ^{59}Fe, and that the stable-tracer technique can be used for plasma iron clearance studies. In such cases when the concentration of the element being studied is relatively constant, it is not necessary to measure the total element concentration to correct for the natural abundance of the tracer.

Since activation analysis has extremely high detection sensitivity for many elements, the stable tracer technique can be used to study many elements of biological interest. Elements presently being studied by the use of enriched isotopic tracers include calcium, strontium, chromium, and selenium in addition to iron. As many as 40 elements may be amenable to similar studies.

Many of the 20 monoisotopic elements may be useful as biological tracers, especially when they are normally present in the body at very low concentrations. The stable tracer can be given in amounts that do not upset homeostatic equilibrium. One such application is the use of stable colloidal ^{197}Au to measure liver blood flow (Yasukochi and Watanabe, 1965; Yasukochi, 1966).

OTHER STUDIES

Biological tissues and fluids have been analyzed for specific trace elements by the activation technique in attempts to elucidate their role in normal and abnormal states. In some studies, the concentrations of a number of elements have been observed to be significantly different from normal in persons with certain diseases. Some typical examples are given in Table 20-11. The medical significance of these observations, if any, is not yet understood.

In conclusion, the neutron activation technique has been used in biomedical studies: (1) to measure the normal elemental content of biological tissues and fluids; (2) to determine whether the trace elemental contents are altered in diseases of unknown etiology, in metabolic diseases, or after industrial exposures; and (3) to measure metabolic functions with stable isotopic tracers. It is likely that its use will increase as the field of nuclear medicine grows.

TABLE 20-11. CONCENTRATIONS OF ELEMENTS IN BIOLOGICAL SUBSTANCES IN VARIOUS DISEASES

CONDITION	MATRIX ANALYZED	ELEMENT*	REFERENCE
Myocardial infarction	Serum	Mn ↑	Kanabrocki et al., 1964
	Urine	Mn ↑, Cu ↑	Kanabrocki, 1965
	Tissue	As ↑, Mo ↓, Cu ↓, Ce ↑	Wester, 1965
Uremia	Blood	As ↑, Mo ↑	Brune et al., 1966
Chronic myelogenous leukemia	Leukocytes	Cu ↓, Mn ↓	Frischauf, 1963
Rheumatoid arthritis	Blood	Cu ↑	Plantin and Strandberg, 1965
Cancer	Tissues	↓ (many)	Samsahl and Brune, 1965
Muscular dystrophy	Skeletal muscle	K ↓, Na ↑	Williams et al., 1957
Melanoma	Tissue	Se ↑, Sc ↑, Cu ↑	Kramer and Wahl, unpublished
Wilson's disease	Serum	Cu ↓	Fell, 1965
Hyperphagia and obesity	Tissue	Au ↑	Debons et al., 1960
Fatty cirrhosis	Tissue	Mn ↓	Barak and Beckenhauer, 1966

* Arrows pointing up indicate an elevated concentration; arrows pointing down, a decreased concentration.

REFERENCES

Applications of Computers to Nuclear and Radiochemistry. NAS–NS–3107. Office of Technical Services, Department of Commerce, Washington, D.C., 1962.

Babb, A. L., et al.: The Use of Neutron Activation Analysis in the Early Diagnosis of Cystic Fibrosis in Children. Trans. Amer. Nuc. Soc. 9:591, 1966.

Barak, A. J., and Beckenhauer, H. C.: Liver and Serum Manganese, Magnesium and Zinc in Fatty Cirrhosis. J. Nucl. Med. 7:358, 1966.

Brune, D., Samsahl, K., and Wester, P. O.: A Comparison Between the Amount of As, Au, Br, Cu, Fe, Mo, Se, and Zn in Normal and Uraemic Human Whole Blood by Means of Neutron Activation Analysis. Clin. Chim. Acta 13:285, 1966.

Comar, C. L., and Bronner, F.: Mineral Metabolism. Academic Press, New York, 1964.

Comar, D.: Activation Analysis as a Tool for Medical Research. Nucleonics 24:54, 1966.

Crouthamel, C. E.: Applied Gamma-Ray Spectrometry. Pergamon Press, New York, 1960.

Dearnaley, G., and Northrop, D. C.: Semiconductor Counters for Nuclear Radiations. John Wiley and Sons, New York, 1963.

Debons, A. F., et al.: Localization of Hypothalamic Centers Regulating Appetite. Physiologist 3:48, 1960.

Fell, G. S.: Wilson's Disease: Comparison of Copper Levels by Neutron Activation and Chemical Methods. Proc. Ass. Clin. Biochem. 3:287, 1965.

Frischauf, H.: Studies on the Content of Trace Elements in Leukocytes with Neutron Activation Analysis. Folia Haemat. (Frankfurt) 7:291, 1963.

Hughes, D. J.: Pile Neutron Research. Addison-Wesley Publishing Co., Reading, Mass., 1953.

Hughes, D. J., and Harvey, J. A.: Neutron Cross Sections. USAEC Report, BNL 325, 1958 (and Supplements 1 and 2, 1960, 1964).

Kanabrocki, E. L.: Manganese and Copper Levels in Human Urine. J. Nucl. Med. 6:780, 1965.

Kanabrocki, E. L., et al.: Neutron Activation Studies of Biological Fluids: Manganese and Copper. Int. J. Appl. Radiat. 15:175, 1964.

Kopito, L., et al.: Studies in Cystic Fibrosis—Analysis of Nail Clippings for Sodium and Potassium. New Eng. J. Med. 272:504, 1965.

Kopito, L., and Shwachman, H.: Spectroscopic Analysis of Tissues from Patients with Cystic Fibrosis and Controls. Nature 202:501, 1964.

Kramer, H. H., and Wahl, W. H.: Unpublished Data.

Lenihan, J. M. A.: Trace Elements in Biomedical Research. Nucleonics 23:50, 1965a.

Lenihan, J. M. A.: Activation Analysis in Clinical Science. In Lenihan, J. M. A., and Thomson,

S. J.: Activation Analysis—Principles and Applications. Academic Press, New York, 1965b, pp. 119–124.

Loveridge, B. A., and Smales, A. A.: Activation Analysis and Its Application in Biochemistry. *Meth. Biochem. Anal.* 5:225, 1957.

Lowman, J. T., and Krivit, W.: Activation Analysis: A New Stable Isotope Method for Tracer Studies. *Univ. Minn. Med. Bull.* 33:203, 1962.

Lowman, J. T., and Krivit, W.: New In Vivo Tracer Method with the Use of Nonradioactive Isotopes and Activation Analysis. *J. Lab. Clin. Med.* 61:1042, 1963.

Plantin, L. O., and Strandberg, P. O.: Whole Blood Concentrations of Copper and Zinc in Rheumatoid Arthritis Studied by Activation Analysis. *Acta Rheum. Scand.* 11:30, 1965.

Rubinson, W.: The Equations of Radioactive Transformation in a Neutron Flux. *J. Chem. Phys.* 17:542, 1949.

Samsahl, K., and Brune, D.: Simultaneous Determination of 30 Trace Elements in Cancerous and Non-Cancerous Human Tissue Samples by Neutron Activation Analysis. *Int. J. Appl. Radiat.* 16:273, 1965.

Schroeder, H. A., and Balassa, J. J.: Abnormal Trace Metals in Man: Arsenic. *J. Chronic Dis.* 19:85, 1966.

Schütte, K. H.: The Biology of the Trace Element. J. B. Lippincott Co., Philadelphia, 1964.

Smith, H.: Biological Applications of Activation Analysis. *In* Curry, A. S.: Methods of Forensic Science. Vol. 3. Interscience Publishers, New York, 1964, pp. 70–111.

Subcommittee on Radiochemistry, National Academy of Sciences, National Research Council, Office of Technical Services, Department of Commerce. NAS–NS–3000 Series. Washington, D. C., 1960.

Taylor, T. I., and Havens, W. W., Jr.: Neutron Spectroscopy and Neutron Interactions in Chemical Analysis. *In* Berl, W. G. (ed.): Physical Methods in Chemical Analysis. Vol. 3. Academic Press, New York, 1956.

Tipton, I. H., et al.: Trace Elements in Human Tissue. *Health Phys.* 11:403, 1965.

Underwood, E. J.: Trace Elements in Human and Animal Nutrition. Academic Press, New York, 1962.

Wagner, H. N., Jr., Nelp, W. B., and Dowling, J. H.: Use of Neutron Activation Analysis for Studying Stable Iodine Uptake by the Thyroid. *J. Clin. Invest.* 40:1984, 1961.

Wahl, W. H., Nass, H. W., and Kramer, H. H.: Use of Stable Isotopes and Activation Analysis for In Vivo Diagnostic Studies. *In* Radioactive Pharmaceuticals. CONF-651111, U.S. Department of Commerce, Washington, D.C., 1965, pp. 191–204.

Wester, P. O.: Trace Elements in Human Myocardial Infarction Determined by Neutron Activation Analysis. *Acta Med. Scand.* 178:765, 1965.

Williams, J. D., et al.: Electrolyte Levels in Normal and Dystrophic Muscle Determined by Neutron Activation. *Lancet* 1:464, 1957.

Yasukochi, H.: Liver Flow Index Determined by Activation Analysis. *J. Nucl. Med.* 7:357, 1966.

Yasukochi, H., and Watanabe, N.: Some Applications of the Activation Analysis to Medicine. *Nippon Acta Radiol.* 25:137, 1965.

GENERAL REFERENCES

Bowen, H. J. M., and Gibbons, D.: Radioactivation Analysis. Oxford University Press, London, 1963.

Crouthamel, C. E.: Applied Gamma-Ray Spectrometry. Pergamon Press, New York, 1960.

Friedlander, G., Kennedy, J. W., and Miller, J. M.: Nuclear and Radiochemistry. John Wiley and Sons, New York, 1964.

Koch, R. C.: Activation Analysis Handbook. Academic Press, New York, 1960.

Lenihan, J. M. A., and Thomson, S. J.: Activation Analysis. Academic Press, New York, 1965.

Lyon, W. S., Jr.: Guide to Activation Analysis. D. Van Nostrand Company, Princeton, 1964.

Proceedings of the International Conference on Modern Trends in Activation Analysis. Texas A&M University, College Station, Texas, 1961, 1965.

Taylor, D.: Neutron Irradiation and Activation Analysis. George Newnes Ltd., London, 1964.

Taylor, T. I., and Havens, W. W., Jr.: *In* Berl, W. G. (ed.): Physical Methods in Chemical Analysis. Vol. 3. Academic Press, New York, 1956.

CHAPTER XXI

TECHNICAL DETAILS OF
COMMON PROCEDURES

HENRY N. WAGNER, Jr.

INTRODUCTION

In this chapter some of the step-by-step procedures of various tests are outlined. We hope that the information will be particularly useful to technicians and others responsible for performing the procedures. Certain general principles will be considered first.

CONTAMINATION

Contamination of samples and equipment with radioactivity must be scrupulously avoided. A contaminated test tube, syringe, or pipette can make a whole study worthless or, even worse, yield misleading results. Disposable test tubes, syringes, and needles should be used whenever possible. Separate glassware should be used for each radionuclide and it should be washed separately. Immediately after use, the glassware should be placed in water containing detergent. Pipettes should be washed continuously overnight in commercially available pipette washers. If washing fails to remove all activity, it is often helpful to soak the glassware in a solution of the stable substance. Glassware used for short-lived isotopes can be further decontaminated after washing by storage for five or more half-lives of the nuclide.

The outside as well as the inside of tubes used for counting must be clean, since radioactivity of both is often measured in a well-counter. Inexpensive disposable plastic gloves minimize contamination. Steel or plastic trays covered with absorbent paper should be used to confine possible spillage to a small area. The crystal of a well-counter should be lined with plastic sheets that can be changed if a spill occurs.

STANDARDS

In many tests, an unknown sample is compared to a standard which contains a known fraction of the injected radioactive substance. The standard is usually prepared at the same time as the dose to be injected, using a calibrated syringe or even the same syringe used for the dose. Suitable dilutions of the dose are made, depending on the sensitivity of the radiation detection system. In counting the standard and unknown, it is important to compare the same volume of both under exactly the same geometric and other conditions affecting counting efficiency. Usually the sample and standard are counted in the same counter, one after the other. This avoids the necessity of correction for physical decay, as for example in long-term studies. Red blood cells should be hemolyzed by freezing and thawing or by exposure to saponin; this prevents settling of the red cells to the bottom of the tubes, which affects the conditions of counting.

RADIATION PROTECTION

The reader is referred to Chapter XVIII, entitled Principles of Radiation Safety, for guidance in this area. High levels of activity should be kept behind lead shielding. A lead-lined refrigerator is useful for storage of radiopharmaceuticals. In working with volatile substances a hood with suitable flow rates of air should be used.

THYROID STUDIES

PREPARATION OF STANDARD SOLUTIONS OF ^{131}I

A nonsterile stock solution of sodium iodide (^{131}I), for use in several different studies of the thyroid, is prepared once a week at a concentration of 1 μc. per milliliter on the day of preparation. In preparing doses of ^{131}I for oral administration, the required volume of the stock solution is pipetted into a waxed paper or plastic cup which contains several ounces of tap water. Before drinking, the patient is warned not to spill the contents or wet the upper lip, and he is asked to drink two subsequent rinsings of the cup.

In measurements of thyroid uptake, the standard is measured in a "phantom" constructed to simulate the neck in the region of the thyroid. We follow the standardized procedure of Brucer and use a Lucite cylinder which contains receptacles for 5 ml. test tubes. Two and a half milliliters of stock solution is pipetted into each of two disposable test tubes. These tubes are then filled with water, closed with stoppers, and placed in the appropriate positions in the phantom.

Thyroid uptake

Gamma radiation from the neck in the thyroid region is measured 2 and 24 hours after oral administration of 5 ml. of stock solution containing 5 μc. of radioiodine; the data are corrected for extrathyroidial radioactivity with a lead filter as will be described. The results obtained in the patient are compared with a thyroid phantom containing an amount of radioactivity equal to the dose, and the uptake is expressed as a percentage of the administered dose.

The patient omits breakfast on the morning of the test and eats nothing for 2 hours after drinking the dose. He is asked to return for uptake measurements at 2 and 24 hours after administration of the dose. The percentage uptake is measured as follows: the patient is placed on the examining couch in the recumbent position with slight hyperextension of the neck. Radioactivity is measured in the region of the thyroid with and without a 4 by 4 by 1-in. thick lead filter between the detector and the thyroid gland. This lead filter should be placed as close to the surface of the neck as possible, since its purpose is to eliminate thyroidal activity and permit measurement of extrathyroidal radioactivity. The phantom containing the standard is then counted at the same distance with and without the lead filter. The distance between the crystal face of the detector and the anterior surface of the neck or phantom is 25 cm. Patients who have previously received radioactive materials must have measurements before the dose of ^{131}I is given. Background counts, which may include activity resulting from previous administration of radiopharmaceuticals, are subtracted in calculating the accumulation of the ^{131}I dose.

The uptake is expressed as a percentage of the administered dose according to the formula:

$$\% \text{ uptake} = \frac{\text{Gross counts/min. patient's neck minus gross counts/min. patient's neck with lead filter}}{\text{Gross counts/min. standard minus gross counts/min. standard with lead filter}} \times 100$$

Normal values for the percentage uptake are: 2 hours, 5 to 12 per cent; 6 hours, 8 to 25 per cent; and 24 hours, 15 to 40 per cent. An uptake value is obtained at 6 hours only if the 2 hour uptake is greater than 12 per cent.

Many medications interfere with the uptake of iodine by the thyroid; therefore it is advisable to ask the patient about previous radiosotope studies, radiographic studies such as those of the kidneys or gallbladder, thyroid medications, iodine-containing medication such as Lugol's solution, potassium iodide, cough medicine, antithyroid drugs such as thiocyanate, perchlorate, cortisone, ACTH, estrogens, and other drugs.

Thyroid uptake and scan

This procedure differs from the procedure previously described in that the patient is given a 25 ml. dose of stock solution containing 25 μc. of ^{131}I sodium iodide. Preparation of the stock solution and dose as well as uptake measurements are identical to the usual thyroid uptake procedure. If a 5 μc. ^{131}I standard is used when a 25 μc. dose is given, a correction is made by multiplying the background-corrected count rate of the standard by 5.

Thyroid suppression test

This test is useful when the results of the uptake test are at the boundary between the normal and hyperthyroid categories. A 25 μg. dose of l-triiodothyronine is given orally three times a day for 8 days. After the residual radio-activity in the thyroid is counted, another dose of ^{131}I is administered and the rate of accumulation is measured in the usual fashion. In hyperthyroidism, uptake values fail to show as much depression as in normal persons, who usually have a decrease to less than 50 per cent of the control value.

THYROID STIMULATION TEST

This test is performed when the initial uptake value is abnormally low, suggesting hypothyroidism. Thyrotropin (Thyrotropar, Armour Laboratories) is available in a vial containing 10 U.S.P. units of lyophilized hormone, to which is added 21 ml. of sterile sodium chloride solution. Ten units of TSH (thyroid-stimulating hormone) is given intramuscularly the evening before and the morning of the test. The residual radioactivity in the thyroid gland is counted before the ^{131}I dose is given. A double dose (10 ml.) of ^{131}I is given from the stock solution, and measurements are performed 2 and 24 hours later.

In hypothyroidism secondary to hypopituitarism, or when the thyroid is suppressed by exogenous thyroid medication, the percentage uptake is increased by the administration of TSH, usually by at least 20 per cent of the administered dose. In primary hypothyroidism, after radioiodine therapy, or in thyroiditis, TSH usually fails to increase radioiodine uptake.

Thyroid-stimulating hormone begins to be effective about 8 hours after injection. There are usually no serious side effects with TSH, but occasional transient inflammatory reactions at the site of injection and generalized urticaria may occur and require antihistamine drugs. Some clinicians give 5 to 10 units of TSH on each of 3 successive days to insure maximum response and give the radioiodine 24 hours after the last dose of TSH.

THYROID UPTAKE AND URINARY EXCRETION

This examination is useful in patients with thyroid carcinoma, particularly after total thyroidectomy and radioiodine therapy. After an overnight fast, an oral dose of 50 ml. of stock solution of ^{131}I sodium iodide is given. The total urinary output is collected for 48 hours in two large plastic containers, one for each 24 hour period. The patient is instructed to collect carefully all urine specimens and to avoid losing urine during defecation. The radioiodine uptake over the region of the thyroid is measured at 48 hours.

The total urinary volume for each 24 hour period and the radioactivity in 2.0 ml. aliquots of urine from each specimen is measured together with a 2 ml. standard from the ^{131}I stock solution, diluted to a suitable volume for counting. The urinary excretion is expressed as a percentage of the administered dose.

The urinary excretion over the 2 day period and the percentage uptake by the thyroid are added. The sum is subtracted from 100 per cent to determine the amount of ^{131}I retained in other sites. If less than 90 per cent is excreted over the 2 day period, the presence of functioning thyroidal tissue within the body is suspected. Search for the site of the tissue can be made by scanning.

PROTEIN-BOUND ^{131}I

This test is an index of the rate of incorporation of iodide into hormonal iodine, which, in hyperthyroidism, occurs at a rapid rate. Forty-eight hours after an oral dose of radioiodine the amount of protein-bound radioactivity per liter of plasma is measured and expressed as a percentage of the administered dose. The tracer dose is administered in the form of 15 ml. of the stock solution of ^{131}I sodium iodide. Twenty-five milliliters is given if a scan is to be done. A standard is made from the ^{131}I stock solution, and 5 ml. aliquots are pipetted into two test tubes. Forty-eight hours after administration of the dose a blood sample is withdrawn into a heparinized syringe (12 ml. of blood is usually needed to provide 5 ml. of plasma). The blood should be centrifuged gently to avoid hemolysis; precisely 5.0 ml. of plasma is removed. Plasma ^{131}I is calculated. In hyperthyroid patients, more than 0.20 per cent of the dose per liter of plasma will usually be found after 48 hours.

If the value for total plasma radioiodine is less than 0.20 per cent, the procedure is terminated without further determinations. If the result is greater than 0.20 per cent, 5 ml. plasma samples are passed through resin columns (Amberlite IRA-400 in chloride form) to remove any unbound ^{131}I, i.e., in the form of iodide. The resin columns are placed over empty test tubes marked at a level of 10 ml. The 5 ml. plasma samples are passed through the resin beds. Precisely ½ minute later, 5 ml. of distilled water is pipetted into the empty test tube that contained the plasma and this washing is poured onto the same column. After 1 minute, the receptacle test tube will contain nearly 10 ml. Water is added to the 10 ml. mark and mixed well. The volume of the sample and the standard should both equal 10 ml. before measurement of radioactivity.

An alternate method is to precipitate the protein from plasma using trichloroacetic acid (TCA) instead of the resin. To a known volume of plasma, 1½ volumes of 20 percent TCA is added. The supernatant is removed after centrifugation and counted along with a standard. The result is expressed as percentage of administered radioactivity per liter of plasma.

Triiodothyronine (T3) resin test

A measured amount of ^{131}I or ^{125}I T3 is incubated with plasma. Radioactive T3 not bound by plasma proteins is absorbed by means of an anion exchange resin. Ten milliliters of venous blood is withdrawn into a syringe and transferred to a test tube. Two plasma aliquots of 1 ml. each are pipetted into two special test tubes; radioactive T3 is added by means of a syringe. The time is noted and a resin sponge is added to the plasma mixture. Air is expressed from the sponge with a plastic plunger. The plunger is washed with running tap water before it is used from one tube to the next. The sponges are added serially to all tubes at 1 minute intervals in order to keep the time of incubation exactly 60 minutes for each tube. The radioactivity in each tube is measured and recorded as "total activity."

Sixty minutes after the addition of the resin sponges, the plasma is aspirated and 5 ml. of tap water is added to each tube containing a sponge; the sponges are squeezed with the plunger several times and the water is aspirated. This step is repeated three times, the entire procedure being performed within 1 minute. The time of incubation with the sponge before the first washing of the sponge (60 minutes) and the room temperature (20 ± 3° C.) must be controlled.

In order to check the temperature of the incubation tubes, 5 ml. of water is added to an extra tube at the beginning of the procedure; a thermometer is inserted and checked for significant deviation from room temperature (20° C. or 68° F.). Deviations greater than $\pm$ 3° C. are excessive. The [131]I T3 solution is stored in a refrigerator at 4° C. and must be allowed to come to room temperature before use.

The following data are recorded: background radioactivity in the duplicate samples, the average value of uptake of the particular lot of resin sponges determined by the manufacturers, and the duration of incubation.

The radioactivity bound by the sponge is expressed as a percentage of the total incubated dose of [131]I T3, according to the formula:

$$\% \text{ radioactivity bound} = \frac{\text{Counts/min. in sponge after washing}}{\text{Total counts/min. before washing}} \times 100$$

Hyperthyroid range: above 35 per cent
Nonhyperthyroid range: below 35 per cent

THYROIDAL CLEARANCE OF PLASMA [131]I

A sterile stock solution of [131]I (iodide) is prepared by adding 30 μc. of ^{131}I to a sterile, rubber-capped vial containing 30 ml. of isotonic saline. With a sterile syringe, approximately 15 ml. of stock solution is removed from the vial for preparation of standards. Exactly 10 ml. of the sterile stock solution is measured in a 10 ml. syringe and injected intravenously into the patient. The exact time of the injection is noted and thyroid uptake is measured either continuously or at $\frac{1}{2}$ and 1 hour intervals following injection; counting is done with and without a lead filter covering the thyroid gland.

Forty-five minutes after the injection, 5 ml. of blood is withdrawn. The specimen is centrifuged at 2000 rpm for 5 minutes. Two milliliters of plasma is pipetted into a test tube for counting.

$$\text{Thyroidal clearance of } [131]I = \frac{\% \text{ dose in thyroid at 1 hour } - \% \text{ dose in thyroid at } \frac{1}{2} \text{ hour}}{\% \text{ dose/ml. plasma at } \frac{3}{4} \text{ hour} \times 30 \text{ min.}}$$
(ml. plasma/min.)

Normal values: mean—16 ml./min.; range—8–38 ml./min.

This procedure is used chiefly to detect increased thyroid function in patients who have been treated for hyperthyroidism or in patients with severe renal disease.

HEMATOLOGICAL STUDIES

RED CELL VOLUME USING THE PATIENT'S CELLS

Using sterile techniques, we add 30 μc. of sodium chromate (^{51}Cr) to a sterile evacuated, stoppered tube. Ten milliliters of venous blood is withdrawn from the patient into a 20 ml. syringe containing 2 ml. of acid citrate dextrose (ACD) solution and transferred to the tube. The blood, ACD solution, and chromate are incubated for 10 to 15 minutes with occasional gentle shaking of the tube.

If NIH Formula A acid citrate dextrose anticoagulant is used, 85 to 90 per cent of the total ^{51}Cr is bound to the red cells after 10 minutes' incubation at room temperature. If NIH Formula B anticoagulant is used, tagging is slower and less complete. If heparin is used as anticoagulant, adequate tagging of red cells with ^{51}Cr requires about 1 hour.

The residual unbound chromate is reduced to the chromic form by adding 50 mg. of ascorbic acid and allowing it to stand for an additional 3 minutes. If the patient has previously been given radioactive materials, an 8 ml. sample of blood is obtained. The needle is left in place and the syringe containing the 8 ml. of blood is replaced with a syringe containing exactly 5 ml. of the labeled blood (10 μc.). The total volume of blood in the syringe is injected. The syringe is *not* flushed with blood. After 30 minutes, 8 ml. of blood is withdrawn from a vein of the opposite arm and the activity of 1 ml. is measured. Five milliliters of the labeled cells from the original dose is kept as a standard. Hematocrit determinations are made on both the standard blood sample and the sample obtained after 30 minutes. Five milliliters of standard blood and 5 ml. of the 30 minute sample are centrifuged at 2000 rpm for 10 minutes. Two 1 ml. samples of plasma are pipetted for counting. If a blank blood sample was obtained, whole blood and plasma samples are similarly prepared. The calculations are as follows:

$$\text{Blood volume (ml.)} = \frac{\binom{\text{Volume}}{\text{injected}}\left[\binom{\text{Net counts/min./ml.}}{\text{whole blood standard}} - \binom{\text{Net counts/min./ml.}}{\text{plasma standard}}\binom{\text{Standard decimal}}{\text{plasmocrit}}\right]}{\binom{\text{Net counts/min./ml.}}{\text{patient's whole blood}} - \binom{\text{Net counts/min./ml.}}{\text{patient's plasma}}\binom{\text{Patient's decimal}}{\text{plasmocrit}}}$$

Decimal plasmocrit $= 1.00 -$ hematocrit

Using the hematocrit, the red cell volume and the plasma volume may be obtained from the total blood volume.

$$\text{Red cell volume} = \text{Total blood volume} \times \frac{\text{Hct.}}{100}$$

Total plasma volume $=$ Total blood volume $-$ Red cell volume

The results are expressed as milliliters per kilogram body weight.

Normal Values

Total blood volume: 4550 (3850 to 5250) ml.; 55 to 75 ml. per kilogram
Total red cell volume: 1925 (1750 to 2100) ml.; 25 to 30 ml. per kilogram
Total plasma volume: 2625 (2100 to 3150) ml.; 30 to 45 ml. per kilogram

Falsely high results are found if a faulty intravenous injection technique is used, and the entire dose is not injected into a vein. Poorly tagged or damaged red cells, or free ^{51}Cr in the labeling solution, will also yield spuriously high values. Falsely low values are caused by failing to obtain a preinjection blood sample in a patient who has had previous administration of radioactive tracers. Contamination of equipment with radioactivity will also yield spuriously low values.

RED CELL VOLUME WITH ^{51}CR-LABELED O-NEGATIVE RED BLOOD CELLS

Instead of labeling the patient's own red blood cells for each determination, red cells from a Group O, Rh negative donor may be labeled and used in all patients for a 2 week period. The advantage is that the labeled cells are immediately available. The blood should be withdrawn from a known O-negative donor into a plastic bag containing one part of ACD solution for each five parts of blood. Chromium-51 (sodium chromate) is added to yield a specific activity of 2 μc. per milliliter of blood; the bag is gently shaken at intervals for 15 minutes. When using semiautomatic techniques for blood volume determinations, a specific activity of 10 μc. per milliliter is needed. The tagged red blood cells are kept in a refrigerator at 4° C. and settle to the bottom of the storage bag. After 2 weeks, unused labeled cells are discarded.

The labeled red cells must be washed within 48 hours before use. To do this, we puncture the inlet of an empty 150 ml. plastic bag with the sterile tip of its attached tubing. The delivery tube from a bottle of sterile sodium chloride solution is inserted and approximately 20 cc. is poured into the plastic bag. The tubing from the blood storage bag is connected and an equal amount of settled red cells is added. The opening of the 150 ml. bag is closed with a screw clamp and the bag is agitated gently and centrifuged at 2000 rpm for 10 minutes. The bag must be withdrawn carefully from the centrifuge to avoid mixing of the separated plasma and red cells. The supernatant plasma is aspirated with a long sterile spinal needle. The original total volume is reconstituted with sterile saline. A three-way stopcock on an extension tube is inserted into the bag, which should be gently agitated before each use to adequately mix the labeled red cells and saline.

The procedure for administration and measurement of the radioactivity of the O-negative cells is similar to that with the patient's own labeled red cells. A blank of 6 ml. of whole blood must be obtained if the patient has previously received a radioactive substance. Then exactly 5 ml. of the ^{51}Cr-washed O-negative red cells is injected. The patient's vein should be entered with an empty syringe which is replaced by the syringe containing the labeled red cells, which are then injected. Thirty minutes later, a heparinized sample is withdrawn from the opposite arm, a hematocrit is determined, and 5 ml. whole blood is pipetted into a test tube.

A standard is prepared by diluting 5 ml. of the tagged ^{51}Cr red cells in a volumetric flask. Five milliliters of the standard solution and the 5 ml. blood sample are counted in a well scintillation counter together with the blank if necessary. The results are calculated using the equation:

$$\text{Total blood volume} = \frac{\text{Net counts/min./ml. standard} \times \text{dilution factor} \times \text{volume injected}}{\text{Net counts/min./ml. sample}}$$

The red cell volume and plasma volume are obtained using the hematocrit. The normal values are the same as described for the preceding procedures.

PLASMA VOLUME

To determine plasma volume with ^{131}I serum albumin, a stock solution containing approximately 2 μc. per milliliter is prepared for injection by adding 60 μc. of ^{131}I serum albumin to a sterile, rubber-capped 30 cc. vial of sodium chloride solution. The patient should be given 10 drops of Lugol's solution or potassium iodide solution on the day of the study. Exactly 5 ml. of the stock solution, containing 10 μc. or less, is injected intravenously. At 10, 15, and 20 minutes after injection, 5 ml. blood samples are obtained with a heparinized syringe from the opposite arm. The hematocrit is measured and 2 ml. of plasma from each sample is pipetted for counting.

If the patient has previously received radioactive substances, a 5 ml. sample should be obtained before the radioactive albumin is injected. A standard is prepared from the stock solution and the radioactivity in 2 ml. is measured. The plasma radioactivity is plotted on semilog paper as a function of time and the plasma radioactivity is extrapolated from the curve to the time of injection. This extrapolated figure is used to determine the plasma volume, according to the equation:

$$\text{Plasma volume} = \frac{\text{Volume injected} \times \text{counts/min./ml. of stock solution} \times \text{dilution factor}}{\text{Extrapolated counts/min./ml. plasma}}$$

Total blood volume may be obtained from the hematocrit and plasma volume. All results are expressed as milliliters per kilogram body weight.

Normal Values

Total blood volume: 68 to 88 ml. per kilogram

Red cell volume: 30 to 38 ml. per kilogram

Plasma volume: 39 to 44 ml. per kilogram

For simultaneous measurement of red cell volume using ^{51}Cr-labeled red cells and plasma volume using ^{125}I or ^{131}I albumin, the red cell volume is measured first. The serum albumin is injected through the same needle just after withdrawing the 30 minute ^{51}Cr blood sample. Alternatively, ^{131}I or ^{125}I albumin and ^{51}Cr red cells can be injected simultaneously. The radioactivity from each can be differentiated by gamma-ray spectrometry.

Semiautomatic techniques

Commercial equipment is available which eliminates the pipetting, diluting, and calculating steps of the preceding procedures. These instruments may be used for either red blood cell or plasma volume. The manufacturer's instructions should be consulted for recommended doses and details of operation. In essence, the syringe containing the dose to be injected is measured automatically and is stored in a memory unit. The radioactivity of the blank and the sample withdrawn after injection are measured in a like manner and the blood volume, calculated automatically, is indicated on a scale. Special test tubes are supplied that expose a constant volume to the detectors, thus making accurate pipetting unnecessary.

Red cell survival

If the patient is to have a combined blood volume and red cell survival measurement, the labeling is the same as described under Blood Volume Using the Patient's Cells except that 120 μc. of ^{51}Cr is used. When measurement is made only of red cell survival, 5 ml. of the patient's blood is added to 1 cc. of ACD together with 40 μc. of ^{51}Cr. This mixture is incubated 10 to 15 minutes; 50 mg. (1 cc.) ascorbic acid is added and after 3 minutes the total mixture is injected into the patient. Six milliliter samples of blood are withdrawn every other day three times a week for 2 weeks. Five milliliters is pipetted from each sample, hemolyzed with saponin or by freezing and thawing, and stored at 4° C. Hematocrits are obtained on each sample. Counting of all samples is carried out on the day the last blood sample is obtained. The counting rate of each sample is plotted on semilog paper as a function of time to obtain the half-time of disappearance of the labeled red blood cells. Whole blood is counted and the results are expressed as counts per minute per unit volume. If the hematocrit has fallen during the course of the procedure, estimation of the red cell survival is inaccurate.

The normal red cell survival as measured by ^{51}Cr-labeled red blood cells results in a half-time of 25 to 35 days. The results of the test can also be expressed as a percentage decrease per day. The normal values are 1.5 to 2.5 per cent per day.

SPLENIC SEQUESTRATION

While measuring red cell survival, we can also measure the degree of splenic sequestration of red blood cells by measuring the rate of accumulation of ^{51}Cr by the spleen as compared to the liver and precordium. The counting rate is measured by means of an external detector at 24 hours after injection and every other day for 2 weeks.

To measure the precordial radioactivity, the detector is centered over the third costal cartilage on the left side, with the patient in the supine position. To measure liver radioactivity, the detector is placed over the ninth and tenth ribs on the right between the midclavicular and anterior axillary line with the patient in the supine position. For measurement over the spleen, the detector is placed over the ninth and tenth ribs on the left at the posterior axillary line with the patient in the prone position. If the spleen is palpable, the detector is positioned over the palpable mass. The skin is marked with indelible ink to indicate the position of the external detector from one day to the next. The results are expressed as the ratio of the count rate over the spleen to the count rate over the precordium. The count rate over the liver is also expressed relative to the count rate over the precordium. These ratios are graphed as a function of time.

PLASMA IRON CLEARANCE

Twelve microcuries of sterile ferrous citrate (^{59}Fe) with an activity of about 100 μc. per milliliter and 2 to 3.5 μc. per microgram is added to a sterile, rubber-capped vial containing 12 ml. of saline solution to yield a dilution of 1 μc. per milliliter. To prepare a standard solution, exactly 5 ml. of stock solution is removed with a sterile syringe and placed in a 100 ml. volumetric flask. The volume is increased to the 100 ml. mark with tap water. Five milliliters is pipetted into a test tube and kept as a standard equal to 5 per cent of the administered dose. Five milliliters of stock solution containing 5 μc. ^{59}Fe is injected intravenously. To measure the plasma clearance of ^{59}Fe, three 6 ml. blood specimens are obtained with heparinized syringes at 30, 60, and 90 minutes following injection. The radioactivity of a 5 ml. aliquot from each specimen is measured and plotted on semilogarithmic paper. The normal plasma iron disappearance half-time is 60 to 120 minutes.

PLASMA IRON TURNOVER RATE (PIT)

To calculate this rate, it is necessary to perform a chemical determination of the plasma iron concentration. One also has to calculate the plasma volume and measure the plasma iron clearance half-time.

$$\frac{\text{PIT}}{\text{(mg./day)}} = \frac{0.693 \times \text{plasma iron (mg./ml.)} \times \text{plasma vol. (ml.)} \times 24}{\text{T}\frac{1}{2} \text{ (hr.)}}$$

The normal range of value is 27 to 42 mg. per day or

$$\frac{\text{PIT}}{\text{(mg./kg./day)}} = \frac{0.693 \times \text{plasma iron (mg./ml.)} \times \text{plasma vol. (ml.)} \times 24}{\text{T}\frac{1}{2} \text{ (hr.)} \times \text{body wt. (kg.)}}$$

Values from 0.46 to 0.78 mg. per kilogram per day are in the normal range.

INCORPORATION OF IRON INTO RED CELLS

The preparation and injection of the ^{59}Fe standard for this procedure are the same as for the measurement of plasma iron clearance. Six milliliter blood specimens are obtained every other day three times a week for 2 weeks. Five milliliters is pipetted from each sample, hemolyzed with saponin, and stored at 4° C. Hematocrit determinations are made for each sample. After all samples are collected, they are counted along with the standard.

$$\% \text{ RBC incorporation of radioactive iron} = \frac{\text{Counts/ml. blood} \times \text{blood vol. (ml.)} \times 100}{\text{Counts injected}}$$

The percentage of administered iron incorporated into red blood cells is graphed as a function of time. The normal is 60 to 80 per cent of the administered dose in 7 to 10 days.

SITES OF HEMATOPOIESIS

The preparation of the dose of labeled iron is the same as that for the plasma iron clearance. After injection, external counting is carried out over the precordium, liver, spleen, and sacrum. The counting procedure is identical to that used to detect splenic sequestration of labeled red blood cells, except that ^{59}Fe rather than ^{51}Cr is detected. The ratios of liver, spleen, and sacrum to precordial counts are plotted as a function of time. In a normal person, the radioactivity in the sacrum usually rises on the first day or two of the study, and then gradually falls during the subsequent 2 weeks. Usually the accumulation of radioactivity in the sacrum is greater than that of the liver or spleen. The latter organs accumulate iron at an increased rate in patients with extramedullary hematopoiesis.

COMBINED BLOOD VOLUME, RED CELL SURVIVAL, AND FERROKINETICS

The technique outlined in the section on Red Cell Survival is used for the combined measurement of red cell survival and blood volume. After the 30 minute ^{51}Cr blood sample has been obtained for the blood volume determination, the syringe is replaced with one containing 5 ml. of stock solution containing 5 μc. ^{59}Fe. After this is injected intravenously, a plasma iron clearance and iron incorporation determination are done as described previously.

All the samples are counted in a well-type counter using pulse-height analysis. The samples from the blood volume are counted first using an 80 kev. window with the analyzer centered on the 320 kev. peak of ^{51}Cr. The plasma clearance samples are then measured with the lower-level discriminator set to eliminate the ^{51}Cr radioactivity but include the 1.1 and 1.3 Mev. photopeaks of ^{59}Fe. The blood samples of day 1 through 14 along with the ^{59}Fe standard are counted at both the ^{59}Fe and ^{51}Cr settings.

Since some ^{59}Fe is detected at the ^{51}Cr settings, a correction must be made. The ^{51}Cr samples are corrected for the ^{59}Fe contamination as follows:

^{51}Cr activity = counts/min. of sample at ^{51}Cr settings — counts/min. of sample at ^{59}Fe settings $\times$ iron correction factor

$$\text{Iron correction factor} = \frac{\text{Counts/min. } ^{59}Fe \text{ standard at } ^{51}Cr \text{ setting}}{\text{Counts/min. } ^{59}Fe \text{ standard at } ^{59}Fe \text{ setting}}$$

GASTROINTESTINAL STUDIES

VITAMIN B_{12} ABSORPTION

EIGHT HOUR PLASMA TEST

In measuring absorption of tracer doses of vitamin B_{12} from the intestine, it is essential to control the microgram quantity of vitamin B_{12} administered. If the oral dose contains from 0.1 to 0.5 μg. of vitamin B_{12}, approximately 70 per cent is absorbed. With larger doses progressively smaller percentages are absorbed.

A stock solution of cobalt-57 vitamin B_{12} is diluted with tap water so that the 10 ml. test dose contains approximately 0.3 μg. of vitamin B_{12} and 1.0 μc. of ^{57}Co. The dose is given orally after the patient has fasted for 12 hours, and he eats no food for the following 2 hours. Eight hours after administration of the isotope, a 22 ml. blood sample is withdrawn into a heparinized syringe. A 10 ml. plasma sample and standard are counted in a well scintillation detector with a gamma-ray spectrometer. The standard can be prepared to contain 1 per cent of the administered dose by diluting 1 ml. of the prepared solution to 100 ml. in a volumetric flask; 10 ml. aliquots of this solution are counted for the standard. To standardize the results for variation in body weight, the plasma concentration of radioactivity is expressed in relation to the body weight.

$$\% \text{ dose/1 liter plasma} = \frac{\text{Net counts/min./10 ml. plasma}}{\text{Net counts/min./10 ml. standard}} \times 100$$

The normal plasma level after 8 hours is greater than 0.6 per cent of the administered dose per liter of plasma. In pernicious anemia or malabsorption syndrome, less than 0.25 per cent of the administered dose is present per liter of plasma. Since 7 per cent of patients with vitamin B_{12} malabsorption may have plasma values within the normal range, the Schilling test is preferable to the 8 hour plasma test, and is now routine in our laboratory.

URINARY EXCRETION (SCHILLING) TEST

A 1 mg. dose of stable vitamin B_{12} is given intramuscularly to promote renal excretion of absorbed vitamin B_{12}. Usually the stable vitamin is given 1 hour after the oral test dose of labeled vitamin B_{12} which is identical to that used for the 8 hour plasma test. The stable vitamin B_{12} saturates tissue and plasma binding sites prior to the absorption of most of the radioactive vitamin B_{12}. The unbound vitamin B_{12} is excreted by the kidney. Absorption is considered normal if more than 15 per cent of the dose is recovered in the 24 hour urine. Values of less than 6 to 7 per cent excretion indicate significant malabsorption of vitamin B_{12}. In patients with renal insufficiency, the excretion of radioactive vitamin B_{12} may be delayed. In such patients, urine should be collected for an additional 24 hours. Because of the delayed absorption of vitamin B_{12}, even in normal persons, one can perform the urinary excretion test after obtaining the 8 hour plasma sample. One thousand micrograms of stable B_{12} injected 8 hours after the oral tracer will saturate the binding sites of the plasma so that the subsequently absorbed vitamin B_{12} is excreted in the urine. After this injection, patients with normal B_{12} absorption excrete more than 9 per cent of the administered dose in a subsequent 24 hour period. Aliquots of urine may be counted, or alternatively the total radioactivity of the 24 hour specimen can be measured. After dilution to a fixed volume, the total specimen can be counted directly on top of a sodium iodide detector and compared to a standard of identical volume. The most common error is incomplete collection of urine. If the 24 hour urine volume is small (less than 600 ml.) and the excreted radioactivity is low, it is wise to repeat the test to be certain that the urine collection was complete. Otherwise, falsely low absorption results will be obtained.

If less than 6 per cent of the dose is excreted in 24 hours, the test should be repeated with an oral dose of 30 mg. of intrinsic factor. Three to seven days must elapse before the repeat test. A 24 hour urine specimen preceding the repeat dose of radioactive B_{12} must be collected as a "blank." A normal urinary excretion value after the administration of intrinsic factor occurs in pernicious anemia. If the urinary excretion is still abnormally low after intrinsic factor, the patient has either malabsorption from causes other than addisonian pernicious anemia or acquired resistance to intrinsic factor.

FECAL RADIOACTIVITY

To minimize the handling of fecal specimens and to preserve constant geometric counting conditions, the following technique is used: new 1 gallon paint cans are used for each 24 hour collection period, although specimens from longer collection periods can be accumulated in one can. After the fecal specimens have been obtained, approximately 5 ml. of concentrated phenol in water and 300 to 700 ml. of tap water is added and the lid tightly shut. The can is weighed to a precision of 1 g. and is shaken on a commercial paint shaker for about 10 minutes. A second can is filled with water to the same weight as the specimen and is used during measurement of background radioactivity. The standard is pipetted into a third can and tap water is added to equalize the weight to that of the specimen can. An external detector such as that used for thyroid studies or a well scintillation detector is used to measure the radioactivity.

In studies in which fecal collections are made, the patient should be instructed to avoid contaminating the collection with urine. This is particularly important in women.

EXUDATIVE ENTEROPATHY

Fifty or a hundred microcuries of ^{51}Cr serum albumin is administered intravenously, and exactly the same amount is injected into a fecal collection can and used as a standard. Complete fecal collection is made for a period of 4 days. Radioactivity in the specimens is measured by the procedure described in the previous section. Approximately 2.0 per cent of the dose is usually found in a 4 day collection from normal persons. Greater amounts are found in exudative enteropathy.

Fifteen to twenty microcuries of ^{131}I polyvinylpyrrolidone (PVP) can be used instead of ^{51}Cr serum albumin, in which case 10 drops of Lugol's solution is given to block the thyroid. One per cent or less of the dose can be expected in a 4 day collection. A value of 1.5 per cent or greater is abnormal.

GASTROINTESTINAL BLEEDING

Fifteen milliliters of the patient's blood is labeled with 40 to 50 μc. of ^{51}Cr sodium chromate using the ascorbic acid method. The technique used in determining the red cell volume is followed. Two milliliters of a sample of blood obtained 30 minutes after injection is saved for future counting. Twenty-four hour fecal specimens are collected for 4 days. On the fourth day, 5 ml. of heparinized blood is withdrawn. Ten milliliters of whole blood is pipetted into a fecal collection can on the first and on the fourth day of collection. Radioactivity in fecal collections is counted according to the procedure described under Fecal Radioactivity.

The following equation is used:

$$\text{Fecal blood loss} = \frac{\text{Total net counts/min. in fecal specimens} \times 10}{(\text{Net counts/min./10 ml. of 30 min. blood sample} + \text{net counts/min./10 ml. of blood sample on 4th day})/2}$$

GASTROINTESTINAL ABSORPTION

IRON ABSORPTION

Syrup of ferrous sulfate contains approximately 4 g. of iron per 100 ml. plus citric acid in sugar and water. Ferrous sulfate ($FeSO_4 \cdot 7H_2O$) is 20 per cent iron. Two milliliters of syrup is pipetted into a 50 ml. graduate cylinder and diluted with tap water to about 20 ml. Three milliliters of 5 per cent ascorbic acid solution (2 ml. vials contain 100 mg.) and 30 μc. ^{59}Fe citrate are added. The total volume in the graduate cylinder is increased to 30 ml. with tap water. Ascorbic acid in doses of 10 mg. per milligram of iron keeps the iron in the reduced or ferrous form. To prepare the fecal standard, 10 ml. of the labeled ferrous solution is pipetted into a feces container with 200 to 300 ml. of water. This standard contains the same amount of radioactivity as the dose. Ten milliliters of the labeled ferrous solution (equivalent to about 5 mg. of iron) is pipetted into a paper cup. (The patient should not have breakfast before administration of the dose.) After the patient drinks the solution, the cup is rinsed with tap water and he drinks the rinsings. The cup is saved for counting the residual activity. The patient should not eat or drink until 2 hours after the dose. Fecal specimens are collected for 5 days.

The standard and fecal specimens are counted under identical geometrical conditions. The following equations are used:

$$\% \text{ recovered in feces} = \frac{\text{Net counts/min. in all fecal specimens}}{\text{Net counts/min. in standard}} \times 100$$

$$\% \text{ of oral iron absorbed} = 100\% - \% \text{ in feces}$$

In normal persons, less than 40 per cent of the oral iron is absorbed (mean, 20 per cent). In iron deficiency anemia not due to malabsorption, more than 40 per cent of the iron is absorbed (mean, 56 per cent).

ABSORPTION OF LABELED FAT

The patient must fast the night preceding the administration of the test dose and should receive no food for at least 2 hours thereafter. Ten drops of Lugol's solution is given the day of and the day after the test. A commercially available capsule containing 25 to 50 μc. of ^{131}I triolein is given orally to the patient with sips of water. This is followed by a dose of carrier fat containing 1 g. per kilogram body weight and 3 ounces of thin barium. A standard reference solution is supplied with the capsules and is used to prepare the fecal and blood standards. Six milliliter heparinized blood samples are withdrawn at 4, 5, and 6 hours following ingestion of the fat. Five milliliter samples are pipetted and counted with the blood standard. A radiograph of the abdomen is obtained at 6 hours to evaluate the emptying of the stomach and the distribution of the material throughout the bowel. Feces are collected from the patient for at least 48 hours. Radioactivity in the collection is measured and the result compared with a fecal standard. The normal range of blood levels between 4 and 6 hours is 1.4 to 4 per cent of the administered dose per liter of whole blood. If less than 3 per cent of the administered labeled fat is excreted in the feces within 2 to 3 days, the absorption of fat is considered to be normal. In pancreatic insufficiency, or in malabsorption due to disease of the intestines, excretion of the labeled fat in the feces is abnormally high, and the 4 to 6 hour blood levels are low. If gastric emptying is delayed, the 4 to 6 hour blood levels may be low, but the fecal excretion will be normal. If the fecal specimens are contaminated with urine, the value of the fecal excretion will appear abnormally high, but the blood levels will be normal.

If ^{131}I oleic acid is used, the study is done in exactly the same manner as with ^{131}I triolein. In pancreatic insufficiency, the absorption of the oleic acid would be expected to be normal. In malabsorption syndrome due to small bowel disease, absorption of both oleic acid and triolein will tbe poor.

In the past, problems of radiopharmaceutical purity have plagued the use of the radioiodinated fats. This resulted in the procedure falling into disrepute. With improved understanding and better quality control these procedures may eventually be revived for more widespread clinical use. The most promising is the collection of $^{14}CO_2$ in the breath at intervals after ingestion of ^{14}C-labeled triglycerides as described in Chapter XII.

RENAL STUDIES

GENERAL CONSIDERATIONS

In the chlormerodrin accumulation test and the ^{131}I ortho-iodohippurate renogram, the time course of radioactivity in each kidney is measured independently and the results between the two kidneys are compared. Two sodium iodide crystal scintillation detectors are directed at the kidneys. The patient lies in a supine position with the detectors mounted beneath the table. This position is most comfortable for the patient during the hour-long period of observation in the chlormerodrin test. It is essential that the patient not move significantly during the study or the results will be invalid.

For each detector there is a separate power supply, amplifier, pulse-height analyzer, and either a scaler or rate meter connected to a strip chart recorder. The on-line recording makes it easy to detect motion of the patient. Each detection system is calibrated separately. Since these tests involve comparison of one kidney with the other, it is helpful if two detectors are balanced to achieve comparable sensitivity. This is done using standard solutions of the radionuclide being used, adjusting the width of the window of the pulse-height analyzer.

The most frequent source of error is incorrect positioning of the detectors over the kidneys. Errors are minimized by the use of a preliminary radiograph and by checking whether positioning was correct at the end of the study. This is done in two ways: by moving the detector to be certain it was over the area of maximum radioactivity, and by correlating the subsequent scanning image of the kidneys with the selected detector positions.

CHLORMERODRIN ACCUMULATION TEST

The patient lies in a supine position. An abdominal radiograph is taken to locate the kidneys. The center of the outline of each kidney is located by means of a radiopaque centimeter scale on the left side of the patient. Using a corresponding centimeter scale on the side of the table, the detectors are carefully centered beneath the kidneys. The patient must not move after the radiograph is taken.

With the patient on the table and the detection system in operation, mercury-197 chlormerodrin is injected intravenously. A test dose of 30 to 150 μc. is used, depending on whether a renal scan is to follow the uptake study. The time of injection is indicated on the records and measurements are made for 60 minutes.

To calculate the results, the count rates at 5, 10, 20, 30, 40, 50, and 60 minutes are read from rate meter tracings or from scalers. The count rate at each time, t, is divided by the count rate at 5 minutes after injection. These values are referred to as C_t and C_5, respectively, and are compared using the equation:

$$\frac{R}{L} = \frac{\dfrac{C_t}{C_5} \quad \text{Right kidney}}{\dfrac{C_t}{C_5} \quad \text{Left kidney}}$$

The ratios are calculated, rather than the absolute counting rates, to correct for geometric variations between the two sides. Measurement of the relative increase of the radioactivity for each kidney detector tends to correct for geometric differences among patients and between the two sides of the same patient. Normal values have been given in Chapter XIII.

[131]I ORTHO-IODOHIPPURATE RENOGRAM

During the half hour before the study the patient drinks 250 ml. of water. Some clinicians, however, prefer that the patient not be given water. The kidneys are localized by a radiograph and the detectors are positioned in the same manner as for the chlormerodrin test. A time constant of 1 second and a paper speed of 6 inches per minute are usually used initially and changed to 30 seconds and 12 inches per minute 2 minutes after the intravenous injection of 20 to 40 μc. of [131]I Hippuran. The recording is continued for 30 minutes or until the half-time of the decreasing part of the curve is exceeded.

Various means of analyzing these curves have been used. The present state of the art of performing the renogram is such that each laboratory should select a method and establish a normal range by measurements made under standardized conditions. Chapter XIII describes this test in detail and gives the normal values.

GLOMERULAR FILTRATION RATE (G.F.R.)

The patient is given 750 to 1000 ml. of water to drink 1 hour before examination. Five milligrams of stable vitamin B_{12} is injected intravenously, followed 15 minutes later by 1.5 to 2.0 μc. of [57]Co-labeled vitamin B_{12}. A standard is prepared of the injected dose. An external scintillation detection system is used to monitor radioactivity over the precordium. With the patient in the supine position, the detector is positioned over the precordium 1 to 2 cm. above the left fourth and fifth intercostal spaces in the midclavicular line with the main axis of the detector perpendicular to the recumbent patient. Care should be taken not to include the kidneys in the field of the detector.

The counting rate is recorded for 90 to 120 minutes, and the results are graphed on semilog paper as a function of time. The slope of the concentration curve is obtained by subtracting the logarithmic values of two points and dividing by the time interval between the two points. A plasma sample obtained 45 minutes after injection is used to relate the volume being monitored externally to the concentration per milliliter of plasma. With this known, the expression for the clearance which equals the G.F.R. becomes:

$$\text{G.F.R. (ml./min.)} = \frac{\text{Vol. of distribution (ml.)} \times 0.693}{T\frac{1}{2} \text{ (min.)}}$$

The concentration in plasma at 45 minutes is extrapolated back to the time of injection using the slope of the precordial tracing. The total dose injected divided by the concentration at $T = 0$ yields the volume of distribution of the tracer. Iothalamate labeled with ^{131}I and ^{51}Cr ethylenediamine tetraacetic acid (EDTA) have also been used.

SCANNING TECHNIQUES

GENERAL CONSIDERATIONS

The patient should be made as comfortable as possible and instructed to remain immobile during the procedure. For small children or uncooperative adults, sedation may be necessary. Head clamps for brain scanning and compression bands are helpful.

Whenever a focusing collimator is used, the operator must position the detector so that the region of interest is as close as possible to the focal plane. The detector is then moved to outline the field of interest and to locate the regions of highest and lowest count rates. This facilitates selection of optimum operational parameters. Small pieces of lead are placed on the body surface to orient the scan to a radiograph taken after the completion of the scanning procedure. The radiograph is obtained with the patient in the same position as for the scan. Ideally the x-ray tube should be 6 feet away to reduce image magnification.

Confusion in the interpretation of scans may arise if the images are not marked according to the orientation of the patient. To evaluate the scan properly, the following information should be indicated:

TABLE 21-1. USEFUL DATA FOR SCANNING

ORGAN TO BE SCANNED	SUBSTANCE USED	DOSE	TIME BETWEEN ADMINISTRATION OF DOSE AND START OF SCAN	HALF-LIFE OF ISOTOPE	ENERGY OF ISOTOPE'S MOST USEFUL PHOTOPEAK KEV	WINDOW SETTING	COLLIMATOR RESOLUTION
Thyroid	Na [131]I	15–25 μc.	24 hr.	8.1 days	364	324–404	Fine
	99mTcO₄⁻	1 mc.	30 to 60 min.	6.0 hr.	140	135–170	
Kidneys	197Hg chlormerodrin	300 μc.	1 hr.	65 hr.	77	65–95	Fine
	203Hg chlormerodrin	150 μc.	1 hr.	47 days	280	239–309	
Lungs	131I MAA	150–300 μc. Not over 0.1 mg. protein/ kg. body weight	Immediate	8.1 days	364	324–404	Medium
	113mIn iron hydroxide	1 mc.	Immediate	1.7 hr.	390	350–410	Fine
Spleen	197Hg MHP-tagged and damaged erythrocytes	300 μc.	1 hr.	65 hr.	77	65–95	Fine
	51Cr heat-treated erythrocytes	300 μc.	24 hr.	28 days	320	280–360	
Brain	99mTcO₄⁻	15 mc.	1–3 hr.	6.0 hr.	140	135–170	Fine
	131I serum albumin	5.5 μc./kg. but not over 500 μc.	24–48 hr.	8.1 days	364	324–404	
	113m In DTPA	15 mc.	Immediate	1.7 hr.	390	350–410	Fine
Heart	99mTc serum albumin	2 mc.	5–10 min.	6.0 hr.	140	135–170	Fine to medium
	131I Cholografin	150 μc.		8.1 days	364	324–404	
	131I serum albumin	150 μc.		8.1 days	364	324–404	
Placenta	99mTc serum albumin	1 mc.	5–10 min.	6.0 hr.	140	135–170	Coarse
Liver	99mTc sulfur colloid	2 mc.	5–30 min.	6.0 hr.	140	135–170	Fine
	131I AA	500 μc.	5–10 min.	8.1 days	364	324–404	
Bones	85Sr (NO₃)₂	100–200 μc.	At least 48–72 hr.; optimal: 5–7 days	64 days	513	474–554	Medium to coarse

1. The side of the patient (right or left).

2. The surface of the body that was scanned, i.e., the surface of the body closest to the detector. This is indicated by either "anterior" or "posterior" or "right lateral" or "left lateral."

3. The position of the patient during the scan: either "recumbent prone" or "recumbent supine," or "right decubitus" or "left decubitus."

THYROID SCANNING

Twenty-five microcuries of the ^{131}I sodium iodide stock solution prepared as for the ^{131}I thyroid uptake studies is given orally from a paper cup. Twenty-four hours later, the anterior aspect of the hyperextended neck is scanned. The usual borders of the scan are 1 inch above the laryngeal prominence and 1½ inch below the suprasternal notch. The lateral margins of the neck should be included. The radiograph should include the manubrium.

One millicurie of technetium-99m pertechnetate given intravenously can be used instead of ^{131}I. In this case, the scan is performed 30 to 60 minutes after the intravenous dose.

SPLEEN SCANNING

The compound 1-mercuri-2-hydroxypropane (MHP) labeled with ^{197}Hg simultaneously tags and moderately damages red blood cells. One milligram of MHP is reacted with 1 to 2 ml. of blood to produce the optimum degree of damage. To obtain 300 μc. of ^{197}Hg together with a concentration of 1 mg. of MHP per milliliter of packed cells, it is necessary to vary the volume of blood to correct for the decrease in specific activity that results from radioactive decay of the ^{197}Hg. In preparing the dose for the procedure, the weight of stable MHP in the volume of MHP that contains 300 μc. of ^{197}Hg is calculated. This volume is placed in a sterile evacuated test tube. If the patient's hematocrit is unknown, it is assumed to be 40 per cent. The amount of blood that will yield 1 mg. of MHP for each milliliter of packed cells is added to the evacuated test tube containing the ^{197}Hg MHP. After inverting the sterile tube several times, the labeled blood is drawn into a sterile syringe and is reinjected into the patient.

The scan is usually performed 1 hour later but can be delayed several hours. Posterior and left lateral views are obtained. The scan should cover a broad area around the region of the spleen. A radiograph including the left lung base, the left hemidiaphragm, the air bubble of the stomach, and the left iliac crest is taken.

An alternative, but in our experience, less satisfactory method of splenic scanning is the heat treatment of ^{51}Cr-labeled red blood cells to induce their sequestration in the spleen. The first step is to withdraw 5 ml. of the patient's blood into a syringe containing 1 ml. anticoagulant solution (ACD–NIH Formula A) using sterile technique. The blood is injected into a evacuated tube. Three hundred microcuries of sterile ^{51}Cr sodium chromate is added and the tube is incubated at room temperature for 15 minutes. Fifty milligrams of ascorbic acid is added to reduce the residual chromate to chromic ion. The tube is incubated at 49.5° ± 1° for 1 hour in a water bath. After incubation, the tube is cooled in cold water to room temperature and the labeled, heated cells are injected intravenously. The scan may be performed within 1 hour, but best results are obtained by waiting 24 hours. This procedure is preferred to the MPH method in searching for an accessory spleen. Renal uptake of ^{197}Hg may obscure the splenic remnant in the MHP method.

RENAL SCANNING

Three hundred microcuries of ^{197}Hg chlormerodrin is injected intravenously 1 hour before scanning. A posterior scan of the lumbar region of the body is performed, and should include the pelvis if both kidneys are not seen in the usual position. The radiograph should include the pelvis and bladder area.

PREPARATION OF ^{99m}TC PERTECHNETATE FOR BRAIN SCANNING

Technetium-99m pertechnetate is obtained from a molybdenum-99–technetium-99m generator, which consists of a shielded aluminum oxide column ("the cow") from which pertechnetate can be eluted ("milked") daily. For protection of the laboratory personnel, the generator is mounted on a stand behind a shield of lead and lead-glass bricks. Each morning the column is eluted with 20 ml. of sterile, nonpyrogenic, physiological sodium chloride solution. Only 3 per cent of the available activity is eluted with the first 5 ml., but 60 to 85 per cent is eluted from the subsequent 5 to 20 ml. The pH of the eluate is checked with pH paper, and if found to be below 5.5, is adjusted with 0.1 N NaOH prepared with pyrogen-free water. A preliminary elution of 8 to 10 ml. is discarded from each generator before use. The eluate is sterilized by autoclaving under pressure in a rubber-capped 30 cc. vial at 260° F. for 20 minutes.

Radioassay must be carried out routinely before human use. This can be done without dilution of the eluate by using a large well-type ionization chamber and electrometer, and comparing the eluate with a standard of ^{57}Co. Before the ionization chamber is used the first time, it should be calibrated against a scintillation counter with diluted solutions. Calibrations with a Lauritsen electroscope using a radium standard are less desirable since the assay of technetium is approximately 30 per cent too high with this method.

PREPARATION OF ^{113m}IN CHELATE FOR BRAIN SCANNING

Indium-113m is obtained from a ^{113}Sn-^{113m}In generator which consists of a shielded zirconium oxide column from which ^{113m}In(Cl)$_3$ can be eluted several times a day. The column is eluted with 10 ml. sterile, nonpyrogenic dilute hydrochloric acid (0.04 to 0.06 N). To 8 ml. of the eluted ^{113m}In is added 0.2 ml. (200 micrograms) of ferric ion as ferric chloride, 1 ml. diethyltriamine-pentaacetic acid (1.6 mg.), 60 mg. sodium chloride; titrate with dilute sodium hydroxide to pH 6.5 to 7.5. The yellow complex that is formed is sterilized by autoclaving at 15 p.s.i. for 20 minutes.

BRAIN SCANNING

Two hundred microcuries per kilogram body weight of ^{99m}Tc pertechnetate or ^{113m}In DTPA is given intravenously 1 hour before the scanning procedure. The front and back, vertex, and both sides of the skull are scanned. To aid in position-ing, the chin is supported with a sponge and the head is placed without flexion or hyperextension of the neck. For the anterior view, the head is flexed slightly forward. A radiograph is made in each position after the scanning before the patient is allowed to move.

Technetium-99m pertechnetate or Indium-113m DTPA is the agent of choice for brain scanning although ^{131}I serum albumin, [203]Hg or [197]Hg chlormerodrin, and other agents have also been used. Although investigation with [113m]In chelates have not allowed us to accumulate as much data as with ^{99m}Tc pertechnetate, there is evidence that the quality of scans and delineation of lesion with [113m]In compare favorably with [99m]Tc. A laboratory performing fewer than seven brain scans a week should consider using [113m]In for economic reasons. The scanning dose is the same as that used for ^{99m}Tc pertechnetate (200 μc. per kg. body weight) and gives an equal radiation dose to the patient. Scanning can be started within 10 minutes of injection.

PREPARATION OF ^{99m}Tc-LABELED HUMAN SERUM ALBUMIN
FOR MEDIASTINAL, CARDIAC, AND PLACENTAL SCANNING

All reagents must be made with pyrogen-free water and stored at 4° C. Resin batches must be washed with five different 50 ml. portions of sterile pyrogen-free water before making the column. After the column is made, it is washed with an additional 250 ml. of sterile pyrogen-free water.

The desired quantity of ^{99m}Tc pertechnetate is eluted from a molybdenum generator with sterile, pyrogen-free physiological sodium chloride solution. The solution is acidified with six drops of 2 N HCl. Five to 8 milligrams of ascorbic acid and 5 to 8 mg. of $FeCl_3 \cdot 6H_2O$ are added to the eluted acidified ^{99m}Tc pertechnetate as solids. The pH of this solution is adjusted to 5.5 by adding 1 N NaOH drop by drop. A purple color is observed at pH 5.5.

Into a separate beaker we place 5 ml. of 0.1 N acetate buffer (pH 5.6), 3 ml. of 10 per cent dextrose, 2 ml. of 25 per cent certified human serum albumin, and one drop of anifoam. While the albumin solution is being stirred, the tagging solution is slowly added. When the addition is complete, the pH is adjusted to 2.5 with 1 N HCl (dropwise). The solution is then incubated several minutes.

A column 14 mm. wide is prepared to approximately 15 cm. height with anion exchange resin, chloride form, 50 to 100 mesh. The column is washed with *water for injection*. The incubated protein solution is passed over the resin col-umn and collected at a rate of 8 to 12 drops a minute. The first 10 ml. is discarded; approximately 20 ml. is then collected as more *water for injection* is added. After mixing, the pH is adjusted to pH 5.5 to 7.5 with dilute NaOH. The solution is filtered through a sterile, 0.45 μ Millipore filter into a previously sterilized vial. A sterile rubber stopper is attached and crimped. The contents are then ready for assay of the radioactivity.

PREPARATION OF STABILIZED [113m]IN FOR MEDIASTINAL,
CARDIAC AND PLACENTAL SCANNING

To the desired quantity of [113m]In (in approximately 8 ml. of 0.05 N hydro-chloric acid) is added 1 ml. 20 per cent gelatin, U.S.P. (sterile, nonpyrogenic) and 60 mg. sodium chloride in 0.5 ml. sterile water; titrate to pH 3.5 with dilute sodium hydroxide (approximately 0.2 N). The product is sterilized by autoclaving at 15 p.s.i. for 20 minutes.

Mediastinal and Cardiac Scanning

Thirty microcuries of ^{99m}Tc serum albumin per kilogram body weight is given intravenously immediately before the scan. The scanning area extends from the jugular notch to 1 inch below the xiphoid process and includes the top third of the liver. The lateral border of the scan is the midclavicular line on the right and the anterior axillary line on the left. To decrease magnification of the radiographic image of the cardiovascular silhoutte, the radiograph is taken in two halves. The first half is taken with the x-ray tube over the right midclavicular line at the fourth interspace, with the left side of the chest shielded by the use of a square collimator. The x-ray tube is then moved to a position over the left midclavicular line, and the left hemithorax is x-rayed on the same film.

Iodine-131 Cholografin or ^{131}I serum albumin are also used, but are inferior to ^{99m}Tc serum albumin. All are given intravenously immediately before the scan.

Although ^{99m}Tc serum albumin has been the agent of choice in several laboratories, the fact that the preparation takes approximately 1 hour to complete and requires sterilization by Millipore filtration may be disadvantageous to some investigators. The ^{113m}In preparation just described can be prepared in approximately 30 minutes; this includes terminal sterilization by autoclaving (15 p.s.i. for 20 minutes), a distinct advantage. The usual doses are *2 mc. for cardiac scanning and 1 mc. for placental scanning.* Scanning is begun immediately after intravenous injection.

Placental Scanning

One millicurie of ^{99m}Tc serum albumin is injected intravenously immediately before scanning. The anterior surface of the body is scanned, beginning slightly below the perineum. It is continued upward until the liver is clearly shown. A radiograph is not taken. A lateral scan is helpful.

One millicurie of stabilized ^{113m}In is used for placental scanning. An advantage is the absence of radioactivity in the urine, excretion being only 0.08 to 0.1 per cent of the administered dose in 2 hours.

Preparation of ^{99m}Tc-sulfur colloid for liver and bone marrow scanning

The following solutions are made with sterile, pyrogen-free water, placed in serum vials, and sterilized by autoclaving at 15 p.s.i. for 20 minutes.

Sodium thiosulfate, 8 mg. per ml. (anhydrous equivalent).

1 N hydrochloric acid.

1 N sodium hydroxide.

6 per cent dextran, high-molecular-weight.

Sodium phosphate buffer, 38.07 g. $Na_2HPO_4 \cdot 7\ H_2O$ + 2.30 g. $NaH_2PO_4 \cdot H_2O$ dissolved in 250 ml. sterile, pyrogen-free water.

Other materials and equipment needed are:

Teflon-coated bar magnet, ½ in. by ⅛ in.

Hot plate and magnetic stirrer combination.

Paper chromatographic analysis system—Whatman No. 1 paper and 85 per cent methanol.

The procedure is as follows:

1. A 20 to 30 ml. serum vial is washed with pyrogen-free water and dried. A Teflon-coated bar magnet is placed inside.

2. The following reagents are added in order

   a. 0.5 ml. sodium reagents are added in order

   b. 2 ml. 6 per cent dextran solution.

   c. 1 ml. 1 N hydrochloric acid.

3. Heat in a boiling water bath (100° C.), while stirring, for 3.5 to 4.0 minutes.

4. Remove the reactive mixture and, while stirring, titrate to pH 5.5 with a 1 to 2 mixture of 1 N sodium phosphate batter mixture. Precaution: If the pH of the colloid becomes greater than pH 6.5, dissolution will take place, making it impossible to readjust to a lower pH without changing the nature of the product.

5. Seal, cap, and autoclave at 15 p.s.i. for 20 minutes.

6. Assay as described for ^{99m}Tc pertechnetate.

7. Quality control is established by descending chromatography on Whatman No. 1 paper with 85 per cent methanol as the developing solvent. The chromatogram is allowed to develop over approximately 22 to 25 cm. After drying, in air, it is cut into 2 cm. strips which are counted in a well scintillation counter. The ^{99m}Tc-sulfur colloid remains at the origin while the free pertechnetate ion migrates with an R_f of approximately 0.6 to 0.65. There should not be more than 2.5 per cent free pertechnetate in the colloid. Because of the short physical half-life of ^{99m}Tc, it is necessary to use the colloid before the chromatograph is completed. However, if the colloid does not concentrate in the liver, this analysis makes it possible to determine whether liver disease or a technical error in the preparation of the radiopharmaceutical is responsible.

Liver scanning

Two millicuries of ^{99m}Tc-sulfur colloid is given intravenously 5 to 30 minutes before the scanning procedure is begun. The anterior, posterior, and right lateral scans are obtained routinely.

The accompanying radiograph must show the diaphragm, the lungs, the lung base, and the air bubble of the stomach. The radiograph should be taken on suspended respiration or expiration, never on inspiration.

An alternative radiopharmaceutical for liver scanning is ^{131}I-labeled aggregated human serum albumin. Five hundred microcuries is given intravenously immediately before the scan. One hundred microcuries of colloidal gold-198 may also be used. Iodine-131 rose bengal is used if hepatocellular function or biliary patency is to be studied.

Lung scanning

Ten drops of Lugol's solution in an ounce of water is given on the day before the scan to block the thyroid gland. If it is impossible to give the Lugol's earlier, 10 drops may be given immediately before the procedure. In any case, administration of Lugol's solution is continued for 3 subsequent days.

The patient lies quietly in the recumbent position before the injection. Three hundred microcuries of ^{131}I MAA (macroaggregated serum albumin) is injected intravenously. The scan is begun immediately thereafter. The dose of MAA should not exceed 0.1 mg. protein per kilogram body weight. The injection is given over a period of from 6 to 10 seconds to average out differences in respiratory cycles. The posterior aspect of the thorax is routinely scanned, but anterior and lateral views increase the value of the examination. A chest radiograph is obtained routinely. Indium-113m in the form of iron hydroxide particles has advantages described in Chapter X.

Indium-113m as ^{113m}In-Fe(OH)$_3$ has been utilized for lung scanning in several laboratories. The material is made in the following manner using sterile, nonpyrogenic reagents:

To 8cc. ^{113m}In eluted from a ^{113m}Sn-^{113m}In generator in 0.05 N hydrochloric acid is added 0.1 ml. Fe(Cl)$_3$ containing 100 micrograms of ferric ion; this is titrated with 0.5 N sodium hydroxide to pH 10.5 to 12.0. Stir for 2 minutes and add 1 ml. 20 per cent gelatin, U.S.P. Titrate with dilute hydrochloric acid to pH 7.5 to 8.0. Sterilize by autoclaving at 15 p.s.i. for 20 minutes. The particle size of the ^{113m}In-Fe(OH)$_3$ compound should be between 20 to 50 microns (with very few large particles) as seen in a hemacytometer. Immediate lung uptake will be of the order of 90 per cent with less than 5 per cent in the liver. The usual dose for lung scanning is 1 to 2 mc. given intravenously. Scanning is begun immediately after injection.

Bone scanning

A dose of 100 to 200 μc. strontium-85 as inorganic strontium nitrate is given intravenously at least 48 to 72 hours before the scan. The radiograph should include the area of the scan and should be taken while the patient is still in the scanning position. Recently 2 mc. of ^{87m}Sr has been found to be more satisfactory. In this case the scan is performed 2 to 4 hours after administration.

PERIPHERAL CIRCULATION

Leg

The patient should receive 10 drops of Lugol's solution on the day of the study and on each of the subsequent 3 days. To produce reactive hyperemia, and increase the difference between normal persons and patients with circulatory diseases, a pneumatic cuff is applied over the lower extremity up to the level of the mid thigh. The inguinal area is draped with sterile towels and swabbed with Merthiolate. The operator, wearing surgical gloves, injects 1 per cent Xylocaine intradermally and subcutaneously at the injection site. A No. 20 needle is inserted into the femoral artery and directed upstream. The cuff is inflated for 5 minutes at a pressure 10 mm. above the mean arterial pressure (diastolic pressure + one third of the pulse pressure = mean arterial pressure).

A syringe containing 400 μc. of MAA ^{131}I is attached to the No. 20 needle and the contents are injected 20 seconds after release of the cuff. Just before injection, the syringe is shaken to insure uniform mixing of the MAA particles. After injection, blood is withdrawn into the syringe, which is flushed several times.

Marks are made on the lower extremity of the patient at the medial malleolus, mid patella, and upper limits of the cuff. The posterior aspect of the lower extremity is scanned and total counts recorded from below the toes up to the medial malleolus. The radioactivity at 4 cm. intervals above the medial malleolus to the mid thigh is also measured.

The volume of each 4 cm. segment of the leg is found by recording the volume of water displaced as the leg is progressively immersed in a water-filled container.

In addition to obtaining an image of the distribution of the radioactivity by scanning, the data are quantified as follows: All recorded radioactivity in the hyperemic zone from foot to mid thigh is considered as 100 per cent. The percentage of blood flow to segments within the hyperemic zone is calculated by dividing the counts recorded from each 4 cm. segment by the total radioactivity in the entire hyperemic zone.

$$\% \text{ blood flow} = \frac{\text{Counts per 4 cm. segment} \times 100}{\text{Total counts foot to mid thigh}}$$

The percentage of blood flow per unit volume is obtained by dividing the percentage of blood flow in each segment by the volume of that segment. A correction is made for differences in the lengths of legs among different persons by dividing the distance between the medial malleolus and the mid patella into 10 equal units and calculating the percentage blood flow per unit volume for each of these units.

Arm

The patient is given 10 drops of Lugol's solution on each of 4 days beginning the day of the study. The antecubital area of the patient's arm is draped with sterile towels and swabbed with Merthiolate. One per cent Xylocaine is injected intradermally and into deeper tissues at the injection site. A No. 18 arterial needle is inserted into the brachial artery and directed upstream. A stylet is placed inside the arterial needle. A syringe containing 300 μc. of ^{131}I MAA is shaken to insure mixing and attached to the arterial needle after removal of the stylet. The MAA ^{131}I is then injected. The syringe is flushed three times with blood. To prevent bleeding, local pressure is applied to the injection site for 5 to 10 minutes after the arterial needle is removed.

The arm is marked at the mid forearm (midway between the olecranon and ulnar styloid), the ulnar styloid, and the metacarpal heads. An image of the distribution of radioactivity is made by scanning the posterior aspect of the arm. Care is taken to keep the hand and fingers in the focal plane of the collimator. The scan is obtained from mid forearm to fingertips; total counts are determined in the regions demarcated by mid forearm, ulnar styloid, metacarpal heads, and fingertips.

The volume of each segment is measured by displacement of water, as in the leg studies. The calculations of the percentage of blood flow per segment are also made as in the leg studies. In the case of the arms, the total radio-activity from mid forearm to fingertips is considered as 100 per cent.

ACCRETION OF ^{87m}Sr IN EPIPHYSES AND METAPHYSES AS AN INDEX OF GROWTH

The patient is given an intravenous injection of approximately 1 mc. of ^{87m}Sr in an accurately measured volume. Using an external detector, we measure the rate of accumulation of radioactivity over the knees, mid shaft, and ankles immediately after injection and every half hour during the first 6 hours and several times on the following day. A standard solution of ^{87m}Sr containing a known amount of activity is prepared. Because of the short half-life of ^{87m}Sr (2.8 hours), the standard should be counted at the beginning and end of each measurement, and the average of these two count rates used in the calculation. The results are expressed as the percentage of the injected dose in each region at various times after injection. These values are graphed as a function of time. The scanning image of the joints is also obtained.

CISTERNOGRAPHY

A 1 per cent solution of ^{131}I serum albumin with a specific activity of 250 to 500 μc. per cubic centimeter is used. One hundred microcuries of the ^{131}I serum albumin is diluted to 5 cc. with saline and injected into the subarachnoid space, the usual site of lumbar puncture. At 2, 4, 7, and 24 hours after the injection, a lateral view of the brain is obtained by scanning. Cotton plugs are placed in the nose at the time the radioactivity is seen at the region of the skull. These are changed every hour for 3 hours and are then counted in a well scintillation counter. In a normal person no radioactivity will be found on the cotton. If there is radioactivity present, it suggests a leakage of spinal fluid. Contamination of the cotton plugs with saliva or blood should be avoided.

APPENDIX

GREEK ALPHABET

ALPHA	A	α		NU	N	ν
BETA	B	β		XI	Ξ	ξ
GAMMA	Γ	γ		OMICRON	O	o
DELTA	Δ	δ		PI	Π	π
EPSILON	E	ϵ		RHO	P	ρ
ZETA	Z	ζ		SIGMA	Σ	σ
ETA	H	η		TAU	T	τ
THETA	Θ	θ		UPSILON	Y	υ
IOTA	I	ι		PHI	Φ	ϕ
KAPPA	K	κ		CHI	X	χ
LAMBDA	Λ	λ		PSI	Ψ	ψ
MU	M	μ		OMEGA	Ω	ω

FUNDAMENTAL PHYSICAL CONSTANTS AND CONVERSION FACTORS

CHARGE

e.s.u.	= 1 electrostatic unit
Electron charge	= 4.803×10^{-10} e.s.u.
	= 1.602×10^{-19} coulombs

MASS

a.m.u.	= 1 atomic mass unit
	= 1.66×10^{-24} grams
	= 1/12 the weight of 1 atom of ^{12}C
Electron	= 9.1×10^{-28} g. = .000549 a.m.u.
Proton	= 1.6725×10^{-24} g. = 1.00758 a.m.u.
Neutron	= 1.6757×10^{-24} g. = 1.00893 a.m.u.
Hydrogen atom	= 1.6734×10^{-24} g. = 1.00814 a.m.u.
Alpha particle	= 6.598×10^{-24} g. = 4.0028 a.m.u.

ENERGY

1 electron volt (e.v.)	= 1.602×10^{-12} ergs
1 kilo electron volt (kev.)	= 1.602×10^{-9} ergs
1 million electron volt (Mev.)	= 1.602×10^{-6} ergs
1 watt	= 10^7 ergs/second

MASS-ENERGY RELATIONSHIPS

E (ergs)	= mc^2
1 a.m.u.	= 931 Mev.
Electron rest mass m_o	= 0.511 Mev.

FUNDAMENTAL PHYSICAL CONSTANTS AND CONVERSION FACTORS
(*Continued*)

ACTIVITY UNITS

1 curie (c., Ci)	$= 3.7 \times 10^{10}$ atoms disintegrating/second
1 millicurie (mc., mCi)	$= 3.7 \times 10^{7}$ atoms disintegrating/second
1 microcurie (μc., μCi)	$= 3.7 \times 10^{4}$ atoms disintegrating/second
1 nanocurie (nc., nCi)	$= 37$ atoms disintegrating/second
1 picocurie (pc., pCi)	$= 0.037$ atoms disintegrating/second
1 rutherford (rd.)	$= 10^{6}$ atoms disintegrating/second
1 millicurie	$= 37$ rutherfords
1 roentgen (R)	$= 1$ e.s.u. per cc. standard dry air
1 rad	$= 100$ ergs per g.

EQUIVALENTS OF THE ROENTGEN

1 roentgen = 1 e.s.u. per cc. standard dry air (0.001293 g. air)
= 2.08×10^{9} ion pairs/cc. standard dry air
= 1.61×10^{12} ion pairs/g. dry air
at 33.7 **e.v./ion** pair, 1 roentgen = 7.01×10^{4} Mev./cc. standard dry air
= 5.43×10^{7} Mev./g. dry air
= 86.9 ergs/g. dry air

SOME FUNDAMENTAL CONSTANTS AND FORMULAE

1. **Angstrom unit (Å)** $= 10^{-8}$ cm.
2. Avogadro's number (N_0) $= 6.025 \times 10^{23}$ molecules per gram-mole
3. Compton wavelength (h/mc) $= 0.02426$ Å
4. Change in wavelength of a photon scattered in a Compton interaction is given by:
$$\Delta\lambda = 0.02426 \, (1 - \text{Cos } \theta)$$
where: $\Delta\lambda$ = change in wavelength in angstrom units;
θ = the scattering angle formed by the path of the primary gamma-ray and the path of the scattered gamma-ray
5. Euler's number: e = 2.718281828459045 . . .
6. Molar volume: V_0 = 22.42 liters/gram molecular weight
7. Planck's constant: h = 6.625×10^{-27} erg sec./cycle
8. Velocity of light: c = 2.998×10^{10} cm./sec.
9. Energy-frequency: E = hf; where E is in ergs, h is Planck's constant, and f is frequency in cycles/second

10. Energy-wavelength: $E = h \frac{c}{\lambda}$; where c is velocity of light and λ is wavelength in units of length reciprocal to those used for stating c. Converting energy from ergs to kev., and wavelength to angstrom units, we get: E in kev. $\times \lambda$ in Å = 12.4 kev. Å.

TABLE FOR COMPUTATION OF $\dfrac{A}{A_0} = e^{-.693 \frac{t}{T_{\frac{1}{2}}}}$

$\dfrac{A}{A_0}$	$\dfrac{t}{T_{\frac{1}{2}}}$	$\dfrac{A}{A_0}$	$\dfrac{t}{T_{\frac{1}{2}}}$	$\dfrac{A}{A_0}$	$\dfrac{t}{T_{\frac{1}{2}}}$	$\dfrac{A}{A_0}$	$\dfrac{t}{T_{\frac{1}{2}}}$
.00	0	.75	0.415	.50	1.000	.25	2.000
.99	0.014	.74	0.435	.49	1.030	.24	2.060
.98	0.029	.73	0.454	.48	1.060	.23	2.121
.97	0.044	.72	0.474	.47	1.090	.22	2.187
.96	0.055	.71	0.494	.46	1.121	.21	2.252
.95	0.074	.70	0.515	.45	1.153	.20	2.321
.94	0.089	.69	0.535	.44	1.185	.19	2.400
.93	0.105	.68	0.556	.43	1.218	.18	2.478
.92	0.120	.67	0.578	.42	1.252	.17	2.560
.91	0.136	.66	0.600	.41	1.287	.16	2.648
.90	0.152	.65	0.622	.40	1.323	.15	2.740
.89	0.168	.64	0.644	.39	1.360	.14	2.840
.88	0.184	.63	0.667	.38	1.397	.13	2.946
.87	0.201	.62	0.690	.37	1.445	.12	3.060
.86	0.218	.61	0.713	.36	1.475	.11	3.188
.85	0.235	.60	0.737	.35	1.515	.10	3.325
.84	0.252	.59	0.762	.34	1.557	.09	3.478
.83	0.269	.58	0.786	.33	1.600	.08	3.649
.82	0.286	.57	0.811	.32	1.645	.07	3.840
.81	0.304	.56	0.836	.31	1.691	.06	4.060
.80	0.322	.55	0.863	.30	1.739	.05	4.325
.79	0.340	.54	0.889	.29	1.787	.04	4.650
.78	0.359	.53	0.916	.28	1.839	.03	5.060
.77	0.377	.52	0.944	.27	1.890	.02	5.640
.76	0.396	.51	0.972	.26	1.945	.01	6.640

PHYSICAL DATA FOR A NUMBER OF RADIOACTIVE NUCLIDES[*]

In this table are listed a large number of the radioactive nuclides currently used in medical practice or in research. The data represent a collection from a number of published sources. Most of the radioactive decay data are from the Table of Isotopes by Strominger, Hollander, and Seaborg, in Reviews of Modern Physics, April, 1958. Values for average beta energies and for Γ have been either taken from Radiation Dosimetry, by Hine and Brownell, Academic Press, 1956, National Bureau of Standards Handbook 78 (Report of International Commission on Radiological Units and Measurements, 1959), or computed by Quimby and Feitelberg.

---

[*] From Quimby, E. H., and Feitelberg, S.: Radioactive Isotopes in Medicine and Biology. Lea & Febiger, Philadelphia, 1963.

ELEMENT	ATOMIC NUMBER Z	MASS NUMBER A	HALF PERIOD	RADIATION	$\bar{E}_\beta$ MEV.	Γ† Γ PER MC.-HR. AT 1 CM.
Antimony	51	122	67 hr	β^-,γ	0.566	2.7
		124	60 da	β^-,γ	0.35	9.8
Argon	18	37	35 da	EC	0 003	
Arsenic	33	74	17.5 da	β^+,β^-,γ	0.37	5.1
		76	26.8 hr	β^-,γ	1.14	3.1
Beryllium	4	7	53 da	EC,γ	0.00005	0.3
Bismuth	83	210	5 da	β^-	0.375	
Bromine	35	82	35.7 hr	β^-,γ	0.142	14.6
Cadmium	48	109	1.3 yr	EC	0.023	
Calcium	20	45	164 da	β^-	0.077	
(with scandium 47)		47	4.7 da	β^-,γ	0.553	5.95
Carbon	6	11	20.4 min	β^+	0.380	6.2
		14	5570 yr	β^-	0.050	
Cerium	58	141	33 da	β^-,γ	0.150	0.5
Cesium	55	134	2.3 yr	β^-,γ	0.116	8.0
(with barium 137m)		137	30 yr	β^-,γ	0.242	3.0
Chlorine	17	38	37.3 min	β^-,γ	1.50	8.64
Chromium	24	51	27.8 da	EC,γ	0.005	0.18
Cobalt	27	57	270 da	EC	0.007	
		58	72 da	EC,β^+,γ	0.035	5.4
		60	5.2 yr	β^-,γ	0.093	12.9
Copper	29	64	12.8 hr	EC,β^+,β^-,γ	0 130	1.1
Gallium	31	72	14.3 hr	β^-,γ	0.475	13.6
Gold	79	198	2.69 da	β^-,γ	0.328	2.27
		199	3.15 da	β^-,γ	0.13	0.42
Hydrogen	1	3	12.26 yr	β^-	0.006	
Iodine	53	125	60 da	EC,γ	0.027	0.6
		130	12.6 hr	β^-,γ	0.285	12.1
		131	8.1 da	β^-,γ	0.188	2 20
		132	2.33 hr	β^-,γ	0.483	12.3
Iron	26	55	2 94 yr	EC	0.006	
		59	45 da	β^-,γ	0.118	6.8
Indium	49	113m	1.7 hr	EC,γ	0.113	1.75
Krypton	36	85	10.3 yr	β^-,γ	0.224	0.02
Lanthanum	57	140	40 hr	β^-,γ	0.54	12.0
Magnesium	12	28	21.2 hr	β^-,γ	1.38	10.2
(with aluminium 28)						
Manganese	25	52	5.8 da	EC,β^+,γ	0.072	18.5
		54	320 da	EC,γ	0.006	4.7

† For positron emitters the energy of the annihilation radiation is included in Γ.

PHYSICAL DATA FOR A NUMBER OF RADIOACTIVE NUCLIDES
(*Continued*)

ELEMENT	ATOMIC NUMBER Z	MASS NUMBER A	HALF PERIOD	RADIATION	$\overline{E}_\beta$ MEV.	Γ† Γ PER MC.-HR. AT 1 CM.
Mercury	80	197	2.7 da	EC,γ	0.08	0.4
		203	47.9 da	β⁻,γ	0.10	1.2
Molybdenum	42	99	66 hr	β⁻,γ	0.400	1.29
Nickel	28	56	6.4 da	EC	0.007	
		63	125 yr	β⁻	0.018	
Niobium	41	95	35 da	β⁻,γ	0.043	4.5
Phosphorus	15	32	14.3 da	β⁻	0.70	
Potassium	19	42	12.5 hr	β⁻,γ	1.45	1.4
Praesodymium	59	142	19.3 hr	β⁻,γ	0.79	0.64
		143	13.7 da	β⁻	0.315	
Promethium	61	147	2.5 yr	β⁻	0.062	
Radium (in equilibrium with Rn, Ra A, B, and C)	88	226	1620 yr	α,β⁻,γ	No β with filter	8.25 with 0.5 mm Pt filter
Rubidium	37	86	18.6 da	β⁻,γ	0.68	0.49
Scandium	21	46	85 da	β⁻,γ	0.12	11.0
		47	3.4 da	β⁻,γ	0.146	0.48
Selenium	34	75	127 da	EC,γ	0.011	1.84
Silver	47	111	7.5 da	β⁻,γ	0.34	0.17
Sodium	11	22	2.6 yr	β⁺,γ	0.193	13.2
		24	15 hr	β⁻,γ	0.56	18.7
Strontium	38	85	65 da	EC,γ	0.014	3.2
		89	54 da	β⁻	0.56	
(with yttrium-90)		90	28 yr	β⁻	0.20 + 0.93	
Sulfur	16	35	87 da	β⁻	0.049	
Technetium	43	99	6 hr	EC,γ	0.014	0.56
Tellurium	52	121	17 da	EC,γ	0.027	3.4
Thallium	81	204	4.1 yr	β⁻,EC	0.234	
Thulium	69	170	125 da	β⁻,γ	0.32	0.01
Tin (with indium-113m)	50	113	115 da	EC,γ	0.025	3.5
Tungsten	74	185	74 da	β⁻	0.130	
Vanadium	23	48	16 da	β⁺,EC,γ	0.14	10.0
Xenon	54	133	5.27 da	β⁻,γ	0.110	0.44
Yttrium	39	90	64.6 hr	β⁻	0.93	
		91	58 da	β⁻,γ	0.585	0.21
Zinc	30	65	245 da	EC,β⁺,γ	0.010	2.9
Zirconium (with niobium-95)	40	95	65 da	β⁻,γ	0.163	9.0

Iridium-192 and tantalum-182, which are being used in interstitial therapy, have not been included in this table because of uncertainties in the value of Γ and $\overline{E}_\beta$. At present treatments are usually based on rather empirically determined "radium equivalents."

SUMMARY OF DOSE LIMITS FOR INDIVIDUALS*

ORGAN OR TISSUE	MAXIMUM PERMISSIBLE DOSES FOR ADULTS EXPOSED IN THE COURSE OF THEIR WORK	DOSE LIMITS FOR MEMBERS OF THE PUBLIC
Gonads, red bone-marrow	5 rems in a year	0.5 rem in a year
Skin, bone, thyroid	30 rems in a year	3 rems in a year†
Hands and forearms; feet and ankles	75 rems in a year	7.5 rems in a year
Other single organs	15 rems in a year	1.5 rems in a year

* From Recommendations of the International Commission on Radiological Protection. (Adopted September 17, 1965.) Publication 9. Pergamon Press, New York, 1966.

† 1.5 rems in a year to the thyroid of children up to 16 years of age.

THE GONAD DOSE PER EXAMINATION ACCORDING TO MEASUREMENTS ON PATIENTS BY HAMMER-JACOBSEN, AND BY LARS-ERIC LARSSON*

(Exposure of Man to Ionizing Radiation Arising from Medical Procedures, a report of ICRP and ICRU, 1957.)

EXAMINATION	GONAD DOSE PER EXAMINATION (MRAD) (MINIMUM AND MAXIMUM VALUES) †	
	MALE	FEMALE
Intravenous pyelography	20–3900	60–4100
Urethrocystography	200–17000	200–1600
Hip	20–3600	30–450
Femur	50–3500	20–100
Pelvimetry		400–2500
Pelvis	50–2800	70–300
Lumbar and sacral spine	70–1200	500–900
Abdomen	40–2700	20–1300
Hysterosalpingography		140–6700
Barium enema	50–500	1100–2900
Barium meal	2–30	8–80
Chest	1–3	3–10
Cholecystography	1–10	10–40

* From Recommendations of the International Commission on Radiological Protection. Publication 3. Pergamon Press, New York, 1960.

† The great spread of the values for the gonad dose per examination is mainly due to wide variations in techniques used.

865

LEAD HALF VALUE LAYERS AND GAMMA RAY DOSE FACTORS FOR VARIOUS RADIOACTIVE NUCLIDES*

ISOTOPE	HALF VALUE LAYER CM. LEAD	Γ Γ PER MC.-HR. AT 1 CM.
Bromine-82	1.0	14.6
Cesium-137	0.5	3.0
Chromium-51	0.2	0.18
Cobalt-60	1.2	12.9
Copper-64	0.4	1.1
Gold-198	0.3	2.27
Iodine-130	0.7	12.1
Iodine-131	0.3	2.20
Iodine-132	1.0	12.3
Iron-59	1.1	6.8
Manganese-52	1.0	18.5
Potassium-42	1.2	1.40
Sodium-22	1.0	13.2
Sodium-24	1.5	18.7
Tin-113	0.3	3.5
Zinc-65	1.0	2.9

* From Quimby, E. H., and Feitelberg, S.: Radioactive Isotopes in Medicine and Biology. Lea & Febiger, Philadelphia, 1963.

AVERAGE DOSES TO SELECTED ORGANS FOR VARIOUS AGES IN RADS/MICROCURIE ADMINISTERED FOR DIAGNOSTIC TESTS EMPLOYING RADIOACTIVE ISOTOPES*

ORGAN	RADIONUCLIDE	ROUTE OF ADMINISTRATION	DOSE					
			NEWBORN RADS/ MICROCURIE	1 YR. RADS/ MICROCURIE	5 YR. RADS/ MICROCURIE	10 YR. RADS/ MICROCURIE	15 YR. RADS/ MICROCURIE	STANDARD MAN RADS/ MICROCURIE
Liver	$Na_2H^{32}PO_4$	Intravenous	0.55	0.17	0.10	0.06	0.04	0.03
	Colloidal ^{198}Au	Intravenous	0.49	0.20	0.12	0.08	0.05	0.04
	^{57}Cobalt-labeled vitamin B_{12}	Oral	1.5	0.68	0.41	0.28	0.21	0.16
	^{58}Cobalt-labeled vitamin B_{12}	Oral	2.3	1.2	0.76	0.54	0.42	0.33
	^{60}Cobalt-labeled vitamin B_{12}	Oral	30.0	15.0	10.0	6.9	5.3	4.2
Spleen	$Na_2H^{32}PO_4$	Intravenous	0.55	0.17	0.10	0.06	0.04	0.03
	Colloid ^{198}Au	Intravenous	0.49	0.20	0.12	0.08	0.05	0.04
	$Na_2^{51}Cr_2O_4$ "altered red cell"	Intravenous	0.49	0.16	0.10	0.05	0.04	0.04
Bone and marrow	$Na_2H^{32}PO_4$	Intravenous	0.55	0.17	0.10	0.06	0.04	0.03
Thyroid	$Na^{131}I$	Oral	32.0	10.0	4.3	3.1	1.7	1.3
	$Na^{125}I$	Oral	19.0	6.1	2.6	1.8	1.0	0.82
	$Na^{132}I$	Oral	1.2	0.40	0.17	0.12	0.07	0.05
Kidney	Chlormerodrin	Intravenous	0.66	0.22	0.14	0.09	0.07	0.06
	Hippuran ^{131}I	Intravenous	0.01	0.004	0.003	0.002	0.001	0.001
	Hippuran ^{125}I	Intravenous	0.002	0.0006	0.0004	0.0002	0.0002	0.0002

* From Seltzer, R. A., Kereiakes, J. G., and Saenger, E. L.: Radiation Exposure from Radioisotopes in Pediatrics. *New England J. Med.* 271:84, 1964. Reproduced with permission of The New England Journal of Medicine.

AVERAGE WHOLE-BODY DOSES FOR VARIOUS AGES IN
MILLIRADS/MICROCURIE ADMINISTERED FOR DIAGNOSTIC
TESTS EMPLOYING RADIOACTIVE ISOTOPES*

RADIONUCLIDE	ROUTE OF ADMINISTRATION	PURPOSE OF PROCEDURE	DOSE					
			NEWBORN MILLIRADS/MICROCURIE	1 YR. MILLIRADS/MICROCURIE	5 YR. MILLIRADS/MICROCURIE	10 YR. MILLIRADS/MICROCURIE	15 YR. MILLIRADS/MICROCURIE	STANDARD MAN MILLIRADS/MICROCURIE
$^{55}Fe_2Cl_6$	Oral	Iron absorption	12.0	3.4	2.0	1.2	0.75	0.59
$^{59}Fe_2Cl_6$	Oral		40.0	15.0	9.1	5.9	3.9	3.3
$^{55}Fe_2Cl_6$	Intravenous	Plasma iron transport	120.0	34.0	20.0	12.0	7.5	5.9
$^{59}Fe_2Cl_6$	Intravenous	Degree and site of erythropoiesis	290.0	110.0	65.0	42.0	27.0	23.0
$Na_2{}^{51}CrO_4$	Intravenous	Red-cell volume, survival, gastrointestinal blood loss, and splenic scan	4.5	1.6	0.98	0.63	0.41	0.34
$^{51}CrCl_3$	Intravenous	Plasma volume, gastrointestinal protein loss	2.3	0.80	0.40	0.31	0.20	0.17
^{57}Cobalt-labeled vitamin B_{12}		Vitamin B_{12} absorption	54.0	22.0	14.0	9.1	6.1	5.3
^{58}Cobalt-labeled vitamin B_{12}			210.0	85.0	54.0	35.0	24.0	21.0
^{60}Cobalt-labeled vitamin B_{12}			2400.0	1000.0	630.0	410.0	270.0	240.0
$Na_2H^{32}PO_4$	Intravenous	Tumor localization	170.0	48.0	29.0	17.0	11.0	8.4
Colloidal ^{198}Au	Intravenous	Liver blood flow, scan	5.4	2.2	1.4	0.92	0.62	0.54
Chlormerodrin	Intravenous	Kidney scan, brain scan	2.1	0.84	0.53	0.36	0.23	0.20
Na ^{131}I	Oral		10.0	2.0	1.3	0.81	0.53	0.45
Na ^{125}I	Oral	Thyroid function, scan	9.4	1.6	1.0	0.67	0.44	0.39
Na ^{132}I	Oral		1.1	0.44	0.27	0.17	0.11	0.09
R ^{131}ISA	Intravenous	Plasma volume, cardiac output, gastrointestinal protein loss, and brain scan	28.0	8.9	5.4	3.4	2.1	1.7
Oleic acid ^{131}I or Triolein ^{131}I	Oral or intravenous	Lipid absorption, blood clearance	10.0	3.3	2.0	1.2	0.78	0.65
PVP ^{131}I	Intravenous	Gastrointestinal protein loss, brain scan	18.0	5.8	3.5	2.2	1.4	1.1
Rose Bengal ^{131}I	Intravenous	Liver blood flow, scan, function	3.7	1.5	0.92	0.61	0.40	0.36
Hippuran ^{131}I	Intravenous	Kidney function	0.33	0.13	0.08	0.06	0.04	0.03
Hippuran ^{125}I	Intravenous		0.09	0.04	0.02	0.02	0.01	0.01

* From Seltzer, R. A., Kereiakes, J. G., and Saenger, E. L.: Radiation Exposure from Isotopes in Pediatrics. *New England J. Med.* 271:84, 1964. Reproduced with permission of The New England Journal of Medicine.

BODY WEIGHTS, ORGAN WEIGHTS, AND CALCULATED GEOMETRICAL FACTORS FOR VARIOUS AGES*

AGE	WHOLE BODY WEIGHT GM.	$\bar{g}$ CM.	KIDNEY WEIGHT GM.	$\bar{g}$ CM.	LIVER WEIGHT GM.	$\bar{g}$ CM.	SPLEEN WEIGHT GM.	$\bar{g}$ CM.
Newborn	3,540	64	23	16	136	27	9.4	12
1 yr.	12,100	89	72	22	333	36	31.0	17
5 yr.	20,300	94	112	25	591	44	54.0	20
10 yr.	33,500	102	187	30	918	50	101.0	25
15 yr.	55,000	112	247	33	1289	55	138.0	28
Standard man	70,000	126	300	35	1700	59	150.0	29

* From Seltzer, R. A., Kereiakes, J. G., and Saenger, E. L.: Radiation Exposure from Radioisotopes in Pediatrics. *New England J. Med.* 271:84, 1964. Reproduced with permission of The New England Journal of Medicine.

ABSORBED FRACTIONS FOR CENTRAL POINT SOURCE GAMMA EMITTERS IN SPHERES*

MASS IN KG.	ENERGIES IN MEV. 0.020	0.030	0.040	0.060	0.100	0.140	0.160	0.279	0.662	2.75
2	0.989	0.794	0.548	0.322	0.243	0.233	0.239	0.241	0.239	0.171
4	0.996	0.878	0.669	0.421	0.317	0.301	0.303	0.302	0.298	0.213
6	0.999	0.916	0.736	0.488	0.370	0.348	0.349	0.344	0.336	0.242
8	0.999	0.938	0.782	0.540	0.413	0.386	0.387	0.377	0.365	0.264
10	0.999	0.952	0.815	0.581	0.448	0.418	0.418	0.405	0.388	0.282
20	0.999	0.982	0.901	0.709	0.569	0.529	0.527	0.500	0.463	0.345
30	0.999	0.991	0.938	0.780	0.644	0.600	0.598	0.562	0.522	0.386
40	0.999	0.995	0.957	0.826	0.698	0.652	0.650	0.608	0.562	0.418
50	0.999	0.996	0.969	0.859	0.738	0.692	0.690	0.644	0.595	0.443
60	0.999	0.997	0.976	0.882	0.770	0.725	0.722	0.675	0.622	0.464
70	0.999	0.998	0.981	0.900	0.796	0.752	0.749	0.700	0.646	0.483
80	0.999	0.998	0.985	0.915	0.818	0.775	0.772	0.722	0.666	0.500
90	0.999	0.999	0.987	0.926	0.836	0.794	0.791	0.741	0.684	0.514
100	0.999	0.999	0.989	0.935	0.851	0.811	0.808	0.758	0.700	0.528
120	0.999	0.999	0.992	0.948	0.876	0.839	0.835	0.786	0.728	0.552
140	0.999	0.999	0.994	0.958	0.895	0.860	0.857	0.809	0.751	0.572
160	0.999	0.999	0.996	0.965	0.910	0.878	0.874	0.829	0.770	0.580
180	0.999	0.999	0.997	0.971	0.923	0.892	0.889	0.845	0.786	0.606
200	0.999	0.999	0.998	0.976	0.933	0.904	0.901	0.858	0.800	0.621

* Data from Ellett, W. H., Callahan, A. B., and Brownell, G. L.: Gamma-Ray Dosimetry of Internal Emitters. Monte Carlo Calculations of Absorbed Dose from Point Sources. *Brit. J. Radiol.* 37:45, 1964; II. Monte Carlo Calculations of Absorbed Dose from Uniform Sources. *Brit. J. Radiol.* 38:541, 1965; III. Monte Carlo Calculations of Absorbed Dose for Low-Energy Gamma-Rays. *Brit. J. Radiol.* Submitted for publication, Jan. 1967.

ABSORBED FRACTIONS FOR CENTRAL POINT GAMMA EMITTERS IN ELLIPTICAL CYLINDERS AND ELLIPSOIDS*†

MASS IN KG.	ENERGIES IN MEV.												
	0.020	0.030	0.040	0.060	0.080	0.100	0.140	0.160	0.279	0.364	0.662	1.460	2.75 Radium
2	0.924	0.605	0.374	0.203	0.169	0.159	0.160	0.164	0.171	0.180	0.179	0.160	0.127	0.166
4	0.956	0.697	0.461	0.263	0.217	0.202	0.200	0.205	0.214	0.221	0.220	0.196	0.157	0.205
6	0.971	0.749	0.518	0.305	0.253	0.233	0.229	0.235	0.242	0.250	0.247	0.221	0.178	0.231
8	0.980	0.785	0.560	0.340	0.283	0.258	0.252	0.258	0.265	0.272	0.268	0.240	0.194	0.251
10	0.985	0.811	0.594	0.368	0.308	0.280	0.272	0.277	0.283	0.290	0.285	0.256	0.207	0.267
20	0.995	0.881	0.698	0.468	0.397	0.358	0.342	0.347	0.348	0.354	0.345	0.311	0.255	0.325
30	0.998	0.914	0.757	0.534	0.456	0.413	0.341	0.394	0.391	0.396	0.385	0.347	0.287	0.363
40	0.998	0.934	0.796	0.581	0.501	0.456	0.429	0.431	0.424	0.428	0.415	0.374	0.311	0.391
50	0.999	0.946	0.824	0.619	0.537	0.491	0.460	0.461	0.450	0.454	0.439	0.396	0.331	0.414
60	0.999	0.956	0.845	0.649	0.567	0.520	0.487	0.487	0.473	0.476	0.460	0.415	0.348	0.433
70	0.999	0.963	0.862	0.674	0.593	0.545	0.511	0.509	0.493	0.496	0.478	0.431	0.362	0.450
80	0.999	0.968	0.875	0.696	0.616	0.567	0.532	0.529	0.511	0.513	0.493	0.445	0.375	0.465
90	0.999	0.972	0.886	0.715	0.636	0.587	0.551	0.547	0.527	0.528	0.507	0.458	0.386	0.478
100	0.999	0.976	0.896	0.731	0.654	0.604	0.568	0.564	0.542	0.542	0.520	0.470	0.397	0.490
120	0.999	0.981	0.911	0.759	0.685	0.634	0.597	0.592	0.567	0.567	0.543	0.490	0.416	0.512
140	0.999	0.985	0.922	0.782	0.710	0.660	0.622	0.617	0.589	0.588	0.562	0.508	0.432	0.530
160	0.999	0.987	0.932	0.801	0.731	0.681	0.644	0.639	0.609	0.606	0.580	0.523	0.446	0.547
180	0.999	0.989	0.940	0.818	0.750	0.700	0.662	0.658	0.627	0.623	0.595	0.537	0.458	0.562
200	0.999	0.990	0.948	0.833	0.765	0.717	0.678	0.675	0.643	0.638	0.610	0.550	0.470	0.576

* The elliptical cylinders and ellipsoids have their principal axes in the ratios of 1/1.8/6.19 and 1/1.8/9.27, respectively.
† Data from Ellett, Callahan, and Brownell.

ABSORBED FRACTIONS FOR CENTRAL POINT SOURCE GAMMA EMITTERS IN STRAIGHT CYLINDERS*†

MASS IN KG.	ENERGIES IN MEV.					
	0.040	0.080	0.160	0.364	0.662	1.460
2	0.538	0.264	0.229	0.245	0.234	0.205
4	0.655	0.344	0.297	0.301	0.294	0.258
6	0.721	0.400	0.342	0.339	0.331	0.291
8	0.766	0.445	0.378	0.369	0.360	0.317
10	0.798	0.481	0.407	0.394	0.382	0.337
20	0.884	0.604	0.510	0.480	0.461	0.407
30	0.922	0.679	0.578	0.537	0.512	0.453
40	0.944	0.732	0.629	0.578	0.552	0.487
50	0.958	0.771	0.669	0.614	0.584	0.516
60	0.967	0.802	0.702	0.643	0.611	0.541
70	0.974	0.827	0.730	0.667	0.634	0.562
80	0.979	0.848	0.753	0.688	0.655	0.580
90	0.983	0.865	0.774	0.707	0.673	0.597
100	0.986	0.879	0.791	0.724	0.689	0.612
120	0.990	0.901	0.820	0.751	0.717	0.638
140	0.993	0.917	0.842	0.774	0.739	0.659
160	0.994	0.928	0.859	0.793	0.757	0.678
180	0.994	0.937	0.872	0.808	0.772	0.693
200	0.994	0.942	0.883	0.821	0.784	0.706

* The principal axes of the straight cylinders are in the ratio of 1/1/0.75.
† Data from Ellett, Callahan, and Brownell.

ABSORBED FRACTIONS FOR A UNIFORM DISTRIBUTION OF ACTIVITY IN ELLIPSOIDS*†

MASS IN KG.	ENERGIES IN Mev.										
	0.020	0.030	0.040	0.060	0.080	0.100	0.160	0.364	0.662	1.46	2.75
2	0.702	0.407	0.316	0.131	0.0771	0.0987	0.116	0.115	0.135	0.0992	0 100
4	0.762	0.485	0.327	0.176	0.131	0.133	0.147	0.151	0.157	0.136	0.122
6	0.795	0.529	0.349	0.206	0.162	0.155	0.166	0.174	0.176	0.158	0.137
8	0.815	0.560	0.371	0.228	0.184	0.172	0.181	0.191	0.192	0.174	0.150
10	0.830	0.583	0.391	0.247	0.201	0.185	0.194	0.204	0.206	0.186	0.160
20	0.868	0.649	0.467	0.308	0.255	0.233	0.238	0.249	0.254	0.227	0.191
30	0.884	0.685	0.515	0.346	0.289	0.265	0.268	0.277	0.284	0.252	0.211
40	0.893	0.709	0.548	0.374	0.316	0.290	0.292	0.299	0.305	0.271	0.227
50	0.900	0.727	0.572	0.397	0.338	0.312	0.311	0.317	0.321	0.286	0.240
60	0.905	0.741	0.591	0.416	0.357	0.330	0.327	0.332	0.335	0.299	0.252
70	0.909	0.753	0.606	0.432	0.375	0.346	0.341	0.345	0.346	0.310	0.263
80	0.912	0.763	0.618	0.446	0.390	0.361	0.353	0.356	0.356	0.321	0.272
90	0.916	0.772	0.629	0.459	0.404	0.374	0.365	0.367	0.365	0.330	0.281
100	0.918	0.780	0.640	0.471	0.417	0.386	0.375	0.377	0.373	0.339	0.290
120	0.924	0.793	0.659	0.492	0.439	0.407	0.394	0.395	0.390	0.355	0.305
140	0.929	0.804	0.678	0.511	0.458	0.425	0.412	0.411	0.406	0.370	0.317
160	0.933	0.814	0.698	0.528	0.473	0.440	0.429	0.426	0.423	0.384	0.328
180	0.937	0.821	0.720	0.544	0.486	0.454	0.445	0.440	0.441	0.398	0.338
200	0.940	0.828	0.744	0.559	0.497	0.466	0.461	0.453	0.460	0.410	0.347

* The principal axes of the ellipsoids are in the ratio of 1/1.8/9.27.
† Data from Ellett, Callahan, and Brownell.

ABSORBED FRACTIONS FOR A UNIFORM DISTRIBUTION OF ACTIVITY IN SMALL SPHERES AND THICK ELLIPSOIDS*†

MASS IN KG.	ENERGIES IN Mev.										
	0.020	0.030	0.040	0.060	0.080	0.100	0.160	0.364	0.662	1.460	2.750
0.3	0.684	0.357	0.195	0.109	0.0880	0.0850	0.0891	0.101	0.0988	0.0937	0.0780
0 4	0.712	0.388	0.216	0.121	0.0980	0.0930	0.0988	0.110	0.111	0.100	0.0850
0.5	0.731	0.412	0.234	0.131	0.106	0.0990	0.106	0.118	0.119	0.106	0.0900
0.6	0.745	0.431	0.249	0.140	0.114	0.105	0.113	0.124	0.126	0.111	0.0952
1.0	0.780	0.486	0.295	0.167	0.138	0.125	0.132	0.144	0.146	0.127	0.107
2.0	0.818	0.559	0.366	0.212	0.177	0.160	0.165	0.177	0.176	0.156	0.129
3.0	0.840	0.600	0.412	0.245	0.205	0.188	0.190	0.201	0.198	0.177	0.145
4.0	0.856	0.629	0.445	0.271	0.247	0.227	0.210	0.220	0.217	0.194	0.159
5.0	0.876	0.671	0.492	0.312	0.264	0.241	0.227	0.236	0.232	0.208	0.171
6.0							0.241	0.250	0.244	0.220	0.180

* The principal axes of the small spheres and thick ellipsoids are in the ratios of 1/1/1 and 1/0.667/1.333.

† Data from Ellett, Callahan, and Brownell.

ABSORBED FRACTIONS FOR A UNIFORM DISTRIBUTION OF ACTIVITY IN FLAT ELLIPSOIDS*†

MASS IN KG.	ENERGIES IN MEV.								
	0.020	0.030	0.040	0.060	0.080	0.100	0.160	0.662	2.750
0.3	0.627	0.306	0.167	0.0900	0.0760	0.0720	0.0793	0.0865	0.0630
0.4	0.654	0.334	0.182	0.0980	0.0830	0.0790	0.0859	0.0968	0.0700
0.5	0.674	0.356	0.196	0.106	0.0890	0.0850	0.0918	0.105	0.0760
0.6	0.690	0.374	0.208	0.112	0.093	0.0900	0.0971	0.111	0.0800
1.0	0.731	0.423	0.248	0.134	0.111	0.106	0.114	0.130	0.0940
2.0	0.779	0.492	0.311	0.173	0.143	0.133	0.143	0.156	0.114
3.0	0.803	0.533	0.350	0.200	0.166	0.154	0.162	0.174	0.127
4.0	0.820	0.564	0.378	0.221	0.185	0.171	0.177	0.188	0.139
5.0	0.833	0.588	0.400	0.238	0.202	0.185	0.190	0.201	0.149
6.0	0.844	0.608	0.421	0.254	0.216	0.198	0.202	0.213	0.159

* The principal axes of the flat ellipsoids are in the ratio of 1/0.5/2.0.
† Data from Ellett, Callahan, and Brownell.

ABSORBED FRACTIONS FOR SMALL STRAIGHT CYLINDERS— CENTRAL POINT SOURCE AT CENTER*†

RADIUS (CM.)	1.342	1.897	2.324	2.683	3.000
HEIGHT (CM.)	2.263	3.160	3.871	4.470	5.000
MASS (G.)	12.64	35.74	65.66	101.1	141.3
ENERGY (MEV.)					
0.040	0.0902	0.1316	0.1650	0.1936	0.2193
0.080	0.0387	0.0557	0.0695	0.0814	0.0916
0.160	0.0412	0.0587	0.0730	0.0849	0.0953
0.364	0.0471	0.0660	0.0804	0.0924	0.1029
0.662	0.0475	0.0671	0.0812	0.0936	0.1042
1.460	0.0426	0.0595	0.0728	0.0834	0.0926

* Rossi tissue formula ($C_5H_{40}O_{18}N$) is used in these calculations. It has an electron density of 3.41×10^{23} electrons/cm.^{3}.
† Data from Ellett, Callahan, and Brownell and from personal communications from J. G. Kereiakes and G. K. Bahr, Radioisotope Laboratory, Cincinnati General Hospital, Cincinnati, Ohio.

ABSORBED FRACTIONS FOR STRAIGHT CYLINDERS—CENTRAL POINT SOURCE AT CENTER*†

RADIUS (CM.)	HEIGHT (CM.)	ENERGIES (MEV.)					
		0.040	0.080	0.160	0.364	0.662	1.460
3	5	0.219	0.0916	0.0953	0.103	0.104	0.0926
	10	0.266	0.1134	0.1148	0.124	0.124	0.111
	15	0.279	0.1195	0.1216	0.131	0.131	0.117
	20	0.283	0.1225	0.1243	0.134	0.134	0.120
5	5	0.299	0.128	0.128	0.137	0.140	0.124
	10	0.403	0.179	0.170	0.180	0.181	0.160
	15	0.442	0.200	0.189	0.199	0.199	0.175
	20	0.458	0.210	0.198	0.208	0.208	0.184
10	5	0.379	0.174	0.168	0.183	0.185	0.165
	10	0.582	0.292	0.261	0.268	0.265	0.234
	15	0.682	0.365	0.318	0.318	0.311	0.273
	20	0.731	0.409	0.353	0.348	0.339	0.298

* Rossi tissue formula ($C_5H_{40}O_{18}N$) is used in these calculations. It has an electron density of 3.41×10^{23} electrons/cm.^{3}.

† Data from Ellett, Callahan, and Brownell.

AVERAGE GEOMETRICAL FACTOR, $\bar{g}$, FOR CYLINDERS CONTAINING A UNIFORMLY DISTRIBUTED γ-RAY EMITTER ($\mu = 0.028$)*

LENGTH OF CYLINDER (CM.)	RADIUS OF CYLINDER (CM.)										
	1	2	3	5	7	10	15	20	25	30	35
1	3.8	7.5	10.2	13.0	13.5	13.8	15.1	16.0	17.5	18.0	19.0
2	6.5	11.7	15.7	21.6	23.2	25.2	28.1	30.5	32.8	35.4	37.3
3	8.4	14.7	19.8	27.7	31.0	34.5	39.2	42.9	46.5	49.5	52.5
5	10.6	18.8	25.6	36.0	42.4	48.5	56.1	62.6	68.2	73.0	77.2
7	11.6	21.4	29.3	41.4	50.0	59.0	68.7	77.8	84.7	90.2	93.8
10	12.7	23.6	33.0	47.1	57.8	70.2	83.2	94.0	103	109	113
15	13.7	25.6	36.4	53.2	66.1	81.4	99.7	113	123	130	135
20	14.2	26.7	38.0	56.3	72.2	89.6	111	127	139	147	152
30	14.5	27.6	39.7	59.9	76.8	98.8	124	144	159	172	179
40	14.8	28.2	40.7	62.4	80.0	103	133	156	175	187	197
50	14.8	28.4	41.3	64.1	82.2	106	139	165	185	199	208
60	14.8	28.7	41.7	65.5	84.0	109	143	171	193	206	216
70	14.8	28.8	41.9	65.6	85.3	111	146	174	196	212	222
80	14.8	28.8	42.1	65.8	86.0	112	148	176	198	214	226
90	14.8	28.9	42.3	66.0	86.5	113	149	177	199	216	228
100	14.8	29.2	42.5	66.2	86.8	114	150	179	201	218	230

* From Focht, E. F., Quimby, E. H., and Gershowitz, M.: Revised Average Geometric Factors for Cylinders in Isotope Dosage. Part I. *Radiology* 85:151, 1965.

PHOTON MASS ATTENUATION COEFFICIENT μ_o/ρ,[a] AND PHOTON MASS ENERGY–ABSORPTION COEFFICIENT μ_{en}/ρ FOR WATER*

E MEV.	μ_o/ρ G./CM.^{2}	μ_{en}/ρ G./CM.^{2}
0.01	4.99	4.79
0.015	1.48	1.28
0.02	0.711	0.512
0.03	0.337	0.149
0.04	0.248	0.0677
0.05	0.214	0.0418
0.06	0.197	0.0320
0.08	0.179	0.0262
0.10	0.168	0.0256
0.15	0.149	0.0277
0.2	0.136	0.0297
0.3	0.119	0.0319
0.4	0.106	0.0328
0.5	0.0966	0.0330
0.6	0.0894	0.0329
0.8	0.0785	0.0321
1.0	0.0706	0.0309[b]
1.5	0.0575	0.0282[b]
2	0.0493	0.0260[b]
3	0.0396	0.0227[b]

a. Does not include Rayleigh (coherent) scattering and the photonuclear effect.

b. Other values of μ_{en}/ρ same as μ_a/ρ (mass absorption coefficient).

* From Hubbell, J. H., and Berger, M. J.: Sections 4.1 and 4.2. *In* Jaeger, R. G. (ed.): Engineering Compendium on Radiation Shielding. International Atomic Energy Agency, Vienna. Springer-Verlag, Berlin (in press).

K-SHELL FLUORESCENT YIELD (ω_k)*

ELEMENT	ATOMIC NO.	ω_k	ELEMENT	ATOMIC NO.	ω_k
O	8	0.005	Zr	40	0.735
Ne	10	0.02	Mo	42	0.775
Mg	12	0.035	Rh	45	0.81
Si	14	0.06	Ag	47	0.835
S	16	0.09	Sb	51	0.865
A	18	0.13	Ba	56	0.90
Ca	20	0.17	Nd	60	0.915
Sc	21	0.195	Tb	65	0.93
V	23	0.24	Tm	69	0.94
Mn	25	0.29	Ta	73	0.95
Co	27	0.345	Re	75	0.95
Cu	29	0.40	Au	79	0.96
Ga	31	0.46	Bi	83	0.965
As	33	0.535	Fr	87	0.965
Kr	36	0.64	Th	90	0.965
Sr	38	0.695			

* From Fink, R. W., Jopson, R. C., Mark, H., and Swift, C. D.: Atomic Fluorescence Yields. *Rev. Modern Physics* 38:513, 1966.

GASTROINTESTINAL TRACT OF THE STANDARD MAN*

PORTION OF GI TRACT THAT IS THE CRITICAL TISSUE	MASS OF CONTENTS (G.)	TIME FOOD REMAINS, τ (DAY)	FRACTION FROM LUNG TO GI TRACT, f_a (SOL.)	(INSOL.)
Stomach (S)	250	1/24	0.50	0.625
Small intestine (SI)	1100	4/24	0.50	0.625
Upper large intestine (ULI)	135	8/24	0.50	0.625
Lower large intestine (LLI)	150	18/24	0.50	0.625

* From International Commission on Radiological Protection, Committee II, 1959: Permissible Dose for Internal Radiation. *Health Phys.* 3:1, 1960.
See also:

Eve, I. S.: A Review of the Physiology of the Gastrointestinal Tract in Relation to Radiation Doses from Radioactive Materials. *Health Phys.* 12:131, 1966.

Dolphin, G. W., and Eve, I. S.: Dosimetry of the Gastrointestinal Tract. *Health Phys.* 12:163, 1966.

ORGANS OF STANDARD MAN

See Table 17–2, page 747.

INTAKE AND EXCRETION OF THE STANDARD MAN[*]

WATER BALANCE			
INTAKE (cm.³/day)		EXCRETION (cm.³/day)	
Food	1000	Urine	1400
Fluids	1200	Sweat	600
Oxidation	300	From lungs	300
		Feces	200
Total	2500	Total	2500

AIR BALANCE			
	O₂ (VOL. %)	CO₂ (VOL. %)	N₂ + OTHERS (VOL. %)
Inspired air	20.94	0.03	79.03
Expired air	16	4.0	80
Alveolar air (inspired)	15	5.6	—
Alveolar air (expired)	14	6.0	—

Vital capacity of lungs	3–4 liters (men)
	2–3 liters (women)
Air inhaled during 8 hr. work day	10^7 cm.³/day
Air inhaled during 16 hr. not at work	10^7 cm.³/day
Total	2×10^7 cm.³/day
Interchange area of lungs	50 m.²
Area of upper respiratory tract, trachea, bronchi	20 m.²
Total surface area of respiratory tract	70 m.²

[*] From International Commission on Radiological Protection, Committee II, 1959: Permissible Dose for Internal Radiation. *Health Phys.* 3:1, 1960.

INDEX

Page numbers in *italic* type indicate illustrations.